Insurance
Handbook for the
Medical
Office

Insurance Handbook for the Medical Office

Ninth Edition

Marilyn Takahashi Fordney, CMA-AC, CMT

Formerly Instructor of Medical Insurance, Medical Terminology,
Medical Machine Transcription, and Medical Office Procedures
Ventura College
Ventura, California

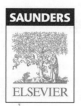

**Technical Collaborator
and Contributing Author:**

Brenda K. Burton, CCP
Director, MEDEXTEND
Fayetteville, Georgia

SAUNDERS
ELSEVIER

11830 Westline Industrial Drive
St. Louis, Missouri 63146

INSURANCE HANDBOOK FOR
THE MEDICAL OFFICE, Ninth Edition

ISBN 13   978-1-4160-0100-3
ISBN 10   1-4160-0100-X

ISBN 13   978-1-4160-0100-3
ISBN 10   1-4160-0100-X

Acquisitions Editor: Susan Cole
Associate Developmental Editor: Colin Odell
Publishing Services Manager: Patricia Tannian
Senior Project Manager: Anne Altepeter
Design Coordinator: Teresa McBryan

Printed in China

Last digit is the print number: 9   8   7   6   5   4   3   2   1

This book is dedicated to insurance billing and coding specialists throughout the nation, to insurance billing and coding instructors, and to new and former students who motivate me to continue writing in this challenging and ever-changing career field.

"I hear and I forget, I see and I remember, I do and I understand."

Chinese Proverb

ABOUT THE AUTHOR

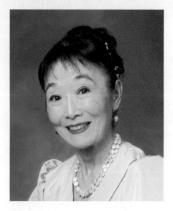

A dedicated professional, Marilyn Takahashi Fordney worked as a medical assistant for 14 years in various settings. During her 19-year teaching career, she taught courses in administrative medical assisting, medical insurance, and medical terminology at many community colleges and in adult education schools. Fordney is a Certified Medical Assistant and Certified Medical Transcriptionist. In 1977 she was named Woman of the Year by the Business and Professional Women's Club of Oxnard, California. In June 2005 Fordney was inducted into the Council of Fellows by the Text and Academic Authors Association in Las Vegas, Nevada.

Fordney's books have won national awards. This textbook, *Insurance Handbook for the Medical Office*, won the William Holmes McGuffey Award in Life Sciences for its excellence and longevity in the field. *Medical Insurance Billing and Coding: An Essentials Worktext*, a spin-off of the *Handbook*, won the Texty Excellent Award in its first edition.

Preface

Welcome to the Ninth Edition

When this book was first published in 1977, few people were aware of how important the subject of health insurance would become. *Insurance Handbook for the Medical Office* now celebrates its 29th year. Through the years it has become the leading textbook in its field because of its interactive learning system. The *Handbook* has gained wide acceptance across the nation among educators and working insurance billers and coders.

Because many legislative mandates and technological advances have occurred since the previous edition, it has been challenging and exciting to put the ninth edition together. Since changes take place daily in the insurance industry, *Insurance Handbook for the Medical Office* will be revised every 2 years to keep the information current.

PURPOSE

The goals of this text are to prepare students to excel as insurance billers and to increase efficiency and streamline administrative procedures for one of the most complex tasks of the physician's business: insurance coding and billing.

In the past 15 years, health care professionals and the community have witnessed the emergence of an administrative medical specialty known variously as insurance billing specialist, medical biller, or reimbursement specialist. Several national organizations offer certification in the field, which is quickly achieving recognition and professionalism. Thus the *Handbook* has been written to address this specialty as another branch of the administrative medical assistant profession. Health care reform is leading to an explosion of jobs in the medical field, especially for those trained in coding and processing insurance claims, electronically as well as manually. Training in this area is necessary because it is common to find medical practices either undercharging or not charging for billable services as a result of a lack of knowledge among office personnel.

Insurance claims are being submitted for patients on recommendation of management consultants to control cash flow, obtain correct reimbursement amounts, honor insurance contracts, compete with other medical practices, and maintain a good relationship with patients. Even offices that do not routinely complete insurance claims for patients will make exceptions for the aged or those patients with mental incompetence, illiteracy, diminished eyesight, or a poor command of the English language. When the amount of the bill is hundreds or thousands of dollars or when a surgical report is required, the physician's office should submit the bill to obtain maximum reimbursement. Those who administer the federal government's Medicare program increasingly promote electronic transmission of insurance claims. Because of these factors, as well as the requirement to document care, the amount of paperwork has increased by leaps and bounds, becoming burdensome and unwieldy. This text addresses all clerical functions of the medical biller, and illustrations throughout the text feature generic forms created to help simplify billing procedures.

Numerous schools and colleges have established one-year certification programs for those interested in a career as an insurance billing specialist, and many existing programs offer medical insurance as a full-semester, 18-week course. Community college extension divisions also offer community service classes and short courses in this subject. Some schools include it as part of a medical assisting program's curriculum so the individual has knowledge in all administrative functions of a physician's office. The text may be used as a learning tool and resource guide in all of those programs as well as in vocational or commercial training institutes and welfare-work programs. It also serves as a text for in-service training in the private medical office. It may be used for independent home study if no formal classes are available in the community. The lay reader who is not pursuing a career in the medical field will find the text useful when working with a claims assistance professional or for billing his or her insurance plans. Insurance companies and their agents have found this a valuable reference book when answering clients' questions.

The text is designed primarily for the student who plans to seek employment in an outpatient setting (physician's office or clinic) or wishes to establish an independent billing business and needs a good understanding of the reimbursement process. Because many types of insurance coverage are available in the United States, those types most commonly encountered in physicians' offices and clinics have been emphasized in this text in simple, nontechnical explanations and tables. Documentation in the medical record is the key to substantiating procedure and diagnostic code selections for proper reimbursement. Thus, in this edition, Chapter 4, Medical Documentation, has been further updated and enhanced. In recent years, the federal government targeted this issue with the introduction of Medicare compliance policies related to documentation and confidentiality; such issues are therefore covered to help physicians comply with possible reviews or audits of their billing practices. Finally, the text may be used as a stand-alone reference source or as an educational tool to increase the knowledge of someone currently working as an insurance billing specialist in a private medical office.

CONTENT

New Features

Each chapter has been updated to reflect 2005 policies and procedures.

- All chapters have been completely restructured for better organization and flow of content, with legal information included where applicable to insurance billing and coding. The information presented is not a substitute for legal advice, and the physician and his or her insurance billing specialist should always seek legal counsel about specific questions of law as they relate to medical practice.
- SERVICE boxes: A color screened box at the beginning of each chapter highlights patient service with regard to the topic being discussed.

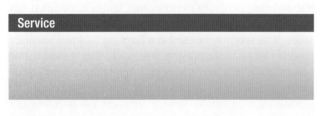

- HIPAA Compliance Alerts are interspersed throughout all of the chapters for emphasis.

- Figures: Most figures have been labeled and highlighted to quickly guide the reader for clearer and better understanding.
- Chapter 2, Compliance and the E-Health Initiative, is new to this edition and focuses on the Health Insurance Portability and Accountability Act (HIPAA). The chapter explains HIPAA's impact on insurance reform and administrative simplification.
- Chapter 8, Electronic Data Interchange: Transactions and Security, has been completely rewritten and updated. It contains additional HIPAA information on requirements for electronic transmission of insurance claims and explains the security rules.

General Features

Experts in the field reviewed the chapters in the eighth edition so that improvements in content, clarity of topics, and deletions could be considered. A unique color-coded icon feature used throughout the book denotes and clarifies information specific to each type of payer. This system makes the learning process more effective by helping students identify each insurance payer with a specific color and graphic. These icons follow:

 All payers: All payer guidelines, including all private insurance companies and all federal and state programs.

 All Private Payers: All private insurance companies.

 Medicaid: State Medicaid programs.

 Medicare: Federal Medicare programs, Medicare/Medicaid, Medicare/Medigap, and Medicare Secondary Payer (MSP).

 TRICARE: TRICARE Standard (formerly CHAMPUS), TRICARE Prime, TRICARE Extra.

 CHAMPVA: Civilian Health and Medical Program of the Department of Veterans Affairs.

 Workers' Compensation: State workers' compensation programs.

Additional features of this textbook include the following:
- Objectives are presented at the beginning of each chapter to guide instructors in preparing lecture

material and inform readers about what will be presented. By reviewing the key terms introducing each chapter, students are alerted to important words for the topic.

OBJECTIVES

- Basic health insurance information and coding examples are shown for persons who are studying for a certification examination. Special emphasis is placed on correct and incorrect procedural codes and appropriate documentation—the keys to obtaining maximum reimbursement.

Example   Office Emergency

Incorrect Coding

99212 Office visit, level 2, established patient
12005 Simple repair of scalp laceration, 12.6 cm
99070 Surgical tray (itemized)

Correct Coding

99212 Office visit, level 2, established patient
99058 *Office services provided on an emergency basis*
12005 Simple repair of scalp laceration, 12.6 cm

- Chapter 7, The Paper Claim: CMS-1500, uses a unique block-by-block approach specific to each different payer that denotes and clarifies information about the CMS-1500 insurance claim form. The icons and graphics system is used to help students retain information. Templates illustrate placement of information on the form.

---

33. PHYSICIAN'S, SUPPLIER'S BILLING NAME, ADDRESS, ZIP CODE
& PHONE #
JOHN DOE MD 555 486 9001
123 ANY STREET
ANYTOWN XY 12345
PIN# 70 98765XX   GRP#

- Chapters 8 through 16: Many specific quick-action solutions for insurance problems, tracing delinquent claims, and appealing denied claims are provided. Thorough up-to-date information is presented for Medicare, Medicaid, TRICARE, private plans, workers' compensation, managed care plans, disability income insurance, and disability benefit programs. Helpful billing tips and guidelines for submitting insurance claims are given for each type of insurance program covered.
- Chapter 17, Hospital Billing, is intended especially for those students interested in pursuing a career in the hospital setting.
- Chapter 18: This final chapter provides information pertinent to seeking a position as an insurance billing specialist, a self-employed claims assistance professional,

or an electronic claims processor. It explains the impact of HIPAA compliance policies when working as a business associate to a medical practice when processing insurance claims.
- Appendix A assists the insurance billing specialist in locating audiotapes, books, newsletters, periodicals, software, and videotapes from various resources. It lists names, addresses, toll-free telephone numbers, and Web sites.
- An extensive glossary of basic medical and insurance terms and abbreviations is included.

SUPPLEMENTAL MATERIAL

Workbook

Users of the *Workbook* that accompanies this edition of the textbook will find the following new features:

- Competency-based education: A point system has been applied to code and claims completion for *Workbook* assignments for instructors who need to document and gather statistics for competency-based education. *Handbook* learning objectives, *Workbook* performance objectives for all assignments, use of the tutorial software and text with reinforcement by *Workbook* assignments, the test section at the end of the *Workbook* and the quizzes of key terms featured on the Web site, and incorporation of classroom activities and suggestions from the *Instructor's Electronic Resource Guide on CD-ROM* provide a complete competency-based educational program.
- Patient records and ledgers have been updated and reworded to correspond with the 2005 procedural and diagnostic code books.
- Chapters 2 and 8 have new review questions and many new assignments added.

General Features

For students, the *Workbook* that accompanies the text is a practical approach to learning insurance billing. It progresses from easy to more complex issues within each chapter and advances as new skills are learned and integrated. Chapter outlines serve as a lecture guide. Each chapter has performance objectives for assignments that indicate to students what will be accomplished. Key terms are repeated for quick reference when studying. Patients' medical records, financial accounting statements, and encounter forms are presented as they might appear in the physician's files, so the student may learn how to abstract information to complete claim forms properly and accurately. For this edition, the patient records and ledgers have been completely updated for technical clinical content and reworded to correspond with the 2005 procedural and diagnostic code books. Easily removable insurance claim forms and other sample documents are included in the *Workbook* for completion and to enhance keying skills. Some assignments give students hands-on experience in keying forms for optical character recognition (OCR) computer equipment, which is used in many states for insurance claims processing and payment. Current procedural and diagnostic code exercises are used throughout the *Workbook* to facilitate and enhance coding skills for submitting a claim or posting to a patient's financial account statement. Critical thinking problems are presented in each chapter. Special appendices are included at the end of the *Workbook*. These include a simulated practice, the College Clinic, with a group of physicians who employ the student; a mock fee schedule with codes and fees (including Medicare); and an abbreviated Medicare Level II HCPCS alphanumeric code list. The appendices may be used as reference tools to complete the procedural code problems. These appendixes include the following:

● Appendix A: details information for a simulated practice called College Clinic. Information is provided about the group of physicians, and a mock fee schedule is included with codes and fees (including Medicare).
● Appendix B: provides an abbreviated Medicare Level II HCPCS alphanumeric code list with a list of modifiers.
● Appendix C: provides Medi-Cal information and review questions.
● Appendix D: contains the answers to the self-study review questions for each chapter.

AltaPoint Student Software Challenge

Most medical practices use computer technology to perform financial operations; therefore, a user-friendly health care practice management software program accompanies the *Handbook* and *Workbook*. The goal is to give the learner a hands-on, realistic approach as though working in a medical office setting. This software, AltaPoint, allows the student to generate paper CMS-1500 forms and build electronic insurance claim files.

The user completes assignments by accessing the data files in AltaPoint. The database includes patient demographic information, patient health records, and financial accounts for each patient. Encounter forms for 10 patients appear in the *Workbook*. The skill of extracting data from the encounter form to input into the AltaPoint practice management software is developed. Reading data from the patient files to ensure that the data are accurate and correspond to the assigned diagnostic and procedural code numbers when the CMS-1500 claim form is generated allows the user to experience the common tasks performed by a billing specialist.

A hard copy of all work may be printed to submit to the instructor for a score.

Additional features of the AltaPoint software for the 2005 edition of this text are:

● Complete fee schedule, which may be accessed electronically for inputting fees on financial accounting records, which then are included on corresponding insurance claims that are generated.
● Computerized practice management system that includes full accounting records that allows the user to post service dates and automatically view the patient's outstanding balance.
● Pop-up messages that appear for immediate help when a case requires additional or corrected data to be entered.
● Lists of patients, insurance companies, providers and, in addition, enhanced reporting (e.g., insurance aging or batch summary reports) that allow the user to track and review entered data on screen or in hard copy.
● Transaction screen that allows the user to search for claims by service data, date billed, account number, patient name, or insurance carrier.
● Electronic claim submission screens that simulate the process of sending electronic claims to insurance carriers.

Instructors may wish their students to work through the first case or basic cases 1 through 4 strictly for learning and to use case 5 for testing and grading. Cases 6 through 10, which are advanced and insurance specific (e.g., Medicare, TRICARE), may be used for practice or testing. This simulated learning methodology makes possible an easier transition from classroom to workplace.

Instructor's Resource Manual

The *Instructor's Resource Manual* is available in printed form and on CD-ROM. This resource allows the instructor the flexibility to quickly adapt the textbook for his or her individual classroom needs and to gauge students' understanding. The *Instructor's Resource Manual* features the following:

● Guidelines for establishing a medical insurance course
● Answer keys to the *Workbook* and software assignments and tests with rationales, optional codes, and further explanations for most of the code problems
● Render ideas on how to use the text as an adjunct to a medical office procedures course
● Lesson plans for each chapter
● Suggested classroom activities
● Ideas on how to use the text as an adjunct to an administrative medical assisting or medical office procedures course

The CD-ROM includes all of the information in the printed *Instructor's Resource Manual*, plus the following:

- An image collection of forms and summaries of important chapter concepts from the textbook for use as overheads or as PowerPoint slides. A PowerPoint presentation will capture attention and create lively lectures to assist in learning and retention.
- A test bank with more than 1000 questions to assist instructors in test construction. The test provides various testing formats, such as multiple choice, true or false, mix and match, completion of blanks, and labeling of illustrations. Questions are rated (i.e., Difficulty: easy, moderate, or hard) to help instructors with test construction for the topic being taught. The tests can be customized, revised, and printed.

Evolve Course Management System

Evolve is an interactive learning environment that works in coordination with the textbook. It provides Internet-based course management tools that instructors can use to reinforce and expand on the concepts delivered in class. It can be used for the following:

- To publish the class syllabus, outline, and lecture notes
- To set up "virtual office hours" and e-mail communication
- To share important dates and information through the online class calendar
- To encourage student participation through chat rooms and discussion boards

Evolve also provides online access to free Learning Resources designed specifically to give students and instructors the information they need to quickly and successfully learn the topics covered in this textbook. These Learning Resources include:

- Self-assessment quizzes to evaluate students' mastery through multiple choice, true/false, fill-in-the-blank, and matching questions. Instant scoring and feedback are available at the click of a button.
- Weblinks: Hundreds of Web sites have been carefully gathered to supplement the content of the textbook. The Weblinks are regularly updated, with new ones added as they are developed.
- Technical updates to keep up with changes in government regulations, codes, and other industry changes.

Medical Insurance Online

Medical Insurance Online is an exciting resource for instructors and students. It offers a simulated, interactive office externship experience with feedback provided throughout. The following list is a sampling of what students will experience with the innovative Medical Insurance Online program:

- It functions as a "virtual externship" in which users go through an office orientation at which they meet their virtual office manager and medical staff.
- Users gain on-the-job training as they perform a number of true-to-life activities, interacting with virtual patients, troubleshooting claims, maintaining compliance with regulations, meeting insurance payer requirements, and more.
- Users fill in specific portions of the insurance claim form and receive immediate feedback.
- The program provides direct interaction with and constant access to all paperwork relevant to each patient claim.
- After completing each "virtual day," users have a chance to review with the virtual office manager the material they encountered by answering a number of questions and receiving feedback.
- Automatically scored quizzes at the end of each phase and an examination at the end of each module allow students to demonstrate their mastery of the content.
- By the end of the course, the user has followed claims through their life cycle for each of the various insurance payers, including private commercial carriers, Medicare/Medicaid, Medigap, Managed Care (HMOs), and others.

SUMMARY

The *Handbook* and its ancillaries provide a complete competency-based educational program. *Handbook* learning objectives, *Workbook* performance objectives, assignments, tests, AltaPoint tutorial software, the virtual externship available on *Medical Insurance Online*, and incorporation of lesson plans and suggested classroom activities from the *Instructor's Resource Manual* ensure that students know everything they need to succeed in the workforce.

Escalating costs of medical care, the impact of technology, and the explosion of managed care plans have affected insurance billing procedures and claims processing and have necessitated new legislation for government and state programs. Therefore it is essential that all medical personnel handling claims continue to update their knowledge. This may be accomplished by reading bulletins from state agencies and regional insurance carriers, speaking with insurance representatives, or attending insurance workshops offered at local colleges or local chapters of professional associations, such as those mentioned in Chapters 1 and 18. It is hoped that this text will resolve any unclear issues pertaining to current methods and become the framework on which the insurance billing specialist builds new knowledge as understanding and appreciation of the profession are attained.

ACKNOWLEDGMENTS

During my 14 years as a medical assistant, 19 years of teaching, and 29 years of writing, hundreds of students, physicians, friends, colleagues, and instructors have contributed valuable suggestions and interesting material for this book. I wish to express my thanks to all of them, with special emphasis on the following:

- Lois C. Oliver, retired professor, Pierce College, Woodland Hills, California, helped me organize my first medical insurance class in 1969 and offered assistance and encouragement throughout the preparation of the first edition of the *Handbook*.
- Marcia O. "Marcy" Diehl, CMA-A, CMT, a former co-author and retired instructor, Grossmont Community College, El Cajon, California, generously shared her knowledge, ideas, and class materials.
- Members of the California Association of Medical Assistant Instructors (CAMAI) contributed suggestions for improving the text and gave me motivation from time to time to continue the project.
- Mary E. Kinn, CPS, CMA-A, author and retired assistant professor, Long Beach City College, Long Beach, California, provided a perspective review of my syllabus. Without her positive endorsement, the first edition of this book might not have been published.
- Overwhelming thanks to my technical collaborator and contributor, Brenda K. Burton, who helped me with updating each chapter to HIPAA compliance issues and the electronic transmission of insurance claims. Brenda also developed the tutorial AltaPoint software for this edition. Writing has its ups and downs, and she gave me support during many of the difficult periods. Special thanks to the students of Linda French's classes at the Simi Valley Adult School and Career Institute in Simi Valley, California, who contributed their criticisms, lent technical subject matter, offered suggestions, and through voluntary participation helped to enhance and create *Workbook* assignments for the previous edition. A note of appreciation to my assistants, Barbara Evans and Gemma Budie Hiranuma, who did many tasks to allow me free time to research and write.

I gratefully acknowledge the work of Teresa McBryan, Art and Design, Elsevier, for the design of this edition. Jim Woods of Camarillo, California, took the photograph for "About the Author." Jack Foley, photographer, and Nick Kaufmann Productions took the photographs found throughout the text. I wish to acknowledge and thank both of them.

I also thank the print shop staff, Publications Department, Ventura College, Ventura, California, who printed the first California syllabus of this text.

I am indebted to many individuals on the staff at Elsevier for encouragement and guidance. I express particular appreciation to Susan Cole, senior acquisitions editor; Colin Odell, associate developmental editor; and Anne Altepeter, senior project manager, for coordination of the entire project.

Numerous supply companies were kind enough to cooperate by providing forms and descriptive literature of their products, and their names are found throughout the text and *Workbook* figures.

But colleagues, production staff, and editors working as a team do not quite make a book; there are others to whom I must express overwhelming debt and enduring gratitude, and these are the consultants who reviewed some of the chapters or who provided vital information about private, state, and federal insurance programs. Without the knowledge of these advisers, the massive task of compiling an insurance text truly national in scope might never have been completed. Although the names of all those who graciously assisted me are too numerous to mention, I take great pride in listing my principal consultants for this ninth edition.

Marilyn Takahashi Fordney, CMA-AC, CMT
Oxnard, California

Principal Consultants and Reviewers

Conejo Chapter of the American Association
of Professional Coders
Thousand Oaks, California

George S. Conomikes and Staff
President, Conomikes Associates, Inc., Los Angeles,
California

Deborah Emmons, CMA
President, S.T.A.T. Transcription Service,
Port Hueneme, California

Sandy Gutt
Instructor, Southern California Regional Occupational
Center, Torrance, California

Gemma Budie Hiranuma
Accounting/Human Resources
Broccoli International USA, Inc.
Los Angeles, California

Lucille M. Loignon, MD, FACS
Diplomate, American Board of Ophthalmology,
Oxnard, California

Kathy A. McCall, CMA-AC, BS, MA
Retired Professor of Allied Health, Community College
of Allegheny County, Pittsburgh, Pennsylvania

Walter A. Shaff
President, CPR, Lake Oswego, Oregon

Griff Stelzner
Assistant Claims Manager, State Compensation
Insurance Fund, Oxnard, California

Carolyn Talesfore
Advertising and Promotions Manager,
Bibbero Systems, Inc. Petaluma, California

Barbara Warfield
Rhino Graphics, Port Hueneme, California

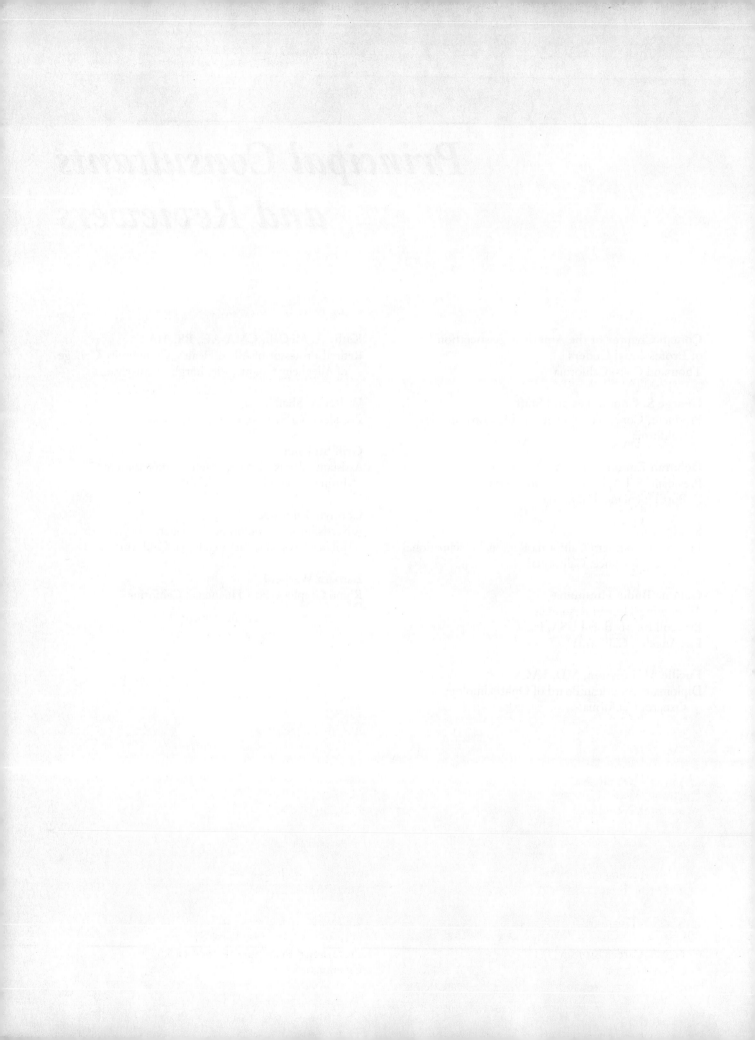

Editorial Review Board

Contents

UNIT 1
Career Role and Responsibilities

1 Role of an Insurance Billing Specialist, 3

Background of Insurance Claims, Coding, and Billing, 4
Role of the Insurance Billing Specialist, 5
Job Responsibilities, 5
Educational and Training Requirements, 14
Career Advantages, 17
Qualifications, 18
Medical Etiquette, 19
Medical Ethics, 20
Confidentiality, 21
Employer Liability, 21
Employee Liability, 22
Scope of Practice, 22
Future Challenges, 22

2 Compliance and the E-Health Initiative, 25

Compliance Defined, 26
Health Information Using Electronic Technologies, 26
E-Health Information Management, 26
National Health Information Infrastructure, 26
Health Level Seven, 26
Systematized Nomenclature of Human and Veterinary Medicine (SNOMED) International, 27
Health Insurance Portability and Accountability Act (HIPAA), 27
Title 1: Health Insurance Reform, 27
Title II: Administrative Simplification, 27
Defining Roles and Relationships: Key Terms, 28
HIPAA in the Practice Setting, 29

The Privacy Rule: Confidentiality and Protected Health Information, 29
Confidential Information, 30
Patients' Rights, 35
Privacy Rules: Patient Rights under HIPAA, 36
Right to Notice of Privacy Practices, 36
Right to Request Restrictions on Certain Uses and Disclosures of PHI, 36
Right to Request Confidential Communications, 36
Right to Access, Inspect, and Obtain PHI, 37
Right to Request Amendment of PHI, 38
Right to Receive an Accounting of Disclosures of PHI, 38
Organization and Staff Responsibilities in Protecting Patient Rights, 39
Verification of Identity and Authority, 39
Validating Patient Permission, 40
Training, 41
Safeguards: Ensuring That Confidential Information Is Secure, 41
Complaints to Health Care Practice and Workforce Sanctions, 41
Mitigation, 41
Refraining from Intimidating or Retaliatory Acts, 41
Transaction and Code Set Regulations: Streamlining Electronic Data Interchange, 41
Standard Unique Identifiers, 42
The Security Rule: Administrative, Physical, and Technical Safeguards, 43
Application to Practice Setting, 43
Guidelines for HIPAA Privacy Compliance, 43
Consequences of Noncompliance with HIPAA, 44
Office of the Inspector General, 45
Fraud and Abuse Laws, 45
Federal False Claims Act (31 US Code §3729-33), 45
Qui Tam "Whistleblower," 46
Civil Monetary Penalties Law (42 US Code §320a-27a), 46

Criminal False Claims Act (18 US Code), 47
Stark Laws (42 US Code §1395), 47
Anti-Kickback Statute, 47
Safe Harbors, 47
Additional Laws and Compliance, 47
Operation Restore Trust, 48
Medicare Integrity Program, 48
Correct Coding Initiative, 48
Increased Staffing and Expanded Penalties for
Violations, 48
Special Alerts, Bulletins, and Guidance
Documents, 48
Exclusion Program, 48
**Compliance Program Guidance for
Individual and Small Group Physician
Practices,** 48
Increased Productivity and Decreased Penalties
with Plan, 49
**Seven Basic Components of a Compliance
Plan,** 49
Conducting Internal Monitoring
and Auditing, 49
Implementing Compliance and Practice
Standards, 49
Designating a Compliance Officer or
Contact, 50
Conducting Appropriate Training and
Education, 50
Responding Appropriately to Detected
Offenses and Developing Corrective
Action, 50
Developing Open Lines
of Communication, 50
Enforcing Disciplinary Standards through
Well-Publicized Guidelines, 51
**What to Expect from Your Health Care
Practice,** 51
Compliance Lessons Learned, 51

UNIT 2
The Claims Process

3 Basics of Health Insurance, 55
History, 56
Insurance in the United States, 56
Legal Principles of Insurance, 56
Insurance Contracts, 57
**Physician–Patient Contracts and Financial
Obligation,** 57
Implied or Expressed Contracts, 57
The Insurance Policy, 58
Policy Application, 58
Policy Renewal Provisions, 58
Policy Terms, 59

Coordination of Benefits, 60
General Policy Limitations, 60
Choice of Health Insurance, 61
Group Contract, 61
Individual Contract, 65
Prepaid Health Plan, 65
Types of Health Insurance Coverage, 65
CHAMPVA, 65
Competitive Medical Plan, 65
Disability Income Insurance, 65
Exclusive Provider Organization, 65
Foundation for Medical Care, 65
Health Maintenance Organizaiton, 65
Independent or Individual Practice
Association, 66
Maternal and Child Health Program, 66
Medicaid, 66
Medicare, 66
Medicare/Medicaid, 66
Point-of-Service Plan, 66
Preferred Provider Organization, 66
TRICARE, 66
Unemployment Compensation Disability, 67
Veterans Affairs Outpatient Clinic, 67
Worker's Compensation Insurance, 67
Examples of Insurance Billing, 67
Keeping Up to Date, 68
**PROCEDURE: Handling and Processing
Insurance Claims,** 68
**PROCEDURE: Prepare and Post to a
Patient's Financial Accounting
Record,** 88

4 Medical Documentation, 91
The Documentation Process, 92
Health Record, 92
Documenters, 92
**General Principles of Health Record
Documentation,** 93
Medical Necessity, 94
External Audit Point System, 94
Legalities of Health Record Documentation, 94
**Documentation Guidelines for Evaluation
and Management Services,** 95
Contents of a Medical Report, 98
Documentation of History, 98
Documentation of Examination, 101
Documentation of Medical Decision-Making
Complexity, 103
Documentation Terminology, 104
Terminology for Evaluation and Management
Services, 104
Diagnostic Terminology and Abbreviations, 107
Directional Terms, 108
Surgical Terminology, 110

Review and Audit of Health Records, 113
  Internal Reviews, 113
  Retention of Records, 119
  Termination of a Case, 120
  Prevention of Legal Problems, 123
  PROCEDURE: **Abstract Data from a Health Record,** 123
  PROCEDURE: **Compose, Format, Key, Proofread, and Print a Letter,** 124

5 *Diagnostic Coding,* 127

The Diagnostic Coding System, 128
  Types of Diagnostic Codes, 128
  Reasons for the Development and Use of Diagnostic Codes, 128
  Physician's Fee Profile, 129
History of Coding Diseases, 129
International Classification of Diseases, 130
  History, 130
  Organization and Format, 130
  Contents, 130
How to Use the Diagnostic Code Books Properly, 130
  Coding Instructions, 132
Rules for Coding, 136
  Signs, Symptoms, and Ill-Defined Conditions, 136
  Sterilization, 137
  Neoplasms, 137
  Circulatory System Conditions, 138
  Diabetes Mellitus, 139
  Pregnancy, Delivery, or Abortion, 140
  Admitting Diagnoses, 141
  Burns, 141
  Injuries and Late Effects, 141
ICD-10-CM Diagnosis and Procedure Codes, 143
PROCEDURE: **Basic Steps in Selecting Diagnostic Coding,** 145

6 *Procedural Coding,* 151

Understanding the Importance of Procedural Coding Skills, 152
Coding Compliance Plan, 152
  Current Procedural Terminology, 152
Methods of Payment, 154
  Fee Schedule, 154
  Usual, Customary, and Reasonable, 155
  Developing a Fee Schedule Using Relative Value Studies Conversion Factors, 157
How to Use the CPT Code Book, 157
  Category I, II, and III Codes, 158
  Code Book Symbols, 158
  Evaluation and Management Section, 159

  Surgery Section, 167
  Unlisted Procedures, 172
  Coding Guidelines for Code Edits, 172
  Code Monitoring, 176
Helpful Hints in Coding, 176
  Office Visits, 176
  Drugs and Injections, 176
  Adjunct Codes, 177
  Basic Life or Disability Evaluation Services, 177
Code Modifiers, 177
  Correct Use of Common CPT Modifiers, 183
  Comprehensive List of Modifier Codes, 190
  PROCEDURE: **Determine Conversion Factors,** 190
  PROCEDURE: **Choose Correct Procedural Codes for Professional Services,** 190

7 *The Paper Claim: CMS-1500,* 195

History, 196
Types of Claims, 196
Compliance Issues Related to Insurance Claim Forms, 197
  Claim Status, 197
Abstracting from Medical Records, 198
  Cover Letter Accompanying Insurance Claims, 198
  Life or Health Insurance Applications, 198
Health Insurance Claim Form (CMS-1500), 202
  Basic Guidelines for Submitting a Claim, 202
  Completion of Insurance Claim Forms, 202
Common Reasons Why Claim Forms Are Delayed or Rejected, 205
  Additional Reasons Why Claim Forms Are Delayed, 207
Optical Scanning Format Guidelines, 207
  Optical Character Recognition, 207
  Do's and Don'ts for Optical Character Recognition, 207
PROCEDURE: **Instructions for the Health Insurance Claim Form (CMS-1500),** 210
  Insurance Program Templates, 257

8 *Electronic Data Interchange: Transactions and Security,* 269

Electronic Data Interchange, 270
Electronic Claims, 270
Advantages of Electronic Claim Submission, 270
Clearinghouses, 270
Transaction and Code Set Regulations: Streamlining Electronic Data Interchange, 271
  Transaction and Code Set Standards, 272

Transition from Paper CMS-1500 to Electronic Standard HIPAA 837, 276
Levels of Information for 837P Standard Transaction Format, 276
Claims Attachments Standards, 277
Standard Unique Identifiers, 277
Practice Management System, 280
Building the Claim, 281
Encounter or Multipurpose Billing Forms, 281
Scannable Encounter Form, 282
Keying Insurance Data for Claim Transmission, 282
Encoder, 287
Clean Electronic Claims Submission, 288
Putting HIPAA Standard Transactions to Work, 288
Interactive Transactions, 288
Electronic Remittance Advice, 289
Driving the Data, 289
Methods for Sending Claims, 289
Computer Claims Systems, 292
Payer or Carrier-Direct, 292
Clearinghouse, 292
Transmission Reports, 292
Electronic Processing Problems, 292
Billing and Account Management Schedule, 292
Administrative Simplification Enforcement Tool (ASET), 292
The Security Rule: Administrative, Physical, and Technical Safeguards, 296
HIPAA: Application to the Practice Setting, 297
Computer Confidentiality, 297
Confidentiality Statement, 297
Prevention Measures, 297
Records Management, 299
Data Storage, 299
Electronic Power Protection, 299

9 Receiving Payments and Insurance Problem Solving, 303
Follow-Up after Claim Submission, 304
Claim Policy Provisions, 304
Insured, 304
Payment Time Limits, 304
Explanation of Benefits, 305
Components of an EOB, 305
Interpretation of an EOB, 305
Posting an EOB, 305
Claim Management Techniques, 307
Insurance Claims Register, 307
Tickler File, 307
Insurance Company Payment History, 308

Claim Inquiries, 308
Problem Paper and Electronic Claims, 310
Types of Problems, 310
Rebilling, 317
Review and Appeal Process, 319
Filing an Official Appeal, 319
Medicare Review and Redetermination Process, 320
TRICARE Review and Appeal Process, 323
State Insurance Commissioner, 328
Commission Objectives, 328
Types of Problems, 328
Commission Inquiries, 329
PROCEDURE: Trace an Unpaid Insurance Claim, 330
PROCEDURE: File an Official Appeal, 330

10 Office and Insurance Collection Strategies, 333
Cash Flow Cycle, 334
Accounts Receivable, 334
Patient Education, 335
Patient Registration Form, 336
Fees, 336
Fee Schedule, 336
Fee Adjustments, 336
Communicating Fees, 340
Collecting Fees, 340
Credit Arrangements, 348
Payment Options, 348
Credit and Collection Laws, 351
Statute of Limitations, 351
Equal Credit Opportunity Act, 351
Fair Credit Reporting Act, 352
Fair Credit Billing Act, 352
Truth in Lending Act, 352
Truth in Lending Consumer Credit Cost Disclosure, 353
Fair Debt Collection Practices Act, 353
The Collection Process, 354
Office Collection Techniques, 354
Insurance Collection, 358
Collection Agencies, 361
Credit Bureaus, 363
Credit Counseling, 363
Small Claims Court, 363
Tracing a Skip, 365
Special Collection Issues, 367
PROCEDURE: Seven-Step Billing and Collection Guidelines, 371
PROCEDURE: Telephone Collection Plan, 372
PROCEDURE: Create a Financial Agreement with a Patient, 373

PROCEDURE: **File a Claim in Small Claims Court,** 373
PROCEDURE: **File an Estate Claim,** 374

UNIT 3

Health Care Payers

11 The Blues Plans, Private Insurance, and Managed Care Plans, 379

Private Insurance, 380
Blue Cross and Blue Shield Plans, 380
Managed Care, 380
Prepaid Group Practice Health Plans, 381
Benefits, 382
Health Care Reform, 382
Managed Care Systems, 383
Health Maintenance Organizations, 383
Exclusive Provider Organizations, 384
Foundations for Medical Care, 384
Independent Practice Associations, 384
Preferred Provider Organizations, 384
Physician Provider Groups, 385
Point-of-Service Plans, 385
Triple-Option Health Plans, 385
Medical Review, 385
Quality Improvement Organization, 385
Utilization Review of Management, 386
Management of Plans, 386
Contracts, 386
Preauthorization or Prior Approval, 387
Diagnostic Tests, 390
Managed Care Guide, 390
Plan Administration, 390
Financial Management, 392
Payment, 392
Statement of Remittance, 394
Accounting, 394
Fee-for-Service, 394
Year-End Evaluation, 395
Bankruptcy, 396
Conclusion, 396

12 Medicare, 401

Background, 402
Policies and Regulations, 402
Eligibility Requirements, 402
Health Insurance Card, 403
Enrollment Status, 404
Benefits and Nonbenefits, 404
Additional Insurance Programs, 409
Medicare/Medicaid, 409

Medicare/Medigap, 409
Medicare Secondary Payer, 410
Automobile or Liability Insurance Coverage, 411
Medicare Managed Care Plans, 411
Health Maintenance Organizations, 411
Carrier Dealing Prepayment Organization, 412
Utilization and Quality Control, 412
Quality Improvement Organizations, 412
Federal False Claims Amendment Act, 413
Medicare Billing Compliance Issues, 413
Clinical Laboratory Improvement Amendment, 413
Payment Fundamentals, 414
Provider, 414
Prior Authorization, 415
Waiver of Liability Provision, 417
Elective Surgery Estimate, 418
Prepayment Screens, 419
Correct Coding Initiative, 420
Medicare Reimbursement, 421
Chronology of Payment, 421
Reasonable Fee, 421
Resource-Based Relative Value Scale, 421
Healthcare Common Procedure Coding System (HCPCS), 421
Claim Submission, 422
Local Coverage Determination, 422
Fiscal Intermediaries and Fiscal Agents, 422
Provider Identification Numbers, 422
Patient's Signature Authorization, 422
Time Limit, 423
Paper Claims, 423
Electronic Claims, 424
Medicare/Medicaid Claims, 424
Medicare/Medigap Claims, 424
Medicare/Employer Supplemental Insurance Claims, 424
Medicare/Supplemental and MSP Claims, 424
Deceased Patients Claims, 424
Physician Substitute Coverage, 425
After Claim Submission, 425
Remittance Advice, 425
Medicare Summary Notice, 425
Beneficiary Representative/Representative Payee, 425
Posting Payments, 426
Review and Redetermination Process, 426
PROCEDURE: **Determine Whether Medicare Is Primary or Secondary and Determine Additional Benefits,** 431
PROCEDURE: **Complete an Advance Beneficiary Notice (ABN) Form,** 432

13 Medicaid and Other State Programs, 435

History, 436
Medicaid Programs, 436
  Maternal and Child Health Program, 436
  Low-Income Medicare Recipients, 437
Medicaid Eligibility, 438
  Verifying Eligibility, 438
  Categorically Needy, 438
  Medically Needy, 438
Maternal and Child Health Program Eligibility, 439
  Accepting Medicaid Patients, 439
  Identification Card, 440
  Point-of-Service Machine, 440
  Retroactive Eligibility, 442
Medicaid Benefits, 442
  Covered Services, 442
  Disallowed Services, 442
Medicaid Managed Care, 442
Claim Procedure, 443
  Copayment, 443
  Prior Approval, 443
  Time Limit, 443
  Reciprocity, 443
  Claim Form, 443
After Claim Submission, 446
  Remittance Advice, 446
  Appeals, 447
Medicaid Fraud Control, 447

14 TRICARE and CHAMPVA, 449

History of TRICARE, 450
TRICARE Programs, 450
  Eligibility, 450
  Nonavailability Statement, 451
TRICARE Standard, 451
  Enrollment, 451
  Identification Card, 451
  Benefits, 451
  Fiscal Year, 452
  Authorized Providers of Health Care, 453
  Preauthorization, 455
  Payment, 455
TRICARE Extra, 456
  Enrollment, 456
  Identification Card, 456
  Benefits, 456
  Network Provider, 456
  Preauthorization, 456
  Payments, 456
TRICARE Prime, 457
  Enrollment, 457
  Identification Card, 457
  Benefits, 457
  Primary Care Manager, 457
  Preauthorization, 457
  Payments, 457
TRICARE for Life, 458
  Enrollment, 458
  Identification Card, 459
  Benefits, 459
  Referral and Preauthorization, 459
  Payment, 459
TRICARE Plus, 459
  Enrollment, 459
  Identification Card, 459
  Benefits, 459
  Payment, 459
TRICARE Prime Remote Program, 461
  Enrollment, 461
  Identification Card, 461
  Benefits, 461
  Referral and Preauthorization, 461
  Payments, 461
Supplemental Health Care Program, 461
  Enrollment, 461
  Identification Card, 461
  Benefits, 461
  Referral and Preauthorization, 461
  Payments, 461
TRICARE Hospice Program, 461
TRICARE and HMO Coverage, 462
CHAMPVA Program, 462
  Eligibility, 462
  Enrollment, 462
  Identification Card, 462
  Benefits, 463
  Provider, 463
  Preauthorization, 463
Claims Procedure, 463
  Fiscal Intermediary, 463
  TRICARE Standard and CHAMPVA, 464
Medical Record Access, 465
  Privacy Act of 1974, 465
  Computer Matching and Privacy Protection Act of 1988, 465
  TRICARE Extra and TRICARE Prime, 466
  TRICARE Prime Remote and Supplemental Health Care Program, 466
  TRICARE for Life, 467
  TRICARE/CHAMPVA and Other Insurance, 467
  Medicaid and TRICARE/CHAMPVA, 467
  Medicare and TRICARE, 467
  Medicare and CHAMPVA, 467
  Dual or Double Coverage, 467
  Third-Party Liability, 468
  Workers' Compensation, 468

After Claim Submission, 468
TRICARE Summary Payment Voucher, 468
CHAMPVA Explanation of Benefits
Document, 468
Quality Assurance, 468
Claims Inquiries and Appeals, 468
PROCEDURE: Completing a CHAMPVA
Claim Form, 471

15 *Workers' Compensation,* 477
History, 478
Workers' Compensation Statutes, 478
Workers' Compensation Reform, 478
Workers' Compensation Laws and
Insurance, 479
Purposes of Workers' Compensation Laws, 479
Self-Insurance, 479
Managed Care, 480
Eligibility, 480
Industrial Accident, 480
Occupational Illness, 480
Coverage, 480
Federal Laws, 480
State Laws, 480
State Disability and Workers'
Compensation, 484
Benefits, 484
Types of State Claims, 485
Nondisability Claim, 485
Temporary Disability Claim, 485
Permanent Disability Claim, 486
Fraud and Abuse, 487
Occupational Safety and Health
Administration Act of 1970, 489
Background, 489
Coverage, 490
Regulations, 490
Filing a Complaint, 490
Inspection, 490
Record Keeping and Reporting, 490
Legal Situations, 491
Medical Evaluator, 491
Depositions, 491
Medical Testimony, 491
Liens, 491
Third-Party Subrogation, 494
Medical Reports, 494
Privacy and Confidentiality, 494
Documentation, 495
Health Information Record Keeping, 495
Terminology, 495
Reporting Requirements, 500
Employer's Report, 500
Medical Service Order, 503

Physician's First Report, 504
Progress or Supplemental Report, 504
Final Report, 504
Claim Submission, 504
Financial Responsibility, 504
Fee Schedules, 506
Helpful Billing Tips, 510
Billing Claims, 510
Out-of-State Claims, 511
Delinquent or Slow Pay Claims, 511
PROCEDURE: Completing the Doctor's
First Report of Occupational Injury or
Illness, 513

16 *Disability Income Insurance and
Disability Benefit Programs,* 519
Disability Claims, 520
History, 520
Disability Income Insurance, 520
Individual, 520
Group, 522
Federal Disability Programs, 522
Workers' Compensation, 522
Disability Benefit Programs, 522
State Disability Insurance, 525
Background, 525
State Programs, 526
Funding, 526
Eligibility, 526
Benefits, 528
Time Limits, 528
Medical Examinations, 529
Restrictions, 529
Voluntary Disability Insurance, 529
Claims Submission, 529
Disability Income Claims, 529
Conclusion, 531

UNIT 4
*Inpatient and Outpatient
Billing*

17 *Hospital Billing,* 541
Patient Service Representative, 542
Qualifications, 542
Primary Functions and Competencies, 542
Principal Responsibilities, 542
Medicolegal Confidentiality Issues, 542
Documents, 542
Verbal Communication, 542
Computer Security, 545

Admissions Procedures, 546
  Appropriateness Evaluation
    Protocols, 546
  Admitting Procedures for Major Insurance
    Programs, 546
  Preadmissions Testing, 548
Compliance Safeguards, 548
Utilization Review, 549
  Quality Improvement Organization Program,
    549
Coding Hospital Procedures, 549
  Outpatient—Reason for Visit, 549
  Inpatient—Principal Diagnosis, 549
Coding Inpatient Procedures, 550
  ICD-9-CM Volume 3 Procedures, 550
Coding Outpatient Procedures, 551
  Current Procedural Terminology, 551
  Health Care Common Procedure Coding
    System, 551
  Modifiers, 552
Inpatient Billing Process, 552
  Admitting Clerk, 552
  Insurance Verifier, 552
  Attending Physician, Nursing Staff, and
    Medical Transcriptionist, 553
  Discharge Analyst, 554
  Charge Description Master, 554
  Code Specialist, 555
  Insurance Billing Editor, 555
  Nurse Auditor, 556
Reimbursement Process, 556
  Reimbursement Methods, 556
  Electronic Data Interchange, 557
  Hard Copy Billing, 558
  Receiving Payment, 558
Outpatient Insurance Claims, 558
  Hospital Professional Services, 558
Billing Problems, 558
  Duplicate Statements, 559
  Double Billing, 559
  Phantom Charges, 559
Hospital Billing Claim Form, 559
  Uniform Bill Inpatient and Outpatient Paper
    or Electronic Claim Form, 559
Diagnosis-Related Groups, 560
  History, 560
  The Diagnosis-Related Groups System, 561
  Diagnosis-Related Groups and the Physician's
    Office, 562
Outpatient Classification, 563
  Ambulatory Payment Classification
    System, 563
**PROCEDURE: New Patient Admission and
  Insurance Verification,** 565
**PROCEDURE: Coding from ICD-9-CM
  Volume 3,** 566

**PROCEDURE: Editing a Uniform Bill
  (UB-92) Paper or Electronic Claim
  Form,** 566
**PROCEDURE: Completing the UB-92 Paper
  or Electronic Claim Form,** 567

UNIT 5

Employment

18 Seeking a Job and Attaining Professional Advancement, 583

Employment Opportunities, 584
  Insurance Billing Specialist, 584
  Claims Assistance Professional, 584
Job Search, 584
  Online Job Search, 585
  Job Fairs, 586
  Application, 586
  Letter of Introduction, 589
  Resume, 589
  Interview, 591
  Follow-Up Letter, 595
Self-Employment, 595
  Setting Up an Office, 595
  Finances to Consider, 596
  Marketing, Advertising, Promotion, and Public
    Relations, 600
  Documentation, 600
  Mentor, 601
  Networking, 601
**PROCEDURE: Creating an Electronic
  Resume,** 605
**PROCEDURE: Preparing a Resume
  in ASCII,** 605

APPENDIX A

**Resources for Audiotapes, Books,
Newsletters, Periodicals, Software, and
Videotapes,** 607

APPENDIX B

Medi-Cal, 613

GLOSSARY, 635

INDEX, 653

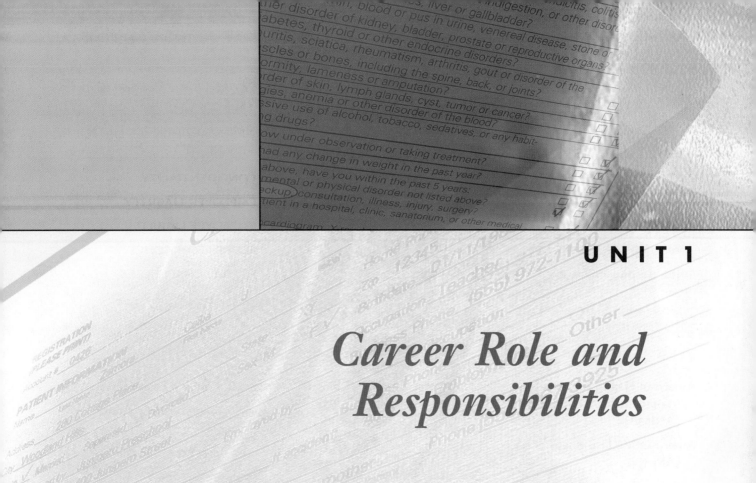

UNIT 1

Career Role and Responsibilities

CHAPTER OUTLINE

BACKGROUND OF INSURANCE CLAIMS, CODING, AND BILLING

ROLE OF THE INSURANCE BILLING SPECIALIST

Job Responsibilities

Educational and Training Requirements

Career Advantages

Qualifications

MEDICAL ETIQUETTE

MEDICAL ETHICS

CONFIDENTIALITY

EMPLOYER LIABILITY

EMPLOYEE LIABILITY

SCOPE OF PRACTICE

FUTURE CHALLENGES

KEY TERMS

American Health Information Management Association (AHIMA)

American Medical Association (AMA)

cash flow

claims assistance professional (CAP)

ethics

etiquette

insurance billing specialist

list service (listserv)

medical billing representative

multiskilled health practitioner (MSHP)

reimbursement specialist

respondeat superior

senior billing representative

1

Role of an Insurance Billing Specialist

OBJECTIVES*

After reading this chapter, you should be able to:

- Identify the background and importance of accurate insurance claims submission, coding, and billing.

- Name at least three skills possessed by insurance billing specialists.

- Describe the variety of career possibilities and areas of specialization open to those trained as insurance billing specialists.

- List personal qualifications and skills to be acquired by an insurance billing specialist.

- State the personal image to be projected as an insurance billing specialist.

- Specify the educational requirements for a job as an insurance billing specialist and a coder.

- Explain how insurance knowledge and medical knowledge can be kept current.

- Differentiate between medical ethics and medical etiquette.

*Performance objectives and exercises for hands-on practical experience for this chapter appear in the *Workbook*.

Service

When choosing a career as an insurance billing specialist, match your talents to the job. An attitude directed at serving the patient's needs should be your priority. Be alert to discover ways you can serve the patient while carrying out your job duties. A medical insurance billing specialist's primary goal is to assist in the revenue cycle, helping both the patient in obtaining maximum insurance plan benefits and ensuring a cash flow to the health care provider. *Revenue* is regular income and the *cycle* is the regularly repeating set of events that produces it. The insurance billing specialist's responsibility is to conduct business in an ethical manner. Service to patients gives the opportunity to show high values, principles, and moral character, which will be appreciated and noticed.

BACKGROUND OF INSURANCE CLAIMS, CODING, AND BILLING

Welcome to the world of insurance billing, an exciting, ever-changing, and fast growing career field. To help you focus on important terms and definitions, some of the basic words in this and subsequent chapters appear in bold or italic type. See the Glossary at the end of this textbook for a comprehensive list of key terms, with detailed definitions to broaden your knowledge.

A physician may have many problems that can affect obtaining maximum payment for services. He or she relies on professionals to handle billing, transmission, and follow-up of claims. The health care industry is one of the most heavily regulated industries in the United States.

A number of billing and payment mechanisms are associated with health insurance carriers, and a number of health insurance policy issues pertaining to compliance are connected with each carrier.

There are two billing components: hospital billing and professional billing. Hospital billing is done for a facility, such as an acute care hospital, a skilled nursing or long-term care facility, a rehabilitation center, or an ambulatory surgical center. Professional billing is done for a physician or *non-physician practitioner* (NPP). An NPP is an individual who has not obtained a medical degree but is allowed to see patients and prescribe medications, such as a nurse practitioner, physical therapist, speech therapist, licensed clinical social worker, or certified registered nurse practitioner. These people are sometimes referred to as *physician extenders*. An insurance billing specialist must realize that NPPs have a provider number and are permitted to submit claims to an insurance carrier. There may be occasions when the patient does not see a doctor but is directed to the NPP. Proper authorization and documentation is required, and then an encounter form

is generated for the NPP. Hence, this course is designed for professional billing.

Payment schedules for payment of professional services are based on the payer type, for example, managed care, workers' compensation, or Medicare. Physicians are paid according to relative value units, which are based on three things: (1) the cost (overhead) of delivering care, (2) malpractice insurance, and (3) the physician's work. A fee schedule is published by the Centers for Medicare and Medicaid Services, a federal organization that sets the mandates for financing and delivery of care in the United States. Managed care organizations establish their own physician fee schedules. Their rates are close to what Medicare pays.

Whether you are employed to perform hospital or professional billing functions, the basic setup of a business office encompasses the following units or combined departments: reception of the patient, rendering of medical services, documentation of the services, and financial accounting. You must understand their function in relation to the business office and the practice as a whole and how they affect payment for services. The flow of information is one of the most vital components of an organization. Knowing the departments within the organization can assist in the effective flow of information, such as by written documents, telephone calls, oral communication among co-workers, or electronic mail (e-mail).

Office procedures performed throughout a workday include the following:

Scheduling appointments involves assigning time slots for patients' visits. Canceling and rescheduling may also be involved. If the time is not properly assigned, there may be an influx or low volume of patients at a given time. Paperwork required for the visit must be obtained. It is important to record why the patient requires a visit.

Registering patients may involve preregistration for visits. Financial and personal data are collected and accurately recorded (input) in a timely manner. Incorrect information affects the back office procedures and submission and payment of claims.

Documenting pertinent clinical notes and assigning a diagnosis and service code to the patient's condition and visit is done by the provider of service. Other forms pertaining to treatment requests by secondary providers are recorded by this team. The insurance billing specialist may be required to contact the insurance company to obtain authorization for treatment by secondary providers. He or she must also ensure that forms are properly completed and data are input into the system.

Proper documentation and assignment of the correct code for service both impact reimbursement.

Charging entries pertain to inputting the patient's services into the system. The charge entry person must ensure that the insurance is correctly sequenced in the system, for example, primary versus secondary health insurance or workers' compensation or automobile insurance versus primary health insurance. This person must ensure that the diagnosis coincides with the service rendered. For example, an obstetrics/gynecology visit should not have a diagnosis related to ophthalmology. Many times individuals have the same names, so billing service dates and the name of the patient seen must be accurate. Charge entry staff must ensure that the correct charge is assigned to the correct patient. Proper charge entry ensures timely billing and reimbursement.

Filing and maintaining health information records and distributing the mail to various departments within the office is done by a file clerk. He or she pulls health records and works with various internal and external forms required by the billing department.

Bookkeeping and accounting is the posting of payments received (cash, checks, electronic funds transfer) to patients' financial accounts. The bookkeeper or accountant must pay special attention to adjustments, denials, and write-offs. These entries may require investigation for validation. He or she may also receive insurance carrier remittance advices and may be assigned to follow up on denials.

ROLE OF THE INSURANCE BILLING SPECIALIST

In the past, administrative front office staff working in a physician's office performed both administrative and clinical duties. As decades passed, staff members' duties entailed either one or the other. Currently, because of changes in government regulations and standards for the insurance industry, specific medical assisting job tasks have become specialized. In a medical practice, it is commonplace to find administrative duties shared by a number of employees (e.g., administrative medical assistant, bookkeeper, file clerk, insurance billing specialist, office manager, receptionist, or transcriptionist). Several job title names are associated with medical billing personnel. The title used may depend on the region within the United States. Some of the most popular titles include **insurance billing specialist,** electronic claims processor, medical biller, **reimbursement specialist, medical billing representative,** and **senior billing representative.** Hence, the title suggests that the employee is proficient in all aspects of medical billing.

In this handbook, the title "insurance billing specialist" is used throughout. In clinics and large practices, it is common to find a billing department made up of many people, and within the department each position is specialized, such as Medicare billing specialist, Medicaid billing specialist, coding specialist, insurance counselor, collection manager, and medical and financial records manager.

Some medical practices and clinics contract with management services organizations (MSOs), which perform a variety of business functions, such as accounting, billing, coding, collections, computer support, legal advice, marketing, payroll, and management expertise. An insurance billing specialist may find a job working for an MSO as a part of this team.

An independent billing company may be a suitable organization for an insurance billing specialist.

Cost pressures on health care providers are forcing employers to reduce personnel costs by hiring **multi-skilled health practitioners** (MSHPs). An MSHP is a person cross-trained to provide more than one function, often in more than one discipline. Knowledge of insurance claims completion and coding enhances skills so that he or she can offer more flexibility to someone hired in a medical setting.

People called **claims assistance professionals** (CAPs) work for the consumer and help patients organize, file, and negotiate health insurance claims of all types. A CAP's primary goals are to assist the consumer in obtaining maximum benefits and to tell the patient how much to pay the providers to make sure there is no overpayment. A medical insurance billing specialist may also function in this role.

Job Responsibilities

Whether you are employed by the medical practice of an academic medical center or a hospital, or if you are a solo practitioner, billing employees should be able to perform any and all duties assigned pertaining to the business office. This includes front and back office responsibilities. Both entities work in conjunction to ensure a strong billing cycle and enhanced reimbursement. Examples of generic job descriptions are shown in Figures 1–1 through 1–4 to illustrate what job duties, skills, and requirements might be encountered for various insurance billing and coding positions. Job descriptions are used as tools by assisting managers, supervisors, and employers in recruiting, supervising, and evaluating individuals in these positions for salary upgrades. Companies have had to modify their job descriptions to address individuals with physical impairments who may fall under the American with Disabilities Act.

GENERIC JOB DESCRIPTION FOR ENTRY LEVEL INSURANCE BILLING SPECIALIST

Knowledge, skills, and abilities:
1. Minimum education level consists of certificate from one-year insurance billing course, associate degree, or equivalent in work experience and continuing education.
2. Knowledge of basic medical terminology, anatomy and physiology, diseases, surgeries, medical specialties, and insurance terminology.
3. Ability to operate computer, printer, photocopy, and calculator equipment.
4. Written and oral communication skills including grammar, punctuation, and style.
5. Ability and knowledge to use procedure code books.
6. Ability and knowledge to use diagnostic code books.
7. Knowledge and skill of data entry.
8. Ability to work independently.
9. Certified Procedural Coder (CPC) or Certified Coding Specialist (CCS) status preferred.

Working conditions:
Medical office setting. Sufficient lighting.

Physical demands:
Prolonged sitting, standing and walking. Use of word processor or computer equipment. Some stooping, reaching, climbing, and bending. Occasional lifting of _____lbs. to a height of 5 feet. Hearing and speech capabilities necessary to communicate with patients and staff in person and on telephone. Vision capable of viewing computer monitors, calculators, charts, forms, text, and numbers for prolonged periods.

Salary:
Employer would list range of remuneration for the position.

Job responsibilities:	**Performance standards:**
1. Abstracts health information from patient records.	1.1 Uses knowledge of medical terminology, anatomy and physiology, diseases, surgeries, and medical specialties.
	1.2 Consults reference materials to clarify meanings of words.
	1.3 Meets accuracy and production requirements adopted by employer.
	1.4 Verifies with physician any vague information for accuracy.
2. Exhibits an understanding of ethical and medicolegal responsibilities related to insurance billing programs.	2.1 Observes policies and procedures related to federal privacy regulations, health records, release of information, retention of records, and statute of limitations for claim submission.
	2.2 Meets standards of professional etiquette and ethical conduct.
	2.3 Recognizes and reports problems involving fraud, abuse, embezzlement, and forgery to appropriate individuals.

FIGURE 1–1   Generic job description for an insurance billing specialist.

3. Operates computer
to transmit insurance claims.

3.1 Operates equipment skillfully
and efficiently.
3.2 Evaluates condition of equipment and
reports need for repair or replacement.

4. Follows employer's policies
and procedures.

4.1 Punctual work attendance and is dependable.
4.2 Answers routine inquiries related to
account balances and dates insurance
forms submitted.

5. Transmits insurance
claims accurately.

5.1 Updates insurance registration and
account information.
5.2 Processes payments and posts to
accounts accurately.
5.3 Handles correspondence related to
insurance claims.
5.4 Reviews encounter forms for accuracy
before submission to data entry.
5.5 Inserts data for generating insurance claims
accurately.
5.6 Codes procedures and diagnoses
accurately.
5.7 Telephones insurance companies with
regard to delinquent claims.
5.8 Traces insurance claims.
5.9 Files appeals for denied claims.
5.10 Documents registration data from patients
accurately.
5.11 Maintains separate insurance files.

6. Enhances knowledge and
skills to keep up-to-date.

6.1 Attends continuing education activities.
6.2 Obtains current knowledge applicable to
state and federal programs as they relate
to insurance claim submission.
6.3 Keeps abreast and maintains files of current
changes in coding requirements from Medicare,
Medicaid, and other third-party payers.
6.4 Assists with updating fee schedules and
encounter forms with current codes.
6.5 Assists in the research of proper coding
techniques to maximize reimbursement.

7. Employs interpersonal
expertise to provide good
working relationships with
patients, employer, employees,
and insurance companies.

7.1 Works with employer and employees
cooperatively as a team.
7.2 Communicates effectively with patients
and insurance companies regarding
payment policies and financial obligations.
7.3 Executes job assignments with diligence
and skill.
7.4 Assists staff with coding and reimbursement problems.
7.5 Assists other employees when needed.
7.6 Assists with giving fee estimates to
patients when necessary.

FIGURE 1–1, cont'd Generic job description for an insurance billing specialist.

GENERIC JOB DESCRIPTION FOR PRIVATE CONTRACTOR AS A CLAIMS ASSISTANCE PROFESSIONAL

Knowledge, skills, and abilities:
1. Minimum education level consists of certificate from one-year insurance billing course, associate degree, or equivalent in work experience and continuing education.
2. Knowledge of basic medical terminology, anatomy and physiology, diseases, surgeries, medical specialties, and insurance terminology.
3. Ability to operate computer and printer, as well as photocopy and calculator equipment.
4. Written and oral communication skills including grammar, punctuation, and style.
5. Ability and knowledge to use procedure code books.
6. Ability and knowledge to use diagnostic code books.
7. Ability to keyboard 45 to 60 wpm.
8. Ability to work independently.
9. Certified Claims Assistance Professional (CCAP) status preferred.

Working conditions:
Home office setting. Sufficient lighting and space to allow for at least 3 or more people.

Physical demands:
Prolonged sitting, standing, and walking. Use of computer equipment. Some stooping, reaching, climbing, and bending. Occasional lifting of ____lbs. to a height of 5 feet. Hearing and speech capabilities necessary to communicate with clients in person and on telephone. Vision capable of viewing computer monitors, calculators, charts, forms, text, and numbers for prolonged periods.

Salary:
Client would pay a percentage of reimbursement or annual salary, hourly wage, or per claim fee.

Job responsibilities:	**Performance standards:**
1. Files secondary insurance claims and maintains insurance files.	1.1 Completes accurately and submits secondary insurance claims.
2. Tracks insurance claim payments received by clients.	2.1 Maintains files and traces insurance claims for clients.
3. Exhibits an understanding of ethical and medicolegal responsibilities related to insurance billing programs.	3.1 Observes policies and procedures related to federal privacy regulations of health records, release of information, retention of records, and statute of limitations for claim submission.

FIGURE 1–2   Generic job description for private contractor as a claims assistance professional.

Administrative front office duties have gained in importance for the following reasons. Documentation is vital to good patient care. It must be done comprehensively for proper reimbursement. Diagnostic and procedural coding must be reviewed for its correctness and completeness. Insurance claims must be promptly submitted, ideally within 1 to 5 business days to ensure continuous cash flow. **Cash flow** is the amount of actual money available to the medical practice. Without money coming in, overhead expenses cannot be met and a practice will face financial difficulties. Data required for billing must be collected from all health care providers as well as from hospitals, outpatient clinics, and laboratories involved in a case.

	3.2 Meets standards of professional etiquette and ethical conduct.
	3.3 Recognizes and reports problems involving fraud, abuse, embezzlement, and forgery to appropriate individuals.
4. Knowledge of medical terminology.	4.1 Explains data on insurance claim forms.
5. Knowledge of procedure and diagnostic code requirements, as well as health insurance terminology.	5.1 Understands procedural and diagnostic codes and checks to see if correct codes were used.
6. Operates computer equipment to complete and submit secondary insurance claims.	6.1 Operates equipment skillfully and efficiently.
	6.2 Evaluates condition of equipment and negotiates repair or replacement.
7. Employs interpersonal expertise to provide good working relationships with clients, medical office personnel, and insurance companies.	7.1 Works with clients, medical office personnel, and insurance companies with efficiency, diligence, and skill.
	7.2 Communicates effectively with clients and insurance companies regarding payment policies.
	7.3 Answers routine inquiries related to status of clients' accounts and dates insurance forms submitted.
8. Assists clients in challenging insurer's denials of payment of claims.	8.1 Handles correspondence related to denial of insurance payment.
	8.2 Telephones insurance companies and medical offices with regard to delinquent claims.
9. Interacts with health personnel to render additional information to appeal a denied claim and obtains payment for clients depending on terms of the health insurance policy or program.	9.1 Files appeals for denied claims.
10. Enhances knowledge and skills to keep up-to-date.	10.1 Attends continuing education activities.
	10.2 Obtains current knowledge applicable to private insurance and the Medicare program related to insurance claim submission and payments.
	10.3 Keeps abreast of current changes in coding requirements from Medicare, Medicaid, and other third-party payers.

FIGURE 1–2, cont'd Generic job description for private contractor as a claims assistance professional.

An insurance billing specialist in a large medical practice may act as an insurance counselor, taking the patient to a private area of the office to discuss the practice's financial policies and the patient's insurance coverage, and to negotiate a reasonable payment plan. The insurance billing specialist discusses claims processing with contracted and noncontracted carriers, the billing of secondary insurances and patients once the carrier pays its portion, self-pay billing, and time payment plans. Federal and state programs require the provider to submit claims for the patient. In other plans, it is the patient's obligation, rather than the provider's, to send the claim to the insurance carrier.

GENERIC JOB DESCRIPTION FOR AN ELECTRONIC CLAIMS PROCESSOR

Knowledge, skills, and abilities:
1. Minimum education level consists of certificate from one-year insurance billing course, associate degree, or equivalent in work experience and continuing education.
2. Knowledge of basic medical terminology, anatomy and physiology, diseases, surgeries, medical specialties, and insurance terminology.
3. Ability to operate computer and printer, as well as photocopy and calculator equipment.
4. Written and oral communication skills including grammar, punctuation, and style.
5. Ability and knowledge to use procedure code books.
6. Ability and knowledge to use diagnostic code books.
7. Knowledge and skill of data entry.
8. Ability to work independently.
9. Certified Electronic Claims Processor (CECP) status preferred.

Working conditions:
Medical office setting. Sufficient lighting.

Physical demands:
Prolonged sitting, standing and walking. Use of computer equipment. Some stooping, reaching, climbing, and bending. Occasional lifting of _____ lbs. to a height of 5 feet. Hearing and speech capabilities necessary to communicate with patients and staff in person and on telephone. Vision capabilities necessary to view computer monitors, calculators, charts, forms, text, and numbers for prolonged periods.

Salary:
Employer would list range of remuneration for the position.

Job responsibilities:	Performance standards:
1. Acts as a link between the medical provider or facility and insurance companies.	1.1 Uses knowledge of medical terminology, anatomy and physiology, diseases, surgeries, and medical specialties. 1.2 Understands computer applications and equipment required to convert and transmit patient billing data electronically. 1.3 Consults reference materials to clarify meanings of words. 1.4 Meets accuracy and production requirements adopted by employer. 1.5 Verifies with physician any vague information for accuracy. 1.6 Reduces volume of paperwork and variety of claim forms providers need to submit claims for payment.
2. Converts patient billing data into electronically readable formats.	2.1 Inputs data and transmits insurance claims accurately, either directly or through a clearinghouse. 2.2 Answers routine inquiries related to account balances and dates insurance data transmitted to insurance carriers.

FIGURE 1–3 Generic job description for an electronic claims processor.

3. Uses software that eliminates common claim filing errors, provides clean claims to insurance carriers, expedites payments to providers or facilities, and follows up on delinquent or denied claims.

4. Exhibits an understanding of ethical and medicolegal responsibilities related to insurance billing programs and plans.

5. Operates computer equipment to complete insurance claims.

6. Follows employer's policies and procedures.

7. Enhances knowledge and skills to keep up-to-date.

8. Employs interpersonal expertise to provide good working relationships with patients, employer, employees, and insurance companies.

2.3 Updates and maintains software applications with requirements of clearinghouses and insurance carriers.

3.1 Codes procedures and diagnoses accurately.
3.2 Telephones insurance companies about delinquent claims.
3.3 Traces insurance claims.
3.4 Files appeals for denied claims.

4.1 Observes policies and procedures related to federal privacy regulations, health records, release of information, retention of records, and statute of limitations for claim submission.
4.2 Meets standards of professional etiquette and ethical conduct.
4.3 Recognizes and reports problems involving fraud, abuse, embezzlement, and forgery to appropriate individuals.

5.1 Operates equipment skillfully and efficiently.
5.2 Evaluates condition of equipment and reports need for repair or replacement.

6.1 Must have punctual work attendance and be dependable.

7.1 Attends continuing education skills activities.
7.2 Obtains current knowledge applicable to state and federal programs as they relate to transmission of insurance claims.
7.3 Keeps abreast and maintains files of current changes in coding requirements from Medicare, Medicaid, and other third-party payers. Assists in the research of proper coding techniques to maximum reimbursement.

8.1 Works with employer and employees cooperatively as a team.
8.2 Communicates effectively with patients and insurance companies regarding payment policies and financial obligations.
8.3 Executes job assignments with diligence and skill.
8.4 Assists staff with coding and reimbursement problems.
8.5 Assists other employees when needed.
8.6 Assists with giving fee estimates to patients when necessary.

FIGURE 1–3, cont'd   Generic job description for an electronic claims processor.

GENERIC JOB DESCRIPTION FOR HOSPITAL CODERS

POSITION TITLE

Health Information/Medical Record Technician; Coder and Specialist for an acute and/or ambulatory care setting.

DEPARTMENT

Health Information/Medical Record.

JOB SUMMARY

Codes information from the medical records of patients to generate a clinical patient care database for the facility. Assures the maintenance and accuracy of diagnostic and procedural statistics for the facility, as well as optimum appropriate reimbursement from third party payers, by the timely coding of diagnoses and procedures using the required classification systems.

SPECIFIC RESPONSIBILITIES

Reviews and screens the entire medical record to abstract medical, surgical, laboratory, pharmaceutical, demographic, social and administrative data from the medical record in a timely manner.

Ensures providers that all diagnoses and procedures that may impact the facility's reimbursement are identified and attested to by the physician, if appropriate, sequenced correctly, and coded in an accurate and ethical manner for optimum reimbursement. Determines correct codes for routine, and/or new or unusual diagnoses and procedures not clearly listed in ICD-9-CM and CPT.

Consults with physicians for clarifications of clinical data when encountering conflicting or ambiguous information. Keeps abreast of regulator changes affecting coded information required by the Health Care Financing Administration, the office of Statewide Health Planning Department, and others, as apropriate; and applies current Uniform Hospital Discharge Data Set (UHDDS) definitions for code selection.

Maintains knowledge of current information related to third-party reimbursement regulations and seeks continuing education in all phases of coding acumen.

Participates in the Coding Team's regular meetings with the objective of solving problems, brain-storming, educating physicians and others as to the coding policies and procedures of the facility, as well as promoting consistency of data collected.

Achieves a balance in quality and quantity, with a goal of maintaining both elements at a prescribed level of efficiency.

Abides by AHIMA's established code of ethical principles to safe guard the public and contribute within the scope of the profession to quality and efficiency in health care, thus promoting ethical conduct.

OTHER SPECIFIC OR POTENTIAL DUTIES/RESPONSIBILITIES FOR THIS POSITION

Identifies any loss of revenue by failure to charge for any procedures, supplies, injections, or other services, and then submits the missed charges.

Verifies all fee sheets to assure that all charges, appropriate modifiers, dates of injury, E code(s), as well as referring physicians' license numbers (when required), have been documented.

Assigns Diagnosis-Related Groups (DRGs) after identifying not only the principal diagnosis (reason for admission) but also significant complications and/or comorbidities, as well as operating room procedures following comparison of relative weights in the DRG GROUPER software, and selection of the highest reimbursement allowable among alternative principal diagnoses documented in the record.

Identifies and abstracts information from medical records for special studies and audits, internal and external.

Assists physicians, ancillary, and administrative personnel with retrieving patient care information for research, planning, and marketing projects.

Answers questions regarding DRGs, as well as disease and procedure classification systems.

FIGURE 1–4   Generic job description for a hospital coder. (*From Stewart SP:* Generic job description for coders. *J CHIA, 1992, California Health Information Association, Fresno, Calif.*)

Generates reports using a computer report-writer to retrieve coded and abstracted information from the provider's data processing system.

Orients and instructs new personnel and/or students from health information/medical record technology/ administration programs, on unit operations, coding and abstracting activities.

DESCRIPTION OF SKILLS
I. TECHNICAL SKILLS REQUIRED:

A. Experience with and knowledge of instructional notations and conventions of ICD-9-CM and CPT HCPCS classification systems; and ability to follow the detailed guidelines related to their use in assigning single, and sequencing multiple, diagnosis and procedure codes for appropriate reimbursement and data collection.

B. Ability to read handwritten and transcribed documents in the health record, interpret information, and enter complete and accurate data into an on-line computer system.

C. Comprehensive knowledge of medical diagnostic and procedural terminology required.

D. College-level understanding of disease processes, anatomy and physiology necessary for assigning accurate numeric and alpha-numeric codes.

E. Knowledge of Federal, state and local government regulations and requirements which pertain to patient care information.

F. Knowledge of legalities and confidentiality issues involved with release of clinical or billing information.

G. Knowledge of third-party payer reimbursement requirements and an understanding of relative values for multimedical specialties, encounters, and procedures in acute care and ambulatory care settings.

II. DECISION-MAKING/
RESEARCH SKILLS REQUIRED:

A. Ability to query, analyze and determine the type of data needed to meet the request for information.

B. Ability to communicate technical and clinical information concerning patient care and classification systems at different levels; i.e., physicians, ancillary, and administrative personnel.

C. Ability to apply policies and procedures regarding data security and confidentiality to protect the inappropriate release of information.

D. Ability to exercise judgment with minimal supervision.

III. ORGANIZATIONAL SKILLS REQUIRED:

A. Ability to assume responsibility for compilation of clinical data related to inpatient and outpatient encounters including diagnoses, procedures, physicians and services.

B. Remains current with periodic updates of all coding manuals and guidelines in accordance with federal, state and local regulations.

C. Ability to manage time schedules, deadlines, multiple requests and priorities, and to maintain productivity.

IV. INTERPERSONAL SKILLS REQUIRED:

A. Communicates effectively, orally and in writing, with physicians, nurses and peers (both inter- and intra-departmentally) and with external organizations.

B. Communicates medical information with consideration of ethical and professional standards.

C. Upholds standards of federal privacy regulations regarding patients, personnel, and physicians.

V. EDUCATION AND
EXPERIENCE REQUIRED:

A. High school diploma.

B. Completion of an accredited program for coding certification or an accredited health information medical record technology program. A Certified Coding Specialist (CCS), a Certified Coding Specialist—Physician (CCSP), a Registered Health Information Technician (RHIT), or a Registered Health Information Administrator (RHIA) preferred, with current affiliation with the American Health Information Management Association.

C. Continuing education in health information management is required.

FIGURE 1–4, cont'd Generic job description for a hospital coder.

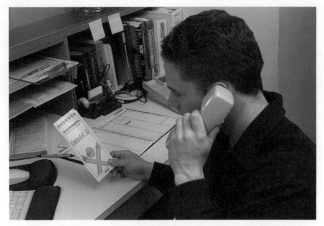

FIGURE 1–5 Insurance biller talking to a patient on the telephone about copayment required for an office visit under the patient's insurance plan.

Any copayments or deductible amounts should be collected from the patient at each visit. Also self-pay patients should be reminded that payment is due at the time of service. This is done to ensure that the physician will be paid for services rendered and to develop good communication lines. Patients who are informed are patients who pay their bills. The counselor learns the deductible amount and verifies with the insurance company whether any preauthorization, precertification, or second-opinion requirements exist. Counseling helps obtain payment in full when expensive procedures are necessary. In some offices, the insurance biller may act as a collection manager who answers routine inquiries related to account balances and insurance submission dates, assists patients in budgeting, follows up on delinquent accounts, and traces denied, "adjusted," or unpaid claims (Figure 1–5).

Large accounts receivable (total amount of money owed for professional services rendered) in a health care practice can be traced to a failure to verify insurance plan benefits, obtain authorization or precertification, or collect copayments and deductibles or inadequate claims filing. The rush to get a claim "out the door" cannot be justified when a practice has thousands or millions of dollars in unpaid or denied claims. Accounts receivables will be low and revenue high if a practice takes the extra time to ensure the claim is 100% accurate, complete, and verified.

In 1997, the American Association of Medical Assistants (AAMA) developed a role delineation study analyzing the many job functions of the medical assistant; it was updated in 2002 and published in 2003. Table 1.1 shows the Medical Assistant Role Delineation Chart, with highlighted areas indicating material covered in this textbook. The topics shown on the role delineation chart must be studied to pass the certification examination offered by the AAMA. Further information about many types of certification and registration is discussed in Chapter 18.

Educational and Training Requirements

Generally, a high school diploma or general equivalency diploma (GED) is required for entry into an insurance billing or coding specialist accredited program.

Table 1.1 | **Medical Assistant Role Delineation Chart**

Administrative		Clinical	
Administrative Procedures	**Practice Finances**	**Fundamental Principles**	**Patient Care**
Perform basic administrative medical assisting functions	Perform procedural and diagnostic coding	Apply principles of aseptic technique and infection control	Prepare patient for examinations, procedures, and treatments
Schedule, coordinate, and monitor appointments	Apply bookkeeping principles	Comply with quality assurance practices	Assist with examinations, procedures, and treatments
Schedule inpatient/outpatient admissions and procedures	Manage accounts receivable	Screen and follow up patient test results	Prepare and administer medications and immunizations
Understand and apply third-party guidelines	Manage accounts payable	**Diagnostic Orders**	Maintain medication and immunization records
Obtain reimbursement through accurate claims submission	Process payroll	Collect and process specimens	Recognize and respond to emergencies
Monitor third-party reimbursement	Document and maintain accounting and banking records	Perform diagnostic tests	Coordinate patient care information with other health care providers
	Develop and maintain fee schedules*		Initiate IV and administer IV medications with appropriate training and as permitted by state law

Table 1.1 Medical Assistant Role Delineation Chart—cont'd

Administrative

Administrative Procedures	Practice Finances	Clinical Fundamental Principles
Understand and adhere to managed care policies and procedures	Manage renewals of business and professional insurance policies*	Adhere to established patient screening procedures
Negotiate managed care contracts	Manage personnel benefits and maintain records*	Obtain patient history and vital signs
	Perform marketing, financial, and strategic planning	Prepare and maintain examination and treatment areas

General

Professionalism	Legal Concepts	Instruction
Display a professional manner and image	Perform within legal and ethical boundaries	Instruct individuals according to their needs
Demonstrate initiative and responsibility	Prepare and maintain medical records	Explain office policies and procedures
Work as a member of the health care team	Document accurately	Teach methods of health promotion and disease prevention
	Follow employer's established policies dealing with the health care contract	Locate community resources and disseminate information
Prioritize and perform multiple tasks	Implement and maintain federal and state health care legislation and regulations	Develop educational materials
Adapt to change	Comply with established risk management and safety procedures	Conduct continuing education activities
Promote the CMA credential	Recognize professional credentialing criteria	**Operational Functions**
Enhance skills through continuing education	Develop and maintain personnel, policy, and procedure manuals*	Perform inventory of supplies and equipment
Treat all patients with compassion and empathy		Perform routine maintenance of administrative and clinical equipment
Promote the practice through positive public relations		Apply computer techniques to support office operations
Communication Skills		
Recognize and respect cultural diversity		Perform personnel management functions
Adapt communications to individual's ability to understand		Negotiate leases and prices for equipment and supply contracts
Use professional telephone technique		
Recognize and respond effectively to verbal, nonverbal, and written communications		
Use medical terminology appropriately		
Use electronic technology to receive, organize, prioritize, and transmit information		
Serve as liaison		

Green colored blocks represent skills taught in this textbook.
Tan colored blocks are additional skills that an insurance billing specialist may need.
Reprinted by permission of the American Association of Medical Assistants from the AAMA Role Delineation Study. Occupational Analysis of the Medical Assisting Profession, 2003.
*Denotes advanced skills.

The accredited program usually offers additional education in medical terminology, insurance claims completion, procedural and diagnostic coding, anatomy and physiology, computer skills, ethics and medicolegal knowledge, and general office skills. Completion of an accredited program for coding certification or an accredited health information technology program is necessary for a job as a coder.

Experience in coding and insurance claim processing or management, completion of a 1-year insurance specialist certificate program at a community college, or both usually is required for a job as an insurance billing specialist. The curriculum that might be offered in a 1-year certificate program is shown in Figure 1–6. You might find that the courses in your locale may be labeled with different titles and time frames; the information contained in Figure 1–6 is specifically from a community college in Pennsylvania. Courses should cover medical terminology, anatomy and physiology, introduction to computer technology, procedural and diagnostic coding, and comprehensive medical insurance billing. A 2-year educational course can result in obtaining an associate's degree. Training prepares an individual for a wide range of employment opportunities. Knowledge of computer hardware and software, electronic data transmission requirements, and health care claim reimbursement is recommended for people planning to become electronic claims processors. Many accredited programs include an externship (on-the-job) period of training that may be paid or unpaid.

The **American Health Information Management Association (AHIMA)** published diagnostic and procedure

---

MEDICAL INSURANCE SPECIALIST CERTIFICATE PROGRAM

PROGRAM DESCRIPTION: The Medical Insurance program prepares you for employment in the area of medical insurance and health care claims processing. This program also serves the needs of health care personnel interested in upgrading their professional skills. Training in computerized medical billing, CPT-4 and ICD-9-CM coding, and processing medical insurance claims are included in the curriculum. Students may be enrolled on a full-time or part-time basis, and may complete the program by attending either day or evening classes. Accelerated or fasttrack courses are also available for those wishing to complete this program within a short time period. The program graduates students with marketable skills that are in demand. They are employed in hospitals, insurance companies, private medical laboratories, billing bureaus, and doctors' offices. Graduates may apply credits toward other certificate or associate degree programs.

The following courses are included in this program:

First Semester

Medical Terminology	3 Credits
Administrative Medical Office Management	4 Credits
Biology	3 Credits
Keyboarding	3 Credits
Computer I	2 Credits
	TOTAL 15 Credits

Second Semester

Principles and Applications of Medical Insurance	3 Credits
Current Issues of Medical Insurance	3 Credits
Medical Financial Management	3 Credits
Word Processing	3 Credits
Basic Principles of Composition	3 Credits
	TOTAL 15 Credits

FIGURE 1–6   Example of a 1-year medical insurance specialist certificate program offered at a community college. Basic coding is taught as a part of the course in Administrative Medical Office Management, and advanced coding is covered in Principles and Applications of Medical Insurance. Biology may be titled Anatomy and Physiology in some colleges. *(Reprinted with permission from Community College of Allegheny County, Pittsburgh, Pa.)*

coding competencies for outpatient services and diagnostic coding and reporting requirements for physician billing. Refer to these competencies for a more inclusive list of educational and training requirements by visiting the Web site listed in the Internet Resources at the end of this chapter.

It is necessary to have a moderate to high degree of knowledge of the health insurance business if your goal is to become a self-employed insurance billing specialist or claims assistance professional. In addition to insurance terminology, claims procedures, and coding, you must know commercial insurance carriers' requirements as well as Medicare and state Medicaid policies and regulations. You also need human relations skills and proficiency in running a business, including marketing and sales expertise.

To reach a professional level, certification is available from many national associations, depending on the type of certification desired. Refer to Chapter 18 for more information on this topic.

Career Advantages

Jobs are available in every state, ranging from non-management to management positions. Insurance billing specialists can receive a salary of $8000 part time to $50,000 or more full time or more per year depending on knowledge, experience, duties, responsibilities, locale, and size of the employing institution. Jobs are available in consulting firms, insurance and managed care companies, clinics, hospitals, multispecialty medical groups, and private physicians' practices, and as instructors or lecturers. You can be your own boss by either setting up an in-home billing service or establishing an office service for billing.

Self-Employment or Independent Contracting

Many people establish independently owned and self-operated businesses within their communities as medical insurance billing specialists, coders, claim assistance professionals, or collectors. However, the responsibilities are greater in this area because such work demands a full-time commitment, a lot of hard work, long hours to obtain clients, and the need to advertise and market the business. This means you are responsible for everything—advertising, billing, bookkeeping, and so on. Some billers work from their homes and others rent or lease an office. If you eventually plan on self-employment and you are weak in an area, such as accounting, then take a bookkeeping course. Chapter 18 discusses setting up your own business.

Flexible Hours

Another advantage of this career field is the opportunity to have flexible hours. Most other employees in the physician's office must adhere to the physician's schedule. However, the medical insurance billing specialist may want to come in early to transmit electronic claims during off-peak hours or stay late to make collection calls. It may be advantageous to both the physician and insurance specialist to vary his or her schedule according to the needs of the practice. In-home or office billing services save a medical practice valuable time, money, and overhead costs because the physician does not have to cover benefits or equipment.

Disabled Workers

A career as an insurance billing specialist or a collector of delinquent accounts can be very rewarding for persons with disabilities. These jobs are for individuals who have current knowledge of health care insurance billing as well as state and federal collection laws. Interacting well with people both in person and by telephone is essential in these roles. The financial management responsibilities and other jobs involving telephone communications are an opportunity for someone who is visually impaired because he or she is usually a good listener when properly and specifically trained. Special equipment may be necessary to enhance job performance, such as Braille keyboard, magnified computer screen, audible scanner, or tape recorder.

Working independently from a home office may appeal to a physically disabled person when there is no need to commute to a physician's office on a daily basis. Accessing information remotely via the computer and fax machine is a manageable method for success. However, it is important first to gain experience before trying to establish a home office business.

The government amended the Rehabilitation Act in 1998 to "require Federal agencies to make their electronic and information technology accessible to people with disabilities" because inaccessible technology may obviously interfere with one's ability to obtain and use information quickly and easily. Section 508 was enacted to diminish barriers in information technology. This makes new opportunities available for people with disabilities. You can learn more by visiting the Section 508 Web site listed in the Internet Resources at the end of this chapter.

Inquire at your local vocational rehabilitation center for training disabled individuals. Specific to being a delinquent account collector, you may contact the American Collectors Association (ACA) in Minneapolis, which has developed a training program for the visually impaired. Chapter 10 is devoted to the topic of collections.

Qualifications

Attributes

An individual must have a variety of characteristics or qualities to function well as an insurance billing specialist. Strong critical thinking and reading skills with good comprehension are a must. It is important to be a logical and practical thinker as well as a creative problem solver. Being meticulous and neat makes it easier to get the job done at the workstation. A person with good organizational skills and who is conscientious and loyal is always an asset to the employer. A person with a curious nature will dig deeper into an issue and not be satisfied with an answer unless the "whys" and "whats" are defined. This also helps one to grow while on the job and not become stagnant. This list is by no means complete; maybe you can think of additional attributes that might lead to a more successful career.

Skills

A person who completes insurance claims must have many skills. One needs the following skills to be proficient:

- Solid foundation and working knowledge of medical terminology, including anatomy, physiology, disease, and treatment terms, as well as the meanings of abbreviations.
  Application: Interpretation of patient's chart notes and code manuals.
  Incorrect: Final diagnosis: ASHD.
  Correct: Final diagnosis: Arteriosclerotic heart disease.
  It is difficult to locate the diagnostic code using an abbreviation; therefore, you must be able to translate it.
- Expert use of procedural and diagnostic code books and other related resources.
  Application: Code manuals and other reference books are used to assign accurate codes for each case billed.
- Precise reading skills.
  Application: Differentiate between a technical description of two different but similar procedures.
  Procedure (CPT) Code No. 43352 Esophagostomy (fistulization of esophagus, external; cervical approach).
  Procedure (CPT) Code No. 43020 Esophagotomy (cervical approach, with removal of foreign body).
  Note that the additional letter "s" to the surgical procedure in the first part of the example changes the entire procedure.
- Basic mathematics.
  Application: Calculate fees and adjustments on the insurance claim forms and enter into the patient accounts. It is essential that these figures be accurate.

- Knowledge of medicolegal rules and regulations of various insurance programs.
  Application: Avoid filing of claims considered fraudulent or abusive because of code selection and program policies.
- Knowledge of compliance issues
  Application: Federal Privacy, Security, Transaction rules in addition to Fraud, Waste and Abuse. For further information, see Chapter 2.
- Basic keyboarding and computer skills.
  Application: Good keyboarding and data entry skills and knowledge of computer programs is essential because the industry increasingly involves practice management software and electronic claims submission; handwritten claims are a format of the past.
- Proficiency in accessing information through the Internet.
  Application: Obtain federal, state, and commercial insurance regulations and current information as needed through the Internet. Sign on as a member of a **list service (listserv),** which is a service run from a Web site where questions may be posted. Find one composed of working coders to obtain answers on how to code complex, rare, or difficult medical cases.
- Knowledge of billing and collection techniques.
  Application: Use latest billing and collection ideas to keep cash flow constant and avoid delinquent accounts.
- Expertise in the legalities of collection on accounts.
  Application: Avoid lawsuits by knowing state and federal collection laws as they apply to medical collection of accounts receivable.
- Generate insurance claims with speed and accuracy.
  Application: If you develop your own business as a medical claims and billing specialist, you may be paid according to the amount of paid claims the health care practice is reimbursed. Because you will rely on volume for an income, the more expeditious you become, the more money you earn. Therefore accuracy in selecting the correct codes, data entry, and motivation in completing claims also become marketable skills. Measure your correct claim productivity for precision and time when you complete the insurance claim forms for this course and see how many accurate claims you can generate.

Personal Image

To project a professional image, be attentive to apparel and grooming (Figure 1–7). If a person works at home, the tendency is to dress casually (e.g., blue jeans, sneakers, shorts, tank tops). In a work setting, however, a uniform may be required or you might be expected to wear business attire that is conservative and stylish but not trendy. For women, this includes a business suit, dress, or skirt of

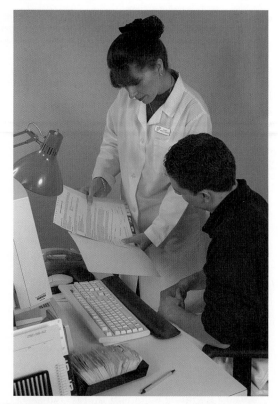

FIGURE 1–7 Male and female medical personnel who project a clean, fresh, and professional image with appropriate hairstyling.

appropriate length; slacks; sweaters; blouses; and dress shoes. For men, a business suit or dress slacks and jacket, shirt, tie (optional), and dress shoes are appropriate.

It is important, upon hire, to discuss with the supervisor appropriate dress code. Keep in mind fragrances can be offensive or cause allergies to some clients and patients; therefore, use good judgment. Fingernails should be carefully manicured and appropriate to dress code. For a woman, subdued eye makeup is appropriate for day use.

Consult the employer for office policy regarding body piercing and tattoos.

Remember you are in a professional environment and must present yourself in such a way.

Behavior

Many aspects make an individual a true professional: getting along with people rates high on the list, as does maintaining confidentiality of patients' medical histories and ongoing medical treatment. An insurance billing specialist depends on many co-workers for information needed to bill claims (e.g., the receptionist who collects the patient information). Therefore it is necessary to be

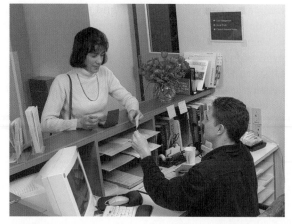

FIGURE 1–8 Interaction of insurance billing specialist with patient depicting medical etiquette.

a team player and treat patients and co-workers with courtesy and respect. Consider all co-workers' duties as important because they are part of the team helping you obtain the goal of processing the billing and obtaining maximum reimbursement for the patient and physician. Communicate effectively. Be honest, dependable, and on time. Never take part in office gossip or politics. Be willing to do the job and be efficient in how you carry it out.

MEDICAL ETIQUETTE

Before beginning work as an insurance billing specialist, it is wise to have a basic knowledge of medical etiquette as it pertains to the medical profession, the insurance industry, and the medical coder (Figure 1–8). Medical **etiquette** has to do with how medical professionals conduct themselves. Customs, courtesy, and manners of the medical profession can be expressed in three simple words: *consideration for others*.

Several points about medical etiquette bear mentioning:

1. Never keep another physician waiting longer than necessary in the reception room. Usher him or her into the physician's office as soon as it is unoccupied.
2. Always connect another physician who is calling on the telephone to your physician immediately, asking as few questions as possible. The only exception is if you know the physician calling is treating one of your patients and you wish to verify the name to pull the chart or other data for your physician.
3. Follow the basic rules of etiquette with co-workers while working in the office, such as acknowledging people who enter your office or come to your desk by saying "I'll be with you in a moment."
4. Identify yourself to callers and people you call.
5. Do not use first names until you know it is appropriate to do so.

6. Keep a professional demeanor and maintain a certain amount of formality when interacting with others. Remember to be courteous and always project a professional image.
7. Observe rules of etiquette when sending e-mail messages and placing or receiving cell phone calls. These rules fall under the Health Insurance Portability and Accountability Act and are stated in detail in Chapter 8.

MEDICAL ETHICS

Medical **ethics** are not laws, but standards of conduct generally accepted as moral guides for behavior by which an insurance billing or coding specialist may determine the propriety of his or her conduct in a relationship with patients, the physician, co-workers, the government, and insurance companies. You are entrusted with holding patients' medical information in confidence, collecting money for your physician, and being a reliable resource for your co-workers. Acting with ethical behavior means carrying out responsibilities with integrity, decency, honesty, competence, consideration, respect, fairness, trust, and courage.

The earliest written code of ethical principles and conduct for the medical profession originated in Babylonia about 2500 BC and is called the Code of Hammurabi. Then, about the fifth century BC, Hippocrates, a Greek physician who is known as the Father of Medicine, conceived the Oath of Hippocrates.

In 1980 the **American Medical Association (AMA)** adopted a modern code of ethics called the Principles of Medical Ethics for the benefit of the health professional and to meet the needs of changing times. The Principles of Medical Ethics of the AMA (Box 1.1) guide physicians' standards of conduct for honorable behavior in the practice of medicine.

It is the coder's responsibility to inform administration or his or her immediate supervisor if unethical or possibly illegal coding practices are taking place. Illegal activities are subject to penalties, fines, and/or imprisonment and can result in loss of morale, reputation, and the good will of the community. Standards of ethical coding developed by the AHIMA are available at their Web site. See Internet Resources at the end of this chapter.

The following are principles of ethics for the medical assistant and insurance billing specialist:

● Never make critical remarks about a physician to a patient or anyone else. Maintain dignity; never belittle patients.

Box 1.1   Principles of Medical Ethics of the American Medical Association

PREAMBLE

The medical profession has long subscribed to a body of ethical statements developed primarily for the benefit of the patient.

As a member of the profession, a physician must recognize responsibility not only to patients, but also to society, to other health professionals, and to self. The following principles adopted by the American Medical Association are not laws, but standards of conduct that define the essentials of honorable behavior for the physician.

I. A physician shall be dedicated to providing competent medical service with compassion and respect for human dignity.
II. A physician shall deal honestly with patients and colleagues, and strive to expose those physicians deficient in character or competence, or who engage in fraud or deception.
III. A physician shall respect the law and also recognize a responsibility to seek changes in those requirements that are contrary to the best interests of the patient.
IV. A physician shall respect the rights of patients, of colleagues and of other health professionals, and shall safeguard patient confidences within the constraints of the law.
V. A physician shall continue to study, apply and advance scientific knowledge, make relevant information available to patients, colleagues, and the public, obtain consultation, and use the talents of other health professionals when indicated.
VI. A physician shall, in the provision of appropriate patient care, except in emergencies, be free to choose whom to serve, with whom to associate, and the environment in which to provide medical services.
VII. A physician shall recognize a responsibility to participate in activities contributing to an improved community.

● Notify your physician if you discover that a patient in your practice may have questionable issues of care, conduct, or treatment with your office or another physician's practice. In certain circumstances, it may be unethical for two physicians to treat the same patient for the same condition.
● Maintain a dignified, courteous relationship with all persons in the office—patients, staff, and the physician—as well as with insurance adjusters, pharmaceutical representatives, and others who come into or telephone the office.
● Do not make critical statements about the treatment given a patient by another physician.

Anyone who uses the Internet for health-related reasons has a right to expect that organizations that provide health products, services, or information online will uphold ethical principles. The Internet Healthcare Coalition has developed eHealth Code of Ethics, which is available at their Web site. See Internet Resources at the end of this chapter.

It is *illegal* to report incorrect information to government-funded programs, such as Medicare, Medicaid, and TRICARE. However, private insurance carriers operate under different laws and it is *unethical, not illegal,* to report incorrect information to private insurance carriers. Incorrect information may damage the individual and the integrity of the database, allow reimbursement for services that should be paid by the patient, or deny payment that should be made by the insurance company.

Examples of illegal and unethical coding follow:

1. Violating guidelines by using code numbers or modifiers to increase payment when the case documentation does not warrant it.
2. Coding services or procedures that were not performed for payment.
3. Unbundling services provided into separate codes when one code is available and includes all the service.
4. Failing to code a relevant condition or complication when it is documented in the health record or, vice versa, assigning a code without documentation from the provider.
5. Coding a service in such a way that it is paid when usually it is not covered.
6. Coding another condition as the principal or primary diagnosis when the majority of the patient's treatment is for the preexisting condition.

The AHIMA has established a code of ethics. This code is appropriate for persons handling health information, whether they are health information specialists, insurance billing specialists, or coders (Figure 1–9).

In the final analysis, most ethical issues can be reduced to right and wrong with the main focus being the moral dictum to do no harm.

CONFIDENTIALITY

An insurance billing specialist must be held responsible for maintaining confidentiality when working with patients and their records. The next chapter presents information related to the privacy issues of the Health Insurance Portability and Accountability Act (HIPAA).

EMPLOYER LIABILITY

As mentioned, insurance billing specialists can be either self-employed or employed by physicians, clinics, or hospitals. Physicians are legally responsible for their own conduct and any actions of their employees performed within the context of their employment. This is referred to as *vicarious liability*, also known as **respondeat superior,** which literally means "let the master answer." However, this does not mean that an employee cannot be sued or brought to trial. Actions of the insurance biller may have

---

Preamble

This Code of Ethics sets forth ethical principles for the health information management profession. Members of this profession are responsible for maintaining and promoting ethical practices. This Code of Ethics, adopted by the American Health Information Management Association, shall be binding on health information management professionals who are members of the Association and all individuals who hold an AHIMA credential.

I. Health Information management professionals respect the rights and dignity of all individuals.
II. Health information management professionals comply with all laws, regulations, and standards governing the practice of health information management.
III. Health information management professionals strive for professional excellence through self-assessment and continuing education.
IV. Health information management professionals truthfully and accurately represent their professional credentials, education, and experience.
V. Health information management professionals adhere to the vision, mission, and values of the Association.
VI. Health information management professionals promote and protect the confidentiality and security of health records and health information.
VII. Health information management professionals strive to provide accurate and timely information.
VIII. Health information management professionals promote high standards for health information management practice, education, and research.
IX. Health information management professionals act with integrity and avoid conflicts of interest in the performance of their professional and AHIMA responsibilities.

FIGURE 1–9 AHIMA Code of Ethics revised and adopted by AHIMA House of Delegates October 4, 1998. American Health Information Management Association, Journal of AHIMA 70, no. 1 (1999) p. 1 of insert before p. 17. Copyright 1999 by the American Health Information Management Association. All rights reserved. No part of this may be reproduced, reprinted, stored in a retrieval system, or transmitted, in any form or by any means, electronic, photocopying, recording, or otherwise, without the prior written permission of the association.

a definite legal ramification on the employer, depending on the situation. For example, if an employee knowingly submits a fraudulent Medicare or Medicaid claim at the direction of the employer and subsequently the business is audited, both the employer and employee can be brought into litigation by the state or federal government. An insurance biller always should check with his or her physician-employer to determine whether he or she is included in the medical professional liability insurance policy, otherwise known as malpractice insurance. If not included, he or she could be sued as an individual. It is the physician's responsibility to make certain all staff members are protected.

EMPLOYEE LIABILITY

Errors and omissions insurance is protection against loss of money caused by failure through error or unintentional omission on the part of the individual or service submitting the insurance claim. Some physicians contract with a billing service to handle claims submission, and some agreements contain a clause stating that the physician will hold the company harmless from "liability resulting from claims submitted by the service for any account." This means the physician is responsible for mistakes made by the billing service. Thus errors and omissions insurance would not be needed in this instance. If a physician asks the insurance biller to do something that is the least bit questionable, such as write off patient balances for certain patients automatically, then make sure you have a legal document or signed waiver of liability relieving you of the responsibility for such actions.

SCOPE OF PRACTICE

An individual who works as a CAP acts as an informal representative of patients (policyholders and Medicare beneficiaries), helping to obtain insurance reimbursement. A CAP reviews and analyzes existing or potential policies; renders advice; and offers counseling, recommendations, and information. A CAP may not interpret insurance policies or act as an attorney. The legal ability of a CAP to represent a policyholder is limited. When a claim cannot be resolved after a denied claim has been appealed to the insurance company, the CAP must be careful in rendering a personal opinion or advising clients that they have a right to pursue legal action. Always check in your state to see if there is a scope of practice. In some states, a CAP could be acting outside the scope of the law by giving advice to clients on legal issues, even if licensed as an attorney but not practicing law full time. If the client wishes to take legal action, it is his or her responsibility to find a competent attorney specializing in contract law and insurance. In some states, giving an insured client advice on purchase or discontinuance of insurance policies is construed as being an insurance agent.

A number of states require CAPs to be licensed, depending on the services rendered to clients. CAPs who perform only the clerical function of filing health insurance claims do not have to be licensed. Check with your state's Department of Insurance and insurance commissioner (see Chapter 9) to determine whether you should be licensed.

If working as a CAP who does not handle checks or cash, inquire about an errors and omissions insurance policy by contacting the Alliance of Claims Assistance Professionals (ACAP).* When employed as a medical assistant who is submitting insurance claims, information on professional liability insurance may be obtained from the American Association of Medical Assistants, Inc.†

FUTURE CHALLENGES

As you begin your study to become an insurance billing specialist, remember that you are expected to profitably manage a medical practice's financial affairs or patient accounts; otherwise, you will not be considered qualified for this position. In subsequent chapters you will learn the important information and skills to help you achieve this goal. You will be expected to

● Know billing regulations for each insurance program and managed care plan in which the practice is a participant.
● Know the aspects of compliance rules and regulations.
● State various insurance rules about treatment and referral of patients.
● Become proficient in computer skills and use of various medical software packages.
● Learn electronic billing software and the variances of each payer.
● Develop diagnostic and procedural coding expertise.
● Know how to interpret third-party remittance advice summary reports, explanation of benefit documents, or both.
● Attain bookkeeping skills necessary to post, interpret, and manage patient accounts.
● Stay up-to-date by reading the latest health care industry association publications, participating in e-mail listserv discussions, and attending seminars on billing and coding.
● Cross-train so you become familiar with other aspects of the medical practice.

---

*ACAP, 873 Brentwood Drive, West Chicago, IL 60185-3743.
†20 North Wacker Drive, Suite 1575, Chicago, IL 60606.

RESOURCES

INTERNET

- For a list of educational and training requirements of the AHIMA diagnostic and procedure coding competencies for outpatient services and diagnostic coding and reporting requirements for physician billing
  Web site: **http://www.ahima.org**

- For standards of ethical coding developed by the American Health Information Management Association, visit
  Web site: **http://www.ahima.org**

- For eHealth Code of Ethics developed by the Internet Healthcare Coalition Organization, visit
  Web site: **http://www.ihealthcoalition.org**

- For Rehabilitation Act in 1998, which makes electronic and information technology accessible to people with disabilities, visit the Web site for Section 508:
  Web site: **http://www.section508.gov**

ASSIGNMENT

STUDENT

✔ Read Introduction in the *Workbook*, which explains how you will be working as an insurance billing specialist during this course.

✔ Study Chapter 1.

✔ Answer the review questions in the *Workbook* to reinforce the theory learned in this chapter and help prepare for a future test.

✔ Complete the assignments in the *Workbook* to help develop critical thinking and writing skills. As you proceed through the assignments in the *Workbook*, you will broaden your knowledge of medical terminology as well as gain an entry-level skill in diagnostic and procedural coding and insurance claim completion.

✔ Turn to the glossary at the end of this textbook for a further understanding of the key terms used in this chapter.

CHAPTER OUTLINE

COMPLIANCE DEFINED
HEALTH INFORMATION USING
   ELECTRONIC TECHNOLOGIES
   E-Health Information
      Management
   National Health Information
      Infrastructure
   Health Level Seven
SYSTEMIZED NOMENCLATURE
   OF HUMAN AND VETERINARY
   MEDICINE (SNOMED)
   INTERNATIONAL
HEALTH INSURANCE
   PORTABILITY AND
   ACCOUNTABILITY ACT (HIPAA)
   Title I: Health Insurance Reform
   Title II: Administrative
      Simplification
   Defining Roles And
      Relationships: Key Terms
   HIPAA in the Practice Setting
THE PRIVACY RULE:
   CONFIDENTIALITY AND
   PROTECTED HEALTH
   INFORMATION
   Confidential Information
   Patients' Rights
   Privacy Rules: Patient Rights
      under HIPAA
   Right to Notice of Privacy
      Practices
   Right to Request Restrictions
      on Certain Uses and
      Disclosures of PHI
   Right to Request Confidential
      Communications
   Right to Access, Inspect, and
      Obtain PHI
   Right to Request Amendment
      of PHI

Right to Receive an Accounting
   of Disclosures of PHI
ORGANIZATION AND STAFF
   RESPONSIBILITIES IN
   PROTECTING PATIENT RIGHTS
   Verification of Identity and
      Authority
   Validating Patient Permission
   Training
   Safeguards: Ensuring That
      Confidential Information is
      Secure
   Complaints to Health Care
      Practice and Workforce
      Sanctions
   Mitigation
   Refraining from Intimidating
      or Retaliatory Acts
TRANSACTION AND CODE SET
   REGULATIONS:
   STREAMLINING ELECTRONIC
   DATA INTERCHANGE
   Standard Unique Identifiers
THE SECURITY RULE:
   ADMINISTRATIVE, PHYSICAL,
   AND TECHNICAL SAFEGUARDS
APPLICATION TO PRACTICE
   SETTING
   Guidelines for HIPAA Privacy
      Compliance
CONSEQUENCES OF
   NONCOMPLIANCE WITH HIPAA
OFFICE OF INSPECTOR GENERAL
   Fraud and Abuse Laws
   Federal False Claims Act
   Qui Tam "Whistleblower"
   Civil Monetary Penalties Law
   Criminal False Claims Act
   Stark Laws
   Anti-Kickback Statute

Safe Harbors
Additional Laws and Compliance
Operation Restore Trust
Medicare Integrity Program
Correct Coding Initiative
Increased Staffing and Expanded
   Penalties for Violations
Special Alerts, Bulletins, and
   Guidance Documents
Exclusion Program
COMPLIANCE PROGRAM
   GUIDANCE FOR INDIVIDUAL
   AND SMALL GROUP
   PHYSICIAN PRACTICES
   Increased Productivity and
      Decreased Penalties with Plan
SEVEN BASIC COMPONENTS OF
   A COMPLIANCE PLAN
   Conducting Internal Monitoring
      and Auditing
   Implementing Compliance and
      Practice Standards
   Designing a Compliance Officer
      or Contact
   Conducting Appropriate
      Training and Education
   Responding Appropriately to
      Detected Offenses and
      Developing Corrective Action
   Developing Open Lines of
      Communication
   Enforcing Disciplinary
      Standards Through Well-
      Publicized Guidelines
WHAT TO EXPECT FROM YOUR
   HEALTH CARE PRACTICE
COMPLIANCE LESSONS LEARNED
INTERNET RESOURCES

KEY TERMS

abuse

authorization form

breach of confidential
   communication

business associate

clearinghouse

code set

compliance

compliance plan

confidential
   communication

confidentiality

consent form

covered entity

disclosure

e-health information
   management (eHIM)

electronic media

embezzlement

fraud

health care provider

individually identifiable
   health information
   (IIHI)

nonprivileged
   information

phantom billing

privacy

privacy officer, privacy
   official (PO)

privileged information

protected health
   information (PHI)

standard

state preemption

transaction

use

2

Compliance and the E-Health Initiative

OBJECTIVES*

After reading this chapter, you should be able to:

- Name the initiative that is working toward development of a personal health record created and controlled by the individual or family.

- Define e-health information management (eHIM).

- Explain the difference between Title I Insurance Reform and Title II Administrative Simplification.

- Describe the federal standards under the Health Insurance Portability and Accountability Act (HIPAA).

- State the fines and penalties imposed by the Civil Monetary Penalties Law.

- Define protected health information (PHI).

- Explain the Privacy Rule as it pertains to protected health information.

- Illustrate the difference between privileged and nonprivileged information.

- Explain the difference between a notice, a consent, and an authorization when disclosing PHI.

- Identify the difference between disclosure and use of PHI.

- List the three major categories of security safeguards under HIPAA.

- List the civil and criminal penalties of noncompliance with HIPAA regulations.

- List various types of insurance fraud.

- Define abuse as it relates to the subject of billing insurance claims.

- State the guidelines for HIPAA privacy compliance.

*Performance objectives and exercises for hands-on practical experience for this chapter appear in the *Workbook*.

Service

The insurance billing specialist has many opportunities to serve patients' needs. When presenting the Notice of Privacy, greet the patient with a smile and a helpful and caring attitude. Be ready to answer questions regarding the notice. Have the notice available in those languages spoken by a significant portion of the medical practice's patient population. Serve patients by respecting their privacy and keeping protected health information confidential, disclosing it only according to the medical practice's correct policies and procedures that comply with federal regulations.

Use of electronic formats in the health care industry is a driving force behind electronic communications that will make a full circle to complete the patient care process. It is your duty to understand how health information and electronic technologies tie together. As an educated and informed employee, you can better serve the patients that visit your office.

COMPLIANCE DEFINED

Compliance in the health care industry is the process of meeting regulations, recommendations, and expectations of federal and state agencies that pay for health care services and regulate the industry. Health care compliance encompasses the claims reimbursement processes, managed care procedures, Occupational Safety and Health Administration (OSHA), Clinical Laboratory Improvement Amendments (CLIA), licensure, and due diligence in obeying the law.

Any business that is involved with the health care industry must conform its practices to follow the principles and practices as identified by state and federal agencies. The professional elements of the principles and practices include:

● Regulations and recommendations to protect individuals
● Streamline processes
● Supporting system-wide stability

A compliance strategy provides a standardized process for handling business functions, much like a "user's manual." This will enable consistent and effective management and staff performance. Failure to comply with mandates leads to sanctions and fines from state and federal agencies. Failure to follow guidelines potentially results in more fraud and abuse in the claims reimbursement cycle.

HEALTH INFORMATION USING ELECTRONIC TECHNOLOGIES

Over the past decade, the United States health care system has undergone rapid change with regard to the separate issues of privacy, security, and claims processing. A number of organizations have participated to help standardize and improve the delivery and quality of health care.

Some code systems and additional terminology have been created by the adoption of the many federal statutes. In this chapter you will learn some important key terms related to health information as it pertains to compliance and its role in electronic technology. You will also get acquainted with important initiatives that control the use of health information. In subsequent chapters, you will learn many more terms and read more in-depth discussion on certain subjects related to compliance with government regulations that affect health care. These appear as color-screened sections entitled "HIPAA Compliance Alert."

E-Health Information Management

E-health information management, more commonly seen as *eHIM*, is a term coined by the American Health Information Management Association's eHealth Task Force to describe any and all transactions in which health care information is accessed, processed, stored, and transferred using electronic technologies.

National Health Information Infrastructure

The National Health Information Infrastructure (NHII) is an initiative set forth to improve patient safety and the quality of health care as well as to better inform individuals regarding their own health information and to help them understand health care costs.

NHII is overseen by the Department of Health and Human Services with the National Committee on Vital and Health Statistics (NCVHS) serving as a public advisory committee (Box 2.1).

Health Level Seven

Health Level Seven (HL7) is a standards developing organization whose mission is "to provide standards for the exchange, management and integration of data that support clinical patient care and the management, delivery, and evaluation of health care services. Specifically, to create flexible, cost effective approaches, standards, guidelines, methodologies, and related services for interoperability between health care information systems." A **standard** means a rule, condition, or requirement.

Data exchanged between systems must share a well-defined knowledge of what meaning is behind the data transferred; therefore, part of HL7 focuses on efforts to manage vocabulary terms used in its messages. For example, this can be thought of as electronic (digital)

- An initiative to improve effectiveness, efficiency, and overall quality of health and health care in the United States
- A comprehensive knowledge-based network of interoperable systems of clinical, public health, and personal health information that would improve decision-making by making health information available when and where it is needed
- The set of technologies, standards, applications, systems, values, and laws that support all facets of individual health, health care, and public health
- Voluntary
- Not a centralized database of medical records or a government regulation

The scope of the initiative, in addition to health care research, is:

- Personal health, which includes a personal health record created and controlled by the individual or family, plus nonclinical information, such as self-care trackers and directories of health care providers
- Health care delivery, which includes information such as provider notes, clinical orders, decision-support programs, digital prescribing programs, and practice guidelines. Health care providers will retain responsibility for their own patients' medical records.
- Public health, which enables sharing of information to improve the clinical management of populations of patients such as vital statistics, population health risks, and disease registries

supporting documentation. This collection of data is a stream of encoded information that translates into understandable language when it is received. For years, the insurance biller has been making a copy of a patient's paper chart note and attaching it to the CMS-1500 paper claim form. The health care industry's future looks to HL7 to expand the capabilities of submitting claims and to enable the transfer of the data contained within the health record without using paper at all! To get a general idea of HL7, look at Example 2.1.

| **Example 2.1** |

To determine the date and time of a patient's birth date, for instance, let's say a neonate for whom the age in hours might be relevant, the time of the birth, using military time, can be recorded with the birth date. From this, the age can be generated from the date of birth (DOB). Baby Jane was born on March 24, 2004, at 8:26 AM.

When the required HL7 format is YYYYMM-DDHHMM, Baby Jane's date and time of birth will be entered for transmission as: **200403240826**

YYYY	MM	DD	HH	MM
2004	03	24	08	26
Year	Month	Day	Hour	Minute

Systematized Nomenclature of Human and Veterinary Medicine (SNOMED) International

SNOMED, a code system that is used for managing patient electronic health records (EHRs), that is, medical records, teaching medical information science (informatics), indexing and managing research data, and billing for laboratory medicine procedures is found in a book entitled *Systematized Nomenclature of Human and Veterinary Medicine (SNOMED) International*, volumes I though IV. This topic is mentioned in Chapter 5.

HEALTH INSURANCE PORTABILITY AND ACCOUNTABILITY ACT (HIPAA)

The *Health Insurance Portability and Accountability Act of 1996* (HIPAA), Public Law 104-191, has significant impact on both individuals and health care providers. There are two provisions of HIPAA, *Title I: Insurance Reform* and *Title II: Administrative Simplification*. HIPAA projects long-term benefits that include lowered administrative costs, increased accuracy of data, increased patient and customer satisfaction, and reduced revenue cycle time, ultimately improving financial management.

Title I: Health Insurance Reform

The primary purpose of HIPAA Title I: *Insurance Reform*, is to provide continuous insurance coverage for workers and their insured dependents when they change or lose jobs. This aspect of HIPAA affects individuals as consumers, not particularly as patients. Previously, when an employee left or lost a job and changed insurance coverage, a "preexisting" clause prevented or limited coverage for certain medical conditions. HIPAA now limits the use of preexisting condition exclusions, prohibits discrimination for past or present poor health, and guarantees certain employers and individuals the right to purchase new health insurance coverage after losing a job. Additionally, HIPAA allows renewal of health insurance coverage regardless of an individual's health condition that is covered under the particular policy.

Title II: Administrative Simplification

The goals of HIPAA Title II: *Administrative Simplification*, focus on the health care practice setting and aim to reduce administrative costs and burdens. Standardizing electronic transmissions of administrative and financial information will reduce the number of forms and methods used in the claims processing cycle and reduce the nonproductive effort that goes into processing paper or nonstandard electronic claims. Additional provisions are meant to ensure the privacy and security of an individual's health data.

Two parts of the Administrative Simplification provisions are as follows:

1. Development and implementation of standardized electronic transactions using common sets of descriptors (i.e., standard code sets). These must be used to represent health care concepts and procedures when performing health-related financial and administrative activities electronically (i.e., standard transactions) (see Box 2.2). HIPAA has been part of a great shift in processing electronic data. Transaction standards apply to the following, which are called covered entities under HIPAA: health care insurance coverage carriers, health care providers, and health care clearinghouses. A **clearinghouse** is a third-party administrator (TPA) that receives insurance claims from the physician's office, performs software edits, and redistributes the claims electronically to various insurance carriers.
2. Implementation of privacy and security procedures to prevent the misuse of health information by ensuring:

   ● Privacy and confidentiality
   ● Security of health information

Administrative simplification has created uniform sets of standards that protect and place limits on how confidential health information can be used. For years, health care providers have locked medical records in file cabinets and refused to share patient health information. Patients now have specific rights regarding how their health information is used and disclosed because federal and state laws regulate the protection of an individual's privacy. Knowledge and attention to the rights of patients are important to the compliance endeavor in a health care practice. Providers are entrusted with health information and are expected to recognize when certain health information can be used or disclosed.

Patients have the legal right to request (1) access and amendments to their health records, (2) an accounting of those who have received their health information, and (3) restrictions on who can access their health records. Understanding the parameters concerning these rights is crucial to complying with HIPAA.

Health care providers and their employer can be held accountable for using or disclosing patient health information inappropriately. HIPAA regulations will be enforced, as clearly stated by the U.S. government. The revolution of HIPAA will take time to understand and implement correctly, but as the standards are put into action, both within the practice setting and across the many different fields comprising the health industry, greater benefits will be appreciated by the health care provider, staff, and patients.

Defining Roles and Relationships: Key Terms

HIPAA legislation required the *U.S. Department of Health and Human Services* (HHS) to establish national standards and identifiers for electronic transactions as well as implement privacy and security standards. In regard to HIPAA, *Secretary* refers to the HHS Secretary or any officer or employee of HHS to whom the authority involved has been delegated.

The *Centers for Medicare and Medicaid Services* (CMS), previously known as the Health Care Financing Administration (HCFA), will enforce the insurance portability and transaction and code set requirements of HIPAA.

The *Office for Civil Rights* (OCR) will enforce privacy standards.

A **covered entity** transmits health information in *electronic form* in connection with a *transaction* covered by HIPAA. The covered entity may be (1) a health care coverage carrier such as Blue Cross/Blue Shield, (2) a health care clearinghouse through which claims are submitted, or (3) a health care provider such as the primary care physician.

A **business associate** is a person who, on behalf of the covered entity, performs or assists in the performance of a function or activity involving the use or disclosure of individually identifiable health information, including claims processing or administration, data analysis, processing or administration, utilization review, quality assurance, billing, benefit management, practice management, and repricing. For example, if a provider practice contracts with an outside billing company to manage its claims and accounts receivable, the billing company would be a business associate of the provider (the covered entity).

Box 2.2	Examples of Administrative and Financial Data	
Administrative Information	**Financial Information**
Referral certification and authorization for services	Health care claim submission for services
Enrollment/disenrollment of individual into health plan	Process health plan premium payment
Health plan eligibility	Check status of a previously submitted claim
	Health care payment and remittance advice
	Coordination of benefits

Electronic media refers to the mode of electronic transmission, including the following:

● Internet (online mode—wide open)
● Extranet or private network using Internet technology to link business parties
● Leased phone or dial-up phone lines, including fax modems (speaking over phone is not considered an electronic transmission)
● Transmissions that are physically moved from one location to another using magnetic tape, disk, or compact disk media

A **health care provider** is a provider of medical or health services and any other person or organization who furnishes bills or is paid for health care in the normal course of business.

Privacy and security officers oversee the HIPAA-related functions. These individuals may or may not be employees of a particular health care practice. A **privacy officer** or **privacy official (PO)** is designated to help the provider remain in compliance by setting policies and procedures (P&P) and by training and managing the staff regarding HIPAA and patient rights, and the PO is usually the contact person for questions and complaints. A *security officer* protects the computer and networking systems within the practice and implements protocols such as password assignment, backup procedures, firewalls, virus protection, and contingency planning for emergencies.

A **transaction** refers to the transmission of information between two parties to carry out financial or administrative activities related to health care. These data transmissions include information that complete the health care claim process and are discussed further in Chapter 8.

HIPAA in the Practice Setting

The previous "roles" create relationships that guide the health care provider and the practice. A health care provider can include a physician's assistant, nurse practitioner, social worker, chiropractor, radiologist, or dentist; HIPAA does not only affect medical physicians. The health care provider is designated as an HIPAA-mandated covered entity under certain conditions. It is important to remember that health care providers who transmit any health information in electronic form in connection with an HIPAA transaction are covered entities. Electronic form or media can include floppy disk, compact disk (CD), or file transfer protocol (FTP) over the Internet. Voice-over-modem faxes, meaning a telephone line, are not considered electronic media, although a fax from a computer (e.g., WinFax program) is considered an electronic medium.

HIPAA requires the designation of a PO to develop and implement the organization's P&P. The PO for an

---

Box 2.3   HIPAA Help

If a health care provider either transmits directly or uses a "business associate" (e.g., billing company or clearinghouse) to transmit information electronically for any of the transactions listed, the health care provider is a "covered entity" and must comply with HIPAA

---

organization may hold another position within the practice or may not be an employee of the practice at all. Often, the PO is a contracted professional and available to the practice through established means of contact.

The business associate often is considered an extension of the provider practice. If an office function is outsourced with use or disclosure of individually identifiable health information, the organization that is acting on behalf of the health care provider is considered a business associate. For example, if the office's medical transcription is performed by an outside service, the transcription service is a business associate of the covered entity (the health care provider/practice). See Box 2.3.

HIPAA privacy regulations as a federal mandate will apply unless the state laws are contrary or more stringent with regard to privacy. A state law is contrary if it is impossible to comply with the state law while complying with federal requirements or if the state law stands as an obstacle to the purposes of the federal law. **State preemption,** a complex technical issue not within the scope of the health care provider's role, refers to instances when state law takes precedence over federal law. The PO determines when the need for preemption arises.

THE PRIVACY RULE: CONFIDENTIALITY AND PROTECTED HEALTH INFORMATION

What I may see or hear in the course of the treatment or even outside of the treatment in regard to the life of men, which on no account one must spread abroad, I will keep to myself holding such things shameful to be spoken about.

Hippocrates, 400 BC

The Hippocratic Oath, federal and state regulations, professional standards, and ethics all address patient privacy. Because current technology allows easy access to health care information, HIPAA imposes new requirements for health care providers. Since computers have become indispensable for the health care office, confidential health data have been sent across networks, e-mailed over the Internet, and even exposed by hackers, with few safeguards taken to protect data and prevent information from being intercepted or lost. With the implementation of standardizing electronic transactions of health care information, the use of technologies will pose new risks for privacy and security. These concerns were addressed under HIPAA, and regulations now closely govern how the industry handles its electronic activities.

Privacy is the condition of being secluded from the presence or view of others. **Confidentiality** is using discretion in keeping secret information. Integrity plays an important part in the health care setting. Staff members of a health care organization need a good understanding of HIPAA's basic requirements and must be committed to protecting the privacy and rights of the practice's patients.

Disclosure means the release, transfer, provision of access to, or divulging in any other manner of information outside the entity holding the information. An example of a disclosure would be if you give information to the hospital's outpatient surgery center about a patient you are scheduling for a procedure.

A **consent form** *is not* required *before* physicians use or disclose protected health information for treatment, payment, or routine health care operations (TPO).

Treatment includes coordination or management of health care between providers or referral of a patient to another provider. Protected health information (PHI) can be disclosed to obtain reimbursement. Other health care operations include performance reviews, audits, training programs, and certain types of fundraising (Figures 2–1 through 2–4).

Keep in mind that an HIPAA privacy consent is not the same as a consent to treat.

Exceptions may be based on specific state law requirements, on an emergency situation, on a language barrier that makes it impossible to obtain, or when treating prison inmates.

For some "extra" activities, including marketing, research, and psychotherapy notes, an **authorization form** is needed for use and disclosure of PHI that is not included in any existing consent form agreements.

Individually identifiable health information (IIHI) is any part of an individual's health information, including demographic information (e.g., address, date of birth) collected from the individual, that is created or received by a covered entity. This information relates to the individual's past, present, or future physical or mental health or condition; the provision of health care to the individual; or the past, present, or future payment for the provision of health care. IIHI data identify the individual or establish a reasonable basis to believe the information can be used to

identify the individual. For example, if you as a health care provider are talking to an insurance representative, you will likely give information such as the patient's date of birth and last name. These pieces of information would make it reasonably easy to identify the patient. If you are talking to a pharmaceutical representative about a drug assistance program that covers a new pill for heartburn and you only say that your practice has a patient living in your town who is indigent and has stomach problems, you are not divulging information that would identify the patient.

Protected health information (PHI) is any data that identifies an individual and describes his or her health status, age, sex, ethnicity, or other demographic characteristics, whether or not that information is stored or transmitted electronically. It refers to IIHI that is transmitted by electronic media, maintained in electronic form or transmitted, or maintained in any other form or medium. PHI does not include IHII in education records covered by the Family Educational Right and Privacy Act.

Traditionally, the focus has been on protecting paper medical records and documentation that held patient's health information, such as laboratory results and radiology reports. HIPAA Privacy Regulation expands these protections to apply to PHI. The individual's health information is protected regardless of the type of medium in which it is maintained. This includes paper, the health care provider's computerized practice management and billing system, spoken words, and x-ray films.

Use means the sharing, employment, application, utilization, examination, or analysis of IHII within an organization that holds such information. When a patient's billing record is accessed to review the claim submission history, the individual's health information is in "use."

HIPAA imposes requirements to protect not only disclosure of PHI outside of the organization, but also for internal uses of health information. PHI may not be used or disclosed without permission of the patient or someone authorized to act on behalf of the patient, unless the use or disclosure is specifically required or permitted by the regulation (e.g., treatment, payment, and health care operations [TPO]). The two types of disclosure required by HIPAA Privacy Rule are to the individual who is the subject of the PHI and to the Secretary or DHHS to investigate compliance with the rule.

Confidential Information

The insurance billing specialist must be responsible for maintaining confidentiality of patients' health information when working with patients and their medical records.

REQUIRED ELEMENTS
OF HIPAA AUTHORIZATION

Identification of person (or class)
authorized to request

Authorization for Release of Information

PATIENT NAME: __Levy__ __Chloe__ __E.__ _____
  LAST   FIRST   MI   MAIDEN OR OTHER NAME
DATE OF BIRTH: _02_ - _12_ - _1950_ SS# _320_ - _21_ - _3408_ MEDICAL RECORD #: _____3075_____
  MO DAY YR
ADDRESS: _____3298 East Main Street_____ CITY: __Woodland Hills__ STATE: _XY_ ZIP: _12345-0001_

DAY PHONE: _____013-340-9800_____ EVENING PHONE: _____013-549-8708_____

I hereby authorize ____Gerald Practon, MD____ **(Print Name of Provider) to release information from my medical record as indicated below to:**

NAME: _____Margaret L. Lee, MD_____

Identification of person (or class)
to whom covered entity is to
use/disclose

ADDRESS: _____328 Seward Street_____ CITY: __Anytown__ STATE: _XY_ ZIP: _45601-0731_

PHONE: _____013-219-7698_____ FAX: _____013-290-9877_____

INFORMATION TO BE RELEASED:
  DATES:

Description of information to be
released with specificity to allow
entity to know which information
the authorization references

☒ History and physical exam ____6-8-20XX____
☐ Progress notes _____
☐ Lab reports _____
☐ X-ray reports _____
☐ Other:_____ _____
_____ _____

I specifically authorize the release of information relating to:
☐ Substance abuse (including alcohol/drug abuse)
☐ Mental health (including psychotherapy notes)
☐ HIV related information (AIDS related testing)
X _____
SIGNATURE OF PATIENT OR LEGAL GUARDIAN   DATE

PURPOSE OF DISCLOSURE: ☐ Changing physicians ☒ Consultation/second opinion ☐ Continuing care
☐ Legal ☐ School ☐ Insurance ☐ Workers Compensation
☐ Other (please specify):_____

Description of each purpose of the
requested use or disclosure

1. I understand that this authorization will expire on _09/01/20XX_ (Print the Date this Form Expires) days after I have signed the form.

2. I understand that I may revoke this authorization at any time by notifying the providing organization in writing, and it will be effective on the date notified except to the extent action has already been taken in reliance upon it.

Expiration date, time period,
or event

Statement that is revocable by
written request

3. I understand that information used or disclosed pursuant to this authorization may be subject to redisclosure by the recipient and no longer be protected by Federal privacy regulations.

4. I understand that if I am being requested to release this information by ____Gerald Practon, MD____ (Print Name of Provider) for the purpose of: _____

a. By authorizing this release of information, my health care and payment for my health care will not be affected if I do not sign this form.
b. I understand I may see and copy the information described on this form if I ask for it, and that I will get a copy of this form after I sign it.
c. I have been informed that ____Gerald Practon, MD____ (Print Name of Provider) will/will not receive financial or in-kind compensation in exchange for using or disclosing the health information described above.

5. I understand that in compliance with ____XY____ (Print the State Whose Laws Govern the Provider) statute, I will pay a fee of $ _5.00_ (Print the Fee Charged). There is no charge for medical records if copies are sent to facilities for ongoing care or follow up treatment.

Individual's (patient's) signature
and date

__Chloe E. Levy__ __6/1/XX__ OR _____
SIGNATURE OF PATIENT   DATE   PARENT/LEGAL GUARDIAN/AUTHORIZED PERSON   DATE

_____ ☐_____
RECORDS RECEIVED BY   DATE   RELATIONSHIP TO PATIENT

FOR OFFICE USE ONLY
DATE REQUEST FILLED_____ BY:_____
IDENTIFICATION PRESENTED_____ FEE COLLECTED $_____

Statement of representative's
authority

FIGURE 2-1 Completed Authorization for Release of Information form for a patient relocating to another city. The figure indicates the required elements for HIPAA authorization. **NOTE:** This form is used on a one-time basis for reasons other than treatment, payment, or health care operations. When the patient arrives at the new physician's office, a consent for treatment, payment, and health care operations form will need to be signed. (*From Federal Register, Vol. 64, No. 212, Appendix to Subpart E of Part 164: Model Authorization Form, November 3, 1999.*)

NAME OF FACILITY
Consent for Release of Information

Date May 16, 20XX

1. I hereby authorize ___College Hospital___ to release the following information from the
   Name of Institution
   health record(s) of __Martha T. Jacobson__
   Patient name

   ___52 East Rugby Street, Woodland Hills, XY 12345___
   Address

   covering the period(s) of hospitalization from:
   Date of Admission __January 3, 20XX__
   Date of Discharge __January 5, 20XX__
   Hospital # ____278-1200____   Birthdate ____June 27, 1960____
2. Information to be released:
   ☐ Copy of (complete) health record(s)   ☑ Discharge summary
   ☐ History and physical   ☐ Operative report
   ☐ Other _____
3. Information is to be released to: ___Michael Hotta, MD___
   ___260 West Main Street, Woodland Hills, XY 12345___
4. Purpose of disclosure ___June 14, 20XX consultation___

5. I understand this consent can be revoked at any time except to the extent that disclosure
   made in good faith has already occurred in reliance to this consent.
6. Specification of the date, event, or condition upon which this consent expires:
   ___December 31, 20XX___
7. The facility, its employees and officers, and attending physician are released from legal
   responsibility or liability for the release of the above information to the extent indicated and
   authorized herein.

Signed ___Martha T. Jacobson___
                    (Patient or Representative)

   _____
                    (Relationship to Patient)
   __May 16, 20XX__
                    (Date of Signature)

FIGURE 2–2 Consent for Release of Information form to a hospital. *(From the American Health Information Management Association, Chicago, Ill.)*

Example 2.2 lists some of the protected health information that is typical in a medical office.

Example 2.2   Protected Health Information in a Medical Office

Intake forms	Encounter sheets
Laboratory work requests	Physician's notes
Physician-patient conversations	Prescriptions
Conversations that refer to patients by name	Insurance claim forms
Physician dictation tapes	X-rays
Telephone conversations with patients	E-mail messages

The patient record and any photographs obtained are confidential documents and require an authorization form that must be signed by the patient to release information (see Figures 2–1 through 2–4). If the form is a photocopy, it is necessary to state that the photocopy is approved by the patient, or write to the patient and obtain an original signed document.

Exceptions to HIPAA

Unauthorized release of information is called **breach of confidential communication** and is also considered an HIPAA violation, which may lead to fines.

Confidentiality between the physician and patient is automatically waived in the following situations:

1. When the patient is a member of a managed care organization (MCO) and the physician has signed a contract with the MCO that has a clause that says "for quality care purposes, the MCO has a right to access the medical records of their patients, and for utilization management purposes," the MCO has a right to audit those patients' financial records. Other managed care providers need to know about the patients if involved in the care and treatment of members of the MCO.
2. When patients have certain communicable diseases that are highly contagious or infectious and state health agencies require providers to report, even if the patient does not want the information reported.

COLLEGE CLINIC
4567 Broad Avenue
Woodland Hills, XY 12345-0001
Phone: 555/486-9002
Fax: 555/487-8976

CONSENT TO THE USE AND DISCLOSURE OF HEALTH INFORMATION

I understand that this organization originates and maintains health records which describe my health history, symptoms, examination, test results, diagnoses, treatment, and any plans for future care or treatment. I understand that this information is used to:

- plan my care and treatment
- communicate among health professionals who contribute to my care
- apply my diagnosis and services, procedures, and surgical information to my bill
- verify services billed by third-party payers
- assess quality of care and review the competence of healthcare professionals in routine healthcare operations

I further understand that:

- a complete description of information uses and disclosures is included in a *Notice of Information Practices* which has been provided to me
- I have a right to review the notice prior to signing this consent
- the organization reserves the right to change their notice and practices
- any revised notice will be mailed to the address I have provided prior to implementation
- I have the right to object to the use of my health information for directory purposes
- I have the right to request restrictions as to how my health information may be used or disclosed to carry out treatment, payment, or health care operations
- the organization is not required to agree to the restrictions requested
- I may revoke this consent in writing, except to the extent that the organization has already taken action in reliance thereon.

☐ I request the following restrictions to the use or disclosure of my health information.

_____

_____   _____
Date   Notice Effective Date

_____   _____
Signature of Patient or Legal Representative   Witness

_____   _____
Signature   Title

Date _____   __ Accepted __ Rejected

FIGURE 2-3 An example of a consent form used to disclose and use health information for treatment, payment, or health care operations. This is not required under HIPAA but you may find that some medical practices may use it. (*From Fordney MT, French L: Medical insurance billing and coding: a worktext, Philadelphia, Elsevier, 2003.*)

3. When a medical device breaks or malfunctions, the Food and Drug Administration requires providers to report certain information.
4. When a patient is suspect in a criminal investigation or to assist in locating a missing person, material witness, or suspect, police have the right to request certain information.

5. When the patient's records are subpoenaed or there is a search warrant. The courts have the right to order providers to release patient information.
6. When the patient is suing someone, such as an employer, and wishes to protect herself or himself.
7. When there is a suspicious death or suspected crime victim, providers must report cases.

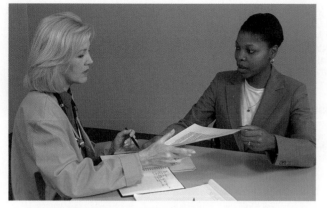

FIGURE 2–4 Patient signing a consent form.

8. When the physician examines a patient at the request of a third party who is paying the bill, as in workers' compensation cases.

9. When state law requires the release of information to police that is for the good of society, such as cases of child abuse, elder abuse, domestic violence, or gunshot wounds.

For information on confidentiality as it relates to computer use, refer to Chapter 8.

The purpose of the privacy rule is so that patients who receive medical treatment may have control in the manner in which specific information is used and to whom it is disclosed. **Confidential communication** is a privileged communication that may be disclosed only

---

EMPLOYEE CONFIDENTIALITY STATEMENT

As an employee of _____ABC Clinic, Inc._____ (employer), having been trained as an insurance billing specialist with employee responsibilities and authorization to access personal medical and health information, and as a condition of my employment, I agree to the following:

A. I recognize that I am responsible for complying with the Health Insurance Portability and Accountability Act (HIPAA) of 1996 policies regarding confidentiality of patients' information, which, if I violate, may lead to immediate dismissal from employment and, depending on state laws, criminal prosecution.

B. I will treat all information received during the course of my employment, which relates to the patients, as confidential and privileged information.

C. I will not access patient information unless I must obtain the information to perform my job duties.

D. I will not disclose information regarding my employer's patients to any person or entity, other than that necessary to perform my job duties, and as permitted under the employer's HIPAA policies.

E. I will not access any of my employer's computer systems that currently exist or may exist in the future using a password other than my own.

F. I will safeguard my computer password and will not show it in public.

G. I will not allow anyone, including other employees, to use my password to access computer files.

H. I will log off of the computer immediately after I finish using it.

I. I will not use e-mail to transmit patient information unless instructed to do so by my employer's HIPAA privacy officer.

J. I will not take patient information from my employer's premises in hard copy or electronic form without permission from my employer's HIPAA privacy officer.

K. Upon termination of my employment, I agree to continue to maintain the confidentiality of any information learned while an employee and agree to relinquish office keys, access cards, or any other device that provides access to the provider or its information.

Mary Doe
Signature

_____Mary Doe_____
Print name

September 14, 20XX
Date

Brenda Shield
Witness

FIGURE 2–5 An example of an employee confidentiality agreement that may be used by an employer when he or she is hiring an insurance billing specialist.

with the patient's permission. Everything you see, hear, or read about patients remains confidential and does not leave the office. Never talk about patients or data contained in medical records where others may overhear. Some employers require employees to sign a confidentiality agreement (Figure 2–5). Such agreements should be updated periodically to address issues raised by the use of new technologies.

Privileged Information

Privileged information is related to the treatment and progress of the patient. The patient must sign an authorization to release this information or selected facts from the medical record. Some states have passed laws allowing certain test results (e.g., disclosure of the presence of the human immunodeficiency virus [HIV] or alcohol or substance abuse) and other information to be placed separate from the patient's medical record. A special authorization form is used to release this information.

Nonprivileged Information

Nonprivileged information consists of ordinary facts unrelated to treatment of the patient, including the patient's name, city of residence, and dates of admission or discharge. This information must be sensitized against unauthorized disclosure under the Privacy section of the HIPAA. The patient's authorization is not needed for the purposes of treatment, payment, or health care operations, unless the record is in a specialty hospital (e.g., alcohol treatment) or a special service unit of a general hospital (e.g., psychiatric unit). Professional judgment is required. The information is disclosed on a legitimate need-to-know basis, meaning that the medical data should be revealed to the attending physician because the information may have some effect on the treatment of the patient.

Patients' Rights

Right to Privacy

All patients have a right to privacy. It is important never to discuss patient information other than with the physician, an insurance company, or individual who has been authorized by the patient. If a telephone inquiry is made and you need to verify that a caller is who they say they are, ask for one or more of the following items: patient's full name, home address, date of birth, social security number, mother's maiden name, or dates of service. Or ask for a call-back number and compare it to the number on file or ask the patient to fax a sheet with their signature on it so you can compare it to one on file. Some hospitals may assign a code word or number that may be a middle name

or date that is easy for patients to remember. If a patient does not know the code word, then ask for personal identifying information as mentioned.

If a telephone inquiry is made about a patient, ask the caller to put the request in writing and include the patient's signed authorization. If the caller refuses, have the physician return the call. If a relative telephones asking about a patient, have the physician return the call. When you telephone a patient about an insurance matter and reach voice mail, use care in the choice of words when leaving the message in the event the call was inadvertently received at the wrong number. Leave your name, the office name, and return telephone number. Never attempt to interpret a report or provide information about the outcome of laboratory or other diagnostic tests to the patient. Let the physician do it (Figure 2–6).

Do not discuss a patient with acquaintances, yours or the patient's. Do not leave patients' records or appointment books exposed on your desk. If confidential documents are on your desk that patients can easily see as they walk by, either turn the documents over or lock them in a secure drawer when you leave your desk, even if you are gone for only a few moments. If patient information is on your computer, either turn the screen off or save it on disk, lock the disk in a secure place, and clear the information from the screen. Never leave a computer screen with patient information visible, even for a moment, if another patient may see the data. Properly dispose of notes, papers, and memos by using a shredding device. Be careful when using the copying machine because it is easy to forget to remove the original insurance claim or medical record from the document glass. Use common sense and follow the guidelines mentioned in this chapter to help you keep your professional credibility and integrity.

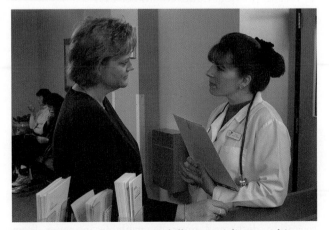

FIGURE 2–6 Insurance billing specialist consulting with the supervisor/office manager about office policies regarding release of a patient's medical record.

Privacy Rules: Patient Rights under HIPAA

Patients are granted the following federal rights that allow them to be informed about PHI and to control how their PHI is used and disclosed:

1. Right to Notice of Privacy Practices
2. Right to request restrictions on certain uses and disclosures of PHI
3. Right to request confidential communications
4. Right to access (inspect and obtain a copy) PHI
5. Right to request an amendment of PHI
6. Right to receive an accounting of disclosures of PHI

Right to Notice of Privacy Practices

Under HIPAA, patients are entitled to receive the written Notice of Privacy Practices (NPP) of their provider, such as at the first visit or at enrollment. If it is an emergency treatment situation, get the acknowledgment signed at the earliest time practicable following the emergency. Getting the patient acknowledgment or documenting that an attempt was made to do so must be done once only.

The NPP outlines the individual's rights and covered entity's legal duties in regard to PHI. The NPP must be provided and written in "plain language" and the staff must make a reasonable "best effort" to obtain a signature from the patient acknowledging receipt. This can be recorded simply as signing a label on the inside cover of the chart. The front desk reception area is an ideal location for distribution of the NPP to the patient with the registration sheet and other required forms. If the patient cannot or will not sign, a staff member should document this in the patient's health record. An NPP will be tailored to each organization and must explain the following:

● How PHI may be used and disclosed by the organization
● Health provider duties to protect PHI
● Patient's rights regarding PHI
● How complaints may be filed with the office and HHS if the patient believes his or her privacy rights have been violated
● Who to contact for further information (usually the PO)
● Effective date of the NPP

You may have already seen these notices posted at a local pharmacy or had to sign an acknowledgment that you read a copy of the NPP at your personal physician's office. The health care provider's patients must have ready access to your organization's NPP. This notice must be posted prominently in the office (e.g., on the wall by the reception desk) and must be available in paper form for patients who request it. If the office has a Web site, the notice must be posted prominently there as well.

HIPAA states that covered entities may not require individuals to waive their rights "as a condition of the provision of treatment or payment." A provider with a Web site that provides information about customer services or benefits must have the NPP placed on the site and must deliver a copy electronically on request.

Right to Request Restrictions on Certain Uses and Disclosures of PHI

Patients do have the right to ask for restrictions on how your office uses and discloses PHI for TPO. The patient may have items in their previous medical history that are not applicable to the current disclosure and may even cause the patient embarrassment; the patient may request that this PHI not be disclosed. (e.g., a patient had a successfully treated sexually transmitted disease many years before and requests that, whenever possible, this material not be disclosed.) The covered entity is not required to agree to these requests but must have a process to review the requests, accept and review any appeal, and give a sound reason for not agreeing to the request. If agreed upon, however, the restrictions must be documented and followed. Such restrictions may be tracked by flagging the patient's medical chart that indicates a restriction applies or by using a pop-up note in the practice management software. There must be an implemented procedure in place to check for any restrictions before PHI is disclosed (Box 2.4).

A practice may disclose confidential information in certain situations *without* a written authorization from the patient (e.g., reporting communicable diseases, reporting about victims of abuse, and law enforcement purposes). You can ask your PO or refer to the medical practice's policy and procedure manual for clarification when disclosures are permissible.

In addition, unless a patient has requested that such disclosures *not* occur and the provider has agreed, health information may be disclosed to a family member, relative, close friend, or any other person identified by the patient.

Right to Request Confidential Communications

A patient can request to receive confidential communications by alternative means or at an alternative location. For example, a patient may ask that the health care provider call the patient at work rather than at the residence or patients may request that their test results be sent to them in writing rather than by telephone. It is the patient's right to request such alternative methods of communication, and the health care office must accommodate *reasonable* requests.

Box 2.4	HIPAA Help

In regard to the patient's right to request restrictions on certain uses and disclosures of PHI, you will find key terms addressed in the NPP that apply to the right.

- **Minimum Necessary.** Privacy regulations require that use or disclosure of only the minimum amount of information necessary to fulfill the intended purpose be permitted. There are some exceptions to this rule. You do not need to limit PHI for disclosures in regard to health care providers for treatment, the patient, HHS for investigations of compliance with HIPAA, or as required by law.

  Minimum necessary determinations for *uses of PHI* must be determined within each organization, and reasonable efforts must be made to limit access to only the minimum amount of information needed by identified staff members. In smaller offices, employees may have multiple job functions. If a medical assistant helps with the patient examination, documents vital signs, and then collects the patient's co-pay at the reception area, the assistant will likely access clinical and billing records. Simple procedure and policy (P&P) about appropriate access to PHI may be sufficient to satisfy the Minimum Necessary requirement. Larger organizations may have specific restrictions on who should have access to different types of PHI, because staff members tend to have a more targeted job role. Remain knowledgeable about your office's policy regarding Minimum Necessary. If you are strictly scheduling appointments, you may not need access to the clinical record. An x-ray technician will likely not need to access the patient billing records.

  Minimum Necessary Determinations for *disclosures of PHI* are distinguished by two categories within the Privacy Rule:

  1. For disclosures made on a routine and recurring basis, you may implement policies and procedures, or standard protocols, for what will be disclosed. These disclosures would be common in your practice. Examples may include disclosures for workers' compensation claims or school physical forms.
  2. For other disclosures that would be considered nonroutine, criteria should be established for determining the Minimum Necessary amount of

PHI and to review each request for disclosure on an individual basis. A staff member (e.g., PO, medical records supervisor) will likely be assigned to determine this situation when the need arises.

As a general rule, remember that you must limit your requests to access PHI to the Minimum Necessary to accomplish the task for which you will need the information.

- **De-identification of Confidential Information.** Other requirement relating to uses and disclosures of PHI include health information that does not identify an individual or leaves no reasonable basis to believe that the information can be used to identify an individual. This "de-identified" information is no longer individually identifiable health information (IIHI). Most providers will never have the need to de-identify patient information, and the requirements for de-identifying PHI are lengthy. The regulations give specific directions on how to ensure all pieces of necessary information are removed to fit the definition. De-identified information is not subject to the privacy regulations because it does not specifically identify an individual.

- **Marketing** refers to communicating about a product or service where the goal is to encourage patients to purchase or use the product or service. For instance, a dermatologist may advertise for a discount on facial cream when you schedule a dermabrasion treatment. You will likely not be involved in marketing, but keep in mind the general rule that PHI (including names and addresses) cannot be used for marketing purposes without specific authorization of the patient. Sending appointment reminders and general news updates about your organization and the services you provide would not be considered marketing and would not require patient authorization.

- **Fundraising.** Again, you will likely not be involved in fundraising activities, but HIPAA allows demographic information and dates of care to be used for fundraising purposes without patient authorization. The disclosure of any additional informat ion requires patient authorization. Your organization's NPP will state that patients may receive fundraising materials and are given the opportunity to opt out of receiving future solicitations.

This can become a serious issue, especially in cases of domestic violence when the individual is at risk for physical harm within the home environment. The patient does not need to explain the reason for the request. The health care office must have a process in place both to evaluate requests and appeals and to respond to the patient.

Patients may be required by the office to make their request in writing. Documenting such requests in writing with the patient's signature is an effective way to protect the practice's compliance endeavors. The office may even condition the agreement by arranging for payment of any additional costs from the patient that the request has created. For example, the patient asks that all correspondence be sent by registered mail; this request may be able to be honored without significant additional staff time but the patient should expect to incur the actual additional mailing costs.

Right to Access, Inspect, and Obtain PHI

A patient has the right to access, inspect, and obtain a copy of his or her confidential health information. Privacy regulations allow the provider to require the patient make the request for access in writing. Generally, a request must be acted on within 30 days. A reasonable, cost-based fee for copies of PHI may only include the costs for the following:

- Supplies and labor for copying
- Postage when mailed
- Preparing a summary of the PHI if the patient has agreed to this instead of complete access

This "fee" for copying varies widely by state and each provider should be aware of the state allowances and conform their fee to that which gives most relief to the patient. The HIPAA-determined fee applies *only* to fees for copies to patients and not copies for other required or allowed disclosures, such as subpoenas. The fee structures for other disclosures are often set by state law. If you are a staff member involved in applying fees for copying, you should seek guidance from your PO.

Under HIPAA Privacy Regulation, patients do not have the right to access the following:

● Psychotherapy notes
● Information compiled in reasonable anticipation of, or for use in, legal proceedings
● Information exempted from disclosure under the Clinical Laboratory Improvements Amendment (CLIA)

The office may deny patient access for the above reasons without giving the patient the right to review the denial. Also, if the PHI was obtained from an individual other than a health care provider under a promise of confidentiality, access may be denied if such access would likely reveal the identity of the source. Other circumstances in which an individual may be denied access will be detailed in the practice's policy manual.

If the health care provider has determined that the patient would be endangered (or cause danger to another person) from accessing the confidential health information, access may be denied. In this case, the patient has the right to have the denial reviewed by another licensed professional who did not participate in the initial denial decision.

Regarding psychotherapy notes, HIPAA gives special protection to PHI. Disclosure of a patient's mental health records requires specific patient permission. This means that when an insurance payer requests the health records to review the claim, a patient authorization is required.

Certain clinical data are excluded from the definition of psychotherapy notes. In other words, when an individual is utilizing the services of a mental health professional, not all information gathered and recorded in the health record of the mental health provider is considered psychotherapy notes. The law lists specific items that are excluded from such notes:

● Medication prescription and monitoring
● Counseling session start and stop times
● Modalities and frequencies of treatment furnished
● Results of clinical tests
● Any summary of the following items: diagnosis, functional status, treatment plan, symptoms, prognosis, and progress to date

In general, the major difference between what are and what are not considered psychotherapy notes is the information that is the *recorded (in any manner) documentation and/or analysis of conversation.* This information should also be kept separate from the medical section of the

---

Box 2.5   HIPAA Help

According to the HIPAA Privacy Rule, the term *psychotherapy notes* means notes recorded (in any medium) by a health care provider who is a mental health professional documenting or analyzing the contents of conversation during a private counseling session or a group, joint, or family counseling session and that are separated from the rest of the individual's medical record.

---

patient health record to be distinguished as psychotherapy notes. For example, Jane Doe tells her psychologist the details of her childhood trauma. The documented conversation specific to her trauma (e.g., what occurred, how she felt) is considered the psychotherapy notes and cannot be released without specific permission from Jane Doe.

It is important also to understand that patients do *not* have the right to obtain a copy of psychotherapy notes under HIPAA. However, the treating mental health provider *may* decide when a patient may obtain access to this health information.

State law must always be considered. Some states allow patients access to their psychotherapy notes; therefore state law would take precedence over HIPAA as a result of the state pre-emption allowance.

Right to Request Amendment of PHI

Patients have the right to request that their PHI be amended. As with the other requests, the provider may require the request be in writing. The provider must have a process to accept and review both the request and any appeal in a timely fashion. The health care provider may deny this request in the following circumstances:

● The provider who is being requested to change the PHI is not the creator of the information (e.g., office has records sent by referring physician).
● The PHI is believed to be accurate and complete as it stands in the provider's records.
● The information is not required to be accessible to the patient (see Right to Access, Inspect, and Obtain PHI).

Generally, the office must respond to a patient's request for amendment within 60 days. If a request is denied, the patient must be informed in writing of the reason for the denial. The patient must also be given the opportunity to file a statement of disagreement. These rules are complex in regard to steps of appeal, rebuttal, and documentation that must be provided if a request for amendment is denied. The PO will instruct providers on additional responsibilities if they are directly involved in this process.

In summary, **patients have the right to:**
- Be informed of the organization's privacy practices by receiving a Notice of Privacy Practices (NPP).
- Have their information kept confidential and secure.
- Obtain a copy of their health record.
- Request to have their health records amended.
- Request special considerations in communication.
- Restrict unauthorized access to their confidential health information.

Patients cannot keep their confidential health information from being used for treatment, payment, or health care operations (TPO) nor may they force amendments to their health record. As you become more acclimated to your organization's policies and procedures regarding the handling of protected health information (PHI), you will be better able to recognize how your position is an important part in HIPAA compliance.

Health care providers and staff will likely not be reading the *Federal Register* and thus will want to familiarize themselves with the general forms used in their practice setting. They should be aware of the following:
- **Written acknowledgment:** After providing the patient with the Notice of Privacy Practices (NPP), a "good faith" effort must be made to obtain written acknowledgment of the patient receiving the document. If the patient refuses to sign or is unable to sign, this must be documented in the patient record.
- **Authorization forms:** Use and disclosure of protected health information (PHI) is permissible for treatment, payment, or health care operations (TPO), because the NPP describes how PHI is used for these purposes. The health care provider is required to obtain signed authorization to use or disclose health information for situations beyond the TPO. This is a protection for the practice. Providers must learn about the particular "authorization" forms used in their office. Psychotherapy notes are handled separately under HIPAA. Such notes have additional protection, specifically, that an authorization for any use of disclosure of psychotherapy notes must be obtained.

Your organization will be expected to handle requests made by patients to exercise their rights. You must know your office's process for dealing with each specific request. With your understanding of HIPAA and your organization's policy manual, you will be guided in procedures specific to your health care practice.

Right to Receive an Accounting of Disclosures of PHI

Providers should maintain a log of disclosures of PHI, either on paper or within the organization's computer system, of all disclosures other than those made for TPO, facility directories, and some national security and law enforcement agencies. The process for providing an accounting should be outlined in the practice's policy manual. Patients may request an accounting (or tracking) of disclosures of their confidential information and are granted the right to receive this accounting once a year without charge. Additional accountings may be assessed a cost-based fee.

These accountings were required to start on April 14, 2003, when privacy regulations became enforceable. Items to be documented must include the following:

- Date of disclosure
- Name of the entity or person who received the PHI, including their address, if known
- Brief description of the PHI disclosed
- Brief statement of the purpose of the disclosure

The patient is entitled to one accounting per year free of charge. Additional accountings may be assessed a cost-based fee. See Boxes 2.6 and 2.7.

ORGANIZATION AND STAFF RESPONSIBILITIES IN PROTECTING PATIENT RIGHTS

The covered entity must implement written *policies and procedures* (P&P) that comply with HIPAA standards. P&P are tailored guidelines established to accommodate each health care practice and designed to address PHI. HIPAA requires each practice to implement P&P that comply with privacy and security rules. The office should have a policy and procedures manual to train providers and staff and to serve as a resource for situations that need clarification. Revisions in P&P must be made as necessary and appropriate to comply with laws as they change. Documentation must be maintained in written or electronic form and retained for 6 years of its creation or when it was last in effect, whichever is later.

Verification of Identity and Authority

Before any disclosure, you must verify the identity of persons requesting PHI if they are unknown to you. You may request identifying information such as date of birth, social security number, or even a code word stored in your practice management system that is unique to each patient. Public officials may show you badges, credentials, official letterheads, and other legal documents of authority for identification purposes. Additionally, you must verify that the requestor has the right and the need to have the PHI.

Exercising professional judgment will fulfill your verification requirements for most disclosures because you are acting on "good faith" in believing the identity of the individual requesting PHI. It is good practice, when making any disclosure to note, to note the "authority" of the person receiving the PHI and how this was determined. This evidence of due diligence on your part would enforce a needed structure on your staff and dampen any complaints that might arise.

Validating Patient Permission

Before making any uses or disclosures of confidential health information other than for the purposes of TPO, your office must have appropriate patient permission. Always check for conflicts between various permissions your office may have on file for a given patient (Table 2.1). This information should be maintained either in your practice management system or in the medical chart, where it can be easily identified and retrieved.

For example, if a covered entity has agreed to a patient's request to limit how much of the PHI is sent to a consulting physician for treatment, but then received the patient's authorization to disclose the entire medical record to that physician, this would be a conflict. In general, the more restrictive permission would be the deciding factor. Privacy regulations allow resolving conflicting permissions by either obtaining new permission from the patient or by communicating orally or in writing with the

Table 2.1 Uses and Disclosures of Protected Health Information	
Permitted Disclosures (no authorization required)	**What It Means for Your Practice**
Disclose PHI to patient	You may discuss the patient's own medical condition with him or her. **Doing so does not require a signed authorization from the patient.**
Disclose PHI for treatment	Treatment includes speaking with the patient, ordering tests, writing prescriptions, coordinating his or her care, and consulting with another health care provider about the patient. **"Treatment" does not require a signed authorization from the patient.**
Disclose PHI for payment	Payment includes obtaining the patient's eligibility or benefits coverage information from the insurance payer, obtaining pre-approval for treatment, and billing and managing the claims process. **"Payment" does not require a signed authorization from the patient.**
Disclose PHI for health care operations	Do not confuse this with performing surgery. The term *health care operations* refers to the business activities in which your organization participates. Examples include case management, certification, accreditation, medical reviews, and audits to detect fraud and abuse. **"Operations" do not require a signed authorization from the patient.**
Disclose PHI for public purposes	PHI may be disclosed for public health purposes such as reporting a communicable disease, injury, child abuse, domestic violence, judicial and administrative proceedings, law enforcement, coroner or medical examiner, or research purposes if PHI is "de-identified." This is not an all-inclusive list, but these examples **do not require a signed authorization from the patient.**
Disclose PHI for workers' compensation	You may disclose PHI as authorized by the laws relating to workers' compensation. Such disclosures to programs that provide benefits for work-related injuries or illness **do not require a signed authorization from the patient.**
Disclosures That Require Patient's Opportunity to Agree or Object	**What It Means for Your Practice**
Disclose PHI to persons involved with the patient	You must provide patients with an opportunity to object to sharing PHI with family, friends, or others involved with their care. The health care provider can use professional judgment when disclosing PHI to a person involved with the patient's care when the patient is not present. **Requires the patient have the opportunity to agree or object.**
Disclosures (authorization required)	**What It Means for Your Practice**
Disclose psychotherapy notes	Psychotherapy notes may not be disclosed without authorization except for use by the originator (therapist) for treatment. **A signed authorization IS required.**
Disclose PHI to a child's school for permission to participate in sports	You may not disclose a child's PHI to the school to permit the student's participation in a sports activity. **A signed authorization IS required.**
Disclose PHI to employer	You may not disclose PHI to a patient's employer unless the information is needed to comply with Occupational Safety and Health Administration (OSHA), Mine Safety and Health Administration (MSHA), or other state laws. **With certain exceptions, a signed authorization IS required.**
Disclose PHI to insurer	You may not disclose PHI to an insurer for underwriting/eligibility without authorization from the patient, for example, if the patient is trying to obtain a life insurance policy. **A signed authorization IS required.**
Disclose PHI for fundraising or marketing	If your health care practice does fundraising or marketing, you may not disclose PHI without prior authorization from the patient. **A signed authorization IS required.**

patient to determine the patient's preference. Be sure to document any form of communication in writing.

Training

Under HIPAA regulations, a covered entity must train all members of its workforce. This training must include the practice's P&P with respect to PHI as "necessary and appropriate for the members of the workforce to carry out their function within the covered entity." This training will address how your role relates to PHI in your office, and you will be instructed on how to handle confidential information. The PO for your health care practice will likely be the instructor for this type of training. HIPAA training focuses on how to handle confidential information securely in the office, as discussed later.

Safeguards: Ensuring That Confidential Information Is Secure

Every covered entity must have appropriate safeguards to ensure the protection of an individual's confidential health information. Such safeguards include administrative, technical, and physical measures that will "reasonably safeguard" PHI from any use or disclosure that violates HIPAA, whether intentional or unintentional (Box 2.8).

Complaints to Health Care Practice and Workforce Sanctions

Individuals, both patients and staff, must be provided with a process to make a complaint concerning the P&P of the covered entity. If a violation involves the misuse of PHI, this incident should be reported to the practice's PO. Should there be further cause, the OCR may also be contacted.

Workforce members are subject to appropriate sanctions for failure to comply with the P&P regarding PHI set forth in the office. Types of sanctions applied will vary depending on factors involved with the violation. Sanctions can range from a warning to suspension to termination. This information should be covered in the P&P manual. Written documentation of complaints and sanctions must be prepared with any disposition.

Mitigation

Mitigation means to "alleviate the severity" or "make mild." In reference to HIPAA, the covered entity has an affirmative duty to take reasonable steps in response to breaches. If a breach is discovered, the health care provider is required to mitigate, to the extent possible, any harmful effects of the breach. For example, if you learn you have erroneously sent medical records by fax to an incorrect party, steps should be taken to have the recipient destroy the PHI. Mitigation procedures also include activities of the practice's business associates. Being proactive and responsible by mitigating will reduce the potential for a more disastrous outcome from the breach or violation.

Refraining from Intimidating or Retaliatory Acts

HIPAA privacy regulations prohibit a covered entity from intimidating, threatening, coercing, discriminating against, or otherwise taking retaliatory action against:

- Individuals for exercising HIPAA privacy rights
- Individuals for filing a complaint with HHS, for testifying, assisting, or participating in an investigation about the covered entity's privacy practices, or for reasonably opposing any practice prohibited by the regulation

TRANSACTION AND CODE SET REGULATIONS: STREAMLINING ELECTRONIC DATA INTERCHANGE

HIPAA *Transaction and Code Set* (TCS) regulation was developed to introduce efficiencies into the health care system. The objectives are to achieve a higher quality of care and to reduce administrative costs by streamlining the processing of routine administrative and financial transactions. HHS has estimated that by implementing TCS, almost $30 billion over 10 years would be saved. A **code set** is any set of codes with their descriptions used to encode data elements, such as tables of terms, medical concepts, medical diagnostic codes, or medical procedure codes.

Technology and the use of *electronic data interchange* (EDI) has made the processing of transactions more efficient and reduced administrative overhead costs in other industries. EDI is the exchange of data in a standardized format through computer systems. Standardizing transactions and code sets is required to use EDI effectively, with the implementation of standard formats, procedures, and data content.

TCS regulation required the implementation of specific standards for transactions and code sets by

Box 2.8	Examples of Safeguards	
Administrative	**Technical**	**Physical**
Verifying the identity of an individual picking up health records	User name/password required to access patient records from computer	Locked, fireproof filing cabinets for storing paper records

October 16, 2003. The intent of TCS requirements is to achieve a single standard. As an example in the pre-HIPAA environment, when submitting claims for payment, health care providers did business with insurance payers who required the use of their own version of local code sets (e.g., state Medicaid programs) or identifiers and paper forms. Before HIPAA, more than 400 versions of a *National Standard Format* (NSF) existed to submit a claim for payment. HIPAA will streamline the standards and enable greater administrative efficiencies throughout the health care system. As these methods are adapted, health care provider offices will benefit from less paperwork, and standardizing data will result in more accurate information and a more efficient organization (Table 2.2).

Medical code sets are data elements used uniformly to document why patients are seen (diagnosis, ICD-9-CM) and what is done to them during their encounter (procedure, CPT-4 and HCPCS). Each covered entity organization is responsible for implementing the updated codes in a timely manner, using the new HIPAA-mandated TCS codes and deleting old or obsolete ones (Table 2.3).

HIPAA also provides standards for the complete cycle of administrative transactions and electronic standard formats, which are presented in detail in Chapter 8 (Box 2.9).

Standard Unique Identifiers

The use of standard unique identifiers will improve efficiency in the management of health care by simplifying administration systems. This will enable the efficient electronic transmission of certain health information used across the industry.

- *Standard Unique Employer Identifier* (use EIN to identify employers; compliance by July 30, 2004). The EIN will be used to identify employers rather than inputting the actual name of the company. Employers can use their EIN to identify themselves in transactions involving premium payments to health plans on behalf of their employees or to identify themselves or other employers as the source or receiver of information about eligibility. Employers can also use EINs to identify themselves in transactions when enrolling or disenrolling employees in a health plan.
- *Standard Unique Health Care Provider Identifier*. This is proposed to be an 8-position alphanumeric identifier for the health care provider and will be assigned permanently, a lifetime number. It is known as the National Provider Identifier (NPI) number and providers may apply for this number no earlier than May 23, 2005.
- *Standard Unique Health Plan Identifier*. Final Rule published January 23, 2004, which is effective May 23, 2005.

Table 2.2   Recognized Benefits of TCS and EDI

Benefit	Result
More reliable and timely processing	Fast eligibility evaluation; reduced accounts receivable cycle; industry averages for claim turnarounds are 9 to 15 days for electronic versus 30 to 45 days for paper claims
Quicker reimbursement from payer	Improves cash flow for the health care organization
Improved accuracy of data	Decreases processing time, increases data quality, and leads to better reporting
Easier and more efficient access to information	Improves patient support
Better tracking of transactions	Facilitates tracking of transactions (i.e., when sent and received), allowing for monitoring (e.g., prompt payments)
Reduction of data entry/manual labor	Electronic transactions facilitate automated processes (e.g., automated payment posting).
Reduction in office expenses	Reduces office supplies, postage, and telephone charges.

EDI, Electronic data interchange; *TCS*, transaction and code set.

Table 2.3   Medical Code Sets

Code Set	Organization	Updates
Common Procedure Terminology (CPT)	American Medical Association (AMA)	Annually; changes go into effect each January 1; Category III codes update in January and July
Code on Dental Procedures and Nomenclature (CDT)	American Dental Association (ADA)	
National Drug Codes (NDC)	Food and Drug Administration (FDA)	Daily; see **http:www.fda.gov/cder** for quarterly updates
Health Care Common Procedure Coding System (HCPCS)	Centers for Medicare and Medicaid Services (CMS)	Major update January 1; periodic updates throughout the year as necessary
International Classification of Diseases Clinical Modification (ICD-9-CM and ICD-10)	U.S. Department of Health and Human Services (DHHS)	Annually; changes go into effect each October 1 for Medicare claims

Box 2.9 ▌HIPAA Help

When a patient comes into your office and is treated, his or her confidential health information is collected and put into the computerized practice management system. The services rendered are assigned a standard code from the HIPAA-required *code sets* (e.g., CPT), and the diagnosis is selected from another code set (e.g., ICD-9-CM), much the same as before HIPAA.

When claims are generated for electronic submission, all data collected are compiled and constructed into an HIPAA *standard transaction*. This electronic data interchange (EDI) is recognized across the health care sector in computer systems maintained by providers, the clearinghouses, and insurance payers. The harmony among the covered entities results in a more efficient claim life cycle.

● *Standard Unique Patient Identifier.* The intention to create a standard for a uniform patient identifier prompted protest among public interest groups, who saw a universal identifier as a civil liberties threat. Therefore the issue of a universal patient identifier is on hold indefinitely.

THE SECURITY RULE: ADMINISTRATIVE, PHYSICAL, AND TECHNICAL SAFEGUARDS

Security measures encompass all the administrative, physical, and technical safeguards in an information system. The Security Rule addresses only *electronic* protected health information (ePHI), but the concept of protecting PHI that will become ePHI makes attention to security for the entire office important. The Security Rule is divided into three main sections: administrative safeguards, technical safeguards and physical safeguards.

Administrative safeguards prevent unauthorized use or disclosure of PHI through administrative actions and P&P to manage the selection, development, implementation, and maintenance of security measures to protect ePHI.

Technical safeguards are technologic controls in place to protect and control access to information on computers in the health care organization.

Physical safeguards also prevent unauthorized access to PHI. These physical measures and P&P protect a covered entity's electronic information systems and related buildings and equipment from natural and environmental hazards and unauthorized intrusion.

More about the Security Rule is discussed in Chapter 8.

APPLICATION TO PRACTICE SETTING

HIPAA affects all areas of the health care office, from the reception area to the provider. In conjunction with being educated and trained in job responsibilities, every staff member must be educated about HIPAA and trained in the P&P pertinent to the organization.

Reasonable safeguards are measurable solutions based on accepted standards that are implemented and periodically monitored to demonstrate that the office is in compliance. Reasonable efforts must be made to limit the use or disclosure of PHI. If you are the front desk receptionist and you close the privacy glass between your desk and the waiting area when you are making a call to a patient, this is a reasonable safeguard to prevent others in the waiting room from overhearing.

Incidental uses and disclosures are permissible under HIPAA only when reasonable safeguards or precautions have been implemented to prevent misuse or inappropriate disclosure of PHI. When incidental uses and disclosures result from failure to apply reasonable safeguards or adhere to the minimum necessary standard, the Privacy Rule has been violated. If you are in the reception area and you close the privacy glass when having a confidential conversation, and you are still overheard by an individual in the waiting room, this would be "incidental." You have applied a reasonable safeguard to prevent this from happening.

Guidelines for HIPAA Privacy Compliance

As an insurance billing specialist, you will likely answer the telephone and speak during the course of your business, and there will be questions about what you can and cannot say. Reasonable and appropriate safeguards must be taken to ensure that all confidential health information in your office is protected from unauthorized and inappropriate access, including both verbal and written forms.

1. Consider that conversations occurring throughout the office could be overheard. The reception area and waiting room are often linked, and it is easy to hear the scheduling of appointments and exchange of confidential information. It is necessary to observe areas and maximize efforts to avoid unauthorized disclosures. Simple and affordable precautions include using privacy glass at the front desk and having conversations away from settings where other patients or visitors are present. Health care providers can move their dictation stations away from patient areas or wait until no patients are present before dictating. Phone conversations by providers in front of patients, even in emergency situations, should be avoided. Providers and staff must use their best professional judgment.

2. Be sure to check in the patient medical record and in your computer system to determine whether there are any special instructions for contacting the patient regarding scheduling or reporting test results. Follow these requests as agreed by the office.

3. Patient sign-in sheets *are* permissible, but limit the information you request when a patient signs in, and change it periodically during the day. A sign-in sheet must not contain information such as reason for visit because some providers specialize in treating patients with sensitive issues. Thus showing that a particular individual has an appointment with your practice may pose a breach of patient confidentiality.

4. Make sure you have patients sign a form acknowledging receipt of the NPP. The NPP allows you to release the patient's confidential information for billing and other purposes. If your practice has other confidentiality statements and policies besides HIPAA mandates, these must be reviewed to ensure they meet HIPAA requirements.

5. Formal policies for transferring and accepting outside PHI must address how your office keeps this information confidential. When using courier services, billing services, transcription services, or e-mail, you must ensure that transferring PHI is done in a secure and compliant manner.

6. Computers are used for a variety of administrative functions, including scheduling, billing, and managing medical records. Computers typically are present at the reception area. Keep the computer screen turned so that viewing is restricted to authorized staff. Screen savers should be used to prevent unauthorized viewing or access. The computer should automatically log off the user after a period of being idle, requiring the staff member to reenter his or her password.

7. Keep your user name and password confidential, and change them often. Do not share this information. An authorized staff member such as the PO will have administrative access to reset your password if you lose it or if someone discovers it. Also, practice management software can track users and follow their activity. Do not set yourself up by giving out your password. Safeguards include password protection for electronic data and storing paper records securely.

8. Safeguard your work area; do not place notes with confidential information in areas that are easy to view by nonstaff. Cleaning services will access your building, usually after business hours; ensure that you safeguard PHI.

9. Place medical record charts face down at reception areas so the patient's name is not exposed to other patients or visitors to your office. Also, when placing medical records on the door of an examination room, turn the chart so that identifying information faces the door. If you keep medical charts in the office on countertops or in receptacles, it is your duty to ensure that nonstaff persons will not access the records. Handling and storing medical records will certainly change because of HIPAA guidelines.

10. Do not post the health care provider's schedule in areas viewable by nonstaff individuals. The schedules are often posted for convenience of the professional staff, but this may be a breach in patient confidentiality.

11. Fax machines should not be placed in patient examination rooms or in any reception area where nonstaff persons may view incoming or sent documents. Only staff members should have access to the faxes.

12. If you open your office mail or take telephone calls pertaining to medical record requests, direct these issues to the appropriate staff member.

13. If you are involved in coding and billing, be sure to recognize, learn, and use HIPAA TCS.

14. Send all privacy-related questions or concerns to the appropriate staff member.

15. Immediately report any suspected or known improper behavior to your supervisor or the PO so that the issue may be documented and investigated.

16. If you have questions, contact your supervisor or the PO.

Health care organizations face challenges in implementing the HIPAA requirements; do not let these overwhelm you. Your office is required to take reasonable steps to build protections specific to your health care organization. Compliance is an ongoing endeavor involving teamwork. Understand your office's established P&P. Monitor your own activities to ensure you are following the required procedures. Do not take shortcuts when your actions involve patient privacy and security.

Be alert to other activities in your office. Help your co-workers change work habits that do not comply with HIPAA. Do not ignore unauthorized uses and disclosures of PHI, and do not allow unauthorized persons to access data. You have an obligation to your employer and the patients you serve.

CONSEQUENCES OF NONCOMPLIANCE WITH HIPAA

The prosecution of HIPAA crimes is handled by different governing bodies. HHS handles issues regarding TCS and security. Complaints can be filed against a covered entity for not complying with these rules. The OCR oversees privacy issues and complaints, referring criminal issues to the Office of Inspector General (OIG). The OIG provides the workup for referral cases, which may involve the Federal Bureau of Investigation (FBI) and other agencies.

Serious civil and criminal penalties apply for HIPAA noncompliance. General noncompliance with the privacy, security, and transaction regulations result in a $100 fine per violation and up to $25,000 per person for identical violations in a given calendar year. Specific to the Privacy Rule is a $50,000 fine and imprisonment for 1 year if one knowingly obtains or discloses IIHI. The person who obtains or discloses such health information under false pretenses is subject to a $100,000 fine. If one obtains or discloses PHI with the intent to sell, transfer, or use it for commercial advantage, personal gain, or malicious harm, a maximum fine of $250,000 and up to 10 years' imprisonment may be applied.

OFFICE OF INSPECTOR GENERAL

The mission of the OIG is to safeguard the health and welfare of the beneficiaries of HHS programs and to protect the integrity of HHS programs (Medicare and Medicaid). The OIG was established to identify and eliminate fraud, abuse, and waste and "to promote efficiency and economy in departmental operations." HIPAA legislation has radically changed the focus and mission within OIG. HIPAA pushed OIG into a new era, guaranteeing funds for the OIG programs and mandating initiatives to protect the integrity of all health care programs. The OIG undertakes nationwide audits, as well as investigations and inspections to review the claim submission processes of providers and reimbursement patterns of the programs. Recommendations are made to the HHS Secretary and the U.S. Congress on correcting problematic areas addressed in the federal programs. According to the OIG:

Efforts to combat fraud were consolidated and strengthened under Public Law 104-191, the Health Insurance Portability and Accountability Act of 1996 (HIPAA). The act established a comprehensive program to combat fraud committed against all health plans, both public and private. The legislation required the establishment of a national Health Care Fraud and Abuse Control Program (HCFAP), under the joint direction of the Attorney General and the Secretary of the Department of Health and Human Services (HHS) acting through the Department's Inspector General (HHS/OIG). The HCFAP program is designed to coordinate federal, state, and local law enforcement activities with respect to health care fraud and abuse. The act requires HHS and Department of Justice (DOJ) to detail in an annual report the amounts deposited and appropriated to the Medicare Trust Fund, as well as the source of such deposits.

Health care providers must be aware of the potential liabilities when submitting claims for payment that are deemed to be "fraudulent" or inappropriate by the government. The government may impose significant financial and administrative penalties when health care claims are not appropriately submitted, including criminal

prosecution against the offending party. Fraud, according to the OIG, can result from deliberate unethical behavior or simply from mistakes and miscues that cause excessive reimbursement. The OIG is the professional health care provider's (and their agents') "partner" in fighting fraud and abuse.

Compliance Program Guidance recommendations from the OIG must be the guiding principle of a health care practice in regard to the potential for unethical behavior or the mistakes that may occur within the organization. The *Individual and Small Group Physician Practices* and the *Compliance Program Guidance for Third-Party Medical Billing Companies* are two publications in a series for the health care industry that provide guidance and acceptable principles for business operations. See Internet Resources at the end of this chapter.

If you are involved in the claims processing procedures in your organization, note the importance and urgency in following the legal and ethical path when performing your duties. Your "honest mistake" could lead to a situation that puts the health care provider at risk for investigation of fraud, waste, or abuse if it continues and is not corrected.

Fraud and Abuse Laws

Fraud can occur when deception is used in a claim submission to obtain payment from the payer. Individuals who knowingly, willfully, and intentionally submit false information to benefit themselves or others commit fraud. Fraud can also be interpreted from mistakes that result in excessive reimbursement. No proof of "specific intent to defraud" is required for fraud to be considered. Fraud usually involves careful planning. Examples are listed in Box 2.10.

Abuse means incidents or practices by physicians, not usually considered fraudulent, which are inconsistent with accepted sound medical business or fiscal practices. Examples are listed in Box 2.11.

In subsequent chapters about various insurance programs, additional information about fraud and abuse pertinent to each program is given.

Federal False Claims Act (31 US Code §3729-33)

"A false claim is a claim for payment for services or supplies that were not provided specifically as presented or for which the provider is otherwise not entitled to payment." Presenting a claim for an item or service based on a code known to result in greater payment or to

Box 2.10 Examples of Fraud

Bill for services or supplies not provided (**phantom billing** or invoice ghosting) or for an office visit if a patient fails to keep an appointment and is not notified ahead of time that this is office policy.

Alter fees on a claim form to obtain higher payment.

Forgive the deductible or copayment.

Alter medical records to generate fraudulent payments.

Leave relevant information off a claim (e.g., failing to reveal whether a spouse has health insurance coverage through an employer).

Upcode (e.g., submitting a code for a complex fracture when the patient had a simple fracture).

Shorten (e.g., dispensing less medication than billed for).

Split billing schemes (e.g., billing procedures over a period of days when all treatment occurred during one visit).

Use another person's insurance card in obtaining medical care.

Change a date of service.

Post adjustments to generate fraudulent payments.

Solicit, offer, or receive a kickback, bribe, or rebate in return for referring a patient to a physician, physical therapist, or pharmacy or for referring a patient to obtain any item or service that may be paid for in full or in part by Medicare or Medicaid.

Restate the diagnosis to obtain insurance benefits or better payment.

Apply deliberately for duplicate payment (e.g., billing Medicare twice, billing Medicare and the beneficiary for the same service, or billing Medicare and another insurer in an attempt to get paid twice).

Unbundle or explode charge (e.g., billing a multichannel laboratory test as if individual tests were performed).

Collusion between a physician and a carrier employee when the claim is assigned (if the physician deliberately overbilled for services, overpayments could be generated with little awareness on the part of the Medicare beneficiary).

Bills based on gang visits (e.g., a physician visits nursing home and bills for 20 visits without furnishing any specific service to, or on behalf of, individual patients).

Knowingly bill for the same item or service more than once or when another party bills the federal health care program for an item or service also billed by the physician.

Box 2.11 Examples of Medical Billing Abuse

Refer excessively to other providers for unnecessary services.

Charge excessively for services or supplies.

Perform a battery of diagnostic tests when only a few are required for services.

Violate Medicare's physician participating agreement.

Call patients back for repeated and unnecessary follow-up visits.

Bill Medicare beneficiaries at a higher rate than other patients.

Submit bills to Medicare instead of to third-party payers (e.g., claims for injury from an automobile accident, in a store, or the workplace).

Breach assignment agreement.

Fail to make required refunds when services are not reasonable and necessary.

Require patients to contract to pay their physician's full charges, in excess of the Medicare charge limits.

Require a patient to waive rights to have the physician submit claims to Medicare and obligate a patient to pay privately for Medicare-covered services.

Require patients to pay for services not previously billed, including telephone calls with the physician, prescription refills, and medical conferences with other professionals.

Require patients to sign a global waiver agreeing to pay privately for all services that Medicare will not cover, and using these waivers to obligate patients to pay separately for a service that Medicare covers as part of a package or related procedures.

submit a claim for services not medically necessary is also a violation of the False Claims Act (FCA). The government uses the FCA as a primary enforcement tool.

Although no proof of specific intent to defraud is required, liability can occur when a person knowingly presents or causes to present such a claim or makes, uses, or causes a false record or statement to have a false or fraudulent claim paid or approved by the federal government.

A coder or biller who has knowledge of fraud or abuse should take the following measures:

1. Notify the provider both personally and with a dated, written memorandum.

2. Document the false statement or representation of the material fact.

3. Send a memorandum to the office manager or employer stating your concern if no change is made.

4. Maintain a written audit trail with dated memoranda for your files.

5. Do not discuss the problem with anyone who is not immediately involved.

Qui Tam "Whistleblower"

Qui Tam in the FCA provisions allows a private citizen to bring a civil action suit for a violation on behalf of the federal government. This involves fraud by government contractors and other entities who receive or use government funds. The Qui Tam "whistleblower" shares in any money recovered.

Civil Monetary Penalties Law (42 US Code §320a-27a)

The U.S. Congress enacted the Civil Monetary Penalty (CMP) statute to provide administrative remediation to combat health care fraud and abuse. The HIPAA's Final Rule includes civil monetary penalties when there is a pattern of upcoded claims or billing for medically unnecessary services. CMP imposes civil monetary penalties and assessments against a person or organization for making false or improper claims against any federal health care program.

Criminal False Claims Act (18 US Code)

The Criminal False Claims Act did not apply specifically to the health care industry before HIPAA. HIPAA amendments to the criminal code include the following:

- Theft or Embezzlement (18 US Code §669). This law brings fines and imprisonment against any individual who "knowingly and willfully embezzles, steals, or otherwise without authority converts to the use of any person other than the rightful owner, or intentionally misapplies any of the moneys, funds, securities, premiums, credits, property, or other assets of a health care benefit program." This law does not just affect Medicare and Medicaid programs. **Embezzlement** means stealing money that has been entrusted in one's care. In many cases of insurance claims embezzlement, the physician is held as the guilty party and has to pay huge sums of money to the insurance carrier when false claims are submitted by an employee. If an undiscovered embezzler leaves the employer and you are hired to replace that person, you could be accused some months down the line of doing something that you did not do. Take precautions as an employee to protect the medical practice. These precautions are discussed in Chapter 4.
- False Statement Relating to Health Care Matters (18 US Code §1035). Any individual who knowingly and willfully "falsifies, conceals, or covers up by any trick, scheme, or device a material fact; or makes any materially false, fictitious, or fraudulent statements or representations, or makes or uses any materially false writing or document knowing the same to contain any materially false, fictitious, or fraudulent statement or entry, in connection with the delivery of or payment for health care benefits, items, or services" is subject to fines and imprisonment.
- Health Care Fraud (18 US Code §1347). Any individual who knowingly and willfully "executes, or attempts to execute, a scheme or artifice to defraud any health care benefit program; or to obtain, by means of false or fraudulent pretenses, representations, or promises, any of the money or property owned by, or under the custody or control of, any health care benefit program, in connection with the delivery of or payment for health care benefits, items, or services" is subject to fines and imprisonment. If serious bodily injury or even death occurs, the person may face life imprisonment.
- Obstruction of Criminal Investigations of Health Care Offenses (18 US Code §1518). An individual is subject to fines and imprisonment when the person "willfully prevents, obstructs, misleads, delays or attempts to prevent, obstruct, mislead, or delay the communication of

information or records relating to a violation of a Federal health care offense to a criminal investigator."

Stark Laws (42 US Code §1395)

Stark laws prohibit the submission of claims for "designated services" or referral of patients if the referring physician has a "financial relationship" with the entity that provides the services. Originally named "Stark I," this law pertained only to clinical laboratories. Stark laws carry exceptions, so it is important to understand the referral processes and in-office ancillary services used by your health care organization.

Anti-Kickback Statute

According to CMS, discounts, rebates, or other reductions in price may violate the Anti-Kickback statute because such arrangements induce the purchase of items or services payable by Medicare or Medicaid. However, some arrangements are clearly permissible if they fall within a "safe harbor." One safe harbor protects certain discounting practices. For purposes of this safe harbor, a "discount" is the reduction in the amount a seller charges a buyer for a good or service based on an "arms-length" transaction. In addition, to be protected under the discount safe harbor, the discount must apply to the original item or service purchased or furnished; that is, a discount cannot be applied to the purchase of a different good or service than the one on which the discount was earned. A "rebate" is defined as a discount that is not given at the time of sale. A "buyer" is the individual or entity responsible for submitting a claim for the item or service that is payable by the Medicare or Medicaid programs. A "seller" is the individual or entity who offers the discount.

Safe Harbors

Safe harbors specify various business and service arrangements that are protected from prosecution under the Anti-Kickback statute. These include certain investments, care in underserved areas, and other arrangements.

Additional Laws and Compliance

Other laws pertaining to fraud and abuse include the Federal Deposit Insurance Corporation (FDIC) Mail and Wire Fraud provisions, as follows:

- §1341. Frauds and swindles. An individual is subject to both fines and imprisonment when having "devised or intending to devise any scheme or artifice to defraud, or for obtaining money or property by means of false or fraudulent pretenses" by use of the U.S. Postal

Service, whether sent by or delivered to the Postal Service.

● §1343. Fraud by wire, radio, or television. An individual will be fined and/or imprisoned "for obtaining money or property by means of false or fraudulent pretenses, representations, or promises, transmits or causes to be transmitted by means of wire, radio, or television communication."

The U.S. government is clearly committed to the investigation and prosecution of health care fraud. As with HIPAA policies and procedures, it is imperative that health care entities develop their own compliance program to identify and prevent fraud.

Operation Restore Trust

Launched in 1995, Operation Restored Trust (ORT) was designed to coordinate the activities of the OIG along with CMS and other HHS entities in identifying and preventing fraud. An established hotline (1-800-HHS-TIPS) for the public allows reporting issues that might indicate fraud, abuse, or waste. ORT has been successful due to planning with the DOJ and other law enforcement agencies, training state and local organizations to detect fraud and abuse, and implementing statistical methods to identify providers for audits and investigations.

Medicare Integrity Program

The goal of the Medicare Integrity Program (MIP) is to identify and reduce Medicare overpayments through a series of audits and reviews of provider claims and cost report data. Initiatives of MIP include identifying plan beneficiaries with additional insurance and educating health care providers. Program integrity contractors help expand the scope of the MIP. This endeavor has recovered several billions of dollars in the fight against fraud waste and abuse in the Medicare program.

Correct Coding Initiative

The Correct Coding Initiative (CCI) was developed to detect improperly coded claims through the use of computer edits. Services that should be grouped together and paid as one item rather than billed separately to obtain higher reimbursement are identified with the computer system.

Increased Staffing and Expanded Penalties for Violations

A significant increase in staffing among the OIG, DOJ, and FBI over the past decade has included prosecutors (over 400% increase since 1993) and FBI agents (over 300% since 1993). With additional employees, the industry has seen the promotion of compliance endeavors across the health care sector. Penalties for violations have increased.

Special Alerts, Bulletins, and Guidance Documents

Special Fraud Alerts are published by the OIG to alert the industry concerning specific patterns or trends related to fraudulent or abusive activities regarding the Medicare and Medicaid programs. *Special Advisory Bulletins* report industry practices and arrangements that may implicate fraud and abuse. *Other guidance documents* include updates, response letters, and alerts important to more specifically targeted matters. All notices are available at the OIG Web site, and you can sign up for their mailing list.

Exclusion Program

According to OIG:

No program payment will be made for anything that an excluded person furnishes, orders, or prescribes. This payment prohibition applies to the excluded person, anyone who employs or contracts with the excluded person, any hospital or other provider where the excluded person provides services, and anyone else. The exclusion applies regardless of who submits the claims and applies to all administrative and management services furnished by the excluded person.

Excluded persons/facilities are convicted for program-related fraud and patient abuse, actions from licensing boards, and defaulting on Health Education Assistance Loans.

Your health care organization must not conduct business with any health care provider or subcontract with any agent who has been listed as an Excluded Individual. Be sure to check the updated listings at the OIG Web site.

COMPLIANCE PROGRAM GUIDANCE FOR INDIVIDUAL AND SMALL GROUP PHYSICIAN PRACTICES

The OIG published the *Individual and Small Group Physician Practices* in September 2000. This guidance recommended by the OIG is voluntary; however, an effective plan reduces the risk of legal action and creates a "good faith" effort in combating fraud, waste, and abuse. A **compliance plan** requires that a health care practice review all billing processes through audits and establish controls that will correct weaknesses and prevent errors.

A well-designed compliance program can (1) speed the claims-processing cycle, (2) optimize proper payment or claims, (3) minimize billing mistakes, (4) reduce the likelihood of a government audit, (5) avoid conflict with Stark laws and the Anti-Kickback statute, (6) show a "good faith" effort that claims will be submitted appropriately, and (7) relay to staff that there is a duty to report mistakes and suspected or known misconduct.

If you are a claims-processing staff member, your organization's claims-processing supervisor should research industry sector program guidance to help with specific concerns regarding the specialty/facility setting. Check the OIG Web site to view addenda, comments, and drafts of additional compliance guidance subjects.

Increased Productivity and Decreased Penalties with Plan

The presence of an OIG compliance program can significantly mitigate imposed penalties in the event of an OIG audit or other discovery of fraudulent billing activities. These P&P can be found in the provider's P&P manual. For those not currently in the role of a Privacy/Security/Compliance Officer, knowledge about P&P as they pertain to both HIPAA and OIG will be invaluable throughout their career.

Because health care providers rely on the expertise of their billing and coding staff to process claims accurately and promptly, they also look to these staff members for advice and guidance. If you are directly involved in this area of your organization, you will likely be expected to understand the complexities of the various laws and regulations governing the medical claims process.

Compliance plans effectively become a "meeting of the minds" among the players; providers, claims-processing staff, and payers all are agreeing to process claims in accordance with shared values. Consider your organization's OIG compliance program as a way to integrate regulatory requirements directly into your claims-processing procedures. OIG views the experienced claims-processing staff as the critical screen for the health care provider's claims. The common denominators in the key benefits identified by OIG are efficiency, consistency, and integrity.

SEVEN BASIC COMPONENTS OF A COMPLIANCE PLAN

OIG outlines the following seven components of an effective program guidance plan specifically for the individual and small group physician practices:

1. Conducting internal monitoring and auditing.

2. Implementing compliance and practice standards.
3. Designating a compliance officer or contact.
4. Conducting appropriate training and education.
5. Responding appropriately to detected offenses and developing corrective action.
6. Developing open lines of communication.
7. Enforcing disciplinary standards through well-publicized guidelines

Conducting Internal Monitoring and Auditing

A comprehensive auditing and monitoring program will not eliminate misconduct within an organization but will minimize the risk of fraud and abuse by identifying the risk areas. OIG does not provide a specific set of guidelines on conducting audits or ongoing monitoring. The compliance officer, with the committee's assistance, should identify problem areas and should have established auditing priorities and procedures as part of the organization's compliance program.

Special attention should be made to the risk areas associated with claims submission and processing. Also, a thorough review of the organization's standards and written P&P should be conducted to ensure proper guidelines for complying with state and federal laws and insurance payer requirements.

Implementing Compliance and Practice Standards

Written standards and procedures address risk areas that an office needs to monitor and follow. Specific risk areas* identified by OIG include the following:

● Billing for items or services not rendered or not provided as claimed
● Submitting claims for equipment, medical supplies, and services that are not reasonable and necessary
● Double billing resulting in duplicate payment
● Billing for noncovered services as if covered
● Knowing misuse of provider identification numbers, which results in improper billing
● Unbundling, or billing for each component of the service instead of billing or using an all-inclusive code
● Failure to use coding modifiers properly
● Clustering
● Upcoding the level of service provided

---

*Data from *Federal Register* 65(194):59439, 2000.

In addition to these risk areas, policies should be developed that address the following:

● Definition of reasonable and necessary
● Proper medical documentation
● Federal sentencing guidelines
● Record retention

You should be able to access your organization's P&P manual to review the standards and protocol for these issues involving your practice.

Designating a Compliance Officer or Contact

As with the HIPAA PO, the compliance officer is the key individual overseeing your organization's compliance program monitoring with the support of the Compliance Committee. Again, as with HIPAA, policies and procedures need to be drafted. These established guidelines identify and prevent fraud and abuse activities as described by OIG.

The number of members on your compliance committee is not important, and prospective staff members from human resources, claims auditing, billing, legal, and medicine departments can ensure a comprehensive mix. You may currently participate on your office's compliance committee or may be asked to do so in the future. The compliance committee acts as a review board. Some committees consist of provider-client office staff and billing company staff. Some committees are simply the provider-client and the billing company staff, or a combination of the provider-client, their practice manager, and the billing company staff. The committee, empowered by management, legitimizes the compliance strategy within your organization. In addition to possessing professional experience in claims processing and auditing, committee members are expected to use good judgment and high integrity to fulfill committee obligations.

Conducting Appropriate Training and Education

Because OIG compliance program guidelines are based on Federal Sentencing Guidelines, significant elements of an effective compliance program involve proper education and training of staff. Every employee and individual who interacts with your health care organization and may be accountable for potential misconduct should be considered in the organization's training sessions.

You should be required to attend training in a "general" compliance training session at least annually. For staff members involved in claims processing (coding and billing),

a separate training session should be held to cover internal procedures, federal and state laws regarding fraud and abuse, and specific government and other payer reimbursement policies. Periodic professional courses in continuing education should be available. Coding and billing personnel should receive training at least annually to remain updated on CPT/HCPCS and ICD-9-CM codes for each year. You will attend training either on site, at a remote location, or both.

Effective training can reduce potential errors, penalties, and fines. An educated staff makes fewer errors, reduces your organization's risks, and requires less micromanagement.

Responding Appropriately to Detected Offenses and Developing Corrective Action

When faced with the discovery of an offense or an error, inaction may be interpreted as indifference. This could impose a potential jeopardy to the reputation of the health care provider's practice. Your office should have a process for investigating problems and taking necessary corrective action. Issues that would raise concern include significant change in claims that are rejected; software edits that show a pattern of misuse of codes or fees; unusually high volume of charges, payments, or rejections; and notices from insurance payers regarding claims submitted by your office.

You and your fellow staff members should be encouraged to report concerns for any suspected or known misconduct, with an established chain of command in the reporting path. Some incidences of misconduct may violate criminal, civil, or administrative law. If the situation warrants, the compliance officer should report the misconduct promptly to the appropriate government authority.

Report fraud and abuse. Contact the HHS OIG as follows:

● Telephone hotline 800-HHS-TIPS (1-800-447-8477)
● TTY 800-377-4950
● Fax 800-223-8164
● Web site **http://oig.hhs.gov/hotline.html**

Developing Open Lines of Communication

Effective lines of communication provide a channel for employees to report suspected or known misconduct without immediately resorting to an external agency. In this way your health care organization can resolve issues internally.

"Open door" policies ensure an environment where staff members feel secure to ask about the organization's existing P&P and to report questionable activities. Your role as a conscientious employee will allow you to know the steps to take in reporting any suspicious business activity.

You will learn your office's procedure for reporting misconduct. It is important to follow these guidelines to protect your reputation and credibility within the workplace. Depending on the size of the practice, the methods for contacting managerial staff may include anonymous telephone calls through a "hotline" or written report forms.

Enforcing Disciplinary Standards through Well-Publicized Guidelines

The unfortunate downside to compliance is that misconduct does occur. For this reason, health care organizations must have established disciplinary guidelines and must make these well known to employees and other agents who contract with the organization. We all want to know what will happen if we "make a mistake" and what progressive forms of discipline await situations involving misconduct. Disciplinary standards include the following:

- Verbal warning
- Written warning
- Written reprimand
- Suspension or probation
- Demotion
- Termination of employment
- Restitution of any damages
- Referral to federal agencies for criminal prosecution

Whether the misconduct was intentional or negligent, all levels of employees need to know what is expected of them. Your office must publish this information and disseminate it to all employees.

WHAT TO EXPECT FROM YOUR HEALTH CARE PRACTICE

Although every health care organization or practice is different in regard to policies and procedures, you now know what to expect in the workplace, as follows:

- Practice adherence to HIPAA and OIG mandates and recommendations
- Privacy/Security/Compliance Officer (even if one person)
- Policy and procedure manual
- Employee training and education (at least annually and whenever there are changes in business operations that affect staff members directly)
- Complaint and sanctions process

COMPLIANCE LESSONS LEARNED

You must strongly consider the lessons learned from the privacy, transaction, and security rules in conjunction with OIG compliance recommendations. The most important points are to read your organization's P&P manual and to ask questions about the many aspects of HIPAA or the general operations of your organization. Always use your ethical and "best practice" approach to be an informed and effective employee.

RESOURCES

INTERNET @

The Internet is a valuable tool for obtaining information on compliance programs.

- American Health Information Management Association
  Web site: **http://www.ahima.org**

- American Medical Association
  Web site: **http://www.ama-assn.org**

- Centers for Medicare and Medicaid Services
  Web site: **http://www.cms.gov/providers/fraud**

- Department of Health and Human Services, Office of Inspector General
  Web site: **http://www.oig.hhs.gov/progorg/org**

- Federal Bureau of Investigation
  Web site: **http://www.oig.hhs.gov**

- MEDEXTEND
  Web site: **http://www.medextend.com**

- National Health Information Structure, resource for ongoing projects, meetings and documents relevant to the NHII initiative
  Web site: **http://aspe.hhs.gov/sp/NHII/**

- Office of Civil Rights
  Web site: **http://www.hhs.gov/ocr/hipaa**

- Office of the Inspector General Red Book, a compendium of significant cost saving recommendations
  Web site: **http://www.dhhs.gov/progorg/oig/redbk/index.htm**

- OIG Compliance Program Guidance for Third-Party Medical Billing Companies, *Federal Register* 63(243):70141, 1998.

- OIG Compliance Program for Individual and Small Group Physician Practices, *Federal Register* 65(194):59439, 2000.

- Phoenix Health Systems: HIPAA Advisory
  Web site: **http://www.hipaadvisory.com**

- U.S. Government Printing Office with link to the online *Federal Register*
  Web site: **http://www.access.gpo.gov/.su_docs/**

- Workgroup for Electronic Data Interchange
  Web site: **http://www.wedi.org**

- National Health Information Infrastructure initiative report "Information for Health: A Strategy for Building the National Health Information Infrastructure"
  Web site: **http://www.ncvhs.hhs.gov/nhiilayo.pdf**

- For up-to-date information on fraud alerts, visit the Office of the Inspector General and Federal Bureau of Investigation
  Web site: **http://www.oig.hhs.gov**
  Web site: **http://www.fbi.gov**

- The national hotline of the Office of the Inspector General is 1-800-HHS-TIPS.
  To obtain current information on fraud in the Medicaid program, visit:
  Web site: **http://www.oig.hhs.gov/hotline.html**

- To obtain current information on fraud in Medicare or Medicaid programs, visit
  Web site: **http://www.cms.hhs.gov/providers/fraud**

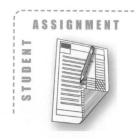

ASSIGNMENT

STUDENT

✔ Study Chapter 2.

✔ Answer the review questions in the *Workbook* to reinforce the theory learned in this chapter and help prepare you for a future test.

✔ Complete the assignments in the *Workbook* to give you experience in making decisions regarding situations of fraud abuse, incidental disclosures or compliance violations, consents, or authorizations.

✔ Turn to the glossary at the end of this textbook for a further understanding of the key terms used in this chapter.

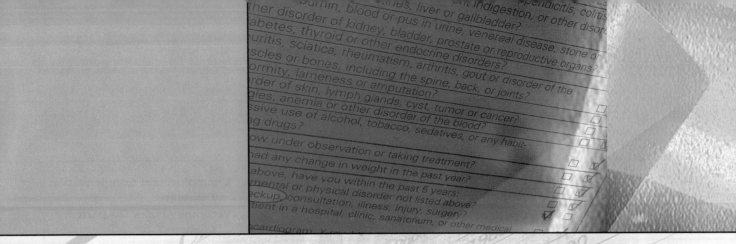

The Claims Process

CHAPTER OUTLINE

HISTORY
INSURANCE IN THE UNITED
  STATES
LEGAL PRINCIPLES OF
  INSURANCE
  Insurance Contracts
PHYSICIAN–PATIENT
  CONTRACTS AND FINANCIAL
  OBLIGATION
  Implied or Expressed Contracts
THE INSURANCE POLICY
  Policy Application
  Policy Renewal Provisions
  Policy Terms
  Coordination of Benefits
  General Policy Limitations
CHOICE OF HEALTH INSURANCE
  Group Contract
  Individual Contract
  Prepaid Health Plan

TYPES OF HEALTH INSURANCE
  COVERAGE
  CHAMPVA
  Competitive Medical Plan
  Disability Income Insurance
  Exclusive Provider Organization
  Foundation for Medical Care
  Health Maintenance
    Organization
  Independent or Individual
    Practice Association
  Maternal and Child Health
    Program
  Medicaid
  Medicare
  Medicare/Medicaid
  Point-of-Service Plan
  Preferred Provider
    Organization
  TRICARE

Unemployment Compensation
  Disability
Veterans Affairs Outpatient
  Clinic
Workers' Compensation
  Insurance
EXAMPLES OF INSURANCE
  BILLING
KEEPING UP TO DATE
PROCEDURE: HANDLING
  AND PROCESSING INSURANCE
  CLAIMS
PROCEDURE: PREPARE
  AND POST TO A PATIENT'S
  FINANCIAL ACCOUNTING
  RECORD

KEY TERMS

accounts receivable management
applicant
assignment
blanket contract
capitation
The Civilian Health and Medical Program of the Department of Veterans Affairs (CHAMPVA)
claim
coinsurance
competitive medical plan (CMP)
conditionally renewable
contract
daysheet
deductible
disability income insurance

electronic signature
eligibility
emancipated minor
encounter form
exclusions
exclusive provider organization (EPO)
expressed contract
extended
financial accounting record
foundation for medical care (FMC)
guaranteed renewable
guarantor
health insurance
health maintenance organization (HMO)
high risk
implied contract
indemnity

independent or individual practice association (IPA)
insured
major medical
Maternal and Child Health Program (MCHP)
Medicaid (MCD)
Medicare (M)
Medicare/Medicaid (Medi-Medi)
member
noncancelable policy
nonparticipating provider (nonpar)
optionally renewable
participating provider (par)
patient registration form
personal insurance

point-of-service (POS) plan
posted
preauthorization
precertification
predetermination
preferred provider organization (PPO)
premium
running balance
State Disability Insurance (SDI)
subscriber
TRICARE
Unemployment Compensation Disability (UCD)
Veterans Affairs (VA) outpatient clinic
Workers' compensation (WC) insurance

Basics of Health Insurance

OBJECTIVES*

After reading this chapter, you should be able to:

- Describe the history of insurance in the United States.

- Distinguish among the three major classes of health insurance contracts.

- State four concepts of a valid insurance contract.

- Explain the difference between an implied and an expressed physician–patient contract.

- Describe in general terms the important federal, state, and private health insurance plans.

- Define common insurance terms.

- List four actions to prevent problems when given signature authorization for insurance claims.

- Explain the administrative life cycle of a physician-based insurance claim from completion to insurance carrier processing and payment.

- Establish an insurance claims register or log.

- Determine the appropriate questions to ask a patient for a complete patient record.

- List the functions of an aging report in a computerized practice management system or a "tickler" file in a paper environment.

- Handle insurance claims in the physician's office to obtain payment and minimize rejection by insurance carriers.

- Record proper information and post to the patient's ledger after claims submission and payment received.

*Performance objectives and exercises for hands-on practical experience for this chapter appear in the *Workbook*.

Service

You must be friendly and courteous when handling insurance claims in order to maintain a harmonious physician–patient relationship. Collections often can be significantly improved and simplified if the patient feels free to discuss personal financial problems at any time and is educated regarding the physician's fees. Quickly obtain precertification, preauthorization, or predetermination so the patient's treatment plan may be carried out without delay. Assist and instruct the patient in filling out a patient information form so data is accurate and complete. Explain and answer the patient's questions about your office's Notice of Privacy Practices (NPP). Remember it is important for you to understand what the NPP states. Promptly transmit accurate insurance claim data to the insurance carrier so reimbursement is received in a timely manner on behalf of the patient.

HISTORY

The insurance industry is among the world's largest businesses. In the 1800s, life insurance came to be widely offered. Health insurance began to be available in the early part of the 20th century because anyone can have an accident or become ill unexpectedly, leading to large expenses. **Health insurance** is a contract between a policyholder and an insurance carrier or government program to reimburse the policyholder for all or a portion of the cost of medically necessary treatment or preventive care based on the contract purchased. Its main purpose is to help offset some of the high costs accrued during sickness or when an injury occurred.

During the Renaissance, when Italian traders insured valuable cargo to be shipped across the Mediterranean, they recorded the insurance agreement on a piece of folded paper called a "polizza." English merchants adapted the term to their insurance practices, modifying the pronunciation to suit the Anglo-Saxon tongue, resulting in the word "policy."

Insurance in the United States

In 1850, the Franklin Health Assurance Company of Massachusetts began offering insurance for nonfatal injury. About 10 years later, the Travelers Insurance Company of Hartford marketed a plan that is similar to today's health insurance. Many other companies began writing health insurance policies, and in 1911 Montgomery Ward and Company offered benefits to its ill or injured employees. This was the first group plan. These commercial plans paid only when an individual was sick or received an injury.

By the 1960s, most private insurance companies sold policies that included hospital care, surgical fees, and physicians' services. In addition to those benefits, many plans now offer catastrophic health insurance coverage, preventive care, dental insurance, disability income insurance, and long-term care and home health care insurance for the chronically ill, disabled, and developmentally disabled. State insurance laws regulate the way policies are written and minimum requirements of coverage.

Medical care costs continuously escalate, forcing insurance companies to reduce the benefits of individual subscribers. Rising costs have caused the federal government to adopt cost-containment policies for the Medicare, Medicaid, and TRICARE programs (TRICARE is a three-option managed health care program offered to active duty uniform service members and their families; military retirees and their families; and survivors of all uniformed services who are not eligible for Medicare.) Although managed care began in the 1930s when Kaiser Industries provided health care to their employees, it was not until the 1980s that many types of plans sprung up across the nation to control the cost of medical care and help those who could not afford health insurance. Because individual needs vary, each patient may have a different type of health insurance policy with various benefits. Patients may be covered under different types of private, state, or federal programs.

LEGAL PRINCIPLES OF INSURANCE

The role of a medical insurance billing specialist is to complete the insurance claim accurately and facilitate claims submission so that optimal accurate reimbursement is received quickly. However, before developing the skill of coding and completing insurance claim forms, it is necessary to know frequently encountered legal problems and how to handle them. Legal situations occur daily in the performance of these job duties and involve confidentiality of medical records, accurate insurance claim completion, fraud and abuse issues, credit and collection laws, and so on. An insurance biller cannot escape liability by pleading ignorance. It cannot be overemphasized that keeping up to date on health care plan policies and procedures is essential. Most legal issues of private health insurance claims fall under civil law and Medicare, Medicaid, and TRICARE programs fall under federal laws. Insurance is regulated by state law and is not considered a federally regulated industry, except that Health Insurance Portability and Accountability Act (HIPAA) and Office of Inspector General (OIG) federal regulations help govern the entire industry.

It is important for an insurance billing specialist to know some basic insurance terms, understand basic insurance concepts, and have a working knowledge of medical terminology.

Insurance Contracts

The first legal item in the business of handling medical insurance is the insurance contract (also known as a policy). There is no standard health insurance contract. Individuals who take out a policy receive an original document composed by the insuring company.

There are four considerations involved in drawing up a valid insurance contract:

1. The person must be a mentally competent adult and not under the influence of drugs or alcohol when signing the contract.
2. The insurance company must make an offer (the signed application), and the person must accept the offer (issuance of the policy), without concealment or misrepresentation of facts on the application.
3. An exchange of value (the first premium payment) submitted with the application, known as a *consideration*, must be present.
4. A legal purpose must exist, which is an insurable interest in the case of a health insurance policy. This means that the policyholder expects to continue in good health, but that the insurance policy will provide something of value if an accident or illness strikes.

A policy can be challenged when a fraudulent statement is made by the subscriber. A challenged policy means that coverage may not be in effect. After a policy has been in force for 2 years (3 years in some states), a policy becomes incontestable (may not be challenged). If the time limit has passed and a policy is guaranteed renewable, the policy becomes incontestable even if false statements were made on the application. Further information and additional insurance terminology concerning contracts is provided in detail in Chapter 4.

PHYSICIAN–PATIENT CONTRACTS AND FINANCIAL OBLIGATION

Implied or Expressed Contracts

A physician and his or her staff must be aware of the physician's obligations to each patient, and his or her liabilities in regard to service, and the patient's obligations to the physician. The physician–patient contract begins when the physician accepts the patient and agrees to treat him or her. This action can be either an implied or expressed contract. An **implied contract** is defined as not manifested by direct words but implied or deduced from the circumstance, the general language, or the conduct of the patient. For example, if Mary Johnson goes to Dr. Doe's office and Dr. Doe gives Ms. Johnson professional services that she accepts, this is an implied contract. If the patient is unconscious when treatment is rendered, treatment is based on an implied-in-fact contract.

An **expressed contract** can be verbal or written. However, most physician–patient contracts are implied.

Private Patients

For a patient who carries private medical insurance, the contract for treatment is between the physician and the patient. The patient is liable for the entire bill. The insurance is meant to help offset the expense. However, for patients who belong to a preferred provider organization (PPO), the patient is not liable for the bill if the physician does not follow his or her contract with the payer.

Guarantor

A **guarantor** is an individual who promises to pay the medical bill. A signed agreement indicating the guarantor is the responsible party constitutes an expressed promise. Usually, a patient is the guarantor and must be of legal age (18 or 21 years, depending on state law). For example, a divorced parent of a child may be the guarantor and, therefore, solely liable for the child's bill. Most laws governing financial responsibility state that a husband is responsible for his wife's debts; a wife is not always responsible for her husband's debts. However, this always depends on the way the contractual application reads and individual state laws. A father is ordinarily responsible for his children's debts if they are minors and are not emancipated (Figure 3–1). Children may or may not be responsible for the debts of their parents, depending on the circumstances and state laws.

Emancipated Minor

An **emancipated minor** is a person younger than 18 years of age who lives independently, is totally self-supporting,

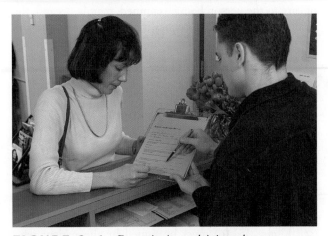

FIGURE 3–1 Receptionist explaining where a guarantor's signature goes on a patient registration form for the medical services rendered to a family member.

is married or divorced, is a parent even if not married, or is in the military and possesses decision-making rights. College students living away from home even when financially dependent on their parents are considered emancipated. Parents are not liable for the medical expenses incurred by an emancipated minor. The patient record should contain the minor's signed statement that he or she is on his or her own.

Managed Care Patients

A physician under contract to a managed care plan may or may not periodically receive an updated list of current enrollees. The physician is obligated to see those individuals who are enrolled if one of them calls for an appointment. However, the contract for treatment occurs when the patient is first seen. If the physician no longer wishes to treat a patient on a managed care plan, termination is handled according to the same method used when discharging patients who are insured under private insurance or state or government programs. The method of how to do this is explained in the next chapter.

An insurance specialist should be able to read and explain managed care plan contracts that the office participates with, but if the specialist is unable to interpret these matters, professional assistance from the physician's attorney, the medical practice's accountant, or the managed care plan should be sought. He or she should understand billing and collection requirements and track payments made by the managed care plan.

Employment and Disability Examinations

Courts in most jurisdictions have ruled that there is no physician–patient relationship in an employment or disability examination and the doctor does not owe a duty of care to the person being examined, mainly because the insurance company is requesting the examination and the patient is not seeking the medical services of the physician.

Workers' Compensation Patients

Workers' compensation cases involve a person being injured on the job. These cases may be referred to as industrial accidents or illnesses. In these types of cases, the contract exists between the physician and the insurance company. When there is a dispute as to whether the injured party was hurt at work, a Patient Agreement form (see Figure 15–16) must be signed by the patient who agrees to pay the physician's fees if the case is declared to be non–work-related.

THE INSURANCE POLICY

Insurance policies are complex and contain a great deal of legalese. This can cause misunderstanding by patients or anyone trying to obtain information from the policy. Basic health insurance coverage includes benefits for hospital, surgical, and other medical expenses. **Major medical** or *extended benefits* contracts are designed to offset large medical expenses caused by prolonged illness or serious injury. Some of these policies include coverage for *extended care* or *skilled nursing facility* benefits. The **insured** is known as a **subscriber** or, in some insurance programs, a **member**, *policyholder*, or *recipient* and may not necessarily be the patient seen for the medical service. The subscriber may or may not be the guarantor. The insured is the individual (enrollee) or organization protected in case of loss under the terms of an insurance policy. In group insurance, the employer is considered the insured, and the employees are the risks. However, when completing an insurance claim form, the covered employee is listed as the insured. A policy might also include *dependents* of the insured. Generally, this term refers to the spouse and children of the insured, but under some contracts, parents, other family members, and domestic partners may be covered as dependents.

Policy Application

Before a policy is issued, the insurance company decides whether it will enter into a contract with the **applicant** who is applying for the insurance coverage. Information is obtained about the applicant so the company can decide whether to accept the risk. Generally, the application form has two sections: part one contains basic information about the application, and part two concerns the health of the individual.

An insurance policy is a legally enforceable agreement, or **contract.** If a policy is issued, the applicant becomes part of the insurance contract or plan. The policy becomes effective only after the company offers the policy and the person accepts it and then pays the initial premium (Figure 3–2). If a premium is paid at the time the application is submitted, then the insurance coverage can be put into force before the policy is delivered. Depending on the laws in some states, the applicant also can have temporary conditional insurance if the agent issues a specific type of receipt.

Policy Renewal Provisions

Health insurance policies may have renewal provisions written into the policy stating the circumstances when the company may refuse to renew, may cancel coverage, or may increase the premium. It is important for the

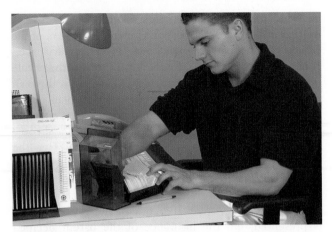

FIGURE 3–2 Insurance billing specialist searching in an index file for an insurance company's telephone number to inquire about a patient's coverage under an insurance policy.

biller to understand that coverage may change from the last time the physician saw the patient for an appointment. It is a good routine always to verify with the patient the insurance information each time he or she comes for an appointment. It may seem redundant but it may avoid a lot of future confusion and delays in payment.

In private health insurance, there are five classifications: (1) cancelable, (2) optionally renewable, (3) conditionally renewable, (4) guaranteed renewable, and (5) noncancelable.

A renewable provision in a *cancelable* policy grants the insurer the right to cancel the policy at any time and for any reason. The company notifies the insured that the policy is canceled and refunds any advance premium the policyholder has paid. In some states, this type of policy is illegal.

In an **optionally renewable** policy, the insurer has the right to refuse to renew the policy on a date (premium due or anniversary date) specified in the contract and may add coverage limitations or increase premium rates.

Conditionally renewable policies grant the insurer a limited right to refuse to renew a health insurance policy at the end of a premium payment period. Reasons stated in the policy may be due to age, employment status, or both but not because of the insured's health status.

The **guaranteed renewable** classification is desirable because the insurer is required to renew the policy as long as premium payments are made. However, these policies may have age limits of 60, 65, or 70 years, or they may be renewable for life.

In a **noncancelable policy,** the insurer cannot increase premium rates and must renew the policy until the insured reaches the age specified in the contract. Some disability income policies have noncancelable terms.

Policy Terms

To keep the insurance in force, a person must pay a monthly, quarterly, or annual fee called a **premium**. If the premium is not paid, a *grace period* of 10 to 30 days is usually given before insurance coverage ceases. Many states have laws that allow the insurance company to apply the provider's payment to the patient's insurance premium. This forces the provider to recoup payment from the patient. In addition, usually a **deductible** (a specific amount of money) must be paid each year before the policy benefits begin. Generally, the higher the deductible, the lower the cost of the policy. Most policies as well as Part B of the Medicare program have a **coinsurance** or *cost-sharing* requirement, which means the insured will assume a percentage of the fee (e.g., 20%) or pay a specific dollar amount (e.g., $5 or $10) for covered services.

Managed care plans use the term *copayment* (copay) when referring to the amount the patient pays at the point of arriving in the office and before he or she sees the physician. It is not advisable to routinely waive copayments because the health care provider has agreed to accept a patient portion. Many insurance companies do not tolerate this practice. Not only would it be a loss of income to the provider but if the provider is audited, the federal government can assess penalties for not collecting coinsurance for patients seen under the Medicare program. Generally, deductibles, coinsurance, and copayments should be collected at the time of service with the exception of the Medicare program, which does not recommend collecting the deductible in advance from the beneficiary. In cases of financial hardship, a discount or waiver may be considered. Be sure to document this and obtain the patient's signature and any document that verifies the patient's financial status.

Health insurance policies consider an *accident* to be an unforeseen and unintended event. Some policies cover accidents occurring from the first day the policy is in force. Others may contain an *elimination period* or a *waiting period* before benefits for sickness or accident become payable.

Generally, it is the patient's responsibility to give a written notice of **claim** to the insurance company within a certain number of days, known as a *time limit*. However, Blue Cross and Blue Shield plans, some managed care plan contracts, and Medicare guidelines require that the provider of service is obligated to submit the claim. Usually as a courtesy, the claim is filed for the patient by the provider of professional services. The insurance billing specialist must be able to abstract proper information from the patient record, which is used to code the diagnoses and services rendered; to complete an insurance claim form; to make entries (post) to a patient's financial accounting record (ledger); and to follow up on unpaid claims. If any one of these procedures is not done properly, correct reimbursement or payment (also called **indemnity**) from the insurance *carrier* will not be generated.

Follow-up on unpaid claims is made by contacting the claims representative, called a *claims adjudicator* or an *adjuster*. If the payment is to go directly from the insurance company to the physician, then the patient must sign a document granting permission.

Coordination of Benefits

A *coordination of benefits* statement is included in most policies and contracts with providers.

When the patient has more than one insurance policy, this clause requires insurance companies to coordinate the reimbursement of benefits to determine which carrier is going to be primary and which secondary, thus preventing the duplication or overlapping of payments for the same medical expense. The combination of payments from the primary and secondary carrier cannot be more than the amount of the provider's charges (Example 3.1).

Example 3.1

Mr. Smith has Insurance A and Insurance B. The claim is for $100. The claim is sent to Insurance A. Insurance A allows $80 for the procedure and pays $80. The claim is then sent to Insurance B. Insurance B also allows $80 for the procedure. The claim that was sent to Insurance B was not for $100, but for the remaining $20. The $20 is within the amount allowed by Insurance B; therefore, Insurance B pays the $20. Some carriers try to play by their own rules by stating that because Insurance A paid $80 and the $80 equals the amount Insurance B pays, Insurance B will pay no more for the claim. These rules were established by the National Association of Insurance Commissioners and approved by every State Insurance Commissioner. Therefore be observant of insurance claims like this.

Most state legislatures have adopted the *birthday law*, which is a change in the order of determination of coordination of benefits regarding primary and secondary carriers for dependent children. Rather than the father's insurance being primary, the father's or mother's carrier may be primary. The health plan of the person whose birthday (month and day, *not* year) falls earlier in the calendar year pays first, and the plan of the other person

covering the dependent is the secondary payer. If both mother and father have the same birthday, the plan of the person who has had coverage longer is the primary payer. If one of the two plans has not adopted this birthday rule (i.e., if one plan is in another state), the rules of the plan without the birthday rule determine which plan is primary and which secondary. In cases of divorce, consider that you are not an enforcer of court laws and the divorce decree is between the parents of the child. Have the parent accompanying the child pay the bill at the time of service. He or she can be reimbursed by the responsible party. Keep issues of divorce a matter of decisions made within the court system. If a copy of the court decision is presented, bill the insurance of the parent deemed responsible.

Unions and companies that self-insure their employees do not fall under this birthday law. The states that do not have birthday laws are Georgia, Hawaii, Idaho, Massachusetts, Mississippi, Vermont, Virginia, and Washington, DC.

Finally, a carrier may delay a claim, stating they are attempting to coordinate benefits with the other carrier. This process can be time consuming and may take 90 days or more to resolve. As a biller, you should be diligent in following up on this situation so that the stalled cash flow issue can be resolved. In some situations, the patient may be ultimately responsible for the bill and if you help them understand that, this will bring payment and help to resolve the account balance quicker.

General Policy Limitations

Health insurance policies contain **exclusions**—some more than others. If a person has an injury or illness that is excluded in his or her policy, then there is no insurance coverage for that injury or illness. These exclusions or limitations of the policy could be such factors as losses resulting from military service, attempted suicide, or self-inflicted injuries; losses caused by an injury on the job; pregnancy; and so on. Be aware that some insurance policies may state that a procedure or service is not covered (excluded) when the state law says the procedure is a "mandated benefit." Some examples are reconstructive breast surgery after mastectomy, surgical procedures affecting the upper and lower jawbones, and infertility coverage under group policies. Thus further investigation is necessary beyond reading the policy.

Many policies do not provide benefits for conditions that existed and were treated before the policy was issued; these are called *preexisting conditions*. In some instances, such conditions might be covered after a specified period of time (12 to 18 months) after the issuance of the policy.

Some policies have a *waiver* or *rider*, which is an attachment to a policy that modifies clauses and provisions of the policy by either adding coverage or excluding certain illnesses or disabilities that would otherwise be covered. Generally, waivers are used to eliminate benefits for specific preexisting conditions.

Case Management Requirements

Preapproval

Many private insurance carriers and prepaid health plans have certain requirements that must be met before they approve hospital admissions, inpatient or outpatient surgeries, and elective procedures. First, **eligibility** requirements must be obtained. These are conditions or qualifying factors that must be met before the patient receives benefits (medical services) under a specified insurance plan, government program, or managed care plan. The carrier can refuse to pay part or the entire fee if these requirements are not met. **Precertification** refers to discovering whether a treatment (surgery, hospitalization, tests) is covered under a patient's contract. **Preauthorization** relates not only to whether a service or procedure is covered, but also to finding out whether it is medically necessary. **Predetermination** means discovering the maximum dollar amount that the carrier will pay for surgery, consulting services, radiology procedures, and so on.

Obtain precertification or predetermination when a procedure is tentatively scheduled. The information that may be required to obtain precertification approval by fax or telephone is shown in Figure 3–3. Use the form shown in Figure 3–4 to obtain predetermination by mail. See Figure 11–1 for an example of a preauthorization form. This form also can be used to document the information received when verifying the patient's insurance coverage by telephone. It should become part of the patient's record and used for reference when billing future insurance claims.

After the information is received from the insurance carrier, give the patient an estimate of fees for the proposed surgery. An example of suggested wording for a letter is given in Figure 3–5. This written estimate makes collection quicker and easier.

CHOICE OF HEALTH INSURANCE

There are three ways in which a person can obtain health insurance: (1) take out insurance through a group plan (contract or policy), (2) pay the premium on an individual basis, or (3) enroll in a prepaid health plan.

Group Contract

A *group contract* is any insurance plan by which a group of employees (and their eligible dependents) or other homogeneous group is insured under a single policy issued to their employer or leader, with individual certificates given to each insured individual or family unit. A group policy usually provides better benefits and offers lower premiums. However, the coverage for each person in the group is the same. If a new employee declines enrollment, he or she must sign a waiver stating this fact.

Conversion Privilege

Many physicians can obtain comprehensive group coverage through plans sponsored by the professional organizations to which they belong. Sometimes this is called a **blanket contract.** If the person leaves the employer or organization or the group contract is terminated, the insured may continue the same or lesser coverage under an individual policy if the group contract has a *conversion privilege.*

Usually, conversion from a group policy to an individual policy increases the premium and could reduce the benefits. However, if the person has a condition that would make him or her ineligible for coverage or is a case considered at **high risk,** it is advantageous to convert to an individual policy because no physical examination is required; therefore a preexisting condition cannot be excluded.

Income Continuation Benefits

According to the Consolidated Omnibus Budget Reconciliation Act of 1985 (COBRA), when an employee is laid off from a company with 20 or more workers, federal law requires that the group health insurance coverage be extended to the employee and his or her dependents at group rates for up to 18 months. This also applies to those workers who lose coverage because of reduced work hours. In the case of death of a covered employee, divorced or widowed spouse, or employee entitled to Medicare, the extension of coverage may be for 36 months. However, the employee must pay for the group policy; this is known as *income continuation benefits.* See the section on COBRA in Chapter 12 for additional information on this topic.

Medical Savings Accounts

The Health Insurance Portability and Accountability Act (HIPAA) of 1996 was federal legislation created to

COLLEGE CLINIC
4567 Broad Avenue
Woodland Hills, XY 12345-0000

Phone: 555/486-9002   Fax: 555/590-2189

Insurance Precertification Form

Date: _5/4/XX_
To: Insurance Carrier ___Cal-Net Care___   From: _Janet_____ Office Mgr.
      Address ____9900 Baker Street_____
      _____Los Angeles, CA 90067_____

Check those that apply: Admission certification ✔   Outpatient___ Inpatient ✔
                           Surgery certification ✔   Emergency situation ✔

Patient's name ____Ronald Stranton_____   Date of Birth: _4-14-49_
Patient's address ___639 Cedar Street____   Sex: Male ✔ Female ____
      _____Woodland Hills, XY 12345_____   Social Security No. _527-XX-7250_
Insured's Name __Same_____   Policy Group ID No. _A59_
Insured's Address _____   Employer: _Aerostar Aviation_

Treating physician ___Clarence Cutler, M.D.___   NPI #: ___430 500 47XX___
Primary Care Physician _Gerald Practon, M.D._   NPI #: ___462 7889 7XX___

Name of Hospital__College Hospital____   Admission Date: _5/4/XX_
                                         Estimated Length of Stay: _3-5 d_
Admitting Diagnosis _____Volvulus_____   Diagnosis Code: _560.2_
Complicating conditions to substantiate need for inpatient hospitalization_____
_____Complete bowel obstruction_____
Date current illness or injury began ___5/2/XX___
Procedure/surgery to be done __Reduction of Volvulus__   Procedure code _44050_

Second opinion needed   Yes ____ No ✔ Date performed _____

Telephone precertification: _____Emergency Cert. 5/4/XX_____
Name of representative certifying____McKenzie Kwan____
Direct-dial telephone number of representative ___1-800-463-9000 ext. 227___

Reason(s) for denial _____
Certification approved   Yes ✔ No ____ Certification approval No. _69874_
Authorization for services Yes ✔ No ____ Authorization No. _69874E_

Note: The information contained in this facsimile message is confidential and privileged information intended only for the use of the individual or entity named above. If the reader of this message is not the intended recipient, you are hereby notified that any dissemination, distribution, or copying of this communication is strictly prohibited. If you have received this communication in error, please immediately notify me by telephone and return the original facsimile to me via the U.S. Postal Service. Thank you.

FIGURE 3–3 Insurance precertification form. This form can be faxed to the insurance company or used when telephoning to obtain approval for hospitalization under a patient's insurance policy or managed care plan.

(1) expand efforts to combat fraud and abuse, as learned in the previous chapter, (2) protect workers and their families so they can obtain and maintain health insurance if they change or lose their jobs, and (3) establish a medical savings account pilot project. An Archer *medical savings account* (MSA) is a type of tax-free savings account that allows individuals and their employers to set aside money to pay for health care expenses. An employer can set up an MSA for his or her employees and make an annual contribution to the MSA, which is tax deductible for both employer and employee. MSA balances accumulate from year to year tax-free, but unused funds may not be carried over in a *flexible spending account* (FSA) (another type

of MSA). Earned interest is not taxed. MSAs are portable, allowing individuals to take their MSA with them when they change jobs or relocate. When health care services are provided, the patient files a claim to receive reimbursement from these funds and uses the explanation of benefits (EOB) from the insurance company as documentation. Processing of the explanation of benefits for insurance claims with large deductibles (e.g., more than $1000), even though you know the insurance company will not be paying for the services, is necessary so that the patient/employee may submit documentation and recoup funds from the MSA. It also may be necessary to provide EOB documents from the insurance company

COLLEGE CLINIC
4567 Broad Avenue
Woodland Hills, XY 12345-0001

Phone: 555/486-9002   Fax: 555/487-8976

INSURANCE PREDETERMINATION FORM

Perry Cardi, MD
Physician

Patient: Leslee Austin   Telephone # (555) 486-8452
Address: 209 Refugio Road   Date of Birth 04-07-44
City Woodland Hills   State XY   ZIP 12345-0001
Social Security # 629-XX-9260   Accident Yes_____ No X
Insurance Company American Insurance   Member # Am 45692
Insurance Co. Address 4040 Broadway Ave   Group # 123P
                     Valley Vista, XY 12345   Telephone # (555) 238-5000
Policy holder Leslee Austin
Relationship to insured: Self X Spouse_____ Child_____ Other_____
Type of coverage: HMO X PPO_____ 80/20_____ 70/30_____ Other:_____
Procedure/Service Cardioversion (CPT 92960)
Diagnosis Atrial fibrillation (ICD–9–CM 427.31)

- -

BENEFITS:
Coverage effective date: From 02/01/XX To 01/31/XX   Maximum benefit or benefit limitation: $1,000,000 lifetime
Pre-existing exclusions: Lupus erythematosus   Second opinion requirements: Yes_____ No X
Major medical   Yes X No_____   Precertification/Preauthorization Yes X No_____
Deductable   Yes_____ No X Amount $_____   Reference # 432786
  Per family: Yes_____ No X Amount $_____   Authorized by: Lucille Vasquez
  Deductible paid to date: Amount $_____
Out of pocket expense limit: Amount $_____
                                  Per:_____

- -

COVERAGE: COVERAGE DETAILS AND LIMITS
  Procedures/Services
    Office visits   YES X   NO _____   Physical exam; one per year
    Consultations   YES X   NO _____   _____
    ER visits   YES X   NO _____   _____
    X-ray   YES X   NO _____   _____
    Laboratory   YES X   NO _____   Need authorization
    Office surgery   YES X   NO _____   Need authorization
    Hospital surgery   YES X   NO _____   _____
    Anesthesia   YES X   NO   Need authorization
  DME   _____
    Physician payment schedule: RVS_____ RBRVS_____ UCR_____ Other X

- -

  Payment sent to: Provider X Patient _____ Time limit after submission? 30 days
  Verification by: Karen Reynolds   Date: 07-14-XX

FIGURE 3–4 Insurance predetermination form. This form can be sent to the insurance company to find out the maximum dollar amount that will be paid for primary surgery, consulting services, postoperative care, and so on.

to patients who do not receive them for this same purpose. Medicare beneficiaries are eligible to enroll in a similar tax-advantaged savings account, which may be referred to as a *Medicare medical savings account.*

Health Savings Accounts

The Medicare reform act was signed into law in December 2003, giving Americans a tool for defraying medical costs called *health savings accounts* (HSAs). HSAs are open to anyone younger than 65 years of age who enrolls in a high-deductible (e.g., more than $1000/individual or $2000/family) health plan (HDHP). Annual out-of-pocket expenses (deductibles and copays) apply and may not exceed $5150 for self-only coverage ($10,200 for family coverage). Employers pay the monthly premiums. Employees pay the deductibles when they receive health care treatment and may share some of the costs of the

COLLEGE CLINIC
4567 Broad Avenue
Woodland Hills, XY 12345-0000

Phone: 555/486-9002   Fax: 555/487-8976

Current date

Patient's name
Address
City, State, ZIP code

Dear

This letter gives you an estimate of the fees for your proposed surgery. Verification of coverage and benefit information has been obtained from your insurance company. Listed are your benefits for the proposed surgical expenses and the estimated balance after your insurance carrier pays.

Surgical procedure   Craniotomy
Date of surgery   February 21, 20XX
Name of hospital   College Hospital
Hospital address   4500 Broad Ave., Woodland Hills, XY 12345

		Insurance pays	Estimated balance
Surgeon's fee	2548.09	1344.24	1203.85
Preoperative visit			
Preoperative tests			

You have a policy deductible of $1000   which____ has ✓ has not been met.

The surgery requires the use of an anesthesiologist, assistant surgeon, and a pathologist. These physicians will bill you separately for their services. The hospital will also bill you separately.

This office will file your insurance claim for the surgical procedure, so the insurance payment should come directly to us. If the insurance carrier sends you the payment, then you are responsible to get the payment to this office within five days. Your balance after surgery should be approximately $1203.85. You are responsible for any remaining balance after our office receives the insurance payment.

Thank you for choosing our medical practice. If you have any questions, please call me.

Sincerely,

Karen Martinez, CMA
Administrative Medical Assistant

FIGURE 3–5   Sample letter to a patient supplying an estimate of the fees for proposed surgery.

plan via payroll deductions. These accounts are a tax-favored savings plan in which a working person can deposit money in an HSA and deduct the amount of the deposits from taxable income. Withdrawals from HSAs are tax-free when used for qualifying medical expenses. Money left unspent in an HSA may be rolled over year after year.

An alternative plan is a *Health Reimbursement Account* (HRA), which has a high deductible and may be better than an HSA for a chronically ill person (e.g., a person with diabetes). However, only employers can contribute to the account and workers do not put their own funds in them. Employers may keep the money if a worker quits.

Individual Contract

Any insurance plan issued to an individual (and dependents) is called an *individual contract*. Usually, this type of policy has a higher premium, and often the benefits are less than those obtainable under a group health insurance plan. Sometimes this is called **personal insurance.**

Prepaid Health Plan

This is a program of health care in which a specified set of health benefits is provided for a subscriber or enrolled group of subscribers who pay a yearly fee or fixed periodic payments. Providers of services are paid by capitation. **Capitation** is a system of payment used by managed care plans in which physicians and hospitals are paid a fixed, per capita amount for each patient enrolled over a stated period of time, regardless of the type and number of services provided. For additional information on this topic, refer to Chapter 11.

TYPES OF HEALTH INSURANCE COVERAGE

Many forms of health insurance coverage are currently in effect in the United States. These are referred to as third-party payers (private insurance, government plans, managed care contracts, and workers' compensation). A brief explanation of the programs to be discussed in this text is given here but, for an in-depth study, refer to the appropriate chapters that follow.

CHAMPVA: The **Civilian Health and Medical Program of the Department of Veterans Affairs** is administered by the Department of Veterans Affairs. This federal program shares the medical bills of spouses and children of veterans with total, permanent, service-connected disabilities or of the surviving spouses and children of veterans who died as a result of service-connected disabilities (see Chapter 14).

Competitive Medical Plan: A **competitive medical plan (CMP)** is a type of managed care organization created by the 1982 Tax Equity and Fiscal Responsibility Act (TEFRA). This federal legislation allows for enrollment of Medicare beneficiaries into managed care plans (see Chapter 12).

Disability Income Insurance: **Disability income insurance** is a form of health insurance that provides periodic payments to replace income when the insured is unable to work as a result of illness, injury, or disease (see Chapter 16). This type of insurance should not be confused with workers' compensation, because those injuries must be work related.

Exclusive Provider Organization: An **exclusive provider organization (EPO)** is a type of managed health care plan in which subscriber members are eligible for benefits only when they use the services of a limited network of providers. EPOs combine features of both HMOs and PPOs. Employers agree not to enter into an agreement with any other plan for coverage of eligible employees. EPOs are regulated under state health insurance laws (see Chapter 11).

Foundation for Medical Care: A **foundation for medical care (FMC)** is an organization of physicians, sponsored by a state or local medical association, concerned with the development and delivery of medical services and the cost of health care (see Chapter 11).

Health Maintenance Organization: A **health maintenance organization (HMO)** is an organization that provides a wide range of comprehensive health care services for a specified group at a fixed periodic payment. The emphasis is on preventive care. Physicians are reimbursed by capitation. An HMO can be sponsored by the government, medical schools, hospitals, employers, labor unions, consumer groups, insurance companies, or hospital medical plans (see Chapter 11).

Independent or Individual Practice Association: An **independent** or **individual practice association (IPA)** is a type of managed care plan in which a program administrator contracts with a number of physicians who agree to provide treatment to subscribers in their own offices or clinics for a fixed capitation payment per month. Subscribers to IPA plans have limited or no choice of physician. IPA physicians continue to see their fee-for-service patients (see Chapter 11).

Maternal and Child Health Program: A **Maternal and Child Health Program (MCHP)** is a state and federal program for children who are younger than 21 years of age and have special health care needs. It assists parents with financial planning and may assume part or all of the costs of treatment, depending on the child's condition and the family's resources (see Chapter 13).

Medicaid: **Medicaid (MCD)** is a program sponsored jointly by federal, state, and local governments to provide health care benefits to medically indigent persons on welfare (public assistance), aged individuals who meet certain financial requirements, and the disabled. Some states have expanded coverage for other medically needy individuals who meet special state-determined criteria. Coverage and benefits vary widely from state to state. In California, this program is known as *Medi-Cal* (see Chapter 13 and Appendix B).

Medicare: **Medicare (M)** is a national four-part program. It consists of a hospital insurance system (Part A), supplementary medical insurance (Part B), Medicare Plus Choice Program (Part C), and the Medicare Prescription Drug benefits (Part D). It is for those at 65 years of age. It was created by the 1965 Amendments to the Social Security Act and is operated under the provisions of the act. Benefits are also extended to certain disabled people (e.g., totally disabled or blind) and coverage and payment are provided for those requiring kidney dialysis and kidney transplant services (see Chapters 12 and 13).

Medicare/Medicaid: **Medicare/Medicaid (Medi-Medi)** is a program that covers those persons eligible for both Medicare and Medicaid (see Chapters 12 and 13).

Point-of-Service Plan: A **point-of-service (POS) plan** is a managed care plan consisting of a network of physicians and hospitals that provides an insurance company or employer with discounts on its services. Patients can refer themselves to a specialist or see a nonprogram provider for a higher copayment (see Chapter 11).

Preferred Provider Organization: A variation of a managed care plan is a **preferred provider organization (PPO).** This is a form of contract medicine by which a large employer (e.g., hospitals or physicians) or any organization that can produce a large number of patients (e.g., union trusts or insurance companies) contracts with a hospital or a group of physicians to offer medical care at a reduced rate (see Chapter 11).

TRICARE: A government-sponsored program called **TRICARE** provides military and nonmilitary hospital and medical services for spouses of active service personnel, dependents of active service personnel, retired service personnel and their dependents, and dependents of members who died on active duty. Active duty service members (ADSMs) are not eligible for TRICARE, but have benefits like TRICARE Prime in which the Department of Defense (DoD) covers all allowable charges for medically necessary care (see Chapter 14).

Unemployment Compensation Disability: Unemployment Compensation Disability (UCD) or State Disability Insurance (SDI) is insurance that covers off-the-job injury or sickness and is paid for by deductions from a person's paycheck. This program is administered by a state agency in only six states (see Chapter 16).

 Veterans Affairs Outpatient Clinic: Veterans Affairs (VA) outpatient clinic is where medical and dental services are rendered to a veteran who has a service-related disability (see Chapter 14).

 Workers' Compensation Insurance: Workers' compensation (WC) insurance is a contract that insures a person against on-the-job injury or illness. The employer pays the premium for his or her employees (see Chapter 15).

EXAMPLES OF INSURANCE BILLING

Sometimes, it is difficult to comprehend the full scale of insurance billing. As an example of total medical billing, six cases are presented to help you understand the entire billing picture from simple to complex.

CASE 1: A new patient comes in with complaints of a sore throat and an infected nail. Evaluation and management (E/M) services are discussed in detail in Chapter 6.

The physician's office bills for:

Evaluation and management services
Penicillin injection
Office surgery for infected nail
Sterile surgical tray (may or may not be billed depending on insurance carrier)

CASE 2: A patient comes in because of an accident and has complaints that require evaluation and management services, x-ray films, and laboratory studies (urinalysis) performed in the physician's office.

The physician's office bills for:

Evaluation and management services
X-ray studies (including interpretation) and laboratory tests (urinalysis; including interpretation)

CASE 3: A patient is seen by the family physician after office hours in the hospital emergency department.

The physician's office bills for evaluation and management services.

The hospital bills for hospital (outpatient) emergency department services (use and supplies).

CASE 4: A physician sends a patient's Papanicolaou smear to a private clinical laboratory.

The physician's office bills for:

Evaluation and management services.
Handling of specimen.
The laboratory bills for the Papanicolaou smear.

CASE 5: A patient is sent to a local hospital for an upper gastrointestinal radiographic series. An x-ray technician obtains the films in the hospital, and a privately owned radiologic group does the interpretation.

The hospital bills for the technical component of the upper gastrointestinal x-ray series (use of equipment).

The radiologic group bills for the professional component of the upper gastrointestinal x-ray series (the interpretation).

CASE 6: A patient is seen in the office and is immediately hospitalized for surgery.

The physician's office bills for initial hospital admission (evaluation and management services) and surgical procedure (e.g., hysterectomy). (The physician is a surgeon.)

The assistant surgeon bills for assisting the surgeon during hysterectomy. (Some insurance carriers do not allow payment.)

The anesthesiologist bills for anesthesia administered during hysterectomy.

The hospital (inpatient) bills for hospital room, operating room, anesthesia supplies, medications, x-ray films, laboratory tests, and medical and surgical supplies (dressings, intravenous lines). The hospital (inpatient) might also bill for blood for transfusions, electrocardiogram, radiation therapy, and respiratory therapy.

A medical assistant or insurance billing specialist in the offices of the attending physician, assistant surgeon, anesthesiologist, radiologic group, and private clinical laboratory submits an itemized statement and/or insurance claim form for reimbursement from the insurance payer or gives the patient the necessary information to submit his or her own claim to the insurance company. EXCEPTION: Medicare patients by federal law may not submit their own claims for physician or hospital services. Exceptions are mentioned in Chapter 12.

In the hospital and hospital emergency department, a member of the hospital staff inputs services into a central computer system that produces an itemized statement and completed insurance claim form via computer to be submitted to the insurance carrier. Hospital billing is explained in Chapter 17.

KEEPING UP TO DATE

- Make a folder or binder of pertinent insurance information. Obtain information booklets and policy manuals from the local offices of the various insurance companies. Obtain sample copies of all the forms required for the insurance plans most used in your physician's office. Keep samples of completed claim forms.
- Changes occur daily and monthly so keep well informed by reading your Medicaid, Medicare, TRICARE, and local medical society bulletins. Maintain a chronologic file on each of these bulletins for easy reference, always keeping the latest bulletin on top.
- Attend any workshops offered in your area on insurance in the medical practice. Network with other insurance specialists to compare policies and discuss common problems. The American Association of Medical Assistants has chapters in many states that feature educational workshops and lectures.
- Become a member of the American Academy of Professional Coders (AAPC), American Association of Medical Billers (AAMB), Medical Association of Billers (MAB), Medical Group Management Association (MGMA), Healthcare Financial Management Association (HFMA), Healthcare Billing and Management Association (HBMA), Professional Association of Health Care Office Management (PAHCOM), and/or American Health Information Management Association (AHIMA). Each of these associations distributes journals or newsletters on a monthly basis featuring current information.
- Make good use of the Internet!

For addresses of the professional associations mentioned in this chapter, refer to Chapter 18, Table 18.1.

PROCEDURE

HANDLING AND PROCESSING INSURANCE CLAIMS

Most offices today are computerized and use practice management software (PMS) for scheduling, **accounts receivable management** (coding and billing) and patient statements, electronic health records, and other administrative functions such as generating patient reminders and letters. However, there are smaller offices that thrive in the paper environment and will continue to do so.

A computerized office may still generate paper insurance claim forms and send to the insurance payer; however, this chapter differentiates health care practices that have computerized operations *OR* are simply using paper ledgers and generating paper-only claims and do not use the computer for any administrative practice management functions.

To help you better understand the differences in methodologies used by paper-based offices versus the computerized office, use the icons as a guide.

Different methods exist for processing insurance claims for the health care practice. The most common ones follow:

1. Posting charges and submitting to the insurance payer on the legacy paper CMS (formerly HCFA) 1500 claim form. This form has been used in the industry since 1975. The CMS 1500 can be prepared manually by filling in the claim information with a pen or be generated by the computer.
2. Electronic claims filing from in-office computers.
3. Contracting with an outside billing service company to prepare and submit claims on behalf of the health care provider's office. Generally, these are filed electronically.
4. Direct data entry (DDE) into the payer's system. The billing specialist logs into the insurance company's system and keys in the data required to process the claim.

Keep in mind that HIPAA regulations will determine whether or not a health care provider is a covered entity and whether or not it is required to submit claims electronically.

In the use of any of these methods, the basic steps (Figure 3–6) in handling and processing insurance claims are as follows:

1. Preregistration—Patient Registration Information Form:
Some medical practices either preregister a new patient

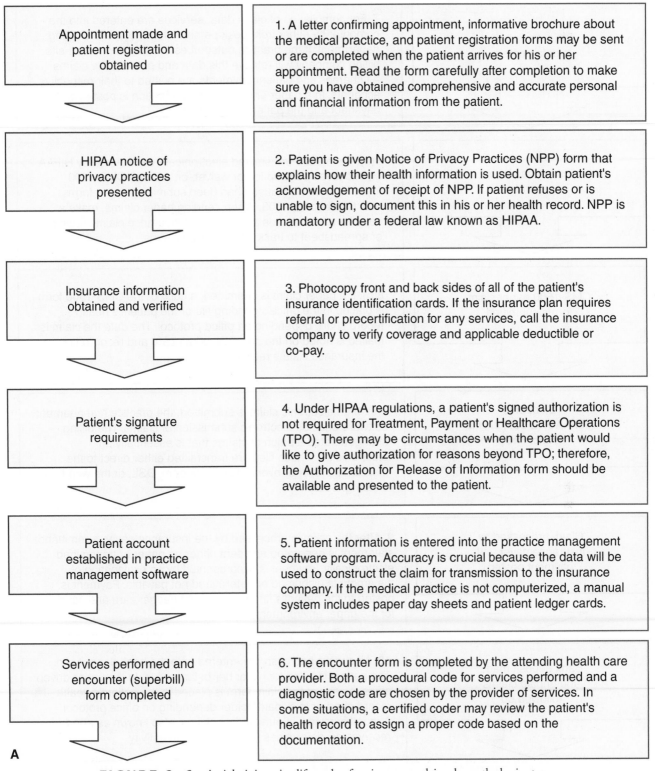

FIGURE 3–6 **A,** Administrative life cycle of an insurance claim shows the basic steps in processing of an insurance claim in a physician's office, to the insurance carrier, and after payment is received.

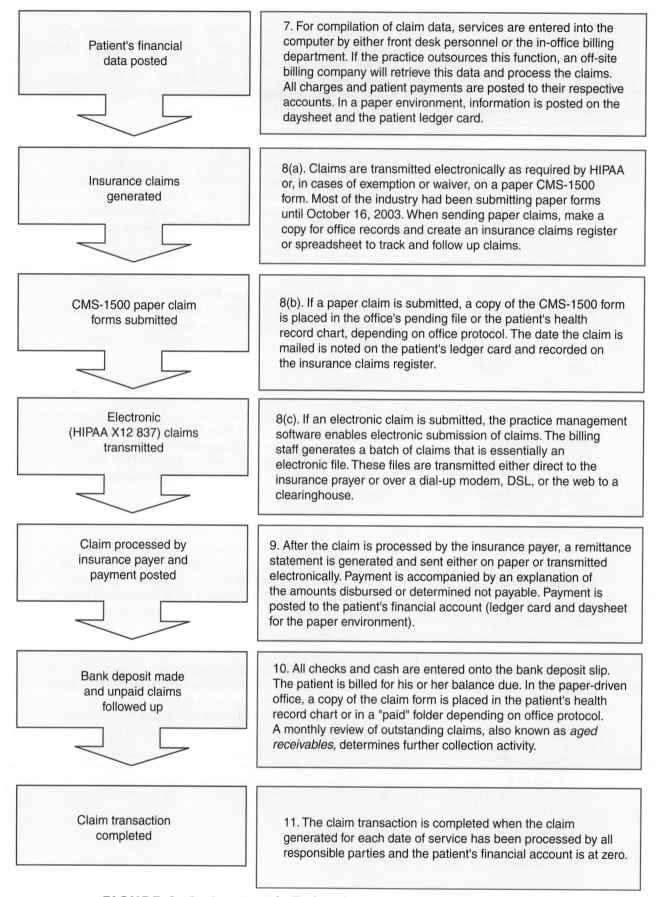

Patient's financial data posted	7. For compilation of claim data, services are entered into the computer by either front desk personnel or the in-office billing department. If the practice outsources this function, an off-site billing company will retrieve this data and process the claims. All charges and patient payments are posted to their respective accounts. In a paper environment, information is posted on the daysheet and the patient ledger card.
Insurance claims generated	8(a). Claims are transmitted electronically as required by HIPAA or, in cases of exemption or waiver, on a paper CMS-1500 form. Most of the industry had been submitting paper forms until October 16, 2003. When sending paper claims, make a copy for office records and create an insurance claims register or spreadsheet to track and follow up claims.
CMS-1500 paper claim forms submitted	8(b). If a paper claim is submitted, a copy of the CMS-1500 form is placed in the office's pending file or the patient's health record chart, depending on office protocol. The date the claim is mailed is noted on the patient's ledger card and recorded on the insurance claims register.
Electronic (HIPAA X12 837) claims transmitted	8(c). If an electronic claim is submitted, the practice management software enables electronic submission of claims. The billing staff generates a batch of claims that is essentially an electronic file. These files are transmitted either direct to the insurance prayer or over a dial-up modem, DSL, or the web to a clearinghouse.
Claim processed by insurance payer and payment posted	9. After the claim is processed by the insurance payer, a remittance statement is generated and sent either on paper or transmitted electronically. Payment is accompanied by an explanation of the amounts disbursed or determined not payable. Payment is posted to the patient's financial account (ledger card and daysheet for the paper environment).
Bank deposit made and unpaid claims followed up	10. All checks and cash are entered onto the bank deposit slip. The patient is billed for his or her balance due. In the paper-driven office, a copy of the claim form is placed in the patient's health record chart or in a "paid" folder depending on office protocol. A monthly review of outstanding claims, also known as *aged receivables,* determines further collection activity.
Claim transaction completed	11. The claim transaction is completed when the claim generated for each date of service has been processed by all responsible parties and the patient's financial account is at zero.

FIGURE 3–6, A, cont'd For legend see p. 69.

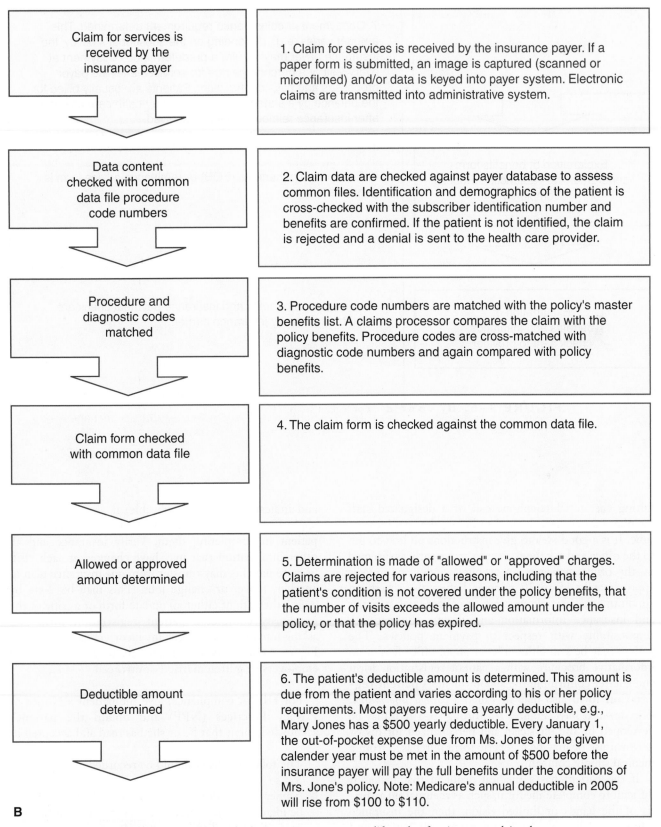

Claim for services is received by the insurance payer

1. Claim for services is received by the insurance payer. If a paper form is submitted, an image is captured (scanned or microfilmed) and/or data is keyed into payer system. Electronic claims are transmitted into administrative system.

Data content checked with common data file procedure code numbers

2. Claim data are checked against payer database to assess common files. Identification and demographics of the patient is cross-checked with the subscriber identification number and benefits are confirmed. If the patient is not identified, the claim is rejected and a denial is sent to the health care provider.

Procedure and diagnostic codes matched

3. Procedure code numbers are matched with the policy's master benefits list. A claims processor compares the claim with the policy benefits. Procedure codes are cross-matched with diagnostic code numbers and again compared with policy benefits.

Claim form checked with common data file

4. The claim form is checked against the common data file.

Allowed or approved amount determined

5. Determination is made of "allowed" or "approved" charges. Claims are rejected for various reasons, including that the patient's condition is not covered under the policy benefits, that the number of visits exceeds the allowed amount under the policy, or that the policy has expired.

Deductible amount determined

6. The patient's deductible amount is determined. This amount is due from the patient and varies according to his or her policy requirements. Most payers require a yearly deductible, e.g., Mary Jones has a $500 yearly deductible. Every January 1, the out-of-pocket expense due from Ms. Jones for the given calender year must be met in the amount of $500 before the insurance payer will pay the full benefits under the conditions of Mrs. Jone's policy. Note: Medicare's annual deductible in 2005 will rise from $100 to $110.

B

FIGURE 3–6 **B,** Adjudication: Insurance payer life cycle of an insurance claim shows the basic steps of an insurance carrier to pay an insurance claim and the documents generated.

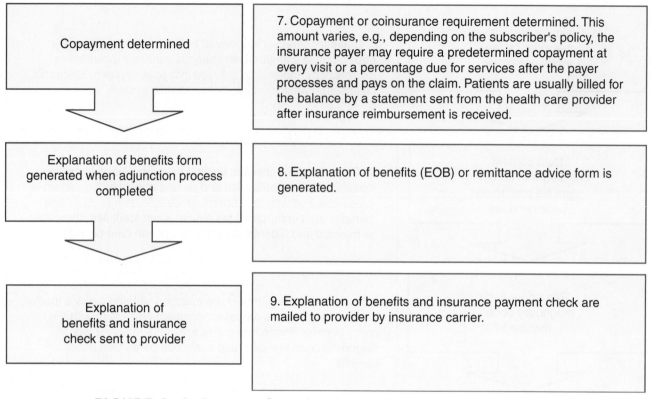

FIGURE 3–6, B, cont'd   For legend see p. 71.

during the initial telephone call or a designated staff member may contact the patient before the appointment time. It is a good idea to give instructions on how to get to the office and ask the patient to arrive early as directed by the office manager. An average window of time is approximately 15 to 20 minutes before the scheduled appointment. This allows time to collect vital statistics and insurance information and discuss the patient's responsibility with respect to payment policies. The patient may be sent either a letter about office fees or an informative brochure with a patient registration form and a letter confirming the appointment. A **patient registration form** also may be called a *patient information form* or *intake sheet* (Figures 3–7 through 3–10). It may be developed by the physician and personalized for his or her own use or may be a generic form purchased from a medical supply company.

If the patient has a medical problem that makes it difficult to complete the form, such as rheumatoid arthritis of the hands or limited vision, then the insurance billing specialist may have to interview the patient and fill in the necessary data. Obtain *complete* information on a new patient by using a form that contains information pertinent to credit and collections. This information must be *accurate*. Instruct the patient to fill in all spaces and indicate N/A (not applicable) if an item does not apply. If the form is returned with blank spaces, assist the patient in completing them. Verify insurance and all other information that may have changed at each visit, because patients may transfer from one insurance plan to another, move, or change jobs. This may be done by giving the patient either an update form or a copy of the previously completed patient registration form and asking him or her to correct any incorrect data in red (see Figure 3–10). Established patients may have changed employers or gotten married or divorced.

For HIPAA compliance, give the patient a Notice of Privacy Practices (NPP) and obtain the patient's acknowledgment that he or she has read and accepted it.

The following facts should be recorded:

● Name: first, middle initial, and last. The name should be identical to the one on the insurance identification card. (Some pediatric patients do not have the same last name as their parents or stepparents.) An insurance check usually is received with the policyholder's name, and it is time-consuming to find and give credit to the patient's account.

Insurance cards copied ☒
Date: Jan. 20, 20XX

Patient Registration Information

Account #: 84516
Insurance #: H-550-64-5172-02
Co-Payment : $OV $10 ER $50

Please PRINT AND complete ALL sections below!

Is your condition the result of a work injury? YES (NO) An auto accident? YES (NO)
Date of injury: _____

PATIENT'S PERSONAL INFORMATION
Marital status ☐ Single ☒ Married ☐ Divorced ☐ Widowed
Sex: ☐ Male ☒ Female
Name: FUHR (last name) LINDA (first name) L. (initial)
Street Address: 3070 Tipper Street (Apt # 4) City: Oxnard State: CA Zip: 93030
Home phone:(555)276-0101 Work phone:(555)372-1151 Social Security # 550-XX-5172
Date of Birth: 11/05/65 Driver's License: (State & Number) G0075012
Employer/Name of School Electronic Data Systems ☒ Full Time ☐ Part Time
Spouse's Name: FUHR (last name) GERALD T. (first name) (initial) Spouse's Work phone:(555) 921-0075
How do you wish to be addressed? LINDA Social Security # 545-XX-2771

PATIENT'S/ RESPONSIBLE PARTY INFORMATION
Responsible party: GERALD T. FUHR Date of Birth: 06-15-64
Relationship to patient: ☐ Self ☒ Spouse ☐ Other Social Security # 545-XX-2771
Responsible party's home phone:(555) 276-0101 Work phone:(555)921-0075
Address: 3070 Tipper Street (Apt # 4) City: Oxnard State: CA Zip: 93030
Employer's Name: General Electric Phone number:(555) 485-0121
Address: 317 East Main City: Oxnard State: CA Zip: 93030
Your occupation: Technician
Spouse's Employer's Name: Electronic Data Systems Spouse's Work phone:(555)372-1151
Address: 2700 West 5th Street City: Oxnard State: CA Zip: 93030

PATIENT'S INSURANCE INFORMATION
Please present insurance cards to receptionist.
PRIMARY insurance company's name: ABC Insurance Company
Insurance address: P.O. Box 12340 City: Fresno State: CA Zip: 93765
Name of insured: Linda L. Fuhr Date of Birth:11/05/65 Relationship to insured: ☒ Self ☐ Spouse ☐ Other ☐ Child
Insurance ID number: H-550-XX-5172-02 Group number: 17098-020-00004
SECONDARY insurance company's name: None
Insurance address: _____ City: _____ State: ____ Zip: _____
Name of insured: _____ Date of Birth: ____ Relationship to insured: ☐ Self ☐ Spouse ☐ Other ☐ Child
Insurance ID number: _____ Group number: _____
Check if appropriate: ☐ Medigap policy ☐ Retiree coverage

PATIENT'S REFERRAL INFORMATION
(Please circle one)
Referred by: Margaret Taylor (Mrs. W. T.) If referred by a friend, may we thank her or him? (Yes) No
Name(s) of other physician(s) who care for you: Jason Smythe, MD

EMERGENCY CONTACT
Name of person not living with you:Hannah Gildea Relationship: Aunt
Address: 4621 Lucretia Avenue City: Oxnard State: CA Zip: 93030
Phone number (home):(555) 274-0132 Phone number (work):(___)_____

Assignment of Benefits • Financial Agreement

I hereby give lifetime authorization for payment of insurance benefits be made directly to Gerald Practon, MD, and any assisting physicians, for services rendered. I understand that I am financially responsible for all charges whether or not they are covered by insurance. In the event of default, I agree to pay all costs of collection, and reasonable attorney's fees. I hereby authorize this healthcare provider to release all information necessary to secure the payment of benefits.
I further agree that a photocopy of this agreement shall be as valid as the original.
Date: Jan 20, 20XX Your signature: *Linda L Fuhr*
Method of payment: ☐ Cash ☒ Check ☐ Credit Card

FIGURE 3–7 Patient registration information form showing a comprehensive listing of personal and financial information obtained from the patient on his or her first visit to the office. (*Courtesy Bibbero Systems, Inc., Petaluma, Calif. Telephone: 800-242-2376; fax: 800-242-9330; Web site: **www.bibbero.com**.*)

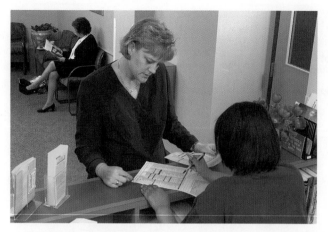

FIGURE 3-8 Receptionist giving instructions to a patient on how to complete the patient registration form.

PATIENT INFORMATION UPDATE

Welcome, we are delighted to see you again!
Please take a few minutes to help us update our records.

Name ___Linda_____L._____Fuhr_____   Today's Date __6-30-XX__
          FIRST   MIDDLE   LAST

1. Has your name changed since your last visit here? ____Yes __X__No
   If yes, what was your old name? __N/A_____
   What name do you use for health insurance if different from above?_N/A_____

2. If you have a new or different address since your initial visit here, please
   indicate below:
   _____2201 West Klein Street_____
   _____Oxnard, CA 93033_____

3. Has your marital status changed? ____Yes __X__No

4. Has your telephone number changed?_X_Yes
   Please indicate your correct telephone number   __555-401-7600_____

5. Has your employment changed? ____Yes _X_ No
   Please indicate your new employer name and address:
   _____N/A_____
   _____
   _____

   New employer telephone #:_____ —— _____

6. Have you changed health insurance companies? ____Yes __X_No
   If yes, please indicate your new health insurance carrier and address.
   Primary _____N/A_____   Secondary _____N/A_____
   _____   _____

   Group Nos. _____   Group Nos. _____
   Subscriber Nos. _____   Subscriber nos. _____

7. Who is responsible for this bill? _Gerald T. Fuhr_____

8. Please note any change in your health since your last visit?
   Illness   _____
   Accident   _____
   Allergies   _____
   Medications being taken _Thyroid_____

   Other   _____
   _____
   _____

9. Signature   _Linda L Fuhr_____

PATIENT INFORMATION UPDATE

FIGURE 3-9 Patient information update form showing questions to ask the patient for updating a previous patient registration information form. *(Courtesy Professional Filing Systems, Inc., Atlanta, Ga.)*

✔ Create and maintain patients' permanent medical records.

✔ Order, review/interpret, document/file, and telephone laboratory test results to the patient.

✔ Order x-rays, review/interpret, compare with previous studies if abnormal, consult with radiologist, document/file, and telephone results to the patient.

✔ Write and send consultation reports/letters to referring or consulting physicians and other providers.

✔ Write letters of referral to specialists.

✔ Create patient education materials.

✔ Conduct medical research pertinent to the patient's case.

✔ Write prescriptions and communicate with pharmacies about patients' prescriptions.

✔ Transmit (or complete) patients' insurance claim forms and complete insurance application forms.

✔ Conduct utilization review negotiations with hospitals and insurance companies.

✔ Review and maintain documentation for patients' hospital medical records.

✔ Write medical orders for hospitalized patients and orders for those in nursing facilities.

✔ Write letters to obtain medical services, instruments, or equipment for patients.

✔ Arrange for hospital admissions and follow-up consultations with nurses and other physicians.

FIGURE 3–10 Details of additional time the provider and staff provide to patients during an office visit or depending on the complexity of a medical problem.

- Practice management systems allow a cross reference of the patient, subscriber, and guarantor's names as well as Social Security number so that when you recall the policyholder's name, the patient's name also appears.
- In a paper or manual system, keep an alphabetic card index of parental or billing names that also lists each patient's name.

● Street address, including apartment number, ZIP code, and telephone number with area code.

● Business address, telephone number with extension, and occupation.

● Date of birth (HIPAA requires eight digits, e.g., January 2, 1936, to be submitted to payers in the format 19360102 [year/month/day]). Your practice management system may collect this data in a different format, but transmit in the required eight-digit format.

● Person responsible for account (guarantor) or insured's name.

● Social Security number.

● Spouse's name and occupation.

● Referring physician's name or other referral source.

● Driver's license number.

● Emergency contact (close relative or friend with name, address, and telephone number).

● Insurance billing information: All insurance company names, addresses, and policy and group numbers. This is important because of the coordination of benefits clause written into some health insurance policies. Elderly patients are given the option of joining managed care programs and are allowed to switch every 30 days. Always ask each elderly patient whether he or she is covered by traditional Medicare or a Medicare HMO. A good patient information sheet has space where this information can be written in by the patient.

2. Insurance Identification Card: Always copy front and back sides of the patient's insurance card and date the photocopy (Figure 3–11). Sometimes the reverse side of the card provides information, such as deductible, copayment, preapproval provisions, and insurance company address and telephone number. A copy produces error-free insurance data and can be used in lieu of completing the insurance section of the patient registration form. On a return visit, ask to see the card and check it with the data on file (Figure 3–12). If it differs, photocopy both sides and write the date on the copy, using this as the base for revising data on file.

3. Patient's Signature Requirements

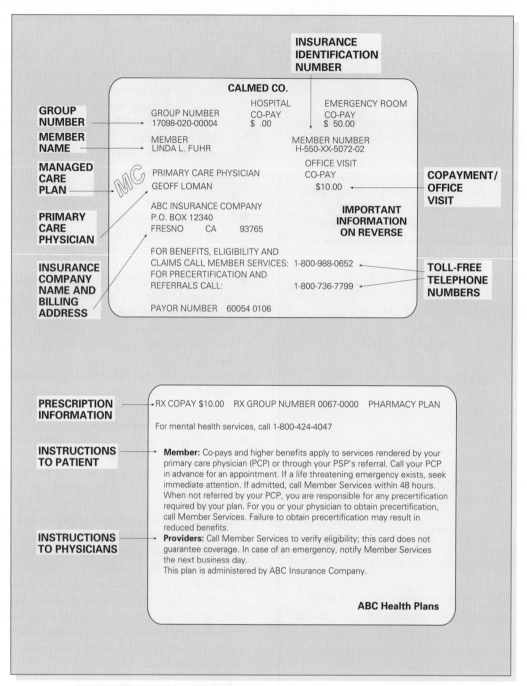

INSURANCE IDENTIFICATION NUMBER

CALMED CO.

GROUP NUMBER
17098-020-00004

HOSPITAL CO-PAY
$ .00

EMERGENCY ROOM CO-PAY
$ 50.00

MEMBER
LINDA L. FUHR

MEMBER NUMBER
H-550-XX-5072-02

PRIMARY CARE PHYSICIAN
GEOFF LOMAN

OFFICE VISIT CO-PAY
$10.00

ABC INSURANCE COMPANY
P.O. BOX 12340
FRESNO   CA   93765

IMPORTANT INFORMATION ON REVERSE

FOR BENEFITS, ELIGIBILITY AND
CLAIMS CALL MEMBER SERVICES: 1-800-988-0652
FOR PRECERTIFICATION AND
REFERRALS CALL: 1-800-736-7799

PAYOR NUMBER   60054 0106

MC

GROUP NUMBER

MEMBER NAME

MANAGED CARE PLAN

PRIMARY CARE PHYSICIAN

INSURANCE COMPANY NAME AND BILLING ADDRESS

COPAYMENT/ OFFICE VISIT

TOLL-FREE TELEPHONE NUMBERS

RX COPAY $10.00   RX GROUP NUMBER 0067-0000   PHARMACY PLAN

For mental health services, call 1-800-424-4047

Member: Co-pays and higher benefits apply to services rendered by your primary care physician (PCP) or through your PSP's referral. Call your PCP in advance for an appointment. If a life threatening emergency exists, seek immediate attention. If admitted, call Member Services within 48 hours. When not referred by your PCP, you are responsible for any precertification required by your plan. For you or your physician to obtain precertification, call Member Services. Failure to obtain precertification may result in reduced benefits.

Providers: Call Member Services to verify eligibility; this card does not guarantee coverage. In case of an emergency, notify Member Services the next business day.
This plan is administered by ABC Insurance Company.

ABC Health Plans

PRESCRIPTION INFORMATION

INSTRUCTIONS TO PATIENT

INSTRUCTIONS TO PHYSICIANS

FIGURE 3–11   Front *(top)* and back *(bottom)* sides of an insurance card.

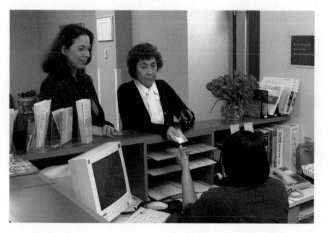

FIGURE 3–12   Patient presenting an insurance identification card to the receptionist for photocopying.

RELEASE OF INFORMATION

If the physician is submitting an insurance claim for the patient, the patient is not required to sign a release of information form before information can be given to an insurance company for obtaining payment for professional services (Figure 3–13). However, some medical practices prefer to operate at a higher level of privacy and continue to obtain patients' signatures on release of information forms.

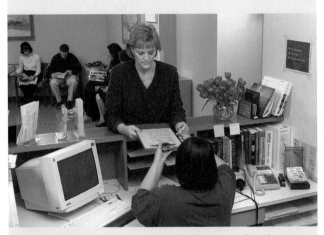

FIGURE 3–13   Insurance billing specialist obtaining the patient's signature on a release of information form.

ASSIGNMENT OF BENEFITS

For the health care provider to receive reimbursement direct from the insurance payer, the patient must sign an assignment of benefits statement for each insurance company. However, before explaining an assignment, it is important to define the difference between participating and nonparticipating providers. A **participating provider (par)** has a contractual agreement with an insurance plan to render care to eligible beneficiaries and bills the insurance carrier directly. The insurance carrier pays its portion of the allowed amount, and the provider bills the patient for the balance not paid by the insurer after the disallowed portion is adjusted off of the account. However, in Blue Plans, the provider is referred to as a *member physician* and may accept the payment as *payment in full* or may bill the patient for any unpaid balance, depending on the contract. Managed care plans also refer to participating providers as member physicians. If the amount of the patient's responsibility can be determined, collect it at the time of the visit. A **nonparticipating provider (nonpar)** is a physician without a contractual agreement with an insurance plan to accept an allowed amount and to render care to eligible beneficiaries. The provider may or may not file an insurance claim as a courtesy to the patient and may obtain full payment at the time of service. The patient should be made aware that his or her insurance plan will cover a considerable amount less on the claim when receiving services from a nonpar provider.

The general definition of **assignment** is the transfer, after an event insured against, of an individual's legal right to collect an amount payable under an insurance contract. Most of the time an agreement is obtained by having the patient sign an assignment of insurance benefits document directing payment to the physician. However, the paper CMS-1500 claim form contains a provision that, when signed by the insured, directs the insurance company to pay benefits directly to the provider of care on whose charge the claim is based. An assignment of benefits becomes a legally enforceable document but must refer to specific hospitalization, course of treatment, or office visits. Each course of treatment needs to have an assignment document executed by the patient unless an annual or lifetime signature authorization is accepted and in the patient's financial file, except when automobile or homeowners' liability insurance is involved.

 Private Carriers: For private insurance companies with whom the provider does not have a contractual agreement, accepting assignment means that the insurance check will be directed to the provider's office instead of to the patient. Because there is no signed agreement with the carrier, the difference between the billed amount and the carrier's allowed amount is not written off but collected from the patient as is any copayment or deductible. In private third-party liability cases, the physician needs to negotiate with the insurance company to make sure benefits are paid to him or her directly.

Managed Care: In managed care plans, a participating provider (also called a *preferred provider*) is a physician who has contracted with a plan to provide medical services to plan members. A nonparticipating provider refers to a physician who has not contracted with a managed care plan to provide medical services to plan members. The assignment is automatic for individuals who have signed with managed care contracts.

Medicaid: For Medicaid cases, there is no assignment unless the patient has other insurance in addition to Medicaid. The Medicaid fiscal intermediary pays the provider directly.

Medicare: The words participating, nonparticipating, and assignment have slightly different meanings in the Medicare program. A physician who accepts assignment on Medicare claims is called a *participating (par) physician* and may not bill, or accept payment for, the amount of the difference between the submitted charge and the Medicare allowed amount. However, an attempt must be made to collect 20% of the allowed charge (coinsurance) and any amount applied to the deductible. A physician who does not participate is called a *nonparticipating (nonpar) physician* and has an option regarding assignment. The physician may either not accept assignment for all services or exercise the option of accepting assignment for some services and collecting from the patient for other services performed at the same time and place. The physician collects the fee from the patient but may bill no more than the Medicare-limiting charge. The check is sent to the patient. When treating federal or state government employees or a Medicare recipient, the physician may lose the fee if government guidelines are not followed.

TRICARE: A provider who accepts TRICARE standard assignment (participates) agrees to accept the allowable charge as the full fee and cannot charge the patient the difference between the provider's charge and the allowable charge. The exception to this is when the provider does not accept assignment on the claim. A provider that participates or does not participate with TRICARE can submit a claim and not accept assignment on a claim-by-claim basis. In the event the provider does not accept assignment, TRICARE sends the sponsor all payments. TRICARE does not communicate with the provider if the provider has questions about the claim. It is up to the provider to bill the sponsor for payment. The provider can collect 115% of the TRICARE allowable from the patient when a CMS-1500 claim form is marked "no" in the accepting assignment block.

Workers' Compensation: There is no assignment for industrial cases. The workers' compensation carrier pays the fee for services rendered according to its fee schedule and the check automatically goes to the physician. The patient is not responsible for payment of services for any work-related injury or illness.

SIGNATURE GUIDELINES

Electronic Environment: Patient signatures cannot be submitted electronically. Use the signature-on-file (SOF) provision to satisfy Medicare's patient signature requirements. Electronic billers are permitted to obtain a lifetime authorization from the beneficiary and retain it in a file for future use on all electronic claims. This authorization allows the office to submit assigned and nonassigned claims on the beneficiary's behalf.

To use this procedure, the patient should sign a brief statement that reads as follows:

(Name of Beneficiary) (Health Insurance Claim Number)

"I request that payment of authorized Medicare benefits be made either to me or on my behalf to (name of physician or supplier) for any services furnished me by physician or supplier. I authorize any holder of medical information about me to release to the Centers for Medicare & Medicaid Services (CMS) and its agents any information needed to determine these benefits or the benefits payable for related services."

Signature Indicator: Patient signature source. Must not be blank. If invalid value is reported, a claim level rejection will occur.

Valid Values:

C = Signed CMS-1500 claim form on file
M = Signed signature authorization form for Block 13 on file
B = Signed signature authorization form for both Blocks 12 and 13 on file
P = Signature generated by provider because the patient was not physically present for service

S = Signed signature authorization form for Block 12 on file
NSF – All versions
ANSI – Versions 30.32 and 30.51
ANSI – Version 4010 (HIPAA)

Most patient registration forms include a statement to sign regarding these two authorizations (bottom of Figure 3–7).

 Paper Environment: Since the enforcement of HIPAA regulations, a patient's signature for the release of information in Block 12 is no longer required. The signature requirement for the assignment of benefits is included in Block 13 of the CMS-1500 insurance claim form (Figure 3-14). If a signature is obtained on a separate form, it may be filed in the patient's health record and the abbreviation "SOF" or spelled-out notation "signature on file" may be used on the insurance claim form.

For a patient on a federal program such as Medicare or TRICARE (see Chapters 12 and 14), acceptance of assignment means not only that the check will come to the physician but also that the physician will accept what the federal program designates as the "allowed amount." The federal program pays a percentage of the allowed amount, and the patient pays a remaining coinsurance (cost-sharing) percentage.

4. Encounter Form: An **encounter form** (also called a *charge slip, multipurpose billing form, patient service slip, routing form, superbill,* or *transaction slip*) is attached to the patient's health record during the visit (Figure 3–15). This contains the patient's name, the date, and, in some instances, the previous balance due. It also contains the procedural and diagnostic codes and the date the patient should return for an appointment. This two- or three-part form is a combination bill, insurance form, and routing document used in both computer and paper-based systems. This also can be a computerized multipurpose billing form that may be scanned to input charges and diagnoses into the patient's computerized account. Time is saved and fewer errors occur because no keystrokes are involved. Medical practices use the encounter form as a communications tool (routing sheet) and as an invoice to the patient. When used as a routing sheet, it becomes a source document for insurance claim data. The encounter form's procedure and diagnostic code sections should be updated annually with correct descriptions because changes, additions, and deletions occur. Remove all codes not used or seldom used and revise and add current valid commonly used codes for the practice. Remember that codes change annually so you must update the encounter form and have different ones printed if changes affect your practice. Because there is no grace period, update

FIGURE 3–14 Section 13 from the health insurance claim form CMS-1500, illustrating authorization for assignment of benefits.

encounter forms twice a year—by October 1 for changes in diagnostic codes and by January 1 for changes in procedural codes. Some practices develop encounter forms for different services (e.g., surgical services, office services [within the facility], and out-of-office service [hospital visits, emergency, outpatient facility, nursing home, or house calls]). Examples of encounter forms are shown in Figure 8–9 and 10–7.

5. Physician's Signature: After examination and treatment, the physician or health care provider rendering services, completes the encounter form by checking off the procedure (services and treatments) codes and diagnostic codes (Figure 3–16). The physician signs the encounter form and indicates whether the patient needs another appointment.

6. Determine Fees: The patient usually carries the encounter form to the reception desk where fees are determined and input for billing (Figure 3–17). He or she is given the opportunity to pay and make a future appointment.

7. Bookkeeping—Financial Accounting Record and Accounts Receivable Management: The value of maintaining careful records of all insurance matters cannot be overemphasized. Accounts receivable (A/R) management breathes life into the practice's cash flow. Encompassed in A/R management is establishing the patient **financial accounting record** and carrying out the claims process.

 A financial account is set up in the practice management system. Data obtained from the patient registration process is keyed into the program and established a patient account. Usually, an account number is automatically assigned by the program and used for tracking and reporting.

Paper Environment: In the paper environment, a ledger card is maintained for each patient who receives professional services (Figure 3–18). An established private patient who is injured on the job requires two ledgers, one for private care and one for posting workers' compensation insurance.

Tax ID # 00-000000

COLLEGE CLINIC
4567 Broad Avenue
Woodland Hills, XY 12345-0001

TELEPHONE: 555/486-9002
FAX: 555/590-2189

1. Medical practice Identifying data

PATIENT'S LAST NAME	FIRST	INITAL	BIRTHDATE	SSN	DATE OF SERVICE
Balanadi	Margarita	S.	2/28/64	034-XX-0121	3/16/XX

2. Patient and insurance data

ADDRESS	CITY	STATE	ZIP	INSURANCE CARRIER
1459 Chestnut	Woodland Hills	XY	12345	Aetna Insurance Co.

3. Type of insurance plan

✓	DESCRIPTION	CPT/MD	FEE	✓	DESCRIPTION	CPT/MD	FEE	✓	DESCRIPTION	CPT/MD	FEE
1.	**OFFICE VISIT, NEW PATIENT**			**5.**	**PROCEDURES (Continued)**			**7.**	**SUPPLIES**		
	Minor (10 min)	99201			Destr.Vular Lession(s), Simple	56501			Cervical Cap	A4261	
	Straightforward (20 min)	99202			Diaphragm / Cervical Cap Fit.	57170			Diaphragm	99070	
✓	Low (30 min)	99203	70.92		Endocervical Curettage	57505			Fentanyl	J3010	
	Moderate (45 min)	99204			Hysterosalpingogram	58340			Flu Vaccine	90658	
	High (60 min)	99205			I & D Bartholin	56420*			IUD		
	WWX (12-17)	99384			I & D Vular or Perineal Abscess	56405*			Pareguard	J7300	
	WWX (18-39)	99385			Injection IM Abx	90788			Mirena	X1532	
	WWX (40-64)	99386			Injection IM	90782			Laminaria Tents #	99070	
	WWX (65-Over)	99387			IUD Insertion	58300*			Norplant	A4260	
2.	**OFFICE VISIT, EST PATIENT**				IUD Removal	58301			Paracervical block	64435	
	Minimal	99211			L. E. E. P.	57522			Rhogam mini dose	J2790	
	Straightforward (10 min)	99212			Normplant, Insertion	11975			full dose	J2790	
	Low (15 min)	99212			Removal	11976			Rocephin	J0696	
	Moderate (20 min)	99214			Ultrasound - Gyn	76857			Supplies	99070	
	High (40 min)	99215		**6.**	**PREGNANCY**				Surgery Tray	A4550	
	WWX (12-17)	99394			Antepartum Care Only				Vaccination		
	WWX (18-39)	99395			(4-6 visits)	59425					
	WWX (40-64)	99396			(7 or more visits)	59426					
	WWX (65-Over)	99397			Circumcision	54150					
3.	**CONSULTATION, NEW OR EST.**				D & C Preg. Rel.	59820		**8.**	**LAB**		
	Low Severity (30 mins)	99242			Delivery Only	59410			Coloscreen (Occult Blood)	82270	
	Moderate (40 min)	99243			High Risk OB Surcharge	58999*			Hemoglobin	85018	
	Moderate-High (80 min)	99244			Laminaria Insertion	59200			Preg. Test Urine	81025	
4.	**HOSPITAL VISIT**				OB Care	59400			Rh factor	86901	
	Admit	9922_			OB Care w/C-S	59510			Urinalysis	81000 81002	
	Visit	9923_			Postpartum Care Only	59430			Wet smear	87210	
5.	**PROCEDURES**				Postpartum TL w/C-S	58611			Collection & Handling	99000	
	Biopsy, Cervical (Polypectomy)	57500*			Prostin gel Insertion	59200			Venipuncture	36415	
	Endometrial	58100*			TAB UP to 10 Weeks	59840		✓	Preg Test	84702	20.00
	Vulva	56605*			10.5 to 14 Weeks	59841					
	Catheterization Urethra	53670*			14.5 to 16 Weeks	59841					
	Colposcopy	57452*			16.5 to 18 Weeks	59841					
	with Biopsy	57454*			18.5 to 20 Weeks	59841					
	Cryo, Simple				20.5 to 22 Weeks	59841					
	D & C GYN	58720*			Ultrasound OB	76815					

4. Codes and fees for professional services

DIAGNOSIS	ICD-9								
☐ Abdominal Pain	789.00	☐ Endometriosis	617.3	☐ Menorrhagia	627.0	☐ Rash	782.1	☐ Fetal Anomaly	759.9
☐ Abnormal Pap Smear	795.00	☐ Endometritis	615.9	☐ Metrorrhagia	626.6	☐ Ret. P.O.C	667.1	☐ Chromosomal Anomaly	655.1
☐ Abortion,Incomplete,Inevitable	637.9	☐ Family Planning	V25.09	☐ Neoplasm, Benign	229.9	☐ Rhogam	656.10	☐ Demise	656.43
☐ Missed	632	☐ Fatigue	780.79	☐ Neoplasm, Malignant	199.1	☐ Skin Lesion	709.9	☐ Distress	656.31
☐ Threatened	640.03	☐ Fever	780.6	☐ Normal Gyn Exam	V72.3	☐ Stress Incont	625.6	☐ Fibroid	654.11
☐ Therapeutic	635.90	☐ Galactorrhea	611.6	☐ Norplant Check, Reinsert, Remove	V25.43	☐ Tubal Occlusion	628.2	☐ Hemorrhage	614.90
☒ Amenorrhea	626.0	☐ Gastrointestine Dis	558.9	☐ Norplant Insert	V25.5	☐ Urinary Tract Infection	599.0	☐ Hyperemesis	643.00
☐ Anemia	285.9	☐ Headache	784.0	☐ Obesity	278.0	☐ Uterus, Myoma	218.9	☐ Hypertension	642._
☐ Barth Gland Abscess	616.3	☐ Hemorrhoids	455.9	☐ Oligomenorrhea	626.1	☐ Vaginal Hematoma	623.6	☐ Large for Dates	656.63
☐ Barth. Cyst	616.2	☐ Herpes, Genitalis	054.10	☐ Osteoporosis	733.00	☐ Vaginitis, Gardnella	616.10	☐ Macrosomia	653.51
☐ Breast Cystic Dis	610.1	☐ Hormone Imbalance	259.9	☐ Ovarian Cyst	620.2	☐ Monilla	112.1	☐ Placenta Previa	641.03
☐ Breast Mass	611.72	☐ Hirsutism	704.1	☐ Pelvic Mass	789.3	☐ Trich	131.01	☐ Poor Reproductive Hist	V23.4
☐ Cervical Dyaplasia	622.1	☐ Hyperlipidemia	272.4	☐ Pelvic Pain	625.9	☐ Vulvo	616.1	☐ Post Partum	V24.2
☐ Cervicitis	616.0	☐ Hypertension	401.9	☐ Pelvic Relaxation	618.8	☐ Venereal Dis. Eposure	V01.6	☐ Post Partum Mastitis	675.22
☐ Circumcision	V50.2	☐ Infertility	628.9	☐ PID	614.9	☐ Vulava, Abscess	616.4	☐ Pre-Eclampsia	642.43
☐ Condyloma	078.1	☐ Irregular Menses	626.4	☐ Polycystic Ovaries	256.4	☐ Dysplasia	623.0	☐ Previous C-section	654.2
☐ Contraception	V25.40	☐ IUD Check, Reinsert remove	V25.42	☐ Polyp Endocervix	622.7	☐ Dystrophy	624.0	☐ Previous Uterine Surgery	654.91
☐ Dysfunc, Bleeding	626.8	☐ Complication	996.32	☐ Post Menopausal Bleed	627.1	☐ LSA	701.0	☐ Prem. Rupt. Memb	658.13
☐ Dyamennorrhea	625.3	☐ Insert	V25.1	☐ Post Menopausal HRT	V07.4	☐ PREGNANCY	V22.2	☐ Preterm Labor	644.03
☐ Dyapareunia	625.0	☐ Labial Cyst	624.8	☐ Post Operative Status	V67.0	☐ Breech	652.21	☐ Small for Dates	656.5_
☐ Elective sterilization	V25.2	☐ Mastodynia	611.71	☐ PMS	625.4	☐ Disproportion	653.4	☐ Twin	651.03
		☐ Menopausal Symptoms	627.2	☐ Pruritis	698.9	☐ Ectopic	633.1		

5. Diagnostic codes

DIAGNOSIS: (IF NOT CHECKED ABOVE)

SURGICAL PROCEDURE

AUTHORIZATION REQUIRED:
Yes ☐
No ☒ #

6. Additional diagnoses

PLACE OF SERVICE: ☒ OFFICE ☐ IN-PT. ☐ OUT-PT. ☐ ER ☐ OBS

DOCTOR'S SIGNATURE
Bertha Caesar, MD

TODAY'S TOTAL FEE 90.92
AMT. RECEIVED —

FACILITY: ☐ CPMC - CA ☐ CPMC - PAC ☐ OTHER

REC'D. BY: ☐ CHECK ☐ CASH ☐ CREDIT CARD #

BALANCE 90.92

7. Total fee charged

FIGURE 3–15 Encounter form: Procedural codes for professional services are taken from the Current Procedural Terminology (CPT) book, and diagnostic codes are taken from the *International Classification of Diseases, Ninth Revision, Clinical Modification* (ICD-9-CM) book. *(Courtesy Bibbero Systems, Inc., Petaluma, Calif. Telephone: 800-242-2376; fax: 800-242-9330; Web site: **www.bibbero.com**.)*

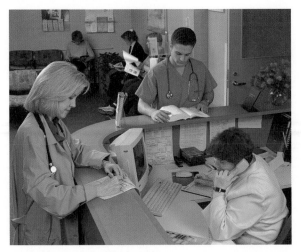

FIGURE 3–16 Physician checking off procedures on the encounter form at the conclusion of a patient's office visit.

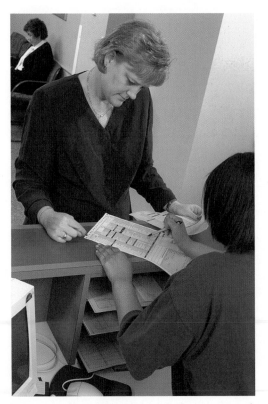

FIGURE 3–17 Patient carrying the encounter form to the medical office's check-up station.

 Using the encounter form, daily transactions are **posted** (recorded) by the billing staff. Professional fees (charges), payments (cash, check, or credit card), adjustments, and balance due are also posted in the practice management software program. Accuracy is important when keying data into the computer especially because this is where the movable data start to build an insurance claim.

At the end of each day, a daysheet is generated and printed. A **daysheet,** or daily record sheet, is a register for recording daily business transactions. The totals from this can be compared with the encounter forms to assure all charges, payments, and adjustments were properly posted. Also, the daysheet is a useful tool for "checks and balances" when assessing the bank deposit slip for accuracy.

All items posted to each patient account are housed in the computer database for accurate and easy retrieval.

 Paper Environment: The paper environment allows transactions to be recorded on the patient ledger cards. All patients seen on one day have their charges (debits) recorded on the daysheet, along with all payments and adjustments (credits). Each day the totals are carried forward and a new daysheet is set up to receive posting for that day (Figure 3–19). The ledger card should show an entry of the date an insurance claim is sent, including the date of services that were billed. Each service must be posted on a single line, and a **running balance** is calculated in the right column. When the ledger is completely filled, the account balance is brought forward (also known as **extended**) to a new card.

Step-by-step instructions for completing a ledger card are given at the end of this chapter in the procedure "Prepare and Post to a Patient's Financial Accounting Record."

8. Insurance Claim: Generally, the insurance billing specialist in the physician's office completes the claim information for the following cases: (1) all hospitalized (both surgical and medical) patients, (2) all claims in which the benefits are assigned to the physician, and (3) special procedures (minor surgery or extensive testing). In these cases, the insurance billing specialist generates an accurate claim to be submitted by using exact procedural and diagnostic codes, including the use of any appropriate documents (operative report or invoice), and mails it to the correct insurance carrier when circumstances call for it to be sent in hardcopy.

The minimum information required by third-party payers is:

● What was done? (services and procedures using procedure codes and appropriate modifiers discussed in Chapter 6)
● Why was it done? (diagnoses using diagnostic codes discussed in Chapter 5)
● When was it performed? (date of service [DOS])
● Where was it received? (place of service [POS])
● Who did it? (provider name and identifying number)

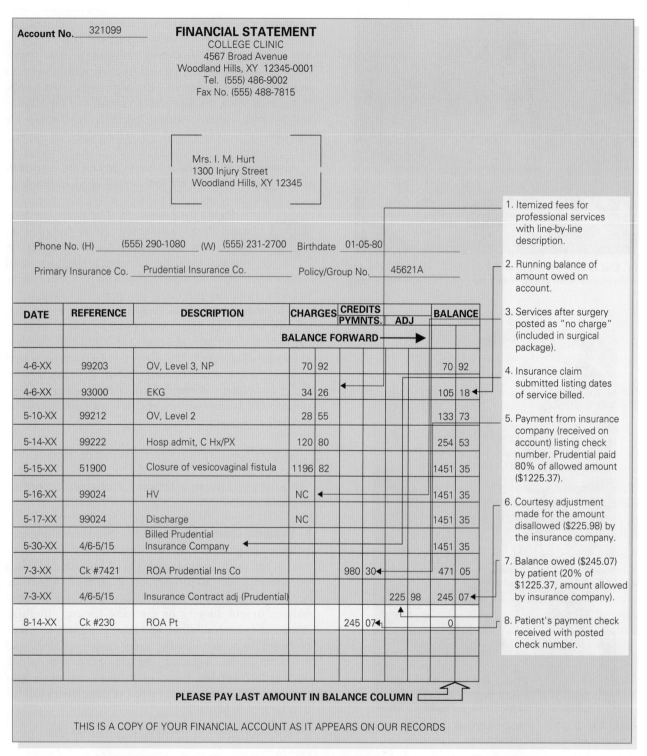

Account No. 321099

FINANCIAL STATEMENT
COLLEGE CLINIC
4567 Broad Avenue
Woodland Hills, XY 12345-0001
Tel. (555) 486-9002
Fax No. (555) 488-7815

Mrs. I. M. Hurt
1300 Injury Street
Woodland Hills, XY 12345

Phone No. (H) _____ (555) 290-1080 _____ (W) (555) 231-2700   Birthdate 01-05-80

Primary Insurance Co. Prudential Insurance Co.   Policy/Group No. 45621A

DATE	REFERENCE	DESCRIPTION	CHARGES	CREDITS PYMNTS.	ADJ	BALANCE
		BALANCE FORWARD ▶				
4-6-XX	99203	OV, Level 3, NP	70 92			70 92
4-6-XX	93000	EKG	34 26			105 18
5-10-XX	99212	OV, Level 2	28 55			133 73
5-14-XX	99222	Hosp admit, C Hx/PX	120 80			254 53
5-15-XX	51900	Closure of vesicovaginal fistula	1196 82			1451 35
5-16-XX	99024	HV	NC			1451 35
5-17-XX	99024	Discharge	NC			1451 35
5-30-XX	4/6-5/15	Billed Prudential Insurance Company				1451 35
7-3-XX	Ck #7421	ROA Prudential Ins Co		980 30		471 05
7-3-XX	4/6-5/15	Insurance Contract adj (Prudential)			225 98	245 07
8-14-XX	Ck #230	ROA Pt		245 07		0

PLEASE PAY LAST AMOUNT IN BALANCE COLUMN

THIS IS A COPY OF YOUR FINANCIAL ACCOUNT AS IT APPEARS ON OUR RECORDS

1. Itemized fees for professional services with line-by-line description.

2. Running balance of amount owed on account.

3. Services after surgery posted as "no charge" (included in surgical package).

4. Insurance claim submitted listing dates of service billed.

5. Payment from insurance company (received on account) listing check number. Prudential paid 80% of allowed amount ($1225.37).

6. Courtesy adjustment made for the amount disallowed ($225.98) by the insurance company.

7. Balance owed ($245.07) by patient (20% of $1225.37, amount allowed by insurance company).

8. Patient's payment check received with posted check number.

FIGURE 3–18 Financial accounting record illustrating posting of professional service descriptions, fees, payments, adjustments, and balance due.

A helpful hint is to group together or batch all outstanding charges to the same type of insurance at one time. This cuts down on errors, allows easier trackability and, in the paper environment, makes manual completion of the forms less tedious.

Submit claims as soon as possible after professional services are rendered. There are time limits (ranging from 30 days to 1½ years) for filing an insurance claim from the date of service. This can vary depending on the commercial carrier, federal or state program, or whether the

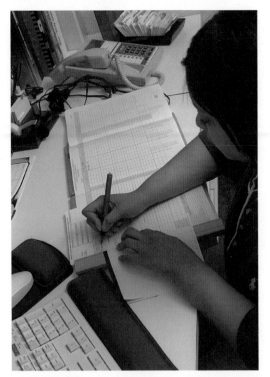

FIGURE 3–19 Medical office employee posting to a patient's financial accounting record or daysheet.

claim is for an illness or accident. Claims filed after the time limit will be denied and a detailed appeal process may be required to have the claim reconsidered. This topic is discussed further within the chapters on Medicare, Medicaid, TRICARE, and workers' compensation.

Financial losses from delay can occur in the following instances. If a patient has had a long-term illness, insurance benefits can expire before a claim is processed. If several physicians treat the same patient, some insurance companies pay only one of the physicians. (Typically, whoever files the claim first is paid first.) In this scenario, the other physicians may have to wait for disbursement by the physician who received the check. Submit hospitalized patients' insurance claim forms promptly upon discharge or on a regular schedule (weekly or twice a month depending on the office protocol) regardless of the discharge date for long-term inpatients.

For patients who pay at time of service and who wish to submit their own insurance claims, they are given two copies of the encounter form. The patient retains one copy for personal records and attaches the second copy to the insurance claim form and forwards it to the insurance company.

9. Provider's Signature: Provider's rarely sign the CMS-1500 insurance claim form. However, when a signature is required, it can be accepted in several formats—handwritten, facsimile stamp, and electronic signature.

State and government programs require a signature. In the Medicare program, certificates of medical necessity require an original signature.

PHYSICIAN'S REPRESENTATIVE

Sometimes a physician gives signature authorization to one person on the staff to sign insurance claims, who then becomes known as the physician's representative, referred to in Figure 3–20 as the "attorney-in-fact." For an authorization of this type, a document should be typed and signed before a notary. This means that whoever signs the form is attesting to it because it is a legal document. If the medical practice is ever audited and fraud or embezzlement is discovered, then the person who had signature authorization can be brought into the case as well as the physician. The federal government will prosecute if this involves a Medicare patient. The state will prosecute if a Medicaid patient is involved.

COMPUTERIZED SIGNATURES

 There are two types of computerized signatures, electronic and digital. An **electronic signature** looks like the signer's handwritten signature. The signer authenticates the document by key entry or with a pen pad using a stylus to capture the live signature.

Example
David Smith, MD

It also can be defined as an individualized computer access and identification system (e.g., a series of numbers, letters, electronic writing, voice, computer key, and fingerprint transmission [biometric system]).

A *digital signature* may be lines of text or a text box stating the signer's name, date, and time and a statement indicating a signature has been attached from within the software application. Refer to Chapter 8 for additional information on computerized signatures.

Example
Electronically signed: David Smith, MD 07/12/2000   10:30:08

SIGNATURE STAMP

 Paper Environment: Some medical practices use a signature stamp so the staff can process insurance forms and other paperwork without interrupting the physician by waiting for her or his signature. For an authorization of this type, a document should be typed and signed before a notary (Figure 3–21).

PROVIDER'S NOTARIZED SIGNATURE AUTHORIZATION

State of ___Iowa___)
)ss
County of ___Des Moines___)

Know all persons by these presents:

     That I, ___John Doe, MD___ have made, constituted, and appointed and by these presents do make, constitute and appoint ___Mary Coleman___ my true and lawful attorney-in-fact for me and in my name place and stead to sign my name on claims, for payment for services provided by me submitted to the ___Blue Cross and Blue Shield of Iowa___. My signature by my said attorney-in-fact includes my agreement to abide by the full payment concept and the remainder of the certification appearing on all ___CMS-1500___ claim forms. I hereby ratify and confirm all that my said attorney-in-fact shall lawfully do or cause to be done by virtue of the power generated herein.

     In witness whereof I have hereunto set my hand this ___20th___ day of ___January___ 20 __XX__.

                ___*John Doe, MD*___
                    (Signature)

Subscribed and sworn to before me this__20th__ day of __January__ 20 __XX__

                        _____
                    Notary Public

My commission expires _____.

FIGURE 3–20 Example of a provider's signature authorization form that can be completed, notarized, and sent to the insurance carrier after a copy is retained for the physician's records.

However, use of this stamp can lead to problems, because it is possible to stamp unauthorized checks, transcribed medical reports, prescriptions, or credit card charge slips. Discontinue the practice if such a stamp is used infrequently. If one is used regularly, prevent problems by doing the following:

● Make only one stamp.
● Allow only long-term, trusted, bonded staff members to have access to the stamp.
● Keep the stamp in a location with a secure lock.
● Limit access to the stamp.

State laws may require that insurance claims or other related documents have an original signature or otherwise bars the use of signature stamps. You must follow those rules regardless of any carrier manual regulations. For information on state laws, contact your state legislature at your state capitol. For data about signatures on hospital medical records, see Chapter 17.

10. Tracking Pending Insurance Claims: In the computerized practice management system, a date is noted each time a claim is generated for submission, whether it is sent electronically or printed on a paper claim form from the computer. A report to determine outstanding balances can be generated using the date claim was filed as a point to assess how many days old the claim is. This report is referred to as an *aging report*. The aging report is used to understand what the bottom line A/R is. In other words, aging report shows a snapshot of how much money is due to the practice from each patient account.

Paper Environment: When submitting paper claims, keep a duplicate of the claim in the office pending file or in the computer system files in the event payment is not received within a predetermined amount of time and the claim must be followed up. This file also may be referred to as a suspense, follow-up, or "tickler" file (Figures 3–22 and 3–23). The term *tickler* came into existence because it tickles or jogs the memory at certain dates in the future. You may be accustomed to hearing the term "aging report" as discussed above.

If not using a computerized system, establish an insurance claims register (tracing file) to keep track of the status of each case that has been billed (Figure 3–24). Record to whom the claim was sent and the submission date on the insurance claims register and the patient's

PROVIDER'S NOTARIZED FACSIMILE OR STAMP SIGNATURE AUTHORIZATION

State of ___Florida___)
)ss
County of ___Jacksonville___)

___John Doe, MD___ being first duty sworn, deposes and says:

I hereby authorize the ___Blue Cross of Florida___
                        (Name of Fiscal Administrator)
to accept my facsimile or stamp signature shown below
_____
               John Doe, MD
          (Facsimile or Stamp Signature)

as my true signature for all purposes under the ___Medicare___
                                          (Name of Insurance Program)
in the same manner as if it were my actual signature, including
my agreeing to abide by the full payment concept and the
remainder of the certification normally signed by the source of
care as it appears on all ___CMS-1500___ claim forms.

                              John Doe, MD
                              (Signature)

Subscribed and sworn to before me this _3rd_ day
of __January__ 20XX.

                    _____
                    Notary Public in and for
_____ County, State of_____
(SEAL)
My commission expires _____ .

FIGURE 3-21 Example of a provider's facsimile or stamp signature authorization form that can be completed, notarized, and sent to the insurance carrier after a copy is retained for the physician's records.

ledger card. The insurance billing specialist handling the insurance forms can see at a glance which claims are becoming delinquent and the amounts owed to the physician. This is an efficient method used for 30- to 60-day follow-up.

Keep two copies of each claim for the physician's records, one to be filed by patient name and the other by carrier name. Or simply record the name of the insurance company on each patient's ledger card and keep a file for each carrier by date of service. Filing by carrier allows all inquiries to be included in a single letter to the insurance company to eliminate having to write to the same company three or four times.

11. Submitting the Claim: When filing claims electronically (details discussed in EDI Chapter 8), a batch will be created and a digital file will be stored in a predetermined directory. Communication with the insurance payer or the clearinghouse will allow transmitting the digital file of claims over a modem, DSL line, or the Internet.

 Mail claims in batches to each carrier to save on postage. You may use a large manila envelope depending on the quantity of claims being submitted or use a window envelope where the insurance address shows through the front so there is no need to address by hand.

Refer to Figure 3-6, *B*, for the phases of adjudication by the insurance carrier of a claim form for payment.

12. Insurance Payments

BANK DEPOSIT AND ANNUAL ALPHA FILE

 After the insurance payer determines reimbursement, a check and corresponding explanation of benefits (EOB)/remittance advice (RA) are sent to the health care provider. Electronic funds transfer (EFT) may be used in place of a mailed paper check. EFT allows the automatic deposit of funds from the payer into the provider's bank account, just as you may have set up with your own paycheck. Electronic EOBs and RA may also be received by modem, downloaded, and printed out.

Payment is posted to the patient's account to reflect amount paid; necessary adjustments and outstanding balance responsibility is transferred to the patient after insurance measures have been exhausted.

 A payment (check) from the insurance carrier should be received in 2 to 8 weeks, accompanied by an EOB or RA document. The duplicate claim form is pulled from the file to verify the payment received against the amount billed.

The payment is posted (credited) to the patient's ledger card and current daysheet indicating the date of posting, name of insurance company, check or voucher number, amount received, and contracted adjustment. After proper payment is received, the duplicate copy of the insurance claim is attached to the explanation of benefits form. These are filed in an annual alpha file according to insurance type, date of service, or patients' names. A date file using the posting date as reference is another option. Some medical practices file claim forms at the back section of the patient's medical record after payment is received and accepted; however, this is an optional but not preferred system.

In either case of electronic or paper office environments, usually all payments received are entered onto a bank deposit slip and may be deposited at the bank.

For further information on improper payments received and tracing delinquent claims, see Chapter 9.

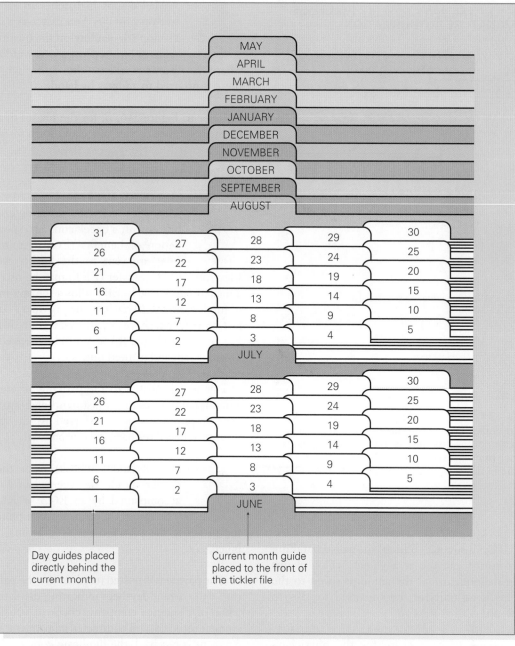

FIGURE 3–22   Example of a 30- to 60-day pending or tickler file for following up on unpaid insurance claims.

13. Monthly Statement: For the patient who has insurance, a monthly statement for all outstanding charges should be sent indicating that insurance has been billed and the amount due is the patient's responsibility. The patient statement should always reflect the same fee as that submitted to the insurance company minus the amount paid by the patient copayment and/or the insurance amount reimbursed. Patients who do not have insurance should receive a monthly statement indicating all outstanding balances due minus any payments or adjustment applied since the last billing statement.

14. Never-Ending Paper Trail: Whether your office is computerized or still operates in a paper-based environment, you will not escape the volumes of paperwork that business produces! Financial records must be retained and may include the following (not an all-inclusive list):

● Copy of the completed patient information form, patient authorization or signature-on-file for assignment of benefits form, copies of insurance identification cards, responsible-party authorization, insurance correspondence.

- Explanation of benefits or remittance advice documents sent from insurance payers.
- Logs of all telephone conversations and actions taken regarding insurance disputes or collection activities. If you do not store these notes in the corresponding patient health record, then you will likely have a master file set up where all logs are kept.
- Encounter forms, referral, and authorization slips.
- Daysheets and deposit slips.

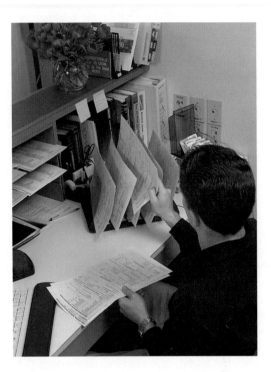

FIGURE 3–23 Insurance billing specialist using a desk sorter to alphabetize insurance claims to make filing easier in the tickler file.

		Claim Submitted		Follow-Up		Claim Paid		
Patient's Name Group/policy No.	Name of Insurance Company	Date	Amount	Date	Date	Date	Amt	Difference
Davis, Bob	BC/BS	1-7-XX	319.37			2/28/XX	294.82	24.55
Cash, David	BC	1-8-XX	268.08	2-10-XX	3-10-XX			
Smythe, Jan	Medicaid	1-9-XX	146.15	2-10-XX				
Phillips, Emma	Medicare	1-10-XX	96.28	2-10-XX				
Perez, Jose	Medi-Medi	1-10-XX	647.09	2-10-XX				
Amato, Joe	Tricare	2-1-XX	134.78	3-10-XX				
Rubin, Billy	Aetna	2-4-XX	607.67	3-10-XX				
Pfeifer, Renee	Travelers	2-10-XX	564.55	3-10-XX				
Tam, Chang	Prudential	2-15-XX	1515.79					
Brown, Harry	Allstate	2-21-XX	121.21					
Park, James	BC	2-24-XX	124.99					

INSURANCE CLAIMS REGISTER Page No. _____

FIGURE 3–24 Insurance claims register. This is an example of how a form can be set up to establish an easy way to follow up on insurance claims.

PROCEDURE

PREPARE AND POST TO A PATIENT'S FINANCIAL ACCOUNTING RECORD

OBJECTIVES: To prepare, insert descriptions, and post fees, payments, credit adjustments, and balances due to a patient's ledger card

EQUIPMENT/SUPPLIES: Typewriter or computer, patient accounts or ledger cards, and calculator

DIRECTIONS: Follow these steps to post charges, payments, adjustments, and balances to a patient's ledger/account (see Figure 3–18) and practice this skill by completing the assignments in the *Workbook*.

1. Personal data: Insert the patient's name and address to prepare the ledger card. Some ledgers may require additional information (attending physician's name, type of insurance, insurance company's name with policy and group numbers, patient's home and work telephone numbers, birth date, Social Security number, driver's license number, spouse's and/or dependents' names, and name, address, and telephone number of nearest relative), depending on the style of card chosen for a medical practice.

2. Date: Post the DOS in the date column, description of the services in the professional service description column, and charge amount in the charge column. The posting date is the actual date the transaction is recorded. If the DOS differs from the posting date, reference the DOS in the description column. This date column should never be left blank.

3. Reference: List a Current Procedural Terminology (CPT) procedure code number in the reference column.

4. Description: Write a brief description of the transaction that is being posted, such as OV for office visit or HV for hospital visit. Indicate the Evaluation and Management service levels (1 through 5) using the last digit of the E/M code (e.g., 99205 = Level **5**). List the name of other services or surgical procedures (e.g., ECG, vaccination, tonsillectomy).

   a. Charges: Add the charge to the running current balance, and enter the current balance in the right column.

   b. Payments: Post the current date the payment is received and indicate ROA (received on account), and who made the payment (e.g., pt [patient] or name of insurance company) in the description column. List the type of payment (cash, check, debit card, money order, or credit card), and voucher or check number (e.g., ck #430) in the reference column.

   c. Adjustments: Post the date the adjustment is being made and indicate the type of adjustment (e.g., insurance plan adj., contract adj., courtesy adj.).

   d. Billing comments: Indicate when the insurance company was billed by posting the current date and name of the insurance company. Include the dates of service being billed in the reference column (e.g., 4/20/XX through 5/1/XX). Indicate when patient statement was sent and amount due if different from the current balance (e.g., Patient billed $45.00 balance after insurance payment).

   e. Other comments: Indicate other comments that pertain directly to the account (e.g., account sent to ABC Collection Agency, account scheduled for small claims court).

5. Charges: Refer to the fee schedule and post each fee (charge) on a separate line in the "charge" column. Charges are debited (subtracted) from the account balance.

6. Payments: Enter the amount paid in the "payment" column and credit (subtract) the payment received from the amount in the running current balance column and enter the current balance.

7. Adjustments: Post the contracted insurance plan discount in the "Adjustment" column by referencing the DOS, insurance company name, and type of contract discount (e.g., HealthNet PPO discount or Medicare courtesy adjustment). Adjustments are credited to the account balance.

8. Current balance: Line by line, credit and debit by adding and subtracting postings to the running balance to determine the amount for the current balance column as shown in Figure 3–18. If a line is used to indicate a date an action was taken (e.g., insurance company or patient billed, account sent to collection), bring down the running balance from the previous line. This column must always contain an amount and should never be left blank. Optional: Post the adjustment on the same line as the payment.

9. Submit an itemized billing statement to the patient for the balance due.

Date	Description	Charge	Payment	Adjustment	Balance
7-3-XX	ROA Prudential Ins #7421		980.30	120.80	1346.17 245.07

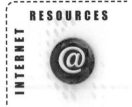

RESOURCES

INTERNET

Web sites for government health insurance programs such as Medicare, TRICARE, and CHAMPVA; state and federal Medicaid and disability benefit programs; and workers' compensation insurance are listed at the end of chapters discussing those topics. Specific health insurance plans may be located by using an Internet search engine and inserting their names.

- America's Health Insurance Plans (for information and links to other health insurance Web sites)
  Web site: **http://www.ahip.org**

Custom forms, such as patient instruction forms, history forms, report forms, patient reminder cards, and others may be designed by office staff and ordered or designed by the medical stationery/supply company after assembling the necessary information. Some of these forms may be available over the Internet from the following supplier's web sites.

- Bibbero Systems, Inc.
  Web site: **http://www.bibbero.com**

- Histacount Medical Practice
  Web site: **http://www.histacount.com**

- Medical Arts Press
  Web site: **http://www.medicalartspress.com**

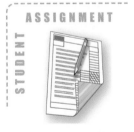

ASSIGNMENT

STUDENT

✔ Study Chapter 3.

✔ Answer the review questions in the *Workbook* to reinforce the theory learned in this chapter and to help prepare you for a future test.

✔ Complete the assignments in the *Workbook* to help reinforce the basic steps in submitting an insurance claim form.

✔ Turn to the glossary at the end of this textbook for a further understanding of the key terms used in this chapter.

CHAPTER OUTLINE

THE DOCUMENTATION PROCESS
   Health Record
   Documenters
   Reasons for Documentation
**GENERAL PRINCIPLES OF
   HEALTH RECORD
   DOCUMENTATION**
   Medical Necessity
   External Audit Point System
   Legalities of Health Record
     Documentation
**DOCUMENTATION GUIDELINES
   FOR EVALUATION AND
   MANAGEMENT SERVICES**

**CONTENTS OF A MEDICAL
   REPORT**
   Documentation of History
   Documentation of Examination
   Documentation of Medical
     Decision-Making Complexity
**DOCUMENTATION
   TERMINOLOGY**
   Terminology for Evaluation and
     Management Services
   Diagnostic Terminology and
     Abbreviations
   Directional Terms
   Surgical Terminology

**REVIEW AND AUDIT OF HEALTH
   RECORDS**
   Internal Reviews
   External Audit
   Retention of Records
   Termination of a Case
   Prevention of Legal Problems
**PROCEDURE: ABSTRACT DATA
   FROM A HEALTH RECORD**
**PROCEDURE: COMPOSE,
   FORMAT, KEY, PROOFREAD,
   AND PRINT A LETTER**

KEY TERMS

acute

attending physician

chief complaint (CC)

chronic

comorbidity

comprehensive (C)

concurrent care

consultation

consulting physician

continuity of care

counseling

critical care

detailed (D)

documentation

electronic health record (EHR)

emergency care

eponym

established patient

expanded problem focused (EPF)

external audit

facsimile (fax)

family history (FH)

health record/medical record

high complexity (HC)

history of present illness (HPI)

internal review

low complexity (LC)

medical necessity

medical report

moderate complexity (MC)

new patient (NP)

ordering physician

past history (PH)

physical examination (PE or PX)

primary care physician (PCP)

problem focused (PF)

prospective review

referral

referring physician

resident physician

retrospective review

review of systems (ROS)

social history (SH)

straightforward (SF)

subpoena

subpoena duces tecum

teaching physician

treating or performing physician

treating practitioner

Medical Documentation

OBJECTIVES*

After reading this chapter, you should be able to:

- Name steps in the documentation process.
- Explain reasons medical documentation is required.
- Identify principles of documentation.
- State contents of a medical report.
- Define common medical, diagnostic, and legal terms.
- List documents required for an internal review of health records.
- Describe the difference between prospective and retrospective review of records.

- State reasons why an insurance company may decide to perform an external audit of medical records.
- Identify principles for retention of health records.
- Explain techniques used for fax confidentiality.
- Respond appropriately to the subpoena of a witness and records.
- Formulate a procedure for termination of a case.
- Prepare legally correct medicolegal forms and letters.

*Performance objectives and exercises for hands-on experience for this chapter appear in the *Workbook*.

Service

Patients are best served by keeping personal health information private and confidential. Following federal HIPAA guidelines for consent and disclosure of information will help keep a medical practice compliant and the patients confident. The physician may send a patient to another doctor for a consultation, see a patient in consultation, or refer a patient to a specialist for the transfer of total or specific care. Written reports or thank you letters may be generated on behalf of the patient to communicate and document good patient care.

THE DOCUMENTATION PROCESS

Health Record

The connection between insurance billing and the health record, also known for decades as "medical" record, should be explained to better understand its importance, as the foremost tool of clinical care and communication. A **health record** can be defined as written or graphic information documenting facts and events during the rendering of patient care. It may be kept in one of the following formats: paper, microfilm, or electronic. Contents of a health record vary from case to case but some of the most common medical office documents are patient registration form, medication record, history and physical, progress or chart notes, consultation reports, imaging and x-ray reports, laboratory reports, immunization record, consent and authorization forms, operative report, and pathology report. In a hospital setting in addition to the aforementioned, there is an identification sheet, physician's orders, and discharge summary.

As learned in Chapter 2, the federal government has set standards to protect the confidentiality, security, and integrity of a patient's protected health information (PHI). Any one of several systems may be used in a medical practice. They are problem-oriented record (POR) system, source-oriented record (SOR) system, integrated record system, or **electronic health record (EHR)** system. A POR system consists of flow sheets, charts, or graphs that allow a physician to quickly locate information and compare evaluations. These data sheets are commonly used to record blood sugar levels for diabetic patients, blood pressure readings for hypertensive patients, weight for obese patients, immunizations, medication refills, and so on. In the SOR system, documents are arranged according to sections, for example, history and physical section, progress notes, laboratory tests, radiology reports, surgical operations, and so on. The integrated record system files all documents in reverse chronologic order and it may be more difficult to locate data because they are scattered throughout the record. An EHR system is created using a computer with software. A template is brought up and by answering a series of questions, data are entered.

ELECTRONIC SECURITY STANDARDS

One provision of the Health Insurance Portability and Accountability Act (HIPAA) directs the adoption of national electronic standards for automatic transfer of certain health care data among health care payers, plans, and providers. This provision encourages medical practices to convert to an electronic record-keeping system or paperless office because this will help transition insurance claim attachments from the paper world into the electronic world. Another provision is that information systems have security safeguards to protect against improper disclosure, unauthorized access, or unintended alteration of information for both data and the system.

A **medical report** is part of the health record and is a permanent legal document that formally states the consequences of the patient's examination or treatment in letter or report form. It is this record that provides the information needed to complete the insurance claim form. When billing the insurance company, the date of service (DOS), point of service (POS), type of service (TOS), diagnosis (dx or Dx), and procedures must be recorded. The TOS can be submitted for HIPAA claims but is no longer required. These data are transferred as codes whether using the paper claim form or sending in electronic format. The codes are used for interpretation by the insurance company when processing a claim.

The key to substantiating procedure and diagnostic code selections for appropriate reimbursement is supporting documentation in the health record. Proper documentation can prevent penalties and refund requests in case the physician's practice is reviewed or audited. Some states or facilities use different terminology when referring to the health record, such as medical information, medical record, progress or chart note, hospital record, or health care record.

Documenters

All individuals providing health care services may be referred to as documenters because they chronologically record pertinent facts and observations about the patient's health. This process is called **documentation** (charting) and may be handwritten or dictated and transcribed. It is the health care provider's responsibility to either hand write the medical information or dictate it for transcription. When voice recognition is used, many practices use a *correctionist* who reviews the computer-generated notes while listening to the physician on tape. The correctionist makes changes related to voice recognition errors. Some practices use printed checklists for typical examinations. The physician notes his or her findings on the checklists and gives this document to an employee for input to the electronic medical record (EMR) system. The EMR system has access to these checklists to minimize typing costs.

The receptionist obtains the first document completed by the patient, called the patient registration information form, as shown in Figure 3–7. The medical assistant or a front desk staff member is often the one to record entries for no-show appointments, prescription refills, and telephone calls in the patients' health records. The insurance billing specialist uses the information in the health record for billing purposes, and it is his or her responsibility to bring any substandard documentation to the physician's attention. In the hospital setting, a trained health information management (HIM) professional maintains the health record for completeness.

When referring to guidelines for documentation of the health record and completion of the insurance claim form, a physician's title may change depending on the circumstances of each patient encounter. This can get confusing at times, so to clarify the physician's various roles and the roles of the practitioners who work for the physician, some of these titles are defined as follows:

- **Attending physician** refers to the medical staff member who is legally responsible for the care and treatment given to a patient.
- **Consulting physician** is a provider whose opinion or advice regarding evaluation or management of a specific problem is requested by another physician.
- **Ordering physician** is the individual directing the selection, preparation, or administration of tests, medication, or treatment.
- **Primary care physician (PCP)** oversees the care of patients in a managed health care plan and refers patients to see specialists for services as needed.
- **Referring physician** is a provider who sends the patient for tests or treatment.
- **Resident physician** is a physician who has finished medical school and is performing one or more years of training in a specialty area on the job at a hospital (medical center). Residents perform the elements required for an evaluation and management (E/M) service in the presence of, or jointly, with the teaching physician, and the resident documents the service.
- **Teaching physician** is a doctor who has responsibilities for training and supervising medical students, interns, or residents and who takes them to the bedsides of patients in a teaching hospital to review course and treatment. Teaching physicians must document that they supervised and were physically present at the time during key portions of the service provided to the patient when performed by a resident.
- **Treating or performing physician** is the provider who renders a service to a patient. In the Medicare program, the definition of a treating physician is a physician who furnishes a consultation or treats a beneficiary for a specific medical problem, and who uses the results of a diagnostic test in the management of the beneficiary's specific medical problem. A radiologist performing a therapeutic intervention procedure is considered a treating physician. A radiologist performing a diagnostic intervention or diagnostic procedure is not considered a treating physician.
- **Treating practitioner** is a nurse practitioner, clinical nurse specialist, or physician assistant who furnishes a consultation or treats a patient for a specific medical problem, pursuant to state law, and who uses the results of a diagnostic test in the management of the patient's specific medical problem.

LEGIBLE DOCUMENTATION

Entries in the patient's record must be legible.

Reasons for Documentation

It is important that every patient seen by the physician has comprehensive legible documentation about what occurred during the visit for the following reasons:

1. Avoidance of denied or delayed payments by insurance carriers investigating the medical necessity of services.
2. Enforcement of medical record-keeping rules by insurance carriers requiring accurate documentation that supports procedure and diagnostic codes.
3. Subpoena of health records by state investigators or the court for review.
4. Defense of a professional liability claim.

GENERAL PRINCIPLES OF HEALTH RECORD DOCUMENTATION

In the early 1990s, the American Medical Association (AMA) modified the terminology "office visits" and used "office and other outpatient services" when coding for those services; the AMA also adopted the phrase "evaluation and management" (E/M) for the name of the section of Current Procedural Terminology (CPT) in which those codes appear. This wording better reflects the components involved when performing an office visit. The AMA and Centers for Medicare and Medicaid Services (CMS) then developed documentation guidelines for

CPT E/M services. These were released to Medicare carriers by CMS in 1995 and then modified and released again in 1997. The guidelines were developed because Medicare has an obligation to those enrolled to ensure that services paid for have been provided and are medically necessary. It was discovered during audits that some medical practices should improve their quality of documentation.

Physicians are not required to use these guidelines but are encouraged to do so for the four reasons stated. Some physicians have adopted the 1995 guidelines, and others use those introduced in 1997. A modification of the 1997 guidelines is under consideration but has not been released as of this edition. Insurance claims processors and auditors may use the 1995 or 1997 guidelines when doing an internal or external chart audit to determine whether the reported services were actually rendered and the level of service was warranted. A variety of formats of documentation are accepted by Medicare fiscal intermediaries (claims processors) as long as the information is discernible. When significant irregular reporting patterns are detected, a review is conducted.

MEDICALLY NECESSARY

The Medicare program has a responsibility to make sure that professional services provided to patients were medically necessary. Documentation must support the level of service and each procedure rendered.

Medical Necessity

Payment may be delayed if the medical necessity of a treatment is questioned. As a rule, **medical necessity** is a criterion used by insurance companies when making decisions to limit or deny payment in which medical services or procedures must be justified by the patient's symptoms and diagnosis. This must be done in accordance with standards of good medical practice, and the proper level of care provided in the most appropriate setting. However, insurers differ on this definition and may or may not cover the services, depending on the benefits of the plan. Inform the patient of this situation with a letter, as shown in Figure 4–1.

External Audit Point System

A point system is used while reviewing each patient's health record during the performance of an audit. Points are awarded only if documentation is present for elements required in the health record. Because every health record is documented differently by each provider of service, a

patient's history may contain details for more than one body area or organ system. Thus when gathering points, it is possible the auditor may shift the points from the history of present illness to those required for the review of the patient's body systems. In addition, when sufficient points have been reached within a section for the level of code used in billing, no further documentation is counted for audit purposes, even though there may be additional comments for other body systems. This point system is used to show where deficiencies occur in health record documentation. It is also used to evaluate and substantiate proper use of diagnostic and procedural codes.

Health maintenance organizations, preferred provider organizations, and all private carriers have the right to claim refunds in the event of accidental (or intentional) miscoding. However, Medicare has the power to levy fines and penalties and exclude providers from the Medicare program. If improper coding patterns exist and are not corrected, then the provider of service will be penalized. Insurance carriers go by the rule "If it is not documented, then it was not performed," and they have the right to deny reimbursement.

Legalities of Health Record Documentation

Insurance carriers have become stricter in enforcing accurate coding substantiated by documentation. It is not uncommon for prepayment and postpayment random audits or reviews by Medicare carriers to occur that monitor the accuracy of physicians' use of E/M services and procedure codes. Medicare fiscal intermediaries have "walk-in rights" (access to a medical practice without an appointment or search warrant) that they may invoke to conduct documentation reviews, audits, and evaluations. Billing patterns that may draw attention to a medical practice for possible audit are as follows:

- Billing intentionally for unnecessary services
- Billing incorrectly for services of *physician extenders* (e.g., nurse practitioner, midwife, physician assistant)
- Billing for diagnostic tests without a separate report in the health record
- Changing dates of service on insurance claims to comply with policy coverage dates
- Waiving copayments or deductibles, or allowing other illegal discounts
- Ordering excessive diagnostic tests (e.g., laboratory tests, x-ray studies)
- Using two different provider numbers to bill the same services for the same patient
- Misusing provider identification numbers, resulting in incorrect billing
- Using improper modifiers for financial gain
- Failing to return overpayments made by the Medicare program

COLLEGE CLINIC
4567 Broad Avenue
Woodland Hills, XY 12345-0001
Phone: 555/486-90020
Fax: 555/487-8976

September 20, 20XX

Dear ABC Managed Care Plan Participant:

This is a quick fact sheet to help our patients understand that some services may not be paid by ABC Managed Care Plan unless there is a *medical* reason to perform them.

The coverage provided by ABC Managed Care Plan, in most instances, includes payment for medically necessary services provided to treat a problem or illness. However, patients who wish their health care providers to perform services outside of those considered a "medical necessity" will be responsible for paying for those services out-of-pocket.

For example, many patients come to our office for the purpose of removing noncancerous facial moles. Although this procedure may be desired by the patient, ABC Managed Care Plan will not pay for the removal without a medical reason for it.

The patient's cost for noncancerous facial mole removal at our practice is approximately $75.

Please understand that, legally, we are required to submit our bill to ABC Managed Care Plan using accurate information about all of the services you received. Using a false medical reason to try to get insurance to pay for a service it otherwise would not cover is considered fraud, and our doctors will not do this. We regret that ABC Managed Care Plan may not wish to pay for a service you desire, but we must follow insurance regulations.

If you would like additional information about payment coverage for these services, you may refer to your ABC Managed Care Plan benefits handbook or call your ABC Managed Care Plan customer service representative at 555-271-0311.

Thank you for choosing us to assist you with your health care needs. As always, providing high-quality health care to you is and remains our primary purpose. If you have any questions about this information, please do not hesitate to telephone and ask our front office staff for more information.

Sincerely,

Mary Anne Mason, CPC

FIGURE 4–1 Letter to a patient who is a member of a managed care plan that provides important information about medical procedures or services that are not covered for payment unless there is a medical necessity.

DOCUMENTATION GUIDELINES FOR EVALUATION AND MANAGEMENT SERVICES

The following is a brief overview of documentation guidelines regarding E/M services:

1. The health record should be accurate, complete (detailed), and legible.
2. The documentation of each patient encounter should include or provide reference to the following:
   a. Chief complaint or reason for the encounter
   b. Relevant history
   c. Examination
   d. Findings
   e. Prior diagnostic test results
   f. Assessment, clinical impression, or diagnosis
   g. Plan for care
   h. Date and legible identity of the health care professional
3. The reason for the encounter or chief complaint should be stated, and the rationale should be documented or inferred for ordering diagnostic and other ancillary services.
4. Past and present diagnoses, including those in the prenatal and intrapartum period that affect the newborn, should be accessible to the treating or consulting physician.

5. Appropriate health risk factors should be identified.

6. The patient's progress, response to and changes in treatment, planned follow-up care and instructions, and diagnosis should be documented.

7. Patient refusal to follow medical advice should be documented and a letter sent to the patient about this noncompliance. Information on termination of a case is found at the end of this chapter.

8. Procedure and diagnostic codes reported on the health insurance claim form or billing statement should be supported by the documentation in the health record and be at a level sufficient for a clinical peer to determine whether services have been coded accurately.

9. The confidentiality of the health record should be fully maintained consistent with the requirements of medical ethics and the law. An authorization form signed by the patient must be obtained to release information to the insurance carrier.

10. Each chart entry should be dated and signed, including the title or position of the person signing. If a signature log has been established, then initials are acceptable, because these would be defined in the log (Figure 4–2). A *signature log* is a list of all staff members' names, job titles, signatures, and initials. In regard to paperless documents, if passwords are used for restricted access, electronic or digital signatures may be acceptable.

11. Charting procedures for progress notes should be standardized. Many physicians use either a method called the SOAP style (Figure 4–3) or the CHEDDAR style (Figure 4–4). However, whatever method is used, make sure it is detailed enough to support current documentation requirements (Figure 4–5).

12. Treatment plans should be written. Include patient/family education and specific instructions for follow-up. Treatment must be consistent with the working diagnosis.

SIGNATURE LOG

Name	Position	Signature or Initials	
Ann M. Arch	Receptionist	Ann M. Arch	AMA
John Bortolonni	Office manager	John Bortolonni	JB
Gerald Practon, MD	Provider	Gerald Practon, MD	GP
Rachel Vasquez, CPC	Insurance billing specialist	Rachel Vasquez, CPC	RV
Mary Ann Worth	Clinical medical assistant	Mary Ann Worth	MAW

FIGURE 4–2 Example of a signature log.

S **Subjective** statements of symptoms and complaints in the patient's own words = chief complaint (CC) *reason for the encounter*

O **Objective** findings = data from physical examination, x-rays, laboratory, and other diagnostic tests *facts and findings*

A **Assessment** of subjective and objective findings = medical decision making *putting all the facts together to obtain a diagnosis*

P **Plan** of treatment = documenting a plan for care to be put into action *recommendations, instructions, further testing, medication*

FIGURE 4–3 Explanation of the acronym "SOAP" used as a format for progress notes defining subjective and objective information, the assessment, and the treatment plan.

C	**Chief complaint**	Stated by the patient as the main reason for seeing the doctor; usually a subjective statement
H	**History of the present illness**	Includes social history and physical symptoms as well as contributing factors
E	**Examination**	Performed by the physician
D	**Details**	List of complaints and problems
D	**Drugs and dosages**	List of the current medications the patient is taking
A	**Assessment**	The diagnostic process and the impression (diagnosis) made by the physician
R	**Return visit information or referral**	Information about return visits or specialists to see for additional tests

FIGURE 4–4 Explanation of the acronym "CHEDDAR" used as a format for progress notes.

13. Medications prescribed and taken should be listed, specifying frequency and dosage.
14. *Request* for a consultation from the attending or treating physician and the *need* for consultation must be documented. The consultant's opinion and any services ordered or performed must be documented and communicated to the requesting physician. Remember the three Rs: There must be a *requesting* physician, and the consultant must *render* an opinion and send a *report*.
15. Record a patient's failure to return for needed treatment by noting it in the health record, in the appointment book, and on the financial record or ledger card. Follow up with a telephone call or send a letter to the patient advising him or her that further treatment is indicated.
16. Use a permanent, not water-soluble, ink pen (legal copy pen) to cross out an incorrect entry on a patient's record. Mark it with a single line and write the correct information, then date and initial the entry. Never erase, white out, or use self-adhesive paper over any information recorded on a patient record (Example 4.1). Maintain the original entry in the electronic file if correcting a computerized document. Note that the section is in error with the date and

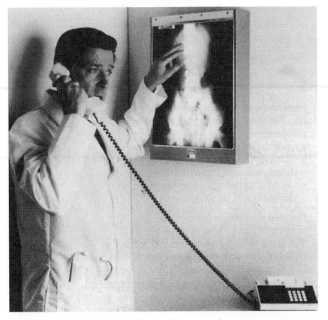

FIGURE 4–5 Physician dictating chart notes. (*From Diehl MO: Diehl and Fordney's medical transcribing techniques and procedures, ed 5, St Louis, Elsevier Science, 2002.*)

Example 4.1

Incorrect	BP 1̶5̶0̶/̶9̶0̶	
	190/70	1/2/20XX
Correct	BP 1̶5̶0̶/̶9̶0̶ *mtf*	
	slightly	
Incorrect	right leg is ~~markedly~~ edematous...	
	slightly	
Correct	right leg is ~~markedly~~ edematous... 1/2/20XX	
	mtf	
Correctly typed:	right leg is slightly edematous...	
	1-2-20XX mtf	

time and enter the correct information with a notation. Never delete or key over incorrect data in a computerized file. Another method for correcting a health record is to create an addendum either typed as a separate document or for a chart note inserted below in the next space available. This is discussed later in this chapter.

17. Document all laboratory tests ordered in the health record. When the report is received, the physician should initial the report, indicating that it has been read. Each documentation is considered an element and allows a point if the record undergoes an external audit.

18. Ask the physician for approval for a different code before submitting the claim to the insurance carrier if the insurance biller questions any procedure or diagnostic codes marked on the encounter form (Figure 4–6).

19. Retain all records until you are positive they are no longer needed by conforming to federal and state laws as well as the physician's wishes. Retention of records is discussed at the end of the chapter and shown in Table 4.2.

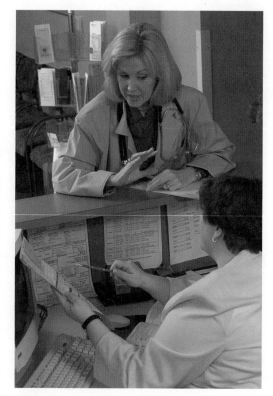

FIGURE 4–6 Insurance billing specialist checking information with physician before recording it on the insurance claim.

SIGNATURE LOG

Make sure all health record entries are signed or electronically verified by the physician (author) and his or her title or position. This provides clear evidence that the physician reviewed the note and/or ensures he or she is aware of all test results (normal and abnormal). Documented physician review of test results can be factored when determining appropriate coding levels for services.

CONTENTS OF A MEDICAL REPORT

The degree of documentation depends on the complexity of the service and the specialty of the physician. For example, a "normal chest examination" may have a different meaning to a cardiologist than it does to a family physician as far as the details of the examination and documentation.

The first time a new patient is seen, a family and social history is taken and updated as needed in subsequent visits. When a new or an established patient comes to see the physician with a new injury or illness, the documentation should also include the patient's health history, the physical examination, results from any tests that are performed, the medical decision-making process, the diagnosis, and the treatment plan.

Documentation of History

The following documentation information for the history and physical examination is based on the 1997 Medicare guidelines.

The history includes the chief complaint (CC); history of present illness (HPI); review of systems (ROS); and past history, family, or social history (PFSH).* The extent of the history is dependent on clinical judgment and on the nature of the presenting problems. Each history includes some or all of the following elements (Figure 4–7).

Chief Complaint

The **chief complaint** (CC) is a concise statement usually in the patient's own words describing the symptom, problem, condition, diagnosis, physician-recommended return, or other factor that is the reason for the encounter. *The CC is a requirement for all levels of history:* problem focused, expanded problem focused, detailed, and comprehensive; these are described at the end of the section on history of present illness.

---

*These abbreviations in the history portion of the report may vary depending on the physician who is dictating (e.g., *PI* for present illness, *PH* for past history, *FH* for family history).

Hospital number: 00-83-06

Scott, Aimee

Rex Rumsey, MD

HISTORY

CHIEF COMPLAINT: Pain and bleeding after each bowel movement for the past 3 to 4 months.

PRESENT ILLNESS: This 68-year-old white female says she usually has three bowel movements a day in small amounts, and there has been a change in the last 3 to 4 months in frequency, size, and type of bowel movement. She has slight burning pain and irritation in the rectal area after bowel movements. The pain lasts for several minutes, then decreases in intensity. She has had no previous anorectal surgery or rectal infection. She denies any blood in the stool itself or associated symptoms. Bright red blood occurs after stools have passed.

PAST HISTORY:
ILLNESSES: The patient had polio at age 8 from which she has made a remarkable recovery. Apparently, she was paralyzed in both lower extremities and now has adequate use of these. She has no other serious illnesses.

ALLERGIES: ALLERGIC TO PENICILLIN. She denies any other drug or food allergies.
MEDICATIONS: None.
OPERATIONS: Right inguinal herniorrhaphy 25 years ago.

SOCIAL HISTORY: She does not smoke or drink. She lives with her husband who is an invalid and for whom she cares. She is a retired former municipal court judge.

FAMILY HISTORY: One brother died of cancer of the throat (age 59), and another has cancer of the kidney (age 63).

REVIEW OF SYSTEMS:
SKIN: No rashes or jaundice.
HEENT: Head normocephalic. Normal TMs. Normal hearing. Pupils equal, round, reactive to light. Deviated septum. Oropharynx clear.
CR: No history of chest pain, shortness of breath, or pedal edema. She has had some mild hypertension in the past but is not under any medical supervision nor is she taking any medication for this.
GI: Weight is stable. See present illness.
OB-GYN: Gravida II Para II. Climacteric at age 46, no sequelae.
EXTREMITIES: No edema.
NEUROLOGIC: Unremarkable.

mtf
D: 5-17-20XX
T: 5-20-20XX

Rex Rumsey, MD

FIGURE 4–7 Example of a medical report done in modified block format showing the six components of a history.

History of Present Illness

The **history of present illness (HPI)** is a chronologic description of the development of the patient's present illness from the first sign or symptom or from the previous encounter to the present. If the physician is unable to obtain a sufficient diagnosis for the patient's condition, the health record documentation must reflect this. The history may include one or more of the following eight descriptive elements:

1. **Location**—Area of the body where the symptom is occurring.
2. **Quality**—Character of the symptom/pain (burning, gnawing, stabbing, fullness).
3. **Severity**—Degree of symptom or pain on a scale from 1 to 10. Severity also can be described with terms such as severe, slight, and persistent.

4. **Duration**—How long the symptom/pain has been present and how long it lasts when the patient has it.

5. **Timing**—When the pain/symptom occurs (e.g., morning, evening, after or before meals).

6. **Context**—The situation associated with the pain/symptom (e.g., dairy products, big meals, activity).

7. **Modifying factors**—Things done to make the symptom/pain worse or better. (For example, "If I eat spicy foods I get heartburn, but if I drink milk afterward the pain is not as bad.")

8. **Associated signs and symptoms**—The symptom/pain and other things that happen when the symptom/pain occurs (e.g., chest pain leads to shortness of breath).

The documented elements are counted and totaled (Figure 4–8, *A*). The health record should describe one

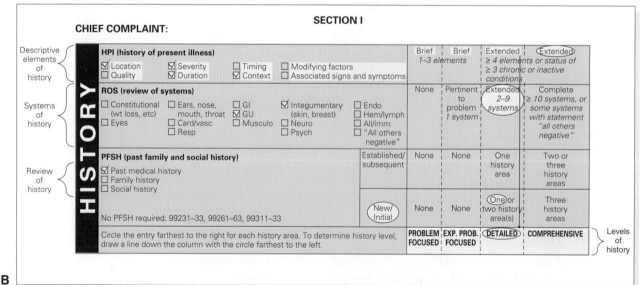

FIGURE 4–8   A, Documentation from a health record highlighting elements required for the history. **B,** Review/audit sheet Section I with check marks and circled elements to show how the history in the example is declared as detailed. This shows two of three history components (*arrow*) used for the purpose of determining the assignment of a procedure code at the appropriate level of service. (*From the Iowa Medical Society, IMS Services, West Des Moines, Iowa, 1998.*)

to three elements of the present illness for a *brief level* of HPI. At least four elements of the HPI or the status of at least three chronic or inactive conditions is required for the *extended level* of HPI. Only two of three history elements are required for certain types of cases, such as newborns or subsequent hospital care. Figure 4–8, *B*, shows Section I of the review/audit sheet that depicts the history containing the HPI, ROS, and PFSH. The check marks and circled element in the HPI (Section I) of the figure relate to the case illustrated.

The types of evaluation and management services for the history are based on four levels of history. However, the ROS and PFSH must be totaled before the final decision on the level of service is assigned. The four levels of history may be defined as follows:

1. **Problem focused (PF)**—Chief complaint; brief history of present illness or problem
2. **Expanded problem focused (EPF)**—Chief complaint; brief history of present illness; problem-pertinent system review
3. **Detailed (D)**—Chief complaint; extended history of present illness; problem-pertinent system review extended to include a review of a limited number of additional systems; *pertinent* past, family, or social history directly related to the patient's problems.
4. **Comprehensive (C)**—Chief complaint; extended history of present illness; review of systems that is directly related to the problem identified in the history of the present illness, plus a review of all additional body systems; *complete* past, family, and social history.

Review of Systems

A **review of systems (ROS)** is an inventory of body systems obtained through a series of questions that is used to identify signs or symptoms that the patient might be experiencing or has experienced. Checklists are permitted, but if a body system is not considered, then it should be crossed out. For an ROS, the following systems are recognized: constitutional symptoms (e.g., fever, weight loss), eyes, ears, nose, mouth, throat, cardiovascular, respiratory, gastrointestinal, genitourinary, musculoskeletal, integumentary (skin or breast), neurologic, psychiatric, endocrine, hematologic/lymphatic, and allergic/immunologic.

The body systems are counted and totaled. The health record should describe one system of the ROS for a *pertinent to problem level*. For an *extended level*, two to nine systems are required. For a *complete level*, at least 10 organ systems must be reviewed and documented. Refer to Figure 4–8, *B* for a visual understanding of Section I of the review/audit sheet. The check marks and circled

element in the ROS (Section I) of the figure relate to the case illustrated.

Past, Family, and Social Histories

The past, family, and social histories (PFSH) consists of a review of three areas:

1. **Past history (PH)**—The patient's past experiences with illnesses, operations, injuries, and treatments
2. **Family history (FH)**—A review of medical events in the patient's family, including diseases that may be hereditary or place the patient at risk
3. **Social history (SH)**—An age-appropriate review of past and current activities (e.g., smokes, consumes alcohol)

The PFSH review areas are counted and totaled. The health record must contain at least one history area for a *detailed extended level* and specific items from two of the three history areas for a *comprehensive level* of PFSH. Refer to Figure 4–8, *B* for a visual guide of the PFSH in Section I of the review/audit sheet. Note the difference in the number of required elements for new versus established patients and the circled element for the case in question.

A vertical line is drawn down the right four columns that contain the most elements to determine the history level. The elements of HPI, ROS, and PFSH must at least be met or may exceed the criteria determined for a PF, EPF, D, or C history level.

Documentation of Examination

Physical Examination

The **physical examination (PE or PX)** is objective in nature; that is, it consists of the physician's findings by examination or test results. Figure 4–9 is an illustration of a single organ system examination from the CMS Documentation Guidelines for 1997 that shows the details (elements) of examination for each body area within the genitourinary system. The three circled elements of the genitourinary system and one circled element of the gastrointestinal system relate to the case in question. For purposes of examination, the following body areas and organ systems are recognized.

Organ Systems/Body Areas—Elements of Examination

Constitutional (vital signs, general appearance)
Eyes
Ears, nose, mouth, and throat
Neck
Respiratory

MULTIORGAN SYSTEM EXAMINATION REQUIREMENTS (SHADED)
CONTENT and DOCUMENTATION

Level of Exam	Perform and Document
(Problem focused)	(One to five elements identified by a bullet.)
Expanded Problem Focused	At least six elements identified by a bullet.
Detailed	At least twelve elements identified by a bullet.
Comprehensive	Perform all elements identified by a bullet; document every element in every shaded box and at least one element in every unshaded box.

Genitourinary

System/Body Area	Elements of Examination
Constitutional	• Measurement of **any three of the following seven** vital signs: 1) sitting or standing blood pressure, 2) supine blood pressure, 3) pulse rate and regularity, 4) respiration, 5) temperature, 6) height, 7) weight (may be measured and recorded by ancillary staff) • General appearance of patient *e.g. development, nutrition, body habitus, deformities, attention to grooming*
Neck	• Examination of neck *e.g. masses, overall appearance, symmetry, tracheal position, crepitus* • Examination of thyroid *e.g. enlargement, tenderness, mass*
Respiratory	• Assessment of respiratory effect *e.g. intercostal retractions, use of accessory muscles, diaphragmatic movement* • Auscultation of lungs *e.g. breath sounds, adventitious sounds, rubs*
Cardiovascular	• Auscultation of heart with notation of abnormal sounds and murmurs • Examination of peripheral vascular system by observation *e.g. swelling, varicosities* and palpation *e.g. pulses, temperature, edema, tenderness*
Chest (breasts)	See genitourinary (female)
Gastrointestinal (abdomen)	⊙ Examination of abdomen with notation of presence of masses or tenderness • Examination for presence or absence of hernia • Examination of liver and spleen • Obtain stool sample for occult blood test when indicated
Genitourinary (male)	• Inspection of anus and perineum Examination (with or without specimen collection for smears and cultures) of genitalia including: • Scrotum *e.g. lesions, cysts, rashes* • Epididymides *e.g. size, symmetry, masses* ⊙ Testes *e.g. size, symmetry, masses* • Urethral meatus *e.g. size, location, lesions, discharge* ⊙ Penis *e.g. lesions, presence or absence of foreskin, foreskin retractability, plaque, masses, scarring, deformities* Digital rectal examination including: ⊙ Prostate gland *e.g. size, symmetry, nodularity, tenderness* • Seminal vesicles *e.g. symmetry, tenderness, masses, enlargement* • Sphincter tone, presence of hemorrhoids, rectal masses
Genitourinary (female) Includes at least seven of the eleven elements to the right identified by bullets:	• Inspection and palpation of breasts *e.g. masses or lumps, tenderness, symmetry, nipple discharge* • Digital rectal examination including sphincter tone, presence of hemorrhoids, rectal masses Pelvic examination (with or without specimen collection for smears and cultures) including: • External genitalia *e.g. general appearance, hair distribution, lesions* • Urethral meatus *e.g. size, location, lesions, prolapse* • Urethra *e.g. masses, tenderness, scarring* • Bladder *e.g. fullness, masses, tenderness* • Vagina *e.g. general appearance, estrogen effect, discharge, lesions, pelvic support, cystocele, rectocele* • Cervix *e.g. general appearance, lesions, discharge* • Uterus *e.g. size, contour, position, mobility, tenderness, descent or support* • Adnexa/parametria *e.g. masses, tenderness, organomegaly, nodularity* • Anus and perineum

Genitourinary (continued)

System/Body Area	Elements of Examination
Lymphatic	• Palpation of lymph nodes in neck, axillae, groin and/or other location
Skin	• Inspection and/or palpation of skin and subcutaneous tissue *e.g. rashes, lesions, ulcers*
Neurological/psychiatric	Brief assessment of mental status including: • Orientation to time, place and person • Mood and affect *e.g. depression, anxiety, agitation*

Skin

System/Body Area	Elements of Examination
Constitutional	• Measurement of **any three of the following seven** vital signs: 1) sitting or standing blood pressure, 2) supine blood pressure, 3) pulse rate and regularity, 4) respiration, 5) temperature, 6) height, 7) weight (may be measured and recorded by ancillary staff) • General appearance of patient *e.g. development, nutrition, body habitus, deformities, attention to grooming*
Eyes	• Inspection of conjuctive and lids
Ears, nose, mouth and throat	• Inspection of lips, teeth and gums • Examination of oropharynx *e.g. oral mucosa, hard and soft palates, tongue, tonsils, and posterior pharynx*
Neck	• Examination of thyroid *e.g. enlargement, tenderness, mass*
Gastrointestinal (abdomen)	• Examination of liver and spleen • Examination of anus for condyloma and other lesions
Lymphatic	• Palpation of lymph nodes in neck, axillae, groin and/or other location
Extremities	• Inspection and palpation of digits and nails *e.g. clubbing, cyanosis, inflammation, petechiae, ischemia, infections, nodes*
Skin	• Palpation of scalp and inspection of hair of scalp, eyebrows, face, chest, pubic area (when indicated) and extremities • Inspection and/or palpation of skin and subcutaneous tissue *e.g. rashes, lesions, ulcers, susceptibility in and presence of photo damage* in **eight of the following ten areas:** 1) head including face, 2) neck, 3) chest including breasts and axilla, 4) abdomen, 5) genitalia, groin, buttocks, 6) back, 7) right upper extremity, 8) left upper extremity, 9) right lower extremity, 10) left lower extremity Note: For the comprehensive level, the examination of all eight anatomic areas must be performed and documented. For the three lower levels of examination, each body area is counted separately. For example, inspection and/or palpation of the skin and subcutaneous tissue of the head and neck extremities constitutes two areas. • Inspection of eccrine and apocrine glands of skin and subcutaneous tissue with identification and location of any hyperhidrosis, chromhidroses or bromhidrosis
Neurological/psychiatric	Brief assessment of mental status including: • Orientation to time, place and person • Mood and affect *e.g. depression, anxiety, agitation*

FIGURE 4–9   Review/audit worksheet of a general multiorgan system physical examination that shows the details (elements) of examination for each body area/system. Circled bullets relate to the example case shown in Figure 4–8, *A*. *(From the Iowa Medical Society, IMS Services, West Des Moines, Iowa, 1998.)*

Cardiovascular
Chest, including breasts and axillae
Gastrointestinal (abdomen)
Genitourinary (male)
Genitourinary (female)
Lymphatic
Musculoskeletal
Skin
Neurologic
Psychiatric

NOTE: In addition, any reasons for not examining a particular body area or system should be listed.

Types of Physical Examination

When performing an internal review of a patient's health record, the number of elements identified by bullets are counted for each system and a total is obtained. The total is circled on Section II of the review/audit sheet as shown for the case illustrated (Figure 4–10).

The levels of evaluation and management services are based on four types of physical examination (PE), as follows:

1. **Problem focused (PF)**—A limited examination of the affected body area or organ system. The health record should describe one to five elements identified by a bullet for a problem-focused level of PE.
2. **Expanded problem focused (EPF)**—A limited examination of the affected body area or organ system and other symptomatic or related organ systems. At least six elements identified by a bullet are required for an expanded problem-focused level of PE.

3. **Detailed (D)**—An extended examination of the affected body areas and other symptomatic or related organ systems. At least two elements identified by a bullet from each of six areas/body systems OR at least 12 elements identified by a bullet in two or more areas/body systems are required for a detailed level of PE.
4. **Comprehensive (C)**—A general multisystem examination or complete examination of a single organ system. For a comprehensive level of PE, all elements must be identified by a bullet and documentation must be present for at least two elements identified by a bullet from each of nine areas/body systems.

The extent of the examination and what is documented range from limited examinations of single body areas to general multisystem or complete single-organ system examinations, depending on clinical judgment and the nature of the presenting problem.

Documentation of Medical Decision-Making Complexity

In the medical decision-making process, the physician must look at the number of diagnoses or treatment options, the amount or complexity of data to be reviewed, and the risk of complications or associated morbidity or mortality. *Morbidity* is a diseased condition or state, whereas *mortality* has to do with the number of deaths that occur in a given time or place.

Number of diagnoses or management options. This is based on the number and types of problems addressed during the visit, the complexity of establishing

SECTION II

Four elements identified

	General Multisystem Exam		Single Organ System Exam
EXAM	1-5 elements identified by •	PROBLEM FOCUSED	1-5 elements identified by •
	≥6 elements identified by •	EXPANDED PROBLEM FOCUSED	≥6 elements identified by •
	≥2 elements identified by • from 6 areas/systems OR ≥12 elements identified by • from at least 2 areas/systems	DETAILED	≥12 elements identified by • EXCEPT ≥ 9 elements identified by • for eye and psychiatric exams
	≥2 elements identified by • from 9 areas/systems	COMPREHENSIVE	Perform all elements identified by • ; document all elements in shaded boxes; document ≥ 1 element in unshaded boxes.

FIGURE 4–10 Review/audit worksheet Section II for a general multisystem physical examination and single organ system examination. The circled item relates to a problem-focused examination for the example case (see Figure 4–8, *A*) for the purpose of coding. *(From the Iowa Medical Society, IMS Services, West Des Moines, Iowa, 1998.)*

a diagnosis, and the number of management options that must be considered by the physician. For the case illustrated, the number of problems is 1, which equals 3 points (Figure 4–11, top section).

Amount or complexity of data to be reviewed. This is based on the types of diagnostic tests ordered or reviewed. A decision to obtain and review old health records or obtain history from sources other than the patient increases the amount and complexity of data to be analyzed. For the case illustrated, no points apply (see Figure 4–11, middle section).

Risk of complications, morbidity, or mortality. This is based on other conditions associated with the presenting problem known as the risk of complications, morbidity, or mortality, as well as comorbidities, the diagnostic procedures, or the possible management options (treatment rendered—surgery, therapy, drug management, services, and supplies). **Comorbidity** means underlying disease or other conditions present at the time of the visit. In determining the level of risk, the element (presenting problem, diagnostic procedure ordered, or management options selected), which has the highest level (minimal, low, moderate, or high) is used.

To discover whether the *level of risk* is minimal, low, moderate, or high, bulleted elements are marked on the review/audit sheet (Figure 4–12, Section III, Part C). For the case illustrated, the elements fall within the moderate level of risk category.

To conclude the internal review of a patient's health record, a level must be determined from one of four types of medical decision making: **straightforward (SF), low complexity (LC), moderate complexity (MC),** and **high complexity (HC).** The bottom portion of Figure 4–11, Section III, shows the results obtained from Parts A, B, and C circled. For the case illustrated, the number of diagnoses is declared *multiple*, there are *no data reviewed*, and the risk of complications is *moderate;* therefore a *moderately complex* level of decision making has been assigned to be used for coding and billing purposes.

DOCUMENTATION TERMINOLOGY

Terminology for Evaluation and Management Services

While learning the complexities of medical documentation and how important it is as it relates to coding and billing, you have discovered that you must have a good foundation of medical terminology. To use the diagnostic and procedure code books efficiently, you must become familiar with their language, abbreviations, and symbols. The first terms introduced are most commonly used for evaluation and management services.

New Versus Established Patient

In coding E/M services, two categories of patients are considered: the new patient and the established patient. A **new patient** is one who *has not received* any professional services from the physician or another physician of the same specialty who belongs to the same group practice *within the past 3 years*. An **established patient** is one who *has received* professional services from the physician or another physician of the same specialty who belongs to the same group practice *within the past 3 years*. Medicare policies regarding the definition of new and established patients may have different requirements and are discussed in Chapter 12.

A physician may provide several types of services to evaluate and manage a patient who is seeking medical care (i.e., consultation, referral, concurrent care, continuity of care, critical care, emergency care, or counseling).

Consultation

A **consultation** includes services rendered by a physician whose opinion or advice is requested by another physician or agency in the evaluation or treatment of a patient's illness or a suspected problem. The requesting physician must document the request in the patient's health record and the consulting physician should state: "Patient is seen at the request of Dr. John Doe for a . . . reason." Consultations may occur in a home, office, hospital, extended care facility, or other location. A physician consultant recommends diagnostic or therapeutic services and may initiate these services if requested by the referring physician. The opinion must be in writing, documented in a consultation report, and communicated to the referring physician. The consultant may order a diagnostic or therapeutic service to formulate the opinion at an initial or subsequent visit. Reimbursement is significantly more than for an equivalent office visit.

Referral

A **referral** is the transfer of the total or specific care of a patient from one physician to another for known problems. It is not a consultation. For example, a patient is sent by a primary case physician to an orthopedist for care of a fracture.

However, when dealing with managed care plans, the term "referral" is also used when requesting an authorization for the patient to receive services elsewhere (e.g., referral for laboratory tests, radiology procedures, specialty care). As a courtesy, the physician may send a thank-you note to the referring physician with comments about the patient's condition.

COMPLEXITY

SECTION III A AND B

A **NUMBER OF DIAGNOSES OR TREATMENT OPTIONS**

Problems to exam physician	Number X points = Result		
Self-limited or minor (stable, improved or worsening)	Max = 2	1	
Est. problem (to examiner); stable, improved		1	
Est. problem (to examiner); worsening		2	
New problem (to examiner); no additional workup planned	Max = 1 1	3	3
New prob. (to examiner); add. workup planned		4	
		TOTAL	3

Bring total to line A in final result for complexity

B **AMOUNT AND/OR COMPLEXITY OF DATA TO BE REVIEWED**

Data to be reviewed	Points
Review and/or order of clinical lab tests	1
Review and/or order of tests in the radiology section of CPT	1
Review and/or order of tests in the medicine section of CPT	1
Discussion of test results with performing physician	1
Decision to obtain old records and/or obtain history from someone other than patient	1
Review and summarization of old records and/or obtaining history from someone other than patient and/or discussion of case with another health care provider	2
Independent visualization of image, tracing or specimen itself (not simply review of report)	2
TOTAL	0

Bring total to line B in final result for complexity

Draw a line down the column with 2 or 3 circles and circle decision making level OR draw a line down the column with the center circle and circle the decision making level.

A	Number diagnoses or treatment options	≤ 1 Minimal	2 Limited	3 Multiple	≥ 4 Extensive
B	Amount and complexity of data	≤ 1 Minimal or low	2 Limited	3 Moderate	≥ 4 Extensive
C	Highest risk	Minimal	Low	Moderate	High
	Type of decision making	Straight-foward	Low complex	Moderate complex	High complex

Note: The wound was not a considering factor in the medical decision making.

FIGURE 4–11 Section III of the review/audit worksheet. Part A: Number of diagnoses or treatment options. Part B: Amount or complexity of data to be reviewed. Lower one third: Used to compile the results obtained from Parts A, B, and C (see Figure 4–10) to determine the level of medical decision making. Circled points and words relate to a moderately complex level of decision making for the example case (see Figure 4–8, *A*) for coding and billing purposes. *(From the Iowa Medical Society, IMS Services, West Des Moines, Iowa, 1998.)*

SECTION III

C

RISK OF COMPLICATIONS AND/OR MORBIDITY OR MORTALITY

Level of risk	Presenting problem(s)	Diagnostic procedure(s) ordered	Management options selected
MINIMAL	• One self-limited or minor problem *(e.g., cold, insect bite, tinea corporis)*	• Laboratory tests requiring venipuncture • Chest x-rays • KOH prep • EKG/EEG • Urinalysis • Ultrasound *e.g. echo*	• Rest • Gargles • Elastic bandages • Superficial dressings
LOW	• Two or more self-limited or minor problems • One stable chronic illness *(e.g., well-controlled hypertension, non-insulin dependent diabetes, cataract, BPH)* • Acute uncomplicated illness or injury *(e.g., cystitis, allergic rhinitis, simple sprain)*	• Physiologic test not under stress *(e.g., pulmonary function tests)* • Non-cardiovascular imaging studies with contrast *(e.g., barium enema)* • Superficial needle biopsies • Clinical laboratory tests requiring arterial puncture • Skin biopsies	• Over-the-counter drugs • Minor surgery with no identified risk factors • Physical therapy • Occupational therapy • IV fluids without additives
MODERATE	• *One* or more *chronic illnesses* with mild exacerbation, progression or side effects of treatment • Two or more stable chronic illnesses • Undiagnosed new problem with uncertain prognosis *(e.g., lump in breast)* • Acute illness with systemic symptoms *(e.g., pyelonephritis, pneumonitis, colitis)* • Acute complicated injury *(e.g., head injury with brief loss of consciousness)*	• Physiologic test under stress *(e.g., cardiac stress test, fetal contraction stress test)* • Diagnostic endoscopies with no identified risk factors • Deep needle or incisional biopsy • Cardiovascular imaging studies with contrast and no identified risk factors *(e.g., arteriogram, cardiac cath)* • Obtain fluid from body cavity *(e.g., lumbar puncture, thoracentesis, culdocentesis)*	• Minor surgery with identified risk factors • Elective major surgery (open percutaneous or endoscopic) with no identified risk factors • *Prescription drug management* • Therapeutic nuclear medicine • IV fluids with additives • Closed treatment of fracture or dislocation without manipulation
HIGH	• One or more chronic illnesses with severe exacerbation, progression or side effects of tx • Acute or chronic illnesses or injuries that may pose a threat to life or bodily function *(e.g., multiple trauma, acute MI, pulmonary embolus, severe respiratory distress, progressive severe rheumatoid arthritis, psychiatric illness with potential threat to self or others, peritonitis, acute renal failure)* • An abrupt change in neurological status *(e.g., seizure, TIA, weakness, sensory loss)*	• Cardiovascular imaging studies with contrast with identified risk factors • Cardiac electrophysiological tests • Diagnostic endoscopies with identified risk factors • Discography	• Elective major surgery (open, percutaneous or endoscopic) with identified risk factor • Emergency major surgery (open, percutaneous or endoscopic) • Parenteral controlled substances • Drug therapy requiring intensive monitoring for toxicity • Decision not to resuscitate or de-escalate care because of poor prognosis

FIGURE 4–12 Section III, Part C, of the review/audit worksheet used for determining the level of risk. The highlighted areas relate to a moderate level of risk for the example case (see Figure 4–8, *A*) for coding purposes. *(From the Iowa Medical Society, IMS Services, West Des Moines, Iowa, 1998.)*

Concurrent Care

Concurrent care is the providing of similar services (e.g., hospital visits) to the same patient by more than one physician on the same day. Usually, such cases involve the presence of a physical disorder (e.g., diabetes) at the same time as the primary admitting diagnosis, and this may alter the course of treatment or lengthen recovery time for the primary condition. For example, two internists (a general internist and a cardiologist) see the same patient in the hospital on the same day. The general internist admitted the patient for diabetes and requested that the cardiologist also follow the patient's periodic chest pain and arrhythmia. If the second doctor is not identified in carrier records as a cardiologist, the claim may be denied. This is because the services appear to be duplicated by physicians of the same specialty. When billing insurance companies, physicians providing concurrent care may be cross-referenced on the claim form. Medicare has a list that includes 62 specialties and subspecialties to help carriers more accurately judge whether concurrent care is necessary. Periodically, the physician should check with the carrier's provider service representative to see if the provider has updated its subspecialty status so that claims for concurrent care are not denied.

Continuity of Care

If a case involves **continuity of care** (e.g., a patient who has received treatment for a condition and is then referred by the physician to a second physician for treatment for the same condition), both physicians are responsible to provide arrangements for the patient's continuing care. In such a case, records must be provided by the referring physician and the insurance billing specialist must obtain summaries or records of the patient's previous treatment. Obtain hospital reports before coding if the patient was seen in the hospital, emergency department, or outpatient department. Contact the hospital's health record department for copies of reports after outpatient treatment or after a patient's discharge. In some cases, coding from hospital reports can increase reimbursement but can delay submission of claims because reports may not be available in a timely manner.

Critical Care

Critical care means the intensive care provided in a variety of acute life-threatening conditions requiring constant "full attention" by a physician. It can be provided in the critical care unit or emergency department (ED) of a hospital. A critical illness or injury acutely impairs one or more vital organ systems such that there is a high probability of imminent or life-threatening deterioration in the patient's condition. Examples of vital organ system failure include, but are not limited to, central nervous system failure, circulatory failure, shock, and renal, hepatic, metabolic, or respiratory failure. Critical care may sometimes, but not always, be rendered in a critical care area, such as a coronary care unit (CCU), intensive care unit (ICU), respiratory care unit (RCU), or ED, also called the emergency room (ER).

Emergency Care

Emergency care differs from critical care in that it may be given by the physician in a hospital emergency department or in a physician's office setting. Emergency care is that provided to acutely ill patients and may or may not involve organ system failure but does require immediate medical attention. In physician-directed emergency care, advanced life support, the physician is located in a hospital emergency or critical care department, and is in two-way voice communication with ambulance or rescue personnel outside the hospital. The physician directs the performance of necessary medical procedures. Physicians who work in the ED of a hospital are not employees of the hospital and bill separately for the services they perform.

In the Medicare program, an emergency medical condition is currently defined as a medical condition manifesting itself by acute symptoms of sufficient severity (including severe pain) such that the absence of immediate medical attention could reasonably be expected to result in placing the patient's health in serious jeopardy, serious impairment to body functions, or serious dysfunction of any body organ or part.

Many states have adopted the prudent lay person definition of an emergency as defined in the Balanced Budget Act of 1996. This is similarly stated as "any medical condition of recent onset and severity, including but not limited to severe pain, that would lead to a prudent lay person, possessing an average knowledge of medicine and health, to believe that his or her condition, sickness, or injury is of such a nature that failure to obtain immediate medical care could result in placing the patient's health in serious jeopardy, serious impairment to bodily functions, or serious dysfunction of bodily organ or part."

Counseling

Counseling is a discussion with a patient, family, or both concerning one or more of the following: diagnostic results, impressions, or recommended diagnostic studies; prognosis; risks and benefits of treatment options; instructions for treatment or follow-up; importance of compliance with chosen treatment options; risk factor reduction; and patient and family education.

Diagnostic Terminology and Abbreviations

When completing the health record, some physicians write "imp" (impression) or "Dx" (diagnosis), which usually serves as the diagnosis when completing the claim. If the diagnosis is not in the chart note and there is doubt about the diagnosis, always pull the chart and request that the physician review it. Attach a note to the insurance claim for the physician to read before signing the form. If the patient has been in the hospital, request a copy of the discharge summary, which contains the admitting and discharge diagnoses.

Official American Hospital Association policy states that "abbreviations should be totally eliminated from the more vital sections of the health record, such as final diagnosis, operative notes, discharge summaries, and descriptions of special procedures." Many physicians are not aware of this policy, and the final diagnosis may appear as an abbreviation on the patient's record. Frequently, an abbreviation translates to several meanings. Use your medical dictionary (most list abbreviations alphabetically with the unabbreviated words) to interpret the abbreviation or ask the physician when clarification is needed.

Refer to Figure 4–13, which indicates commonly used abbreviations that appear in office progress notes. In the *Workbook*, refer to the detailed list of common medical abbreviations in Appendix A. Additional knowledge will be obtained when you complete each assignment involving a patient's health record in the *Workbook* because you must define all of the abbreviations.

If a lay term appears on a patient record, the correct medical term should be substituted to locate the correct diagnostic code (e.g., "contusion" for "bruise").

An **eponym** (term including the name of a person, e.g., Graves' disease) should not be used when a comparable anatomic term can be used in its place (Example 4.2).

Example 4.2

Eponym	Comparable Medical Term
Buerger's disease	Thromboangiitis obliterans
Graves' disease	Exophthalmic goiter
Wilks syndrome	Myasthenia gravis

The word **"acute"** refers to a condition that runs a short but relatively severe course. The word **"chronic"** means a condition persisting over a long period of time. However, the word "recurrent" is preferable for certain conditions and should be used instead of "chronic." For example, if "chronic asthma" is charted, it should be coded as "recurrent asthma." For proper documentation to support chronic conditions, two criteria are that the documentation actually states something about the chronic condition and that the conditions are pertinent to the patient's current treatment. For example, if a physician states "controlled diabetes"; this is a fact. If the physician asks the patient about his or her sugar level and diet and documents the findings, then something specific has been identified about the chronic condition and this would pass an audit for correct documentation.

Whenever the words "question of," "suspected," "rule out," or the abbreviation "R/O" are used in connection with a disease or illness, do not code these conditions as if they existed or were established. Instead, code the chief complaint, sign, or symptom. These are only a few of the many terms used in documentation.

An abnormal or unexpected finding without elaboration in the health record is insufficient documentation and should be described. Commonly used phrases or abbreviations that may not support billing of services are "WNL" (within normal limits), "noncontributory," "negative/normal," "other than the above, all systems were normal," and so on. For example, phrases used to document findings, such as "all extremities are within normal limits," do not indicate how many extremities or which ones were examined. Documentation must indicate exactly what limb was examined, and abbreviated wording would not pass an external audit. If it is determined such phrases are "canned" notes that can mean no assessment was actually performed, then this is fraud.

Another phrase commonly used when examining a patient and the findings are within normal limits is the word, "negative" (e.g., "ears, nose, and throat negative" or "chest x-rays negative"). The physician needs to document that there were no abnormalities in the system being examined. Detailed documentation justifies billed services by providing verification and allows points when an external audit is performed. Thus it should be dictated "Chest film (or report) was reviewed." Or "Chest x-ray report was read."

Directional Terms

The following terms are commonly used to describe location of pain and injuries to areas of the abdomen, as shown in Figure 4-14, *A* (four quadrants) and *B* (nine regions):

Right upper quadrant (RUQ) or right hypochondriac: Liver (right lobe), gallbladder, part of the pancreas, parts of the small and large intestines
Epigastric: Upper middle region above the stomach
Left upper quadrant (LUQ) or left hypochondriac: Liver (left lobe), stomach, spleen, part of the pancreas, parts of the small and large intestines
Right and left lumbar: Middle, right, and left regions of the waist
Umbilical: Central region near the navel
Right lower quadrant (RLQ) or right inguinal: parts of the small and large intestines, right ovary, right uterine (fallopian) tube, appendix, and right ureter
Hypogastric: Middle region below the umbilical region contains urinary bladder and female uterus
Left lower quadrant (LLQ) or left inguinal: Parts of the small and large intestines, left ovary, left uterine tube, and left ureter

GIOVANNI, CARLOS A.

DATE	PROGRESS NOTES
11-11-xx	Pt referred to College Hospital ER by employer for workers' compensation injury. I was called in as on-call
	neurosurgeon to evaluate the pt. Pt states that today at 2 p.m. he fell from the roof of a private home while
	installing an antenna at 2231 Duarte St., Woodland Hills, XY 12345 in Woodland Hills County. He describes the
	incident as follows: "When I was attaching the base of an antenna, the weight of the antenna shifted and knocked
	me off the roof." Pt complains of head pain and indicates brief loss of consciousness. I performed a C HX/PX.
	Complete skull x-rays showed fractured skull. CT of head/brain (without contrast) indicates well-defined R.
	subdural hematoma. Pt suffering from cerebral concussion; no open wound. Tr plan: Adm pt to College
	Hospital (5 p.m.) and schedule R infratentorial craniotomy to evacuate hematoma. (H/MDM). Obtained
	authorization and prepared Dr.'s First Report.
	AP/llf *Astro Parkinson, MD*
11-12-xx	Performed R infratentorial craniotomy and evacuated subdural hematoma. Pt stable and returned to room; will be
	seen daily. TD: Estimated RTW 1-15-xx. Possible cranial defect & head disfigurement resulting. Pt to be
	hospitalized for approx 2 weeks.
	AP/llf *Astro Parkinson, MD*
11-13-xx	HV (EPF HX/PX M/MDM). Pt improving; recommend consult with Dr. Graff for cranial defect. Authorization
	obtained from adjuster (Steve Burroughs) at State Comp.
	AP/llf *Astro Parkinson, MD*
11-14-xx	Pt seen in cons by Dr. Cosmo Graff who stated he does not recommend correcting PO cranial defect. Both
	Dr. Graff and I explained how the defect resulted from the injury; there may be some improvement over time.
	Pt states he is grateful to be alive (EPF HX/PX M/MDM).
	AP/llf *Astro Parkinson, MD*
11-15-xx	Daily HV (EPF HX/PX M/MDM). Pt progressing appropriately; no complications have occurred.
thru	
11-29-xx	AP/llf *Astro Parkinson, MD*
11-30-xx	DC from hosp. Permanent cranial defect resulting from fracture and surgery. RTO 1 wk.
	AP/llf *Astro Parkinson, MD*
12-7-xx	OV (EPF HX/PX LC/MDM) Pt doing very well. No HA or visual disturbances, BP 120/80, alert and oriented.
	He is anxious to return to work. Pt cautioned about maintaining low activity level until released. RTO 2 wks.
	AP/llf *Astro Parkinson, MD*
12-21-xx	OV (PF HX/PX SF/MDM). Pt continues to improve. Suggested he start a walking program 3 x wk and monitor
	symptoms. May do light activity and lifting (10 lbs). Adv to call if any symptoms return. RTO 10 days.
	AP/llf *Astro Parkinson, MD*
12-29-xx	OV (PF HX/PX SF/MDM). Pt did not experience any symptoms with increased activity. No further trt necessary.
	Pt will increase activity and call if any problems occur. Pt scheduled to resume reg W on 1-15-xx. Final report
	submitted to workers' compensation carrier.
	AP/llf *Astro Parkinson, MD*

FIGURE 4–13 Medical office progress notes indicating some common medical abbreviations and symbols used in a patient's health record.

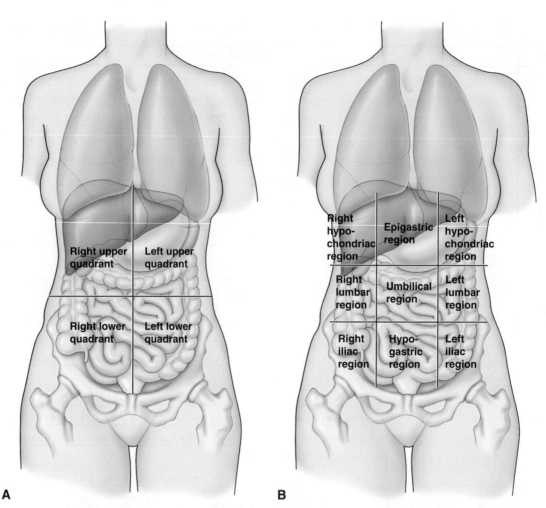

FIGURE 4–14   Regions of the abdomen. **A,** Four quadrants. **B,** Nine regions. (*From Herlihy B, Maebius NK: The human body in health and illness, ed 2, St Louis, Elsevier Science, 2003.*)

Surgical Terminology

Surgical procedures of the integumentary system, such as repair of lacerations, are listed in the procedure code book as *simple, intermediate,* or *complex* repairs. Simple lacerations are superficial, requiring one-layer closure. Intermediate lacerations require layered closure of one or more of the deeper layers of the skin and tissues. Complex lacerations require more than layered closure and may require reconstructive surgery. Documentation should list the length (in centimeters) of all incisions and layers of involved tissues (subcutaneous, fascia, muscle, and grafts) so that correct procedure codes for excision of lesions and type of repair can be determined.

If time is a factor in coding for reimbursement, then D documentation should list the length of time spent on the procedure, especially if of unusual duration, such as, prolonged services, counseling, or team conferences. This should be stated somewhere in the report.

If state-of-the-art instruments or equipment are used, document the equipment as well as the time spent using it.

Therapeutic or cosmetic surgical procedures should be broken down into two categories—state how much of the procedure was functional and how much was cosmetic or therapeutic. Generally, the insurance carrier pays for the functional portion of the procedure even if there is no coverage for cosmetic or therapeutic procedures.

If you type reports to be submitted with insurance claims to help justify the claim, you should also become familiar with the terms for various operational incisions (Figure 4–15). Terms such as *undermining* (cut in a horizontal fashion), *take down* (to take apart), or *lysis of adhesions* (destruction of scar tissue) appear in many operations but should not be coded separately. Note the *position* (e.g., lithotomy, dorsal) of the patient during the operation and the *surgical approach* (e.g., vaginal, abdominal). These help determine the proper code selection. Major errors can occur when an insurance biller is not familiar with the medical terms being used. Ask the physician to clarify the case if there is a question, because medical terminology is very technical and can puzzle even the most knowledge-able insurance billing specialist. Additional key words to

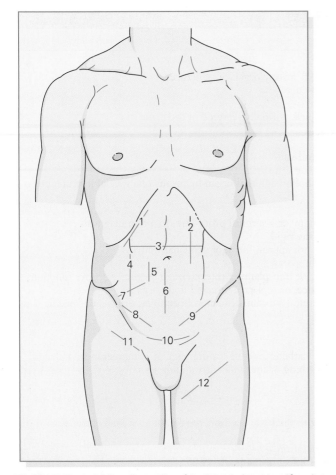

FIGURE 4–15 Operational incisions. Anterior (front) view: *1*, subcostal incision; *2*, paramedian incision; *3*, transverse incision; *4*, upper right rectus incision; *5*, midrectus incision; *6*, midline incision; *7*, lower right rectus incision; *8*, McBurney or right iliac incision; *9*, left iliac incision; *10*, suprapubic incision; *11*, hernia incision; and *12*, femoral incision.

look for that may affect code selection and reimbursement besides terminology listed in Table 4.1 are listed here along with brief definitions:

Bilateral: Pertaining to both sides
Blood loss of more than 600 mL: Severe bleeding
Complete or total: Entire or whole
Complicated by: Involved with other situations at the same time
Hemorrhage: Escape of blood from vessels; bleeding
Initial: First procedure or service
Multiple: Affecting many parts of the body at the same time
Partial: Only a part, not complete
Prolonged procedure due to: Series of steps extended in time to get desired result
Simple: Single and not compound or complex
Subsequent: Second or more procedures or services
Surgical: Pertaining to surgery
Uncomplicated: Not intricately involved; straightforward (procedure)
Unilateral: Pertaining to one side
Unusual findings or circumstances: rare or not usual conclusion
Very difficult: hard to do, requiring extra effort and skill

Additional words used to detail accidents and injuries are shown in Figures 15–5 through 15–9.

If you would like a more thorough discussion of medical terminology, many good books are available.*

*Chabner D-E: *The language of medicine,* ed 7, St Louis, Saunders, 2004; Leonard PC: *Building a medical vocabulary,* St Louis, Elsevier Science, 1997.

Table 4.1 Terminology Used in Coding Procedures

Medical Term	Definition
Ablation	Surgical removal of a body part, as by incision
Acquired	Condition or disorder contracted after birth; not hereditary or innate
Amputation	Removal of a body part, limb, or organ
Anastomosis	Surgical or pathologic connection of two tubular structures
Anomaly	Congenital or developmental defect; deviation from normal
Arthrocentesis	Surgical puncture of a joint to remove fluid
Arthrodesis	To surgically immobilize a joint; fusion
Aspiration	To draw in by inhaling or draw out by suction
Biopsy	Removal of living tissue for microscopic examination
Cauterization	Means of destroying tissue, treating infectious wounds, or stopping bleeding with use of chemicals (silver nitrate), heat, freezing, or electrical current
Chemosurgery	Use of chemicals to destroy tissue
Chemotherapy	Use of chemicals to treat disease
Closed treatment	To treat a condition (e.g., a fracture) without surgically opening the location closure to bring together the edges of a wound
Congenital	Condition present from birth; believed to be inherited
Curettage	Scraping of a cavity to remove tissue, growths, or debris
Débridement	Excision of dead or damaged tissue and foreign matter from a wound

Continued

Table 4.1 Terminology Used in Coding Procedures—cont'd

Medical Term	Definition
Decompression	Removal of pressure
Decortication	Removal of external layer (beneath the capsule) from any organ or structure
Defect	Imperfection, malformation, dysfunction, or absence
Destructive	Causing ruin; opposite of constructive
Dialysis	To separate from the blood harmful waste products normally secreted in the urine
Dilation	Enlargement of a hollow structure or opening
Discission	Incision or cutting into
Dissection	Cutting of parts for the purpose of separation and study
Drainage	Continuous withdrawal of fluid from a wound, sore, or cavity
Endoscopy	Visual examination of the interior of a canal or hollow internal organ by means of a special instrument
Evacuation	Removal of waste material
Excision	The act of cutting out
Exploration	An active examination, usually involving endoscopy or a surgical procedure, to aid in diagnosis
Fixation	The act of holding or fastening; immobilize; make rigid
Foreign body	Any substance or particle in the body that does not appear, form, or grow naturally
Fulguration	Destruction by means of high-frequency electric sparks
Graft	Any organ, tissue, or object used for implanting or transplanting to encourage healing, improve function, safeguard against infection, improve appearance, or replace a diseased body organ
Immunoassay	Any of several methods used for measuring chemical substances such as hormones, drugs, and specific proteins
Implant	Tissue or substance inserted or grafted into body
Incision	To cut into
Indwelling	Located or implanted inside the body, such as a catheter or tube for drainage or administration of drugs
In situ	Localized; in one specific location without disturbing or invading surrounding tissue
Instrumentation	Application or use of instruments or tools
Internal	Within the body
Insertion	To place or implant; site of attachment
Introduction	Device for controlling and directing; to insert into the body via tube, needle, oral, or anal entrance
Ligation	The process of binding or tying a body structure
Lysis	Destruction, decomposition, breakdown, or separation
Manipulation	Use of hands to produce a desired movement or effect in the body
Marsupialization	Surgical conversion of a closed cavity (abscess or cyst) into an open pouch to allow healing
Obstruction	Blockage of a structure that prevents it from functioning normally
Occlusion	Blockage of any passage, canal, opening, or vessel in the body; acquired or congenital
Open treatment	To lay open internal parts to administer treatment
Paring	Surgical removal of foreign material or dead or damaged tissue by cutting or scraping
Percutaneous	Through the skin
Qualitative	Referring to the quality, value, or nature of something
Quantitative	A measurable amount or portion
Radical	Extreme or drastic treatment or surgery aimed at eliminating a major disease by removing all affected tissue and any surrounding tissue that might be diseased
Reconstitution	Returning a substance that has been changed to its original state for preservation and storage
Reconstruction	Repair, mold, change, or alter to effect recovery
Reduction	To restore to a normal position
Repair	To remedy, replace, or heal; restore to a healthy state
Replantation	Surgical replacement of a body part
Revision	To amend or alter; to correct or improve
Resection	Partial excision of a body structure
Shunt	An artificial passage constructed to divert flow from one route to another
Suture	Material (wire, thread, or staples) used in closing or attaching body tissue; to unite body tissue by stitching together; the seam formed by stitching body tissue together; line of union (border or joint) such as between the skull bones
Therapy	Treatment of disease or pathologic conditions
Transection	A cross section; division by cutting transversely
Transposition	Displacement of an organ from one side of the body to the other; congenital anomaly in which a part of the body normally appearing on the right side is located on the left side of the body
Traumatic	Physical or psychological wound or injury

REVIEW AND AUDIT OF HEALTH RECORDS

Internal Reviews

Prospective Review

The first type of **internal review** is **prospective review,** also termed *prebilling audit* or *review*, which is done *before* billing is submitted. This may be done by some medical practices daily, weekly, or monthly.

● Stage one of a prospective review is done to verify that completed encounter forms match patients seen according to the appointment schedule and have been posted on the daysheet. A prospective review is begun by obtaining the encounter forms and locating the dates in question for the review in the appointment schedule, printing the schedule as verification. The appointment schedule is then compared to the encounter forms to match patients for the date in question. Next check to see if all charges (procedures or services) have been posted on the daysheet or daily transaction register.

● Stage two of a prospective review is done to verify that all procedures or services and diagnoses listed on the encounter form match data on the insurance claim form. To perform this stage, use the completed claim form or print an insurance billing worksheet. Match the information on the claim or worksheet with the date of service, procedure or service, and diagnosis on the encounter form. It is possible that one or more diagnoses may not match. A common reason is because an active diagnosis has not been entered into the computer system and the computer defaults to the last diagnosis given for an established patient. Another problem occurs when the diagnosis is not linked to the procedure. Such problems must be found before billing and corrected before claims are printed.

Retrospective Review

The second type of internal review is called **retrospective review,** which is done *after* billing insurance carriers. A coder or insurance biller may be asked to perform a retrospective review to determine whether there is a lack of documentation. To accomplish this, pull 15 to 20 health records per provider from the last 2 to 4 months at random. Recommended internal audit tools are

Pencil
Internal record review worksheets
Current procedure code book
Current diagnostic code book
Current Healthcare Common Procedures Coding System (HCPCS) code book
Medical dictionary
Abbreviation reference book
Drug reference book (e.g., *Physicians' Desk Reference* or drug reference for nurses)
Laboratory reference book
Provider's manual for insurance program or plan
Insurance carrier's newsletters

Forms similar to the Internal Record Review Form shown in Figures 4–8 through 4–12 may be used as tools to gather information from the patient's record, laboratory reports, pathology reports, radiology reports, operative reports, and other diagnostic tests. If the physician's documentation is inadequate, errors or deficiencies will appear as the review is being conducted. You will discover that doing an internal review of this type is not an exact science and critical thinking skills are put into use. Because documentation guidelines and code policies are updated and refined periodically, it is extremely important to read and keep bulletins from all insurance carriers, especially from the local fiscal Medicare intermediary. Advise the physician of any new requirements. This resource may be the only notification of changes unless you routinely attend local or national workshops.

EXTERNAL AUDIT

An **external audit** is a retrospective review of medical and financial records at the request of a physician, an outside contractor, an insurance company, or external reviewer as part of the practice's compliance plan. It may be done by a Medicare representative to investigate suspected fraud or abusive billing practices.

In 1984, Michigan signed into law the Health Care Claim Act with felony penalties ranging to 10 years in prison and fines of up to $50,000 per count for attempting to defraud an insurance company. Other states are following suit in establishing such laws. Another federal law to prevent overuse of services and to spot Medicare fraud is the Federal False Claims Amendment Act of 1986, which is discussed in detail in Chapter 12.

Most insurance companies perform routine audits on unusual billing patterns. Insurance companies have computer software programs capable of editing and screening insurance claims to identify billing excesses or potential abuses before payment is rendered. Insurance carriers may hire undercover agents who visit physicians' offices if overuse and

Continued

EXTERNAL AUDIT—cont'd

abuse of procedure codes are suspected. Physicians who charge excessive fees are routinely audited by most carriers. Carriers spot check by sending questionnaires to patients and asking them if they received medical care from Dr. Doe to verify the services rendered. The answers are then compared with what the physician billed. Many insurance companies have installed antifraud telephone hotlines or billing question telephone lines for patients. Investigations can result from such calls, depending on the circumstances. Tips also come from peer review organizations, state licensing boards, whistle-blowing physicians, ex-staff members, and patients. If there is any suspicion of fraud, the insurance company will notify the medical practice, specify a date and time at which they will come to the office, and indicate which records they wish to audit (Figure 4–16).

Investigators question the patient, look at the documentation in the medical record, and interview the staff and all physicians who have participated in the care of the patient. Points are awarded if documentation is present. Auditors also look at appointment books and add up the hours the physician sees patients on any given day when a medical practice uses time-based procedure codes when submitting insurance claims.

Audit Prevention

Health Insurance Portability and Accountability Act Compliance Program

As mentioned in Chapter 2, the HIPAA was created in 1996 by the Department of Health and Human Services (HHS) Office of the Inspector General (OIG) to combat fraud and

abuse, to protect workers so they could obtain and maintain health insurance if changing or losing a job, and establish a medical savings account. The act also developed the concept of compliance planning as related to clinical documentation. OIG and HHS as well as the Health Care Compliance Association (HCCA) and many other health care agencies have asked physicians to voluntarily develop and implement compliance programs. OIG published guidelines to assist a physician and his or her staff in establishing a medical practice's compliance program to enhance documentation for Medicare cases as well as all patients seen by the physician. Purposes of a compliance program are to reduce fraudulent insurance claims and to provide quality care to patients.

A *compliance program* is composed of policies and procedures to accomplish uniformity, consistency, and conformity in medical record keeping that fulfills official requirements. If a medical practice experiences an external Medicare audit, HHS OIG and the Department of Justice considers that the medical practice made a reasonable effort to avoid and detect misbehavior if a compliance plan has been in place. When errors are found and a determination is made that fraud did occur, an existing compliance program shows a good faith effort that the medical practice is committed to ethical and legal business. There is no single best compliance program because every medical practice is different. However, there are some elements that lead to a successful compliance program. These are

- Written standards of conduct
- Written policies and procedures
- Compliance officer and/or committee to operate and monitor the program
- Training program for all affected employees
- Process to give complaints anonymously
- Internal audit performed routinely
- Investigation and remediation plan for problems that develop
- Response plan for improper or illegal activities

A compliance program must be tailored to fit the needs of each medical practice depending on its corporate structure, mission, size, and employee composition. The statutes, regulations, and guidelines of the federal and state health insurance programs, as well as the policies and procedures of the private health plans should be integrated into every medical practice's compliance program. The ultimate goals are to improve quality of services and control of claims submission, and to reduce fraud, waste, abuse, and the cost of health care to federal, state, and private health insurers.

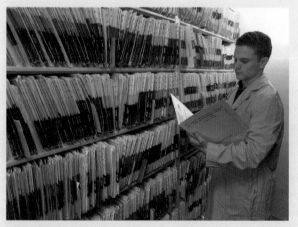

FIGURE 4–16   Insurance billing specialist searching for a patient's chart in the files to pull records for an external audit.

Software Edit Checks

An *edit check* is a good audit prevention measure to have in place because the software program automatically screens transmitted insurance claims and electronically examines them for errors and/or conflicting code entries. Carriers accept a variety of levels of service; however, if only one or two levels are consistently listed, this is usually not realistic and will attract attention and, possibly, an audit. If services are downcoded and the physician neglected to document the correct level of services performed, an addendum to a medical record must be made to justify the level of service reported (Figure 4–17). Amended chart notes must be labeled "Addendum" or "Late entry," dated on the day of the amendment, and signed by the physician.

There must be correct use of diagnostic and procedural codes with modifiers. Modifiers are two digits added onto CPT codes for procedures and services and are not used in diagnostic coding. These are further discussed in Chapter 6. If the diagnosis does not match the service provided, the claim will be thrown out by the edit check of the computer program. It is equally important that everything involved in patient care be well documented so that selected diagnostic and procedural codes are supported (Figure 4–18).

In subsequent chapters, you will obtain further knowledge on what needs to be documented in relationship to diagnostic and procedure codes. Information on the Civil Monetary Penalties Law to prosecute cases of Medicare and Medicaid fraud can be found in Chapter 12.

Once an individual has been found guilty of committing a Medicare or Medicaid program-related crime, 5 to 15 years or lifetime exclusion from program participation is mandatory under Section 1128(a) of the Social Security Act. An individual can be anyone who participates in fraud or abuse, including the physician, nurse, home health aide, insurance billing specialist, claims assistance professional, electronic claims processor, and medical assistants. Being an excluded individual is a serious matter and requires

Yuen Wong DOB: 07-11-XX REF: John Doe, MD

12-03-20XX

Blood:	0		
Sugar:	0		
Ketones:	0	BP:	136/80
Alb:	0	Temp:	98.5°
PH:	6	Weight:	181 lbs.
Bili:	0		

ORIGINAL CHART NOTE

Put him on Vibra-Tabs 100 mg bid for acute bronchitis. He is to return in 1 week. Blood pressure is to be monitored.

Gerald Practon
Gerald Practon, MD

mtf

Addendum to Chart note of 12-03-20XX, prepared 2-10-20XX

Established patient presents with noticeable wheezing and complaining of tightness in chest. Patient has a history of chronic bronchitis and these symptoms have been present in patient's previous episodes of upper respiratory infections. Patient is afebrile. Symptoms first occurred yesterday. Sputum is discolored, slight cough. Patient has a history of chronic urinary tract infection with previous acute episode of pyelonephritis. Urinalysis performed to evaluate chronic urinary tract infection. Noticeable weight gain (10 lbs.) since patient discontinued smoking last fall.

ADDENDUM

Gerald Practon
Gerald Practon, MD

FIGURE 4–17 Example of an addendum to a patient's health record to justify the level of service reported. The insurance carrier downcoded the services from level 99213 to 99212.

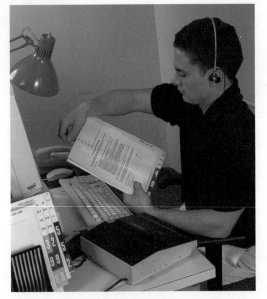

FIGURE 4-18 Medical transcriptionist inserting a transcribed chart note into a patient's health record.

a reinstatement process to work in those environments again. Recovering from your loss of credibility and trustworthiness may be a monumental task. Do not jeopardize your future in the medical field!

Faxing Documents

The common term *fax* is derived from the word **facsimile**, which means transmission of written and graphic matter by electronic means. We know that faxes are an important communication tool. Faxing has been used to transmit insurance claims data directly to an electronic claims processor, resubmit an unpaid insurance claim, send further documentation on a claim to insurance carriers, obtain preauthorization for surgery on a patient, network with other insurance billers, and send medical reports between offices and to other medical facilities across the country. Unless otherwise prohibited by state law, information that is transmitted by fax is acceptable and may be filed with the patient's health record. Documents to be faxed can be a graphic illustration, typewritten, or handwritten with pen. Pencil does not fax to recipient as clearly as does pen. To prevent deterioration of documents faxed on thermal paper (when the machine is not a plain paper fax), photocopy the document onto regular paper before it is filed with health records. Be sure to refer to the HIPAA Privacy Rules in Chapter 2 to refresh your knowledge when faxing protected health information.

Sensitive Information

From the legal standpoint, protecting the patient's confidentiality in the fax process is critical. If, because of circumstances, health records or a medical report must be faxed, you should have the patient sign an authorization to release information via fax equipment. The American Health Information Management Association (AHIMA) advises that fax machines *should not* be used for *routine* transmission of patient information. AHIMA recommends that documents should be faxed *only* when (1) hand or mail delivery will not meet the needs of immediate patient care or (2) required by a third party for ongoing certification of payment for a hospitalized patient.

Documents containing information on sexually transmitted diseases, drug or alcohol treatment, or human immunodeficiency virus (HIV) status should not be faxed. Psychiatric records and psychotherapy notes should not be faxed except for emergency requests. Psychotherapy notes may be defined as notes recorded in any medium that document or analyze the contents of conversation during a private, group, joint, or family counseling session. Psychotherapy notes exclude medication prescription and monitoring, counseling session start and stop times, modalities and frequencies of treatment furnished, results of clinical tests, and any summary of the following items: diagnosis, functional status, treatment plan, symptoms, prognosis, and progress to date.

Fax machines should be located in secure or restricted access areas. Do not fax to machines in mail rooms, office lobbies, or other open areas unless they are secured with passwords. To ensure protection, a cover sheet should be used for all transmissions. This can be a half sheet, full sheet, or small self-adhesive form attached to the top of the first page. It should contain the following information:

● Name of recipient
● Name of sender
● Date
● Total number of pages including the cover sheet
● Fax and telephone numbers of recipient and sender in case of transmittal problems (e.g., lost page or dropped line)
● A statement that it is personal, privileged, and confidential medical information intended for the named recipient only (Figure 4-19).

Transmittal Destination

Noise or interference from telephone lines can be severe enough to distort a fax transmission, so, when it is necessary, verify receipt. There are a number of ways to ensure that a faxed document has reached the correct destination.

● Place a telephone call to the requesting physician's office 10 to 15 minutes after faxing patient records to verify their receipt.

FAX TRANSMITTAL SHEET

To: _____ College Hospital (outpatient surgery) _____ Date 10-21-20XX

Fax Number: (555) 486-8900 Telephone Number (555) 487 6789 Time 10:00 a.m.

Number of pages (including this one): 3

From: Raymond Skeleton, MD _____ Phone (555) 486-9002

Note: This transmittal is intended only for the use of the individual or entity to which it is addressed, and may contain information that is privileged, confidential, and exempt from disclosure under applicable law. If you are not the intended recipient, any dissemination, distribution, or photocopying of this communication is strictly prohibited. If you have received this communication in error, please notify this office immediately by telephone and return the original FAX to us at the address below by U.S. Postal Service. Thank you.

Remarks: _____ Enclosed are Margaret Yont's radiology reports on her _____
_____ L. tibia/fibula and L. foot fractures _____

If you cannot read this FAX or if pages are missing, please contact:

COLLEGE CLINIC
4567 Broad Avenue
Woodland Hills, XY 12345-0001
Phone: 555/486-9002
Fax: 555/487-8976

INSTRUCTIONS TO THE AUTHORIZED RECEIVER: PLEASE COMPLETE THIS STATEMENT OF RECEIPT AND RETURN TO SENDER VIA THE ABOVE FAX NUMBER.
- -

I, Cheryl Watson, CMA , verify that I have received 3
(no. of pages including cover sheet)

from Raymond Skeleton, MD
(sending facility's name)

FIGURE 4–19 Example of a fax cover sheet for medical document transmission.

- Request that the authorized receiver sign and return an attached receipt form at the bottom of the cover sheet on receipt of the faxed information.
- Make arrangements with the recipient for a scheduled time for transmission.
- Send the fax to a coded mailbox. Coded mailboxes require the sender to punch in a code indicating the individual to whom the fax is addressed and the receiver to then punch in his or her own code to activate the printer.
- Ask the receiving party for a patient reference number (e.g., the patient's Social Security number). Blank out the patient's name and write in the reference number on the document before faxing it. Also ask other providers to fax records by reference number rather than by patient name.
- Run a fax transmission confirmation report from your own fax machine. Most current fax machines have this capability. The report will show what number was dialed and whether or not the transmission was successful.

To safeguard against a fax sent to the wrong destination, telephone or fax a request to destroy misdirected information. Note the incident, along with the misdialed number, in the patient's health record and in an HIPAA disclosure log. Program frequently used numbers into the fax machine to avoid misdirecting faxed communications. Edit your release of records authorization form to allow for fax transmission because it is acceptable to honor an authorization sent via this method.

Medicare Guidelines

Check with the Medicare fiscal intermediary to find out whether faxing of claims and documents is acceptable for Medicare patients. The use of a fax transmittal system requires that the physician retain the original facsimile with the signature on it. Further information on digital fax may be found in Chapter 8.

Financial Data

Never fax a patient's financial data. In court, faxing medical information can be justified on the basis of medical necessity, but faxing financial information cannot be justified.

Legal Documents

Consult an attorney to make sure that documents (e.g., contracts, proposals, insurance claims) requiring signatures are legally binding if faxed. To ensure legality, do the following:

● Transmit the entire document, front and back, to be signed and not only the page to be signed so the receiver has full disclosure of the agreement.
● As mentioned above, obtain confirmation that the receiver is in receipt of all pages sent, because an incomplete document may be invalid.
● Insert a clause in the contract stating that faxed signatures will be treated as originals.
● Follow up and obtain the original signature in hard copy form as soon as possible.

Subpoena

Subpoena literally means "under penalty." In legal language, it is a writ requiring the appearance of a witness at a trial or other proceeding. Strictly defined, a *subpoena duces tecum* requires the witness to appear and to bring or send certain records "in his possession." Frequently, however, only the records may be sent, and the physician is not required to appear in court.

A subpoena is a legal document signed by a judge or an attorney in the name of a judge. In cases in which a pretrial of evidence or deposition is set up, the subpoena may be issued by a notary public, in which event it is called a *notary subpoena*. If an attorney signs it, he or she must attest it in the name of a judge, the court clerk, or other proper officer.

It is possible for a state investigator to subpoena patient records and then file administrative charges against the physician, not because of the practice of shoddy medicine but rather because the case was inadequately documented for the treatment provided. Health records also may be subpoenaed as proof in a medical malpractice case. Complete documentation and well-organized patient records help establish a strong defense in a medical professional liability claim.

The Subpoena Process

A subpoena must be personally served or handed to the prospective witness or keeper of the health records.

Neither civil nor criminal subpoenas can be served via the telecopier (fax) machine. The acceptance of a document by someone authorized to accept it is the equivalent of personal service. The subpoena cannot be left on a counter or desk. In a state civil case, a "witness fee" and payment for travel to and from court are given, if demanded, at the time a subpoena is served. The fee is discretionary in criminal cases. In some states, provision is made for substitute service by mail or through newspaper advertisements. This is permitted only after all reasonable efforts to effect personal service have failed.

Never accept a subpoena or give records to anyone without the physician's prior authorization. The medical office should designate one person as keeper of the health records. If the subpoena is only for health records or financial data, the representative for the specific doctor then can usually accept it, and the physician will not be called to court.

If a physician is on vacation and there is no designated keeper of the records, tell the deputy that the physician is not in and cannot be served. Suggest the deputy contact the physician's attorney and relay this information.

When the "witness fee" has been received and the subpoena has been served, pull the chart and place it and the subpoena on the physician's desk for review. Willful disregard of a subpoena is punishable as contempt of court.

The medical office is given a prescribed time in which to produce the records. It is not necessary to show them at the time the subpoena is served unless the court order so states. The attorney usually employs a person or copy service to copy records that are under subpoena. At the time the subpoena is served, a date is usually agreed upon in which the representative will return and copy the portion of the record that is named in the subpoena. Often only the portion of the health record requested is removed from the original chart and put in a copy folder. Items such as the patient registration information sheet, encounter form, and explanation of benefits should not be included. You may also telephone the attorney who sent the subpoena and ask whether the records can be mailed. If so, mail them by certified mail with return receipt requested. Retain a copy of the records released. You will have to appear in court if specified in the subpoena. Verify with the court that the case is actually on the calendar. If you do not appear, you are in contempt of court and subject to a penalty, possibly several days in jail.

If original records are requested, move them to a safe place, preferably under lock and key, so that they cannot be taken away or tampered with before the trial date.

Make photocopies of the original records because this will prevent total loss of the records and facilitate discovery of any altering or tampering while they are out of your custody. Number the pages of the records so you will know if a page is missing.

On the day of your court appearance, comply with all instructions given by the court. *Do not* give up possession of the records unless instructed to do so by the judge. *Do not* permit examination of the records by anyone before their identification in court. *Do not* leave the chart in the court unless it is in the possession of the judge or jury and a receipt for it has been obtained.

When you have questions, call the physician's attorney or the court's information and assistance staff.

Retention of Records

Today, most health records are either stored in color-coded file folders containing a collection of paper documents or reside in multiple electronic databases displayed in a variety of formats via computer access. Regardless of the system used, there are general guidelines that must be followed to record information correctly, use it according to law, and retain it.

Health Records

Preservation of health records is governed by state and local laws. Individual states generally set a minimum of 6 to 10 years for keeping records, but it is the policy of most physicians to retain health records of all living patients indefinitely. With enactment of the Federal False Claims Act, proof materials for the establishment of evidence, such as x-ray films, laboratory reports, and pathologic specimens, probably should be kept indefinitely in the event of a legal inquiry. Calendars, appointment books, and telephone logs also should be filed and stored. Cases that involve radiologic injury claims (e.g., leukemia from radiation) may begin running the statute of limitations after discovery of the injury, which may occur 20 or 30 years after radiation exposure. Recommended retention periods for paper files are shown in Table 4.2. Electronic health records (EHRs) may have different retention periods depending on state law.

A person's health record may be of value not only to himself or herself in later years but also to the person's children. In some states, a minor may file suit, after he or she has attained legal age, for any act performed during childhood that the person believes to be wrong or harmful. Sometimes a suit may be permitted even 2 to 3 years after the child has reached legal age. Thus it is important to

Table 4.2 Records Retention Schedule		
Temporary Record	**Retention Period (yr)**	**Permanent Record (retained indefinitely)**
Accounts receivable (patient ledgers)	7	
Appointment sheets	3	Accounts payable records
Bank deposit slip (duplicate)	1	Bills of sale for important purchases (or until you no longer own them)
		Canceled checks and check registers
Bank statements and canceled checks	7	Capital asset records
		Cash books
Billing records (for outside service)	7	Certified financial statements
Cash receipt records	6	Contracts
		Correspondence, legal
Contracts (expired)	7	Credit history
Correspondence, general	6	Deeds, mortgages, contracts, leases, and property records
Daysheets (balance sheets and journals)	5	Equipment guarantees and records (or until you no longer own them)
Employee contracts	6	Income tax returns and documents
Employee time records	5	Insurance policies and records
Employment applications	4	Journals (financial)
Insurance claim forms (paid)	3	
Inventory records	3	
Invoices	6	Health records (active patients)
Health records (expired patients)	5	Health records (inactive patients)
Medicare financial records	7	
Remittance advice documents	7	Mortgages
Payroll records	7	Property appraisals and records
Petty cash vouchers	3	Telephone records
Postal and meter records	1	X-ray films
Tax worksheets and supporting documents	7	Year-end balance sheets and general ledgers

keep records until patients are 3 to 4 years beyond the age of majority.

Deceased patients' charts should be kept for at least 5 years. Shred documents that are no longer needed. Some practices prefer to use medical record storage companies, which may put records on microfilm before disposal. If records are disposed of by a professional company, be sure to obtain a document verifying method of disposal. Maintain a log of destroyed records showing the patient's name, Social Security number, date of last visit, and treatment.

Financial Documents

According to income tax regulations on record retention, accounting records should be kept a minimum of 4 years (following the due date for filing the tax return or the date the tax is paid, whichever is later). Always contact an accountant before discarding records that may determine tax liability. Suggested retention periods are listed in Table 4.2.

A federal regulation mandates that assigned claims for Medicaid and Medicare be kept for 7 years; the physician is subject to auditing during that period. The Federal False Claims Amendment Act of 1986 allows a claim of fraud to be made up to 10 years from the date a violation was committed. Documentation must be available for inspection and copying by the investigator of the false claim (31 USC§3729-3733).

Termination of a Case

A physician may wish to withdraw formally from further care of a patient because the patient discharged the physician, did not follow instructions, did not take the

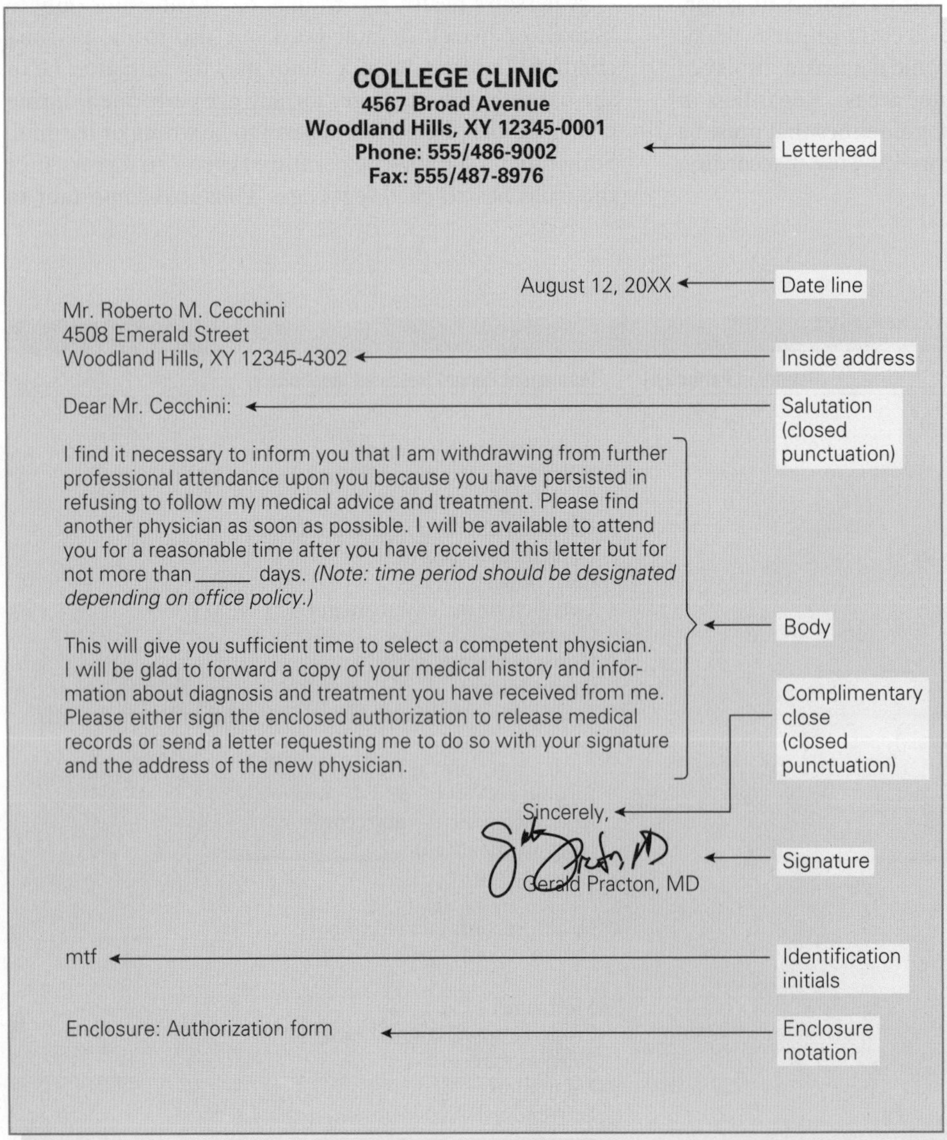

COLLEGE CLINIC
4567 Broad Avenue
Woodland Hills, XY 12345-0001
Phone: 555/486-9002
Fax: 555/487-8976
— Letterhead

August 12, 20XX — Date line

Mr. Roberto M. Cecchini
4508 Emerald Street
Woodland Hills, XY 12345-4302 — Inside address

Dear Mr. Cecchini: — Salutation (closed punctuation)

I find it necessary to inform you that I am withdrawing from further professional attendance upon you because you have persisted in refusing to follow my medical advice and treatment. Please find another physician as soon as possible. I will be available to attend you for a reasonable time after you have received this letter but for not more than _____ days. *(Note: time period should be designated depending on office policy.)*

This will give you sufficient time to select a competent physician. I will be glad to forward a copy of your medical history and information about diagnosis and treatment you have received from me. Please either sign the enclosed authorization to release medical records or send a letter requesting me to do so with your signature and the address of the new physician.

— Body

— Complimentary close (closed punctuation)

Sincerely,

Gerald Practon, MD — Signature

mtf — Identification initials

Enclosure: Authorization form — Enclosure notation

FIGURE 4-20
Example of letter of withdrawal from a case that is typed in modified-block style with closed punctuation and special notations (placement of parts of letter).

recommended medication, failed to return for an appointment, or discontinued payment on an overdue account. A physician may terminate a contract by:

● Sending a letter of withdrawal (Figure 4–20) to the patient by certified mail with return receipt (Figure 4–21), so that proof of termination is in the patient's health record.

● Sending a letter of confirmation of discharge when the patient states that he or she no longer desires care (Figure 4–22). This should also be sent certified mail with return receipt requested.

UNITED STATES POSTAL SERVICE

First-Class Mail
Postage & Fees Paid
USPS
Permit No. G-10

● Sender: Please print your name, address, and ZIP+4 in this box ●

COLLEGE CLINIC
4567 BROAD AVENUE
WOODLAND HILLS, XY 12345 0001

A

SENDER: *COMPLETE THIS SECTION*

■ Complete items 1, 2, and 3. Also complete item 4 if Restricted Delivery is desired.
■ Print your name and address on the reverse so that we can return the card to you.
■ Attach this card to the back of the mailpiece, or on the front if space permits.

1. Article Addressed to:

Mr. John Doe
2761 Fort Street
Woodland Hills, XY 12345

COMPLETE THIS SECTION ON DELIVERY

A. Received by (*Please Print Clearly*) | B. Date of Delivery

C. Signature

X

☐ Agent
☐ Addressee

D. Is delivery address different from item 1? ☐ Yes
If YES, enter delivery address below: ☐ No

3. Service Type
☒ Certified Mail   ☐ Express Mail
☐ Registered   ☐ Return Receipt for Merchandise
☐ Insured Mail   ☐ C.O.D.

4. Restricted Delivery? (*Extra Fee*)   ☐ Yes

2. Article Number (*Copy from service label*)
7000 0520 0020 3886 3129

PS Form 3811, July 1999   Domestic Return Receipt   102595-00-M-0952

B

FIGURE 4–21 **A** and **B** (front and back), A domestic return receipt Postal Service Form 3811.

Continued

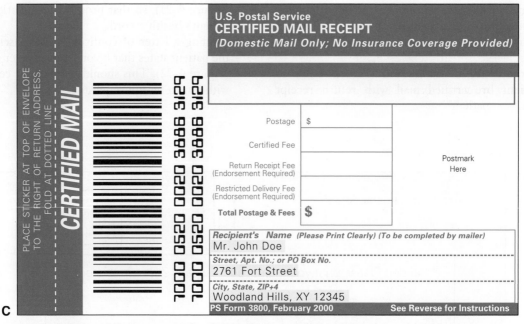

FIGURE 4–21, cont'd **C,** Receipt for certified mail Postal Service Form 3800 (U.S. Government Printing Office) shown completed.

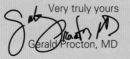

COLLEGE CLINIC
4567 Broad Avenue
Woodland Hills, XY 12345-0001
Phone: 555/486-9002
Fax: 555/487-8976

September 3, 20XX

Mrs. Gregory Putnam
4309 North E Street
Woodland Hills, XY 12345-4398

Dear Mrs. Putnam:

This will confirm our telephone conversation today during which you discharged me from attending you as your physician in your present illness. In my opinion, your medical condition requires continued treatment by a physician. If you have not already obtained the services of another physician, I suggest you do so without further delay.

You may be assured that, upon your written authorization, I will furnish your new physician with information regarding the diagnosis and treatment you have received from me.

Very truly yours

Gerald Procton, MD

mtf

FIGURE 4–22 Letter to confirm discharge by patient. Letter typed in modified block style (dateline, complimentary close, and signature indented) with open punctuation (no commas after salutation or complimentary close).

● Sending a letter confirming that the patient left the hospital against medical advice or the advice of the physician. If there is a signed statement in the patient's hospital records to this effect, it is not necessary to send a letter. If a letter is sent, a copy of the letter and return signature card from the post office must be filed with the patient's records.

Prevention of Legal Problems

After reading Chapters 1 through 4, you have discovered there are many instances in which an insurance biller must be careful in executing job duties to avoid the possibility of a lawsuit. A summary of guidelines for prevention of lawsuits is shown in Box 4.1.

PROCEDURE

ABSTRACT DATA FROM A HEALTH RECORD

OBJECTIVE: To abstract data from a health record for composing a letter or completing an insurance claim form or other related billing document.

EQUIPMENT/SUPPLIES: Patient's health record, form to insert abstracted data, and pen or pencil.

DIRECTIONS: Follow these steps, including rationales, to learn this skill and practice it by completing the *Workbook* assignment.

1. Read and review the patient's health record thoroughly to learn all parts of the case.
2. Answer these questions to assist you in understanding all aspects of the patient's health record.
3. Did the patient undergo surgery? What surgical procedure was performed?
4. What is the patient's diagnosis?
5. What medication was prescribed, if any?
6. Does the patient have any past history indicating anything of importance?
7. Does the patient have any food or drug allergies? If so, what are they?
8. What is the etiology (cause) of the present disease, injury, or illness?
9. What is the prognosis (prediction) for this patient's medical condition?
10. What laboratory tests were ordered or performed?
11. What x-rays were ordered or obtained?
12. Define every abbreviation listed in the patient's chart notes or history and physical examination.
13. What documents assisted you in locating the answers to these questions?

Box 4.1 Prevention of Lawsuits—Guidelines for Insurance Billing Specialists

1. Keep information about patients strictly confidential.
2. Obtain proper instruction and carry out responsibilities according to the employer's guidelines.
3. Keep abreast of general insurance program guidelines, annual coding changes, and medical and scientific progress to help when handling insurance matters.
4. Secure proper written consent in all cases before releasing a patient's health record.
5. Do not refer to consent or acknowledgment forms as "releases." Use the word "consent" or "authorization" forms as required by law. This also produces a better understanding of the document to be signed.
6. Make sure documentation of patient care in the health record corresponds with billing submitted on the insurance claim.
7. Exercise good judgment in what you write and how you word electronic mail because it does not give security against confidentiality.
8. Make every effort to reach an understanding with patients in the matter of fees by explaining what services will be received and what the "extras" may be. For hospital cases, it is advisable to explain that the fee the physician charges is for his or her services only and that charges for the bed or ward room, operating room, laboratory tests, and anesthesia will be billed separately in addition to the physician's charges.
9. Do not discuss other physicians with the patient. Patients sometimes invite criticism of the methods or results of former physicians. Remember that you are hearing only one side of the story.
10. Tell the physician immediately if you learn that a new patient is still under treatment by another physician and did not give this information to the physician during the initial interview.
11. Do not compare the respective merits of various forms of therapy and refrain from discussing patients' ailments with them. Patients come to talk to the physician about their symptoms, and you may give them incorrect information. Let the physician make the diagnosis. Otherwise, you may seriously embarrass the physician, yourself, or both of you.
12. Report a physician who is doing something illegal that you are aware of. You can be held responsible for being silent and failing to report an illegal action.
13. Say nothing to anyone except as required by the attorney of the physician or by the court if litigation is pending.
14. Be alert to hazards that may cause injury to anyone in the office and report such problems immediately.
15. Consult the physician before turning over a delinquent account to a collection agency.
16. Be courteous in dealing with patients and always act in a professional manner.

PROCEDURE

COMPOSE, FORMAT, KEY, PROOFREAD, AND PRINT A LETTER

OBJECTIVE: To compose, format, key, proofread, and print a letter using common business letter style guidelines.

EQUIPMENT/SUPPLIES: Computer, printer, letterhead stationery, envelope, attachments (documents if necessary), thesaurus, English dictionary, medical dictionary, and pen or pencil.

DIRECTIONS: Follow these steps, including rationales, to learn this skill and practice it by completing the *Workbook* assignments.

1. Assemble materials, determine the recipient's address, and decide on modified or full block letter style or format.

2. Turn on the computer and select the word processing program. Open a blank document.

3. Key the date line beginning at least three lines below the letterhead and make certain it is in the proper location for the chosen style.

4. Double-space down and insert the inside address and make certain it is in the proper location for the chosen style. Select a style to insert an attention line, if necessary.

5. Double-space and key the salutation. Use either open or mixed punctuation. A business letter should include a title and the person's last name.

6. Double-space and enter the reference line ("Re:" or "Subject:") in the location for the chosen letter style. This assists the recipient in identifying the contents of the letter immediately.

7. Double-space and key the body (content) of the letter in single-space and make certain the paragraph style is proper for the format chosen. Double-space between paragraphs. Save the letter to the computer hard drive every 15 minutes.

8. Proofread the letter on the computer screen for composition and format.

9. Proofread the letter on the computer screen for typographical, spelling, grammatical, and mechanical errors. Use the spell-check feature of the word processing program and reference books to check for correct spelling, meaning, or usage.

10. Key the second page heading (name, page number, and date) in vertical or horizontal format if a second page is needed.

11. Key a complimentary close and make certain it is in the proper location for the chosen style.

12. Drop down four spaces and key the sender's name and title or credentials as printed on the letterhead because handwritten signatures may be difficult to read.

13. Double-space and insert the sender's and typist's reference initials in lowercase letters, separating the two sets of initials with either a color or slash.

14. Single- or double-space to insert copy ("CC"), or enclosure ("Enclosure" or "Enc"), or attachment notations.

15. Double-space to insert a postscript ("P.S."), if necessary.

16. Save the file before printing a hard copy and proofread the letter once more. Make corrections, if needed.

17. Print the final copy to be sent and proofread. Make a copy to be retained in the files in case it is needed for future reference.

18. Save the file to a CD-ROM to be stored for future reference.

19. Prepare an envelope and use the format for optical scanning recommended by the U.S. Postal Service. Insert special mailing instructions in the correct location on the envelope if sending by certified mail.

20. Clip attachments to the letter and give it to the physician for review and signature.

RESOURCES

INTERNET

@

- A model compliance plan for third-party billing companies can be found at:
  Web site: **http://oig.hhs.gov/ fraud/docs/complianceguidance/thirdparty.pdf**

ASSIGNMENT

STUDENT

✔ Study Chapter 4.

✔ Answer the review questions in the *Workbook* to reinforce the theory learned in this chapter and help prepare you for a future test.

✔ Complete the assignments in the *Workbook* to give you experience in reviewing patients' medical reports and records.

✔ Turn to the glossary at the end of this textbook for a further understanding of the key terms used in this chapter.

CHAPTER OUTLINE

**THE DIAGNOSTIC CODING
SYSTEM**
  Types of Diagnostic Codes
  Reasons for the Development
    and Use of Diagnostic Codes
  Physician's Fee Profile
HISTORY OF CODING DISEASES
**INTERNATIONAL
  CLASSIFICATION OF DISEASES**
  History
  Organization and Format
  Contents

**HOW TO USE THE DIAGNOSTIC
  CODE BOOKS PROPERLY**
  Coding Instructions
RULES FOR CODING
  Signs, Symptoms, and
    Ill-Defined Conditions
  Sterilization
  Neoplasms
  Circulatory System Conditions
  Diabetes Mellitus
  Pregnancy, Delivery, or
    Abortion

  Admitting Diagnoses
  Burns
  Injuries and Late Effects
**ICD-10-CM DIAGNOSIS
  AND PROCEDURE
  CODES**
**PROCEDURE: BASIC STEPS
  IN SELECTING DIAGNOSTIC
  CODES**

KEY TERMS

adverse effect

benign tumor

chief complaint (CC)

combination code

complication

E codes

etiology

in situ

*International Classification of
Diseases, Ninth Revision, Clinical
Modification* (ICD-9-CM)

intoxication

italicized code

late effect

malignant tumor

not elsewhere classifiable (NEC)

not otherwise specified (NOS)

physician's fee profile

poisoning

primary diagnosis

principal diagnosis

secondary diagnosis

slanted brackets

syndrome

V codes

5

Diagnostic Coding

OBJECTIVES*

After reading this chapter, you should be able to:

- State the history of diagnostic coding.
- Explain the purpose and importance of coding diagnoses.
- Use diagnostic code books properly and obtain codes accurately.

- State the meaning of basic abbreviations and symbols in the code books.
- Define diagnostic code terminology.
- Perform diagnostic coding accurately after completing the problems in the *Workbook*.

*Performance objectives and exercises for hands-on practical experience for this chapter appear in the *Workbook*.

Service

Diagnostic coding must be accurate because payment for inpatient services rendered to a patient may be based on the diagnosis. In the outpatient setting, the diagnosis code must correspond to the treatment or services rendered to the patient or payment may be denied.

THE DIAGNOSTIC CODING SYSTEM

This chapter deals with diagnostic coding for outpatient professional services, and the next chapter relates to coding of procedures. Proper coding can mean the financial success or failure of a medical practice. A working knowledge of medical terminology, including a basic course in anatomy and physiology, is essential to becoming a topnotch coder of diagnoses. The coding must be accurate because in many instances, such as with a patient under the Medicare program, payment for outpatient services are related to the procedure codes but must be supported and justified by the diagnosis. Payment for services is based on diagnostic coding in the inpatient setting only. All documented diagnoses that affect the current status of the patient may be assigned a code. This includes conditions that exist at the time of the patient's initial contact with the physician as well as conditions that develop subsequently that affect the treatment received. Diagnoses that relate to a patient's previous medical problem that have no bearing on the patient's present condition are not coded. The American Health Information Management Association (AHIMA) and American Hospital Association (AHA) diagnostic coding guidelines for outpatient services and diagnostic coding and reporting requirements for physician billing may be found by visiting the Web sites listed in the Internet Resources at the end of this chapter.

Types of Diagnostic Codes

Codes must be sequenced correctly on an insurance claim so that the chronology of patient care events (main reason for the office visit) and severity of disease can be understood. The Health Insurance Claim Form CMS-1500 requires that a diagnostic code apply to a procedure code by insertion of the codes in Field 21 on lines 1, 2, 3, or 4 of the form. Also the primary surgical procedure code must always be listed first on the claim form for full reimbursement and the secondary procedures, which are paid at less than 100% of allowable, must be listed in succession. The diagnostic code is matched to the appropriate surgical or medical procedure code.

When submitting insurance claims for patients seen in a physician's office or an outpatient hospital setting,

Box 5.1   Primary versus Principal Diagnosis

PRIMARY DIAGNOSIS

Definition: Main reason (diagnosis, condition, chief complaint) for the encounter/visit in the health record that is responsible for services provided
List first
Location: Outpatient setting only (physician office visits and hospital-based outpatient services)
Diagnosis Code: Code the condition, sign, or symptom to the highest degree of certainty for the encounter/visit. May code signs, symptoms, abnormal test results, or other reason for the visit when a diagnosis has not been confirmed
May not code diagnosis documented as "probable," "suspected," "questionable," "rule out," or "working diagnosis."

PRINCIPAL DIAGNOSIS

Definition: Condition established after study that prompted the hospitalization.
Location: Inpatient setting only
Diagnosis Code: Code the condition as if it existed or was established if at time of discharge documentation lists "probable," "suspected," "likely," "questionable," "possible," or "still to be ruled out."
Diagnosis Related Group (DRG): Assignment of DRG number for hospital reimbursement.

the **primary diagnosis,** which is the main reason for the encounter, must be listed first. In an office setting, this is commonly called the **chief complaint (CC).** The **secondary diagnosis,** listed subsequently, may contribute to the condition or define the need for a higher level of care but is not the underlying cause. The underlying cause of a disease is referred to as the **etiology** and is sequenced in the first position. The **principal diagnosis,** used in inpatient hospital coding, is the diagnosis obtained after study that prompted the hospitalization. It is possible for the primary and principal diagnosis codes to be the same. The concept of a "principal diagnosis" is only applicable to inpatient hospital orders. Box 5.1 outlines the important considerations whenever you come across same or similar phrases related to the diagnosis because they represent two very different coding scenarios in the outpatient versus inpatient settings.

Reasons for the Development and Use of Diagnostic Codes

Diagnostic coding was developed for the following reasons:

1. Tracking of disease processes
2. Classification of causes of mortality
3. Medical research
4. Evaluation of hospital service utilization

Medical practices use diagnostic codes on insurance claims and never write out the diagnostic description.

The consequences of not using ICD-9-CM (*International Classification of Diseases, Ninth Revision, Clinical Modification*) codes are many. For example, claims can be denied, fines or penalties can be levied, sanctions can be imposed, and the physician's level of reimbursement for inpatient claims may be affected. It is required that diagnostic codes be used on all claims; processing is accurate and prompt if coding is correctly done. When insurance claim reimbursement records are comprehensive, statistics can be gathered to make future payments more realistic for the physicians in private practice.

MEDICAL CODE SET

As learned in Chapter 2, a code set is any set of codes with their descriptions used to encode data elements, such as tables of terms, medical concepts, medical diagnostic codes, or medical procedure codes. Each transaction must include the use of medical and other code sets. The ICD-9-CM Official Guidelines for Coding and Reporting must be used when assigning diagnostic codes. HIPAA does not require insurance health plans to change their business rules regarding payment based on the codes. However, insurance payers cannot reject an insurance claim because it includes a valid HIPAA standard code that the payer system does not yet recognize.

Occasionally an insurance company replies to a claim with an explanation of benefits or remittance advice stating, "This procedure or item is not payable for the diagnosis as reported for lack of medical necessity." For example, a patient has undergone magnetic resonance imaging (MRI) of the brain. Medicare will not reimburse for MRI for the diagnosis of transient ischemic attack or Alzheimer's disease but will pay for it with the diagnosis of cerebral insufficiency. The procedures that are diagnosis-related include most imaging services (e.g., radiography, computed tomography, and MRI), cardiovascular services (e.g., electrocardiograms, Holter monitors, echocardiography, Doppler imaging, and stress testing), neurologic services (e.g., electroencephalography and noninvasive ultrasonography), some laboratory services, and vitamin B_{12} injections. It is important to know the procedures that are diagnosis-related and exactly which diagnosis relates to the procedure being billed. A reference book may be helpful in this situation and a number of manuals are available from commercial publishers. For cases dealing with the Centers for Medicare and Medicaid Services, consult the Web site for local medical review policies (LMRP) or obtain the manuals from the Medicare and Medicaid fiscal intermediaries.

Physician's Fee Profile

A **physician's fee profile** is a compilation of each physician's charges and the payments made to him or her over a given period of time for each specific professional service rendered to a patient. Each insurance company keeps a profile on every provider for services that are processed for statistical purposes. As charges are increased, so are payments, and the profile is then updated through the use of statistical computer data gathered from submitted processed claims. Every claim form filed by a third-party payer is entered into permanent computerized records. The compiled data (fees charged; procedure and diagnostic codes) may be used in the future as the basis for the physician's fee profile. To ensure accuracy of future profiles, the insurance billing specialist should use specific diagnostic codes on a routine basis.

There are two types of profiles: *individual customary profile* and *prevailing profile*. Ask each insurance carrier whether the carrier will update the physician's fee profile on an annual basis.

HISTORY OF CODING DISEASES

From the earliest days of medical treatment, people have tried to name and classify diseases. Although many attempts have been made to systematize and clarify disease terminology, no one method has ever been accepted by the entire medical community.

Around 1869, the American Medical Association prepared the *American Nomenclature of Diseases*. In 1903 the *Bellevue Hospital Nomenclature of Diseases* was published; it was subsequently replaced by the *Standard Nomenclature of Diseases and Operations*. In the 1960s, the American Medical Association published *Current Medical Information and Terminology* (CMIT), which used a computer format to make frequent revisions easier. Medical terms were alphabetically arranged and included detailed descriptions of the diseases and two- and four-digit code numbers. Publication of the book ceased in 1991.

Institutions (within a facility), pathologists, and those involved with generating medical reports and billing for laboratory medicine procedures use a system for retrieving types of diagnoses. These codes are found in a comprehensive multilingual clinical terminology book entitled *Systematized Nomenclature of Human and Veterinary Medicine (SNOMED International)*, Volumes I through IV.* In addition, this system is used for managing patient records, teaching medical information science (informatics), and

---

*Available from the College of American Pathologists, 325 Waukegan Road, Northfield, IL, 60093-2750.

indexing and managing research data. SNOMED is also used to compare terminology context or classification description principles with the ICD-9-CM system. This process of linking content from one terminology or classification scheme to another is called *mapping*. This helps minimize duplicating data entry and patient data integration and helps with development of a "crosswalk." For example, when new codes are annually introduced, a crosswalk is made creating a map between the old codes and the new ones.

INTERNATIONAL CLASSIFICATION OF DISEASES

History

The *International Classification of Diseases* (ICD) had its beginnings in England during the 17th century. The United States began using the ICD to report causes of death and prepare mortality statistics in the latter half of the 19th century. Hospitals began using the ICD in 1950 to classify and index diseases. The ninth revision of the *International Classification of Diseases* (ICD-9), published by the World Health Organization, is currently being used by state health departments and the U.S. Public Health service for mortality reporting.

Organization and Format

In 1979 the ***International Classification of Diseases, Ninth Revision, Clinical Modification*** (ICD-9-CM) was published by the Department of Health Services in the United States. It is updated annually and has three volumes. Volume 1 is a Tabular List of Diseases, each having an assigned number. Volume 2 is an Alphabetic Index of Diseases. Volume 3 is a Tabular List and Alphabetic Index of Procedures used primarily in the hospital setting. The systematized arrangement in these books makes it possible to encode, computerize, store, and retrieve large volumes of information from the patient's medical record. ICD-9-CM is used by hospitals, physicians, and other health care providers to code and report clinical information necessary for participation in various government programs, such as Medicare, Medicaid, and quality improvement organizations/professional review organizations.

Volumes 1 and 2 are used in physicians' offices and other outpatient settings to complete insurance claims. These two volumes are almost completely compatible with the original international version (ICD-9). The code numbers have from three to five digits. Although abbreviated versions of the ICD-9-CM are available, it is preferable to obtain the complete ninth revision of Volumes 1 and 2.

Annual updates of the ICD-9-CM are published in three publications: *Coding Clinic*, published by the American Hospital Association; the *American Health Information Management Association Journal*, published by the American Health Information Management Association; and the *Federal Register*, published by the U.S. Government Printing Office. Coding from an out-of-date manual can delay payment or cause costly mistakes that can lead to financial disaster. Annual ICD-9-CM code revisions must be in place and in use by October 1 each year. There is no longer a 3-month grace period to implement these changes and revisions. Effective 2005, changes will occur April 1 and October 1 annually. Thus it is more important than ever to make sure updated codes are used. Refer to Appendix A for the names and addresses of several companies that publish the ICD-9-CM.

Psychiatric disorders are coded using the *Diagnostic and Statistical Manual of Mental Disorders, Fourth Edition* (DSM-IV). Refer to Appendix A for information regarding where to obtain this code book.

Contents

Table 5.1 is an outline of Volumes 1 and 2 of the ICD-9-CM. Volume 1 chapter headings with associated codes are listed. The Supplementary Classifications list V and E codes, which are discussed later. Sections A, B, C, and D of the Appendices are not used in physician outpatient billing. Volume 2 contains three sections: an Alphabetic Index for Diseases and Injuries, a Table of Drugs and Chemicals, and an Alphabetic Index to External Causes of Injuries and Poisonings (E codes). An outline and information on how to find codes in Volume 3 are provided in Chapter 17. This reference is used primarily in the hospital setting. Some publishers place ICD-9-CM Volume 2 before Volume 1 to help the user expedite finding the correct code.

HOW TO USE THE DIAGNOSTIC CODE BOOKS PROPERLY

To become a proficient coder, it is important to develop an understanding of the conventions and terminology of ICD-9-CM. Read all of the information at the introduction or beginning of Volumes 1 and 2 before coding. Volume 1, the Tabular List for the disease classifications, makes use of certain abbreviations, punctuation, symbols, and other conventions, as shown in Box 5.2.

In Volume 2, the Alphabetic Index for Disease Classification, the symbol of **slanted brackets (*[ ]*)** is used to indicate the need for another code. A code is given after a listing followed by slanted brackets enclosing an

Table 5.1 Outline of Volumes 1 and 2 of ICD-9-CM

Volume 1	Chapter Headings	Codes
1	Infectious and Parasitic Diseases	001–139
2	Neoplasms	140–239
3	Endocrine, Nutritional, and Metabolic Diseases and Immunity Disorders	240–279
4	Diseases of the Blood and Blood-Forming Organs	280–289
5	Mental Disorders	290–319
6	Diseases of the Nervous System and Sense Organs	320–389
7	Diseases of the Circulatory System	390–459
8	Diseases of the Respiratory System	460–519
9	Diseases of the Digestive System	520–579
10	Diseases of the Genitourinary System	580–629
11	Complications of Pregnancy, Childbirth, and the Puerperium	630–676
12	Diseases of the Skin and Subcutaneous Tissue	680–709
13	Diseases of the Musculoskeletal System and Connective Tissue	710–739
14	Congenital Anomalies	740–759
15	Certain Conditions Originating in the Perinatal Period	760–779
16	Symptoms, Signs, and Ill-Defined Conditions	780–799
17	Injury and Poisoning	800–999

SUPPLEMENTARY CLASSIFICATIONS

	Classification of Factors Influencing Health Status and Contact with Health Service	V01–V82
	Classification of External Causes of Injury and Poisoning	E800–E999

APPENDICES

A	Morphology of Neoplasms	
B	Glossary of Mental Disorders	
C	Classification of Drugs by American Hospital Formulary Service List Number and Their ICD-9-CM Equivalents	
D	Classification of Industrial Accidents According to Agency	
E	List of Three-Digit Categories	

VOLUME 2

Section 1	Index to Diseases and Injuries, alphabetic	
Section 2	Table of Drugs and Chemicals	
Section 3	Index to External Causes of Injuries and Poisonings	

Box 5.2 Common ICD-9-CM Code Book Conventions*

ABBREVIATIONS

NEC **Not Elsewhere Classifiable** (in the coding books). The category number for the term including NEC is to be used with ill-defined terms and only when the coder lacks the information necessary to code the term in a more specific category.

Example: **Fibrosclerosis** Familial multifocal NEC **710.8**

NOS **Not Otherwise Specified** (by the physician). This abbreviation is the equivalent of "unspecified." It refers to a lack of sufficient detail in the diagnosis statement to be able to assign it to a more specific subdivision within the classification.

Example: **153.9 Colon, unspecified** Large intestine NOS.

PUNCTUATION

[ ]	Brackets are used to enclose synonyms, alternative wordings, or explanatory phrases.
[code]	Italicized (slanted) brackets enclosing a code, used in Volume 2, the Alphabetic Index, indicates the need for another code. Record both codes in the order as indicated in the index.
⊏	Large bracket may signal a new or revised code.
•	A bullet at a code or line of text indicates the entry is new.
( )	Parentheses are used to enclose supplementary words that may be present or absent in the statement of a disease or procedure without affecting the code number to which it is assigned.
▲	A triangle in the Tabular List indicates the code title is revised. In the Alphabetical Index, the triangle indicates the code has changed.
:	Colons are used in the Tabular List after an incomplete term that needs one or more of the modifiers that follow to make it assignable to a given category.
►◄	When two triangle symbols meet at their points, they appear at the beginning and end of a section of new or revised text.
{ }	Braces are used to enclose a series of terms, each of which is modified by the statement appearing at the right of the brace.

*Some publishers use additional and/or other symbols.

Continued

Box 5.2	Common ICD-9-CM Code Book Conventions*—cont'd

SYMBOLS

☐	The lozenge symbol printed in the left margin preceding the disease code indicates that the content of a four-digit category has been moved or modified.
DEF:	This symbol indicates a definition of disease or procedural term.
MSP:	This identifies specific trauma codes that alert the carrier that another carrier should be billed and Medicare billed second if payment from the first payer does not equal or exceed the amount Medicare would pay.
PDx:	This symbol identifies a V code that can only be used as a primary diagnosis.
SDx:	This symbol identified a V code that can only be used as a secondary diagnosis. A V code without a symbol can be used as either a primary or secondary diagnosis.
♂ ♀	Age and sex symbols are used to detect inconsistencies between the patient's age and diagnosis. Examples are: Newborn age: 0 Pediatric age: 0 to 17 Maternity age: 12 to 55 Adult age: 15 to 124
§	The section mark symbol preceding a code denotes the placement of a footnote at the bottom of the page that is applicable to all subdivisions in that code.
④ ✓4th ⑤ ✓5th	Either of these symbols signals that a fourth or fifth digit is required for coding to indicate the highest level of specificity.

additional code. Record both of these codes in the same sequence as indicated in the index.

An **italicized code** in the Tabular List may never be sequenced as principal or primary diagnoses.

Coding Instructions

Code only the conditions or problems that the physician is actively managing at the time of the visit. The CMS-1500 claim form has space for only four diagnostic codes. First always use Volume 2, the Alphabetic Index, and second go to Volume 1, the Tabular (numerical) List before assigning a code. Never use just one volume and never code from the index. Begin with the Alphabetic Index to locate the main term of the diagnosis. The main term is the condition. The primary arrangement of the Alphabetic Index, the disease index, is by *condition*. If you cannot find the condition listed, consider rearranging the word roots (e.g., crypt orchid/o or orchido crypt/o). Then substitute a similar suffix.

Using a medical dictionary aids in accurate coding. Research any unfamiliar terminology, for example, amaurotic idiocy with severe mental retardation; impaludism. Look up the word(s) you do not know in your medical dictionary.

Volume 2 elements are structured as follows:

● Main terms are classifications of diseases and injuries and appear as headings in **bold** type.
● Subterms are listings under main terms and are indented two spaces to the right under main terms.
● Modifiers (often referred to as nonessential modifiers because their presence or absence does not affect the

code assigned) provide additional description and are enclosed in parentheses.
● Carryover lines continue the text and are indented more than two spaces from the level of the preceding line.
● Subterms of subterms are additional listings and are indented two spaces to the right under the subterm (Box 5.3; see also Figure 5–13).

Always code to the highest degree of specificity. The more digits a code has, the more specific the description is. A three-digit code may be used only when the diagnostic statement cannot be further subdivided. When a three-digit code has subdivisions, the appropriate subdivision must be coded. Some insurance carrier computer systems kick out the lower-level codes (three-digit codes) and hold these claims for medical review, thereby delaying payment. *Do not* arbitrarily use a zero as a filler character when typing a diagnostic code number because this may be interpreted as indicating a different disease. The addition of a zero to a code number that does not require an additional digit also can cause a claim to be denied (Example 5.1).

Example 5.1	Valid Codes and Invalid Codes Caused by Added Zero

Valid code	Invalid code caused by zero added
373.2	373.20
496	496.0

Fifth-digit codes can appear as follows:

1. At the beginning of a chapter
2. At the beginning of a section
3. At the beginning of a three-digit category
4. In a four-digit subcategory

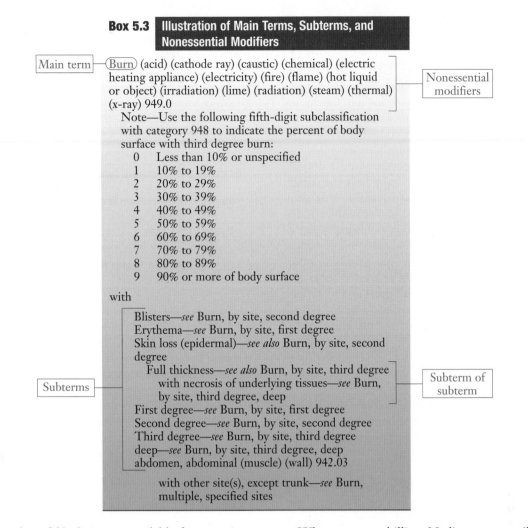

Box 5.3 Illustration of Main Terms, Subterms, and Nonessential Modifiers

Main term—Burn (acid) (cathode ray) (caustic) (chemical) (electric heating appliance) (electricity) (fire) (flame) (hot liquid or object) (irradiation) (lime) (radiation) (steam) (thermal) (x-ray) 949.0 —Nonessential modifiers

Note—Use the following fifth-digit subclassification with category 948 to indicate the percent of body surface with third degree burn:

0 Less than 10% or unspecified
1 10% to 19%
2 20% to 29%
3 30% to 39%
4 40% to 49%
5 50% to 59%
6 60% to 69%
7 70% to 79%
8 80% to 89%
9 90% or more of body surface

with

Blisters—*see* Burn, by site, second degree
Erythema—*see* Burn, by site, first degree
Skin loss (epidermal)—*see also* Burn, by site, second degree
Full thickness—*see also* Burn, by site, third degree —Subterm of subterm
    with necrosis of underlying tissues—*see* Burn, by site, third degree, deep
First degree—*see* Burn, by site, first degree
Second degree—*see* Burn, by site, second degree
Third degree—*see* Burn, by site, third degree
deep—*see* Burn, by site, third degree, deep
abdomen, abdominal (muscle) (wall) 942.03

Subterms

with other site(s), except trunk—*see* Burn, multiple, specified sites

If the fourth or fifth digits are available for a particular three-digit category, then their use is *NOT* optional; therefore select a code book that has the categories marked and color coded so it will not be easy to overlook fifth digits. Near the end of this chapter (accompanying the section Rules for Coding, Diabetes Mellitus) is another example illustrating the use of fifth digits. When the fourth or fifth digit is missing, the code is not complete and technically is not a code but rather a category (Example 5.2). There are some valid three-digit codes (categories) but most have fourth digits (subcategories) and fifth digits (subclassifications). If the base code has a fourth or fifth digit, you must code up to that level.

Example 5.2   Fourth and Fifth Digits

§645   Prolonged pregnancy
[0, 1, 3]   Post-term pregnancy
            Pregnancy which has advanced beyond
            42 weeks of gestation.
The section mark (§) requires a fifth digit; valid digits are in [brackets] under each code. Use 0 as the fourth digit for this category.

When you are billing Medicare, you will find that some diagnostic codes are designated as invalid from year to year. If you work in a medical practice that sees Medicare patients, it is essential to read the regional Medicare bulletins and attend Medicare seminars periodically to keep abreast of these changes, or visit the CMS Web site.

Handy Hints in Diagnostic Coding

If your ICD-9-CM code books are not color-coded, mark manifestation (italicized) codes with a colored highlighter pen (e.g., 608.81 [italicized code]). This will remind you to **always code the underlying disease first.** Also add tabs to main sections of Volume 1 (first page, V codes, E codes, Appendix E) and Volume 2 (Sections 1, 2, and 3). Refer to the end of this chapter for the step-by-step procedures for locating and selecting diagnostic codes.

Many times you locate a diagnostic code in Volume 2 only to find that the cross-referenced code is the same when verified in Volume 1. Indicate these codes in Volume 2 with a colored highlighter pen to remind you that this code is correct as described in Volume 2, which saves the time you would spend checking Volume 1. But, to be sure, always code from the tabular section.

Keep a list of diagnostic and Current Procedural Terminology (CPT) procedure codes commonly encountered by your office, making sure to include fourth and fifth digit specificity. Some insurance companies publish lists of codes specifying diagnostic codes that are acceptable for specific procedures. Consult payer guidelines to determine whether certain procedures are a covered benefit for certain diagnoses and, if not, have the patient sign a waiver. Reference books are available that show codes that link between diagnostic and procedure codes. The American Medical Association publishes a list of the most common diagnostic codes at the end of each of their minispecialty code books. See Appendix B for information on titles and how to obtain reference books that contain such data. If you develop a "cheat sheet," be sure to review, update, and change it on a regular basis (January 1 for procedure codes and in April and October for diagnostic codes).

V Codes

V codes are a supplementary classification of coding located in a separate section at the end of Volume 1, Tabular List. In Volume 2, the Alphabetic Index, the V codes are included in the major section Index of Diseases.

V codes may be used when a person who is not currently sick encounters health services for some specific purpose, such as to act as a donor of an organ or tissue, receive a vaccination, discuss a problem that is not in itself a disease or injury, seek consultation about family planning, request sterilization, or to obtain supervision of a normal pregnancy (Example 5.3). These types of encounters are among the more common services for hospital outpatients and patients of private practitioners, health clinics, and others. In these situations, the V code appears as a primary code and is placed first.

Example 5.3   Supervision of First Pregnancy, Normal

Step 1. Find the heading **pregnancy** in Volume 2.
Step 2. Look for the subheading **supervision.**
Step 3. Look for the second subheading **normal** and a further subheading **first,** which gives you the code V22.0.
Step 4. Find **V22.0** in Volume 1, by where marked Tabular List, and you will see **"Supervision of normal first pregnancy."**

V codes also are used when some circumstance or problem is present that influences the person's health status but is not in itself a current illness or injury, such as when the person is known to have an allergy to a

specific drug. In this instance, the V code cannot be used as a stand-alone code and should be used only as a supplementary code.

Additional code numbers are given for occupational health examinations and routine annual physical examinations; therefore select specific codes depending on the circumstances (Example 5.4).

Example 5.4   Routine Annual Physical Examination

Step 1. Look up **examination,** and notice **annual** as a subterm and the code V70.0
Step 2. Find **V70** in Volume 1, Tabular List, and the wording **"Routine general medical examination at a health facility."**

Sometimes a patient receives a consultation for a preoperative medical evaluation as an inpatient or outpatient (Example 5.5), and the majority of the results are negative for chronic or current illness. A good-health diagnosis code will trigger a rejection by the insurance carrier unless it is mandated by the insurance company. Use an admission (encounter) code from the V72.X code series for "other specified examinations" instead of a treatment code. The term "admission (encounter)" is equivalent to *encounter for* and does not refer to an admission to the hospital.

Example 5.5   Admission (Encounter) Code

A patient to have surgery for gallstones is sent to a cardiologist for evaluation of suspected cardiovascular disease.
Step 1. In Volume 2, look up **admission (encounter) (for) examination, preoperative, cardiovascular V72.81.** Verify it in Volume 2.
Step 2. Code the reason for the surgery—574.xx, cholelithiasis.

When coding a healthy patient examination, V codes (V70.1 and V70.3 through V70.7) should be sequenced as primary diagnoses over all other diagnoses. Be cautious when using V codes as second or third diagnoses because Medicare might automatically reject the claim, and insurance companies that adopt Medicare policies may possibly do so, too.

E Codes

E codes are also a supplementary classification of coding in which you look for external causes of injury rather than disease. The code description states how an injury occurred. E codes are also used in coding adverse reactions to medications (Figure 5–1).

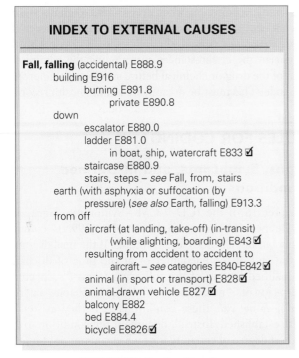

FIGURE 5-1 E coding.

E codes are listed in a separate section of Volume 1, Tabular List, after V codes. To look up E codes, use section 2 in Volume 2. The E codes are also in a separate section, Index to External Causes of Injury and Poisoning, which follows the regular Alphabetic Index. Another quick method of finding E codes is to use Appendix E: List of Three-Digit Categories found in the appendices of the code book.

The use of an E code after the primary or other acute secondary diagnosis explains the mechanism for the injury. For example, if a patient falls and fractures a finger, the fracture code is primary, and an E code following it helps explain how the accident or injury was incurred (Example 5.6). It can help speed the reimbursement process because a payer will see an acute injury code and know a third party is responsible for payment as in a workers' compensation injury or motor vehicle accident. E codes also play a role in gathering data, such as in statistical reporting, credentialing, utilization review, and state injury prevention programs. On the negative side, however, many payers require chart notes to accompany E-code claims, which means generating a paper claim rather than sending it electronically. E codes often trigger a questionnaire to be sent to the beneficiary. This may lead to a delay in reimbursement. Although E codes do not generate revenue, it is recommended that they should be reported in addition to the appropriate procedural and diagnostic codes. This ensures that the most specific information possible is provided in regard to the patient's injury. E codes are billed by the initial entity seeing the patient. If the patient visits the physician's office after hospitalization for injuries sustained in a

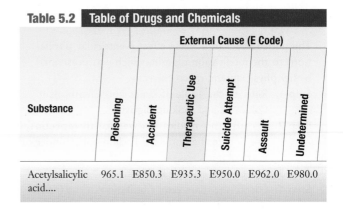

Example 5.6   E Codes

26720 Closed treatment of phalangeal shaft fracture, proximal phalanx, finger; without manipulation, each
816.02 Closed, fracture of one distal phalanx of hand
E880.1 Fall from sidewalk curb

motor vehicle accident, the hospital assigns an E code and there is no requirement for repeating it for the office visit. An E code may never be sequenced in the first position. When using E codes, be sure to list them last on the claim form. Instructions are included here for additional knowledge about the classification system.

The Table of Drugs and Chemicals found in Volume 2 (Table 5.2) contains a classification of drugs and other chemical substances for identifying poisoning states and external causes of adverse effects. Read the foreword at the beginning of this table. Each of the substances listed in the table is assigned a code according to the poisoning classification (960 through 989). These codes are used when there is a state of poisoning, overdose, wrong substance given or taken, or intoxication. If a diagnosis is stated as *possible* or *suspected* suicide attempt, then go to the column entitled "Undetermined" and not "Suicide Attempt."

Adverse effect is defined as an adverse or a pathologic reaction to a drug that occurs when appropriate doses are given to humans for prophylaxis (prevention of disease), diagnosis, and therapy (Example 5.7). When an adverse effect occurs (e.g., drug reaction, hypersensitivity, drug intolerance, idiosyncratic reaction), a code is assigned to the diagnosis that classifies the specific reaction or symptom (e.g., dermatitis, syncope, tachycardia, urticaria). You do not use a code from the 960 to 989 range but do code the specific reaction or symptom from use of the drug followed by a code from the E code column. The E code identifying the agent involved is taken solely from the Therapeutic Use column.

Poisoning is defined as a condition resulting from an intentional overdose of drugs or chemical substances or from the wrong drug or agent given or taken in error (Example 5.8). **Intoxication** is defined as an adverse effect

---

Example 5.7   Coding an Adverse Effect

The patient had an adverse effect (ventricular fibrillation) to the medication digoxin, which was prescribed by her physician and taken correctly.

Step 1. Refer to the Table of Drugs and Chemicals in Volume 2 and look up **digoxin.**

Step 2. Because this medication was for therapeutic use, locate the correct E code number under that column.

Step 3. The correct number is **E942.1.**

Step 4. Locate the main term **fibrillation** in the Index to Diseases.

Step 5. Find the subterm **ventricular.**

Step 6. The correct code number is **427.41.**

Step 7. Verify the code number 427.41 in Volume I, Tabular Listing.

Sequencing: 427.41 Ventricular fibrillation (chief complaint)

E942.1 Therapeutic use, Digoxin

NOTE: For outpatient billing, the E code would not be listed.

Example 5.8   Poisoning Examples

- Taking the wrong medication
- Receiving the wrong medication
- Taking the wrong dose of the right medication
- Receiving the wrong dose of the right medication
- Ingesting a chemical substance not intended for human consumption
- Overdose of a chemical substance (drug)
- Prescription drug taken with alcohol
- Mixing prescription drugs and over-the-counter medications without the physician's advice or consent

Coding a Poisoning

Baby Kathy got into the kitchen cabinet and ingested liquid household ammonia.

Step 1. Refer to the Table of Drugs and Chemicals in Volume 2 and look up **ammonia.**

Step 2. Find the subterm **liquid (household)**

Step 3. Because this is a case of ingesting a chemical substance not intended for human use, locate the correct code number under the **Poisoning** column.

Step 4. Write down the code number **983.2.**

Step 5. Because this is an accident, locate the E code in the **Accident** column **(E861.4).**

Sequencing: 983.2 Poisoning, ammonia

E861.4 Poisoning, accidental, ammonia

NOTE: The manifestation (outcome of the poisoning, e.g., nausea and vomiting) would be coded in the first position if documented in the medical record. For outpatient billing, the E code would not be listed.

---

rather than a poisoning when drugs such as digitalis, steroid agents, and so on are involved. However, whenever the term *intoxication* is used, the biller should clarify with the physician the circumstances surrounding the administration of the drug or chemical before assigning the appropriate code. This must be documented in the health record.

RULES FOR CODING

Signs, Symptoms, and Ill-Defined Conditions

Chapter 16 of the ICD-9-CM—Symptoms, Signs, and Ill-Defined Conditions (codes 780.0 to 799.9)—contains many but not all codes for symptoms. If the final diagnosis at the end of the encounter or at the time of discharge is qualified by any of the following terms ("suspected," "suspicion of," "questionable," "likely," "probable," or "rule out"), *do not code* these conditions as if they existed or were established. Instead, document the condition to the highest degree of certainty for each encounter or visit (e.g., signs, symptoms, abnormal test results, or other reason for the visit) and code the chief complaint, sign, or symptom.

This is contrary to coding practices used by hospital health information management departments for coding the diagnoses of hospital inpatients. If one were to follow hospital coding guidelines and the patient was suspected of having a heart attack, this would be coded as a confirmed case of a myocardial infarction. The same holds true for "possible epilepsy." If the patient had a convulsion and epilepsy was the probable cause but had not been proved, code the convulsion.

The following are instances in which sign and symptom codes can be used:

● No precise diagnosis can be made (Examples 5.9 and 5.10).

Example 5.9   No Precise Diagnosis

The patient has an enlarged liver and further diagnostic studies may or may not be done. Use code 789.10 for hepatomegaly.

Example 5.10   No Precise Diagnosis

The patient complains of painful urination and urinalysis is negative. Use code 788.1 for dysuria.

● Signs or symptoms are transient, and a specific diagnosis was not made (Example 5.11).
● Provisional diagnosis for a patient who does not return for further care (Example 5.12).

Example 5.11   Transient Sign and Symptom Code

The patient complains of **chest pain on deep inspiration.** On examination, the physician finds nothing abnormal and tells the patient to return in 1 week. When the patient returns, the pain has ceased. **Use code 786.52 for painful respiration.**

Example 5.12   Provisional Diagnosis

On examination, the physician documents abnormal percussion of the chest. The patient is sent for a chest x-ray and is asked to return for a recheck. The patient does not have the x-ray and fails to return. Use code **786.7 for abnormal chest sounds.**

● A patient is referred for treatment before a definite diagnosis is made (Example 5.13).

Example 5.13   Sign and Symptom Code before Definite Diagnosis

A patient complains of nausea and vomiting and is referred to a gastroenterologist. Use code **787.01** for nausea with vomiting.

Sterilization

The code V25.2 is used only when the sterilization is performed for the major purpose of contraception rather than being an incidental result of the treatment of a disease. If the sterilization is purely elective, code V25.2 suffices as a single code for the diagnosis. If the sterilization is performed for contraceptive purposes during a current admission for obstetric delivery, sequence code V25.2 in the second position. If the sterilization is the end result of a hysterectomy performed because of injury or damage to the uterus during delivery, do not use code V25.2 but instead code the condition or procedure (i.e., hysterectomy and the diagnosis that precipitated the hysterectomy).

Neoplasms

The main entry "Neoplasm" contains a table with the column headings Malignant, Benign, Uncertain Behavior, and Unspecified. The table is found in the alphabetic index under "Neoplasm" in Volume 2 (Table 5.3). Code numbers for neoplasms are given by anatomic site. For each site, there are six possible code numbers, indicating whether the neoplasm in question is malignant (primary, secondary, or carcinoma in situ), benign, of uncertain behavior, or of unspecified nature. The description of the

---

Example 5.14   Adenocarcinoma of the Breast with Metastases to the Pelvic Bone

Step 1.   Look up **adenocarcinoma** in Volume 2. Do not use the morphology code M8140/3. Notice it states, "see also Neoplasm, by site, malignant."

Step 2.   Locate **neoplasm** in the table in Volume 2. At the top of the page notice the Malignant heading with the subheadings **Primary, Secondary,** and **Ca In Situ. Primary** means the first site of development of the malignancy. **Secondary** means metastasis from the primary site to a second site. **Ca In Situ** means cancer confined to the epithelium of the site of origin without invasion of the basement membrane tissue of the site.

Step 3.   Find the site of the adenocarcinoma (in this case the breast), and look under the Malignant and Primary headings. Note that the code given is **174.9.**

Step 4.   Next, find **bone** as a subterm in the Neoplasm Table and look for the subterm **pelvic.** Now look at the three columns under Malignant and, using the Secondary column, find the **correct code number 198.5.** In listing these diagnoses on the insurance claim, you give the following: **174.9 and 198.5.**

---

neoplasm often indicates which of the six code numbers is appropriate (e.g., malignant melanoma of skin, benign fibroadenoma of breast, or carcinoma in situ of cervix uteri) (Example 5.14). For a tumor that has not been diagnosed as benign or malignant by the pathologist, use the codes in the column labeled "Uncertain Behavior." If a tumor is suspected and not confirmed, use "mass." For example, a breast mass would be coded 611.72. When coding a neoplasm, ask yourself the following questions:

● What is it now?
● Where did it start?
● What happened to it?

Neoplasms are new growths, and they may be benign or malignant tumors. A **benign tumor** is one that does not have the properties of invasion and metastasis (e.g., transfer of disease from one organ to another) and is usually surrounded by a fibrous capsule. Cysts and lesions are *not* neoplasms. A **malignant tumor** has the properties of invasion and metastasis. The term *carcinoma* refers to a cancerous or malignant tumor. Carcinoma **in situ** means cancer confined to the site of origin without invasion of neighboring tissues. A *primary* malignancy means the original neoplastic (malignant) site. A *secondary* neoplasm or malignancy is the site or location to which the original malignancy has spread or metastasized. If the diagnosis does not mention metastasis, then code the case

Table 5.3   Coding for Neoplasms

	MALIGNANT					
	Primary	Secondary	Ca in situ	Benign	Uncertain Behavior	Unspecified
Neoplasm, neoplastic	199.1	199.1	234.9	229.9	238.9	239.9

NOTES:
1. The list below gives the code numbers for neoplasms by anatomic site. For each site there are six possible code numbers according to whether the neoplasm in question is malignant, benign, in situ, of uncertain behavior, or of unspecified nature. The description of the neoplasm will often indicate which of the six columns is appropriate; e.g., malignant melanoma of skin, benign fibroadenoma of breast, carcinoma in situ of cervix uteri.

   Where such descriptors are not present, the remainder of the Index should be consulted where guidance is given to the appropriate column for each morphologic (histologic) variety listed; e.g., Mesonephroma—*see* Neoplasm, malignant; Embryoma—*see also* Neoplasm, uncertain behavior; Disease, Bowen's—*see* Neoplasm, skin, in situ. However, the guidance in the Index can be overridden if one of the descriptors mentioned above is present, e.g., malignant adenoma of colon is coded to 153.9 and not to 211.3 because the adjective "malignant" overrides the Index entry "Adenoma—*see also* Neoplasm benign."
2. Sites marked with an asterisk (*), e.g., face NEC*, should be classified to malignant neoplasm of skin of these sites if the variety of neoplasm is a squamous cell carcinoma or an epidermoid carcinoma and to benign neoplasm of skin of these sites if the variety of neoplasm is a papilloma (any type).

abdomen, abdominal	195.2	198.89	234.8	229.8	238.8	239.8
Cavity	195.2	198.89	234.8	229.8	238.8	238.8
Organ	195.2	198.89	234.8	229.8	238.8	238.8
Viscera	195.2	198.89	234.8	229.8	238.8	239.8
Wall	173.5	198.2	232.5	216.5	238.2	239.2
connective tissue	171.5	198.89	—	215.5	238.1	239.2
abdomino-pelvic accessory sinus—*see* Neoplasm, sinus	195.8	198.89	234.8	229.8	238.8	239.8
acoustic nerve	192.0	198.4	—	225.1	237.9	239.7
acromion (process)	170.4	198.5	—	213.4	238.0	239.2
adenoid (pharynx) (tissue)	147.1	198.89	230.0	210.7	235.1	239.0
adipose tissue (*see also* Neoplasm, connective tissue)	171.9	198.89	—	215.9	238.1	239.2
adnexa (uterine)	183.9	198.82	233.3	221.8	236.3	239.5
adrenal (cortex) (gland) (medulla)	194.0	198.7	234.8	227.0	237.2	239.7
ala nasi (external)	173.3	198.2	232.3	216.3	238.2	239.2
alimentary canal or tract NEC	159.9	197.8	230.9	211.9	235.5	239.0

as a primary neoplasm (Example 5.15). Lymphomas and leukemias are not classified using the primary and secondary terminology.

Example 5.15   Primary and Secondary Cancerous Tumors

Primary   **189**   Malignant neoplasm of cancerous kidney and other and tumor unspecified urinary organs.

      189.0   Kidney, except pelvis
             Kidney NOS
             Kidney parenchyma

Secondary   **198**   Secondary malignant cancerous neoplasm of other tumor specified sites

             Excludes lymph node metastasis (196.0 to 196.9)

      198.0   Kidney

The diagnostic statement "metastatic from" indicates primary stage carcinoma, whereas "metastatic to" indicates secondary stage carcinoma. If the diagnostic statement is "malignant neoplasm spread to," then code it as the primary site spread to the secondary site. The phrase "recurrent malignancy" is new and is coded as a primary neoplasm.

Anatomic sites marked with an asterisk (*) are always considered to be neoplasms of the skin.

In Appendix A of the Tabular List of Volume 2, there is a section entitled Morphology of Neoplasms, which gives M codes. These codes are not used for billing insurance claims by physicians' offices.

Circulatory System Conditions

Diseases of the circulatory system are difficult to code because of the variety and lack of specific terminology used by physicians in stating the diagnoses. Carefully read all inclusion, exclusion, and "use additional code" notations contained in the Tabular List of Volume 1.

Hypertension

The lay term "high blood pressure" is medically termed *hypertension*. Hypertension can cause various forms of heart and vascular disease, or it can accompany some heart conditions. In fact, there is a syndrome called *malignant hypertension* that has nothing to do with tumor formation. It is a condition of very high blood pressure with poor prognosis. A **syndrome** is another name for a symptom complex (a set of complex signs, symptoms, or other manifestations resulting from a common cause or appearing in combination, presenting a distinct clinical picture of a disease or inherited abnormality). Malignant hypertension is a symptom complex of markedly elevated blood pressure (diastolic pressure of more than 140 mm Hg) associated with papilledema. The term *malignant* here means "life threatening." *Benign hypertension* refers to high blood pressure that runs a relatively long and symptomless course. Only a physician can state whether the hypertension is malignant or benign. When in doubt, ask the physician.

When the diagnostic statement indicates a cause by stating "heart condition *due to* hypertension" or "hypertensive heart disease," use codes 402.0X through 402.9X. If the diagnostic statement reads "*with* hypertension" or "cardiomegaly *and* hypertension," you need two separate codes. Elevated blood pressure without mention of hypertension is coded 796.2. Secondary hypertension is coded 405.XX, and the cause of the hypertension should be coded when specified.

Myocardial Infarctions

A separate three-digit category (412) is provided for old myocardial infarction, healed myocardial infarction, or myocardial infarction diagnosed on electrocardiogram. Myocardial infarction of 8 weeks' duration or less (410.xx) is considered acute, if not specified otherwise. Symptoms of more than 8 weeks' duration are coded 414.8, other forms of chronic ischemic heart disease.

Chronic Rheumatic Heart Disease

The conditions presumed to be caused by rheumatic fever are as follows:

● Mitral valve of unspecified etiology 394
● Mitral valve insufficiency 394.1
● Mitral valve and aortic valve disorders of unspecified etiology 396
● Mitral stenosis 394.0

The following condition is not presumed to be caused by rheumatic fever:

● Aortic valve of unspecified etiology 424

Arteriosclerotic Cardiovascular Disease and Arteriosclerotic Heart Disease

Use code 429.2 for a patient who has a diagnosis of arteriosclerotic cardiovascular disease (ASCVD). Code 440.9 excludes ASCVD because it is in conflict with the note given for 429.2. Code 429.2 is primary when the additional code 440.9 is needed. However, a patient with arteriosclerotic heart disease (ASHD) is assigned code 414.0. At code 429.2 in your copy of Volume 1, write in "see code 440" after "use additional code to identify, if desired, the presence of arteriosclerosis." To distinguish between ASCVD and ASHD, cardiovascular means pertaining to heart and blood vessels throughout the body, whereas ASHD means acute or chronic heart disability resulting from an insufficient supply of oxygenated blood to the heart.

Diabetes Mellitus

The two types of diabetes are type I and type II. The following are the clinical features important in the classification of diabetes (Table 5.4).

In type I diabetes (IDDM), the patient's pancreas does not function and produce the necessary insulin. Thus, this patient's body is dependent on insulin. In type II diabetes (NIDDM), the patient's pancreas produces some insulin, but the insulin is ineffective in doing its job, which is removing sugar from the bloodstream. This diabetes may be controlled with diet, oral medication, or insulin.

Table 5.4 Features of Type I and Type II Diabetes	
Type I Diabetes	**Type II Diabetes**
Insulin-dependent diabetes mellitus (IDDM)	Non–insulin-dependent diabetes mellitus (NIDDM)
Patients must be treated with insulin	Patients may be treated with insulin
Insulin levels are very low	Insulin levels may be high "normal," or low
Ketosis prone	Non–ketosis prone
Patients usually are lean	Patients usually are obese
Usually "juvenile onset" (peak onset at early puberty)	Usually "adult onset," although occasionally seen in children
Often little family history of diabetes mellitus	Often strong family history of diabetes mellitus

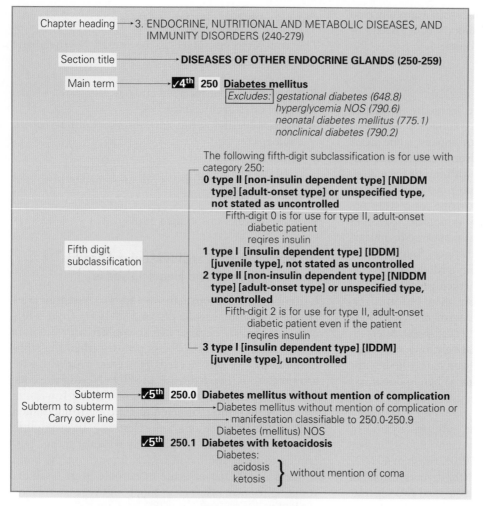

FIGURE 5–2
Classification of diabetes mellitus showing fifth-digit subclassification from *International Classification of Diseases, 9th Revision, Clinical Modification (ICD-9-CM)*, Volume 2.

Table 5.5	Type Grouping for Diabetes
250.00 for non-insulin dependent diabetes (NIDDM) Adult onset Type two, Type II or unspecified Stable or not stated as uncontrolled Non-ketosis prone	**250.02 for non-insulin-dependent diabetes (NIDDM)** Adult onset Type two, Type II or unspecified Uncontrolled
250.01 for insulin-dependent diabetes (IDDM) Juvenile onset Type one, Type I Stable or not stated as uncontrolled Ketosis prone	**250.03 for insulin-dependent diabetes (IDDM)** Juvenile onset Type one, Type I Uncontrolled

Coding *always* requires five digits because of the types and complications that may accompany this disease. Here is the way this classification appears in ICD-9-CM, Volume 2:

Fifth-digit subclassification with code 250 is not based on severity or age grouping of the case (Figure 5–2). It is a type grouping; use Table 5.5 as a guide.

Always ask the physician for further clarification when a medical record contains the statement "discharged on insulin" with no further explanation of the type of diabetes. Do not assume that a patient taking insulin has insulin-dependent diabetes.

Do not use code 250.0X if the diabetes is stated with delivery of a child or as a complication of pregnancy. Use code 648.01.

Pregnancy, Delivery, or Abortion

The following main sections are included:

630 to 633 Ectopic and molar pregnancy

634 to 639 Other pregnancy with abortive outcome (*five-digit subclassifications must be used with categories 634 to 637*)

640 to 648 Complications mainly related to pregnancy (*five-digit subclassifications must be used*)

650 to 659 Normal delivery and other indications for care in pregnancy, labor, and delivery (*five-digit subclassifications must be used in categories 651-659*)

660 to 669 Complications occurring mainly in the course of labor and delivery (*five-digit subclassifications must be used*)

670 to 677 Complications of the puerperium *(five-digit subclassifications must be used for categories 670 to 676)*

The following guidelines are used:

1. Code 650 is used for a completely *normal* delivery. This means normal spontaneous delivery, cephalic (vertex) presentation of one live-born fetus, full-term gestation (with or without episiotomy), no manipulation necessary, and no laceration.
2. A code other than 650 should be used to provide greater detail about a **complication** of abortion, pregnancy, childbirth, or the puerperium when information is available, such as the presence of anemia, diabetes mellitus, or thyroid dysfunction (Example 5.16). Complication of the puerperium is a complication within 6 weeks after labor.

Example 5.16		Complications Related to Pregnancy
648.01	250.00	Pregnancy (delivered) with diabetes mellitus
648.23	282.60	Pregnancy (antepartum) with sickle cell anemia

In most instances, an additional code is added to specify the patient's specific problem.

A multiple gestation (twins, triplets) is a complication of pregnancy and is considered high risk. When a patient delivers and experiences both antepartum and postpartum complications, different fifth digits may be applied on the codes to describe the episodes of care (Example 5.17). In such cases, there is also a need for using a V code to indicate the outcome of delivery of liveborn infants according to type of birth (V30 to V39).

Example 5.17	Multiple Gestation
651.11	Triplet pregnancy (delivered)
675.02	Infection of nipple (postpartum)

Admitting Diagnoses

Some diagnostic codes are considered questionable when used as the first diagnosis on admission of a patient to the hospital (e.g., 278.00 obesity, 401.1 benign hypertension). The inpatient admission diagnosis may be expressed as one of the following:

1. One or more significant findings (symptoms or signs) representing patient distress or abnormal findings on examination.
2. A diagnosis established on an ambulatory care basis or previous hospital admission.

3. An injury or poisoning.
4. A reason or condition not classifiable as an illness or injury, such as pregnancy in labor, follow-up inpatient diagnostic tests, and so on.

When your employer physician makes hospital visits, code the reason for the visit, which may *not* necessarily be the reason the patient was admitted to the hospital.

Burns

To be as specific as possible with coding burns, you need at least two codes. The first code is for the exact site and degree of the burn (940 to 947). The second code found in category 948 describes the percentage of body surface area burned. A fifth digit is included in this category and is necessary to indicate how much of the total body surface had third-degree burns. Think of the body as a whole and not the body parts as a whole. The adult body is divided into regions: head, 9%; arms, 9% each; trunk, 18% front and 18% back; legs, 18% each; and perineum, 1% (Figure 5–3). Children's and infants' bodies have different regional percentages. Burn codes should be sequenced with the highest degree burn first, followed by the other burn codes. However, when a first- and a second-degree burn of the same site are listed, only the highest degree burn of that site is coded, with the fifth digit indicating other anatomic sites of that category.

Injuries and Late Effects

Diagnostic codes for injuries are listed in the Alphabetic Index by the type of injury and are broken down by anatomic site. To code multiple injuries, list the diagnosis for the conditions treated in order of importance, with the diagnosis for the most severe problem listed first. If surgery is involved, the diagnostic code for the surgical problem should be listed first unless there is a severe injury of another part of the body. For example, in the case of an intracranial injury, managed medically, and a fractured phalanx, managed surgically, the intracranial injury is listed as the primary diagnosis and the diagnosis fractured phalanx is sequenced second. The most difficult part of assigning injury codes is knowing what words to look for in the Alphabetic Index. Codes 800 through 959 include fractures, dislocations, sprains, and other types of injury. Injuries are coded according to the general type of injury and broken down within each type by anatomic site. A list of common injury medical terms and the types of injuries included for each is shown in Table 5.6. An injury may have a late effect, which must be coded in a different fashion.

Use the following guides for coding injuries:

1. Decide whether a diagnosis represents a current injury or a late effect of an injury (Example 5.18).

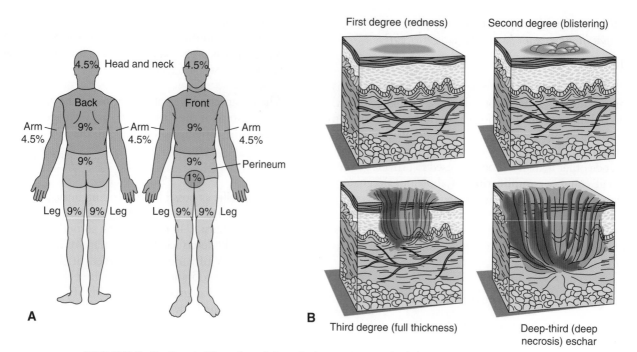

FIGURE 5–3 **A,** The rules of nines for burn injury to the body. **B,** The degrees of burn involving the layers of the skin: first-degree burns include the epidermis (redness), second-degree burns include the epidermis and dermis (blistering), third-degree burns include the first two layers and the subcutaneous tissues (full thickness), and deep-third burns involve all layers of the skin with resulting eschar (deep necrosis).

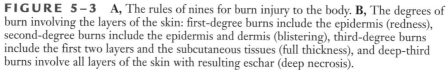

Table 5.6	Common Injury Medical Terms
Contusion	Bruise and hematoma without a fracture or open wound
Crush	Crushing injury not complicated by concussion, fractures, injury to internal organs, or intracranial injury
Dislocation	Displacement and subluxation. Dislocation may be open or closed. Closed dislocation may be complete, partial, simple, or uncomplicated. Open dislocation may be compound, infected, or with foreign body. A dislocation not indicated as closed or open is classified as closed.
Fracture	Fractures may be open or closed. A fracture not indicated as open or closed is classified as closed. An injury described as fracture dislocation is coded as a fracture. Open fractures may be described as compound, infected, missile, puncture, or with foreign body. Closed fractures may be described as comminuted, depressed, elevated, fissured, greenstick, impacted, linear, march, simple, slipped, epiphyseal, or spiral.
Injury, blood vessel	Described as arterial hematoma, avulsion, laceration, rupture, traumatic aneurysm, or traumatic fistula
Injury, internal	Includes all injuries to internal organs such as the heart, lung, liver, kidney, and pelvic organs. Types of injuries to internal organs include laceration, tear, traumatic rupture, penetrating wounds, blunt trauma, crushing, blast injuries, or open wounds to internal organs with or without fracture in the same region.
Injury, intracranial	Includes concussion, cerebral laceration and contusion, or intracranial hemorrhage. These injuries may be open or closed. Intracranial injuries with skull fractures may be found under fracture.
Injury, superficial	Includes abrasion, insect bite (nonvenomous), blister, or scratch.
Sprain/strain	Injury to the joint capsule, ligament, muscle, or tendon described by the following terms: avulsion, hemarthrosis, laceration (closed), rupture, or tear. Open laceration of these structures should be coded as open wounds.
Wound, open	Includes open wounds not involving internal organs. Wounds may be to skin, muscle, or tendon, described as animal bite, avulsion, cut, laceration, puncture wound, or traumatic amputation. Open wounds may be complicated or uncomplicated. Complicated includes injuries with mention of delayed healing, delayed treatment, foreign body, or major infection.

Example 5.18	Current Injury
824.8	**Current injury:** Fracture, left ankle
	OR
733.81 and 905.4	Late effect: Malunion fracture, left ankle

2. Fractures are coded as closed if there is no indication of whether the fracture is open or closed.
3. The word "with" indicates involvement of both sites, and the word "and" indicates involvement of either one or two sites when multiple injury sites are given (Example 5.19).

Example 5.19	Multiple Injury Sites
806	Fracture of the vertebral column **with** spinal cord injury
813	Fracture of radius **and** ulna

Look up code 813 in your diagnostic code book and note that this code section relates to a fracture of the radius, ulna, or both.

A **late effect** means "the residual effect (condition produced) after the acute phase of an illness or injury has terminated." An effect is considered to be late if the diagnosis reads "due to an old injury," "late," "due to" or "following" (previous illness or injury), or "due to an injury or illness that occurred 1 year or more before the current admission of encounter." If time has passed between the occurrence of the acute illness or injury and the development of the residual effect, such as scarring, late effects also may be coded.

Example 5.20 illustrates late effects. Residuals are shown in italics, and the causes are shown in bold print. Code both the residual effect and the cause.

Example 5.20	Late Effects
	A. *Malunion* **fracture,** right tibia
	Traumatic *arthritis* following **fracture** of right knee;
	Hemiplegia following **cerebrovascular thrombosis** 1 year previously
	Scarring caused by third-degree **burn** of right arm
	Contracture of right heel tendons caused by **poliomyelitis**
	B. Traumatic **arthropathy,** shoulder region
	Traumatic **arthritis** of left shoulder due to old **fracture** of left humerus followed by late effect of **fracture of upper extremities**

Use the following guides for coding late effects:

1. Refer to the main term "late" in ICD-9-CM Volume 2 when coding a case with late effects.

2. Use two codes when late effects are involved for both the present condition and the initial condition. The late effect code is usually a secondary diagnosis code, with the primary diagnosis code listed as the current residual condition. In some cases, the late effect is the sole reason for the office visit; in such cases, the late effect code becomes the primary diagnosis.

Now that you have learned the basics of ICD-9-CM coding, the next step is to begin to learn the new system based on ICD-10.

ICD-10-CM DIAGNOSIS AND PROCEDURE CODES

For the past 20 years, the ICD-9-CM diagnosis system has been used. Although it has been updated, the system has outlived its usefulness because of advances in technology, discovery of new diseases, development of new procedures, and the need to report more details for statistical purposes. The time is fast approaching to adopt another system. Actually there are two systems, *International Classification of Diseases, 10th Revision, Clinical Modification* (ICD-10-CM—diagnostic codes) and *ICD-10 Procedure Coding System* (ICD-10-PCS—procedure codes). Both hospital and physician office insurance billers should be concerned with the new diagnosis codes, but only hospital billers need to concern themselves with the procedure codes.

ICD-10 Volume 1: Tabular List was published by the World Health Organization in 1992. It was clinically modified (CM) by the National Center for Health Statistics (NCHS) before code adoption. The CM provides the specifics that the United States needs for collecting data on health status. Reasons for clinical modification are the removal of procedural codes, unique mortality codes, and "multiple" codes. ICD-10-PCS was developed in the mid-1990s by 3M Health Information Systems under contract with the Centers for Medicaid and Medicare Services (CMS). This replaces Volume 3 of ICD-9-CM used in hospital billing but does not replace the CPT code book used in outpatient billing. Reasons for development of ICD-10-PCS are as follows:

● ICD-10 did not have procedure classification.
● ICD-9-CM was not expandable, comprehensive, or multiaxial (broken down into many subdivisions).
● ICD-9-CM did not have standardized terminology and included diagnostic information.
● ICD-10-CM differs from ICD-9-CM in the following ways:
  1. Major changes in code book organization exist.
  2. Many new categories and chapters have been added.
  3. There is a replacement of the traditional numeric coding system with a six-digit and sometimes

seven-digit alphanumeric scheme for ICD-10-CM (Example 5.21). Obstetrics, injuries, and external causes of injuries may have seven-digit codes. Some codes include last-digit alpha characters "a," "b," "d," "g," "j," or "q" to identify initial encounter, subsequent encounter, or sequelae.

Example 5.21   Alphanumeric Codes for ICD-10-CM

FRACTURE OF UPPER LIMB (810-819)

810   Fracture of clavicle
    Includes: collar bone
            interligamentous part of clavicle
    The following fifth-digit subclassification is for
    use with category 810:

        0   unspecified part
            Clavicle NOS
        1   sternal end of clavicle
        2   shaft of clavicle
        3   acromial end of clavicle

✓5ᵗʰ   **810.0   Closed**

ICD-10-CM

  S42.00 Closed fracture of clavicle
    S42.001 Closed fracture of right clavicle
    S42.002 Closed fracture of left clavicle
    S42.009 Closed fracture of clavicle, unspecified side

---

4. Old injury (800 to 999) codes have been changed to S and T codes. Currently coding is done by type of injury, such as fractures, dislocations, and sprains/strains, but in ICD-10 coding is by injury site (injuries to neck, injuries to thorax).
5. Explanatory notes and instructions for use have been greatly expanded.
6. The dagger-and-asterisk system of dual classification in ICD-10 has been considerably expanded for ICD-10-CM (Example 5.22). Note: Some publishers may use different symbols.
7. The E and V codes in ICD-9-CM are now Chapters XX and XXI.

Example 5.22   Symbols used in ICD-10-CM

ICD-10

A39.5†   **Meningococcal Heart Disease**
        Meningococcal:
            Carditis NOS (I52.0*)
            Endocarditis (I39.8*)

ICD-10-CM

A39.5   **Meningococcal Heart Disease**
            A39.50 Meningococcal Carditis . . .
            A39.51 Meningococcal Endocarditis

---

8. The coding system allows for assignment of unique codes as new procedures are developed.
9. Combination diagnosis/symptom codes have been added, e.g., poisoning/external cause codes have been combined.
10. Postoperative complication codes describe both the type and site of complication, e.g., accidental puncture or laceration of the ear during an ear procedure.
11. An activity code category that describes activities in which a patient was engaged when he or she was injured, e.g., horseback riding Y93.013.
12. ICD-10-PCS is much more specific than the CPT coding system when making a comparison.

The second part, section, or volume of the ICD-10-CM is an instruction manual that provides definitions, standards, and rules for the tabular list. The last part or volume is an alphabetical index. These systems allow more code choices and require greater documentation in the medical record. An experienced coder should develop a proactive, positive attitude toward accepting and learning the ICD-10-CM. A coder must have a higher level of clinical knowledge. It is wise to attend an anatomy and physiology course a year before the new system is adopted if you have not already done so. There has been a monumental change from ICD-9-CM to ICD-10-CM. After coding guidelines have been developed, training workshops will be offered. To gain knowledge and proficiency, many hours of instruction may be needed to learn the new system. Even after a person learns how to code, it takes a longer time to code under the new system.

Publishers of ICD-10-CM may use different styles and format so it is important to study and compare the features of several books before making a decision to purchase. When choosing a book, the following questions should be asked: Is color coding being used for emphasis in locating items quickly? Are definitions or notes included to help one interpret and gain a better understanding of difficult medical terms and phrases? Are coding guidelines boxed for easy reference? All of these benefit the coder.

Possible errors may occur when using the Tabular List and when coding diseases or conditions that begin with categories "O" and "I." These can look like the numbers "zero" and "one" (e.g., I00 and O99 are correct and not 100 and 099). In these categories, special attention must be given.

As of the date of the printing of this textbook, guidelines have not been adopted, so training has not begun. The next edition of this textbook will feature how to code using ICD-10-CM.

INDEX TO DISEASES   Anemia

ICD Volume 2
ALPHABETIC INDEX

Anemia 285.9

Anemia-*continued*	**Anemia**-*continued*	Anemia-*continued*
glutathione-reductase deficiency 282.2	hemolytic-*continued*	megaloblastic-*continued*
goat's milk 281.2	resulting from presence of shunt or other	of infancy 281.2
granulocytic 288.0	internal prosthetic device 283.19	of or complicating pregnancy 648.2 ✓5th
Heinz-body, congenital 282.7	secondary 283.19	refractory 281.3
hemoglobin deficiency 285.9	autoimmune 283.0	specified NEC 281.3
hemolytic 283.9	sickle-cell – *see* Disease, sickle-cell	megalocytic 281.9
acquired 283.9	Stransky-Regala type (Hb-E) (*see also*	microangiopathic hemolytic 283.19
with hemoglobinuria NEC 283.2	Disease, hemoglobin) 282.7	microcytic (hypochromic) 280.9
autoimmune (cold type) (idiopathic)	symptomatic 283.19	due to blood loss (chronic) 280.0
(primary) (secondary) (symptomatic)	autoimmune 283.0	acute 285.1
(warm type) 283.	toxic (acquired) 283.19	familial 282.4
due to	uremic (adult) (child) 283.11	hypochromic 280.9
cold reactive antibodies 283.0	warm type (secondary) (symptomatic) 283.0	microdrepanocytosis 282.4
drug exposure 283.0	hemorrhagic (chronic) 280.0	miners' (*see also* Ancylostomiasis) 126.9
warm reactive antibodies 283.0	acute 285.1	myelopathic 285.8
	HEMPAS 285.8	

Main term
Subterm

Subsubterm
Diagnostic code

FIGURE 5–4 Excerpt from the Alphabetic Index of *International Classification of Diseases, 9th Revision, Clinical Modification (ICD-9-CM)*, Volume 2.

PROCEDURE

BASIC STEPS IN SELECTING DIAGNOSTIC CODES

OBJECTIVE: Accurately select and insert diagnostic codes for electronic transmission of an insurance claim.
EQUIPMENT/SUPPLIES: Diagnostic code book (Volumes 1 and 2), medical dictionary, and pen or pencil.
DIRECTIONS: Use a standard method and establish a routine for locating a code. Follow these recommended steps for coding the first diagnosis. There are no shortcuts. For each subsequent diagnosis in a patient's medical record, repeat these steps. Refer to Figure 5-4 as you go through Step 1.
DIAGNOSIS: Refractory megaloblastic anemia, with chronic alcoholic liver disease

1. Locate the main term or condition (not the anatomic site) in the Alphabetic Index, Volume 2 (anemia). To identify the main term, ask what is wrong with the patient.
2. Refer to any notes under the main term (none shown).
3. Read any notes or terms enclosed in parentheses after the main term (nonessential modifiers) (none shown).
4. Look for appropriate subterm (megaloblastic). *Do not* skip over any subterms indented under the main term.
5. Look for appropriate sub-subterm (refractory). Follow any cross-reference instructions (none given).

6. Write down the code (281.3).
7. Verify the code number in the Tabular List, Volume 1 (Figure 5-5).
8. Read and be guided by any instructional terms in the Tabular List. In this example, there are none given.
9. Read complete description and then code to the highest specificity; that is, code to the highest number of digits (three, four, or five) in the classification (refractory megaloblastic anemia, 281.3). When a fourth or fifth digit is listed, its use is *NOT* optional. A three-digit code is considered a category unless no fourth or fifth digit appears after it. Fifth-digit codes appear either at the beginning of a chapter, section, or three-digit category, or within the four-digit subcategory. To facilitate locating those codes that require a fourth or fifth digit, some publishers may insert a symbol (e.g., ⑤) in the codebook. Do not arbitrarily use a zero as a filler character when listing a diagnostic code number. This may nullify the code or indicate a different disease. The code book includes decimal points, but these are not required for transmission of insurance claims.
10. Assign the code.

Now use a step-by-step approach to code chronic alcoholic liver disease and refer to each volume as shown in Example 5.23.

Code initially from the Alphabetic Index, Volume 2. Then go to the Tabular List, Volume 1, to *verify* that the code number selected is in accord with the desired classification of the diagnosis. Look for important instructions that often appear. Check for exclusion notes, which refer to terms or conditions that are not included within the code. These may further direct the coder to the correct ICD-9-CM code assignment (Figure 5–6).

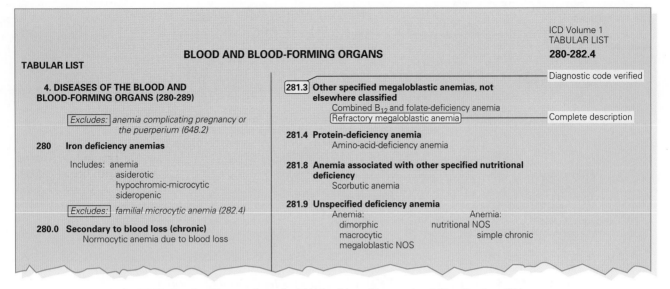

FIGURE 5-5 Excerpt from the Tabular List of *International Classification of Diseases, 9th Revision, Clinical Modification (ICD-9-CM),* Volume 1.

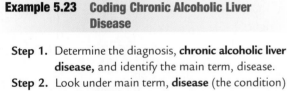

Example 5.23 **Coding Chronic Alcoholic Liver Disease**

Step 1. Determine the diagnosis, **chronic alcoholic liver disease,** and identify the main term, disease.

Step 2. Look under main term, **disease** (the condition) in Volume 2.
   a. A note states "see also Syndrome" and would be followed if you cannot locate the code.
   b. There are no nonessential modifiers to read.
   c. Find the subterm **liver.**
   d. Locate the sub-subterm **chronic.**
   e. There are no cross-references listed.
   f. Write down the code number **571.3.**

Step 3. Verify the code number, not the page number in Volume 1.
   a. Verify you are in the correct chapter, "Diseases of the Digestive System."
   b. The three-digit code category is **Chronic liver disease and cirrhosis (571).**
   c. Note, there are no 5th-digit code requirements.
   d. The complete description reads "571.3 Alcoholic liver damage, unspecified." The code and its title refer to any liver damage caused by alcoholism, without specification as to the nature of the disorder. Because there are no exclusion notes, this is the correct code.

Step 4. Assign and record the correct code, **571.3.**

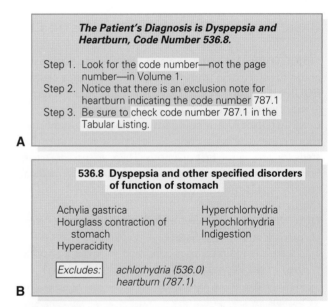

FIGURE 5-6 A, Example of a disease to look up in the Tabular List. **B,** Illustration of coding showing an exclusion note from the Tabular List of *International Classification of Diseases, 9th Revision, Clinical Modification (ICD-9-CM),* Volume 1.

An "excludes" box may appear listing diagnoses and additional codes to research to ensure that the correct code is assigned. As shown in Figure 5-7, this example appears on the insurance claim keyed without the decimal as **5368.**

NOTE: Heartburn is not coded because it is a symptom of dyspepsia and appears as an exclusion under dyspepsia in Volume 1.

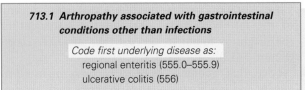

> **713.1 Arthropathy associated with gastrointestinal conditions other than infections**
>
> Code first underlying disease as:
> regional enteritis (555.0–555.9)
> ulcerative colitis (556)

FIGURE 5-7 Coding by etiology.

Certain conditions are classified according to etiology (cause) of the disorder (Figure 5–7). In these cases, you should follow the instructions "Code first underlying disease..." Code the etiology in the first position. Code the disorder in the second position. Words to look for in the diagnostic statement include "acquired," "congenital," "associated with," "obstetric," "nonobstetric," "transmissible," "not transmissible," "traumatic," and "nontraumatic."

When the patient's medical record states a "versus" diagnosis, such as "peptic ulcer versus gastroesophageal reflux," code the presenting symptoms. When a specific condition is stated in the diagnosis as acute (or subacute) and chronic, and the Alphabetic Index provides separate codes at either the third-, fourth-, or fifth-digit level for acute and chronic, use both codes with the acute code given first (Example 5.24).

Example 5.24	**Acute and Chronic Pelvic Inflammatory Disease**
Condition:	Disease
Subcategories:	Pelvis, Pelvic
Sub-subcategory:	Inflammatory
	Acute 614.3
	Chronic 614.4

Four-digit subcategories .8 and .9 usually, but not always, are reserved for "other specified" and "unspecified" conditions, respectively. "Other specified" and "unspecified" subcategories are referred to as residual subcategories (Figure 5–8). Residual subcategories are used for conditions that are specifically named in the medical record but not specifically listed under a code description. If there is a lack of details in the medical record and you cannot match to a specific subdivision, research the medical record for a qualifying statement in the physician's progress notes or history and physical examination report that will allow you to use a more specific diagnostic code (Figure 5–9).

Diagnostic codes must match the age and gender of the patient. If an adult female patient with breast cancer is seen (excluding carcinoma in situ and skin cancer of breast), a code from 174.0 through 174.9 must be used. If a male with breast cancer is treated, a code from 175.0 through 175.9 must be chosen. Some codes apply only to newborns, such as code 775.10 for neonatal diabetes mellitus.

Special Points to Remember in Volume 1

● Use two or more codes if necessary to completely describe a given diagnosis. Example: Arteriosclerotic cardiovascular *disease* (429.2) with congestive heart *failure* (428.0).
● Search for one code when two diagnoses or a diagnosis with an associated secondary process (manifestation) or complication is present. There are instances when two diagnoses are classified with a single code number called a **combination code** (Figure 5–10).
● Use category codes (three-digit codes) only if there are no subcategory codes (fourth-digit subdivisions) (Figure 5–11).

Special Points to Remember in Volume 2

● Notice that appropriate sites or modifiers are listed in alphabetic order under the main terms, with further subterm listings as necessary.
● Examine all modifiers that appear in parentheses next to the main term.

710.4 Polymyositis ← ┐
                         ├── Specified
710.5 Eosinophilia myalgia syndrome ← ┘
      Toxic oil syndrome
      Use additional E code to identify drug if drug induced

710.8 Other specified diffuse diseases of connective tissue ← Other specified
      Multifocal fibrosclerosis (idiopathic) NEC
      Systemic fibrosclerosing syndrome

710.9 Unspecified diffuse connective tissue disease ← Unspecified
      Collagen disease NOS

FIGURE 5-8 Four-digit residual subcategories: specified, other specified, and unspecified disease conditions.

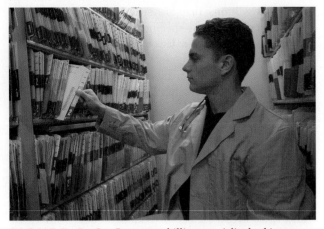

FIGURE 5-9 Insurance billing specialist looking up a patient's medical record file to verify documentation for a diagnostic code.

- Check for nonessential modifiers that apply to any of the qualifying terms used in the statement of the diagnosis found in the patient's medical record (Figure 5–12).
- Notice that eponyms appear as both main term entries and modifiers under main terms such as "disease" or "syndrome" and "operation." As mentioned in Chapter 4 and shown in Example 4.2, an *eponym* is the name of a disease, structure, operation, or procedure, usually derived from the name of a place or a person who discovered or described it first.
- Look for sublisted terms in parentheses that are associated with the eponym (Figure 5–13).
- Locate closely related terms, code categories, and cross-referenced synonyms indicated by *see* and *see also* (Figure 5–14).

491.2 Obstructive chronic bronchitis

Bronchitis:
   emphysematous
   obstructive (chronic) (diffuse)
Bronchitis with:
   chronic airway obstruction
   emphysema

EXCLUDES *asthmatic bronchitis (acute) NOS (493.9) chronic obstructive asthma (493.2x)*

491.20 Without mention of acute exacerbation

Emphysema with chronic bronchitis

491.21 With acute exacerbation

Combination code ⟶ Acute bronchitis with chronic obstructive pulmonary disease [COPD]
Disease combinations ⟶ Acute and chronic obstructive bronchitis
Acute exacerbation of chronic obstructive pulmonary disease [COPD]
Emphysema with both acute and chronic bronchitis

FIGURE 5-10 Combination coding.

---

430 Subarachnoid hemorrhage

   Meningeal hemorrhage
   Ruptured:
      berry aneurysm
      (congenital) cerebral aneurysm NOS

   | Excludes: | *syphilitic ruptured cerebral aneurysm (094.87)*

FIGURE 5-11 Three-digit coding.

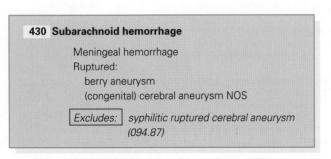

Obesity (constitutional) (exogenous) ◄——— Nonessential
   (familial) (nutritional) (simple) 278.0   modifiers
   adrenal 255.8
   due to hyperalimentation 278.00
   endocrine NEC 259.9
   endogenous 259.9
   Fröhlich's (adiposogenital dystrophy) 253.8
   glandular NEC 259.9
   hypothyroid (*see also* Hypothyroidism) 244.9
   morbid 278.01
   of pregnancy 646.1
   pituitary 253.8
   thyroid (*see also* Hypothyroidism) 244.9

FIGURE 5-12 Coding with modifiers in parentheses.

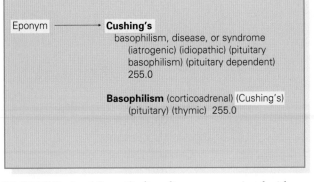

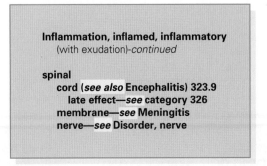

FIGURE 5–13 Coding diagnoses associated with an eponym.

FIGURE 5–14 Cross-referencing synonyms, closely related terms, and code categories from the Alphabetic Index of the *International Classification of Diseases, Ninth Revision, Clinical Modification (ICD-9-CM)*, Volume 2.

INTERNET RESOURCES

For AHIMA diagnostic code guidelines for outpatient services and diagnostic coding and reporting requirements for physician billing:

• Web site: **http://www.ahacentraloffice.com**
  Web site: **http://www.ahima.org**

• For code guidelines for the Center for Medicare and Medicaid Services:
  Web site: **http://www.cms.hhs.gov/medlearn/matters/2004/mm3094.pdf**

• For downloading a prerelease draft of ICD-10-CM from June 2003:
  Web site: **http://www.cdc.gov/nchs/about/otheract/icd9/icd10cm.htm**

• For downloading the November 2003 final draft of ICD-10-PCS:
  Web site: **http://www.cms.hhs.gov/paymentsystem/icd9/icd10.asp?**

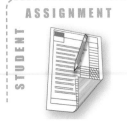

STUDENT ASSIGNMENT

✔ Study Chapter 5.

✔ Answer the review questions in the *Workbook* to reinforce theory learned in this chapter and to help prepare you for a future test.

✔ Complete the assignments in the *Workbook* to gain hands-on experience in diagnostic coding.

CHAPTER OUTLINE

UNDERSTANDING THE IMPORTANCE OF PROCEDURAL CODING SKILLS

CODING COMPLIANCE PLAN
  Current Procedural Terminology

METHODS OF PAYMENT
  Fee Schedule
  Usual, Customary, and Reasonable
  Developing a Fee Schedule Using Relative Value Studies
    Conversion Factors

HOW TO USE THE CPT CODE BOOK
  Category I, II, and III Codes
  Code Book Symbols
  Evaluation and Management Section
  Surgery Section
  Unlisted Procedures
  Coding Guidelines for Code Edits
  Code Monitoring

HELPFUL HINTS IN CODING
  Office Visits
  Drugs and Injections

  Adjunct Codes
  Basic Life or Disability Evaluation Services

CODE MODIFIERS
  Correct Use of Common CPT Modifiers
  Comprehensive List of Modifier Codes

PROCEDURE: DETERMINE CONVERSION FACTORS

PROCEDURE: CHOOSE CORRECT PROCEDURAL CODES FOR PROFESSIONAL SERVICES

KEY TERMS

alternative billing codes (ABCs)

bilateral

bundled codes

comprehensive code

conversion factor

Current Procedural Terminology (CPT)

customary fee

downcoding

fee schedule

global surgery policy

Healthcare Common Procedure Coding System (HCPCS)

modifier

procedure code numbers

professional component (PC)

reasonable fee

relative value studies (RVS)

relative value unit (RVU)

resource-based relative value scale (RBRVS)

surgical package

technical component (TC)

unbundling

upcoding

usual, customary, and reasonable (UCR)

6

Procedural Coding

OBJECTIVES*

After reading this chapter, you should be able to:

- Explain the purpose of coding for professional services.

- Use procedure code books properly.

- Define procedure code terminology.

- Explain the importance and usage of modifiers in procedure coding.

- Code the *Workbook* problems using the CPT manual.

- Describe the differences between CPT and RVS coding systems.

- Describe various methods of payment by insurance companies and state and federal programs.

*Performance objectives and exercises for hands-on practical experience for this chapter appear in the *Workbook*.

Service

Procedure codes must reflect the services rendered to the patient so that payment by an insurance plan is optimal based on the supporting health record documentation and appropriate based on correct code selection.

UNDERSTANDING THE IMPORTANCE OF PROCEDURAL CODING SKILLS

Now that you have learned some terminology and the basics of diagnostic coding, the next step is to learn how to code procedures.

Procedure coding is the transformation of written descriptions of procedures and professional services into numeric designations (code numbers). The physician rendering medical care either writes or dictates this information into the patient's health record. Then the insurance billing specialist abstracts pertinent information and assigns procedure codes. Routine office visits and procedures usually are listed with codes and brief descriptions on the encounter form. These services are documented in the record and circled or checked off on the encounter form by the physician when they are performed during the patient's visit.

With the implementation of computer technology and stricter adherence to federal regulations, more emphasis is being placed on correct procedural coding. Coding must be correct if claims are to be paid promptly and optimally. Every procedure or service must be assigned correct and complete code numbers. Because of the complexity of procedural coding, a working knowledge of medical terminology, including anatomy and physiology, is essential.

Procedure codes are a standardized method used to precisely describe the services provided by physicians and allied health care professionals. They allow claim forms to be optically scanned by insurance companies. The general acceptance of the codes by insurance carriers and government agencies assures the physician who uses a standardized coding system that the services and procedures he or she performs can be objectively identified and priced. The American Hospital Association (AHA) and American Health Information Management Association (AHIMA) guidelines for outpatient services and procedure coding and reporting requirements for physician billing may be found by visiting the Web sites listed in the Internet Resources at the end of this chapter.

The primary coding system used in physicians' offices for professional services and procedures is

Current Procedural Terminology (CPT),* published and updated annually by the American Medical Association (AMA). A relative value scale, called relative value studies (RVS), is also used for services and procedures; it is the system used by Medicare called resource-based relative value scale (RBRVS). RVS and RBRVS provide values for CPT codes that can then be converted into dollars by use of geographic and conversion factors.

Some managed care plans develop a few internal codes for use by the plan only. Sometimes the codes are used for tracking; other times, they are used to provide reimbursement for a service not defined within CPT based on their benefit structure and internal needs.

CODING COMPLIANCE PLAN

Because the government is more involved in health care, each medical practice should construct and maintain a policy and procedure manual in regard to coding guidelines for their medical practice so they are in compliance with HIPAA. Establishing coding and billing policies and procedures helps physicians and their office staff address potential risk areas for fraud and abuse. A plan should include the medical practice's basic ethical philosophy, outline policies, detail coding procedures, and create an environment of confidentiality. Billers and coders should sign a statement annually indicating that they have read, understand, and agree with the medical practice's standards of conduct (see Figure 1–6). The plan should provide coders with the framework for correct coding and indicate that health record documentation must support the codes billed. An internal audit should be done on a regular basis and action taken to correct the offense if noncompliance is discovered. Such plans must have a compliance officer or a committee that oversees the audits, monitors compliance issues, and trains employees in compliance issues.

Current Procedural Terminology

The first edition of *Physicians' Current Procedural Terminology* appeared in 1966, and the book was subsequently revised in 1970, 1973, and 1977. Since 1984, *Current Procedural Terminology* (CPT), fourth edition, has been updated

---

*Available from Book and Pamphlet Fulfillment: OP-3416, American Medical Association, P.O. Box 10946, Chicago, IL 60610-0946, or visit CPT on the Internet at Web site: www.ama-assn.org/cpt.

and revised annually. Code numbers are added or deleted as new procedures are developed or existing procedures are modified. These changes are shown in each edition by the use of symbols, which are described and shown later in this chapter in Figure 6–2. The symbols with their meanings are located at the bottom of each page of code numbers in the CPT code book.

CPT uses a basic five-digit system for coding services rendered by physicians and two-digit add-on modifiers to indicate complications or special circumstances. **Procedure code numbers** represent diagnostic and therapeutic services on medical billing statements and insurance forms (Example 6.1).*

Example 6.1   Current Procedural Terminology Procedure Code Numbers

A 45-year-old woman is seen for an initial office visit for evaluation of recurrent right shoulder pain. The examination required a detailed history and physical examination (D HX & PX) with low complexity medical decision making (LCMDM). Patient complains of pain radiating down right arm. A complete radiographic study of the right shoulder is obtained in the office and read by the physician. A corticosteroid solution is injected into the shoulder joint.

CPT Code	Description of Services
99203	Office visit, new patient
	(E/M service)
73030	Radiologic examination, shoulder, two views
	(Diagnostic service)
20610	Arthrocentesis inj.; major joint, shoulder
	(Therapeutic service)

CPT emerged as the procedural coding of choice when the federal government developed the Health Care Financing Administration (HCFA) Common Procedure Coding System (HCPCS) (pronounced "hick-picks") for the Medicare Program. The HCFA changed its acronym to CMS (Centers for Medicare and Medicaid Services); therefore the HCPCS acronym is translated as **Healthcare Common Procedure Coding System.** The Medicare HCPCS consists of two levels of coding:

● Level I: the AMA CPT codes and modifiers (national codes)
● Level II: CMS-designated codes and alpha modifiers (national codes). Examples of this level may be found at the end of Appendix B of the *Workbook.*

---

*Examples shown in this chapter reflect wording pertinent to coding a specific procedure and may be missing complete chart entries; therefore there may be a gap of information for the reader.

You may discover that one case can be coded in two coding levels. The CPT code should be used when both a CPT and level II code have the same description. The level II code should be used if the descriptions are not identical (e.g., if the CPT code narrative is generic and the HCPCS level II code is specific).

The formula for selecting a code that most accurately identifies the service is as follows:

CPT code = Physician or provider service (PPS)
HCPCS national code = Ambulance, medical and surgical supplies, enteral and parenteral therapy, outpatient PPS, dental procedures, durable medical equipment, procedures/professional services, alcohol and drug abuse treatment services, drugs administered other than oral method, orthotic procedures, prosthetic procedures, other medical services, pathology and laboratory services, casting and splinting supplies, diagnostic radiology services, temporary non-Medicare codes, T codes for state Medicaid agencies, and vision and hearing services

Some private insurance companies have begun to accept level II HCPCS codes. It is wise to check the carrier's provider manual or telephone the carrier before sending in claims for medications and durable medical equipment. The HCPCS is updated each January 1 with periodic updates made throughout the year as necessary. (See Chapter 12 for additional information on coding for Medicare cases.) In some states, the TRICARE and Medicaid programs accept HCPCS codes. Most commercial insurance companies have adopted the level I (CPT) and level II (HCPCS) code systems.

Alternative Billing Codes

Alternative billing codes (ABCs) are five-character alphabetic symbols with appended two-character practitioner modifiers that represent the practitioner type. These codes represent more than 4000 integrative health care products and services (Example 6.2). *Integrative health*

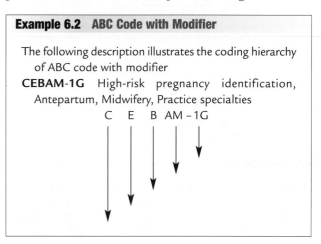

Example 6.2   ABC Code with Modifier

The following description illustrates the coding hierarchy of ABC code with modifier
CEBAM-1G High-risk pregnancy identification, Antepartum, Midwifery, Practice specialties
C   E   B   AM – 1G

---

care is care that incorporates the best approaches from conventional and from complementary and alternative medicine. The following areas of health care are represented by the ABC codes and are within specialty areas:

Acupuncturist	Ayurvedic medicine
Body work	Botanical medicine
Chiropractic	Clinical nutrition
Conventional nursing	Holistic dentists and
Indigenous medicine	physicians
Mental health care	Homeopathy
Minority health care	Massage therapy
Oriental medicine	Midwifery
Physical medicine	Naturopathic medicine
Spiritual and prayer-	Osteopathic medicine
based healing	Somatic educational

Anyone can use ABC codes for research, management, and manual or paper-based commerce. The use of these code sets is unregulated, so they fall outside of the HIPAA regulations of 1996. For electronic commerce, which is a federally regulated use of code sets under HIPAA, ABC codes may be used by any of more than 10,000 entities that secured rights to use the codes under section 45CFR162.940 of the Code of Federal Regulations and their contractual trading partners. Some coded procedures require additional certification or training, and those codes may be used if a practitioner can supply the documentation.

ABC codes may become mandatory. Sandia Health System in New Mexico has been paying ABC-coded claims since 1999. Numerous payers are in the process of implementing the ABC codes for payment. For current information on this subject, to order code resources, or to file a petition for the rights to use the codes, visit Web site: www.alternativelink.com.

METHODS OF PAYMENT

Private insurance companies as well as federal and state programs adopt different methods for establishing payment rates for outpatient services; they are (1) fee schedules; (2) usual, customary, and reasonable (UCR); and (3) relative value scales or schedules. Additional methods of payment for inpatient hospital claims are discussed in Chapter 17.

Fee Schedule

A **fee schedule** is simply a listing of accepted charges or established allowances for specific medical procedures. A medical practice can have more than one fee schedule unless specific state laws restrict this practice because

this might be interpreted as a form of price fixing. Charges refer to the regular rates established by the provider for services rendered to both Medicare beneficiaries and to other paying patients. Charges should be related consistently to the cost of the services and uniformly applied to all patients whether inpatient or outpatient. The following situations can occur:

1. Providers *participating* in the Medicare program would typically be paid by the fiscal agent an amount from a fee schedule for Medicare patients.
2. Providers *not participating* in the Medicare program would be paid by the fiscal agent an amount based on limiting charges for each service set by the Medicare program.
3. Providers having a contractual arrangement with a managed care plan (e.g., health maintenance organization, individual practice association, or preferred provider organization) would be paid based on the fee schedule written into the negotiated contract.
4. Providers rendering services to those who have sustained industrial injuries use a separate workers' compensation fee schedule (see Chapter 15).

Section 1128(b) of the Social Security Act states that a physician may risk exclusion or suspension from the Medicare program if his or her Medicare charges are "substantially in excess of such individual's or entity's usual charges." An exception is charges negotiated for managed care contracts that are not considered the physician's usual charges. In those cases, it is possible that Medicare patients may be charged more than managed care patients. By implementing multiple fee schedules, a provider may risk charging federal or state health programs a fee that might be construed as more than the provider's "usual" charge for a given service. This could potentially result in a violation of the Social Security Act and managed care agreements.

To prevent a possible violation of Section 1128(b) of the Social Security Act, it is suggested that the provider assign one set fee or amount for each procedure code when establishing a fee schedule. This is the fee billed to all carriers and to self-pay patients. Instead of different charges for different carriers, the provider can establish different reimbursement fees based on the amount that the carrier reimburses, which is based on the contract with the carrier. By establishing one fee instead of multiple fees for each procedure, the provider helps establish the usual and customary fee for his or her geographic area. It is also possible to observe when carriers raise their allowable rates, which cannot be done if sending a claim based on the carrier's allowable. It is important as well to monitor carrier adjustments to determine how much revenue is lost because of poor contracts and to monitor employee theft.

Because mistakes can be costly in terms of lost revenue and possible violations, one fee schedule for all patients, with provisions for financial hardship cases, is usually the safest course for health care providers. The physician may want to evaluate the fee schedule in use to annually increase fees due to cost of living and cost of supply increases. Such a process is discussed later under Developing a Fee Schedule Using Relative Value Studies Conversion Factors.

Usual, Customary, and Reasonable

Usual, customary, and reasonable (UCR) is a complex system in which three fees are considered in calculating payment. UCR is used mostly in reference to fee-for-service reimbursement. Figure 6–1 illustrates how a surgeon's payment is determined under this method. The usual fee is the fee that a physician usually charges (submitted fee) for a given service to a private patient. A fee is a **customary fee** if it is in the range of usual fees charged by providers of similar training and experience in a geographic area (e.g., the history of charges for a given service). The **reasonable fee** is the fee that meets the aforementioned criteria or is, in the opinion of the medical review committee, justifiable considering the special circumstances of the case. Reimbursement is based on the lower of the two fees (usual and customary) and determines the approved or allowed amount. In a UCR system, payment can be extremely low for a rarely performed but highly complex procedure because there may be no history of billed charges from other physicians on which to base payment. Many private health insurance plans use this method and pay a physician's full charge if it does not exceed UCR charges. Depending on the policies of each insurance company, the UCR system is periodically updated. UCR is a method chosen by insurance carriers and not the provider. If the physician has a UCR that is significantly lower than those of other practices in his or her area, document this and ask the insurance carrier for a review and possible adjustment. Increasing numbers of plans are beginning to discontinue the UCR system and are adopting the Medicare RBRVS method for physician reimbursement. A description of this system is found under Relative Value Studies, which follows.

To be considered *customary* for Medicare reimbursement, a provider's charges for like services must be imposed on most patients regardless of the type of patient treated or the party responsible for payment of such services. Customary charges are those uniform charges listed in a provider's established charge schedule which is in effect

PARTICIPATING SURGEON
UCR CALCULATION

Four Example Cases

Surgeon's bill	Usual fee	compared to	Customary fee		Payment
1) $400	$350	→	$350	→ declared reasonable (extenuating circumstances)	$400
2) $400	$350	→	$350	→ declared customary (no unusual circumstances)	$350
3) $375	$350	→	$400	→ declared customary (does not exceed customary level)	$375
4) $350	$350	→	$400	→ declared customary (falls within customary range)	$350

Usual Fee– usual submitted fee for a given service to patient.

Customary Fee– in the range of usual fees charged by providers of similar training and experience in a geographical area (i.e., the history of charges for a given service).

Reasonable Fee– meets the aforementioned criteria or is, in the opinion of the medical review committee, justifiable considering the special circumstances of the case.

Payment– based on the lower of usual and customary fees.

FIGURE 6–1 Usual, customary, and reasonable calculation for four participating surgeons' cases.

and applied consistently to most patients and recognized for Medicare program reimbursement.

Relative Value Studies

In 1956, the California Medical Association Committee on Fees published the first edition of the *California Relative Value Studies* (CRVS).

CRVS was subsequently revised and published in 1957, 1960, 1964, 1969, and 1974. **RVS,** referred to as either **relative value studies** or scale, is a coded listing of procedure codes with unit values that indicate the relative value of the various services performed, taking into account the time, skill, and overhead cost necessary for each service (Example 6.3).

Example 6.3   Relative Value Scale

Procedure Code	Description	Units
10060	Incision & drainage of cyst	0.8

Using a hypothetical figure of **$153/unit,** this procedure is valued at $122.40.

Math: $153.00 × 0.8 = $122.40

Units in RVS are based on the median charges of all physicians during the time period in which the RVS was published. A **conversion factor** is used to translate the abstract units in the scale to dollar fees for each service.

The RVS is a sophisticated system for coding and billing of professional services. After the successful use of the California RVS, many state and medical specialty associations adopted the CRVS method. In 1975, the Federal Trade Commission (FTC) challenged the legality of using the RVS as a fee schedule stating it could be interpreted as a form of price fixing in violation of antitrust laws. Since that time, many medical societies and medical specialty associations issued new publications that omitted unit values for the procedures listed, but retained the procedure code portion of RVS.

Some states passed legislation mandating the use of RVS codes for procedures and the unit values as the schedule of fees for workers' compensation claims. In these states, the conversion factor to be used in applying the units is also stated in the law. The insurance carrier pays a specific dollar amount for each unit listed for each procedure in the RVS code book.

An insurer or other third party could devise an RVS based on its own data. This type of RVS would not be created by physicians in an effort to regulate fees and, therefore, would be acceptable based on FTC guidelines.

An example is *Ingenix Relative Values for Physicians* (RVP) (refer to Appendix A for information on where to obtain this book). Additionally, a national RVS developed under a government contract may be acceptable and would not be in violation of antitrust laws.

Resource-Based Relative Value Scale

The **resource-based relative value scale (RBRVS)** is an RVS developed for CMS by William Hsiao and associates of the Harvard School of Public Health. Centers for Medicaid and Medicare Services used it to devise the Medicare fee schedule that was phased in from 1992 through 1996. This approach to fees was developed to redistribute Medicare dollars more equitably among physicians and to control escalating fees that were out of control using the UCR system. This became the basis for physicians' payments nationwide for a 5-year phase-in that began on January 1, 1992. This system consists of a fee schedule based on relative values. The formula for obtaining relative value units is somewhat complex and involves a bit of mathematics in computing three components: a **relative value unit (RVU)** for the service, a geographic adjustment factor (GAF), and a monetary conversion factor (CF).

RELATIVE VALUE UNIT FORMULA:

RVU × GAF × CF = Medicare $ per service

RVUs are based on the physician work RVU, the practice expense RVU, and the malpractice insurance RVU. To bring the fees in line for the region where the physician practices and to adjust for regional overhead and malpractice costs, each of the RVUs is adjusted for each Medicare local carrier by geographic practice cost indices (GPCIs), pronounced "gypsies."

A CF is used to convert a geographically adjusted relative value into a payment amount. This CF is updated to a new amount each year. Figure 6–2 provides an example of calculating payment for one procedure code.

HCPCS/CPT CODE	WORK RVUs	PRACTICE EXPENSE RVUs	MALPRACTICE RVUs	
91000 RVUs	1.04	0.70	0.06	
GPCI*	×1.028	+ ×1.258	+ ×1.370	= Total adjusted
	1.07	0.88	0.08	RVUs, 2.03

For 2005, the conversion factor for nonsurgical care is $37.8975 × 2.03 = Allowed amount $76.93

*The geographical practice cost indices (GPCI) for the medical practice whose location in the example is Oakland, California.

F I G U R E   6 – 2   Formula used to calculate the fee for a specific procedure using the resource-based relative value scale system.

Table 6.1	RBRVS Crosswalk						
A	B	C	D	E	F	G	H
CPT Code	Code Description	RBRVS/RVUs	Conversion Factor	Fee	Contract Conversion Factor	Contract Fee	% Contract Payment
99212	Ofc Visit	0.68	72.06	$49	64.71	$44.00	90%

The figures to work out this formula in the chart for each service are published annually in the *Federal Register*.

RVUs help when determining cost accounting because they take into account the practice expense, malpractice expense, work effort, and cost of living. They also are helpful when negotiating the best contract available with managed care plans; therefore office managers or individuals assisting physicians should know and understand RBRVS data. A crosswalk is an effective way to see how the practice may be affected by an RBRVS contract (Table 6.1). To develop one, make several columns using spreadsheet software. In column A, list common procedure codes used by the practice; column B, the code description; and column C, the RBRVS RVUs. Leave column D blank to insert a conversion factor. In column E, put in the present fee-for-service rate (rounded-out figure). Divide the fee in column E by column C to get the conversion factor. Leave a blank for column F to insert a conversion factor for the contract. List the managed care contract payment in column G. Divide column G by column C to get the conversion factor for column F. Then divide the plan's contract fee by the physician's fee for column H to work out the percentage being paid at the contract rate.

Medicare Fee Schedule

Beginning in 1996, each Medicare local carrier annually sends each physician a Medicare fee schedule for his or her area or region number listing three columns of figures: participating amount, nonparticipating amount, and limiting charge for each procedure code number. To see an example of this, either refer to the Mock Fee Schedule shown in Appendix A of the *Student Workbook for the Insurance Handbook for the Medical Office* or go to your local Medicare fiscal agent's Web site.

Developing a Fee Schedule Using Relative Value Studies Conversion Factors

A physician's fees can be adjusted if they are too high or low; but doing this can present a problem. It is legal to use an RVS guide for setting, realigning, or evaluating fees as long as the physician does not enter into any price-fixing agreements. There are a number of ways to update or establish a fee schedule, ranging from easy to difficult.

They are as follows:

1. Use the RBRVS fee profile sent to each physician's practice in the latter part of each year. This lists the codes most frequently used by the practice with their allowable charges and limiting charge amounts for the coming year. This is used for billing patients under the Medicare program. However, it can help you update the office fee schedule but you must make sure the charges are above the allowances on that schedule and above the allowances of the majority of the other third-party payers to whom the medical practice generally sends insurance claims.

2. Obtain the *Federal Register* with the printed relative values for most of the CPT code numbers and geographic cost indices for the region of service. Using a simple formula, calculate the actual Medicare reimbursement for the procedures the physician most frequently performs, making up a set of separate conversion factors for the Evaluation and Management (E/M), Anesthesia, Surgery, Radiology, Pathology, and Medicine sections. A fee schedule can either be updated or established from the calculations. Take into consideration that the fees should be above the maximums paid by the third-party payers to whom the practice generally bills. This procedure is detailed at the end of this chapter to assist you in gaining experience and skill if choosing to use this method.

3. A more time-consuming method is to review the medical practice's patient mix, that is, those patients with Medicare, the Blue Plans, Medicaid, managed care, private pay, workers' compensation, TRICARE, CHAMPVA, and so on. This may involve a detailed chart review of a large representative sampling of patients seen in the medical practice. Next, review the current fee schedule and current reimbursement amounts for the most commonly billed codes and the payments generated from each insurance in the study. A new fee schedule can be created from these data. See Appendix A for information on how to obtain the code books mentioned in this chapter.

HOW TO USE THE CPT CODE BOOK

The following are guidelines for the 2005 edition of the CPT. There are three categories of CPT codes: I, II, and III. This code book is a systematic listing of five-digit code numbers with no decimals. CPT I is divided into eight code sections with categories and subcategories. The main CPT code sections and appendices are as follows:

Evaluation and Management (E/M)   99201 to 99499
Anesthesia   00100 to 01999
Surgery   10021 to 69990
Radiology, Nuclear Medicine, and   70010 to 79999
　Diagnostic Ultrasound
Pathology and Laboratory   80048 to 89356
Medicine   90281 to 99602
Category II Codes   0001F to 4011F
Category III Codes   0003T to 0088T
Appendix A Modifiers
Appendix B Summary of Additions,
　Deletions, and Revisions
Appendix C Clinical Examples
Appendix D Summary of CPT
　Add-on Codes
Appendix E Summary of CPT Codes
　Exempt from Modifier 51
Appendix F Summary of CPT Codes
　Exempt from Modifier 63
Appendix G Summary of CPT Codes,
　which include Conscious Sedation
Appendix H Alphabetic Index of
　Performance Measures by Clinical
　Condition or Topic
Appendix I Genetic Testing Code
　Modifiers

Each main section is divided into categories and sub-categories according to anatomic body systems, procedure, condition, description, and specialty.

Read through the clinical examples presented in Appendix C. These examples will help you become familiarized with some common case scenarios that might occur for the codes that appear in the E/M section of the CPT.

When on the job, you might want to make your CPT into a reference manual by customizing it. This can help you find codes, modifiers, and rules, making your job easier. Break apart the manual into as many sections as necessary based on specialty, three-hole punch it, and place it into a binder. You may want to add indexes with tabs to the frequently used sections. You can also add coding edits, Medicare updates, and notes at any place in the binder. Color code any codes to which you usually add modifiers or that should not be used until you have reviewed certain data. For example, use red to highlight codes, descriptions, or entire sections, to alert you or anyone using the reference to codes that are often denied. Use yellow to highlight a code that needs to be checked before using it in combination with other codes. Use a symbol (e.g., * or ?) to identify services not covered under certain conditions. Appendix A of the CPT code book is a comprehensive list of the modifiers, so you might want

to add any insurance plan bulletins pertinent to modifiers that affect the specialty you bill for in this section of the binder. Customizing the CPT code book with a reference like this can save time and reduce coding errors.

Category I, II, and III Codes

To improve the existing CPT code system, a CPT-5 Project has been implemented, which includes two new code sets: category II codes, intended for performance measurement; and category III codes, intended for new and emerging technology. Existing CPT codes are considered category I.

Category II codes appear in CPT 2005 in a separate section located immediately after the Medicine section. They also have an alphanumeric identifier with a letter in the last field (e.g., 0502F Subsequent prenatal care visit) to distinguish them from category I codes. Two modifiers are used to indicate that a service specified by a performance measure was considered but, because of either medical or patient circumstance(s) documented in the medical record, the service was not provided. The modifiers are 1P and 2P.

Use of these codes is optional for correct coding.

Category III codes are a temporary set of tracking codes used for emerging technologies. They are intended to expedite data collection and assessment of new services and procedures to substantiate widespread use and clinical effectiveness. A category III code may become a category I code. When it is deleted from category III and adopted as category I code, the CPT book provides clear indication of this change by inserting a cross reference in place of the former category III code; for example, ▶(0025T has been deleted. To report use 76514)◀. The American Medical Association Web site posts updates to this category in July and January every year.

Code Book Symbols

With each new issuance of CPT, deletions and new codes and description changes are added. Become familiar with the new codes and any description changes or deleted codes for codes that may exist on your medical practice's fee schedule. Figure 6–3 shows how to identify new codes and description changes by following the symbols that are used.

When using a new code, marked with a bullet (•), it may take as long as 6 months before an insurance carrier has a mandatory value assignment; therefore reimbursements are received in varying amounts during that time. An exception is in the Medicare program, which has a value assignment published annually in the fall in the *Federal Register*. For revised codes or revised text, marked with a triangle (▲) or (▶◀), highlight what is new or deleted.

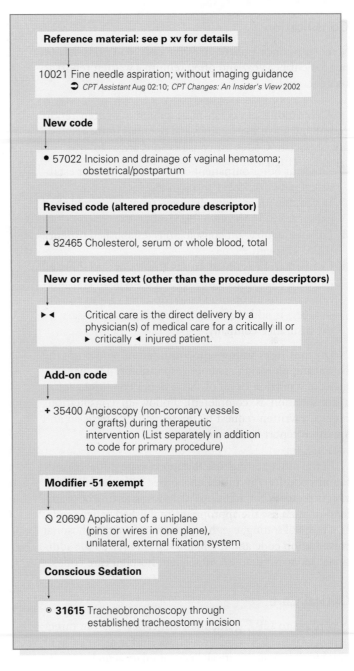

FIGURE 6–3 Symbols that appear in the 2005 *Current Procedural Terminology* (CPT) code book. These symbols and their meanings appear at the bottom of each page of codes in the CPT code book.

This saves time in trying to figure out what was changed and prevents using these codes incorrectly. The symbol "⊃" placed below many codes throughout the code book indicates that the American Medical Association has published reference material on that particular code. The reference citation is also provided. Appendices B and C in the CPT code book provides a summary of code additions, deletions, and revisions. Add-on codes, shown with a plus sign (+), and modifier -51 exempt codes, shown with a symbol (⊘), are explained at the end of this chapter. These symbols are located at the bottom of each page of codes in the CPT code book.

Evaluation and Management Section

The insurance billing specialist must become familiar with the terminology in the procedure code book to use it efficiently. Basic procedural code terminology is reviewed in Chapter 4 to give you a good foundation to begin coding. By now you should know the difference between a new and an established patient, a consultation and a referral, and concurrent care versus continuity of care. This section familiarizes you with specific coding policies in relation to some of the terminology you have learned thus far.

Consultation

Some insurance policies pay for only one consultation per patient per year and often require a written report to be generated.

A consulting physician must submit a written report containing his or her findings and opinions to the requesting physician. Codes for consultations are as follows:

- Office or other outpatient consultations (new or established patient): 99241 through 99245.
- Initial inpatient consultations (new or established patient): 99251 through 99255.
- Follow-up inpatient consultations (established patient): 99261 through 99263.
- Confirmatory consultations (new or established patient): 99271 through 99275. This type of consultation calls for an opinion only. Modifier -32 (mandated services) is added if a second opinion is necessary by the insurance company.

Do not use follow-up consultation codes if the consulting physician assumes responsibility for management of a portion or all of the patient's conditions (after a consultation is completed). Follow-up consultations require a written request by the requesting physician and a written report by the consultant.

In the office setting, use the appropriate initial consultation code for the initial encounter and if a follow-up visit is required for additional diagnostic testing or examination, then use the appropriate established patient code. In a hospital setting, use the appropriate inpatient hospital consultation code and if a follow-up is required for additional services, then use subsequent hospital care codes.

Critical Care

According to CPT guidelines, critical care is the direct delivery of medical care by a physician for a critically ill or injured patient. A critical illness or injury acutely impairs one or more vital organ systems that makes imminent or life-threatening deterioration in the patient's condition highly probable. Critical care involves high complexity decision making to assess, manipulate, and support vital system functions to treat single or multiple vital organ system failure or prevent further life-threatening deterioration of the patient's condition. Examples of vital organ system failure include, but are not limited to, central nervous system failure; circulatory failure; and shock, renal, hepatic, metabolic, or respiratory failure.

Although critical care typically requires interpretation of multiple physiologic parameters or application of advanced technologies, critical care may be provided in life-threatening situations when these elements are not present. Critical care may be provided on multiple days, even if no changes are made in the treatment rendered to the patient, as long as the patient's condition continues to require the level of physician attention described in the preceding paragraph.

Providing medical care to a critically ill, injured, or postoperative patient qualifies as a critical care service only if both the illness or injury and the treatment being provided meet the preceding requirements. Critical care is usually, but not always, given in a critical care area, such as the coronary care unit, intensive care unit, pediatric intensive care unit, respiratory care unit, or emergency care facility. It could occur in the patient's room or in the emergency department.

Critical care services provided to infants 31 days through 24 months of age are reported with pediatric critical care codes 99293 and 99294. The pediatric critical care codes are reported as long as the infant or young child qualifies for critical care services during the hospital stay. Critical care services provided to neonates (30 days of age or younger) are reported with the neonatal critical care codes 99295 and 99296. The neonatal critical care codes are reported as long as the neonate qualifies for critical care services through the 30th postnatal day. The reporting of the pediatric and neonatal critical care services is not based on time or the type of unit (e.g., pediatric or neonatal critical care unit) and it is not dependent on the type of provider delivering the care. For additional instructions on reporting these services, see the Neonatal and Pediatric Critical Care section and codes 99293 through 99296.

Services for a patient who is not critically ill but is in a critical care or intensive care unit are reported by use of other appropriate in-hospital E/M codes.

Critical care and other E/M services may be provided to the same patient on the same date by the same physician.

The following services are included in critical care codes used to report critical care when performed during the critical period by the physician providing critical care: the interpretation of cardiac output measurements (93561, 93562); chest radiographs (71010, 71015, 71020); pulse oximetry (94760, 94761, 94762); blood gases and information data stored in computers (e.g., electrocardiograms, blood pressures, hematologic data [99090]); gastric intubation (43752, 91105); temporary transcutaneous pacing (92953); ventilator management (94656, 94660, 94662); and vascular access procedures (36000, 36400, 36405, 36406, 36410, 36415, 36540, 36600). These services are *not* coded in addition to the critical care codes.

Any services performed in excess of those listed above should be reported separately. Many carriers attempt to downcode claims by stating the procedure is included with critical care. If denied, these claims should be appealed by attaching supporting documentation, such as a copy of the critical care guidelines. The carrier may tell you the codes are inclusive or that they are not a covered benefit. Continue to dispute the denials for these separately payable services until you get paid.

Codes 99289 through 99290 should be reported for the physician's attendance during the transport of critically ill or injured pediatric patients more than 24 months of age to or from a facility or hospital. For physician transport services of critically ill or injured pediatric patients 24 months of age or younger, see 99289 and 99290.

Critical care codes 99291 and 99292 are used to report the total duration of time spent by a physician providing critical care services to a critically ill or injured patient, even if the time spent by the physician on that date is not continuous. For any given period of time spent providing critical care services, the physician must devote his or her full attention to the patient, and therefore cannot provide services to any other patient during the same period of time.

Time spent with the individual patient must be recorded in the patient's record. Time spent engaged in work directly related to the individual patient's care, whether that time was spent at the immediate bedside or elsewhere on the floor or unit even if not continuous, is reported as critical care. For example, time spent on the unit or at the nursing station on the floor reviewing test results or imaging studies, discussing the critically ill patient's care with other medical staff, or documenting critical care services in the medical record is reported as critical care, even though it does not occur at the bedside. Also, when the patient is unable or clinically incompetent to participate in discussions, time spent on the floor or unit with family members or surrogate decision makers obtaining a medical history, reviewing the patient's condition or prognosis, or discussing treatment or limitations of treatment may be reported as critical care, as long as the conversation bears directly on the management of the patient.

Time spent in activities that occur outside of the unit or off the floor (e.g., telephone calls, whether taken at home, in the office, or elsewhere in the hospital) may not be reported as critical care because the physician is not immediately available to the patient.

Time spent in activities that do not directly contribute to the treatment of the patient may not be reported as critical care, even if they are performed in the critical care unit (e.g., participation in administrative meetings or telephone calls to discuss other patients). Time spent performing separately reportable procedures or services should not be included in the time reported as critical care time.

Code 99291 is used to report the first 30 to 74 minutes of critical care on a given date. It should be used only once per date even if the time spent by the physician is not continuous on that date. Critical care of less than 30 minutes total duration on a given date should be reported with the appropriate E/M code.

Code 99292 is used to report additional blocks of time, of up to 30 minutes each, beyond the first 74 minutes. This code has a plus sign (+) and is an "add-on" code. It is never used alone.

Neonatal and Pediatric Critical Care

According to CPT guidelines, the codes 99293 through 99296 are used to report inpatient services provided by a physician directing the care of a critically ill neonate or infant. The same definitions for critical care services apply for the adult, child, and neonate.

The initial day neonatal critical care code (99295) can be used in addition to codes 99360 Physician standby service, 99436 Attendance, or 99440 Newborn resuscitation as appropriate, when the physician is present for the delivery and newborn resuscitation is necessary. Other procedures performed as a necessary part of the resuscitation (e.g., endotracheal intubation) are also reported separately when performed as part of the preadmission delivery room care. They must be performed as a necessary component of the resuscitation and not done for convenience.

Codes 99295 and 99296 are used to report services provided by a physician directing the care of a critically ill neonate through the first 30 days of life. These codes describe care for the date of admission (99295) and subsequent days (99296) and should be reported only once per day per patient. Once the neonate is no longer considered critically ill, the Intensive Low Birth Weight Services codes for those with present body weight of less than 2500 grams (99298 and 99299) or the codes for Subsequent Hospital Care (99231 through 99233) for those with present body weight more than 2500 grams should be used.

Codes 99293 and 99294 are used to report services provided by a physician directing the care of a critically ill infant or young child from 31 days of postnatal age up through 24 months of age. These codes represent care for the date of admission (99293) and subsequent days

(99294) and should be reported by a single physician only once per day per patient in a given setting. The critically ill or injured child older than 2 years of age when admitted to an intensive care unit is reported with hourly critical care service codes (99291 and 99292). When an infant is no longer considered critically ill but continues to require intensive care, the Intensive Low Birth Weight Services codes (99298 and 99299) should be used to report services for infants with a body weight of less than 2500 grams. When the body weight of those infants exceeds 2500 grams, the Subsequent Hospital Care (99231 through 99233) codes should be used.

Care rendered under 99293 through 99296 includes management, monitoring, and treatment of the patient, including:
- Respiratory and pharmacologic control of the circulatory system
- Enteral and parenteral nutrition
- Metabolic and hematologic maintenance
- Parent and family counseling, case management services
- Personal direct supervision of the health care team in the performance of cognitive and procedural activities

The pediatric and neonatal critical care codes include those procedures previously listed for the hourly critical care codes (99291 and 99292). In addition, the following procedures also are included in the bundled (global) pediatric and neonatal critical care service codes (99293 to 99296):
- Umbilical venous (36510) and umbilical arterial (36660) catheters
- Central (36555 and 36556) or peripheral vessel catheterization (36568 through 36571)
- Other arterial catheters (36140 and 36620)
- Oral or nasogastric tube placement (43752)
- Endotracheal intubation (31500)
- Lumbar puncture (62270)
- Suprapubic bladder aspiration (51000)
- Bladder catheterization (51701)
- Initiation and management of mechanical ventilation (94656, 94657) or continuous positive airway pressure (94660)
- Surfactant administration
- Intravascular fluid administration (90780 and 90781)
- Transfusion of blood components (36430 and 36440)
- Vascular punctures (36420 and 36600)
- Invasive or noninvasive electronic monitoring of vital signs
- Respiratory flow volume loop (94375)
- Monitoring or interpretation of blood gases for oxygen saturation (94760 through 94762)

Any services performed that are not listed in the preceding should be reported separately.

Emergency Care

Codes 99281 through 99285 describe various levels of emergency care provided in an emergency department. An *emergency department* (ED) is defined as an organized hospital-based facility for the provision of unscheduled episodic services to patients who present for immediate medical attention. However, some facilities must use the ED to accommodate after-hours patients, overflow clinic patients, or administer minor procedures in the absence of a clinic. When a patient is seen in the ED for a scheduled procedure, he or she must have a valid order for services. The patient should be registered as a clinic patient because his or her visit is not deemed an emergency. Medical necessity rules apply and the hospital should screen the procedure and diagnosis. As learned in Chapter 4, *medical necessity* is services provided that are consistent with the diagnosis. This type of patient falls under the regulations of the Emergency Medical Treatment and Active Labor Act (EMTALA). The facility may either perform an EMTALA screening for the patient or have the patient sign a document indicating he or she is not in the ED for emergency services. In these cases, there is a charge for the scheduled service provided but it is usually inappropriate to charge an E/M visit in addition to the procedure charge.

Code 99288 is used when advanced life support is necessary during emergency care and the physician is located in a hospital emergency or critical care department and is in two-way voice communication with ambulance or rescue personnel outside the hospital.

If office services are provided on an emergency basis, code 99058 (office services provided on an emergency basis—found in the Medicine Section) may be used when billing private insurance cases. CPT codes 99281 through 99285 should not to be used to report emergency care provided in an office setting. Medicare does not pay when code 99058 is used, and other carriers also may deny this code. When a physician spends several hours attending to a patient, coding for prolonged services (modifier -21), in addition to an E/M service office visit, might be indicated. See the section on modifiers for further explanation. Other prolonged services code numbers are 99354 through 99357 and 99358 through 99359.

If a patient comes into the office requiring emergency care for a wound trauma, you might bill for the office visit, suturing of the laceration, and the surgical tray. Most insurance carriers only pay for suturing. Typically, the carrier will state that the office visit is included or bundled (codes grouped together that are related to a procedure) into the suture procedure. The carrier will also typically state that surgical trays/supplies are included or bundled into the suture procedure. If you view the CMS National Correct

Coding Initiative (NCCI) edits, you can see which codes are normally considered part of another procedure. If the NCCI edits do not show the codes as being inclusive, you should appeal the carrier's decision or bill the patient if allowed by federal or state law. This topic is explained in more detail later in this chapter under Coding Guidelines for Code Edits. However, if documentation supports coding the claim for office services provided on an emergency basis (99058), most carriers will reimburse for the office visit in addition to the repair (Example 6.4). For example, if a patient has an extensive open wound of the arm, a bill should be submitted only for the wound repair but if a patient has an extensive wound of the arm with abrasions of the shoulder, contusions of the ribs, and a sprained finger, then a bill should be submitted for the wound repair and an E/M code. The wound diagnosis would be associated to the wound repair, and the diagnosis for the injuries would support the E/M visit. Make sure the appropriate modifiers are appended to the CPT codes on the claim. For example, modifier -25 is used to report a significant and separate procedure that was performed in addition to an E/M. A -25 modifier should be appended to the E/M in the previous example. But, the documentation in the chart must support the reasons for the codes.

Example 6.4 Office Emergency

Incorrect Coding

99212 Office visit, level 2, established patient
12005 Simple repair of scalp laceration, 12.6 cm
99070 Surgical tray (itemized)

Correct Coding

99212 Office visit, level 2, established patient
99058 *Office services provided on an emergency basis*
12005 Simple repair of scalp laceration, 12.6 cm

Miscellaneous service codes 99050 through 99054 can be used depending on the hour at which the patient is seen as an emergency in the physician's office. Most carriers, including Medicare, do not pay for these codes. Some carriers might pay for these codes and require documentation from the provider to support the code. Other codes under Miscellaneous Services in the Medicine Section may be applicable for a patient receiving emergency care, so these should be scrutinized carefully.

Preventive Medicine

Counseling

Codes 99381 through 99397 include counseling that is provided at the time of the initial or periodic comprehensive preventive medicine examination. Codes 99401 through 99412 should be used for reporting counseling given at an encounter separate from the preventive medicine examination.

Sometimes a Medicare patient may have an annual checkup but while having the examination he or she tells the physician of experiencing pain. The physician provides both the preventive and problem-focused services at the same time. You may bill Medicare only for covered screenings or services (such as problem-focused E/M, Pap smear, colon/rectal cancer screening, prostate cancer screening, and so on) and must properly carve out the rest of the noncovered and/or preventive services (codes 99381 through 99397) to bill to the patient. *Carve out* refers to medical services not included as benefits and this term may also be seen in managed care billing and is further discussed in Chapter 11. For preventive medicine when billing a Medicare case, an Advanced Beneficiary Notice is not required.

Categories and Subcategories

The E/M section of CPT has categories and subcategories that have from three to five levels for reporting purposes. These levels are based on key components, contributory factors, and face-to-face time with the patient or family. To begin the coding process, the provider of service must identify the category (e.g., office, hospital inpatient or outpatient, or consultation) and then select the subcategory (e.g., new patient or established patient). The description should be read thoroughly to note the key components (e.g., history, examination; medical decision making) and the contributory factors (e.g., counseling; coordination of care; nature of the presenting problem) and the face-to-face time of the service should be noted. Review the sample in Figure 6–4 illustrating an E/M code for a new patient seen in the office or in an outpatient or ambulatory setting.

Because key components are clinical in nature, the physician must document these factors in the patient's record. In a case in which counseling and coordination of care dominate (more than 50%) the face-to-face physician–patient encounter, then time is considered the key component to qualify for a particular level of E/M services. Tables 6.2 and 6.3 give a concise view of the components for each code number.

Many physicians refer to the E/M codes as level 5 for the most complex to level 1 as the lowest, least complex. These levels coincide with the fifth or last digit of the CPT code, e.g., 99201. It is common to hear a physician say "Ted Brown was seen for a level 4 today." This terminology may appear on encounter forms with five-digit CPT code numbers and be referred to as levels 1 through 5 (Example 6.5).

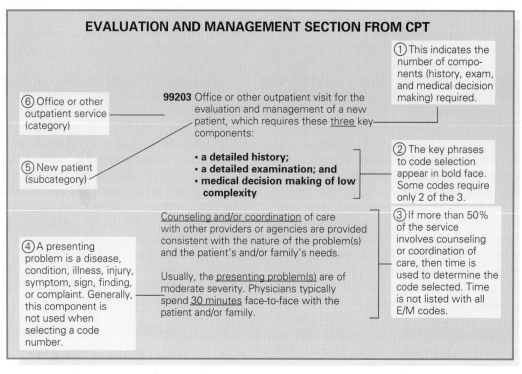

FIGURE 6-4 Evaluation and Management code 99203 defining the main words and phrases. This code is used for a new patient seen in the office or in an outpatient or ambulatory setting.

Table 6.2	Selection of Evaluation and Management Codes					
Code	History	Examination	Medical Decision Making	Problem Severity	Coordination of Care and Counseling	Time Spent (avg)
	OFFICE OR OTHER OUTPATIENT SERVICES (INCLUDES HOSPITAL OBSERVATION AREA)					
New Patient*						
99201	Problem focused	Problem focused	Straightforward	Minor or self-limited	Consistent with problem(s) and patient's needs	10 min face to face
99202	Expanded problem focused	Expanded problem focused	Straightforward	Low to moderate	Consistent with problem(s) and patient's needs	20 min face to face
99203	Detailed	Detailed	Low complexity	Moderate	Consistent with problem(s) and patient's needs	30 min face to face
99204	Comprehensive	Comprehensive	Moderate complexity	Moderate to high	Consistent with problem(s) and patient's needs	45 min face to face
99205	Comprehensive	Comprehensive	High complexity	Moderate to high	Consistent with problem(s) and patient's needs	60 min face to face
Established Patient*†						
99211	—	—	Physician supervision, but presence not required	Minimal	Consistent with problem(s) and patient's needs	5 min face to face
99212	Problem focused	Problem focused	Straightforward	Minor or self-limited	Consistent with problem(s) and patient's needs	10 min face to face

*Key component: For new patients for initial office and other outpatient services, all three components (history, physical examination, and medical decision making) are required in selecting the correct code. For established patients, at least two of these three components are required.
†Includes follow-up, periodic reevaluation, cand management of new problems.

Table 6.2	Selection of Evaluation and Management Codes—cont'd					
Code	History	Examination	Medical Decision Making	Problem Severity	Coordination of Care and Counseling	Time Spent (avg)
OFFICE OR OTHER OUTPATIENT SERVICES (INCLUDES HOSPITAL OBSERVATION AREA)—cont'd						
Established Patient*†—cont'd						
99213	Expanded problem focused	Expanded problem	Low complexity	Low to moderate	Consistent with problem(s) and patient's needs	15 min face to face
99214	Detailed	Detailed	Moderate complexity	Moderate to high	Consistent with problem(s) and patient's needs	25 min face to face
99215	Comprehensive	Comprehensive	High complexity	Moderate to high	Consistent with problem(s) and patient's needs	40 min face to face
HOSPITAL OBSERVATION SERVICES						
99217	—	—	—	—	—	—
99218	Detailed or comprehensive	Detailed or comprehensive	Straightforward or low complexity	Low	Consistent with problem(s) and patient's needs	—
99219	Comprehensive	Comprehensive	Moderate complexity	Moderate	Consistent with problem(s) and patient's needs	—
99220	Comprehensive	Comprehensive	High complexity	High		—
HOSPITAL INPATIENT SERVICES						
Initial Care‡						
99221	Detailed or comprehensive	Detailed or comprehensive	Straightforward or low complexity	Low	Consistent with problem(s) and patient's needs	30 min unit/ floor
99222	Comprehensive	Comprehensive	Moderate complexity	Moderate	Consistent with problem(s) and patient's needs	50 min unit/ floor
99223	Comprehensive	Comprehensive	High complexity	High	Consistent with problem(s) and patient's needs	70 min unit/ floor
Subsequent Care‡§						
99231	Problem focused interval	Problem focused	Straightforward or low complexity	Stable, recovering or improving	Consistent with problem(s) and patient's needs	15 min unit/ floor
99232	Expanded problem focused interval	Expanded problem focused	Moderate complexity	Inadequate response to treatment; minor complication	Consistent with problem(s) and patient's needs	25 min unit/ floor
99233	Detailed interval	Detailed	High complexity	Unstable; significant new problem(s) or complication(s)	Consistent with problem(s) and patient's needs	35 min unit/ floor
99238	Hospital discharge day management					

CPT codes, descriptions, and material are taken from *Current Procedural Terminology*, CPT 2005, Standard Edition, © 2004, American Medical Association. All Rights Reserved.

‡Key components: For initial care, all three components (history, physical examination, and medical decision making) are required in selecting the correct code. For subsequent care, at least two of these three components are required.

§All subsequent levels of service include a review of the medical record, diagnostic studies, and changes in the patient's status, such as history, physical condition, and response to treatment since the last assessment.

Table 6.3 **Code Selection Criteria for Consultations**

E/MCode	History*	Examination	Medical Decision Making*	Problem Severity	Coordination of Care; Counseling	Time (avg)
			OFFICE AND OTHER OUTPATIENT			
99241	Problem focused	Problem focused	Straightforward	Minor or self-limited	Consistent with problem(s) and patient's needs	15 min face to face
99242	Expanded problem focused	Expanded problem focused	Straightforward	Low	Consistent with problem(s) and patient's needs	30 min face to face
99243	Detailed	Detailed	Low complexity	Moderate	Consistent with problem(s) and patient's needs	40 min face to face
99244	Comprehensive	Comprehensive	Moderate complexity	Moderate to high	Consistent with problem(s) and patient's needs	60 min face to face
99245	Comprehensive	Comprehensive	High complexity	Moderate to high	Consistent with problem(s) and patient's needs	80 min face to face
			INITIAL INPATIENT†			
99251	Problem focused	Problem focused	Straightforward	Minor or self-limited	Consistent with problem(s) and patient's needs	20 min unit/floor
99252	Expanded problem focused	Expanded problem focused	Straightforward	Low	Consistent with problem(s) and patient's needs	40 min unit/floor
99253	Detailed	Detailed	Low complexity	Moderate	Consistent with problem(s) and patient's needs	55 min unit/floor
99254	Comprehensive	Comprehensive	Moderate complexity	Moderate to high	Consistent with problem(s) and patient's needs	80 min unit/floor
99255	Comprehensive	Comprehensive	High complexity	Moderate to high	Consistent with problem(s) and patient's needs	110 min unit/floor
			FOLLOW-UP INPATIENT†			
99261	Problem focused	Problem focused	Straightforward or low complexity	Stable, recovering or improving	Consistent with problem(s) and patient's needs	10 min unit/floor
99262	Expanded problem focused	Expanded problem focused	Moderate complexity	Inadequate response to treatment; minor complication	Consistent with problem(s) and patient's needs	20 min unit/floor
99263	Detailed interval	Detailed	High complexity	Unstable; significant new problem(s) and complication	Consistent with problem(s) and patient's needs	30 min unit/floor
			CONFIRMATORY			
99271	Problem focused	Problem focused	Straightforward	Minor or self-limited	Consistent with problem(s) and patient's needs	—
99272	Expanded problem focused	Expanded problem focused	Straightforward	Low	Consistent with problem(s) and patient's needs	—

*Key component: For office and initial inpatient consultations, all three components (history, physical examination, and medical decision making) are required for selecting the correct code. For follow-up consultations, two of these three components are required.
†These codes also are used for residents of nursing facilities.

Table 6.3	Code Selection Criteria for Consultations—cont'd					
E/MCode	History	Examination	Medical Decision Making	Problem Severity	Coordination of Care; Counseling	Time (avg)
			CONFIRMATORY—cont'd			
99273	Detailed	Detailed	Low complexity	Moderate	Consistent with problem(s) and patient's needs	—
99274	Comprehensive	Comprehensive	Moderate	Moderate to high	Consistent with problem(s) and patient's needs	—
99275	Comprehensive	Comprehensive	High	Moderate to high	Consistent with problem(s) and patient's needs	—

CPT codes, descriptions, and material are taken from *Current Procedural Terminology*, CPT 2005, Standard Edition, © 2004, American Medical Association. All Rights Reserved.

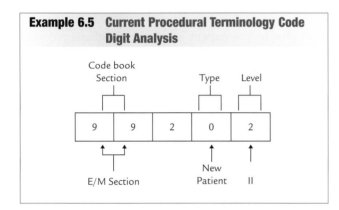

Example 6.5 Current Procedural Terminology Code Digit Analysis

Alternatively, this terminology may be seen abbreviated as L-1, L-2, and so on, but this usage is not preferred because it can be confused with the nomenclature for the sections of the lumbar vertebrae. The level also may be written out as level one, level two, and so on, depending on the complexity of the case. A breakdown of the E/M levels with code numbers is shown in Table 6.4.

In some cases, it is necessary to use a two-digit modifier to give a more accurate description of the services rendered. This is used in addition to the procedure code. Refer to the comprehensive list of modifiers at the end of this chapter for more information.

Table 6.4	Levels with Code Numbers			
	Office Visits		Consultations	
	New	Established	Office	Hospital
Level 1	99201	99211	99241	99251
Level 2	99202	99212	99242	99252
Level 3	99203	99213	99243	99253
Level 4	99204	99214	99244	99254
Level 5	99205	99215	99245	99255

Surgery Section

Coding from an Operative Report

It is best to obtain a copy of the patient's operative report from the hospital when coding surgery. A photocopy can be used so that you can make notes right on the document. When reviewing the report, use a ruler or highlighter pen. Use the ruler to read the report line by line. Highlight words that could indicate that the procedure performed may be altered by specific circumstances and to remind you that a code modifier may be needed. Look up any unfamiliar terms using a medical dictionary or anatomic reference book and write the definition in the margin.

Assign the code for the postoperative diagnosis shown at the beginning of the operative report. Also search for additional diagnoses in the body of the report that you can add as secondary diagnostic codes to support medical necessity, especially if the case is complex.

If the complex surgical procedure is not accurately described in the procedure code nomenclature, include an operative report and list "Attachment" in Block 19 of the insurance claim form so that the claims adjuster clearly understands the case and maximum payment is generated.

Code numbers that describe a part of the body treated render higher reimbursement depending on their location (e.g., suturing of a facial laceration pays a higher rate than suturing of an arm laceration).

Code only the procedures that actually were documented in the report. Check to make sure they neither a part of the main procedure nor bundled by

National Correct Coding Initiative (NCCI) edits, which is discussed later in this chapter. Do not code using only the name of the procedure as it is given in the heading of the operative report. Read the report thoroughly before coding to see whether additional procedures were performed and whether they were part of the main procedure, performed independently, or were unrelated. If the surgical position is noted, this can help you identify the right approach code and a good medical dictionary has illustrations of the various surgical positions. All codes include approach and closure except some skull base surgery codes. Information on how to code multiple procedures that are not inherent in a major procedure may be found at the end of this chapter under modifier -51.

Check to see how many surgeons were involved in the operative procedure and their roles (assistant surgeon, cosurgeon, team surgeon).

Reread the report to make certain that all procedural and diagnostic codes have been identified. Compare the content with the codes you are using. You cannot code circumstances that the physician relays to you verbally. Be sure the words "extensive complications" are in the report if there are such complications.

Look for unusual details, such as special instruments used, unusually long or complex procedures, rare approach techniques, reoperation, or extensive scarring encountered. These conditions may need one or more modifiers appended to the code.

Surgical code descriptions may define a correct coding relationship wherein one code is part of another based on the language used in the description (Example 6.6). An explanation of how to read a description for standalone codes and indented codes is presented at the end of

this chapter under Procedure: Choose Correct Procedural Codes for Professional Services.

Confirm that the report findings agree with the procedure codes on the claim.

Surgical Package

Surgical package is a phrase commonly encountered when billing. Generally, a surgical procedure includes:

- The operation
- Local infiltration; topical anesthesia or metacarpal, metatarsal, or digital block
- Subsequent to the decision for surgery, one related E/M encounter on the date immediately before or on the date of procedure (including history and physical)
- Immediate postoperative care, including dictating operative notes and talking with the family and other physicians
- Writing orders
- Evaluating the patient in the postanesthesia recovery area
- Typical postoperative follow-up care (hospital visits, discharge, or follow-up office visits)

This is referred to as a "surgical package" for operative procedures, and one fee covers the entire set of services (Figure 6-5, *A*). The majority of surgical procedures, including fracture care, are handled in this manner. The global period under CPT is not specifically stated, that is, open-ended, which differs from Medicare postoperative global periods of 0, 10, 30, or 90 days, but most third-party insurance companies apply the same criteria.

Visits not related to the original surgery and complications of the surgery (infection of the wound) are billable. Preoperative services such as consultations, office visits, and initial hospital care are often billed separately. An appropriate five-digit E/M code should be selected for these type services. Payment of these services depends on third-party payment policy and the documentation—some are paid separately; some are not.

Insurance policies and managed care plans vary in what is included in the surgical package fee. Most follow Medicare guidelines; some do not. Plans may include all visits several weeks before surgery, or they may include only visits that occur 1 day before the surgery. When a decision is made for surgery, a commonly asked question is whether a charge may be made for the consultation or office visit and admission if done on the same day. In most cases, the admission should be charged listing initial hospital care codes 99221 through 99223. However, the guidelines are different for surgeons. For example, surgical package rules apply if a surgeon sees a patient in

---

Example 6.6   Integral Code Descriptions

Partial and complete, which means the partial procedure is included in the complete procedure.

56620   Vulvectomy simple; partial
56625   complete

Partial and total, which means the partial procedure is included in the total procedure.

58940   Oophorectomy, partial or total, unilateral
            or bilateral

Unilateral and bilateral, which means the unilateral procedure is included in the bilateral procedure.

58900   Biopsy of ovary, unilateral or bilateral

Single and multiple, which means the single procedure is included in the multiple procedure.

49321   Laparoscopy, surgical, with biopsy (single
            or multiple)

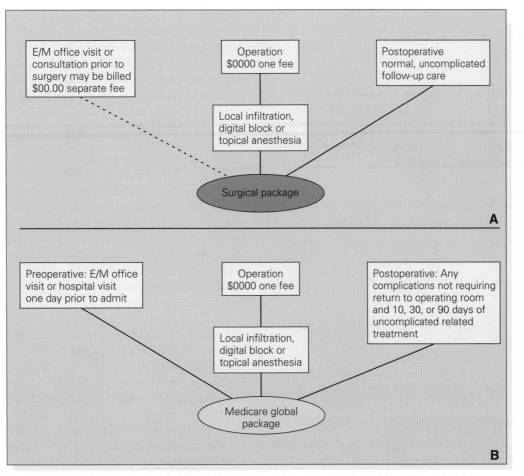

FIGURE 6–5 **A,** Surgical package concept. **B,** Medicare global package.

consultation and recommends that the patient receive immediate transfer of care to the surgeon and admission for surgery. The consultation that resulted in the decision for surgery may be billed by adding modifier -57 (decision for surgery) to the consultation procedure code number. The surgeon may not charge for an admission because all E/M services provided within 24 hours of surgery are included in (bundled) the surgical fee. Most third-party reimbursement systems will not pay medical and surgical services to the same physician on the same date of service.

> **Remember the rule: Not documented, not done.**

Medicare Global Package

Medicare has a **global surgery policy** for major operations that is similar to the surgical package concept. The Medicare global fee is a single fee for all necessary services normally furnished by the surgeon before, during, and after the procedure. This became effective January 1, 1992 (see Figure 6-5, *B*). Included in the package are:

● Preoperative visits (1 day before or day of surgery)
● Intraoperative services that are a usual and necessary part of the surgical procedure

● Complications after surgery that do not require additional trips to the operating room (medical and surgical services)
● Postoperative visits including hospital visits, discharge, and office visits for variable postoperative periods: 0, 10, or 90 days
● Writing orders
● Evaluating the patient in the recovery area
● Normal postoperative pain management

In addition, procedures shown in the global period column of the *Federal Register* may show one of the following alpha codes:

MMM This is a service furnished in uncomplicated maternity cases, which includes prenatal care, delivery, and postnatal care.
XXX No global period. Visits, procedures, and follow-up services may be charged separately.

YYY The global period will be determined by the local Medicare carrier because the code is for an unlisted procedure.
ZZZ The code is part of another service and falls within that service's global period.

Understanding which services are included, what constitutes the global surgical period, and how to code related or unrelated services in the global surgical package for Medicare patients is critical in ensuring correct payment and meeting compliance guidelines.

Services provided for a Medicare patient *not included* in the global surgery package are the following:

● Initial consultation or evaluation (regardless of when it occurs)
● Postoperative visits unrelated to the diagnosis for which the surgical procedure was performed (modifier -24 applies)
● Treatment necessary to stabilize a seriously ill patient before surgery
● Diagnostic tests and procedures
● Related procedure for postoperative complications that requires a return trip to the operating room (modifier -78 applies)
● Immunosuppressive therapy after transplant surgery

If a Medicare patient is discharged from one hospital facility and admitted to a different hospital or facility on the same day, a provider may get paid for both, depending on the circumstances of the case. A low-level admission code (e.g., 99221) is used for the second hospital admission. A higher level admission code may be used when the patient goes from a regular room status to a type of specialized hospital. Two separate CMS-1500 claim forms, one for the discharge and another for the admission, must be used because two different locations of service (hospital names) must appear on the claim forms.

Follow-up Days

The number of follow-up days that are included in the surgical package varies. The CPT code book does not specify how many days should be given, so an additional reference manual is needed. Most states use an RVS for workers' compensation cases, which lists the follow-up days allowed for most surgical procedures. Another source that lists surgical follow-up days for Medicare services is published in the *Federal Register* at the end of each year. Locate Appendix B (the Medicare Fee Schedule) and follow-up days are listed as a global fee period in the ninth column. Obtain the RVS used in your state or a copy of the *Federal Register* for this information.

Medicare lists a 90-day global period for all major procedures and 10 days for minor procedures. Some commercial

insurance carriers have a 45-day global period for all or some major procedures. A few commercial carriers treat major procedures like minor procedures in the surgical package by allowing 10 follow-up days instead of 90. But most third-party insurance companies follow Medicare guidelines and adhere to the 10- and 90-day global periods. To obtain specific carrier information, send the insurance company a list of the most common surgical procedures and ask for the surgical package rules and the number of global days that apply to each code. If this information is not available, it is wise to bill the private carrier for the preoperative and all postoperative visits. When this information is received, a table should be created that shows global days on a payer-by-payer and procedure-by-procedure basis. On the chart of each patient scheduled for surgery, the type of surgery and how many days the insurance policy allows should be indicated. A bill should be submitted for all visits after the surgical package period expires.

For office visits by the physician during the postoperative period, use CPT code number 99024 on the patient's financial account to indicate "No Charge." This code is located in the Medicine Section under Special Services and Reports; Miscellaneous Services. It has no value, is unbundled with other codes, and is used for tracking purposes. Code number 99024 on itemized billing statements lets the patient know how many office visits after surgery have been provided at no charge. There is no Medicare guideline for this code. It is not necessary to list this code when completing an insurance claim unless the insurance carrier has specific instructions requesting that it be shown. If the patient has to be seen beyond the normal postoperative period, the reason must be documented in the patient's medical record and an applicable procedure code and fee for this service should be indicated on the claim form. A bill may be submitted for the office visit if the patient returns to the provider for treatment of an unrelated illness or injury during the postoperative (global) period. The diagnosis codes should support the reason for the visit. If the provider did not perform the surgery but is performing the postoperative care, the provider can charge for the visits but must use the appropriate modifier (-55) to explain the charge.

Repair of Lacerations

If multiple lacerations are repaired with the same technique and are in the same anatomic category, the insurance billing specialist should add up the total length of all the lacerations and report one code to obtain maximum reimbursement. Anatomic categories are the scalp, neck, axillae, external genitalia, trunk, extremities (hands or feet), face, ears, eyelids, nose, lips, or mucous membranes. If the patient had three repairs and each was listed with a different code, the second and third codes are downcoded (coded down one level) by the insurance carrier so a smaller payment is generated. If a patient has lacerations on both sides of the face, the lengths of all the lacerations should be combined because the anatomic region is the same, and a claim should be submitted for the total length. No modifier is used, and the right and left side of the face are not billed separately (Example 6.7).

Example 6.7 Repair of Multiple Lacerations

Three lacerations of the face totaling 8.2 cm

Incorrect Coding

12011	Repair 2.5-cm laceration of face
12013	Repair 2.7-cm laceration of face
12013	Repair 3-cm laceration of face

Correct Coding

12015	Repair 8.2-cm laceration of face

Multiple Lesions

The descriptions for the surgical codes that relate to accessory structures (e.g., scalp, arms, legs) and lesions found in the integumentary system (pertaining to the skin) can cause confusion. Code descriptions, including indentations, should be read completely with attention paid to terms such as *complex, complicated, extensive*, and *multiple* (lesions). Lesion excision code selection is not based on lesion diameter but on excised diameter and the character of the lesion—benign or malignant. Excised diameter is the greatest clinical diameter of the apparent lesion plus the margin necessary for complete excision. Example 6.8 is a guide to obtain maximum reimbursement for paring of seven corns.

Example 6.8 Paring of Seven Corns

Incorrect Coding

11055	Paring; single lesion
11056-51	Two to four lesions
11057-51	More than four lesions
or	
11055 × 7	Paring; single lesion (× seven corns)

Correct Coding

11057	Paring; more than four lesions (seven corns)

If possible, delay submission of the insurance claim for removal of a lesion or lesions until the pathology report is received. Usually, a malignant lesion is reimbursed at a higher rate because of the more detailed nature of the procedure.

Supplies

When billing for office surgery and supplies used, checklists for the items used on the sterile tray (Figure 6–6, *A*) and for determining complete and incomplete records (see Figure 6–6, *B*) should be used. These items can only be charged for if the surgery required the use of *additional* items not normally used for this type of surgery. Medicare pays for trays with some procedure codes but not for others.

Incident-to Services

According to federal Medicare billing guidelines, physicians can bill for services provided by allied health professionals who are members of their practice, such as physician assistants, therapists, nurses, and nurse practitioners, as

---

**MINOR OPERATING ROOM
INSTRUMENT TRAY SUPPLY CHECKLIST**

1 Adson Brown tissue forceps _____
1 Adson tissue forceps with teeth _____
1 long tissue forceps _____
2 mosquito clamps _____
1 Peck Joseph dissecting scissors _____
1 Kahn dissecting scissors _____
1 Reynolds dissecting scissors _____
1 Stratte needle holder _____
1 Webster needle holder _____
4 small piercing towel clips _____
2 double-skin hooks _____
2 single-skin hooks _____
1 knife handle _____
1 #15 blade _____
10 4 x 4s _____
2 cotton-tipped applicators _____
1 small basin _____
3 sterile towels (drapes) _____
1 Bovie pencil _____
Sutures:_____ _____ _____
Dressings: ½-inch Steri-strips _____

**OFFICE SURGERY MEDICAL RECORD
CHECKLIST**

Patient information sheet _____
H and P or progress note _____
Consent form _____
Diagnostic studies _____
Pathology report(s) _____
Anesthesia record _____
Circulating nurse's note _____
Doctor's orders _____
Discharge note _____
Operative report _____
Signature/operative report _____

FIGURE 6–6 *Top*, Checklist to document supplies used when billing for office surgery. This list can be kept with the patient's medical record. *Bottom*, Checklist for identifying complete and incomplete medical records used for a patient receiving office surgery. As each item or document is completed, it is checked off so that the person reviewing the chart can see at a glance what needs to be finalized.

---

long as the services relate to the professional services that the physician provides and direct supervision occurs. Examples for using E/M code 99211 (established patient office visit) not requiring the presence of a physician might include:

● Rechecking a patient for conjunctivitis
● Reading a tuberculin test result
● Checking blood pressure for a patient who is being treated for high blood pressure
● Checking a wound beyond the global period
● Recheck for issuing a return-to-work certificate

The physician must be present in the office suite; thus being available by telephone does not count as direct supervision of the allied health professional. It is important that documentation includes the date of service, reason for the visit, medical necessity, patient encounter information, and signature of the practitioner. To verify that there was a supervising physician, add a place for the physician to countersign that he or she was available and directly supervised the visit.

Prolonged Services, Detention, or Standby

Code numbers 99354 through 99359 should be used to indicate prolonged services with direct face-to-face patient contact; for example, the physician has spent time beyond the usual amount allotted for the service (e.g., 30 to 60 minutes). There are specific codes for services with face-to-face contact and without face-to-face contact. Prolonged service that is less than 30 minutes should not be billed using these codes because the time is included in the E/M code. Time should be documented in the health record to justify use of these codes. Reimbursement for prolonged attendance in the hospital is higher than payment for many other types of care, and reimbursement for critical care is even higher.

Physician standby services are billed using code 99360. Some insurance programs or plans (e.g., Medicare) do not pay for physician standby services, so be sure to check before billing to see whether the commercial carrier will pay. The charge for this type of service is based on what the physician believes is the value of an hour of his or her time. An example of this might be when a pediatrician is on standby during a high-risk cesarean section performed on a pregnant woman.

Unlisted Procedures

When an unusual service is rendered, an unlisted code (Example 6.9) should be used rather than guessing or using an incorrect code. Supporting documentation (letter and copy of operative report) should be sent

Example 6.9   Unlisted Procedure Code
31599   Unlisted procedure, larynx

explaining the service. Since the development of Category III codes, it is important to double check that section of the CPT code book to verify whether a code exists before using an unlisted code. Unlisted codes end in -99 and are found at the end of each section or subsection. A comprehensive listing of unlisted codes is found at the beginning of each section. Some Medicare fiscal agents do not pay for any of the special -99 adjunct codes. The following are guidelines for submitting a claim with an unlisted code to obtain maximum payment:

● Always send supporting documentation with the claim to clearly identify the procedure performed and the medical necessity. If detailed documentation cannot be electronically submitted or faxed to the carrier, send a paper claim with supporting documentation in a large envelope so it is not folded. Do not use paper clips, staples, or tape to affix the attachments to the claim. Mark each attachment with the patient's name, insurance identification number, date of service, page number of the attachment, and total number of pages submitted (e.g., page 2 of 3). This helps the claim's processor match the documentation to the claim in case they are separated. Do not use highlighter to point out the pertinent operative note sections because it may not show up when payers scan the claim. Instead either underline, star, or bracket the applicable sections for quick identification.
● File claims with unlisted procedure codes in a separate "tickler" file. Follow up the status of the claim if there is no response within 1 month.

Coding Guidelines for Code Edits

In 1996 the Medicare program implemented a National Correct Coding Initiative (NCCI). This initiative involves a code editing system consistent with Medicare policies to eliminate inappropriate reporting of CPT codes. *Code editing* is a computer software function that performs online checking of codes on an insurance claim to detect unbundling, splitting of codes, and other types of improper code submissions. NCCI edits are updated quarterly. Such software is used by private payers, federal programs, and state Medicaid programs. Some code pairs in the NCCI edits are followed by a 0 and others by a 1. If the superscript 0 appears with a code pair, it means Medicare never allows a modifier to be used with the codes, so the code pair could never be reported together. The superscript 1 means that you may use a modifier under certain circumstances with appropriate documentation to get both codes reimbursed.

Because every medical practice has billing problems and questions unique to its specialty that arise because of denial or reduction in payment of claims, the billing specialist must become a detective and discover how to obtain maximum reimbursements in the appropriate specialty. The best way is to telephone the insurance carrier inquiring about new coding options and by noting improvements in reimbursement. Coding takes expertise. It is an art, not an exact science. The following explanations of various ways of coding claims assist in obtaining maximum reimbursement for each service rendered and avoiding denials, lowered reimbursement, and possible audit.

Comprehensive and Component Edits

A **comprehensive code** means a single code that describes or covers two or more component codes that are bundled together as one unit. A component code is a lesser procedure and is considered part of the major procedure. Each component code represents a portion of the service described in the comprehensive code and should be used only if a portion of the comprehensive service was performed (Example 6.10).

Example 6.10 Comprehensive and Component Codes

Comprehensive code	93015	Cardiovascular stress test
Component codes	93016, 93017, 93018	

93015 Cardiovascular stress test using maximal or submaximal treadmill or bicycle exercise, continuous electrocardiographic monitoring, or pharmacological stress; with physician supervision, with interpretation and report

93016 Physician supervision only, without interpretation and report

93017 Tracing only, without interpretation and report

93018 Interpretation and report only

Under the Medicare program, NCCI *component code edits* involve procedures that meet any of the following criteria:

1. Code combinations that are specified as "separate procedures" by CPT
2. Codes that are included as part of a more extensive procedure
3. Code combinations that are restricted by the guidelines outlined in CPT
4. Component codes that are used incorrectly with the comprehensive code

If any one of these restricted code combinations is billed, Medicare allows payment for only the procedure with the highest relative value (Example 6.11).

Example 6.11 Separate Procedure

Separate procedure example: Inguinal hernia repair with lesion excised from spermatic cord
Comprehensive code: 49505 Repair initial hernia age 5 years or older; reducible
Component code: 55520 Excision of lesion of spermatic cord **(separate procedure)**

For example, when performing an inguinal hernia repair, the surgeon makes an incision in the groin and dissects tissue to expose the hernia sac, internal oblique muscle, and spermatic cord. If a lesion is excised from the spermatic cord, it is considered a component of the comprehensive hernia repair procedure and is not separately billable. Medicare will deny code 55520 (lesion excision) as a component of procedure code 49505 (hernia repair) when performed during the same operative session.

Mutually Exclusive Code Denials

Mutually exclusive code edits relate to procedures that meet any of the following criteria:

1. Code combinations that are restricted by the guidelines outlined in CPT
2. Procedures that represent two methods of performing the same service
3. Procedures that cannot reasonably be done during the same session
4. Procedures that represent medically impossible or improbable code combinations

In Example 6.12, if one were to submit both codes 47605 and 47653, both of the procedures noted in the example are different methods of accomplishing the same result (removal of the gallbladder with cholangiography). They represent a duplication of efforts and an overlap of services; therefore Medicare would deny code 47563 (laparoscopy) as mutually exclusive to code 47605 (the excision).

Example 6.12 Mutually Exclusive Code

47605 **Excision**, cholecystectomy; with cholangiography

47563 **Laparoscopy**, surgical; cholecystectomy with cholangiography

Note: Different methods of accomplishing same procedure.

Bundled Codes

For insurance claim purposes, **bundled codes** means to group related codes together. To completely understand bundled codes, one must have a thorough knowledge of the service or procedure that is being provided or use an unbundling book as a reference guide.

Example 6.13 illustrates one type of bundling found in the CPT code book. Because code 19271 (excision of chest wall tumor without mediastinal lymphadenectomy) does not include mediastinal lymphadenectomy and code 19272 (with mediastinal lymphadenectomy) does include it, reporting both codes together would be a contradiction in the actual performance of the services at the same session. Hence, when mediastinal lymphadenectomy is part of the procedure, submit code 19272 because code 19271 is bundled with it.

Example 6.13   Bundled Code

Component code	19271	Excision of chest wall tumor code involving ribs, with plastic reconstruction; without mediastinal lymphadenectomy
Comprehensive code	19272	with mediastinal lymphadenectomy

In the Medicare program, a number of services may be affected because CMS considers the services bundled. Because many commercial carriers may follow Medicare guidelines, an understanding of this bundling concept is necessary. When dealing with private insurance, an explanation of benefits (EOB) document may print out with a statement "Benefits have been combined," which means the same thing as bundling.

For example, when listing a sterile tray for an in-office surgical procedure, the tray is bundled with the procedure unless additional supplies are needed in addition to those usually used. CPT code 99070 (supplies and materials) is not reimbursed by Medicare; however, HCPCS level II alphanumeric codes may be used in such cases. The cost of some services and supplies are bundled into E/M codes (e.g., telephone services and reading of test results). However, Medicare pays for slings, splints, rib belts, cast supplies, Hexcelite and light casts, pneumatic ankle-control splints, and prosthetics, but a supplier (provider) number is needed to bill for take-home surgical supplies and durable medical equipment (DME). Medicare claims for supplies and DME go to one of four regional DME carriers whose addresses are listed in Internet Resources at the end of this chapter. A reference book published by Ingenix has comprehensive list of the codes that CMS considers bundled for the Medicare program. (See Appendix A for further information.)

When appealing a claim, a great deal of time may be spent on paperwork only to discover that the code is bundled and denial is imminent. When in doubt about whether services are combined or not, contact the insurance carrier and ask.

Unbundling

Unbundling is coding and billing numerous CPT codes to identify procedures that usually are described by a single code. It is also known as *exploding* or *á la carte* medicine.

Some practices do this unwittingly, but it is considered fraud if it is done intentionally to gain increased reimbursement. Unbundling can lead to downward payment adjustments and possible audit of claims.

Types of unbundling are shown in Examples 6.14 through 6.17:

● Fragmenting one service into component parts and coding each component part as if it were a separate service (see Example 6.14)

Example 6.14   Unbundled Code

Incorrect Coding

43235	Upper gastrointestinal (GI) endoscopy
43600	Biopsy of stomach

Correct Coding

43239	Upper GI endoscopy with biopsy of stomach

● Reporting separate codes for related services when one comprehensive code includes all related services (see Example 6.15)

Example 6.15   Unbundling (Comprehensive Code)

Unbundled Claim

58150	Total abdominal hysterectomy (corpus and cervix) with removal of tubes and with removal of ovary ($1200)
58700	Salpingectomy ($650)
58940	Oophorectomy ($685)

Total Charge: $2535

Claim Coded Correctly

58150	Comprehensive code for all three services Total charge: $1200

● Coding **bilateral** (both sides of the body) procedures as two codes when one code is proper (see Example 6.16)

Example 6.16   Unbundling (Bilateral)

Incorrect Coding

76090-RT	Right mammography
76090-LT	Left mammography

Correct Coding

76091	Mammography, bilateral

● Separating a surgical approach from a major surgical service that includes the same approach (see Example 6.17)

Example 6.17   Bundling (Surgical Approach)

Incorrect Coding

49000   Exploratory laparotomy

44150   Colectomy, total, abdominal

Correct Coding

44150   Colectomy, total, abdominal (correct since it includes exploration of the surgical field)

Insurers use special software designed to detect unbundling. To avoid this problem, always use a current CPT code book. The use of outdated codes often inadvertently results in unbundling. A new technology or technique may have its own code when it is developed, but may be bundled with another code as it becomes commonplace. If the practice uses a billing service, request in writing that its computer system include no unbundling programming.

Always submit current CPT codes because if outdated codes are used, it could red flag a provider with Medicare as being in noncompliance.

Downcoding

Downcoding occurs when the coding system used on a claim submitted to an insurance carrier does not match the coding system used by the company receiving the claim. The computer system converts the code submitted to the closest code in use, which is usually down one level from the submitted code. Therefore, the payment that is generated is usually less. In many states, it is illegal for an insurance company to downcode a claim. Insurance commissioners have published bulletins warning carriers to cease this claims adjudication practice. When a carrier receives a claim, the carrier is allowed to pay or deny the claim. If additional information is needed to adjudicate the claim, it should be requested from the patient or provider. The carrier is limited by the number of days it has to review the claim. At completion of the review, the carrier must pay or deny the claim

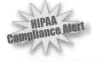

Make sure that the documentation from the provider supports the code that is being submitted to prevent downcoding.

Use current CPT manuals. Review all Medicare updates for changes to HCPCS codes. Always monitor reimbursements and look for downcoding so that you become knowledgeable about which codes are affected. (Example 6.18).

Example 6.18   Downcoding

Incorrect Coding

20010   Incision of abscess with suction irrigation

(Note: 20010 has been deleted from CPT and would result in downcoding.)

Correct Coding

20005   Incision of abscess, deep or complicated

Downcoding also occurs when a claims examiner converts the CPT code submitted to a code in the RVS being used by the carrier. This can occur in workers' compensation claims. When there is a choice between two or three somewhat similar codes, the claims examiner chooses the lowest paying code. Any time the code that was submitted is changed, appeal the change immediately.

Downcoding also may occur when a claims examiner compares the code used with the written description of the procedure included in an attached document. If the two do not match, the carrier will reimburse according to the lowest paying code that fits the description given (Example 6.19). In this example, the word "bone" is a clue to go to the musculoskeletal section of the code book and *not* the integumentary section. See Chapter 9 for additional information and solutions to downcoding.

Example 6.19   Downcoding

Document states: Excision of bone tumor from anterior tibial shaft.

Pathology report states: Tibia bone tumor; benign

Incorrect Coding

11400   Excision of benign lesion including margins except skin tag, trunk, arms or legs; excised diameter 0.5 cm or less

Correct Coding

27635   Excision of bone tumor of tibia, benign

Upcoding

The term **upcoding** is used to describe deliberate manipulation of CPT codes for increased payment. This practice can be spotted by Medicare fiscal agents and insurance carriers using prepayment and postpayment screens or "stop alerts," which are built into most computer coding software programs. An example of intentional upcoding might be a physician who selects one level of service code for all visits with the theory that the costs even out, such as always using code 99213. This opens the door to audits and in the end may cost the practice money. Upcoding may occur unintentionally if the coder is ill informed or does not keep current. Join a free list service (listserv) to keep current, make national coding contacts, and post questions to others who may know the answer to a current coding or billing dilemma; for example, if you wish to join a free listserv go to the Web site: www.partbnews.com/enroll, fill out the enrollment form, and click "Done."

Code Monitoring

Monitoring of CPT codes is done to maximize reimbursement from all insurance carriers. First determine which codes are used most often in the physician's practice. Many computer programs can generate a list of codes, ranking them according to frequency of use. If the practice does not have a computer, take a sampling of the charge slips to find out the prevalent codes. Once the high volume codes are known, focus on coding strategies for the best possible reimbursement (Figure 6–7).

Monitor every Remittance Advice/Explanation of Benefits that comes in directly or via patients. Every private insurance, Medicare, Medicaid, and TRICARE payment received should be checked for accuracy to see whether it is consistently the same or if coding changes have occurred. Incorrect payments should be investigated and appealed. Examine all payments made for codes that do not match those submitted. Be sure to appeal every payment that is less than half of what the physician bills. An example of a code and payment tracking log to help monitor payments received is shown in Figure 6–7.

HELPFUL HINTS IN CODING

Office Visits

When an established patient is seen for an office visit and the medical assistant incidentally takes the patient's blood pressure per the physician's standing order, the physician includes that service with the appropriate level of E/M code number (e.g., 99213 or 99214). If the medical assistant takes the blood pressure and the patient is not seen by the physician but the physician reviews the results, the appropriate E/M code number is 99211 (presence of physician not necessary). If more than one office visit is necessary per day, the requirements for use of modifiers -25 and -59 should be read before submitting a claim to determine whether one of them may be applicable.

Some insurance policies allow only two moderate- or high-complexity office visits per patient per year. Therefore contact the insurance company to learn about any limitations. A physician's practice should have a system in place to track this.

Drugs and Injections

If the insurance claim has a description section (Block 19 on the CMS-1500 claim form), give the name, amount, and strength of the medication as well as how it was administered. This information must be documented in the patient's health record. If a drug is experimental or expensive, you need to include a copy of the invoice when sending in the insurance claim. CPT codes for immunization administration for vaccines are 90471 through 90474, and for therapeutic or diagnostic are 90780 through 90799. Separate codes are used to identify the product being administered. These codes may be either CPT codes 90281 through 90399 and 90476 through 90749 or when billing a Medicare case, level II HCPCS national alphanumeric codes A0000 or J0000. Separate codes are available for combination vaccines. See CPT codes 95004 through

CPT CODE	Practice fee	Medicare date and amount paid	Medicaid date and amount paid	TRICARE date and amount paid	Blue Shield date and amount paid
99201	$00.00	11-XX $00.00	8-XX $00.00	7-XX $00.00	4-XX $00.00
99202	$00.00	12-XX $00.00	9-XX $00.00	10-XX $00.00	6-XX $00.00
99211	$00.00	12-XX $00.00			11-XX $00.00
99212	$00.00				12-XX $00.00
99221	$00.00				
99231	$00.00				
99232	$00.00				
99241	$00.00				

CODE/PAYMENT TRACKING LOG Date: 1-XX

FIGURE 6–7 Example of a code/payment tracking log.

95199 for allergy testing and immunotherapy. If an anesthetic agent is being used, determine whether it is diagnostic, therapeutic, or prophylactic for pain. Medicare bills for immunosuppressive therapy are submitted to durable medical equipment carriers.

Adjunct Codes

Adjunct codes are referred to in the Medicine Section of the CPT as Special Services and Reports and fall under the category of Miscellaneous Services. They are important to consider when billing because these codes provide the reporting physician with a means of identifying special services and reports that are provided in addition to the basic services provided. The circumstances that are covered under these codes (99000 through 99091) include handling of laboratory specimens, telephone calls, seeing patients after hours, office emergency services, supplies and materials, special reports, travel, and educational services rendered to patients. Explain the circumstances on an attached document to justify the use of these codes when submitting an insurance claim. Some insurance companies pay for these services, but others do not.

Basic Life or Disability Evaluation Services

Use code 99450 when reporting examinations done on patients for the purpose of trying to obtain life or disability insurance. Codes 99455 and 99456 may be used for work-related or medical disability examinations. Additional information about life or health insurance examinations is given in Chapter 7.

CODE MODIFIERS

The use of a CPT code's two-digit add-on **modifier** permits the physician to indicate circumstances in which a procedure as performed differs in some way from that described by its usual five-digit code (Example 6.20).

Example 6.20 **Code Modifier for Assistant Surgeon**

27590-**80** Amputation, thigh

A modifier can indicate:

- A service or procedure has either a professional or technical component.
- A service or procedure was performed by more than one physician or in more than one location.
- A service or procedure has been increased or reduced.
- A service or procedure was provided more than once.
- Only part of a service was performed.
- An adjunctive service was performed.
- A bilateral procedure was performed.
- Unusual events occurred.

Modifiers should be considered an exception when coding services or procedures. The majority of professional services or procedures rendered are performed exactly as described by the CPT codes. Modifiers do not change the definition of a code but are used to describe modifying circumstances. It may be necessary when using a modifier to include an operative, pathology, x-ray, or special report to justify its use to an insurance carrier. For each modifier listed in Table 6.5, there is a statement as to when it is appropriate to include a report.

Table 6.5	CPT Modifier Codes

Modifier Code	Explanation
-21	**Prolonged Evaluation and Management Services:** When the face-to-face or floor/unit service(s) provided is prolonged or otherwise greater than that usually required for the highest level of evaluation and management service within a given category, it may be identified by adding modifier -21 to the evaluation and management code number. A report may also be appropriate.* **Example:** A physician spends an hour with a spouse and hospital inpatient, then an additional hour reviewing laboratory studies and x-ray films and reports, setting up a treatment plan with nurses, and coordinating care by two other specialists. **Medicare Payment Rule:** No effect on payment.
-22	**Unusual Procedural Services:** When the services provided are greater than that usually required for the listed procedure, they may be identified by adding modifier-22 to the usual procedure number. A report may also be appropriate.† **Example:** Removal of foreign body from stomach, which usually takes about 45 minutes, takes 2 hours on a particular patient; use modifier -22. A discharge summary or specially dictated statement should be attached to the claim form. This modifier increases the payment. **Medicare Payment Rule:** May result in increased payment based on supporting documentation of the unusual circumstances and complexity of the procedure performed.

*This modifier may affect reimbursement.
†This modifier may affect reimbursement, depending on the payer.

Continued

Table 6.5	CPT Modifier Codes—cont'd

Modifier Code	Explanation
-23	**Unusual Anesthesia:** Occasionally a procedure that usually requires either no anesthesia or local anesthesia must be done under general anesthesia because of unusual circumstances. This circumstance may be reported by adding the modifier -23 to the procedure code of the basic service.[†] **Examples:** A proctoscopy might require no anesthesia. A skin biopsy or excision of a subcutaneous tumor might require local anesthesia. If general anesthesia is needed, append the procedure code with -23.
-24	**Unrelated Evaluation and Management Service by the Same Physician During a Postoperative Period:** The physician may need to indicate that an evaluation and management service was performed during a postoperative period for a reason(s) unrelated to the original procedure. This circumstance may be reported by adding the modifier -24 to the appropriate level of E/M service.[†] **Example:** A patient seen for a postoperative visit after an appendectomy complains of a lump on the leg. The physician takes a history and examines the site, and a biopsy is scheduled. The E/M code 99024 is used for the postsurgery examination and the modifier -24 is added for unrelated service rendered during a postoperative period. **Medicare Payment Rule:** No effect on payment: however, failure to use this modifier when appropriate may result in denial of the E/M service. CMS memo FQA-541 reads "a documented, separately identifiable related service is to be paid for. We would define 'related' as being caused or prompted by the same symptoms or conditions." Make sure to document that the E/M service was related to the procedure.
-25	**Significant, Separately Identifiable Evaluation and Management Service by the Same Physician on the Day of a Procedure or Other Service:** The physician may need to indicate that on the day a procedure or service identified by a CPT code was performed, the patient's condition required a significant, separately identifiable E/M service above and beyond the other service provided or beyond the usual preoperative and postoperative care associated with the procedure that was performed. The E/M service may be prompted by the symptom or condition for which the procedure and/or service was provided. As such, different diagnoses are not required for reporting the E/M service on the same date. **Example:** A patient is seen for a diabetic follow-up and the physician discovers a suspicious mole on the patient's neck (0.4 cm), which is removed. The physician makes a minor adjustment of the oral diabetes medication. This case illustrates a significant E/M service provided on the same day as a procedure, so -25 is added to the E/M code. Code 11420 is used for removal of the benign lesion. **Note:** This modifier is not used to report an E/M service that resulted in a decision to perform surgery. See modifier -57.[†] **Medicare Payment Rule:** No effect on payment; however, failure to use this modifier when appropriate may result in denial of the E/M service.
-26	**Professional Component:** Certain procedures are a combination of a professional physician component and a technical component. When the professional (physician) component is reported separately, the service may be identified by adding the modifier -26 to the usual procedure number.* **Note:** The **professional component** comprises only the professional services performed by the physician during radiologic, laboratory, and other diagnostic procedures. These services include a portion of a test or procedure that the physician does, such as interpretation of the results. The **technical component** includes personnel, materials, including usual contrast media and drugs, film or xerograph, space, equipment, and other facilities but excludes the cost of radioisotopes. When billing for the technical component, use the usual five-digit procedure number with modifier -TC. **Example:** 70450-26 Computerized axial tomography, head or brain; without contrast material. *The modifier -26 indicates the physician interpreted this test only.* 70450-TC Computerized axial tomography, head or brain; without contrast material. *The modifier indicates the facility is billing only for the use of the equipment.*
-27	**Multiple Outpatient Hospital E/M Encounters on the Same Date:** For hospital outpatient reporting purposes, utilization of hospital resources related to separate and distinct E/M encounters performed in multiple outpatient hospital settings on the same date may be reported by adding the modifier -27 to each appropriate level outpatient and/or emergency department E/M code(s). This modifier provides a means of reporting circumstances involving E/M services provided by physician(s) in more than one (multiple) outpatient hospital setting(s) (e.g., hospital emergency department, clinic). Do not use this modifier for physician reporting of multiple E/M services performed by the same physician on the same date. See E/M, emergency department, or preventive medicine services codes. **Example:** Patient is seen in a hospital outpatient clinic. The patient falls in the treatment room and receives a cut on the right arm. The patient is taken to the emergency department for two stitches and a dressing. **Medicare Payment Rule:** Do not use modifier -27 for Medicare outpatients. Continue to use the -G0 (G-zero) modifier that HCFA established to cover multiple procedures, same patient, same day.
-32	**Mandated Services:** Services related to mandated consultation and/or related services (e.g., PRO, third-party payer, governmental, legislative or regulatory requirement), may be identified by adding the modifier -32 to the basic procedure.[‡]

[‡]Modifier is informational in nature. Do not ask for an adjustment in reimbursement. Monitor reimbursement when using this modifier.

Table 6.5	CPT Modifier Codes—cont'd

Modifier Code | **Explanation**

	Example: A patient is referred to the physician by an insurance company for an unbiased opinion regarding permanent disability after a year of treatment following an accident. Add modifier -32 to the E/M code because the second opinion is mandated by the insurance company.
	Medicare Payment Rule: No effect on payment
-47	**Anesthesia by Surgeon:** Regional or general anesthesia provided by the surgeon may be reported by adding the modifier -47 to the basic service (this does not include local anesthesia).†
	Note: Modifier -47 would not be used for anesthesia procedures 00100 through 01999.
	Example: A gastroenterologist performs an endoscopy for removal of esophageal polyps using the snare technique. The physician sedates the patient with Versed to perform the procedure.
	43217 Esophagoscopy with removal of polyps by snare technique
	43217-47 Administered Versed
	Medicare Payment Rule: Medicare will not reimburse the surgeon to administer anesthesia (any type).
-50	**Bilateral Procedure:** Unless otherwise identified in the listings, bilateral procedures requiring a separate incision performed during the same operative session should be identified by the appropriate five-digit code describing the first procedure. The second (bilateral) procedure is identified either by adding modifier -50 to the procedure number.
	Note: It is important to read each surgical description carefully to look for the word "bilateral." A bilateral modifier on a unilateral procedure code indicates that the procedure was performed on both sides of a paired organ during the same operative session.
	Example A: 71060 Bronchography, bilateral (would be listed with no modifier)
	Example B: 19200 mastectomy, radical
	19200-50 mastectomy, radical; bilateral
	Medicare Payment Rule: Payment is based on 150% (200% for x-rays) of the fee schedule amount.
-51	**Multiple Procedures:** When multiple procedures, other than E/M services, are performed at the same session by the same provider, the primary procedure or service may be reported as listed. The additional procedure(s) or service(s) may be identified by adding the modifier -51 to the additional procedure or service code(s).
	Note: This modifier should not be appended to designated "add-on" codes (see Appendix E of CPT). Always list the procedure of highest dollar value first.
	Example: Patient had herniated disk in lower back with stabilization of the area where the disk was removed.
	63030 Lumbar laminectomy with disk removal
	22612-51 Arthrodesis (modifier used after the lesser of the two procedures)
	Medicare Payment Rules: Standard multiple surgery policy—100% of the fee schedule amount is allowed for the highest valued procedure, 50% for the second through fifth procedures, and "by report" for subsequent procedures.
-52	**Reduced Services:** Under certain circumstances a service or procedure is partially reduced or eliminated at the physician's election. Under these circumstances the service provided can be identified by its usual procedure number and the addition of the modifier -52 signifying that the service is reduced. This provides a means of reporting reduced services without disturbing the identification of the basic service.§
	Note: This means there will be no effect on the physician's fee profile in the computer data. It is not necessary to attach a report to the claim when using this modifier, because it indicates a reduced fee. When a physician performs a procedure but does not charge for the service, such as a postoperative follow-up visit that is included in a global service, remember to use code 99024. Some physicians prefer to bill the insurance carrier the full amount and accept what the carrier pays as payment in full. In such cases, a modifier would not be used. If only part of a procedure is performed and the physician feels a reduction in the service is warranted, to develop a reduced fee try calculating the reduced service by time. Calculate the amount (cost) per minute of the complete procedure by dividing the amount (cost) by the usual time it takes to complete the procedure. To determine how long the reduced procedure took, multiply the amount (cost) per minute by the time it took to do the reduced procedure.
	Example: A patient is not able to participate or cooperate in a minimal psychiatric interview (90801) and the physician decides to attempt this at a later date. Modify the code with -52.
	Medicare Payment Rule: Payment is based on the extent of the procedure or service performed. Submit documentation with the claim.
-53	**Discontinued Procedure:** Under certain circumstances, the physician may elect to terminate a surgical or diagnostic procedure. Due to extenuating circumstances or those that threaten the well-being of the patient, it may be necessary to indicate that a surgical or diagnostic procedure was started but discontinued. This circumstance may be reported by adding the modifier "-53" to the code for the discontinued procedure.
	Note: This modifier is not used to report the elective cancellation of a procedure before the patient's anesthesia induction and/or surgical preparation in the operating suite. For outpatient hospital/ambulatory surgery center (ACS), see modifiers -73 and -74.

§This modifier affects reimbursement but not the physician's fee profile.

Continued

Table 6.5	CPT Modifier Codes—cont'd
Modifier Code	**Explanation**

	Example: The physician is beginning a cholecystectomy on a patient. An earthquake of great magnitude occurs and the electricity is shut off. The backup generator comes on and electricity is restored; however, because of the disarray in the operative suite, the physician decides to discontinue the surgery. Code 47562 is used with -53 appended to it.
	Medicare Payment Rule: The carrier will determine the amount of payment "by report." Submit documentation with the claim identifying the extent of the procedure performed and the extenuating circumstances.
-54	**Surgical Care Only:** When one physician performs a surgical procedure and another provides preoperative and/or postoperative management, surgical services may be identified by adding the modifier -54 to the usual procedure number.*
	Note: Because many surgical procedures encompass a "package" concept that includes normal uncomplicated follow-up care, the surgeon will be paid a reduced fee when using this modifier.
	Example: A patient presents in the emergency department with severe abdominal pain. Dr. A, the on-call surgeon, examines the patient and performs an emergency appendectomy. Dr. A is leaving on vacation the next morning so he calls his friend and colleague Dr. B. He asks him to visit the patient in the hospital the following day and take over the postoperative care. Dr. A bills using the appendectomy procedure code 44950 and modifies it with -54.
	Medicare Payment Rule: Payment is limited to the amount allotted for intraoperative services only.
-55	**Postoperative Management Only:** When one physician performs the postoperative management and another physician performs the surgical procedure, the postoperative component may be identified by adding the modifier -55 to the usual procedure number.
	Note: The fee to list would be approximately 30% of the surgeon's fee.
	Example: The Dunmires are relocating to Memphis, Tennessee, when Mrs. Dunmire discovers a lump on her arm. She visits her family physician, Dr. A, who tells her it needs to be excised. She wants her physician (Dr. A) to do the surgery and Dr. A agrees if she promises to arrange for a physician in Memphis to follow up postoperatively. She makes arrangements with Dr. B in Memphis. Dr. B bills using the correct excision code that he obtained from Dr. A and modifies it with -55.
	Medicare Payment Rule: Payment will be limited to the amount allotted for postoperative services only. Payment to more than one physician for split surgical care of a patient will not exceed the amount paid for the total global surgical package.
-56	**Preoperative Management Only:** When one physician performs the preoperative care and evaluation and another physician performs the surgical procedure, the preoperative component may be identified by adding the modifier -56 to the usual procedure number.†
	Example: Dr. A sees Mrs. Jones and determines she needs to have a lung biopsy. He admits her to the hospital and Dr. A becomes ill. Dr. B is called in and performs the surgery. Dr. A bills for the preoperative care using the surgical code he obtained from Dr. B and modifies it with -56.
	Medicare Payment Rule: Payment for this component is included in the allowable for the surgery. If another physician performed the surgery, use an appropriate E/M code to bill for the preoperative service.
-57	**Decision for Surgery:** An evaluation and management service that resulted in the initial decision to perform the surgery may be identified by adding the modifier -57 to the appropriate level of E/M service.‡
	Example: A trauma patient is seen in the emergency department by an orthopedic surgeon for a consultation to determine whether surgery on a fractured femur is necessary. The surgeon subsequently performs surgery 24 hours later in order to provide time for the patient to clear his intestinal contents. The surgeon bills the E/M consultation code and adds the -57 modifier. By adding this modifier, the third-party payer is informed that the consultation is not part of the global surgical procedure. Medicare will pay if it is for major surgery that requires a 90-day postoperative follow-up but not for a minor surgical procedure (0- to 10-day postoperative follow-up).
	Medicare Payment Rule: Payment will be made for the E/M service in addition to the global surgery payment.
-58	**Staged or Related Procedure or Service by the Same Physician During the Postoperative Period:** The physician may need to indicate that the performance of a procedure or service during the postoperative period was (a) planned prospectively at the time of the original procedure (staged); (b) more extensive than the original procedure; or (c) for therapy after a diagnostic surgical procedure. This circumstance may be reported by adding the modifier -58 to the staged or related procedure.‡
	Note: This modifier is not used to report the treatment of a problem that requires a return to the operating room. See modifier -78.
	Example: A patient has breast cancer and a surgeon performs a mastectomy. During the postoperative global period, the surgeon inserts a permanent prosthesis. The -58 modifier is added to the code for inserting the prosthesis, indicating that this service was planned at the time of the initial operation. If the modifier is not used, the insurance carrier may reject the claim because surgery occurred during the surgery's global period.

Table 6.5	**CPT Modifier Codes—cont'd**
Modifier Code	**Explanation**

Modifier Code	Explanation
-59	**Distinct Procedural Service:** Under certain circumstances, the physician may need to indicate that a procedure or service was distinct or independent from other services performed on the same day. Modifier -59 is used to identify procedures/services that are not normally reported together but are appropriate under the circumstances. This may represent a different session or patient encounter, different procedure or surgery, different site or organ system, separate incision/excision, separate lesion, or separate injury (or area of injury in extensive injuries) not ordinarily encountered or performed on the same day by the same physician. However, when another already established modifier is appropriate it should be used rather than modifier -59. Only if no more descriptive modifier is available, and the use of modifier -59 best explains the circumstances, should modifier -59 be used. **Example:** A patient is seen at their physician's office in the morning and the doctor orders a single view (71010) chest x-ray because the patient is complaining of a cough and chest congestion. The physician treats the patient for pneumonia. Later that same day, the patient is seen in the physician's office complaining of chest pain. The physician again orders a chest x-ray, but this time a two-view x-ray (71020). Ordinarily, the single-view chest x-ray will deny as a component of the two-view chest x-ray. However, since they were obtained at separate encounters, addition of the -59 modifier will indicate that these services are not combination components and should be paid for separately. **Medicare Payment Rule:** No effect on payment amount; however, failure to use modifier when appropriate may result in denial of payment for the services.
-62	**Two Surgeons:** When two surgeons work together as primary surgeons performing distinct parts of a single reportable procedure, each surgeon should report his or her distinct operative work using the same procedure code and adding the modifier -62. If additional procedures (including add-on procedures) are performed during the same surgical session, separate codes may be reported without the modifier -62. **Note:** If the cosurgeon acts as an assist in the performance of additional procedure(s) during the same surgical session, those services may be reported using separate procedure code(s) with modifier -80 or -81. **Example:** A procedure for scoliosis is performed by a thoracic surgeon who does the anterior approach and an orthopedic surgeon who does the posterior approach and repair. **Medicare Payment Rule:** Medicare allows 125% of the approved fee schedule amount for the -62 modifier if reported by both surgeons. That total fee is divided in half and dispersed to each surgeon at 62.5% of the approved amount.
-63	**Procedure Performed on Infants less than 4 kg:** Procedures performed on neonates and infants up to a present body weight of 4 kg may involve significantly increased complexity and physician work commonly associated with these patients. This circumstance may be reported by adding the modifier -63 to the procedure number. **Note:** Unless otherwise designated, this modifier may only be appended to procedures/services listed in the 20000-69999 code series. Modifier -63 should not be appended to any codes listed in the Evaluation and Management Services, Anesthesia, Radiology, Pathology/Laboratory, or Medicine sections.
-66	**Surgical Team:** Under some circumstances, highly complex procedures (requiring the concomitant services of several physicians, often of different specialties, plus other highly skilled, specially trained personnel and various types of complex equipment) are carried out under the "surgical team" concept. Such circumstances may be identified by each participating physician with the addition of the modifier -66 to the basic procedure number used for reporting services.* **Example:** A kidney transplant, requiring use of a vascular surgeon, urologist, and nephrologist, with the assistance of anesthesiologist and pathologist, or open heart surgery using perfusion personnel, three cardiologists, and an anesthesiologist. **Medicare Payment Rule:** Carrier medical staff will determine the payment amounts for team surgeries on a report basis. Submit supporting documentation with the claim.
-73	**Discontinued Outpatient Hospital/Ambulatory Surgery Center (ASC) Procedure Before the Administration of Anesthesia:** Because of extenuating circumstances or those that threaten the well being of the patient, the physician may cancel a surgical or diagnostic procedure subsequent to the patient's surgical preparation (including sedation when provided, and being taken to the room where the procedure is to be performed), but prior to the administration of anesthesia (local, regional block[s] or general). Under these circumstances, the intended service that is prepared for but canceled can be reported by its usual procedure number and the addition of modifier -73. **Note:** The elective cancellation of a service before the administration of anesthesia and/or surgical preparation of the patient should not be reported. For physician reporting of a discontinued procedure, see modifier -53.
-74	**Discontinued Outpatient Hospital/Ambulatory Surgery Center (ASC) Procedure After Administration of Anesthesia:** Because of extenuating circumstances or those that threaten the well-being of the patient, the physician may terminate a surgical or diagnostic procedure after the administration of anesthesia (local, regional block[s] or general) or after the procedure was started (incision made, intubation started, scope inserted). Under these circumstances, the procedure started but terminated can be reported by its usual procedure number and the addition of modifier -74.

Continued

Table 6.5	CPT Modifier Codes—cont'd
Modifier Code	**Explanation**
	Note: The elective cancellation of a service before the administration of anesthesia and/or surgical preparation of the patient should not be reported. For physician reporting of a discontinued procedure, see modifier -53.
-76	**Repeat Procedure by Same Physician:** The physician may need to indicate that a procedure or service was repeated subsequent to the original service. This circumstance may be reported by adding modifier -76 to the repeated service.[†]
	Example: A patient is seen by his family physician in the morning for his regular appointment. At that time, his doctor orders an ECG (93000). The patient calls in to his doctor's office in the afternoon to state that he is having some odd chest pain. The physician may request that the patient return to the office for another ECG (93000). The second ECG should be billed with a -76 modifier.
	Medicare Payment Rule: Failure to use this modifier when appropriate (and to submit supporting documentation) may result in denial of the subsequent procedure.
-77	**Repeat Procedure by Another Physician:** The physician may need to indicate that a basic procedure performed by another physician had to be repeated. This situation may be reported by adding modifier -77 to the repeated service.[†]
	Example: A femoral–popliteal bypass graft (35556) is performed in the morning and in the afternoon it becomes clotted. The original surgeon is not available, and a different surgeon performs the repeat operation later in the day. The original surgeon reports 35556. The second surgeon reports 35556-77.
	Medicare Payment Rule: Failure to use this modifier when appropriate (and to submit supporting documentation) may result in denial of the subsequent surgery.
-78	**Return to the Operating Room for a Related Procedure During the Postoperative Period:** The physician may need to indicate that another procedure was performed during the postoperative period of the initial procedure. When this subsequent procedure is related to the first, and requires the use of the operating room, it may be reported by adding the modifier -78 to the related procedure. (For repeat procedures on the same day, see -76.)[†]
	Example: A patient has an open reduction with fixation of a fracture of the elbow. While still hospitalized, the patient develops an infection and is returned to surgery for removal of the pin because it appears to be the cause of an allergic reaction. The original procedure would be billed for the open treatment of the fracture. The pin removal would be billed with modifier -78 because it is a related procedure.
	Medicare Payment Rule: Medicare will pay the full value of the intraoperative portion of a given procedure. Documentation should be submitted with the claim to describe the clinical circumstances.
-79	**Unrelated Procedure or Service by the Same Physician During the Postoperative Period:** The physician may need to indicate that the performance of a procedure or service during the postoperative period was unrelated to the original procedure. This circumstance may be reported by using the modifier -79. (For repeat procedures on the same day, see -76).[†]
	Example: A patient in the hospital has colon resection surgery and is discharged home. After 7 days, the patient develops acute renal failure, is hospitalized, does not recover renal function, and hemodialysis is ordered. A nephrologist inserts a cannula for the dialysis. When billing for the nephrologist, the code for hemodialysis is shown with a -79 modifier indicating that this is unrelated to the initial surgery. If modifier -79 is not used, the insurance carrier may not realize the service is not related to the initial surgery and may reject the claim.
	Medicare Payment Rule: No effect on payment; however, failure to use this modifier when appropriate may result in denial of the subsequent surgery. Specific diagnostic codes will substantiate the medical necessity of the unrelated procedure. Documentation may be required to describe the clinical circumstances. A new global period begins for any procedure modified by -79.
-80	**Assistant Surgeon:** Surgical assistant services may be identified by adding the modifier -80 to the usual procedure number(s).*
	Note: Some insurance policies do not include payment for assistant surgeons, such as for 1-day surgery, but do pay for major or complex surgical assistance. In some instances, prior approval may be indicated owing to the patient's physiologic condition. Medicare will not pay assistant surgeons for operations that are not life threatening. Therefore Medigap insurance will not pay on this service because the service is nonallowable. Assisting surgeons usually charge 16% to 30% of the primary surgeon's fee.
	Example: The primary surgeon performs a right ureterectomy submitting code 50650-RT. The assistant surgeon would bill using the primary surgeon's code with modifier -80 (50650-80).
	Medicare Payment Rule: Payment is based on the billed amount or 16% of the global surgical fee, whichever is lower, for procedures approved for assistant-at-surgery. Medicare will deny payment for an assistant-at-surgery for surgical procedures in which a physician is used as an assistant in less than 5% of the cases nationally.

Table 6.5	CPT Modifier Codes—cont'd
Modifier Code	**Explanation**
-81	**Minimum Assistant Surgeon:** Minimum surgical assistant services are identified by adding the modifier -81 to the usual procedure number. **Note:** Payment is made to physicians but not registered nurses or technicians who assist during surgery.* **Example:** A primary surgeon plans to perform a surgical procedure but during the operation circumstances arise that require the services of an assistant surgeon for a relatively short period. In this scenario, the second surgeon provides minimal assistance and may report using the procedure code with the -81 modifier appended.
-82	**Assistant Surgeon:** (When qualified resident surgeon is not available.) The unavailability of a qualified resident surgeon is a prerequisite for use of modifier -82 appended to the usual procedure code number(s).* **Note:** This modifier is usually used for services rendered at a teaching hospital. **Example:** A resident surgeon is scheduled to assist with an anorectal myomectomy (45108). Surgery is delayed due to the previous surgery, the shift rotation changes, and the resident is not available. A nonresident assists with the surgery and reports the procedure, appending it with modifier -82 (45108-82).
-90	**Reference (Outside) Laboratory:** When laboratory procedures are performed by a party other than the treating or reporting physician, the procedure may be identified by adding the modifier -90 to the usual procedure number.† **Note:** Use this modifier when the physician bills the patient for the laboratory work and the laboratory is not doing its own billing. **Example:** Dr. Input examines the patient, performs venipuncture, and sends the specimen to an outside laboratory for a liver panel. The physician has an arrangement with the laboratory to bill for the test, and, in turn, he bills the patient. Dr. Input bills for the examination (E/M code), venipuncture (36415 or for Medicare 0001), and acute hepatitis panel (80074), using modifier -90 (80074–90) to append to the hepatitis panel code.
-91	**Repeat Clinical Diagnostic Laboratory Test:** In the course of treatment of the patient, it may be necessary to repeat the same laboratory test on the same day to obtain subsequent (multiple) test results. Under these circumstances, the laboratory test performed can be identified by its usual procedure number and the addition of modifier -91. **Note:** This modifier may not be used when tests are rerun to confirm initial results; due to testing problems with specimens or equipment; or for any other reason when a normal, one-time, reportable result is all that is required. This modifier may not be used when other code(s) describe a series of test results (e.g., glucose tolerance tests, evocative/suppression testing). This modifier may only be used for laboratory test(s) performed more than once on the same day on the same patient. **Example:** A patient is scheduled for a nonobstetric dilation and curettage for dysfunctional uterine bleeding. When the patient arrives at the office, a routine hematocrit is obtained. During the procedure, the patient bleeds excessively. After the procedure, the physician orders a second hematocrit to check the patient for anemia due to blood loss. The first hematocrit is billed using CPT code 85013. The second hematocrit is billed using the same code appended with modifier -91 (85013-91).
-99	**Multiple Modifiers:** Under certain circumstances, two or more modifiers may be necessary to delineate a service completely. In such situations modifier -99 should be added to the basic procedure, and other applicable modifiers may be listed as part of the description of the service.‡ **Example:** An assistant surgeon helps repair an enterocele where unusual circumstances appear because of extensive hemorrhaging. 57270-99 Repair of enterocele -22 Extensive hemorrhaging (unusual service) -80 Assistant surgeon **Medicare Payment Rule:** No effect on payment; however, the individual modifier payment policies apply, including any inherent effect they may have on payment.

Modified with permission from the American Medical Association, Chicago, Illinois.

Correct Use of Common CPT Modifiers

A choice of any modifier that fits the situation that is being coded may be used except when the modifier definition restricts the use of specific codes; for example, modifier -51, Multiple Procedures, states that -51 is to be appended for "multiple procedures, other than Evaluation and Management Services…" Discussion of the most commonly used modifiers follows.

-21 Prolonged Evaluation and Management Services

This modifier is used to report a service longer than or greater than that described in the highest level evaluation and management service code (e.g., 99205, 99215, or 99223). In addition, there are some five-digit codes for prolonged services involving direct (face-to-face) patient contact in either the inpatient or outpatient setting

(99354 through 99357) and without direct (face-to-face) contact (99358 and 99359). Prolonged service of less than 30 minutes is not reported separately so these codes are used to report for time beyond that. Refer to the CPT for an illustration of correct reporting for these codes. Example 6.21 shows use of this modifier.

Example 6.21   Prolonged E/M Service

An 80-year-old diabetic woman is seen in a skilled nursing facility (SNF) by her internist for stage II decubitus ulcer with cellulitis. A revision in the treatment plan is indicated because of her condition. The physician performs a detailed interval history and a comprehensive physical examination, and the medical decision making is of moderate complexity. The physician meets with the patient's family to discuss treatment plans and future care (55 minutes).

99313-**21** Subsequent nursing facility care–prolonged E/M service

---

-22 Unusual Procedural Service

Modifier -22 is used when the service provided is greater than that usually necessary for the listed procedure. If you add modifier -22 for unusual service, then the documentation in the health record, such as operative report and/or chart note, must state that unusual service was performed within the context of the normal procedure. Encourage your physician to use appropriate descriptions in the report, and call these words to his or her attention. Three guidelines are (1) the complications cannot be indicated by a separate code; (2) the procedure is lengthy and unusual; and (3) the services provided by the physician are increased because of unusual circumstances or complexities. This modifier may not be used with E/M services. Most insurance carriers send an insurance claim to medical review before payment is made if modifier -22, indicating unusual services, appears on the claim. Because payments may be delayed, be cautious when using this modifier. An operative report should be submitted with the claim. If the insurance carrier routinely denies the claim with modifier -22, an appeal for review should be made. See Chapter 9 for details on the Medicare redetermination (appeal) process.

-25 Significant, Separately Identifiable Evaluation and Management Service by the Same Physician on the Same Day of the Procedure or Other Service

For information on this modifier, see the explanation of modifier -57.

-26 Professional Component

Certain procedures are a combination of a **professional component (PC)** and a **technical component (TC)**. Usually these involve radiology and pathology procedures. The professional (physician) component refers to a portion of a test or procedure that the physician does, such as interpreting an electrocardiogram (ECG), reading an x-ray film, or making an observation and determination using a microscope. The technical component refers to the use of the equipment, the supplies, and the operator who performs the test or procedure, such as ECG machine and technician, radiography machine and technician, and microscope and technician. Do not modify procedures that are either 100% technical or 100% professional or when the physician performs both the professional and technical components. Modifier -26 represents the professional component only. Use of this modifier alerts the insurance company to expect a separate claim from another provider or facility for the technical component (TC).

In Example 6.22, the physician is performing only one of two services—he or she is interpreting the results of bilateral hip x-ray films.

Example 6.22   Professional/Technical Components

73520-**26**	**Professional component** only for a radiograph of both hips. Use to bill physician's fee for interpretation and of X-ray film.	$
73520-**TC**	**Technical component** only for a radiograph of both hips. Use to bill facility fee that owns equipment and employs technician.	$
73520	Radiologic examination, hips, bilateral. Minimum of two views of each hip. Use to bill complete fee when physician owns equipment, employs technician, and interprets x-ray film.	$

The facility where the patient had the x-ray bills only for the technical component by modifying the same code with a -TC (73520-TC). If the physician owns the equipment and reads the x-ray film, there is no need to modify the x-ray code (73520) because both the professional and technical components were done in the office.

-51 Multiple Procedures

Multiple procedures are when more than one surgical service and/or related surgical service is performed on the same day or at the same surgical session by the same physician. In such cases, report the primary service or procedure, which can be determined easily by highest dollar value.

Identify all additional services or procedures by appending codes with modifier -51 (Example 6.23).

Example 6.23   Multiple Procedure Modifier -51

Excision of 2.0-cm benign lesion on the nose and at the same session a biopsy of the skin and subcutaneous tissue of the forearm.

Code	Fee	Description of Services
11442	$	Excision, other benign lesion including margins, face, ears, eyelids, nose, lips, mucous membrane; excised diameter 1.1 to 2.0 cm
11100-**51**		Biopsy of skin, subcutaneous tissue, or mucous membrane (including simple closure), unless otherwise listed; single lesion **(second; multiple procedure)**

The operative report should clearly state which procedures were done through separate incisions and which were done through the same incision. There are many circumstances when multiple procedures are performed. Modifier -51 may be used to identify the following:

● Multiple surgical procedures performed at the same session by the same provider
● Multiple related surgical procedures performed at the same session by the same provider
● Surgical procedures performed in combination at the same session, whether through the same or another incision or involving the same or different anatomy
● A combination of medical and surgical procedures performed at the same session by the same provider

Usually payment for the primary code is 100% of the allowable charge, second code 50%, third code 25%, fourth and remaining codes 10%. However, Medicare pays 50% of the allowable for two to five secondary procedures and does not require the assignment of modifier -51. There are computer systems that can determine code order and automatically make the code adjustment for you. Always bill the full amount and let the insurance carrier make the payment adjustments for percentage considerations. For all insurance carriers, it is recommended that you monitor the Remittance Advice/Explanation of Benefits to ensure correct payment. A decision flow chart is provided for reference to help simplify the modifier decision process (Figure 6–8). As you read through the remainder of this chapter, follow the steps by answering the questions in Figure 6–8, *A*, as they apply to your billing scenario and refer to Figure 6–8, *B*, for key information and descriptions.

If multiple procedures are done as in-office procedures or services and one is using E/M codes, it may be possible to bill a higher level E/M visit because the -51 modifier is not used with E/M services. Do not use the -51 modifier with, add-on codes designated with a "□"

(see Appendix D in CPT), or codes listed as exempt to modifier -51 (see Appendix E in CPT). Add-on codes are codes that cannot stand alone. When billing with add-on codes, you always have to first list another code referred to as the "parent code" to give full description for service billed (Example 6.24).

Example 6.24   Add-on Code

Parent code	11000	Biopsy of skin . . . single lesion each separate/additional lesion (list separately in addition to code for primary procedure)
Add-on code	+11101	

When making a decision about when to use an add-on code, look for a clue phrase that indicates additional procedures, such as "each additional," "list in addition to," and "second lesion."

-52 Reduced Services

Use of this modifier indicates that under certain circumstances a service or procedure is partially reduced or eliminated at the physician's discretion. It is wise to provide an explanation of why the service was reduced. A cover letter or a copy of the operative report should not accompany these claims because usually they are not sent to medical review and attached documents may impede processing. Never use this modifier if the fee is reduced because of a patient's inability to pay.

-57 Decision for Surgery

This modifier is used strictly to report an E/M service that resulted in the initial decision to perform a major surgical procedure within 24 hours of the office visit (e.g., those with a 90-day follow-up period); see Examples 6.25 and 6.26. A -57 modifier may be used for inpatient or outpatient consultations, inpatient hospital visits, and new or established patient visits that occur the day of or the day before surgery. Do not attach modifier -57 to a hospital visit code for the day before surgery or the day of surgery when a decision for a major surgical procedure was made

---

Example 6.25   Decision for Surgery

A new patient is seen in the office complaining of a great deal of pain. Cholangiography is done and reveals blocked bile ducts. The patient is scheduled for surgery the next day.

| 8-1-20xx | 99204-**57** | New patient office visit | $00.00 |
| 8-2-20xx | 47600 | Cholecystectomy | $000.00 |

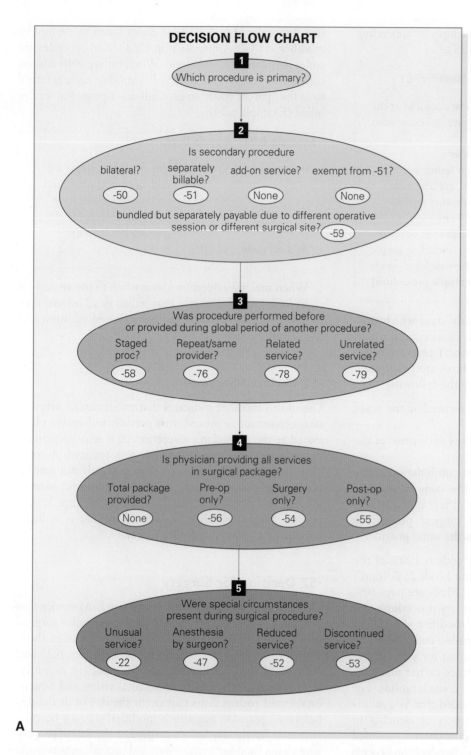

FIGURE 6–8 A, Decision flow chart for surgical procedures.

a week before surgery. Think of -57 as telling the insurance company that the office visit is not part of the global fee.

-25 Significant Separately Identifiable E/M Service

In some cases, you may be confused whether to assign modifier -25 or -57. Modifier -25 is defined as "Significant, separately identifiable evaluation and management service

by same physician on the same day of the procedure or other service." The industry standard is to use -25 when a diagnostic procedure or minor procedure is involved (e.g., those with a 0- to 10-day follow-up period). Typically, E/M services that are modified with -25 are office visits performed on the day of a minor procedure for an established patient. However, the confusion results because the CPT code book states, "This modifier is not used to report an E/M service that resulted in a decision to perform surgery. See modifier -57."

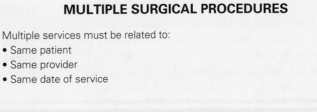

MULTIPLE SURGICAL PROCEDURES

Multiple services must be related to:
- Same patient
- Same provider
- Same date of service

1

- List all procedures in order of reimbursement, highest to lowest
- Most comprehensive service brings greatest reimbursement and is considered primary
- Check all procedures to make sure there is no unbundling, i.e., using two codes when one code describes procedure
- Decision making expands at this point. Follow numbered question to determine correct modifier usage

2

-50 bilateral procedure, not described by code
-51 not bundled, separately billable
-59 ordinarily bundled, separately payable due to special circumstance

3

- The term "primary procedure" can also refer to the first procedure initiating a global surgical period
-58 Current service was planned prospectively at time of first service
-76 Physician repeats procedure subsequent to original procedure
-78 Return to operating room for subsequent procedure, complication relating to original procedure
-79 Unrelated procedure performed during global period of previous surgery

4

- Surgical package means one fee covers the whole package, surgical procedure and postoperative care

5

-22 An extremely difficult procedure due to altered anatomy or unusual circumstances (add 10% to 30% reimbursement)
-47 When the surgeon administers regional or general anesthesia
-52 Procedure/service reduced or eliminated at the discretion of the physician
-53 Procedure is discontinued due to extenuating circumstances or because of threat to the patient

FIGURE 6–8, cont'd B, Guidelines and description of modifiers for multiple surgical procedures.

B

Consult Figure 6–9 when making the decision about which modifier to use for a surgical procedure that is performed within 24 hours of an office visit.

In Medicare cases, the CMS has published in the *National Correct Coding Initiative* (NCCI) the specific codes for modifier -25 use after October 2000. Refer to the bulletin or newsletter pertinent to this update.

-58 Staged or Related Procedure

This modifier is used to indicate that the performance of a procedure or service during the postoperative period was

- Planned (staged) at the time of the original procedure
- More extensive than the original procedure
- For therapy after a diagnostic surgical procedure

Example 6.26   Decision for Surgery

A new patient comes to the office after sustaining a fall while in-line skating. She is in distress, complaining of right wrist pain and swelling of the joint. The injury is evaluated **(1)** with an x-ray film. **(2)** It is determined that the patient has a Smith fracture and manipulation is performed. A long-arm cast is applied **(3)** using fiberglass (Hexcelite) material **(4)**.

(1) 99203-**57** Initial office evaluation (detailed) **with decision for surgery**

(2) 73100-RT Radiologic examination, right wrist, anteroposterior (AP) and lateral (lat) views

(3) 25605 Closed treatment of distal radial fracture (e.g., Colles or Smith type), with manipulation

(4) 99070 Supplies: Casting material (private carrier) Medicine Section code

or

Supplies: Hexcelite material (Medicare carrier)

A4590 HCPCS Level II code

The patient returns in 4 weeks for follow-up care **(1)**. The wrist is radiographed again **(2)**, the long-arm cast is removed **(3)**, and a short-arm cast is applied **(4)** using plaster material **(5)**.

(1) No code Follow-up care included in global fee

(2) 73100-RT Radiologic examination, right wrist, AP and lat views

(3) No code Cast removal included in original fracture care (25605)

(4) 29075-**58** Application, plaster, elbow to finger (short arm) **staged procedure**

(5) 99070 Supplies: Casting material (private carrier)

Medicine Section code

or

Supplies: Plaster material (Medicare carrier)

A4580 HCPCS Level II code

Such circumstances should be reported by adding modifier -58 to the staged or related procedure. The use of this modifier requires accurate documentation of events leading up to the initial surgery and any subsequent surgery. It is only possible to modify procedures if the coder has all of the relevant facts and circumstances. In Example 6.26, the fracture is considered surgery because it is in the surgery section of the CPT book. All fracture codes have 90-day postoperative periods.

-62, -66, -80, -81, -82 More than One Surgeon

If more than one surgeon is involved, clarify for whom you are billing by using the appropriate two-digit modifier as follows:

-62, Cosurgeon, which is when two surgeons work together as primary surgeons performing distinct parts of a procedure. Each physician reports his or her distinct operative work by adding this modifier.

-66, Team surgery is when a group of surgeons work together. Each participating physician adds this modifier to the basic procedure number for the service.

-80, Assistant at surgery.

-81, minimum assistant surgeon.

-82, assistant surgeon (when a qualified resident surgeon is not available) is when a surgeon helps during a surgical procedure.

The assistant physician adds one of these modifiers to the usual procedure number. (See Examples 6.20 and 6.27.)

Modifier -80 (assistant at surgery) is commonly used when billing for a physician who assists the primary physician in performing a surgical procedure (see Example 6.27).

The assisting doctor is paid a reduced fee of 16% to 30% of the allowed fee the primary surgeon receives for performing the surgery based on the patient's contract. The assisting physician uses the same surgical code as the primary surgeon and adds the -80 modifier to it. The fee indicating a reduced percentage typically is listed as the

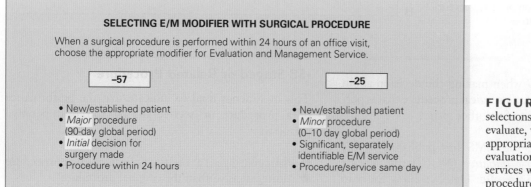

SELECTING E/M MODIFIER WITH SURGICAL PROCEDURE

When a surgical procedure is performed within 24 hours of an office visit, choose the appropriate modifier for Evaluation and Management Service.

–57	–25

- New/established patient
- *Major* procedure (90-day global period)
- *Initial* decision for surgery made
- Procedure within 24 hours

- New/established patient
- *Minor* procedure (0–10 day global period)
- Significant, separately identifiable E/M service
- Procedure/service same day

FIGURE 6–9 Two selections, with criteria to evaluate, when choosing the appropriate code or modifier for evaluation and management services when a surgical procedure is performed within 24 hours of an office visit.

Example 6.27   Assistant at Surgery

Closure of intestinal cutaneous fistula

Operating surgeon bills	44640	**No modifier**
Assistant surgeon bills	44640-**80**	**With modifier**

Example 6.28   Multiple Modifiers

A physician sees a patient who is grossly obese. The operative report documents that a bilateral sliding-type inguinal herniorrhaphy was performed, and the procedure took 2 hours 15 minutes.

49525-**99**	Bilateral repair sliding inguinal hernia requiring 2 hours 15 minutes
-**50**	
-**22**	

---

fee on the claim form. However, some insurance carriers may prefer having the full fee listed and making the reduction themselves. Under some insurance contracts, there may be some surgical procedures that restrict payment for an assistant surgeon, so contact the insurance company to find out if there is any limitation.

-99 Multiple Modifiers

If a procedure requires more than one modifier code, use the two-digit modifier -99 after the usual five-digit CPT code number, all typed on one line; then list each modifier on a separate line (Example 6.28). Some insurance companies require -99 with a separate note in Block 19 of the CMS-1500 claim form or in the freeform area of electronic submissions, indicating which two or more modifiers are being used.

HCPCS

Besides CPT modifiers, HCPCS level II modifiers are used by Medicare and may be used by some commercial carriers. HCPCS level II modifiers may be two

alpha digits (Example 6.29), two alphanumeric characters (Figure 6–10), or a single alpha digit used for reporting ambulance services or results of positron emission tomography scans. A brief list of these modifiers may be found in Appendix A of the CPT code book. They also appear on the inside cover of the CPT code book. A comprehensive list may be found in an HCPCS national level II code book. HCPCS reference books may be obtained from resources listed in Appendix A.

Example 6.29   HCPCS Modifiers

When taking x-ray films of both feet, the billing portion of the insurance claim appears as follows:

05/06/XX	73620 **RT**	Radiologic examination, foot—right
05/06/XX	73620 **LT**	Radiologic examination, foot—left

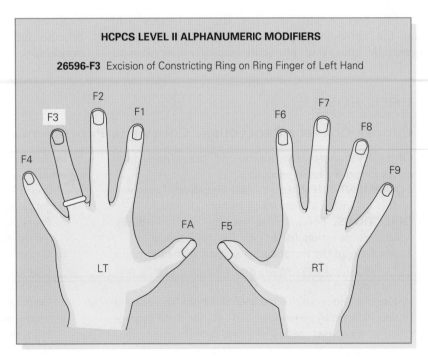

HCPCS LEVEL II ALPHANUMERIC MODIFIERS

26596-F3 Excision of Constricting Ring on Ring Finger of Left Hand

FIGURE 6–10 HCPCS level II alpha modifiers (LT and RT used to identify left and right hands) and alphanumeric modifiers (FA through F9) used to identify digits (fingers) of left and right hands.

Use the two-digit HCPCS modifiers whenever they are necessary. HCPCS modifiers further describe the services provided and can increase or decrease the physician's fee. If not used properly, they can drastically affect the physician's fee profile by reducing future payments to the physician.

Comprehensive List of Modifier Codes

Now that you have learned about some basic modifiers, read through the comprehensive list shown in Table 6.4 to gain information on additional modifiers and their use illustrated by clinical examples.

PROCEDURE

DETERMINE CONVERSION FACTORS

OBJECTIVE: To determine the conversion factors for several procedure codes.

EQUIPMENT/SUPPLIES: *Current Procedural Terminology* code book, geographic practice cost indices and relative value unit pages from the *Federal Register,* calculator, and pen or pencil.

DIRECTIONS: Follow these step-by-step procedures, which include rationales, to practice this job skill.

1. Choose 10 or more procedure codes commonly used in the medical practice and in the same section (E/M, Anesthesia, Surgery, Radiology, Pathology, or Medicine) and list the code numbers, at least 60 code numbers.

2. Use the relative value unit formula: RVU × GAF × CF = Medicare $ per service, and the geographic practice cost indices and relative value unit pages from the *Federal Register.* From the 60 or more codes you have assembled, locate the first procedure code from the Relative Value Units page of the *Federal Register.*

3. For the work amount, obtain the dollar amount from the Work RVUs and multiply that by the GPCI of the locality name of where the medical practice is located.

4. For the overhead amount, obtain the dollar amount from the Practice expense RVUs and multiply that by the figure in the GPCI practice expense column.

5. For the malpractice amount, obtain the dollar amount from the Malpractice RVUs and multiply that by the figure in the GPCI malpractice column.

6. Take the three results and add them together to obtain the total adjusted RVUs.

7. Use the current year Medicare conversion factor amount and multiply that by the total adjusted RVUs amount and that will give the allowed amount for the procedure code.

8. Repeat steps 2 through 7 for all additional procedure codes commonly used by the medical practice for each section of the CPT code book.

9. Look at all the dollar figures that you have determined for all of the procedure codes selected. For each section of the CPT code book, they should fall within the same general range. If they do not, reevaluate those fees that are too high or low and readjust them depending on the service descriptions and market competition comparisons.

The fees should be above the maximums paid by the third-party payers to whom the practice generally bills. Your physician employer may wish to evaluate the fee schedules annually to decide whether fees should be raised for certain procedures or services.

PROCEDURE

CHOOSE CORRECT PROCEDURAL CODES FOR PROFESSIONAL SERVICES

OBJECTIVE: Accurately locate and select procedural codes for professional services.

EQUIPMENT/SUPPLIES: *Current Procedural Terminology* code book, medical dictionary, and pen or pencil.

DIRECTIONS: Follow these step-by-step procedures, which include rationales, to practice this job skill.

1. Always read the Introduction section at the beginning of the code book, which may change annually with each edition.

2. Use the index at the back of the book to locate a specific item by generalized code numbers, *not* by page numbers. Never code from the index. Listings may

be looked up according to names of procedures or services, organs, conditions, synonyms, eponyms, and abbreviations; for example, some primary entries might be as follows:

a. Procedure or service
    Example: Anastomosis; Endoscopy; Splint

b. Organ or other anatomic site
    Example: Salivary Gland; Tibia; Colon

c. Condition
    Example: Abscess; Entropion; Tetralogy of Fallot

d. Synonyms, eponyms, and abbreviations
    Example: EEG; Bricker operation; Clagett procedure

PROCEDURE—CONT'D

If the procedure performed is not listed, check for the organ involved. If the procedure or organ is difficult to find, look up the condition. Key words, such as synonyms or eponyms, and abbreviations will help you find the appropriate code.

3. Locate the code number in the code section for the code range given in the index.

4. Turn to the beginning of the section for the code range given in the index and read the Guidelines at the beginning of the section. This gives general information and instructions on coding certain procedures within the section, defines commonly used terms, explains classifications within the section, and gives instructions specific to the section.

5. Turn to the correct section, subsection, category, or subcategory, and read through the narrative description to locate the most appropriate code to apply to the patient's procedure. Look at the size of the title to find out the area you are in. Some code books have color-coded titles, making this determination easier. In the surgery section, each subsection is further divided into categories based on anatomic site. Within each category are subcategories listed by type of procedure (e.g., excision, repair, destruction, graft) or condition (burn, fracture). Read the notes and special subsection information throughout the section.

11040	Debridement; skin, partial thickness
11041	skin, full thickness
11042	skin, and subcutaneous tissue
11043	skin, subcutaneous tissue, and muscle
11044	skin, subcutaneous tissue, muscle, and bone

FIGURE 6–11 Use of a semicolon.

6. Notice punctuation and indentions. Descriptions for stand-alone codes begin at the left margin and have a full description. No matter how many indented codes are listed, always go back to the stand-alone code to begin reading the description. A semicolon (;) separates common portions from subordinate designations; subterms are indented (Figure 6–11). Any terminology after the semicolon has a dependent status, as do the subsequent indented entries. In Figure 6–12, *A,* the procedure code number 11044 should read as follows: Debridement; skin, subcutaneous tissue, muscle, and bone. Figure 6–12, *B,* shows an insurance claim for a patient who has had six corns pared.

7. When trying to locate an E/M code, identify the place or type of service rendered. Then identify whether the patient is new or established and locate the category or subcategory. Review any guidelines or instructions

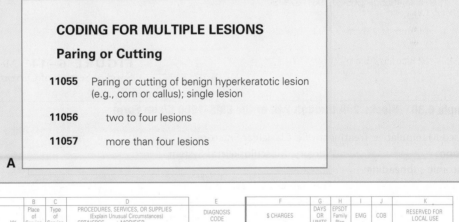

CODING FOR MULTIPLE LESIONS

Paring or Cutting

11055 Paring or cutting of benign hyperkeratotic lesion (e.g., corn or callus); single lesion

11056 two to four lesions

11057 more than four lesions

A

24.	A DATE(S) OF SERVICE					B Place of Service	C Type of Service	D PROCEDURES, SERVICES, OR SUPPLIES (Explain Unusual Circumstances) CPT/HCPCS | MODIFIER	E DIAGNOSIS CODE	F $ CHARGES		G DAYS OR UNITS	H EPSDT Family Plan	I EMG	J COB	K RESERVED FOR LOCAL USE
	MM	DD	YY	MM	DD	YY										
1	05	11	2001				11		99203		1	00	00	1			46	27889700
2	05	11	2001				11		11057		1	00	00	1			46	27889700
3																	
4																	
5																	

B

FIGURE 6–12 **A,** Procedure codes from the Surgery Section of *Current Procedural Terminology.* **B,** Blocks 24A through 24K of the CMS-1500 insurance claim form showing placement of the code on Line 2.

Continued

pertaining to the category or subcategory. Read the descriptors of the levels of E/M service. Identify the requirements necessary for code assignment. Make sure the components necessary were performed by the physician and documented in the chart, and then assign the E/M code. Commercial templates are available to aid in E/M code selection and help tremendously.

8. Select the code. Note the following:
   - Parentheses ( ) further define the code and tell where other services are located (Figure 6–13).
   - Measurements throughout the code book are based on the metric system (Figure 6–14).
   - All anesthesia services are reported by use of the five-digit anesthesia code plus a physical status modifier. The use of other modifiers to explain a procedure further is optional. Example: Patient is a healthy 23-year-old Caucasian woman. Anesthesia is given for a vaginal delivery. The procedure code with modifier is 00946-P1.
   - The Surgery section is the largest segment of the code book. It has many subsections and subheadings. You must be able to break down a procedure and identify various terms that will direct you to the correct code. Blocks 24A through 24K of the CMS-1500 insurance claim form show placement of the code on Line 2 (Example 6.30, bottom).

9. Determine if one or more modifiers are needed to give a more accurate description of the services rendered or the circumstances in which they were performed.

10. Enter the five-digit code number and modifier to the proper field on the insurance claim form exactly as given for each procedure or service rendered. Be careful not to transpose code numbers.

BIOPSY

Defining further ——— **11100** Biopsy of skin, subcutaneous tissue and/or mucous membrane (including simple closure), unless otherwise listed (separate procedure); single lesion

11101 each separate/additional lesion

Location of other services ——— (For biopsy of conjuctiva, see 68100; eyelid, see 67810)

FIGURE 6–13 Use of parentheses in the Surgery Section of *Current Procedural Terminology*.

13150 Repair, complex, eyelids, nose, ears and/or lips; 1.0 cm or less (See also 40650–40654, 67961–67975)

13151 1.1 cm to 2.5 cm

13152 2.6 cm to 7.5 cm

FIGURE 6–14 Metric measurements from the Surgery Section of *Current Procedural Terminology*.

Example 6.30   Blocks 24A through 24K of the CMS-1500 Claim Form

Closed Manipulative Treatment of a Clavicular Fracture
Section: Surgery, Musculoskeletal System
Anatomic subheading: Shoulder
Condition: Fracture or Dislocation
Code: 23505

Thus when completing an insurance claim form for closed manipulative treatment, clavicular fracture, the billing portion appears as follows:

24. A DATE(S) OF SERVICE						B Place of Service	C Type of Service	D PROCEDURES, SERVICES, OR SUPPLIES (Explain Unusual Circumstances) CPT/HCPCS | MODIFIER	E DIAGNOSIS CODE	F $ CHARGES		G DAYS OR UNITS	H EPSDT Family Plan	I EMG	J COB	K RESERVED FOR LOCAL USE
From MM	DD	YYYY	To MM	DD	YYYY											
01	07	20XX				11		99203 |	1	00	00	1			46	27889700
01	07	20XX				11		23505 |	1	00	00	1			46	27889700
								|								
								|								
								|								

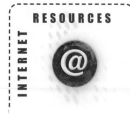

RESOURCES

INTERNET

For AHIMA and AHA diagnostic code guidelines for outpatient services and diagnostic coding and reporting requirements for physician billing:

- Web site: **http://www. ahima.org**
  Web site: **http://www.aha.centraloffice.com**

- To locate the four regional durable medical equipment carriers:
  Web site: **http://www.cms.hhs.gov/suppliers/dmepos**

ASSIGNMENT

STUDENT

✔ Study Chapter 6.

✔ Answer the review questions in the *Workbook* to reinforce the theory learned in this chapter and help prepare you for a future test.

✔ Complete the assignments in the *Workbook* to assist you in hands-on practical experience in procedural coding as well as learning medical abbreviations.

✔ Assignments related to the resource-based relative value scale (RBRVS) because of the complexity of that subject are presented later in the course when studying the chapter about Medicare.

✔ Turn to the glossary at the end of this textbook for a further understanding of the key terms used in this chapter.

CHAPTER OUTLINE

HISTORY
COMPLIANCE ISSUES RELATED
  TO INSURANCE CLAIM FORMS
TYPES OF CLAIMS
  Claim Status
ABSTRACTING FROM MEDICAL
  RECORDS
  Cover Letter Accompanying
    Insurance Claims
  Life or Health Insurance
    Applications

HEALTH INSURANCE CLAIM
  FORM (CMS-1500)
  Basic Guidelines for Submitting
    a Claim
  Completion of Insurance Claim
    Forms
COMMON REASONS WHY CLAIM
  FORMS ARE DELAYED OR
  REJECTED
  Additional Reasons Why Claim
    Forms Are Delayed

OPTICAL SCANNING FORMAT
  GUIDELINES
  Optical Character
    Recognition
  Do's and Don'ts for Optical
    Character Recognition
PROCEDURE: INSTRUCTIONS
  FOR THE HEALTH INSURANCE
  CLAIM FORM (CMS-1500)
  Insurance Program
    Templates

KEY TERMS

clean claim

dirty claim

durable medical equipment
  (DME) number

electronic claim

employer identification number
  (EIN)

facility provider number

group provider number

Health Insurance Claim Form
  (CMS-1500)

incomplete claim

intelligent character recognition
  (ICR)

invalid claim

National Provider Identifier (NPI)

optical character recognition
  (OCR)

"other" claims

paper claim

pending claim

physically clean claim

provider identification number
  (PIN)

rejected claim

Social Security number (SSN)

state license number

unique provider identification
  number (UPIN)

7

The Paper Claim: CMS-1500

OBJECTIVES*

After reading this chapter, you should be able to:

- Give the history of the Health Insurance Claim Form (CMS-1500).

- State when the CMS-1500 claim form may or may not be used.

- Expedite the handling and processing of the CMS-1500 insurance claim form.

- Define two types of claims submission.

- Explain the difference between clean, pending, rejected, incomplete, and invalid claims.

- Abstract from the patient record relevant information for completing the CMS-1500 insurance claim form.

- Describe reasons why claims are rejected.

- Minimize the number of insurance forms returned because of improper completion.

- Identify techniques required for optically scanned insurance claims.

- Execute general guidelines for completing the CMS-1500 claim form for federal, state, and private payer insurance contracts.

*Performance objectives and exercises for hands-on practical experience for this chapter appear in the *Workbook*.

HISTORY

In 1958, the Health Insurance Association of America (HIAA) and the American Medical Association (AMA) attempted to standardize the insurance claim form by jointly developing the Standard Form. It was not universally accepted by all third-party payers, and as the types of coverage became more variable, new claim forms were instituted that required more information than the original Standard Form. The form eventually became known as COMB-1, or Attending Physician's Statement. In 1968, the HIAA decided to revamp the form so that it would be more adaptable to electronic data processing.

In April 1975, the AMA approved a "universal claim form," called the **Health Insurance Claim Form,** referred to as the HCFA-1500, which was an acronym for the Health Care Financing Administration. In July, 2001, HCFA became the Centers for Medicare and Medicaid Services (CMS); thus the form is currently referred to as **CMS-1500.** CMS adopted the form because of the need for a standard format and to quicken claims processing. The CMS-1500 claim form answered the needs of many health insurers processing claims manually. The National Association of Blue Shield Plans Board of Directors adopted a motion supporting the concept of a uniform national claim form.

In 1990, the CMS-1500 was revised and printed in red ink, which allowed claims to be optically scanned by the insurance carriers. Beginning on May 1, 1992, all services for Medicare patients from physicians and suppliers, except for ambulance services, had to be billed on the scannable CMS-1500 form.

The revised form was adopted by TRICARE Management Activity (TMA), formerly known as the Office of Civilian Health and Medical Programs of the Uniformed Services (OCHAMPUS). It also received the approval of the AMA Council on Medical Services. The HIAA endorsed and recommended that their members (private insurance companies) accept the form. In some states, the Medicaid program, as well as industrial (workers' compensation) cases, use this form to process claims. After October 16, 2003, Health Insurance Portability and Accountability Act (HIPAA) required that claims be transmitted electronically in the HIPAA format by providers who are not small providers (institutional organizations with fewer than 25 full-time employees or physicians with fewer than 10 full-time employees).

Widespread use of this form has saved time and simplified processing of claims for both physicians and carriers because it has eliminated the need to complete the many various insurance forms brought into the office by patients. Another way of billing that may be accepted by insurance companies is to complete the CMS-1500 and attach it to the patient's form. The patient's and employer's portions of the private insurance form should be complete and accurate, and the patient should sign the release of information box and the assignment of benefits, if applicable. Both forms are sent directly to the insurance carrier. If the patient is insured by two companies, release of information and assignment for both insurance carriers should be obtained. Most offices use a standard release of information form and assignment of benefits form combined on one page, which becomes part of the patient's health record. The primary carrier should be determined and the claim submitted to that carrier first. After the primary insurance carrier has paid out, a claim should be submitted to the secondary carrier with a copy of the payment check voucher (or patient's explanation of benefits document) attached.

Insurance carriers with various computer programs and equipment that optically scan claims may have instructions on completion of the form that vary by locality and program. Local representatives of insurance carriers should always be contacted to find out whether the form is acceptable before any claims are submitted. A photocopy is not acceptable if the form is processed by the insurance carrier through scanning equipment because the statements on the back of the form are critical to the statements on the claim form side. Quantities of the CMS-1500 can be purchased from many medical office supply companies or from the AMA by calling toll free to 800-621-8335. In many cases, the computerized practice management system will produce the CMS-1500 claim form but an original claim form is required for submission. Also, the CMS-1500 claim form may be downloaded from the CMS Web site but may not be used for submission of claims (see Internet Resources at the end of this chapter).

In this chapter, instructions for completing a paper claim using optical character recognition (OCR) format is emphasized. HIPAA allows small providers with fewer than 10 full-time employees to continue to send paper claims. Medicare advised that the purchased red ink versions of the CMS-1500 claim form with the bar code cannot be duplicated by computer printer; therefore, if the Medicare carrier uses OCR scanning technology, the claims must be originals and not photocopies or they will not be processed. This chapter focuses on the paper claim and Chapter 8 explains the intricacies of transmitting electronic claims as mandated by HIPAA.

TYPES OF CLAIMS

A **paper claim** is one that is submitted on paper, including optically scanned claims that are converted to electronic

COMPLIANCE ISSUES RELATED TO INSURANCE CLAIM FORMS

HIPAA federal laws affect insurance claim submission. The provider rendering the service or procedure must be properly identified with the correct provider number. Claims must only show services rendered that have been properly documented and are medically necessary without evidence of fraud or abuse issues. HIPAA mandates use of electronic standards for automated transfer of certain health care data between health care payers, plans, and providers. The National Provider Identifier (NPI) system for health care providers must be used by May 27, 2007, in connection with the electronic transactions identified in HIPAA. Refer to Chapters 2 and 8 for a complete discussion about health care providers that are required to submit claims electronically.

form by insurance companies. Paper claims may be typed or generated via computer.

An **electronic claim** is one that is submitted to the insurance carrier via dial-up modem (telephone line or computer modem), direct data entry, or over the Internet by way of digital subscriber line (DSL) or file transfer protocol (FTP). Electronic claims are digital files that are not printed on paper claim forms when submitted to the payer.

Claim Status

Paper or electronic claims can be designated as clean, rejected, or pending (suspended).

A **clean claim** means that the claim was submitted within the program or policy time limit and contains all necessary information so it can be processed and paid promptly. A **physically clean claim** is one that has no staples or highlighted areas and on which the bar code area has not been deformed.

A rejected claim means that the claim has not been processed or cannot be processed for various reasons, such as the patient is not identified in the payer system, the provider of services is not active in the insurance company payer records, or the claim was not submitted in a timely manner.

A **pending claim** is an insurance claim that is held in suspense for review or other reason. These claims may be cleared for payment or denied.

Medicare Claim Status

In the Medicare program, besides the phrase "clean claims," specific terms, such as *incomplete*, *rejected*, and *dirty*, are used to describe various claim-processing situations. These terms may or may not be used by other insurance programs.

A *clean claim* means the following:

1. The claim has no deficiencies and passes all electronic edits.
2. The carrier does not need to investigate outside of the carrier's operation before paying the claim.
3. The claim is investigated on a postpayment basis, meaning a claim is not delayed before payment and may be paid. After investigation, payments may be considered "not due" and a refund may be requested from the provider.
4. The claim is subject to medical review with attached information or forwarded simultaneously with electronic medical claim (EMC) records.

Further information on the many methods to ensure clean claims is given in the next chapter.

Medicare claims not considered "clean" claims, which require investigation or development on a prepayment basis (developed for Medicare Secondary Payer information), are known as **"other" claims.**

Participating provider electronic submissions are processed within approximately 14 days of receipt. Participating provider paper submissions and nonparticipating provider claims are not processed until at least 27 days after receipt.

An **incomplete claim** is any Medicare claim missing required information. It is identified to the provider so it can be resubmitted as a new claim.

A **rejected claim,** as mentioned earlier, is one that requires investigation and needs further clarification and possibly answers to some questions. Such a claim should be resubmitted after proper corrections are made.

An **invalid claim** is any Medicare claim that contains complete, necessary information but is illogical or incorrect (e.g., listing an incorrect provider number for a referring physician). An invalid claim is identified to the provider and may be resubmitted.

A **dirty claim** is a claim submitted with errors, one requiring manual processing for resolving problems, or one rejected for payment. Pending or suspense claims are placed in this category because something is holding the claim back from payment, perhaps review or some other problem.

ABSTRACTING FROM MEDICAL RECORDS

Abstraction of technical information from patient records may be requested for three situations: (1) to complete insurance claim forms, (2) when sending a letter to justify a health insurance claim after professional services are rendered, or (3) when a patient applies for life, mortgage, or health insurance. Abstracting to complete insurance claims is discussed later in this chapter.

Cover Letter Accompanying Insurance Claims

A letter accompanying insurance claims should include the patient's name, subscriber's name if different, subscriber identification number, date and type of service, total amount of the claim, a short history, and a clear but concise explanation of the medical necessity, difficulty or complexity, or unusual circumstance (e.g., emergency). The letter and insurance claim should be sent to the attention of the claims supervisor so it may be directed to the appropriate person for processing.

Life or Health Insurance Applications

When a patient applies for insurance, the insurance company may request information from the patient's private physician, require a physical examination, or both.

On some application forms (Figure 7–1), the release of medical information signed by the patient may appear as a separate sheet or as a perforated attachment to a multiple-paged form. In the latter, page 1 is completed by the insurance agent when interviewing the client, page 2 is filled in by the prospective insured, and page 3 is completed by the physician at the time of the physical examination of the prospective insured. Sometimes a form is sent to the client's attending physician along with a check requesting medical information (Figure 7–2). The amount of the check may vary, depending on how much information is requested. If the check is not included, the physician should request a fee based on the length of the report before sending in the completed report form. The fee is required before completion of the form or payment may not be received.

Be extremely accurate when abstracting medical information from the patient's record. Figure 7–3 is a chart note identifying important abstracting components.

Abbreviations on the chart must be understood, and only the requested information should be provided. If the form has questions about high blood pressure, kidney infection, or heart problems, the patient could be prohibited from obtaining life, health, or mortgage insurance if the answers are derogatory. Part of HIPAA laws (Insurance Portability, Part I) provides guidance on circumstances when an individual can be excluded from health insurance benefits coverage. Be sure to check with the insurance company for more information. Because this part of HIPAA is more involved than would apply in the role of a billing specialist, this topic is not discussed in depth here.

If a patient tests positive for human immunodeficiency virus (HIV), legal counsel may be necessary because some state laws allow information on HIV infection and acquired immunodeficiency syndrome (AIDS) to be given only to the patient or to the patient's spouse. In some states, it is illegal to require a blood test for HIV antibodies, a urinalysis for HIV, or an HIV antigen test as a condition of coverage. It also may be illegal to question applicants about HIV status or prior symptoms of and treatment for AIDS or other forms of immune deficiency. Sometimes, private group plans allow medical coverage for people testing positive for HIV or an AIDS-related illness through a state major risk medical insurance program. However, the waiting period may exceed 1 year if the maximum enrollment number has been reached. A separate release of information statement in addition to that previously described is necessary before any information can be released regarding an HIV/AIDS patient.

In some situations, it is preferable to submit a narrative report dictated by the physician instead of completing the form, which has numerous check-off columns and no space for comments. It may be necessary to attach a copy of an operative, pathology, laboratory, or radiology report and an electrocardiogram (ECG) tracing.

A "Please Read" note should be placed on the insurance questionnaire to have the physician check it over thoroughly before signing it and to make sure that the information is accurate and properly stated.

An insurance company may ask a copy service to come to your office to photocopy the patient's record. Usually this is done at the office's convenience, and an appointment should be made. The insurance company should be reminded that an authorization form signed by the patient is necessary to release medical information. An appropriate fee for this service is charged and quoted at the time of the telephone request. The physician should review the records in advance to see that they are in proper order.

PART II of Application to the MASSACHUSETTS INDEMNITY AND LIFE INSURANCE COMPANY

PROPOSED
INSURED
OR ANNUITANT: *Jason F. Reed*

Date of Birth: *March 10, 1972*
Mo.   Day   Year

1. a. Name and address of your personal physician? *Gerald Practon, MD 4567 Broad Ave.,*
   (If none, so state)
   b. Date and reason last consulted? *November 4, 1999*   *Woodland Hills, XY 12345*
   c. What treatment was given or medication prescribed? *Rx flumadine*

		Yes	No
2. Have you ever been treated for or ever had any known indication of:			
a. Disorder of eyes, ears, nose, or throat?		☐	☑
b. Dizziness, fainting, convulsions, recurrent headache, speech defect, paralysis or stroke, mental or nervous disorder?		☐	☑
c. Shortness of breath, persistent hoarseness or cough, blood spitting, bronchitis, pleurisy, asthma, emphysema, tuberculosis or chronic respiratory disorder?		☐	☑
d. Chest pain, palpitation, high blood pressure, rheumatic fever, heart murmur, heart attack or other disorder of the heart or blood vessels?		☐	☑
e. Jaundice, intestinal bleeding, ulcer, hernia, appendicitis, colitis, diverticulitis, hemorrhoids, recurrent indigestion, or other disorder of the stomach, intestines, liver or gallbladder?		☐	☑
f. Sugar, albumin, blood or pus in urine, venereal disease, stone or other disorder of kidney, bladder, prostate or reproductive organs?			
g. Diabetes, thyroid or other endocrine disorders?		☐	☑
h. Neuritis, sciatica, rheumatism, arthritis, gout or disorder of the muscles or bones, including the spine, back, or joints?		☐	☑
i. Deformity, lameness or amputation?		☐	☑
j. Disorder of skin, lymph glands, cyst, tumor or cancer?		☐	☑
k. Allergies, anemia or other disorder of the blood?		☐	☑
l. Excessive use of alcohol, tobacco, sedatives, or any habit-forming drugs?		☐	☑
3. Are you now under observation or taking treatment?		☐	☑
4. Have you had any change in weight in the past year?		☐	☑
5. Other than above, have you within the past 5 years:		☐	☑
a. Had any mental or physical disorder not listed above?		☑	☐
b. Had a (checkup) consultation, illness, injury, surgery?			
c. Been a patient in a hospital, clinic, sanatorium, or other medical facility?		☐	☑
d. Had electrocardiogram, X-ray, blood sugar, basal metabolism, other (diagnostic test)?		☑	☐
e. Been advised to have any diagnostic test, hospitalization, or surgery which was not completed?		☐	☑
6. Have you ever had military service deferment, rejection or discharge because of a physical or mental condition?		☐	☑
7. Have you ever requested or received a pension, benefits, or payment because of an injury, sickness or disability?		☐	☑
8. Family History: Tuberculosis, (diabetes) cancer, high blood pressure, heart or kidney disease, mental illness or suicide?		☑	☐

DETAILS of "Yes" answers. (IDENTIFY QUESTION NUMBER, CIRCLE APPLICABLE ITEMS: Include diagnoses, dates, duration and names and addresses of all attending physicians and medical facilities.)

5b. Last checkup 1997
(G. Practon MD)

5d. Blood serology

8. Father is diabetic

	Age if Living	Cause of Death?	Age at Death?
Father	55		
Mother	54		
Brothers and Sisters	2		
No. Living			
No. Dead			

(For non-medical cases only)
Height _____ Weight _____

9. Females only: Yes No
   a. Have you ever had any disorder of menstruation, pregnancy or of the female organs or breasts? ☐ ☐
   b. To the best of your knowledge and belief are you now pregnant? ☐ ☐

I HEREBY DECLARE that, to the best of my knowledge and belief, the statements and answers in Part II of this Application are full, complete, and true. These statements and answers are to be considered as the basis for any insurance written hereon.

Signed at: (City & State) *Woodland Hills, XY*   Dated: *January 25, 20XX*

x *Jason F. Reed*

_____
Signature of witness   Signature of PROPOSED INSURED

Form MD (70)a

FIGURE 7–1 The prospective insured completes this side of the insurance application form.

PART III—PHYSICIAN'S EXAMINATION REPORT

Acct. No. _145_   District or Agency _____   Name of Agent _James Santor_

Date _Jan. 25, 20xx_   Name of Insuring Company _Hartman Insurance Company_

PROPOSED INSURED: _Reed_ (Last Name)   _Jason_ (First Name)   _F._ (Middle Initial)   Date of Birth _3_ Mo. _10_ Day _1972_ Year

10a.

Height (In Shoes)	Weight (Clothed)	Chest (Full Inspiration)	Chest (Forced Expiration)	Abdomen, at Umbilicus
_5_ ft. _11_ in.	_180_ lbs.	_43_ in.	_42_ in.	_38_ in.

Details of "Yes" answers. (Identify item.)

b. Did you weigh?...... ☒ Yes ☐ No   Did you measure?.................... ☒ Yes ☐ No

c. Is appearance unhealthy or older than stated age?.............. ☐ Yes ☒ No

11. Blood Pressure (Record ALL readings)

Systolic	120		
Diastolic {4th phase	80		
5th phase			

12. Pulse:

	At Rest	After Exercise	3 minutes later
Rate	60	86	66
Irregularities per min.			

13. Heart: Is there any:

Enlargement.............. ☐ Yes ☒ No   Dyspnea.................... ☐ Yes ☒ No

Murmur(s)................. ☐ Yes ☒ No   Edema.................... ☐ Yes ☒ No

(describe below—if more than one, describe separately)

MCL

Location

Constant	☐ ☐
Inconstant	☐ ☐
Transmitted	☐ ☐
Localized	☐ ☐
Systolic	☐ ☐
Presystolic	☐ ☐
Diastolic	☐ ☐
Soft (Gr. 1–2)	☐ ☐
Mod. (Gr. 3–4)	☐ ☐
Loud (Gr. 5–6)	☐ ☐
After Exercise:	
Increased	☐ ☐
Absent	☐ ☐
Unchanged	☐ ☐
Decreased	☐ ☐

Indicate:
Apex by X
Murmur area by ↻
Point of greatest intensity by O
Transmission by ▶

For comments and your impression?

14. Is there on examination any abnormality of the following: Yes No
(Circle applicable items and give details.)

(a) Eyes, ears, nose, mouth, pharynx? _____ ☐ ☒
(If vision or hearing markedly impaired, indicate degree and correction)

(b) Skin (incl. scars); lymph nodes; varicose veins or peripheral arteries?.................... ☐ ☒

(c) Nervous system (include reflexes, gait, paralysis)?......... ☐ ☒

(d) Respiratory system? .... ☐ ☒

(e) Abdomen (include scars)? .... ☐ ☒

(f) Genitourinary system (include prostate)?.............. ☐ ☒

(g) Endocrine system (include thyroid and breasts)? .... ☐ ☒

(h) Musculoskeletal system (include spine, joints, amputations, deformities)?...................... ☐ ☒
(A confidential report may be sent to the Medical Director)

15. (a) Are there any hernias? .... ☐ ☒
(b) Any hemorrhoids? .... ☐ ☒

16. Are you aware of any additional medical history?.............. ☐ ☒

17. Was the examination conducted in the English language?.... ☒ ☐
If No, complete the following:
a. Was an interpreter used?.................. ☐ ☒
b. What language was used? _____
c. Relationship of interpreter to proposed insured?_____

Urinalysis: Specific Gravity

Albumin	Sugar
0	trace

Is specimen being sent?.................... ☒ Yes ☐ No
If Yes, where? _ABC laboratory_

Send Specimen: (Details according to Company) _____

Date: _1-25-20xx_   Time: _10_ (A.M.) P.M.   City: _Woodland Hills_   State: _XY_

Signature of Medical Examiner: _Gerald Practon_ M.D.   Physical Measurements Information _____

PMI-188R—1-88

FIGURE 7–2 Sample of a life insurance application form with the check to the physician omitted. The physician completes this side of the form at the time of the examination of the patient, the prospective insured.

Block 24A Dates of service	Block 24D Documentation of professional services rendered	Block 14 Date of last menstrual period	Block 21 Primary and secondary diagnoses

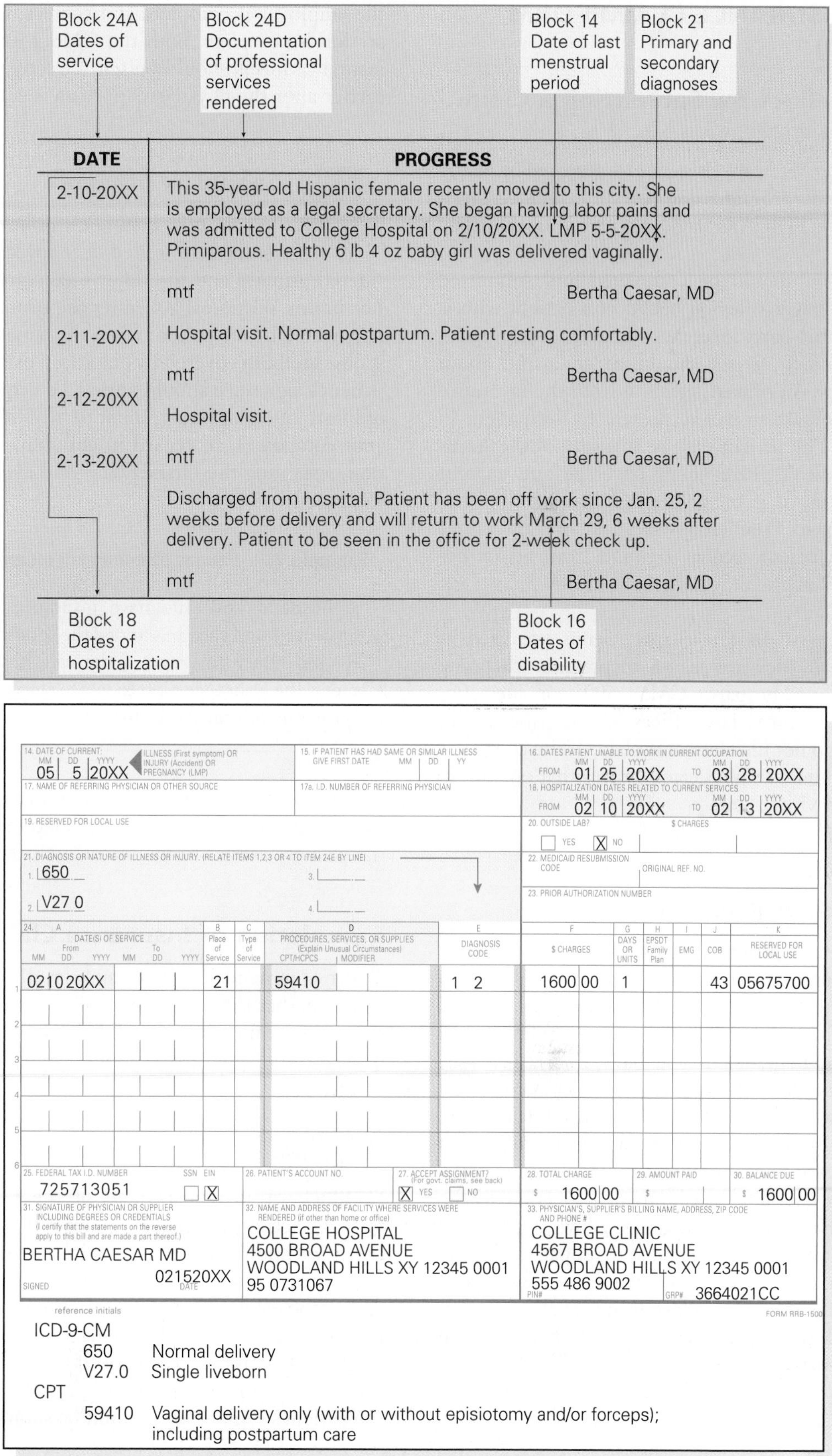

DATE	PROGRESS
2-10-20XX	This 35-year-old Hispanic female recently moved to this city. She is employed as a legal secretary. She began having labor pains and was admitted to College Hospital on 2/10/20XX. LMP 5-5-20XX. Primiparous. Healthy 6 lb 4 oz baby girl was delivered vaginally.
	mtf Bertha Caesar, MD
2-11-20XX	Hospital visit. Normal postpartum. Patient resting comfortably.
	mtf Bertha Caesar, MD
2-12-20XX	Hospital visit.
2-13-20XX	mtf Bertha Caesar, MD
	Discharged from hospital. Patient has been off work since Jan. 25, 2 weeks before delivery and will return to work March 29, 6 weeks after delivery. Patient to be seen in the office for 2-week check up.
	mtf Bertha Caesar, MD

Block 18 Dates of hospitalization

Block 16 Dates of disability

A

B

ICD-9-CM
650   Normal delivery
V27.0   Single liveborn
CPT
59410   Vaginal delivery only (with or without episiotomy and/or forceps); including postpartum care

FIGURE 7-3 **A,** Example of a chart note illustrating important information to read through and abstract for insurance claim completion. **B,** The location of the abstracted information placed in the blocks on a CMS-1500 insurance claim form in OCR format.

HEALTH INSURANCE CLAIM FORM (CMS-1500)

Basic Guidelines for Submitting a Claim

The CMS-1500 insurance claim form is the form required when submitting Medicare claims and is accepted by nearly all state Medicaid programs and private insurance carriers as well as by TRICARE and workers' compensation.

A claim form should be completed and submitted as required by payer rules on behalf of a patient who is covered by a third-party insurance. If coverage is in question, the insurance carrier should be contacted about eligibility status. An official rejection from the insurance company is the best answer to present to the patient in this situation. The patient may be unaware of the status of his or her health care policy coverage and current deductible status. It is recommended that you bill and get paid for services rendered if there is coverage rather than have the patient receive payment from his or her insurance company.

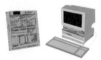

In this chapter, icons are used as they are shown in previous chapters. The paper CMS-1500 icon identifies physicians' offices that are paper based, meaning they do not file electronic claims. The computer icon is used to indicate physicians' offices that operate in an electronic environment.

Individual Insurance

When a patient brings in a form from a private insurance plan that is not a CMS-1500 claim form, he or she should sign it. In addition, the patient should sign the CMS-1500 claim form in Block 13 (Assignment of Benefits). If you have a signed assignments of benefits form in the patient's health record, you can state "signature on file" on the CMS-1500 claim form. The patient's portion of the private insurance form should be checked to ensure that it is complete and accurate. The forms should then be mailed together to the insurance carrier. Some companies allow staples and some do not. It is not recommended to let patients direct their own forms to insurance companies or employers. Patients have been known to lose forms or alter data on documents before mailing, forget to send them, or mail them to an incorrect address.

Group Insurance

When a patient has group insurance through an employer, be sure all the information about the employer is complete and correct. If the employer's section is complete, both the CMS-1500 and the group insurance forms should be sent directly to the insurance carrier after the physician's portion is completed.

Secondary Insurance

When two insurance policies are involved (sometimes called dual coverage), one is considered primary and the other secondary (Example 7.1). For billing purposes, generally the primary policy is the policy held by the patient when the patient and his or her spouse are both covered by employer-paid insurance. The patient's signature should always be acquired for release of information and assignment of benefits for both insurance companies. In regard to children, refer to the section explaining the birthday law and divorced parents in Chapter 3.

Example 7.1   Primary/Secondary Insurance Plans

A husband and wife have insurance through their employers and each has added the spouse to their plans for secondary coverage. If the wife is seen for treatment, the insurance plan to which she is the subscriber is the primary carrier for her.

After payment is made by the primary plan, a claim is submitted with a copy of the explanation of benefits from the primary carrier to the secondary carrier.

Completion of Insurance Claim Forms

The recommendation is to answer all questions on the form whether the form is optically scanned or not. If any questions are unanswerable, DNA (Does Not Apply), NA, or N/A (Not Applicable) should be typed or a dashed line inserted.

Diagnosis

In Block 21, diagnosis field of the CMS-1500 claim form, all accurate diagnostic codes that affect the patient's condition should be inserted, with the primary diagnosis code listed first followed by any secondary diagnosis codes. A diagnosis should never be submitted without supporting documentation in the medical record. The diagnosis must agree with the treatment. If there is no formal diagnosis at the conclusion of an encounter, the code(s) for the patient's symptom(s) should be submitted.

To avoid confusion, it is best to list only one illness or injury and its treatment per form, unless there are concurrent conditions.

24. A		B	C	D	E	F	G	H	I	J	K
DATE(S) OF SERVICE From To MM DD YY MM DD YY		Place of Service	Type of Service	PROCEDURES, SERVICES, OR SUPPLIES (Explain Unusual Circumstances) CPT/HCPCS MODIFIER	DIAGNOSIS CODE	$ CHARGES	DAYS OR UNITS	EPSDT Family Plan	EMG	COB	RESERVED FOR LOCAL USE
1	10 04 20XX 10 08 20XX	21		99232	1	55	56 5			32	783127XX
2											

Service Dates

Insertion of ditto marks (") to indicate repetition of dates for services performed should not be used. Charges for services rendered in different years on the same claim form should not be submitted. Sometimes such practices can be affected by deductible and eligibility factors, thereby delaying reimbursement.

Consecutive Dates

Some carriers allow medical services or hospital or office visits to be grouped if each visit is consecutive, occurs in the same month, uses the same procedure code, and results in the same fee. The fee for a single procedure should be listed in Block 24F, and the number of times the procedure was performed or service supplied should be listed in Block 24G as illustrated in the graphic at the top of this page. However, private insurance carriers should be contacted because some carriers require a total fee listed in Block 24F rather than the fee for a single procedure. If there is a difference in the procedure code or fee for several visits listed on the claim, each separately coded hospital or office visit must be itemized and each procedure or service code and charge entered on a separate line.

No Charge

Insurance claims should not be submitted for services that have no charge, such as global or surgical package postoperative visit, unless the patient requests that it be sent. These services should appear documented in the patient's health and financial records.

Physicians' Identification Numbers

Insurance companies and federal and state programs require certain identification numbers on claim forms be submitted from health care providers and facilities who provide and bill for services to patients. This can be confusing to the beginner as well as to someone experienced in insurance billing procedures, because there are so many different numbers.

● *State license number.* To practice within a state, each physician must obtain a physician's **state license number.** Sometimes this number is requested on forms and is used as a provider number.

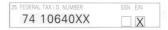

E	F	G	H	I	J	K
DIAGNOSIS CODE	$ CHARGES	DAYS OR UNITS	EPSDT Family Plan	EMG	COB	RESERVED FOR LOCAL USE
						C16021

● *Employer identification number.* In a medical group or solo practice, each physician must have his or her own federal tax identification number, known as an **employer identification number (EIN).** This is issued by the Internal Revenue Service for income tax purposes.

25. FEDERAL TAX I.D. NUMBER	SSN EIN
74 10640XX	☐ ☒

● *Social security number.* In addition, each physician has a **Social Security number (SSN)** for other personal use and may have one or more *tax identification numbers (TINs)* for financial reasons. These are not typically used on the claim form unless the provider does not have an EIN, then the Social Security number may be required.

25. FEDERAL TAX I.D. NUMBER	SSN EIN
082 XX 1707	☒ ☐

Provider Numbers

Claims may require three provider identification numbers: one for the referring physician, one for the ordering physician, and one for the performing physician (billing entity). It is possible that the ordering physician and the performing physician are the same. On rare occasions, the number may be the same for all three, but more frequently three different numbers are required, depending on the circumstances of the case. For placement of the provider number on the CMS-1500 claim form, refer to the block-by-block instructions for Blocks 17a and 24J through K. Keep in mind what role the physicians and their numbers represent in relationship to the provider listed in Block 33. The following examples of blocks from the CMS-1500 insurance claim form show where these numbers are commonly placed. Insurance billing manuals from major insurers give specific directions.

When a nonphysician practitioner (NPP) bills incidentto a physician in the same group, but that physician is out of the office on a day the NPP sees the patient, another physician in the same group can provide direct supervision to meet the incident-to requirements. Incident-to services are discussed in Chapter 6. When the ordering and supervising doctors are different individuals, the ordering doctor's name goes in Block 17 and his or her UPIN (not PIN) goes in Block 17a. The PIN of the supervising doctor goes in Block 24K and the supervising physician signs the form in Block 31. The group's PIN goes in Block 33.

To assist with claims completion, a reference list of provider numbers should be compiled for all ordering physicians and physicians who frequently refer patients. For Medicare claims, physicians' provider numbers can be obtained by calling their offices, contacting the Medicare carrier, or searching the UPIN Registry on the Internet. For license numbers, search the state licensing board on the Internet. Refer to Appendix A for all physician provider numbers when completing *Workbook* assignments.

● *Provider identification number.* Every physician who renders services to patients may be issued a carrier-assigned **provider identification number (PIN)** by the insurance company. With the implementation of the national provider identifier for compliance by May 23, 2007, PINs will no longer be used.

> 33. PHYSICIAN'S, SUPPLIER'S BILLING NAME, ADDRESS, ZIP CODE & PHONE #
> JOHN DOE MD 555 486 9001
> 123 ANY STREET
> ANYTOWN XY 12345
> PIN# 70 98765XX   GRP#

● *Unique provider identification number.* The Medicare program issues each physician a **unique provider identification number (UPIN).** With the implementation of the National Provider Identifier on May 23, 2007, UPINs will no longer be used.

> 17a. I.D. NUMBER OF REFERRING PHYSICIAN
> 46278897XX

● *Group provider number.* The **group provider number** is used instead of the individual PIN for the performing provider who is a member of a group practice that submits claims to insurance companies under the group name.

> 33. PHYSICIAN'S, SUPPLIER'S BILLING NAME, ADDRESS, ZIP CODE & PHONE #
> COLLEGE CLINIC 555 486 9002
> 4567 BROAD AVENUE
> WOODLAND HILLS XY 12345 0001
> PIN#   GRP# 3664021CC

● *National Provider Identifier.* The **National Provider Identifier (NPI)** is a lifetime 10-digit number that will replace all other numbers assigned by various health plans. It will be recognized by state (Medicaid), federal (Medicare, TRICARE, and CHAMPVA), and private programs. Most providers required to submit

standard electronic transactions under HIPAA must apply for an NPI from the National Provider System beginning May 23, 2005. Each provider must begin using the NPI on May 23, 2007, except for small health plans whose compliance date is May 23, 2008. A health care provider will be assigned only one NPI, which is retained for a lifetime even if he or she moves to another state.

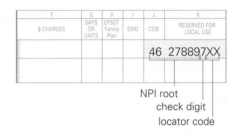

● *Durable medical equipment number.* Medicare providers who charge patients a fee for supplies and equipment, such as crutches, urinary catheters, ostomy supplies, surgical dressings, and so forth must bill Medicare using a **durable medical equipment (DME) number.** These claims are not sent to the regional fiscal intermediary but to another specific location.

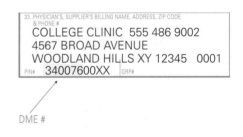

● *Facility provider number.* Each facility (e.g., hospital, laboratory, radiology office, skilled nursing facility) is issued a **facility provider number** to be used by the performing physician to report services done at the location.

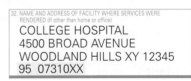

A FINAL NOTE:

AN NPI NUMBER PAYS! BECAUSE IT'S UNIVERSAL

Physician's Signature

The physician should sign the insurance claim form above or under the typed or preprinted physician's name. A stamped signature is allowed in some instances and discussed later in this chapter. A removable indicator "Sign Here" tag may be used to help the physician locate where to sign the claim.

 In the computerized office environment, the practice management system will generate a paper CMS-1500 form. The participating contract with the third-party payer (including Medicare, Medicaid, and the Blue Plans) that is signed by the physician allows the physician's name to be printed in the signature block as it would normally be signed. This is an acceptable method for provider's signature.

Insurance Biller's Initials

The insurance billing specialist should place his or her initials in the bottom left or top right corner of the claim form. Placement of this reference should be consistent. There are three good reasons to adopt this habit:

● To identify who in the office is responsible for the insurance form
● To decrease errors
● To avoid being accused of someone else's error, especially if the previous biller submitted a fraudulent claim

Proofread

Every claim should be proofread for transposition of numbers (group, policy, physician's ID, procedure, and diagnostic codes), misspelled name, missing date of birth, blanks, and attachments. Larger, more complex claims require special attention because they involve greater sums of money and may be more difficult to complete.

Supporting Documentation

Occasionally claims need supporting documents to further explain services billed and to obtain maximum reimbursement.

On any submitted supplemental document, the patient's name, subscriber's name (if different from that of the patient), date of service, and insurance identification number should be included in case the document becomes separated from the claim during processing. This same information should be placed on each page of the document, front and back if two-sided.

If a medication is expensive or experimental, a copy of the invoice received from the supply house or pharmacy should be sent.

When a procedure is complicated, a copy of all pertinent reports (operative, radiology, laboratory, pathology, and discharge summary) should be included.

For a treatment not listed in the procedure code book, a detailed report should be sent that gives the nature, extent, and need for the services. The correct code number should be used for unlisted services or procedures, which usually end in "99" (Example 7.2).

Example 7.2   Unlisted Procedure

Unlisted Allergy Testing Procedure 951**99**

Office Pending File

As mentioned in Chapter 3, the office copy of the insurance form should be filed in a separate alpha (tickler) file for insurance claim copies or in the back of the patient's medical chart, unless the computer system maintains files. The tickler file should be reviewed for followup every 30 days.

The practice management system will keep an accurate record of all patients and activity on their accounts.

COMMON REASONS WHY CLAIM FORMS ARE DELAYED OR REJECTED

It is wise to be aware of common billing errors and how to correct them for quicker claim settlements and to reduce the number of appeals. This may help avoid additional administrative burdens, such as telephone calls, resubmission of claims, appeal letters, and so on. Also see Chapter 9 for information on solutions to denied or delayed claims as well as prevention measures. The following is a list of some reasons why claims are rejected or delayed and suggested solutions when completing the CMS-1500 insurance claim form blocks.

PROBLEM: **Block 1.** Wrong block is checked (i.e., claim submitted to the secondary insurer instead of the primary insurer).

SOLUTION: Obtain data from the patient during the first office visit as to which company is the primary insurer, depending on illness, injury, or accident. Submit the claim to the primary carrier and then send in a claim with a copy of the primary carrier's explanation of benefits (EOB) to the secondary carrier.

PROBLEM: **Blocks 1 to 13.** Information missing on patient portion of the claim form.

SOLUTION: Obtain a complete patient registration form from which information can be extracted. Educate patients on data requirements at the time of the first visit to the physician's office if patients are filling out their portion. Be sure to ask if there have been any changes on subsequent office visits.

PROBLEM: Block 1a. Patient's insurance number is incorrect or transposed (especially in Medicare and Medicaid cases).

SOLUTION: Proofread numbers carefully from source documents. Always photocopy front and back sides of insurance identification cards.

PROBLEM: Block 2. Patient's name and insured's name are entered as the same when the patient is a dependent. A common error seen is the patient listed as insured even when he or she is not the insured (e.g., spouse or child). Block 4 is used for listing the insured's name.

SOLUTION: Verify the insured party and check for Sr., Jr., and correct birth date.

PROBLEM: Block 3. Incorrect gender identification, resulting in a diagnosis or procedure code that is inconsistent with patient's gender.

SOLUTION: Proofread claim before mailing and review patient's medical record to locate gender, especially if the patient's first name could be male or female.

PROBLEM: Blocks 9a through d. Incomplete entry for other insurance coverage.

SOLUTION: Accurately abstract data from the patient's registration form. Telephone the patient if information is incomplete.

PROBLEM: Block 10. Failure to indicate whether patient's condition is related to employment or an "other" type of accident.

SOLUTION: Review patient's medical history to find out details of injury or illness and proofread claim before mailing. Telephone the employer to see if permission was given to treat the patient as a workers' compensation case.

PROBLEM: Block 14. Date of injury is missing, date of last menstrual period (LMP), or dates of onset of illness are omitted. This information is important for determining whether accident benefits apply, patient is eligible for maternity benefits, or there was a preexisting condition.

SOLUTION: Do not list unless dates are clearly documented in the patient's medical record. Read the patient's medical history and call the patient to obtain the date of accident or LMP. Compose an addendum to the record, if necessary. Always proofread the claim before mailing so no data are missing.

PROBLEM: Blocks 17 through 17a. Incorrect or missing name or UPIN/NPI of referring physician on claim for consultation or other services requiring this information.

SOLUTION: Check the patient registration form and the chart note for reference to the referring physician. Develop a list of UPIN/NPI numbers for all physicians in the area.

PROBLEM: Block 19. Attachments (e.g., prescription, operative report, manufacturer's invoice) or Medicaid verification (e.g., labels, identification numbers) is missing.

SOLUTION: Submit all information required for pricing or coverage on an 8.5- × 11-inch paper with the patient's name, subscriber name (if other than patient), and insurance identification number on each attachment (enclosure). Type the word "ATTACHMENT" in Block 19 or 10d. Never staple or clip documentation to a claim.

PROBLEM: Block 21. The diagnostic code is missing, incomplete, invalid, not in standard nomenclature (e.g., missing fourth or fifth digit), includes a written description, or does not correspond to the treatment (procedure code) rendered by the physician.

SOLUTION: Update encounter forms twice a year (October 1 and January 1). Verify and submit correct diagnostic codes by referring to an updated diagnostic code book and reviewing the patient record. Check with the physician if the diagnosis code listed does not go with the procedure code shown.

PROBLEM: Block 24A. Omitted, incorrect, overlapping, or duplicate dates of service.

SOLUTION: Verify against the encounter form or medical record that all dates of service are listed and accurate and appear on individual lines. Date spans for multiple services must be adequate for the number and types of services provided. Each month should be on a separate line and each year should be on a separate claim.

PROBLEM: Block 24B. Missing or incorrect place of service code.

SOLUTION: Verify the place of service from the encounter form or medical record and list the correct code for place of service and submitted procedure.

PROBLEM: Block 24C. Missing or incorrect type of service code for Medicaid, TRICARE, or workers' compensation claims.

SOLUTION: Verify and list the type of service code and confirm that it is correct for the submitted procedure code(s).

PROBLEM: Block 24D. Procedure codes are incorrect, invalid, or missing.

SOLUTION: Verify the coding system used by the insurance company and submit correct procedure code(s) by referring to a current procedure code book. For Medicare patients and certain private insurance plans, check the HCPCS manual for CMS national and local procedure codes.

PROBLEM: **Block 24D.** Incorrect or missing modifier(s).

SOLUTION: Verify usage of modifiers by referring to a current procedure code book and HCPCS manual. Submit valid modifiers with the correct procedure codes (Chapter 6).

PROBLEM: **Block 24F.** Omitted or incorrect amount billed.

SOLUTION: Be certain the fee column is filled in. Check the amounts charged with the appropriate fee schedule.

PROBLEM: **Block 24G.** Reasons for multiple visits made in 1 day are not stated on an attachment sheet.

SOLUTION: Depending on insurance guidelines, submit documentation explaining reason for multiple visits. Use appropriate modifiers or upcode evaluation and management services to include all visits.

PROBLEM: **Block 24G.** Incorrect quantity billed.

SOLUTION: Verify charge amounts. Make sure that the number of units listed is equal to the date span when more than one date of service is billed (e.g., hospital visits).

PROBLEM: **Blocks 24J through K.** Provider's identification number is missing.

SOLUTION: Verify and insert the required provider's number in these blocks.

PROBLEM: **Blocks 24A through K, Line 6.** More than six lines entered on one claim form.

SOLUTION: Insert service date and corresponding procedure on lines one to six only. Complete an additional claim form if more services should be billed.

PROBLEM: **Block 28.** Total amounts do not equal itemized charges.

SOLUTION: Total charges for each claim and verify amounts with patient account. If number of units listed in 24G is more than 1, multiply the units by the fee listed in 24F and add to all other charges listed.

PROBLEM: **Block 31.** Physician's signature is missing.

SOLUTION: Have the physician or physician's representative sign the claim using a removable indicator "Sign Here" tag to indicate the correct location or key in "SOF" or "signature on file."

PROBLEM: **Block 32.** Information is not centered in block as required.

SOLUTION: Enter data **centered** in block.

PROBLEM: **Block 33.** Provider's address, PIN, or group number is missing.

SOLUTION: Obtain provider's data from a list that contains all physicians' professional information.

Additional Reasons Why Claim Forms Are Delayed

PROBLEM: No record of the claim at the insurance company.

SOLUTION: Always keep copies of paper claims or electronic transmission receipts. Send claims with large dollar amounts by certified mail, return receipt requested. Another option is to request that the customer service representative search the insurance carrier's imaging file for the period beginning on the date of service forward until the date you are calling. Sometimes the claim was received and scanned but was never crossed over to the processing unit.

PROBLEM: Claim form submitted is illegible.

SOLUTION: Never hand write a claim form. Check printer ink, toner, or typewriter ribbon and replace when necessary.

PROBLEM: Untimely or lack of response to claim development letters.

SOLUTION: Pay close attention to the due date shown in the letter, and reply to development letters (insurance company's request for additional information) as soon as possible. Send a copy of the claim with the letter and appropriate medical documentation listing the claim control number, if assigned.

OPTICAL SCANNING FORMAT GUIDELINES

Optical Character Recognition

Optical character recognition (OCR), also less commonly referred to as **intelligent character recognition (ICR)** or *image copy recognition (ICR)*, devices (scanners) are being used across the nation in processing insurance claims because of their speed and efficiency. A scanner can transfer printed or typed text and bar codes to the insurance company's computer memory. Scanners read at such a fast speed that they reduce data entry cost and decrease processing time.

More control is gained over data input by using OCR. It improves accuracy, thus reducing coding errors because the claim is entered exactly as coded by the insurance biller.

Do's and Don'ts for Optical Character Recognition

The CMS-1500 form was developed so insurance carriers could process claims efficiently by OCR. Keying a form for OCR scanning requires different techniques than preparing one for standard claims submission. Because the majority of insurance carriers accept the OCR format, it is suggested that it be routinely used. Basic do's and don'ts for completing claims using OCR format follow:

DO: Use original claim forms printed in red ink; photocopies and forms generated from ink jet or laser printers cannot be scanned.

Don't: Hand write information on the document. Handwriting is only accepted for signatures. Handwritten claims require manual processing.

2 nd request

HEALTH INSURANCE CLAIM FORM PICA
FECA BLK LUNG (SSN) OTHER (ID) 1a. INSURED'S I.D. NUMBER (FOR PROGRAM IN ITEM 1)
111704521 A482

DO: Align the printer correctly so characters appear exactly in the proper fields. Enter all information within designated fields.

PICA
1. MEDICARE (Medicare #) MEDICAID (Medicaid #) CHAMPUS (Sponsor's SSN) CHAMPVA (VA File #) GROUP HEALTH PLAN [X] (SSN or ID) FECA BLK LUN (SSN)
2. PATIENT'S NAME (Last Name, First Name, Middle Initial) FOREHAND HARRY N
3. PATIENT'S BIRTH DATE MM 01 DD 06 YY 1946 M [X]
5. PATIENT'S ADDRESS 1456 MAIN STREET
6. PATIENT RELATIONSHIP TO INSURED Self [X] Spouse Child
CITY WOODLAND HILLS STATE XY
8. PATIENT STATUS Single Married [X]
ZIP CODE 12345 0000 TELEPHONE (Include Area Code) (555) 490 9876
Employed [X] Full-Time Student

Don't: Allow characters to touch lines.

Correct

HEALTH INSURANCE CLAIM FORM PICA
FECA BLK LUNG (SSN) OTHER (ID) 1a. INSURED'S I.D. NUMBER (FOR PROGRAM IN ITEM 1)
123456789

Incorrect

HEALTH INSURANCE CLAIM FORM PICA
FECA BLK LUNG (SSN) OTHER (ID) 1a. INSURED'S I.D. NUMBER (FOR PROGRAM IN ITEM 1)
123456789

Don't: Use script, slant, minifont, or italicized fonts or expanded, compressed, bold, or proportional print. Use fonts that have the same width for each character.

DO: Enter all information in upper case (CAPITAL) letters. Keep characters within the borders of each field.

Correct

2. PATIENT'S NAME (Last Name, First Name, Middle Initial)
DOE JANE E

Incorrect

2. PATIENT'S NAME (Last Name, First Name, Middle Initial)
Doe, Jane E.

Don't: Strike over any errors when correcting or crowd preprinted numbers; OCR equipment does not read corrected characters on top of correction tape or correction fluid.

Correct

3. PATIENT'S BIRTH DATE
MM 01 DD 06 YY 1946 M [X] SEX F

Incorrect

3. PATIENT'S BIRTH DATE
MM 01 DD 06 YY 1946 M [X] SEX F

DO: Indicate a deletion for a delete field and go to the next line to insert the data if an optically scanned form has a delete field. Lines, marks, or characters entered in a delete field cause deletion of the entire line.

DO: Complete a new form for additional services if the case has more than six lines of service.

Correct

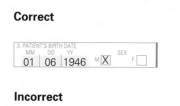

Don't: Use highlighter pens or colored ink on claims because OCR equipment will not recognize these.

DO: Use alpha or numeric symbols.

Don't: Use symbols (#, -, /), periods (.), ditto marks ("), parentheses, or commas (,).

Correct

25. FEDERAL TAX I.D. NUMBER	SSN EIN
123 XX 6789	☒ ☐

Incorrect

25. FEDERAL TAX I.D. NUMBER	SSN EIN
123-XX-6789	☐ ☐

Don't: Use decimals in Block 21 or dollar signs ($) in the money column.

Correct

F
$ CHARGES
10000

Incorrect

F
$ CHARGES
$10000

Don't: Use narrative descriptions of procedures, modifiers, or diagnoses; code numbers are sufficient.

Correct

D
PROCEDURES, SERVICES, OR SUPPLIES
(Explain Unusual Circumstances)
CPT/HCPCS ¦ MODIFIER
42820 ¦

Incorrect

D
PROCEDURES, SERVICES, OR SUPPLIES
(Explain Unusual Circumstances)
CPT/HCPCS ¦ MODIFIER
42820 ¦ tonsill-ectomy

Don't: Use N/A or DNA when information is not applicable. Leave the space blank.

Correct

17. NAME OF REFERRING PHYSICIAN OR OTHER SOURCE

Incorrect

17. NAME OF REFERRING PHYSICIAN OR OTHER SOURCE
DNA

DO: Enter comments in Block 19 (e.g., ATTACH-MENT) for primary EOB submitted with claim to secondary insurance company.

Correct

19. RESERVED FOR LOCAL USE
ATTACHMENT

Incorrect

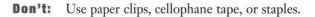

PRIMARY EOB ATTACHED

1. MEDICARE	MEDICAID	CHAMPUS	CHAMPVA
☐ (Medicare #)	☐ (Medicaid #)	☐ (Sponsor's SSN)	☐ (VA File #)

2. PATIENT'S NAME (Last Name, First Name, Middle Initial)
FOREHAND HARRY N

5. PATIENT'S ADDRESS
1456 MAIN STREET

CITY	STATE
WOODLAND HILLS	XY

ZIP CODE	TELEPHONE (Include Area Code)
12345 0000	(555) 555 9876

Don't: Use paper clips, cellophane tape, or staples.

Don't: Staple over the bar code area of the claim form.

DO: Enter eight-digit date formats: 060120XX or 06 01 20XX, depending on the block instructions.

Correct

24.	A				
	DATE(S) OF SERVICE				
	From		To		
	MM	DD	YY	MM	DD	YY
1	03	03	20XX			
2						

Incorrect

24.	A				
	DATE(S) OF SERVICE				
	From		To		
	MM	DD	YY	MM	DD	YY
1	03	03	XX			
2						

DO: Keep signature within signature block. Rubber stamps may be used if they are accepted by insurance carrier and produce complete, clean images, without smudges or missing letters.

Correct

31. SIGNATURE OF PHYSICIAN OR SUPPLIER
INCLUDING DEGREES OR CREDENTIALS
(I certify that the statements on the reverse
apply to this bill and are made a part thereof.)
CONCHA ANTRUM MD
030320XX
SIGNED *Concha Antrum MD* DATE

reference initials

Incorrect

31. SIGNATURE OF PHYSICIAN OR SUPPLIER
INCLUDING DEGREES OR CREDENTIALS
(I certify that the statements on the reverse
apply to this bill and are made a part thereof.)
CONCHA ANTRUM MD
030320XX
SIGNED DATE

Concha Antrum MD
reference initials

Don't: Overtrim or undertrim forms when bursting (taking apart multipage computer printouts). Use care in separating forms and discard any forms with tears or holes.

Don't: Fold or spindle forms when mailing because they will not feed into OCR equipment properly if creased or torn.

DO: Enter information via computer keyboard. Use clean equipment and quality ink jet or laser printers, if possible, not dot matrix.

PROCEDURE

INSTRUCTIONS FOR THE HEALTH INSURANCE CLAIM FORM (CMS-1500)

The Health Insurance Claim Form is divided into two major sections: patient information and physician information. The Patient and Insured (Subscriber) Information section is the upper portion of the claim form and contains 13 blocks numbered 1 through 13 (11 data elements and two signature blocks). The Physician or Supplier Information section is the lower portion of the claim form and consists of 20 blocks numbered 14 through 33 (19 data elements and 1 signature block). Some of the blocks are subdivided, with the subdivisions labeled a, b, c, d, and so forth. There are a total of more than 100 places to enter specific information.

The instructions are straightforward and contain all pertinent information needed to complete a claim (see Figures 7–6 through 7–15). Much information on specific coverage guidelines, program policies, and practice specialties could not be included here.

A brief description of each block and of its applicability to the requirements of private insurance payers, Medicaid, Medicare, TRICARE, CHAMPVA, and workers' compensation is presented. Because guidelines vary at the state and local levels for completing the CMS-1500 claim form for the aforementioned insurance plans, consult your local intermediary or private carriers. For completing Medi-Cal claims in California, refer to Appendix B.

 When completing a claim form, type the insurance carrier's name and address in the top right corner of the CMS-1500 form.

 When generating paper claims via computer, the practice management system will insert the insurance carrier's name and address in the top right corner of the CMS-1500 claim form.

Block numbers match those on the Health Insurance Claim Form. Italicized sections refer students to guidelines in completing the *Workbook* assignments when there are optional ways of completing a block. Icon meanings are as follows:

 All Payers: All payer guidelines including all private insurance companies and all federal and state programs.

 All Private Payers: All private insurance companies.

 Medicaid: State Medicaid programs.

QUESTION: DO THE HIPAA TRANSACTIONS AND CODE SETS STANDARDS APPLY TO PAPER CLAIMS AND OTHER NON-ELECTRONIC TRANSACTIONS?

Answer: No. The HIPAA transactions and code sets standards only apply to electronic transactions conducted by covered entities. Other entities, such as employers or casualty insurance plans, may decide to use them voluntarily but are not required to do so.

For paper transactions, health plans are free to set their own data requirements. Other federal or state laws may require plans or providers to use specific code sets for certain paper transactions. All covered health plans and providers must, however, be able to use the HIPAA standards for electronic transactions. Health plans may choose to require that paper claims include the same data elements, codes, and identifiers that are required by the HIPAA regulations for electronic transactions.

Medicare: Federal Medicare programs, Medicare/Medicaid, Medicare/Medigap, and Medicare Secondary Payer (MSP).

 CHAMPVA: Civilian Health and Medical Program of the Department of Veterans' Affairs.

 TRICARE: TRICARE Standard (formerly CHAMPUS), TRICARE Prime, TRICARE Extra.

 Worker's Compensation: State workers' compensation programs.

Top of Form

Enter name and address of insurance company in the top right corner of the insurance form using all capital letters and no punctuation.

NOTE: This format is being used to demonstrate that the student knows where to direct the claim even though some carriers (e.g., Medicare) do not follow this guideline.

PLEASE
DO NOT
STAPLE
IN THIS
AREA

PRUDENTIAL INSURANCE COMPANY
5450 WILSHIRE BOULEVARD
WOODLAND HILLS XY 12345 0000

HEALTH INSURANCE CLAIM FORM

	PICA								PICA	
1. MEDICARE	MEDICAID	CHAMPUS	CHAMPVA	GROUP HEALTH PLAN	FECA BLK LUNG	OTHER	1a. INSURED'S I.D. NUMBER		(FOR PROGRAM IN ITEM 1)	
(Medicare #)	(Medicaid #)	(Sponsor's SSN)	(VA File #)	X (SSN or ID)	(SSN)	(ID)	111704521		A482	
2. PATIENT'S NAME (Last Name, First Name, Middle Initial)			3. PATIENT'S BIRTH DATE MM DD YY		SEX		4. INSURED'S NAME (Last Name, First Name, Middle Initial)			
FOREHAND HARRY N			01 06 1946	M X	F		SAME			

Block 1

PLEASE
DO NOT
STAPLE
IN THIS
AREA

PRUDENTIAL INSURANCE COMPANY
5450 WILSHIRE BOULEVARD
WOODLAND HILLS XY 12345 0000

HEALTH INSURANCE CLAIM FORM

	PICA								PICA	
1. MEDICARE	MEDICAID	CHAMPUS	CHAMPVA	GROUP HEALTH PLAN	FECA BLK LUNG	OTHER	1a. INSURED'S I.D. NUMBER		(FOR PROGRAM IN ITEM 1)	
(Medicare #)	(Medicaid #)	(Sponsor's SSN)	(VA File #)	X (SSN or ID)	(SSN)	(ID)	111704521		A482	
2. PATIENT'S NAME (Last Name, First Name, Middle Initial)			3. PATIENT'S BIRTH DATE MM DD YY		SEX		4. INSURED'S NAME (Last Name, First Name, Middle Initial)			
FOREHAND HARRY N			01 06 1946	M X	F		SAME			

 All Private Payers: Check the name of the insurance plan or type of insurance for where you are sending the form to and do not check the secondary coverage.

Individual Health Plan: Check "Other" for an individual who is covered under an individual policy.

Group Health Plan: Check this box for those covered under any group contract insurance (e.g., insurance obtained through employment); also for patients who receive services paid by managed care programs (e.g., HMOs, PPOs, IPAs). Some Blue Plans prefer that "other" be checked even if the patient has a group plan. If in doubt, check with the insurance carrier for their preference.

➡ *When completing the **Workbook** assignments, if the insured is employed, assume the insurance is through the employer and is "group" insurance; otherwise assume it is an individual policy and enter "other."*

 Medicaid: Check for person receiving Medicaid benefits.

Medicare: Check for patient who receives Medicare benefits.

Medicare/Medicaid: Check "Medicare" and "Medicaid" if the patient is covered under Medicare and Medicaid programs. Some reference manuals state that when there is secondary insurance, check the insurance plan on the claim form for the one you are sending that form to and insert the secondary insurance information in the correct location on the form.

Medicare/Medigap: Check "Medicare" and, if the patient has group or individual or Medigap coverage, check "Group" or "Other," depending on health plan. Some reference manuals state that when there is secondary insurance, check the insurance plan on the claim form for the one you are sending that form to and insert the secondary insurance information in the correct location on the form.

➡ *When completing the **Workbook** assignments, if the insured is employed, assume the insurance is through the employer and is "group" insurance; otherwise assume it is an individual policy and enter "other."*

MSP: Check "Group" or "Other" (depending on health plan) and "Medicare" when a Medicare patient has insurance primary to Medicare coverage. Some reference manuals state that when there is secondary insurance, check the insurance plan on the claim form for the one you are sending that form to and insert the secondary insurance information in the correct location on the form.

TRICARE: Check "CHAMPUS" for individual receiving TRICARE benefits.

CHAMPVA: Check "CHAMPVA" for individual receiving CHAMPVA benefits.

Workers' Compensation: Check "Other" for all workers' compensation claims except FECA Black Lung. Check "FECA Black Lung" for patients who receive black lung benefits under the Federal Employee Compensation Act.

Block 1a

PLEASE
DO NOT
STAPLE
IN THIS
AREA

PRUDENTIAL INSURANCE COMPANY
5450 WILSHIRE BOULEVARD
WOODLAND HILLS XY 12345 0000

	PICA			HEALTH INSURANCE CLAIM FORM			PICA	

1. MEDICARE	MEDICAID	CHAMPUS	CHAMPVA	GROUP HEALTH PLAN	FECA BLK LUNG	OTHER	1a. INSURED'S I.D. NUMBER	(FOR PROGRAM IN ITEM 1)
(Medicare #)	(Medicaid #)	(Sponsor's SSN)	(VA File #)	X (SSN or ID)	(SSN)	(ID)	111704521	A482

2. PATIENT'S NAME (Last Name, First Name, Middle Initial)	3. PATIENT'S BIRTH DATE MM DD YY	SEX	4. INSURED'S NAME (Last Name, First Name, Middle Initial)
FOREHAND HARRY N	01 06 1946	M X F ☐	SAME

All Private Payers: Enter the patient's policy (identification or certificate) number in the left portion of the block and the group number, if applicable, in the right portion of the block as it appears on the insurance card, without punctuation.

Medicaid: Enter the Medicaid number in the left portion of the block. Do not enter dashes or other special characters in this block.

Medicare: Enter the patient's Medicare Health Insurance Claim (HIC) number from the patient's Medicare card in the left portion of this block, regardless of whether Medicare is the primary or secondary payer.
Medicare/Medicaid: Enter the patient's Medicare number in the left portion of this block.
Medicare/Medigap: Enter the patient's Medicare number in the left portion of this block.
MSP: Enter the patient's Medicare number in the left portion of this block. Refer to Block 11 for primary insurance.

 TRICARE: First enter sponsor's Social Security number (SSN) in the left portion of this block. Then, if the patient is a NATO beneficiary, add "NATO" or, if sponsor is a security agent, add "SECURITY." Do not provide the patient's SSN unless the patient and sponsor are the same.

 CHAMPVA: Enter the Veterans Affairs file number (omit prefix or suffix) or sponsor's Social Security number in the left portion of this block. Do not use any other former service numbers.

 Workers' Compensation: Enter the claim number. If none is assigned, enter the employer's policy number or patient's Social Security number.

Block 2

PLEASE
DO NOT
STAPLE
IN THIS
AREA

PRUDENTIAL INSURANCE COMPANY
5450 WILSHIRE BOULEVARD
WOODLAND HILLS XY 12345 0000

	PICA			HEALTH INSURANCE CLAIM FORM			PICA	

1. MEDICARE	MEDICAID	CHAMPUS	CHAMPVA	GROUP HEALTH PLAN	FECA BLK LUNG	OTHER	1a. INSURED'S I.D. NUMBER	(FOR PROGRAM IN ITEM 1)
(Medicare #)	(Medicaid #)	(Sponsor's SSN)	(VA File #)	X (SSN or ID)	(SSN)	(ID)	111704521	A482

2. PATIENT'S NAME (Last Name, First Name, Middle Initial)	3. PATIENT'S BIRTH DATE MM DD YY	SEX	4. INSURED'S NAME (Last Name, First Name, Middle Initial)
FOREHAND HARRY N	01 06 1946	M [X] F [ ]	SAME

 All Players: Enter the last name, first name, and middle initial of the patient—in that order—as shown on the patient's identification card, even if it is misspelled. Do not use nicknames or abbreviations. Do not use commas. A hyphen may be used if a name is hyphenated (Example 7.3).

Example 7.3 Surname Format

Hyphenated name: Smith-White = SMITH-WHITE
Prefixed name: MacIverson = MACIVERSON
Seniority Name with Numeric Suffix: John R. Ellis, III = ELLIS III JOHN R

Block 3

PLEASE
DO NOT
STAPLE
IN THIS
AREA

PRUDENTIAL INSURANCE COMPANY
5450 WILSHIRE BOULEVARD
WOODLAND HILLS XY 12345 0000

HEALTH INSURANCE CLAIM FORM

PICA

PICA									

1. MEDICARE MEDICAID CHAMPUS CHAMPVA GROUP HEALTH PLAN FECA BLK LUNG OTHER | 1a. INSURED'S I.D. NUMBER (FOR PROGRAM IN ITEM 1)

(Medicare #) (Medicaid #) (Sponsor's SSN) (VA File #) [X] (SSN or ID) (SSN) (ID) **111704521** **A482**

2. PATIENT'S NAME (Last Name, First Name, Middle Initial)   3. PATIENT'S BIRTH DATE   4. INSURED'S NAME (Last Name, First Name, Middle Initial)

FOREHAND HARRY N   MM 01 DD 06 YY 1946 SEX M [X] F [ ]   SAME

All Payers: Enter the patient's birth date using eight digits (01272000). The patient's age must be as follows to correlate with the diagnosis in Block 21:
- *Birth: Newborn diagnosis*
- *Birth to 17 years: Pediatric diagnosis*
- *12 to 55 years: Maternity diagnosis*
- 15 to 124 years: Adult diagnosis

Check the appropriate box for the patient's sex. If left blank, gender block defaults to "female."

Block 4

PLEASE
DO NOT
STAPLE
IN THIS
AREA

PRUDENTIAL INSURANCE COMPANY
5450 WILSHIRE BOULEVARD
WOODLAND HILLS XY 12345 0000

HEALTH INSURANCE CLAIM FORM

PICA

PICA									

1. MEDICARE MEDICAID CHAMPUS CHAMPVA GROUP HEALTH PLAN FECA BLK LUNG OTHER | 1a. INSURED'S I.D. NUMBER (FOR PROGRAM IN ITEM 1)

(Medicare #) (Medicaid #) (Sponsor's SSN) (VA File #) [X] (SSN or ID) (SSN) (ID) **111704521** **A482**

2. PATIENT'S NAME (Last Name, First Name, Middle Initial)   3. PATIENT'S BIRTH DATE   4. INSURED'S NAME (Last Name, First Name, Middle Initial)

FOREHAND HARRY N   MM 01 DD 06 YY 1946 SEX M [X] F [ ]   SAME

All Private Payers: Enter "SAME" when the insured is also the patient. If the insured is not the patient, enter the name of the insured (last name first).

Medicaid: Refer to Medicare guidelines.

Medicare: Leave blank if the insured is also the patient. Enter the insured's name, if different from the patient's.

Medicare/Medicaid: Refer to Medicare guidelines.

Medicare/Medigap: Refer to Medicare guidelines.

MSP: Enter the name of the insured (last name first) which is the subscriber to the primary insurance coverage.

TRICARE: Enter the sponsor's last name, first name, and middle initial, not a nickname or abbreviation. Enter "SAME" if the sponsor and patient are the same.

 CHAMPVA: Enter the veteran's name, last name first.

 Workers' Compensation: Enter the employer's name. If the employer is a large corporation, enter the name of the insured corporation in Block 4 and the local employer in Block 11b (e.g., Elsevier is the insured corporation [4] and Saunders is the employer and would be listed in Block 11b).

Block 5

5. PATIENT'S ADDRESS 1456 MAIN STREET		6. PATIENT RELATIONSHIP TO INSURED Self [X] Spouse [ ] Child [ ] Other [ ]	7. INSURED'S ADDRESS (No., Street)	
CITY WOODLAND HILLS	STATE XY	8. PATIENT STATUS Single [ ] Married [X] Other [ ]	CITY	STATE
ZIP CODE 12345 0000	TELEPHONE (Include Area Code) (555) 490 9876	Employed [X] Full-Time Student [ ] Part-Time Student [ ]	ZIP CODE	TELEPHONE (Include Area Code) ( )

 All Private Payers: Enter the patient's mailing address and residential telephone number.

 Medicaid: Enter the patient's mailing address and residential telephone number.

 Medicare: Enter the patient's mailing address and residential telephone number. On the first line, enter the street address; on the second line, the city and two-character state code (e.g., AZ = Arizona); on the third line, the ZIP code and residential telephone number. Punctuation is not necessary (e.g., ST LOUIS, no period after ST).
Medicare/Medicaid: Enter the patient's mailing address and residential telephone number.
Medicare/Medigap: Enter the patient's mailing address and residential telephone number.
MSP: Enter the patient's mailing address and residential telephone number.

 TRICARE: Enter the patient's mailing address and residential telephone number. Do not enter a post office box number; provide the actual place of residence. If a rural address, the address must contain the route and box number. An APO/FPO address should not be used unless that person is residing overseas.

 CHAMPVA: Enter the patient's mailing address and residential telephone number. Do not enter a post office box number; provide the actual place of residence. If a rural address, the address must contain the route and box number. An APO/FPO address should not be used unless that person is residing overseas.

Workers' Compensation: Enter the patient's mailing address and residential telephone number.

Block 6

5. PATIENT'S ADDRESS 1456 MAIN STREET		6. PATIENT RELATIONSHIP TO INSURED Self ☒ Spouse ☐ Child ☐ Other ☐	7. INSURED'S ADDRESS (No., Street)	
CITY WOODLAND HILLS	STATE XY	8. PATIENT STATUS Single ☐ Married ☒ Other ☐	CITY	STATE
ZIP CODE 12345 0000	TELEPHONE (Include Area Code) (555) 490 9876	Employed ☒ Full-Time Student ☐ Part-Time Student ☐	ZIP CODE	TELEPHONE (Include Area Code) ( )

All Private Payers: Check the patient's relationship to the insured. If the patient is an unmarried "domestic partner," check "Other."

Medicaid: Leave blank. Check appropriate box only if there is third party coverage.

Medicare: Indicate relationship to insured when Block 4 is completed; otherwise, leave blank.
Medicare/Medicaid: Refer to Medicare guidelines.
Medicare/Medigap: Refer to Medicare guidelines.
MSP: Indicate patient's relationship to insured.

TRICARE: Check the patient's relationship to the sponsor. If patient is the sponsor, check "self" (e.g., retiree). If the patient is a child or stepchild, check the box for child. If "other" is checked, indicate how the patient is related to the sponsor in Block 19 or on an attachment (e.g., former spouse).

CHAMPVA: Indicate the patient's relationship to the sponsor. If the patient is the sponsor, check "self." If the patient is a child or stepchild, check the box for child. If "other" is checked, indicate how the patient is related to the sponsor (e.g., former spouse) in Block 19 or on an attachment.

Workers' Compensation: Check "Other."

Block 7

5. PATIENT'S ADDRESS 1456 MAIN STREET		6. PATIENT RELATIONSHIP TO INSURED Self ☒ Spouse ☐ Child ☐ Other ☐	7. INSURED'S ADDRESS (No., Street)	
CITY WOODLAND HILLS	STATE XY	8. PATIENT STATUS Single ☐ Married ☒ Other ☐	CITY	STATE
ZIP CODE 12345 0000	TELEPHONE (Include Area Code) (555) 490 9876	Employed ☒ Full-Time Student ☐ Part-Time Student ☐	ZIP CODE	TELEPHONE (Include Area Code) ( )

All Private Payers: Leave blank if Block 4 indicates "same." Enter "SAME" if Block 4 is completed and the address is identical to that listed in Block 5. Enter address if different from that listed in Block 5.

Medicaid: Refer to Medicare guidelines.

Medicare: Leave blank if Block 4 is blank. Enter "SAME" if Block 4 is completed and the address is identical to that listed in Block 5. Enter address if different from that listed in Block 5.
Medicare/Medicaid: Refer to Medicare guidelines.
Medicare/Medigap: Refer to Medicare guidelines.
MSP: Complete only when Block 4 is completed. If insured is other than the patient, list insured's address and if the address is the same as in Block 5, enter "SAME."

TRICARE: Enter "SAME" if address is the same as that of the patient listed in Block 5. Enter the sponsor's address (e.g., an APO/FPO address or active duty sponsor's duty station or the retiree's mailing address) if different from the patient's address.

CHAMPVA: Enter "SAME" if address is the same as that of the patient. Enter the sponsor's address if different from the patient's address.

Workers' Compensation: Enter the employer's address.

Block 8

5. PATIENT'S ADDRESS (No., Street)		6. PATIENT RELATIONSHIP TO INSURED	7. INSURED'S ADDRESS (No., Street)	
1456 MAIN STREET		Self [X] Spouse [ ] Child [ ] Other [ ]		
CITY	STATE	8. PATIENT STATUS	CITY	STATE
WOODLAND HILLS	XY	Single [ ] Married [X] Other [ ]		
ZIP CODE TELEPHONE (Include Area Code)		Employed [X] Full-Time Student [ ] Part-Time Student [ ]	ZIP CODE TELEPHONE (Include Area Code)	
12345 0000 (555) 490 9876			( )	

All Private Payers: Check the appropriate box for the patient's marital status and whether employed or a student. The "other" box should be checked when a patient is covered under his or her children's health insurance plan or for a domestic partner. For individuals between the ages of 19 and 23, some insurance carriers require documentation from the school verifying full-time student status. This may be obtained as a signed letter from the school or by using a special form supplied by the insurance company.

Medicaid: Leave blank.

Medicare: Check the appropriate box or boxes for the patient's marital status and whether employed or a student (e.g., a beneficiary may be employed, a student, and married). Check "single" if widowed or divorced. In some locales, this block is not required by Medicare.

Medicare/Medicaid: Check appropriate box for the patient's marital status and whether employed or a student. Check "single" if widowed or divorced.

Medicare/Medigap: Check appropriate box for the patient's marital status and whether employed or a student. Check "single" if widowed or divorced.

MSP: Check appropriate box for the patient's marital status and whether employed or a student. Check "single" if widowed or divorced.

TRICARE: Check the appropriate box for the patient's marital status and whether employed or a student.

CHAMPVA: Check the appropriate box for the patient's marital status and whether employed or a student.

Workers' Compensation: Check "Employed." Some workers' compensation carriers may have requirements for marital status; otherwise, leave blank.
*When completing the **Workbook** assignments, leave marital status blank.*

Block 9

9. OTHER INSURED'S NAME (Last Name, First Name, Middle Initial)	10. IS PATIENT'S CONDITION RELATED TO:	11. INSURED'S POLICY GROUP OR FECA NUMBER
a. OTHER INSURED'S POLICY OR GROUP NUMBER	a. EMPLOYMENT? (CURRENT OR PREVIOUS) ☐ YES ☒ NO	a. INSURED'S DATE OF BIRTH MM DD YY M ☐ SEX F ☐
b. OTHER INSURED'S DATE OF BIRTH MM DD YY M ☐ SEX F ☐	b. AUTO ACCIDENT? PLACE (State) ☐ YES ☒ NO	b. EMPLOYER'S NAME OR SCHOOL NAME
c. EMPLOYER'S NAME OR SCHOOL NAME	c. OTHER ACCIDENT? ☐ YES ☒ NO	c. INSURANCE PLAN NAME OR PROGRAM NAME
d. INSURANCE PLAN NAME OR PROGRAM NAME	10d. RESERVED FOR LOCAL USE	d. IS THERE ANOTHER HEALTH BENEFIT PLAN? ☐ YES ☒ NO *If yes*, return to and complete item 9 a-d.

All Private Payers: For submission to primary insurance, leave blank. If patient has secondary insurance, enter patient's full name in last name, first name, and middle initial order.

Medicaid: For primary insurance, leave blank. For secondary insurance, enter patient's full name in last name, first name, and middle initial order.

Medicare: For primary insurance, leave blank. Do not list Medicare supplemental coverage (private, not Medigap) on the primary Medicare claim. Beneficiaries are responsible for filing a supplemental claim if the private insurer does not contract with Medicare to send claim information electronically.
Medicare/Medicaid: Enter Medicaid patient's full name in last name, first name, and middle initial order.
Medicare/Medigap: Enter the last name, first name, and middle initial of the Medigap enrollee if it differs from that in Block 2; otherwise enter "SAME." Only Medicare participating physicians and suppliers should complete Block 9 and its subdivisions, and only when the beneficiary wishes to assign his or her benefits under a Medigap policy to the participating physician or supplier. If no Medigap benefits are assigned, leave blank.
MSP: Leave blank.

 TRICARE: For primary insurance, leave blank. For secondary insurance held by someone other than the patient, enter the name of the insured. Blocks 11a through d should be used to report *other health insurance held by the patient.*

 CHAMPVA: For primary insurance, leave blank. For secondary insurance held by someone other than the patient, enter the name of the insured. Blocks 11a through d should be used to report *other health insurance held by the patient.*

 Workers' Compensation: Leave blank. If case is pending and not yet declared workers' compensation, insert other insurance.

Block 9a

 All Private Payers: Enter the policy and/or group number of the other (secondary) insured's insurance coverage.

 Medicaid: Leave blank.

 Medicare: Refer to appropriate secondary coverage guidelines.
Medicare/Medicaid: Enter Medicaid number here or in Block 10d. However, some states may have different guidelines, so check with your local fiscal intermediary if in doubt.
➡ *When completing the **Workbook** assignments, enter the Medicaid policy number in Block 10d.*
Medicare/Medigap: Enter the policy or group number of the Medigap enrollee preceded by the word "MEDIGAP," "MG," or "MGAP." In addition to Medicare/Medigap, if a patient has a third insurance (e.g., employer-supplemental), all information for the third insurance should be submitted on an attachment.
➡ *When completing the **Workbook** assignments, enter the word "MEDIGAP."*
MSP: Leave blank.

TRICARE: Enter the policy or group number of the other (secondary) insured's insurance policy.

 CHAMPVA: Enter the policy or group number of the other (secondary) insured's insurance policy.

 Workers' Compensation: Leave blank.

Block 9b

 All Private Payers: Enter the other insured's date of birth and gender.

 Medicaid: Leave blank.

 Medicare: Refer to appropriate secondary coverage guidelines.
Medicare/Medicaid: Enter the Medicaid enrollee's birth date, using eight digits (e.g., 030620XX), and gender. If same as patient's, leave blank.
Medicare/Medigap: Enter the Medigap enrollee's birth date, using eight digits (e.g., 030620XX), and gender. If same as patient's, leave blank.
MSP: Leave blank.

 TRICARE: For secondary coverage held by someone other than the patient, enter the other insured's date of birth and check the appropriate box for gender.

 CHAMPVA: For secondary coverage held by someone other than the patient, enter the other insured's date of birth and check the appropriate box for gender.

 Workers' Compensation: Leave blank.

Block 9c

 All Private Payers: For secondary coverage, enter employer's name, if applicable.

 Medicaid: Leave blank.

 Medicare: Refer to appropriate secondary coverage guidelines.
Medicare/Medicaid: Leave blank.
Medicare/Medigap: Enter the Medigap insurer's claims processing address. Ignore "employer's name or school name." Abbreviate the street address to fit in this block by deleting the city and using the two-letter state postal code and ZIP code. For example, 1234 Wren Drive, Any City, Pennsylvania 19106 would be typed "1234 WREN DR PA 19106." *Note: If a carrier-assigned unique identifier (sometimes called "Other Carrier Name and Address," or OCNA) for a Medigap insurer appears in Block 9d, then Block 9c may be left blank.*
MSP: Leave blank.

 TRICARE: For secondary coverage held by someone other than the patient, enter the name of the other insured's employer or name of school.

 CHAMPVA: For secondary coverage held by someone other than the patient, enter the name of the other insured's employer or name of school.

 Workers' Compensation: Leave blank.

Block 9d

 All Private Payers: Enter name of secondary insurance plan or program.

Medicaid: Leave blank.

Medicare: Refer to appropriate secondary coverage guidelines.

Medicare/Medicaid: Leave blank.

Medicare/Medigap: Enter the Medigap insurer's nine-digit alphanumeric PAYERID number if known (often called the OCNA key), and Block 9c may be left blank. If not known, enter the name of the Medigap enrollee's insurance company. If you are a participating provider, all of the information in Blocks 9 through 9d must be complete and correct or the Medicare carrier cannot electronically forward the claim information to the Medigap insurer. For multiple insurance information, enter "ATTACHMENT" in Block 10d and provide information on an attached sheet.

MSP: Leave blank.

TRICARE: For secondary coverage held by someone other than the patient, insert name of insured's other health insurance program. On an attached sheet, provide a complete mailing address for all other insurance information and enter the word "ATTACHMENT" in Block 10d. If the patient is covered by a health maintenance organization (HMO), attach a copy of the brochure showing that the service is not covered by the HMO.

CHAMPVA: For secondary coverage held by someone other than the patient, insert name of insured's other health insurance program. On an attached sheet, provide a complete mailing address for all other insurance information and enter the word "ATTACHMENT" in Block 10d. If the patient is covered by an HMO, attach a copy of the brochure showing that the service is not covered by the HMO.

Workers' Compensation: Leave blank.

Block 10a

9. OTHER INSURED'S NAME (Last Name, First Name, Middle Initial)	10. IS PATIENT'S CONDITION RELATED TO:	11. INSURED'S POLICY GROUP OR FECA NUMBER
a. OTHER INSURED'S POLICY OR GROUP NUMBER	a. EMPLOYMENT? (CURRENT OR PREVIOUS) ☐ YES ☒ NO	a. INSURED'S DATE OF BIRTH MM DD YY SEX M ☐ F ☐
b. OTHER INSURED'S DATE OF BIRTH MM DD YY SEX M ☐ F ☐	b. AUTO ACCIDENT? PLACE (State) ☐ YES ☒ NO	b. EMPLOYER'S NAME OR SCHOOL NAME
c. EMPLOYER'S NAME OR SCHOOL NAME	c. OTHER ACCIDENT? ☐ YES ☒ NO	c. INSURANCE PLAN NAME OR PROGRAM NAME
d. INSURANCE PLAN NAME OR PROGRAM NAME	10d. RESERVED FOR LOCAL USE	d. IS THERE ANOTHER HEALTH BENEFIT PLAN? ☐ YES ☒ NO *If yes*, return to and complete item 9 a-d.

All Payers: Check "yes" or "no" to indicate whether patient's diagnosis described in Block 21 is the result of an accident or injury that occurred on the job or an industrial illness.

Block 10b

All Private Payers: A "yes" checked in Block 10b indicates a third party liability case; file the claim with the other liability insurance or automobile insurance company. List the abbreviation of the state in which the accident took place (e.g., CA for California).

Medicaid: Check appropriate box.

Medicare: Check "no." If "yes," bill the liability insurance as primary insurance and Medicare as secondary insurance.
Medicare/Medicaid: Refer to Medicare guidelines.
Medicare/Medigap: Refer to Medicare guidelines.
MSP: Refer to Medicare guidelines.

TRICARE: Check "yes" or "no" to indicate whether automobile liability applies to one or more of the services described in Block 24. If "yes," provide information concerning potential third-party liability. If a third party is involved in the accident, the beneficiary must complete Form DD 2527 (Statement of Personal Injury—Possible Third-Party Liability) and attach it to the claim.

CHAMPVA: Check "yes" or "no" to indicate whether automobile liability applies to one or more of the services described in Block 24. If "yes," provide information concerning potential third party liability.

Workers' Compensation: Check "yes" to indicate an automobile accident that occurred while the patient was on the job.

Block 10c

All Private Payers: Check "yes" or "no" to indicate whether the patient's condition is related to an accident other than automobile or employment. Verify primary insurance.

Medicaid: Check if applicable.

Medicare: Check "yes" or "no" to indicate whether the patient's condition is related to an accident other than automobile or employment. Verify primary insurance.
Medicare/Medicaid: Refer to Medicare guidelines.
Medicare/Medigap: Refer to Medicare guidelines.
MSP: Refer to Medicare guidelines.

TRICARE: Check "yes" or "no" to indicate whether another accident (not work related or automobile) applies to one or more of the services described in Block 24. If so, provide information concerning potential third party liability. If third party is involved in the accident, the beneficiary must complete Form DD 2527 (Statement of Personal Injury—Possible Third-Party Liability) and attach it to the claim.

CHAMPVA: Refer to TRICARE guidelines.

Workers' Compensation: Check "no."

Block 10d

All Private Payers: Leave blank.

Medicaid: Generally, this block is used exclusively for Medicaid as a secondary payer. Enter the patient's Medicaid (MCD) number preceded by "MCD." Note, however, that this guideline is under discussion, so carriers may not yet notify providers of a usage change for this block. Some carriers state that if more than one type of other insurance applies to the claim, the identifiers for each type should be shown, for example:
Medicare/Medigap and Medicaid coverage = MG/MCD
Medicare/Medigap and Employer-Supp coverage = MG/SP
Medicaid and Employer-Supp coverage = MCD/SP
Primary (MSP) and Medicaid Secondary coverage = MSP/MCD
Two primary insurance plans = 2MSP
→ *When completing the **Workbook** assignments, enter the patient's Medicaid number preceded by "MCD."*

Medicare: Leave blank.
Medicare/Medicaid: Enter the patient's Medicaid (MCD) number preceded by "MCD."
Medicare/Medigap: Leave blank.
MSP: Leave blank.

TRICARE: Generally, leave blank unless regional fiscal intermediary gives special guidelines. However, if Block 11d is checked "yes," the mailing address of the insurance carrier must be attached to the claim form, and in this block enter "ATTACHMENT."
→ *When completing the **Workbook** assignments, leave blank.*

CHAMPVA: Generally, leave blank unless regional fiscal intermediary gives special guidelines. If Block 11d is checked "yes," the mailing address of the insurance carrier must be attached to the claim form, and in this block enter "ATTACHMENT."
→ *When completing the **Workbook** assignments, leave blank.*

Workers' Compensation: Leave blank.

Block 11

9. OTHER INSURED'S NAME (Last Name, First Name, Middle Initial)	10. IS PATIENT'S CONDITION RELATED TO:	11. INSURED'S POLICY GROUP OR FECA NUMBER
a. OTHER INSURED'S POLICY OR GROUP NUMBER	a. EMPLOYMENT? (CURRENT OR PREVIOUS) ☐ YES ☒ NO	a. INSURED'S DATE OF BIRTH MM DD YY SEX M ☐ F ☐
b. OTHER INSURED'S DATE OF BIRTH MM DD YY SEX M ☐ F ☐	b. AUTO ACCIDENT? PLACE (State) ☐ YES ☒ NO	b. EMPLOYER'S NAME OR SCHOOL NAME
c. EMPLOYER'S NAME OR SCHOOL NAME	c. OTHER ACCIDENT? ☐ YES ☒ NO	c. INSURANCE PLAN NAME OR PROGRAM NAME
d. INSURANCE PLAN NAME OR PROGRAM NAME	10d. RESERVED FOR LOCAL USE	d. IS THERE ANOTHER HEALTH BENEFIT PLAN? ☐ YES ☒ NO *If yes*, return to and complete item 9 a-d.

 All Private Payers: Leave Blocks 11 through 11c blank if no private secondary coverage. If (private) secondary insurance, see Blocks 9 through 9d.

 Medicaid: Generally, leave blank. Enter a rejection code if the patient has other third party insurance coverage and the claim was rejected.

 Medicare: If other insurance is not primary to Medicare, enter "NONE" and go to Block 12. Block 11 must be completed. By completing this block, the physician/supplier acknowledges having made a good faith effort to determine whether Medicare is the primary or secondary payer.
Medicare/Medicaid: Refer to Medicare guidelines.
Medicare/Medigap: Refer to Medicare guidelines.
MSP: When insurance is primary to Medicare, enter the insured's policy or group number, or both, and complete Blocks 11a through 11c.

 TRICARE: Leave blank.

 CHAMPVA: Enter the three-digit number of the VA station that issued the identification card.

 Workers' Compensation: Leave blank.

Block 11a

All Private Payers: Leave blank.

Medicaid: Leave blank.

Medicare: Leave blank.
Medicare/Medicaid: Leave blank.
Medicare/Medigap: Leave blank.
MSP: Enter the insured's eight-digit date of birth (061220XX) and gender if different from that listed in Block 3; otherwise, leave blank.

TRICARE: Enter sponsor's date of birth and gender, if different from that listed in Block 3; otherwise, leave blank.

CHAMPVA: Enter sponsor's date of birth and gender, if different from that listed in Block 3.

Workers' Compensation: Leave blank.

Block 11b

All Private Payers: When submitting to secondary insurance, enter the name of the employer, school, or organization if primary policy is a group plan; otherwise, leave blank.

Medicaid: Leave blank.

Medicare: Leave blank.
Medicare/Medicaid: Leave blank.
Medicare/Medigap: Leave blank.
MSP: Enter the employer's name of primary insurance. Also use this block to indicate a change in the insured's insurance status (e.g., "RETIRED" and the eight-digit retirement date). Submit paper claims with a copy of the primary payer's Remittance Advice (RA) document to be considered for Medicare Secondary Payer benefits. Instances when Medicare may be secondary include the following:
    1. Group health plan coverage
        a. Working aged
        b. Disability (large group health plan)
        c. End-stage renal disease
    2. No fault, other liability, or both
        a. Automobile
        b. Homeowner
        c. Commercial
    3. Work-related illness, injury, or both
        a. Workers' compensation
        b. Black lung
        c. Veterans' benefits

TRICARE: Indicate sponsor's branch of service, using abbreviations (e.g., United States Navy = USN).

CHAMPVA: Indicate sponsor's branch of service, using abbreviations (e.g., United States Army = USA).

Workers' Compensation: If a large corporation's name is listed in Block 4, enter the name of the patient's local employer; otherwise, leave this block blank.

Block 11c

All Private Payers: When submitting to secondary insurance, enter the name of the primary insurance plan; otherwise, leave this block blank.

Medicaid: Leave blank.

Medicare: Leave blank.
Medicare/Medicaid: Leave blank.
Medicare/Medigap: Leave blank.
MSP: Enter the complete name of the insurance plan or program that is primary to Medicare. Include the primary payer's claim processing address directly on the EOB.

TRICARE: Enter TRICARE.

CHAMPVA: Indicate name of the secondary coverage held by the patient, if applicable; otherwise, leave this block blank.

Workers' Compensation: Leave blank.

Block 11d

All Private Payers: Check "yes" or "no" to indicate if there is another health plan. If "yes," Blocks 9a through 9d must be completed.

Medicaid: Leave blank.

Medicare: Generally, leave blank; some regions require "yes" or "no" checked, so verify this requirement with your local fiscal intermediary.
*When completing the **Workbook** assignments, leave blank.*
Medicare/Medicaid: Refer to guidelines for Medicare.
Medicare/Medigap: Refer to guidelines for Medicare.
MSP: Leave blank.

TRICARE: Check "yes" or "no" to indicate if there is another health plan. If "yes," Blocks 9a through 9d must be completed.

CHAMPVA: Check "yes" or "no" to indicate if there is another health plan. If "yes," Blocks 9a through 9d must be completed.

Workers' Compensation: Leave blank.

Block 12

READ BACK OF FORM BEFORE COMPLETING & SIGNING THIS FORM.	13. INSURED'S OR AUTHORIZED PERSON'S SIGNATURE I authorize payment of medical benefits to the undersigned physician or supplier for services described below.
12. PATIENT'S OR AUTHORIZED PERSON'S SIGNATURE I authorize the release of any medical or other information necessary to process this claim. I also request payment of government benefits either to myself or to the party who accepts assignment below.	
SIGNED *Harry N. Forehand* DATE *March 3, 20XX*	SIGNED *Harry N. Forehand*

or

READ BACK OF FORM BEFORE COMPLETING & SIGNING THIS FORM.	13. INSURED'S OR AUTHORIZED PERSON'S SIGNATURE I authorize payment of medical benefits to the undersigned physician or supplier for services described below.
12. PATIENT'S OR AUTHORIZED PERSON'S SIGNATURE I authorize the release of any medical or other information necessary to process this claim. I also request payment of government benefits either to myself or to the party who accepts assignment below.	
SIGNED _____ SOF _____ DATE _____	SIGNED _____ SOF _____

All Private Payers: Medical office policy varies for obtaining the patient's signature for release of medical information, but know this is *not* a HIPAA compliance requirement. For offices that prefer the patient's signature in this block, a signature here authorizes the release of medical information for claims processing. Have the patient or authorized representative sign and date this block. If the patient has signed a consent form, "Signature on File" or "SOF" can be entered here. The consent form must be current, possibly may be lifetime, and must be in the medical practice's office files for the patient. Many offices routinely annually renew consent forms. When the patient's representative signs, that person's relationship to the patient must be indicated. If the signature is indicated by a mark (X), a witness must sign his or her name and enter the address next to the mark. If a patient is seen in the hospital and never comes to the doctor's office, the signature forms obtained by the hospital cover the physician.

→ *When completing the **Workbook** assignments, enter "SOF" in this block.*

Medicaid: Leave blank.

Medicare: A signature here authorizes payment of benefits to the physician (if the physician accepts assignment). Have the patient or authorized representative sign and date this block. If the patient has signed a consent form, "Signature on File" or "SOF" can be typed here. The form must be current, may be lifetime, and must be in the physician's file. When the patient's representative signs, that person's relationship to the patient *must* be indicated. If the signature is by mark (X), a witness must sign his or her name and enter the address next to the mark.

→ *When completing the **Workbook** assignments, enter "SOF" in this block.*

Medicare/Medicaid: Refer to Medicare guidelines.

Medicare/Medigap: Refer to Medicare guidelines.

MSP: Guidelines for this block are the same as for Medicare.

TRICARE: A signature here authorizes payment of benefits to the physician (if the physician accepts assignment). Have the patient or the authorized representative sign and date this block. If the patient has signed a consent form, "Signature on File" or "SOF" can be typed here. The form must be current, may be lifetime, and *must* be in the physician's file. When the patient's representative signs, that person's relationship to the patient must be indicated. If the signature is by mark (X), a witness must sign his or her name and enter the address next to the mark.

→ *When completing the **Workbook** assignments, enter "SOF" in this block.*

CHAMPVA: Refer to TRICARE guidelines.

Workers' Compensation: No signature is required.

Block 13

READ BACK OF FORM BEFORE COMPLETING & SIGNING THIS FORM.	13. INSURED'S OR AUTHORIZED PERSON'S SIGNATURE I authorize
12. PATIENT'S OR AUTHORIZED PERSON'S SIGNATURE I authorize the release of any medical or other information necessary to process this claim. I also request payment of government benefits either to myself or to the party who accepts assignment below.	payment of medical benefits to the undersigned physician or supplier for services described below.
SIGNED _Harry N. Forehand_ DATE _March 3, 20XX_	SIGNED _Harry N. Forehand_

or

READ BACK OF FORM BEFORE COMPLETING & SIGNING THIS FORM.	13. INSURED'S OR AUTHORIZED PERSON'S SIGNATURE I authorize
12. PATIENT'S OR AUTHORIZED PERSON'S SIGNATURE I authorize the release of any medical or other information necessary to process this claim. I also request payment of government benefits either to myself or to the party who accepts assignment below.	payment of medical benefits to the undersigned physician or supplier for services described below.
SIGNED _____ SOF _____ DATE _____	SIGNED _____ SOF _____

 All Private Payers: Patient's signature is necessary when benefits are assigned. "SOF" may be listed if the patient's signature is on file.
→ *When completing the **Workbook** assignments, enter "SOF" in this block.*

 Medicaid: Leave blank.

 Medicare: Leave blank.
Medicare/Medicaid: Leave blank.
Medicare/Medigap: For participating provider, a signature here authorizes payment of "mandated" Medigap benefits when required Medigap information is included in Blocks 9 through 9d. List the signature of the patient or authorized representative, or list "SOF" if the signature is on file as a separate Medigap authorization.
→ *When completing the **Workbook** assignments, enter "SOF" in this block.*
MSP: The signature of the patient or authorized representative should appear in this block, or list "SOF" if the signature is on file for benefits assigned from the primary carrier.
→ *When completing the **Workbook** assignments, enter "SOF" in this block.*

 TRICARE: Leave blank.

CHAMPVA: Leave blank.

Workers' Compensation: Leave blank. All payment goes directly to the physician.

Block 14

14. DATE OF CURRENT: ◀ ILLNESS (First symptom) OR INJURY (Accident) OR PREGNANCY (LMP)	15. IF PATIENT HAS HAD SAME OR SIMILAR ILLNESS. GIVE FIRST DATE MM DD YY	16. DATES PATIENT UNABLE TO WORK IN CURRENT OCCUPATION MM DD YY MM DD YY FROM TO
MM DD YY 03 01 20XX		
17. NAME OF REFERRING PHYSICIAN OR OTHER SOURCE PERRY CARDI MD	17a. I.D. NUMBER OF REFERRING PHYSICIAN 67805027XX	18. HOSPITALIZATION DATES RELATED TO CURRENT SERVICES MM DD YY MM DD YY FROM TO
19. RESERVED FOR LOCAL USE		20. OUTSIDE LAB? $ CHARGES ☐ YES ☒ NO

All Private Payers: Enter the eight-digit date the patient's first symptoms occurred from the current illness, if stated in the medical record; date of injury or accident; or for pregnancy, first day of last menstrual period. For chiropractic treatment, enter the eight-digit date that treatment began.

Medicaid: Leave blank.

Medicare: Enter the eight-digit date the patient's first symptoms occurred from the current illness, if stated in the medical record; date of injury or accident; or for pregnancy, first day of last menstrual period. For chiropractic treatment, enter the eight-digit date that treatment began.
Medicare/Medicaid: Refer to Medicare guidelines.
Medicare/Medigap: Refer to Medicare guidelines.
MSP: Refer to Medicare guidelines.

TRICARE: Enter the eight-digit date the patient's first symptoms occurred from the current illness, if stated in the medical record; date of injury or accident; or for pregnancy, first day of last menstrual period. For chiropractic treatment, enter the eight-digit date that treatment began.

CHAMPVA: Refer to TRICARE guidelines.

Workers' Compensation: Enter first date of injury, accident, or industrial illness; it should coincide with the date specified in the Doctor's First Report of Injury.

Block 15

14. DATE OF CURRENT: ◀ ILLNESS (First symptom) OR INJURY (Accident) OR PREGNANCY (LMP)	15. IF PATIENT HAS HAD SAME OR SIMILAR ILLNESS. GIVE FIRST DATE MM DD YY	16. DATES PATIENT UNABLE TO WORK IN CURRENT OCCUPATION MM DD YY MM DD YY FROM TO
MM DD YY 03 01 20XX		
17. NAME OF REFERRING PHYSICIAN OR OTHER SOURCE PERRY CARDI MD	17a. I.D. NUMBER OF REFERRING PHYSICIAN 67805027XX	18. HOSPITALIZATION DATES RELATED TO CURRENT SERVICES MM DD YY MM DD YY FROM TO
19. RESERVED FOR LOCAL USE		20. OUTSIDE LAB? $ CHARGES ☐ YES ☒ NO

All Private Payers: Enter date when patient had same or similar illness, if applicable, and documented in the medical record.

Medicaid: Leave blank.

Medicare: Leave blank.
Medicare/Medicaid: Leave blank.
Medicare/Medigap: Leave blank.
MSP: Leave blank.

TRICARE: Enter date when patient had same or similar illness, if applicable and documented in the medical record.

CHAMPVA: Refer to TRICARE guidelines.

Workers' Compensation: Enter date if appropriate and documented in the medical record.

Block 16

14. DATE OF CURRENT: ◀ ILLNESS (First symptom) OR INJURY (Accident) OR PREGNANCY (LMP)	15. IF PATIENT HAS HAD SAME OR SIMILAR ILLNESS. GIVE FIRST DATE MM DD YY	16. DATES PATIENT UNABLE TO WORK IN CURRENT OCCUPATION
MM DD YY 03 01 20XX		MM DD YY MM DD YY FROM TO
17. NAME OF REFERRING PHYSICIAN OR OTHER SOURCE PERRY CARDI MD	17a. I.D. NUMBER OF REFERRING PHYSICIAN 67805027XX	18. HOSPITALIZATION DATES RELATED TO CURRENT SERVICES MM DD YY MM DD YY FROM TO
19. RESERVED FOR LOCAL USE		20. OUTSIDE LAB? $ CHARGES ☐ YES ☒ NO

All Private Payers: Enter dates patient is employed but cannot work in current occupation. *From:* Enter first *full* day patient was unable to perform job duties. *To:* Enter last day patient was disabled before returning to work.

Medicaid: Leave blank.

Medicare: Enter eight-digit dates patient is employed but cannot work in current occupation. *From:* Enter first *full* day patient was unable to perform job duties. *To:* Enter last day patient was disabled before returning to work.
Medicare/Medicaid: Refer to Medicare guidelines.
Medicare/Medigap: Refer to Medicare guidelines.
MSP: Refer to Medicare guidelines.

TRICARE: Refer to Medicare guidelines.

CHAMPVA: Refer to Medicare guidelines.

Workers' Compensation: May be completed but is not mandatory and must be verified with documentation in Doctor's First Report of Injury. *From:* Enter first *full* day patient was unable to perform job duties. *To:* Enter last day patient was disabled before returning to work.
→ *When completing the **Workbook** assignments, enter information when documented in the medical record.*

Block 17

14. DATE OF CURRENT: ILLNESS (First symptom) OR INJURY (Accident) OR PREGNANCY (LMP)	15. IF PATIENT HAS HAD SAME OR SIMILAR ILLNESS. GIVE FIRST DATE	16. DATES PATIENT UNABLE TO WORK IN CURRENT OCCUPATION
MM DD YY 03 01 20XX	MM DD YY	MM DD YY FROM TO MM DD YY
17. NAME OF REFERRING PHYSICIAN OR OTHER SOURCE PERRY CARDI MD	17a. I.D. NUMBER OF REFERRING PHYSICIAN 67805027XX	18. HOSPITALIZATION DATES RELATED TO CURRENT SERVICES MM DD YY FROM TO MM DD YY
19. RESERVED FOR LOCAL USE		20. OUTSIDE LAB? [ ] YES [X] NO $ CHARGES

All Private Payers: Enter complete name and degree of referring physician, when applicable. Do not list other referrals (i.e., family or friends).

Medicaid: Enter complete name and degree of referring physician, when applicable. Do not list other referrals (i.e., family or friends).

Medicare: Enter the name and degree of the referring or ordering physician on all claims for Medicare-covered services and items resulting from a physician's order or referral. Use a separate claim form for each referring or ordering physician.
Surgeon: A surgeon must complete this block. When the patient has not been referred, enter the surgeon's name. On an assistant surgeon's claim, enter the primary surgeon's name.
Referring physician: A physician who requests a service for the beneficiary for which payment may be made under the Medicare program. When a physician extender (e.g., nurse practitioner) refers a patient for a consultative service, enter the name of the physician supervising the physician extender.
Ordering physician: A physician who orders a consultation or nonphysician services for the patient, such as diagnostic radiology, laboratory, or pathology tests; pharmaceutical services; durable medical equipment (DME); parenteral and enteral nutrition; or immunosuppressive drugs.
When the ordering physician is also the performing physician (e.g., the physician who actually performs the in-office laboratory tests), the performing physician's name and assigned UPIN/NPI number must appear in Blocks 17 and 17a.
When a patient is referred to a physician who also orders and performs a diagnostic service, a separate claim form is necessary for the diagnostic service.
Enter the original referring physician's name and NPI in Blocks 17 and 17a of the first claim form.
Enter the ordering (performing) physician's name and NPI in Blocks 17 and 17a of the second claim form.
Medicare/Medicare: Refer to Medicare guidelines.
Medicare/Medigap: Refer to Medicare guidelines.
MSP: Refer to Medicare guidelines.

TRICARE: Enter name, degree, and address of referring provider. This is required for all consultation claims. If the patient was referred from a Military Treatment Facility (MTF), enter the name of the MTF and attach DD Form 2161 or SF 513, "Referral for Civilian Medical Care."

CHAMPVA: Refer to TRICARE guidelines.

Workers' Compensation: Indicate name and degree of referring provider.

Block 17a

14. DATE OF CURRENT: ILLNESS (First symptom) OR INJURY (Accident) OR PREGNANCY (LMP) MM DD YY 03 01 20XX	15. IF PATIENT HAS HAD SAME OR SIMILAR ILLNESS. GIVE FIRST DATE MM DD YY	16. DATES PATIENT UNABLE TO WORK IN CURRENT OCCUPATION MM DD YY FROM TO MM DD YY
17. NAME OF REFERRING PHYSICIAN OR OTHER SOURCE PERRY CARDI MD	17a. I.D. NUMBER OF REFERRING PHYSICIAN 67805027XX	18. HOSPITALIZATION DATES RELATED TO CURRENT SERVICES MM DD YY FROM TO MM DD YY
19. RESERVED FOR LOCAL USE		20. OUTSIDE LAB? ☐ YES ☒ NO $ CHARGES

All Private Payers: Enter the referring physician's UPIN/NPI number.

Medicaid: Enter the referring physician's UPIN/NPI number.

Medicare: Enter the CMS-assigned UPIN/NPI of the referring or ordering physician (or the supervising physician for a physician extender) as detailed in Medicare Block 17. Temporary "surrogate" NPIs are issued until permanent ones are assigned for physicians in the following categories: residents and interns, retired physicians, nonphysicians (nurse practitioners, clinical nurse specialists, and other state licensed nonphysicians), Veterans Affairs/U.S. Armed Services, Public Health/Indian Health Services, and any physician not meeting the described criteria for a surrogate who has not been issued an NPI.
Medicare/Medicaid: Refer to Medicare guidelines.
Medicare/Medigap: Refer to Medicare guidelines.
MSP: Refer to Medicare guidelines.

TRICARE: Enter the referring physician's state license number. If the patient is referred from a Military Treatment Facility (MTF), leave blank.

CHAMPVA: Refer to TRICARE guidelines.

Workers' Compensation: Leave blank.

Block 18

14. DATE OF CURRENT:	15. IF PATIENT HAS HAD SAME OR SIMILAR ILLNESS.	16. DATES PATIENT UNABLE TO WORK IN CURRENT OCCUPATION
MM DD YY ILLNESS (First symptom) OR INJURY (Accident) OR 03 01 20XX PREGNANCY (LMP)	GIVE FIRST DATE MM DD YY	MM DD YY MM DD YY FROM TO
17. NAME OF REFERRING PHYSICIAN OR OTHER SOURCE PERRY CARDI MD	17a. I.D. NUMBER OF REFERRING PHYSICIAN 67805027XX	18. HOSPITALIZATION DATES RELATED TO CURRENT SERVICES MM DD YY MM DD YY FROM TO
19. RESERVED FOR LOCAL USE		20. OUTSIDE LAB? $ CHARGES ☐ YES ☒ NO

All Payers: Complete this block when a medical service is furnished as a result of, or subsequent to, a related (inpatient) hospitalization, skilled nursing facility, or nursing home visit. Do not complete for outpatient hospital services, ambulatory surgery, or emergency department services. Enter eight-digit admitting and discharge dates. If the patient is still hospitalized at the time of the billing, enter eight zeros in the "TO" field.

Block 19

14. DATE OF CURRENT:	15. IF PATIENT HAS HAD SAME OR SIMILAR ILLNESS.	16. DATES PATIENT UNABLE TO WORK IN CURRENT OCCUPATION
MM DD YY ILLNESS (First symptom) OR INJURY (Accident) OR 03 01 20XX PREGNANCY (LMP)	GIVE FIRST DATE MM DD YY	MM DD YY MM DD YY FROM TO
17. NAME OF REFERRING PHYSICIAN OR OTHER SOURCE PERRY CARDI MD	17a. I.D. NUMBER OF REFERRING PHYSICIAN 67805027XX	18. HOSPITALIZATION DATES RELATED TO CURRENT SERVICES MM DD YY MM DD YY FROM TO
19. RESERVED FOR LOCAL USE		20. OUTSIDE LAB? $ CHARGES ☐ YES ☒ NO

All Private Payers: This block may be completed in a number of different ways depending on commercial carrier guidelines. Some common uses are:

- Enter the word "ATTACHMENT" when an operative report, discharge summary, invoice, or other attachment is included.
- Enter an explanation about unusual services or unlisted services.
- Enter all applicable modifiers when modifier -99 is used in Block 24D (e.g., 99-80 51). If -99 appears with more than one procedure code, list the line number (24-1, -2, -3, and so on) for each -99 listed (Example 7.4).
- Enter the drug name and dosage when submitting a claim for Not Otherwise Classified (NOC) drugs. Enter the word "ATTACHMENT" and attach the invoice.
- Describe the supply when the code 99070 is used.
- Enter the x-ray date for chiropractic treatment.

Example 7.4 Multiple Modifier Format
2-80 51   3-80 51

Medicaid: Check with the regional fiscal intermediary who may have special guidelines for entries in this block.

➤ *When completing the **Workbook** assignments, refer to private payer guidelines.*

Medicare: Although the block is labeled "Reserved for Local Use," CMS guidelines state it may be completed in a number of different ways depending on the circumstances of the services provided to the patient. This block can only contain up to three conditions per claim. Some common uses are:

- Enter the attending physician's NPI and the eight-digit date of the patient's latest visit for claims submitted by a physical or occupational therapist, psychotherapist, chiropractor, or podiatrist.
- Enter the drug's name and dosage when submitting a claim for Not Otherwise Classified (NOC) drugs. Enter the word "ATTACHMENT" and include a copy of the invoice.
- Describe the procedure for unlisted procedures. If there is not sufficient room in this block, send an attachment.
- Enter all applicable modifiers when modifier -99 is used in Block 24D (e.g., 99-80 51). If -99 appears with more than one procedure code, list the line number (24–1, –2, –3, and so on) for each -99 listed (see Example 7.4).
- Enter "Homebound" when an independent laboratory renders an electrocardiogram or collects a specimen from a patient who is homebound or institutionalized.
- Enter the statement "Patient refuses to assign benefits" when a Medicare beneficiary refuses to assign benefits to a participating provider. No payment to the physician will be made on the claim in this case.
- Enter "Testing for hearing aid" when submitting a claim to obtain an intentional denial from Medicare as the primary payer for hearing aid testing and a secondary payer is involved.
- Enter the specific dental surgery for which a dental examination is being performed.
- Enter the name and dosage when billing for low osmolar contrast material for which there is no level II HCPCS code.
- Enter the eight-digit assumed and relinquished dates of care for each provider when providers share postoperative care for global surgery claims.
- Enter the statement "Attending physician, not hospice employee" when a physician gives service to a hospice patient but the hospice in which the patient resides does not employ the physician.

Medicare/Medicaid: Refer to Medicare guidelines.
Medicare/Medigap: Refer to Medicare guidelines.
MSP: Refer to Medicare guidelines.

TRICARE: Generally this block is reserved for local use (e.g., to indicate referral number or enter x-ray date for chiropractic treatment).

CHAMPVA: Refer to TRICARE guidelines.

Workers' Compensation: Leave blank.

Block 20

14. DATE OF CURRENT: MM DD YY	ILLNESS (First symptom) OR INJURY (Accident) OR PREGNANCY (LMP)	15. IF PATIENT HAS HAD SAME OR SIMILAR ILLNESS. GIVE FIRST DATE MM DD YY	16. DATES PATIENT UNABLE TO WORK IN CURRENT OCCUPATION MM DD YY MM DD YY
03 │ 01 │ 20XX			FROM TO
17. NAME OF REFERRING PHYSICIAN OR OTHER SOURCE		17a. I.D. NUMBER OF REFERRING PHYSICIAN	18. HOSPITALIZATION DATES RELATED TO CURRENT SERVICES MM DD YY MM DD YY
PERRY CARDI MD		67805027XX	FROM TO
19. RESERVED FOR LOCAL USE			20. OUTSIDE LAB? $ CHARGES ☐ YES ☒ NO

All Private Payers: Enter "yes" or "no" when billing diagnostic laboratory tests. *NO* means the tests were performed by the billing physician/laboratory. *YES* means that the laboratory test was performed *outside* of the physician's office and that the physician is billing for the laboratory services. If "yes," enter purchase price of the test in the Charges portion of this block and complete Block 32.

Medicaid: Check "no"; outside laboratories must bill directly.

Medicare: Enter "yes" or "no" when billing diagnostic laboratory tests. *NO* means the tests were performed by the billing physician or laboratory. *YES* means that the laboratory test was performed outside of the physician's office and that the physician is billing for the laboratory services. If "yes," enter purchase price of the test in the Charges portion of this block and complete Block 32. *Clinical laboratory services must be billed to Medicare on an assigned basis.*
Medicare/Medicaid: Refer to Medicare guidelines.
Medicare/Medigap: Refer to Medicare guidelines.
MSP: Refer to Medicare guidelines.

TRICARE: Refer to Medicare guidelines.

CHAMPVA: Refer to Medicare guidelines.

Workers' Compensation: Refer to Medicare guidelines.

Block 21

21. DIAGNOSIS OR NATURE OF ILLNESS OR INJURY. (RELATE ITEMS 1,2,3 OR 4 TO ITEM 24E BY LINE)		22. MEDICAID RESUBMISSION CODE ORIGINAL REF. NO.
1. 382 00	3. └──.──┘	
2. └──.──┘	4. └──.──┘	23. PRIOR AUTHORIZATION NUMBER

24.	A		B	C	D	E	F	G	H	I	J	K
	DATE(S) OF SERVICE From	To	Place of Service	Type of Service	PROCEDURES, SERVICES, OR SUPPLIES (Explain Unusual Circumstances) CPT/HCPCS │ MODIFIER	DIAGNOSIS CODE	$ CHARGES	DAYS OR UNITS	EPSDT Family Plan	EMG	COB	RESERVED FOR LOCAL USE
	MM DD YY	MM DD YY										
1												

All Payers: Enter up to four diagnostic codes in priority order, with the primary diagnosis in the first position. Codes must be carried out to their highest degree of specificity. Do not use decimal points or add any code narratives unless required in your locale. Code only the conditions or problems that the physician is actively treating and that relate directly to the services billed.

Block 22

21. DIAGNOSIS OR NATURE OF ILLNESS OR INJURY. (RELATE ITEMS 1,2,3 OR 4 TO ITEM 24E BY LINE)							22. MEDICAID RESUBMISSION CODE	ORIGINAL REF. NO.				
1. ⌊ 382 00			3. ⌊___.___									
2. ⌊___.___			4. ⌊___.___				23. PRIOR AUTHORIZATION NUMBER					

24. A DATE(S) OF SERVICE						B Place of Service	C Type of Service	D PROCEDURES, SERVICES, OR SUPPLIES (Explain Unusual Circumstances) CPT/HCPCS | MODIFIER	E DIAGNOSIS CODE	F $ CHARGES	G DAYS OR UNITS	H EPSDT Family Plan	I EMG	J COB	K RESERVED FOR LOCAL USE
From MM	DD	YY	To MM	DD	YY										
1									1						

All Private Payers: Leave blank.

Medicaid: Complete for resubmission.

Medicare: Leave blank.
Medicare/Medicaid: Refer to Medicaid guidelines.
Medicare/Medigap: Leave blank.
MSP: Leave blank.

TRICARE: Leave blank.

CHAMPVA: Leave blank.

Workers' Compensation: Leave blank.

Block 23

21. DIAGNOSIS OR NATURE OF ILLNESS OR INJURY. (RELATE ITEMS 1,2,3 OR 4 TO ITEM 24E BY LINE)							22. MEDICAID RESUBMISSION CODE | ORIGINAL REF. NO.				
1. | 382 00			3. |___|___								
2. |___|___			4. |___|___				23. PRIOR AUTHORIZATION NUMBER				

24.	A DATE(S) OF SERVICE						B Place of Service	C Type of Service	D PROCEDURES, SERVICES, OR SUPPLIES (Explain Unusual Circumstances) CPT/HCPCS | MODIFIER		E DIAGNOSIS CODE	F $ CHARGES	G DAYS OR UNITS	H EPSDT Family Plan	I EMG	J COB	K RESERVED FOR LOCAL USE
	From MM	DD	YY	To MM	DD	YY											
1											1						

 All Private Payers: Enter the professional or peer review organization (PRO) 10-digit prior authorization number.

 Medicaid: Enter the Professional (Peer) Review Organization (PRO) 10-digit prior authorization or precertification number for procedures requiring PRO prior approval. If billing for an investigational device, enter the Investigational Device Exemption (IDE) number.

 Medicare: Although this block is labeled "Prior Authorization Number," CMS guidelines state it may be completed in a number of different ways depending on the circumstances of the services provided to the patient. Some common uses are:
- Enter the Professional (Peer) Review Organization (PRO) 10-digit prior authorization or precertification number for procedures requiring PRO prior approval.
- Enter the Investigational Device Exemption (IDE) number if billing for an investigational device.
- Enter the 10-digit Clinical Laboratory Improvement Amendments (CLIA) federal certification number when billing for laboratory services billed by a physician office laboratory.
- Enter the six-digit Medicare provider number of the hospice or home health agency (HHA) when billing for care plan oversight services.

Medicare/Medicaid: Refer to Medicare guidelines.
Medicare/Medigap: Refer to Medicare guidelines.
MSP: Refer to Medicare guidelines.

 TRICARE: Enter the Professional (Peer) Review Organization (PRO) 10-digit prior authorization or precertification number for procedures requiring PRO prior approval. If billing for an investigational device, enter the Investigational Device Exemption (IDE) number. Attach a copy of the authorization.

 CHAMPVA: Refer to TRICARE guidelines.

 Workers' Compensation: Leave blank.

Blocks 24A through 24K may not contain more than six detail lines. If the case requires more than six detail lines, put the additional information on a separate claim form, treat it as an independent claim, and total all charges on each claim. Claims cannot be "continued" from one to another. Do not list a procedure on the claim form for which there is no charge.

Block 24A

24. A DATE(S) OF SERVICE						B Place of Service	C Type of Service	D PROCEDURES, SERVICES, OR SUPPLIES (Explain Unusual Circumstances) CPT/HCPCS MODIFIER		E DIAGNOSIS CODE	F $ CHARGES		G DAYS OR UNITS	H EPSDT Family Plan	I EMG	J COB	K RESERVED FOR LOCAL USE
From MM	DD	YY	To MM	DD	YY												
1	030320XX					11		99203		1	70	92	1			12	458977XX
2																	
3																	
4																	
5																	
6																	

25. FEDERAL TAX I.D. NUMBER	SSN	EIN	26. PATIENT'S ACCOUNT NO.	27. ACCEPT ASSIGNMENT? (For govt. claims, see back)	28. TOTAL CHARGE	29. AMOUNT PAID	30. BALANCE DUE
74 10640XX	☐	☒	010	☒ YES ☐ NO	$ 70 92	$	$ 70 92

24. A DATE(S) OF SERVICE						B Place of Service	C Type of Service	D PROCEDURES, SERVICES, OR SUPPLIES (Explain Unusual Circumstances) CPT/HCPCS MODIFIER		E DIAGNOSIS CODE	F $ CHARGES		G DAYS OR UNITS	H EPSDT Family Plan	EMG	Initials COB	Date RESERVED FOR LOCAL USE
From MM	DD	YY	To MM	DD	YY												
1	113020XX					21		99231		1	37	74	1			32	783127XX
2	120120XX		120320XX			21		99231		1	37	74	3			32	783127XX
3																	
4																	
5																	
6																	

25. FEDERAL TAX I.D. NUMBER	SSN	EIN	26. PATIENT'S ACCOUNT NO.	27. ACCEPT ASSIGNMENT? (For govt. claims, see back)	28. TOTAL CHARGE	29. AMOUNT PAID	30. BALANCE DUE
75 67210XX	☐	☒	102	☒ YES ☐ NO	$ 150 96	$	$ 150 96

All Private Payers: Enter the month, day, and year (eight digits with no spaces) for each procedure, service, or supply reported in Block 24D. Make sure the dates shown are no earlier than the date of the current illness if listed in Block 14. If the "from" and "to" dates are the same, enter only the "from" date. Enter the "to" date when reporting a consecutive range of dates for the same procedure code. Use a separate line for each month. Some third-party payers may use different date formats (e.g., December 4, 20XX = 20XX1204).

Medicaid: Enter an eight-digit "from" date (month, day, and year with no spaces) for each service or supply. Leave "to" date blank. No date ranging is allowed for consecutive dates.

Medicare: Enter the month, day, and year (eight digits with no spaces) for each procedure, service, or supply reported in Block 24D. Make sure the dates shown are no earlier than the date of the current illness if listed in Block 14. If the "from" and "to" dates are the same, enter only the "from" date. Enter the "to" date when reporting a consecutive range of dates for the same procedure code. Use a separate line for each month except when reporting weekly radiation therapy, durable medical equipment, or oxygen rental.
Medicare/Medicaid: Refer to Medicare guidelines.
Medicare/Medigap: Refer to Medicare guidelines.
MSP: Refer to Medicare guidelines.

TRICARE: Enter the month, day, and year (eight digits with no spaces) for each procedure, service, or supply reported in Block 24D. Make sure the dates shown are no earlier than the date of the current illness if listed in Block 14. If the "from" and "to" dates are the same, enter only the "from" date. Enter the "to" date when reporting a consecutive range of dates for the same procedure code. Use a separate line for each month.

CHAMPVA: Refer to TRICARE guidelines.

Workers' Compensation: Enter the month, day, and year (eight digits with no spaces) for each procedure, service, or supply reported in Block 24D. Date ranging is not the preferred format for consecutive dates.

Block 24B

24. A DATE(S) OF SERVICE From MM DD YY	To MM DD YY	B Place of Service	C Type of Service	D PROCEDURES, SERVICES, OR SUPPLIES (Explain Unusual Circumstances) CPT/HCPCS | MODIFIER	E DIAGNOSIS CODE	F $ CHARGES	G DAYS OR UNITS	H EPSDT Family Plan	I EMG	J COB	K RESERVED FOR LOCAL USE
1	030320XX		11		99203	1	70 | 92	1			12	458977XX
2												
3												
4												
5												
6												

25. FEDERAL TAX I.D. NUMBER	SSN EIN	26. PATIENT'S ACCOUNT NO.	27. ACCEPT ASSIGNMENT? (For govt. claims, see back)	28. TOTAL CHARGE	29. AMOUNT PAID	30. BALANCE DUE
74 10640XX	☐ ☒	010	☒ YES ☐ NO	$ 70 | 92	$	$ 70 | 92

All Payers: Enter the appropriate "Place of Service" code shown in Figure 7–4. Identify by location where the service was performed or an item was used. Use the inpatient hospital code only when a service is provided to a patient admitted to the hospital for an overnight stay. Enter the name, address, and provider number of the hospital in Block 32.
Medical practices that have multiple offices must show the address of where the service was rendered in Block 32.

Block 24C

24. A DATE(S) OF SERVICE From MM DD YY	To MM DD YY	B Place of Service	C Type of Service	D PROCEDURES, SERVICES, OR SUPPLIES (Explain Unusual Circumstances) CPT/HCPCS | MODIFIER	E DIAGNOSIS CODE	F $ CHARGES	G DAYS OR UNITS	H EPSDT Family Plan	I EMG	J COB	K RESERVED FOR LOCAL USE
1	030320XX		11		99203	1	70 | 92	1			12	458977XX
2												
3												
4												
5												
6												

25. FEDERAL TAX I.D. NUMBER	SSN EIN	26. PATIENT'S ACCOUNT NO.	27. ACCEPT ASSIGNMENT? (For govt. claims, see back)	28. TOTAL CHARGE	29. AMOUNT PAID	30. BALANCE DUE
74 10640XX	☐ ☒	010	☒ YES ☐ NO	$ 70 | 92	$	$ 70 | 92

BLOCK 24B
PLACE OF SERVICE CODES

- 00-02 Unassigned
- 03 School
- 04 Homeless shelter
- 05 Indian health service free-standing facility
- 06 Indian health service provider-based facility
- 07 Tribal 638 free-standing facility
- 08 Tribal 638 provider-based facility
- 09-10 Unassigned
- 11 Doctor's office
- 12 Patient's home
- 13 Assisted living facility
- 14 Group home
- 15 Mobile unit
- 16-19 Unassigned
- 20 Urgent care facility
- 21 Inpatient hospital
- 22 Outpatient hospital
- 23 Emergency department—hospital
- 24 Ambulatory surgical center
- 25 Birthing center
- 26 Military treatment facility/uniformed service treatment facility
- 27-30 Unassigned
- 31 Skilled nursing facility (swing bed visits)
- 32 Nursing facility (intermediate/long-term care facilities)
- 33 Custodial care facility (domiciliary or rest home services)
- 34 Hospice (domiciliary or rest home services)
- 35-40 Unassigned
- 41 Ambulance—land
- 42 Ambulance—air or water
- 43-48 Unassigned
- 49 Independent clinic
- 50 Federally qualified health center
- 51 Inpatient psychiatric facility
- 52 Psychiatric facility—partial hospitalization
- 53 Community mental health care (outpatient, twenty-four-hours-a-day services, admission screening, consultation, and educational services)
- 54 Intermediate care facility/mentally retarded
- 55 Residential substance abuse treatment facility
- 56 Psychiatric residential treatment center
- 58-59 Unassigned
- 60 Mass immunization center
- 61 Comprehensive inpatient rehabilitation facility
- 62 Comprehensive outpatient rehabilitation facility
- 63-64 Unassigned
- 65 End-stage renal disease treatment facility
- 66-70 Unassigned
- 71 State or local public health clinic
- 72 Rural health clinic
- 73-80 Unassigned
- 81 Independent laboratory
- 82-98 Unassigned
- 99 Other place of service

FIGURE 7–4   Block 24B Place of Service Codes.

All Private Payers: Leave blank.

Medicaid: Enter the appropriate "Type of Service" code from Figure 7.5.

BLOCK 24C
TYPE OF SERVICE CODES FOR MEDICAID,
TRICARE, AND WORKERS' COMPENSATION

These codes should be selected depending on the procedure code used on each line. Codes may vary according to regions and claim administrators.

1 Medical care (e.g., evaluation and management services)
2 Surgery
3 Consultation
4 Diagnostic x-ray (e.g., ultrasound and nuclear testing)
5 Diagnostic laboratory
6 Radiation therapy
7 Anesthesia
8 Assistant at surgery
9 Other medical service (e.g., venipuncture, handling of specimen)
0 Blood or packed red cells
A DME rental/purchase
B Drugs
C Ambulatory surgery
D Hospice
E Second opinion on elective surgery
F Maternity
G Dental
H Mental health care
I Ambulance
J Program for persons with disabilities
L Renal supply in home
M Alternate payment for maintenance
N Kidney donor
P Prosthesis, orthotics
V Pneumococcal vaccine
Z Third opinion on elective surgery

FIGURE 7-5 Block 24C Type of Service Codes for Medicaid, TRICARE, and Workers' Compensation.

Medicare: Leave blank. "Type of Service" codes are used on Medicare Remittance Advice (RA) documents and electronic claims.
Medicare/Medicaid: Refer to Medicare guidelines.
Medicare/Medigap: Refer to Medicare guidelines.
MSP: Refer to Medicare guidelines.

TRICARE: Enter the appropriate "Type of Service" code from Figure 7–5. Codes may vary according to regions and claim administrators.
When completing the Workbook assignments, use the codes shown in Figure 7–5.

CHAMPVA: Refer to TRICARE guidelines.

Workers' Compensation: Enter the appropriate "Type of Service" code shown in Figure 7–5. These codes may not be used or may vary according to regions and claim administrators.
When completing the Workbook assignments, use the codes shown in Figure 7–5.

Block 24D

24.	A DATE(S) OF SERVICE			B Place of Service	C Type of Service	D PROCEDURES, SERVICES, OR SUPPLIES (Explain Unusual Circumstances)		E DIAGNOSIS CODE	F $ CHARGES		G DAYS OR UNITS	H EPSDT Family Plan	I EMG	J COB	K RESERVED FOR LOCAL USE
	From MM DD YY	To MM DD YY				CPT/HCPCS	MODIFIER								
1	030320XX			11		99203		1	70	92	1			12	458977XX
2															
3															
4															
5															
6															

25. FEDERAL TAX I.D. NUMBER	SSN EIN	26. PATIENT'S ACCOUNT NO.	27. ACCEPT ASSIGNMENT? (For govt. claims, see back)	28. TOTAL CHARGE	29. AMOUNT PAID	30. BALANCE DUE
74 10640XX	☐ ☒	010	☒ YES ☐ NO	$ 70 92	$	$ 70 92

CPT   99203   Office visit, new patient

All Private Payers: Enter the appropriate CPT/HCPCS code for each procedure, service, or supply and applicable modifier without a hyphen. If it is necessary to use more than two modifiers with a procedure code, enter modifier -99 in Block 24D and list applicable modifiers in Block 19.

Medicaid: Enter the appropriate CPT/HCPCS code for each procedure, service, or supply and applicable modifier without a hyphen.

Medicare: Enter CPT/HCPCS code and applicable modifiers without a hyphen for procedures, services, and supplies without a narrative description. When procedure codes do not require modifiers, leave modifier area blank—do not enter 00 or any other combination. For multiple surgical procedures, list the procedure with the highest fee first. For unlisted procedure codes, include a narrative description in Block 19 (e.g., 99499, "Unlisted Evaluation and Management Service"). If information does not fit in Block 19, include an attachment. When entering an unlisted surgery code, submit the operative notes with the claim as an attachment.
Medicare/Medicaid: Refer to Medicare guidelines.
Medicare/Medigap: Refer to Medicare guidelines.
MSP: Refer to Medicare guidelines.

TRICARE: Enter the appropriate CPT/HCPCS code for each procedure, service, or supply and applicable modifier without a hyphen. If it is necessary to use more than two modifiers with a procedure code, enter modifier -99 in Block 24D and list applicable modifiers in Block 19. When Not Otherwise Classified (NOC) codes are submitted (e.g., supplies and injections), provide a narrative of the service in Block 19 or on an attachment.

CHAMPVA: Refer to TRICARE guidelines.

Workers' Compensation: Enter appropriate RVS codes and applicable modifiers (without a hyphen) used in your state or region.
*When completing the **Workbook** assignments, use appropriate CPT codes.*

Block 24E

21. DIAGNOSIS OR NATURE OF ILLNESS OR INJURY (RELATE ITEMS 1,2,3 OR 4 TO ITEM 24E BY LINE)	22. MEDICAID RESUBMISSION CODE	ORIGINAL REF. NO.
1. 382 00	3.	
	23. PRIOR AUTHORIZATION NUMBER	
2.	4.	

24. A DATE(S) OF SERVICE		B Place of Service	C Type of Service	D PROCEDURES, SERVICES, OR SUPPLIES (Explain Unusual Circumstances) CPT/HCPCS | MODIFIER	E DIAGNOSIS CODE	F $ CHARGES	G DAYS OR UNITS	H EPSDT Family Plan	I EMG	J COB	K RESERVED FOR LOCAL USE
From MM DD YY	To MM DD YY										
1	030320XX	11	99203	1	70 92	1			12	458977XX
2										
3										
4										
5										
6										

25. FEDERAL TAX I.D. NUMBER	SSN EIN	26. PATIENT'S ACCOUNT NO.	27. ACCEPT ASSIGNMENT? (For govt. claims, see back)	28. TOTAL CHARGE	29. AMOUNT PAID	30. BALANCE DUE
74 10640XX	☐ [X]	010	[X] YES ☐ NO	$ 70 92	$	$ 70 92

All Private Payers: Enter all of the diagnosis code reference "pointer" numbers (1, 2, 3, 4) per line item that apply to the CPT code. This links the diagnostic code(s) listed in Block 24E to Block 21. When multiple services are performed, enter the corresponding diagnostic reference number for each service (e.g., 1, 2, 3, or 4). DO NOT USE ACTUAL ICD-9-CM CODES IN THIS BLOCK.
→ *When completing Workbook assignments, more than one diagnosis reference "pointer" number per line item is allowed.*

Medicaid: Refer to Medicare guidelines. In some states, completion may not be required.

Medicare: Enter only one diagnosis code reference "pointer" number per line item linking the diagnostic codes listed in Block 21. When multiple services are performed, enter the corresponding diagnostic reference number for each service (e.g., 1, 2, 3, or 4). DO NOT USE ACTUAL ICD-9-CM CODES IN THIS BLOCK.
Medicare/Medicaid: Refer to Medicare guidelines.
Medicare/Medigap: Refer to Medicare guidelines.
MSP: Refer to Medicare guidelines.

TRICARE: Enter the diagnosis reference number (e.g., indicating up to four ICD-9-CM codes) as shown in Block 21 to relate the date of service and the procedures performed to the appropriate diagnosis. If multiple procedures are performed, enter the diagnosis code reference number for each service.

CHAMPVA: Refer to TRICARE guidelines.

Workers' Compensation: Enter all appropriate diagnosis code reference "pointer" numbers from Block 21 to relate appropriate diagnosis to date of service and procedures performed. A maximum of four diagnosis pointers may be referenced. Place commas between multiple diagnosis reference pointers on the same line.

Block 24F

24.	A					B	C	D		E		F		G	H	I	J	K
	DATE(S) OF SERVICE					Place	Type	PROCEDURES, SERVICES, OR SUPPLIES		DIAGNOSIS		$ CHARGES		DAYS	EPSDT	EMG	COB	RESERVED FOR
	From			To		of	of	(Explain Unusual Circumstances)		CODE				OR	Family			LOCAL USE
	MM DD YY			MM DD YY		Service	Service	CPT/HCPCS | MODIFIER						UNITS	Plan			
1	030320XX					11		99203		1		71	00	1			12	458977XX
2																		
3																		
4																		
5																		
6																		

25. FEDERAL TAX I.D. NUMBER	SSN EIN	26. PATIENT'S ACCOUNT NO.	27. ACCEPT ASSIGNMENT? (For govt. claims, see back)	28. TOTAL CHARGE	29. AMOUNT PAID	30. BALANCE DUE
74 10640XX	☐ [X]	010	[X] YES ☐ NO	$ 71 00	$	$ 71 00

All Private Payers: Enter the fee for each listed service from the appropriate fee schedule. DO NOT ENTER DOLLAR SIGNS OR DECIMAL POINTS. ALWAYS INCLUDE CENTS. If the same service is performed on consecutive days, list the fee for one service in this block and the number of units (times it was performed) in Block 24G. The total for consecutive services should be computed and added into the claim total shown in Block 28.

→ *When completing the **Workbook** assignments for private, Medicaid, TRICARE, and workers' compensation cases, use the Mock Fee. For Medicare participating provider cases, use the Participating Provider Fee. For nonparticipating provider cases, use the Limiting Charge.*

Block 24G

24.	A					B	C	D		E		F		G	H	I	J	K
	DATE(S) OF SERVICE					Place	Type	PROCEDURES, SERVICES, OR SUPPLIES		DIAGNOSIS		$ CHARGES		DAYS	EPSDT	EMG	COB	RESERVED FOR
	From			To		of	of	(Explain Unusual Circumstances)		CODE				OR	Family			LOCAL USE
	MM DD YY			MM DD YY		Service	Service	CPT/HCPCS | MODIFIER						UNITS	Plan			
1	030320XX					11		99203		1		70	92	1			12	458977XX
2																		
3																		
4																		
5																		
6																		

25. FEDERAL TAX I.D. NUMBER	SSN EIN	26. PATIENT'S ACCOUNT NO.	27. ACCEPT ASSIGNMENT? (For govt. claims, see back)	28. TOTAL CHARGE	29. AMOUNT PAID	30. BALANCE DUE
74 10640XX	☐ [X]	010	[X] YES ☐ NO	$ 70 92	$	$ 70 92

All Private Payers: Enter the number of days or units that apply to each line of service. This block is important for calculating multiple visits, anesthesia minutes, or oxygen volume.

Medicaid: Each service must be listed on separate lines (no date ranging). Indicate that each service was performed one time by listing "1" in this block. List number of visits in 1 day.

Medicare: Enter the number of days or units that apply to each line of service. This block is important for calculating multiple visits, number of miles, units of supplies including drugs, anesthesia minutes, or oxygen volume. See the Medicare Manual for reporting anesthesia time or units and for rounding out figures when billing gas and liquid oxygen units.
Medicare/Medicaid: Refer to Medicare guidelines.
Medicare/Medigap: Refer to Medicare guidelines.
MSP: Refer to Medicare guidelines.

TRICARE: Refer to Medicare guidelines.

CHAMPVA: Refer to Medicare guidelines.

Workers' Compensation: Refer to Medicare guidelines.

Block 24H

24. A DATE(S) OF SERVICE		B Place of Service	C Type of Service	D PROCEDURES, SERVICES, OR SUPPLIES CPT/HCPCS | MODIFIER	E DIAGNOSIS CODE	F $ CHARGES	G DAYS OR UNITS	H EPSDT Family Plan	I EMG	J COB	K RESERVED FOR LOCAL USE
From MM DD YY	To MM DD YY										
030320XX		11		99203	1	70 92	1			12	458977XX

25. FEDERAL TAX I.D. NUMBER	SSN EIN	26. PATIENT'S ACCOUNT NO.	27. ACCEPT ASSIGNMENT? (For govt. claims, see back)	28. TOTAL CHARGE	29. AMOUNT PAID	30. BALANCE DUE
74 10640XX	☐ ☒	010	☒ YES ☐ NO	$ 70 92	$	$ 70 92

All Private Payers: Leave blank.

Medicaid: EPSDT means early, periodic, screening, diagnosis, and treatment, and refers to a Medicaid service program for children 12 years of age or younger. Enter "E" for EPSDT services or "F" for family planning services, if applicable.

Medicare: Leave blank.
Medicare/Medicaid: Leave blank.
Medicare/Medigap: Leave blank.
MSP: Leave blank.

TRICARE: Leave blank.

CHAMPVA: Leave blank.

Workers' Compensation: Leave blank.

Block 24I

24.	A DATE(S) OF SERVICE						B Place of Service	C Type of Service	D PROCEDURES, SERVICES, OR SUPPLIES (Explain Unusual Circumstances) CPT/HCPCS	MODIFIER	E DIAGNOSIS CODE	F $ CHARGES		G DAYS OR UNITS	H EPSDT Family Plan	I EMG	J COB	K RESERVED FOR LOCAL USE
	From MM	DD	YY	To MM	DD	YY												
1	03	03	20XX				11		99203		1	70	92	1			12	458977XX
2																		
3																		
4																		
5																		
6																		

25. FEDERAL TAX I.D. NUMBER	SSN EIN	26. PATIENT'S ACCOUNT NO.	27. ACCEPT ASSIGNMENT? (For govt. claims, see back)	28. TOTAL CHARGE	29. AMOUNT PAID	30. BALANCE DUE
74 10640XX	☐ ☒	010	☒ YES ☐ NO	$ 70 92	$	$ 70 92

All Private Payers: Leave blank.

Medicaid: EMG stands for the word "emergency" and means that the service was rendered in *hospital emergency department*. Enter "X" if emergency care is provided in an emergency department.

Medicare: Leave blank.
Medicare/Medicaid: Leave blank.
Medicare/Medigap: Leave blank.
MSP: Leave blank.

TRICARE: Enter "X" in this block to indicate that the service was provided in a hospital emergency department.

CHAMPVA: Enter "X" in this block to indicate that the service was provided in a hospital emergency department.

Workers' Compensation: Leave blank.

Block 24J

24. A DATE(S) OF SERVICE		B Place of Service	C Type of Service	D PROCEDURES, SERVICES, OR SUPPLIES (Explain Unusual Circumstances)	E DIAGNOSIS CODE	F $ CHARGES	G DAYS OR UNITS	H EPSDT Family Plan	I EMG	J COB	K RESERVED FOR LOCAL USE
From MM DD YY	To MM DD YY			CPT/HCPCS | MODIFIER							
030320XX		11		99203 |	1	70 92	1			12	458977XX

25. FEDERAL TAX I.D. NUMBER	SSN EIN	26. PATIENT'S ACCOUNT NO.	27. ACCEPT ASSIGNMENT? (For govt. claims, see back)	28. TOTAL CHARGE	29. AMOUNT PAID	30. BALANCE DUE
74 10640XX	☐ ☒	010	☒ YES ☐ NO	$ 70 92	$	$ 70 92

All Private Payers: Refer to the note for Block 24K.

Medicaid: COB means "coordination of benefits." Check, if applicable, when the patient has other insurance.

Medicare: Refer to the note for Block 24K.
Medicare/Medicaid: Refer to the note for Block 24K.
Medicare/Medigap: Refer to the note for Block 24K.
MSP: Refer to the note for Block 24K.

TRICARE: Leave blank.

CHAMPVA: Leave blank.

Workers' Compensation: Leave blank.

Block 24K

24. A DATE(S) OF SERVICE From MM DD YY	To MM DD YY	B Place of Service	C Type of Service	D PROCEDURES, SERVICES, OR SUPPLIES (Explain Unusual Circumstances) CPT/HCPCS | MODIFIER	E DIAGNOSIS CODE	F $ CHARGES	G DAYS OR UNITS	H EPSDT Family Plan	I EMG	J COB	K RESERVED FOR LOCAL USE
1 030320XX		11		99203	1	70 92	1			12	458977XX
2											
3											
4											
5											
6											

25. FEDERAL TAX I.D. NUMBER SSN EIN	26. PATIENT'S ACCOUNT NO.	27. ACCEPT ASSIGNMENT? (For govt. claims, see back)	28. TOTAL CHARGE	29. AMOUNT PAID	30. BALANCE DUE
74 10640XX ☐ ☒	010	☒ YES ☐ NO	$ 70 92	$	$ 70 92

All Private Payers: Enter the CMS-assigned provider identification number (PIN) or national provider identifier (NPI) for each line of service when the performing physician or supplier is in a group practice and billing under a group ID number. An individual physician's PIN/NPI is not required if he or she is in solo practice or when billing under his or her individual ID number. **Note:** *Enter the first two digits of the NPI in Block 24J. Enter the remaining eight digits of the NPI in Block 24K, including the two-digit location identifier.*

Medicaid: Leave blank.

Medicare: Enter the CMS-assigned provider identification number (PIN) or national provider identifier (NPI) for each line of service when the performing physician or supplier is in a group practice and billing under a group ID number. An individual physician's PIN/NPI is not required if he or she is in solo practice or when billing under his or her individual ID number. **Note:** *Enter the first two digits of the NPI in Block 24J. Enter the remaining eight digits of the NPI in Block 24K, including the two-digit location identifier.*
Medicare/Medicaid: Refer to Medicare guidelines.
Medicare/Medigap: Refer to Medicare guidelines.
MSP: Refer to Medicare guidelines.

TRICARE: Enter the physician's state license number when billing for a group practice using one group ID number. The state license number is an alpha character followed by six numeric digits. If there are not six digits, enter appropriate number of zeros after the alpha character (e.g., A1234 would be A001234).

CHAMPVA: Refer to TRICARE guidelines.

Workers' Compensation: Leave blank.

Block 25

25. FEDERAL TAX I.D. NUMBER	SSN	EIN	26. PATIENT'S ACCOUNT NO.	27. ACCEPT ASSIGNMENT? (For govt. claims, see back)	28. TOTAL CHARGE	29. AMOUNT PAID	30. BALANCE DUE
74 10640XX	☐	☒	010	☒ YES ☐ NO	$ 70 92	$	$ 70 92

31. SIGNATURE OF PHYSICIAN OR SUPPLIER INCLUDING DEGREES OR CREDENTIALS (I certify that the statements on the reverse apply to this bill and are made a part thereof.)	32. NAME AND ADDRESS OF FACILITY WHERE SERVICES WERE RENDERED (If other than home or office)	33. PHYSICIAN'S, SUPPLIER'S BILLING NAME, ADDRESS, ZIP CODE & PHONE #
CONCHA ANTRUM MD 030320XX	SAME	COLLEGE CLINIC 4567 BROAD AVENUE WOODLAND HILLS XY 12345 0001 555 486 9002
SIGNED *Concha Antrum MD* DATE		PIN# GRP# 3664021CC

reference initials

All Payers: Enter the physician or supplier's federal tax ID. This number may be the Employer Identification Number (EIN) or Social Security Number (SSN). Check the corresponding box.
- A Medicaid case may or may not require a physician's tax ID number, depending on individual state guidelines.
- In a Medicare/Medigap case, the physician's federal tax ID number is necessary for Medigap transfer.

→ *When completing the **Workbook** assignments, enter the physician's EIN number and check the appropriate box.*

Block 26

25. FEDERAL TAX I.D. NUMBER	SSN	EIN	26. PATIENT'S ACCOUNT NO.	27. ACCEPT ASSIGNMENT? (For govt. claims, see back)	28. TOTAL CHARGE	29. AMOUNT PAID	30. BALANCE DUE
74 10640XX	☐	☒	010	☒ YES ☐ NO	$ 70 92	$	$ 70 92

31. SIGNATURE OF PHYSICIAN OR SUPPLIER INCLUDING DEGREES OR CREDENTIALS (I certify that the statements on the reverse apply to this bill and are made a part thereof.)	32. NAME AND ADDRESS OF FACILITY WHERE SERVICES WERE RENDERED (If other than home or office)	33. PHYSICIAN'S, SUPPLIER'S BILLING NAME, ADDRESS, ZIP CODE & PHONE #
CONCHA ANTRUM MD 030320XX	SAME	COLLEGE CLINIC 4567 BROAD AVENUE WOODLAND HILLS XY 12345 0001 555 486 9002
SIGNED *Concha Antrum MD* DATE		PIN# GRP# 3664021CC

reference initials

All Payers: Enter the patient's account number assigned by the physician's accounting system. Do not use dashes or slashes. When Medicare is billed electronically, this block must be completed.
→ *When completing the **Workbook** assignments, list the patient account number when provided.*

Block 27

25. FEDERAL TAX I.D. NUMBER	SSN	EIN	26. PATIENT'S ACCOUNT NO.	27. ACCEPT ASSIGNMENT? (For govt. claims, see back)	28. TOTAL CHARGE	29. AMOUNT PAID	30. BALANCE DUE
74 10640XX	☐	☒	010	☒ YES ☐ NO	$ 70 92	$	$ 70 92

31. SIGNATURE OF PHYSICIAN OR SUPPLIER INCLUDING DEGREES OR CREDENTIALS (I certify that the statements on the reverse apply to this bill and are made a part thereof.)	32. NAME AND ADDRESS OF FACILITY WHERE SERVICES WERE RENDERED (If other than home or office)	33. PHYSICIAN'S, SUPPLIER'S BILLING NAME, ADDRESS, ZIP CODE & PHONE #
CONCHA ANTRUM MD 030320XX	SAME	COLLEGE CLINIC 4567 BROAD AVENUE WOODLAND HILLS XY 12345 0001 555 486 9002
SIGNED *Concha Antrum MD* DATE		PIN# GRP# 3664021CC

reference initials

All Private Payers: Check "yes" or "no" to indicate whether the physician accepts assignment of benefits. If "yes," then the physician agrees to accept the amount allowed by the third party. You may need to bill the patient for any copayment or deductible amount.
→ *When completing the **Workbook** assignments, check "yes."*

Medicaid: Check "Yes."

Medicare: Check "yes" or "no" to indicate whether the physician accepts assignment of benefits. If "yes," then the physician agrees to accept the allowed amount paid by the third party plus any copayment or deductible as payment in full. If this field is left blank, "no" is assumed, and a participating physician's claim will be denied. The following provider or supplier must file claims on an assignment basis:

- Clinical diagnostic laboratory services performed in physician's office.
- Physicians wishing to accept assignment on clinical laboratory services but not other services should submit two separate claims, one "assigned" for laboratory and one "nonassigned" for other services. Submit all charges on a nonassigned claim, as indicated in Block 27, and write "I accept assignment for the clinical laboratory tests" at the bottom of Block 24.
- Participating physician or supplier services.
- Physician's services to Medicare/Medicaid patients.
- Services of: physician assistants, nurse practitioners, clinical nurse specialists, nurse midwives, certified registered nurse anesthetists, clinical psychologists, and clinical social workers.
- Ambulatory surgical center services.
- Home dialysis supplies and equipment paid under Method II (monthly capitation payment).

→ *When completing the **Workbook** assignments, check "yes."*

Medicare/Medicaid: Check "yes."

Medicare/Medigap: Check "yes."

MSP: Check "yes" or "no" to indicate whether the physician accepts assignment of benefits for primary insurance and Medicare.

→ *When completing the **Workbook** assignments, check "yes."*

TRICARE: Refer to Medicare guidelines. However, participation in TRICARE may be made on a case-by-case basis.

CHAMPVA: Refer to Medicare guidelines.

Workers' Compensation: Leave blank.

Block 28

25. FEDERAL TAX I.D. NUMBER	SSN EIN	26. PATIENT'S ACCOUNT NO.	27. ACCEPT ASSIGNMENT? (For govt. claims, see back)	28. TOTAL CHARGE	29. AMOUNT PAID	30. BALANCE DUE
74 10640XX	☐ ☒	010	☒ YES ☐ NO	$ 71 00	$	$ 70 92

31. SIGNATURE OF PHYSICIAN OR SUPPLIER INCLUDING DEGREES OR CREDENTIALS (I certify that the statements on the reverse apply to this bill and are made a part thereof.)	32. NAME AND ADDRESS OF FACILITY WHERE SERVICES WERE RENDERED (If other than home or office)	33. PHYSICIAN'S, SUPPLIER'S BILLING NAME, ADDRESS, ZIP CODE & PHONE #
CONCHA ANTRUM MD 030320XX	SAME	COLLEGE CLINIC 4567 BROAD AVENUE WOODLAND HILLS XY 12345 0001 555 486 9002
SIGNED *Concha Antrum MD* DATE		PIN# GRP# 3664021CC

reference initials

All Payers: Enter total charges for services listed in Block 24F. If more than one unit is listed in Block 24G, multiply the number of units by the charge and add the amount into the total charge. Do not enter dollar signs or decimal points. Always include cents.

Block 29

25. FEDERAL TAX I.D. NUMBER	SSN EIN	26. PATIENT'S ACCOUNT NO.	27. ACCEPT ASSIGNMENT? (For govt. claims, see back)	28. TOTAL CHARGE	29. AMOUNT PAID	30. BALANCE DUE
74 10640XX	☐ ☒X	010	☒ YES ☐ NO	$ 70 | 92	$	$ 70 | 92

31. SIGNATURE OF PHYSICIAN OR SUPPLIER INCLUDING DEGREES OR CREDENTIALS (I certify that the statements on the reverse apply to this bill and are made a part thereof.)	32. NAME AND ADDRESS OF FACILITY WHERE SERVICES WERE RENDERED (If other than home or office)	33. PHYSICIAN'S, SUPPLIER'S BILLING NAME, ADDRESS, ZIP CODE & PHONE #
CONCHA ANTRUM MD 030320XX	SAME	COLLEGE CLINIC 4567 BROAD AVENUE WOODLAND HILLS XY 12345 0001 555 486 9002
SIGNED *Concha Antrum MD* DATE		PIN# GRP# 3664021CC

reference initials

 All Private Payers: Enter only the amount paid for the charges listed on the claim.

 Medicaid: Enter only the payment on claim by a third-party payer, excluding Medicare.

 Medicare: Enter only the amount paid for the charges listed on the claim.
Medicare/Medicaid: Refer to Medicare guidelines.
Medicare/Medigap: Enter only the amount paid for the charges listed on the claim.
MSP: Enter only the amount paid for the charges listed on the claim. It is mandatory to enter amount paid by primary carrier and attach an explanation of benefits document when billing Medicare.

 TRICARE: Enter only amount paid by other carrier for the charges listed on the claim. If the amount includes payment by any other health insurance, the other health insurance explanation of benefits, work sheet, or denial showing the amounts paid must be attached to the claim. Payment from the beneficiary should not be included.

 CHAMPVA: Refer to TRICARE guidelines.

 Workers' Compensation: Leave blank.

Block 30

25. FEDERAL TAX I.D. NUMBER	SSN EIN	26. PATIENT'S ACCOUNT NO.	27. ACCEPT ASSIGNMENT? (For govt. claims, see back)	28. TOTAL CHARGE	29. AMOUNT PAID	30. BALANCE DUE
74 10640XX	☐ ☒	010	☒ YES ☐ NO	$ 70 | 92	$	$ 71 | 92

31. SIGNATURE OF PHYSICIAN OR SUPPLIER INCLUDING DEGREES OR CREDENTIALS (I certify that the statements on the reverse apply to this bill and are made a part thereof.)	32. NAME AND ADDRESS OF FACILITY WHERE SERVICES WERE RENDERED (If other than home or office)	33. PHYSICIAN'S, SUPPLIER'S BILLING NAME, ADDRESS, ZIP CODE & PHONE #
CONCHA ANTRUM MD 030320XX	SAME	COLLEGE CLINIC 4567 BROAD AVENUE WOODLAND HILLS XY 12345 0001 555 486 9002
SIGNED *Concha Antrum MD* DATE		PIN# GRP# 3664021CC

reference initials

 All Private Payers: Enter balance due on claim (Block 28 less Block 29).

 Medicaid: Leave blank or enter balance due on claim depending on individual state guidelines.
→ *When completing the **Workbook** assignments, enter the balance due.*

 Medicare: Leave blank.
Medicare/Medicaid: Leave blank.
Medicare/Medigap: Leave blank.
MSP: Leave blank.

 TRICARE: Enter balance due on claim (Block 28 less Block 29).

 CHAMPVA: Enter balance due on claim (Block 28 less Block 29).

 Workers' Compensation: Enter balance due on claim (Block 28 less Block 29).

Block 31

25. FEDERAL TAX I.D. NUMBER	SSN EIN	26. PATIENT'S ACCOUNT NO.	27. ACCEPT ASSIGNMENT? (For govt. claims, see back)	28. TOTAL CHARGE	29. AMOUNT PAID	30. BALANCE DUE
74 10640XX	☐ ☒	010	☒ YES ☐ NO	$ 70 | 92	$	$ 70 | 92

31. SIGNATURE OF PHYSICIAN OR SUPPLIER INCLUDING DEGREES OR CREDENTIALS (I certify that the statements on the reverse apply to this bill and are made a part thereof.)	32. NAME AND ADDRESS OF FACILITY WHERE SERVICES WERE RENDERED (If other than home or office)	33. PHYSICIAN'S, SUPPLIER'S BILLING NAME, ADDRESS, ZIP CODE & PHONE #
CONCHA ANTRUM MD 030320XX	SAME	COLLEGE CLINIC 4567 BROAD AVENUE WOODLAND HILLS XY 12345 0001 555 486 9002
SIGNED *Concha Antrum MD* DATE		PIN# GRP# 3664021CC

reference initials

All Payers: Type the provider's name and show the signature of the physician or the physician's representative above or below the name. Enter the eight-digit date the form was prepared. Most insurance carriers will accept a stamped signature, but the stamp must be completely inside the block. Do not type the name of the association or corporation.

In a computerized office environment, the participating contract with the third-party payer, including Medicare, Medicaid, and the Blue Plans, signed by the physician allows the physician's name to be printed in the signature block as it would normally be signed.

Block 32

25. FEDERAL TAX I.D. NUMBER	SSN EIN	26. PATIENT'S ACCOUNT NO.	27. ACCEPT ASSIGNMENT? (For govt. claims, see back)	28. TOTAL CHARGE	29. AMOUNT PAID	30. BALANCE DUE
74 10640XX	☐ ☒	010	☒ YES ☐ NO	$ 70 | 92	$	$ 70 | 92

31. SIGNATURE OF PHYSICIAN OR SUPPLIER INCLUDING DEGREES OR CREDENTIALS (I certify that the statements on the reverse apply to this bill and are made a part thereof.)	32. NAME AND ADDRESS OF FACILITY WHERE SERVICES WERE RENDERED (If other than home or office)	33. PHYSICIAN'S, SUPPLIER'S BILLING NAME, ADDRESS, ZIP CODE & PHONE #
CONCHA ANTRUM MD 030320XX SIGNED *Concha Antrum MD* DATE	SAME	COLLEGE CLINIC 4567 BROAD AVENUE WOODLAND HILLS XY 12345 0001 555 486 9002 PIN# GRP# 3664021CC

reference initials

All Private Payers: Enter the word "SAME" in the center of the block if the facility furnishing services is the same as that of the biller listed in Block 33. If other than home, office, nursing facility, or community mental health center, enter the name, address, and provider number of the facility (e.g., nursing home, rehabilitation center, or hospital name for physician's hospital services). For durable medical equipment, enter the location where the order is taken. If a test is performed by a mammography screening center, enter the six-digit certification number approved by the Food and Drug Administration (FDA). When billing for purchased diagnostic tests performed outside the physician's office but billed by the physician, enter the facility's name, address, and CMS-assigned NPI where the test was performed.

Medicaid: Refer to Medicare guidelines when completing this block; however, use Medicaid facility provider number.

Medicare: Enter "SAME" in the center of the block only if the facility furnishing services is the actual place of service. Medical practices that have multiple offices must show the address of where the service was rendered in Block 32. If other than home, office, nursing facility, or community mental health center, enter the name, address, and provider number of the facility (e.g., hospital name for physician's hospital services). For hospital services performed by a physician, the Medicare provider number must be preceded by "HSP." For durable medical equipment, enter the location where the order is taken. If the test is performed by a mammography screening center, enter the six-digit FDA-approved certification number. When billing for purchased diagnostic tests performed outside the physician's office but billed by the physician, enter the facility's name, address, and CMS-assigned NPI where the test was performed.
Medicare/Medicaid: Refer to Medicare guidelines.
Medicare/Medigap: Refer to Medicare guidelines.
MSP: Refer to Medicare guidelines.

TRICARE: Refer to private payer guidelines. For partnership providers, indicate the name of the Military Treatment Facility.

CHAMPVA: Refer to private payer guidelines.

Workers' Compensation: Refer to private payer guidelines.

Block 33

25. FEDERAL TAX I.D. NUMBER		SSN EIN	26. PATIENT'S ACCOUNT NO.	27. ACCEPT ASSIGNMENT? (For govt. claims, see back)	28. TOTAL CHARGE	29. AMOUNT PAID	30. BALANCE DUE
74 10640XX		☐ ☒	010	☒ YES ☐ NO	$ 70 | 92	$ |	$ 70 | 92
31. SIGNATURE OF PHYSICIAN OR SUPPLIER INCLUDING DEGREES OR CREDENTIALS (I certify that the statements on the reverse apply to this bill and are made a part thereof.)			32. NAME AND ADDRESS OF FACILITY WHERE SERVICES WERE RENDERED (If other than home or office)		33. PHYSICIAN'S, SUPPLIER'S BILLING NAME, ADDRESS, ZIP CODE & PHONE #		
CONCHA ANTRUM MD 030320XX			SAME		COLLEGE CLINIC 4567 BROAD AVENUE WOODLAND HILLS XY 12345 0001 555 486 9002		
SIGNED *Concha Antrum MD* DATE					PIN#	GRP# 3664021CC	

reference initials

All Private Payers: Refer to Medicare guidelines.

Medicaid: Refer to Medicare guidelines, except use Medicaid's facility provider number.

Medicare: Enter the name, address, and telephone number for the physician, clinic, or supplier billing for services. This is the address that the payment will be mailed to. Either enter the PIN/NPI for a performing physician or supplier who is not a member of a group practice in the lower left section of the block or enter the group number for a performing physician or supplier who belongs to a group practice and is billing under the group ID number in the right lower section of the block.
Medicare/Medicaid: Refer to Medicare guidelines.
Medicare/Medigap: Refer to Medicare guidelines.
MSP: Refer to Medicare guidelines.

TRICARE: Enter the name, address, and telephone number for the physician, clinic, or supplier billing for services. Radiologists, pathologists, and anesthesiologists may use their billing address if they have no physical address. Enter the physician's tax identification number (TIN) in the lower left section of the block; *the group number is not required.*

→ *When completing the Workbook assignments, enter the performing physician's NPI in the lower left section of the block.*

CHAMPVA: Refer to TRICARE guidelines.

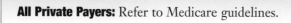

Workers' Compensation: Enter the name, address, and telephone number of the physician. Individual or group provider numbers or state license number generally are required depending on the insurance carrier's requirements.

→ *When completing Workbook assignments, follow Medicare guidelines.*

Bottom of Form Enter insurance billing specialist's initials in lower left corner of the insurance claim form.

Insurance Program Templates

The following pages show completed CMS-1500 insurance claim forms and templates for the most common insurance programs encountered in a medical practice. Screened areas on each form do not apply to the insurance program example shown and should be left blank. Add a tab at the page margin for ease in flipping to this reference section when completing *Workbook* assignments. Examples illustrating entries for basic cases are:

Figure 7–6 Private payer.

Figure 7–7 Back of CMS-1500 insurance claim form.

Figure 7-8 Medicaid.

Figure 7–9 Medicare.

Figure 7–10 Medicare/Medicaid—a crossover claim.

Figure 7–11 Medicare/Medigap—a crossover claim.

Figure 7–12 MSP—other insurance primary and Medicare secondary.

Figure 7–13 TRICARE—Standard.

Figure 7–14 CHAMPVA.

Figure 7–15 Workers' compensation.

INTERNET RESOURCES

Resources for audio tapes, books, newsletters, periodicals, software, and videotapes may be found in Appendix A.

- HIPAA regulations (information)
  Web site: **http://www.hhs.gov**

- Standard Code Set (rules and information for electronic claim submission)
  Web site: **http://www.aspe.hhs.gov/**

- UPIN access: Click "Professionals," click "UPIN Search," scroll down the list of states, enter the physician's name, and submit.
  Web site: **http://www.hgsa.com**

- Center for Medicare and Medicaid Services
  Web site: **http://www.cms.gov**

COMPUTER ASSIGNMENT

Do the exercises for Cases 1 through 6 using the AltaPoint software to review concepts you have learned for this chapter. These cases increase in difficulty. The cases use encounter forms from which you are required to abstract information. These forms are located in the *Workbook*.

STUDENT ASSIGNMENT

✔ Study Chapter 7.

✔ Answer the review questions in the *Workbook* to reinforce the theory learned in this chapter and to help prepare you for a future test.

✔ Complete the assignments in the *Workbook* to give you hands-on experience in abstracting information from case histories and financial accounting record cards as well as completing insurance claim forms.

✔ Study the claim sample in the *Workbook* and try to locate as many errors as possible based on the instructions you have been given in this chapter.

✔ Turn to the glossary at the end of this textbook for a further understanding of the key terms used in this chapter.

PRIVATE PAYER
No secondary coverage

PRIVATE INSURANCE COMPANY NAME
MAILING ADDRESS
CITY STATE ZIP CODE

1. MEDICARE	MEDICAID	CHAMPUS	CHAMPVA	GROUP HEALTH PLAN	FECA BLK LUNG	OTHER	1a. INSURED'S I.D. NUMBER	(FOR PROGRAM IN ITEM 1)
(Medicare #)	(Medicaid #)	(Sponsor's SSN)	(VA File #)	[X] (SSN or ID)	(SSN)	(ID)	111704521	A482

2. PATIENT'S NAME (Last Name, First Name, Middle Initial)
FOREHAND HARRY N

3. PATIENT'S BIRTH DATE MM 01 DD 06 YYYY 1946 SEX M [X] F ☐

4. INSURED'S NAME (Last Name, First Name, Middle Initial)
SAME

5. PATIENT'S ADDRESS (No., Street)
1456 MAIN STREET

6. PATIENT RELATIONSHIP TO INSURED
Self [X] Spouse ☐ Child ☐ Other ☐

7. INSURED'S ADDRESS (No., Street)

CITY WOODLAND HILLS   STATE XY

8. PATIENT STATUS
Single ☐ Married [X] Other ☐

CITY   STATE

ZIP CODE 12345 0000   TELEPHONE (include Area Code) (555) 490 9876

Employed [X] Full-Time Student ☐ Part-Time Student ☐

ZIP CODE   TELEPHONE (include Area Code) ( )

9. OTHER INSURED'S NAME (Last Name, First Name, Middle Initial)

10. IS PATIENT'S CONDITION RELATED TO:

11. INSURED'S POLICY GROUP OR FECA NUMBER

a. OTHER INSURED'S POLICY OR GROUP NUMBER

a. EMPLOYMENT? (CURRENT OR PREVIOUS)
YES ☐ NO [X]

a. INSURED'S DATE OF BIRTH MM DD YYYY   M ☐ SEX F ☐

b. OTHER INSURED'S DATE OF BIRTH MM DD YYYY   M ☐ SEX F ☐

b. AUTO ACCIDENT? PLACE (State)
YES ☐ NO [X]

b. EMPLOYER'S NAME OR SCHOOL NAME

c. EMPLOYER'S NAME OR SCHOOL NAME

c. OTHER ACCIDENT?
YES ☐ NO [X]

c. INSURANCE PLAN NAME OR PROGRAM NAME

d. INSURANCE PLAN NAME OR PROGRAM NAME

10d. RESERVED FOR LOCAL USE

d. IS THERE ANOTHER HEALTH BENEFIT PLAN?
YES ☐ NO [X]   If yes, return to and complete item 9 a-d.

READ BACK OF FORM BEFORE COMPLETING AND SIGNING THIS FORM.
12. PATIENT'S OR AUTHORIZED PERSON'S SIGNATURE I authorize the release of any medical or other information necessary to process this claim. I also request payment of government benefits either to myself or to the party who accepts assignment below.

SIGNED *Harry N. Forehand*   DATE *March 3, 20XX*

13. INSURED'S OR AUTHORIZED PERSON'S SIGNATURE I authorize payment of medical benefits to the undersigned physician or supplier for services described below.

SIGNED *Harry N. Forehand*

14. DATE OF CURRENT: MM 03 DD 01 YYYY 20XX   ILLNESS (First symptom) OR INJURY (Accident) OR PREGNANCY (LMP)

15. IF PATIENT HAS HAD SAME OR SIMILAR ILLNESS GIVE FIRST DATE MM DD YYYY

16. DATES PATIENT UNABLE TO WORK IN CURRENT OCCUPATION MM DD YYYY FROM   TO MM DD YYYY

17. NAME OF REFERRING PHYSICIAN OR OTHER SOURCE
PERRY CARDI MD

17a. I.D. NUMBER OF REFERRING PHYSICIAN
67805027XX

18. HOSPITALIZATION DATES RELATED TO CURRENT SERVICES MM DD YYYY FROM   TO MM DD YYYY

19. RESERVED FOR LOCAL USE

20. OUTSIDE LAB? $ CHARGES
YES ☐ NO [X]

21. DIAGNOSIS OR NATURE OF ILLNESS OR INJURY (RELATE ITEMS 1,2,3 OR 4 TO ITEM 24E BY LINE)
1. 38200   3.
2.   4.

22. MEDICAID RESUBMISSION CODE   ORIGINAL REF. NO.

23. PRIOR AUTHORIZATION NUMBER

24. A DATE(S) OF SERVICE From MM DD YYYY	To MM DD YYYY	B Place of Service	C Type of Service	D PROCEDURES, SERVICES, OR SUPPLIES (Explain Unusual Circumstances) CPT/HCPCS | MODIFIER	E DIAGNOSIS CODE	F $ CHARGES	G DAYS OR UNITS	H EPSDT Family Plan	I EMG	J COB	K RESERVED FOR LOCAL USE
030320XX		11		99203	1	71 00	1			12	45897700

25. FEDERAL TAX I.D. NUMBER SSN ☐ EIN [X]
74 1064090

26. PATIENT'S ACCOUNT NO.
010

27. ACCEPT ASSIGNMENT? (For govt. claims, see back)
YES [X] NO ☐

28. TOTAL CHARGE
$ 71 00

29. AMOUNT PAID
$

30. BALANCE DUE
$ 71 00

31. SIGNATURE OF PHYSICIAN OR SUPPLIER INCLUDING DEGREES OR CREDENTIALS (I certify that the statements on the reverse apply to this bill and are made a part thereof.)
CONCHA ANTRUM MD 030320XX

SIGNED *Concha Antrum MD* DATE

32. NAME AND ADDRESS OF FACILITY WHERE SERVICES WERE RENDERED (if other than home or office)
SAME

33. PHYSICIAN'S, SUPPLIER'S BILLING NAME, ADDRESS, ZIP CODE AND PHONE #
COLLEGE CLINIC
4567 BROAD AVENUE
WOODLAND HILLS XY 12345 0001
555 486 9002
PIN#   GRP# 3664021CC

reference initials

FIGURE 7–6 Front side of the scannable (red ink) Health Insurance Claim Form approved by the American Medical Association's Council on Medical Service. This form is also known as the CMS-1500 and is shown illustrating completion to a private insurance company with no secondary coverage. Third-party payer, state, and local guidelines vary and may not always follow the visual guide presented here. Screened blocks should not be completed for this type of case.

BECAUSE THIS FORM IS USED BY VARIOUS GOVERNMENT AND PRIVATE HEALTH PROGRAMS, SEE SEPARATE INSTRUCTIONS ISSUED BY APPLICABLE PROGRAMS.

NOTICE: Any person who knowingly files a statement of claim containing any misrepresentation or any false, incomplete or misleading information may be guilty of a criminal act punishable under law and may be subject to civil penalties.

REFERS TO GOVERNMENT PROGRAMS ONLY

MEDICARE AND TRICARE PAYMENT: A patient's signature requests that payment be made and authorizes release of any information necessary to process the claim and certifies that the information provided in Blocks 1 through 12 is true, accurate and complete. In the case of a Medicare claim, the patient's signature authorizes any entity to release to Medicare medical and nonmedical information, including employment status, and whether the person has employer group health insurance, liability, no-fault, worker's compensation or other insurance which is responsible to pay for the services for which the Medicare claim is made. See 42 CFR 411.24(a). If item 9 is completed, the patient's signature authorizes release of the information to the health plan or agency shown. In Medicare assigned or TRICARE participation cases, the physician agrees to accept the charge determination of the Medicare carrier or TRICARE fiscal intermediary as the full charge determination of the Medicare carrier or TRICARE fiscal intermediary if this is less than the charge submitted. TRICARE is not a health insurance program but makes payment for health benefits provided through certain affiliations with the Uniformed Services. Information on the patient's sponsor should be provided in those items captioned in "Insured', i.e., items 1a, 4, 6, 7, 9, and 11.

BLACK LUNG AND FECA CLAIMS

The provider agrees to accept the amount paid by the Government as payment in full. See Black Lung and FECA instructions regarding required procedure and diagnosis coding systems.

SIGNATURE OF PHYSICIAN OR SUPPLIER (MEDICARE, TRICARE, FECA AND BLACK LUNG)

I certify that the services shown on this form were medically indicated and necessary for the health of the patient and were personally furnished by me or were furnished incident to my professional service by my employee under my immediate supervision, except as otherwise expressly permitted by Medicare or TRICARE regulations.

For services to be considered as "incident" to a physician's professional service, 1) they must be rendered under the physician's immediate personal supervision by his/her employee, 2) they must be an integral, although incidental part of a covered physician's service, 3) they must be of kinds commonly furnished in physician's offices, and 4) the services of nonphysicians must be included on the physician's bills.

For TRICARE claims, I further certify that I (or any employee) who rendered services am not an active duty member of the Uniformed Services or a civilian employee of the United States Government or a contract employee of the United States Government, either civilian or military (refer to 5 USC 5536). For Black-Lung claims, I further certify that the services performed were for a Black Lung-related disorder.

No Part B Medicare benefits may be paid unless this form is received as required by existing law and regulations (42 CFR 424.32).

NOTICE: Any one who misrepresents or falsifies essential information to receive payment from Federal funds requested by this form may upon conviction be subject to fine and imprisonment under applicable Federal laws.

NOTICE TO PATIENT ABOUT THE COLLECTION AND USE OF MEDICARE, TRICARE, FECA, AND BLACK LUNG INFORMATION
(PRIVACY ACT STATEMENT)

We are authorized by CMS, TRICARE and OWCP to ask you for information needed in the administration of the Medicare, TRICARE, FECA, and Black Lung programs. Authority to collect information is in section 205(a), 1862, 1872 and 1874 of the Social Security Act as amended, 42 CFR411.24(a) and 424.5(a) (6), and 44 USC 3101; CFR 101 et seq and 10 USC 1079 and 1086; 5 USC 8101 et seq; and 30 USC 901 et seq; 38 USC 613; E.O. 9397.

The information we obtain to complete claims under these programs is used to identify you and to determine your eligibility. It is also used to decide if the services and supplies you received are covered by these programs and to insure that proper payment is made.

The information may also be given to other providers of services, carriers, intermediaries, medical review boards, health plans, and other organizations or Federal agencies, for the effective administration of Federal provisions that require other third parties payers to pay primary to Federal program, and as otherwise necessary to administer these programs. For example, it may be necessary to disclose information about the benefits you have used to a hospital or doctor. Additional disclosures are made through routine uses for information contained in systems of records.

FOR MEDICARE CLAIMS: See the notice modifying system No. 09-70-0501, titled 'Carrier Medicare Claims Record,' published in the Federal Register, Vol. 55 No. 177, page 37549, Wed., Sept. 12, 1990, or as updated and republished.

FOR OWCP CLAIMS: Department of Labor, Privacy Act of 1974, "Republication of Notice of Systems of Records," Federal Register, Vol. 55 No. 40, Wed., Feb. 28, 1990, See ESA-5, ESA-6, ESA-12, ESA-13, ESA-30, or as updated and republished.

FOR TRICARE CLAIMS: PRINCIPLE PURPOSE(S): To evaluate eligibility for medical care provided by civilian sources and to issue payment upon establishment of eligibility and determination that the services/supplies received are authorized by law.

ROUTINE USE(S): Information from claims and related documents may be given to the Dept. of Veterans Affairs, the Dept. of Health and Human Services and/or the Dept. of Transportation consistent with their statutory administrative responsibilities under TRICARE/CHAMPVA; to the Dept. of Justice for representation of the Secretary of Defense in civil actions; to the Internal Revenue Service, private collection agencies, and consumer reporting agencies in connection with recoupment claims; and to Congressional Offices in response to inquiries made at the request of the person to whom a record pertains. Appropriate disclosures may be made to other federal, state, local, foreign government agencies, private business entities, and individual providers of care, on matters relating to entitlement, claims adjudication, fraud, program abuse, utilization review, quality assurance, peer review, program integrity, third-party liability, coordination of benefits, and civil and criminal litigation related to the operation of TRICARE.

DISCLOSURES: Voluntary; however, failure to provide information will result in delay in payment or may result in denial of claim. With the one exception discussed below, there are no penalties under these programs for refusing to supply information. However, failure to furnish information regarding the medical services rendered or the amount charged would prevent payment of claims under these programs. Failure to furnish any other information, such as name or claim number, would delay payment of the claim. Failure to provide medical information under FECA could be deemed an obstruction.

It is mandatory that you tell us if you know that another party is responsible for paying for your treatment. Section 1128B of the Social Security Act and 31 USC 3801-3812 provide penalties for withholding this information.

You should be aware that P.L. 100-503, the "Computer Matching and Privacy Protection Act of 1988," permits the government to verify information by way of computer matches.

MEDICAID PAYMENTS (PROVIDER CERTIFICATION)

I hereby agree to keep such records as are necessary to disclose fully the extent of services provided to individuals under the State's Title XIX plan and to furnish information regarding any payments claimed for providing such services as the State Agency or Dept. of Health and Humans Services may request.

I further agree to accept, as payment in full, the amount paid by the Medicaid program for those claims submitted for payment under that program, with the exception of authorized deductible, coinsurance, co-payment or similar cost-sharing charge.

SIGNATURE OF PHYSICIAN (OR SUPPLIER): I certify that the services listed above were medically indicated and necessary to the health of this patient and were personally furnished by me or my employee under my personal direction.

NOTICE: This is to certify that the foregoing information is true, accurate and complete. I understand that payment and satisfaction of this claim will be from Federal and State funds, and that any false claims, statements, or documents, or concealment of a material fact, may be prosecuted under applicable Federal or State laws.

Public reporting burden for this collection of information is estimated to average 15 minutes per response, including time for reviewing instructions, searching existing date sources, gathering and maintaining data needed, and completing and reviewing the collection of information. Send comments regarding this burden estimate or any other aspect of this collection of information, including suggestions for reducing the burden, to CMS, Office of Financial Management, P.O. Box 26684, Baltimore, MD 21207; and to the Office of Management and Budget, Paperwork Reduction Project (OMB-0938-0008), Washington, D.C. 20503.

FIGURE 7–7 Back side of the CMS-1500 Health Insurance Claim Form approved by the American Medical Association's Council on Medical Service.

MEDICAID
No secondary coverage

MEDICAID FISCAL INTERMEDIARY NAME
MAILING ADDRESS
CITY STATE ZIP CODE

1. MEDICARE ☐ (Medicare #) MEDICAID ☒ (Medicaid #) CHAMPUS ☐ (Sponsor's SSN) CHAMPVA ☐ (VA File #) GROUP HEALTH PLAN ☐ (SSN or ID) FECA BLK LUNG ☐ (SSN) OTHER ☐ (ID)	1a. INSURED'S I.D. NUMBER (FOR PROGRAM IN ITEM 1) 276835090

2. PATIENT'S NAME (Last Name, First Name, Middle Initial) ABRAMSON ADAM	3. PATIENT'S BIRTH DATE MM 02 DD 12 YYYY 1995 SEX M ☒ F ☐
	4. INSURED'S NAME (Last Name, First Name, Middle Initial)
5. PATIENT'S ADDRESS (No., Street) 760 FINCH STREET	6. PATIENT RELATIONSHIP TO INSURED Self ☐ Spouse ☐ Child ☐ Other ☐
	7. INSURED'S ADDRESS (No., Street)
CITY WOODLAND HILLS STATE XY	8. PATIENT STATUS Single ☐ Married ☐ Other ☐
	CITY STATE
ZIP CODE 12345 TELEPHONE (include Area Code) (555) 482 6789	Employed ☐ Full-Time Student ☐ Part-Time Student ☐
	ZIP CODE TELEPHONE (include Area Code) ( )
9. OTHER INSURED'S NAME (Last Name, First Name, Middle Initial)	10. IS PATIENT'S CONDITION RELATED TO:	11. INSURED'S POLICY GROUP OR FECA NUMBER

a. OTHER INSURED'S POLICY OR GROUP NUMBER	a. EMPLOYMENT? (CURRENT OR PREVIOUS) YES ☐ NO ☒	a. INSURED'S DATE OF BIRTH MM DD YY SEX M ☐ F ☐
b. OTHER INSURED'S DATE OF BIRTH MM DD YYYY SEX M ☐ F ☐	b. AUTO ACCIDENT? PLACE (State) YES ☐ NO ☒	b. EMPLOYER'S NAME OR SCHOOL NAME
c. EMPLOYER'S NAME OR SCHOOL NAME	c. OTHER ACCIDENT? YES ☒ NO ☐	c. INSURANCE PLAN NAME OR PROGRAM NAME
d. INSURANCE PLAN NAME OR PROGRAM NAME	10d. RESERVED FOR LOCAL USE	d. IS THERE ANOTHER HEALTH BENEFIT PLAN? YES ☐ NO ☐ If yes, return to and complete item 9 a-d.

READ BACK OF FORM BEFORE COMPLETING AND SIGNING THIS FORM.

12. PATIENT'S OR AUTHORIZED PERSON'S SIGNATURE I authorize the release of any medical or other information necessary to process this claim. I also request payment of government benefits either to myself or to the party who accepts assignment below. SIGNED _____ DATE _____	13. INSURED'S OR AUTHORIZED PERSON'S SIGNATURE I authorize payment of medical benefits to the undersigned physician or supplier for services described below. SIGNED _____

14. DATE OF CURRENT: ILLNESS (First symptom) OR INJURY (Accident) OR PREGNANCY (LMP) MM DD YYYY	15. IF PATIENT HAS HAD SAME OR SIMILAR ILLNESS GIVE FIRST DATE MM DD YYYY	16. DATES PATIENT UNABLE TO WORK IN CURRENT OCCUPATION FROM MM DD YYYY TO MM DD YYYY
17. NAME OF REFERRING PHYSICIAN OR OTHER SOURCE	17a. I.D. NUMBER OF REFERRING PHYSICIAN	18. HOSPITALIZATION DATES RELATED TO CURRENT SERVICES FROM MM DD YYYY TO MM DD YYYY
19. RESERVED FOR LOCAL USE		20. OUTSIDE LAB? YES ☐ NO ☒ $ CHARGES
21. DIAGNOSIS OR NATURE OF ILLNESS OR INJURY (RELATE ITEMS 1,2,3 OR 4 TO ITEM 24E BY LINE) 1. 931 3. 2. 4.		22. MEDICAID RESUBMISSION CODE ORIGINAL REF. NO. 23. PRIOR AUTHORIZATION NUMBER

24. A. DATE(S) OF SERVICE				B. Place of Service	C. Type of Service	D. PROCEDURES, SERVICES, OR SUPPLIES (Explain Unusual Circumstances) CPT/HCPCS	MODIFIER	E. DIAGNOSIS CODE	F. $ CHARGES		G. DAYS OR UNITS	H. EPSDT Family Plan	I. EMG	J. COB	K. RESERVED FOR LOCAL USE
From MM DD YYYY		To MM DD YYYY													
07 14 20XX				23	1	99282		1	37	00	1		X		
07 14 20XX				23	2	69200		1	49	00	1		X		

25. FEDERAL TAX I.D. NUMBER 71 32061XX SSN ☐ EIN ☒	26. PATIENT'S ACCOUNT NO. 030	27. ACCEPT ASSIGNMENT? (For govt. claims, see back) YES ☒ NO ☐	28. TOTAL CHARGE $ 86 00	29. AMOUNT PAID $	30. BALANCE DUE $ 86 00
31. SIGNATURE OF PHYSICIAN OR SUPPLIER INCLUDING DEGREES OR CREDENTIALS (I certify that the statements on the reverse apply to this bill and are made a part thereof.) PEDRO ATRICS MD 071420XX SIGNED Pedro Atrics MD DATE	32. NAME AND ADDRESS OF FACILITY WHERE SERVICES WERE RENDERED (if other than home or office) COLLEGE HOSPITAL 4500 BROAD AVENUE WOODLAND HILLS XY 12345 0001 HSC 43700F		33. PHYSICIAN'S, SUPPLIER'S BILLING NAME, ADDRESS, ZIP CODE AND PHONE # COLLEGE CLINIC 4567 BROAD AVENUE WOODLAND HILLS XY 12345 0001 555 486 9002 PIN# GRP# HSC12345F

reference initials

FIGURE 7–8   A Medicaid case with no secondary coverage emphasizing basic elements and screened blocks that do not require completion.

MEDICARE
NO SECONDARY COVERAGE

MEDICARE FISCAL INTERMEDIARY NAME
MAILING ADDRESS
CITY STATE ZIP CODE

1. MEDICARE [X] (Medicare #) MEDICAID [ ] (Medicaid #) CHAMPUS [ ] (Sponsor's SSN) CHAMPVA [ ] (VA File #) GROUP HEALTH PLAN [ ] (SSN or ID) FECA BLK LUNG [ ] (SSN) OTHER [ ] (ID)	1a. INSURED'S I.D. NUMBER (FOR PROGRAM IN ITEM 1) 123 XX 6789A

2. PATIENT'S NAME (Last Name, First Name, Middle Initial)
HUTCH   BILL

3. PATIENT'S BIRTH DATE
MM 05 DD 07 YYYY 1910   SEX M [X] F [ ]

4. INSURED'S NAME (Last Name, First Name, Middle Initial)

5. PATIENT'S ADDRESS (No., Street)
8888 MAIN STREET

6. PATIENT RELATIONSHIP TO INSURED
Self [ ] Spouse [ ] Child [ ] Other [ ]

7. INSURED'S ADDRESS (No., Street)

CITY
WOODLAND HILLS   STATE XY

8. PATIENT STATUS
Single [X] Married [ ] Other [ ]
Employed [ ] Full-Time Student [ ] Part-Time Student [ ]

CITY   STATE

ZIP CODE 12345   TELEPHONE (include Area Code) (555) 732 1544

ZIP CODE   TELEPHONE (include Area Code) (   )

9. OTHER INSURED'S NAME (Last Name, First Name, Middle Initial)

10. IS PATIENT'S CONDITION RELATED TO:

11. INSURED'S POLICY GROUP OR FECA NUMBER
NONE

a. OTHER INSURED'S POLICY OR GROUP NUMBER

a. EMPLOYMENT? (CURRENT OR PREVIOUS)
YES [ ] NO [X]

a. INSURED'S DATE OF BIRTH
MM DD YY   SEX M [ ] F [ ]

b. OTHER INSURED'S DATE OF BIRTH
MM DD YYYY   SEX M [ ] F [ ]

b. AUTO ACCIDENT?   PLACE (State)
YES [ ] NO [X]

b. EMPLOYER'S NAME OR SCHOOL NAME

c. EMPLOYER'S NAME OR SCHOOL NAME

c. OTHER ACCIDENT?
YES [ ] NO [X]

c. INSURANCE PLAN NAME OR PROGRAM NAME

d. INSURANCE PLAN NAME OR PROGRAM NAME

10d. RESERVED FOR LOCAL USE

d. IS THERE ANOTHER HEALTH BENEFIT PLAN?
YES [ ] NO [ ] If yes, return to and complete item 9 a-d.

READ BACK OF FORM BEFORE COMPLETING AND SIGNING THIS FORM.
12. PATIENT'S OR AUTHORIZED PERSON'S SIGNATURE I authorize the release of any medical or other information necessary to process this claim. I also request payment of government benefits either to myself or to the party who accepts assignment below.

SIGNED   SOF   DATE

13. INSURED'S OR AUTHORIZED PERSON'S SIGNATURE I authorize payment of medical benefits to the undersigned physician or supplier for services described below.

SIGNED

14. DATE OF CURRENT: ILLNESS (First symptom) OR INJURY (Accident) OR PREGNANCY (LMP)
MM DD YYYY

15. IF PATIENT HAS HAD SAME OR SIMILAR ILLNESS GIVE FIRST DATE   MM DD YYYY

16. DATES PATIENT UNABLE TO WORK IN CURRENT OCCUPATION
FROM MM DD YYYY   TO MM DD YYYY

17. NAME OF REFERRING PHYSICIAN OR OTHER SOURCE
GERALD PRACTON MD

17a. I.D. NUMBER OF REFERRING PHYSICIAN
46278897XX

18. HOSPITALIZATION DATES RELATED TO CURRENT SERVICES
FROM MM DD YYYY   TO MM DD YYYY

19. RESERVED FOR LOCAL USE

20. OUTSIDE LAB?   YES [ ] NO [X] $ CHARGES

21. DIAGNOSIS OR NATURE OF ILLNESS OR INJURY (RELATE ITEMS 1,2,3 OR 4 TO ITEM 24E BY LINE)
1. 487 0   3.
2.   4.

22. MEDICAID RESUBMISSION CODE   ORIGINAL REF. NO.

23. PRIOR AUTHORIZATION NUMBER

24. A DATE(S) OF SERVICE From MM DD YYYY — To MM DD YYYY	B Place of Service	C Type of Service	D PROCEDURES, SERVICES, OR SUPPLIES (Explain Unusual Circumstances) CPT/HCPCS | MODIFIER	E DIAGNOSIS CODE	F $ CHARGES	G DAYS OR UNITS	H EPSDT Family Plan	I EMG	J COB	K RESERVED FOR LOCAL USE
03 10 20XX	11		99205	1	132 00	1			64	211067XX

25. FEDERAL TAX I.D. NUMBER   75 67321XX   SSN [ ] EIN [X]

26. PATIENT'S ACCOUNT NO.   040

27. ACCEPT ASSIGNMENT? (For govt. claims, see back)   YES [X] NO [ ]

28. TOTAL CHARGE $ 132 00

29. AMOUNT PAID $

30. BALANCE DUE $

31. SIGNATURE OF PHYSICIAN OR SUPPLIER INCLUDING DEGREES OR CREDENTIALS (I certify that the statements on the reverse apply to this bill and are made a part thereof.)
BRADY COCCIDIOIDES   031020XX
SIGNED   Brady Coccidioides MD   DATE

32. NAME AND ADDRESS OF FACILITY WHERE SERVICES WERE RENDERED (if other than home or office)
SAME

33. PHYSICIAN'S, SUPPLIER'S BILLING NAME, ADDRESS, ZIP CODE AND PHONE #
COLLEGE CLINIC
4567 BROAD AVENUE
WOODLAND HILLS XY 12345 0001
555 486 9002
PIN#   GRP# 3664021CC

reference initials

FIGURE 7-9 Example of a completed CMS-1500 Health Insurance Claim Form for a basic Medicare case with no other insurance coverage. The physician has accepted assignment. Screened blocks should not be completed for a Medicare case with no other insurance.

MEDICARE/MEDICAID
(primary) (secondary)
Crossover claim

MEDICARE FISCAL INTERMEDIARY NAME
MAILING ADDRESS
CITY STATE ZIP CODE

1. MEDICARE	MEDICAID	CHAMPUS	CHAMPVA	GROUP HEALTH PLAN	FECA BLK LUNG	OTHER	1a. INSURED'S I.D. NUMBER	(FOR PROGRAM IN ITEM 1)
X (Medicare #)	X (Medicaid #)	(Sponsor's SSN)	(VA File #)	(SSN or ID)	(SSN)	(ID)	660 XX 2715A	

2. PATIENT'S NAME (Last Name, First Name, Middle Initial)
JOHNSON KATHRYN

3. PATIENT'S BIRTH DATE MM 09 DD 07 YYYY 1937 M☐ SEX F ☒

4. INSURED'S NAME (Last Name, First Name, Middle Initial)

5. PATIENT'S ADDRESS (No., Street)
218 VEGA DRIVE

6. PATIENT RELATIONSHIP TO INSURED
Self☐ Spouse☐ Child☐ Other☐

7. INSURED'S ADDRESS (No., Street)

CITY WOODLAND HILLS STATE XY

8. PATIENT STATUS
Single☐ Married☒ Other☐
Employed☐ Full-Time Student☐ Part-Time Student☐

CITY   STATE

ZIP CODE 12345   TELEPHONE (include Area Code) (555) 482 9112

ZIP CODE   TELEPHONE (include Area Code) ( )

9. OTHER INSURED'S NAME (Last Name, First Name, Middle Initial)

10. IS PATIENT'S CONDITION RELATED TO:

11. INSURED'S POLICY GROUP OR FECA NUMBER
NONE

a. OTHER INSURED'S POLICY OR GROUP NUMBER

a. EMPLOYMENT? (CURRENT OR PREVIOUS)
☐YES ☒NO

a. INSURED'S DATE OF BIRTH MM DD YY   M☐ SEX F☐

b. OTHER INSURED'S DATE OF BIRTH MM DD YYYY   M☐ SEX F☐

b. AUTO ACCIDENT? PLACE (State)
☐YES ☒NO

b. EMPLOYER'S NAME OR SCHOOL NAME

c. EMPLOYER'S NAME OR SCHOOL NAME

c. OTHER ACCIDENT?
☐YES ☒NO

c. INSURANCE PLAN NAME OR PROGRAM NAME

d. INSURANCE PLAN NAME OR PROGRAM NAME

10d. RESERVED FOR LOCAL USE
MCD016745289

d. IS THERE ANOTHER HEALTH BENEFIT PLAN?
☐YES ☐NO If yes, return to and complete item 9 a-d.

READ BACK OF FORM BEFORE COMPLETING AND SIGNING THIS FORM.
12. PATIENT'S OR AUTHORIZED PERSON'S SIGNATURE I authorize the release of any medical or other information necessary to process this claim. I also request payment of government benefits either to myself or to the party who accepts assignment below.

SIGNED *Kathryn Johnson*   DATE *10/1/XX*

13. INSURED'S OR AUTHORIZED PERSON'S SIGNATURE I authorize payment of medical benefits to the undersigned physician or supplier for services described below.

SIGNED

14. DATE OF CURRENT: MM DD YYYY ◀ ILLNESS (First symptom) OR INJURY (Accident) OR PREGNANCY (LMP)

15. IF PATIENT HAS HAD SAME OR SIMILAR ILLNESS GIVE FIRST DATE MM DD YYYY

16. DATES PATIENT UNABLE TO WORK IN CURRENT OCCUPATION FROM MM DD YYYY TO MM DD YYYY

17. NAME OF REFERRING PHYSICIAN OR OTHER SOURCE
BRADY COCCIDIOIDES MD

17a. I.D. NUMBER OF REFERRING PHYSICIAN
64211067XX

18. HOSPITALIZATION DATES RELATED TO CURRENT SERVICES FROM MM DD YYYY TO MM DD YYYY

19. RESERVED FOR LOCAL USE

20. OUTSIDE LAB? ☐YES ☒NO $ CHARGES

21. DIAGNOSIS OR NATURE OF ILLNESS OR INJURY (RELATE ITEMS 1,2,3 OR 4 TO ITEM 24E BY LINE)
1. 172 7
2.
3.
4.

22. MEDICAID RESUBMISSION CODE   ORIGINAL REF. NO.

23. PRIOR AUTHORIZATION NUMBER
7680560012

24. A DATE(S) OF SERVICE From MM DD YYYY To MM DD YYYY	B Place of Service	C Type of Service	D PROCEDURES, SERVICES, OR SUPPLIES (Explain Unusual Circumstances) CPT/HCPCS MODIFIER	E DIAGNOSIS CODE	F $ CHARGES	G DAYS OR UNITS	H EPSDT Family Plan	I EMG	J COB	K RESERVED FOR LOCAL USE
100120XX	24		11600	1	195 00	1			50	307117XX

25. FEDERAL TAX I.D. NUMBER 74 6078 9XX SSN☐ EIN☒

26. PATIENT'S ACCOUNT NO. 050

27. ACCEPT ASSIGNMENT? (For govt. claims, see back) ☒YES ☐NO

28. TOTAL CHARGE $ 195 00

29. AMOUNT PAID $

30. BALANCE DUE $

31. SIGNATURE OF PHYSICIAN OR SUPPLIER INCLUDING DEGREES OR CREDENTIALS (I certify that the statements on the reverse apply to this bill and are made a part thereof.)
COSMO GRAFF MD
SIGNED *Cosmo Graff, MD* DATE 100320XX

32. NAME AND ADDRESS OF FACILITY WHERE SERVICES WERE RENDERED (if other than home or office)
WOODLAND HILLS AMBULATORY CENTER
1229 CENTER STREET
WOODLAND HILLS XY 12345 0001
95 0513700

33. PHYSICIAN'S, SUPPLIER'S BILLING NAME, ADDRESS, ZIP CODE AND PHONE #
COLLEGE CLINIC
4567 BROAD AVENUE
WOODLAND HILLS XY 12345 0001
555 486 9002
PIN#   GRP# 3664021CC

reference initials

FIGURE 7–10   Example of a Medicare/Medicaid crossover claim. The CMS-1500 claim form is sent to Medicare (primary payer) and then processed automatically by Medicaid (secondary payer). Screened blocks should not be completed for this type of case.

MEDICARE/MEDIGAP
(primary) (secondary)
Crossover claim

MEDICARE FISCAL INTERMEDIARY NAME
MAILING ADDRESS
CITY STATE ZIP CODE

1. MEDICARE	MEDICAID	CHAMPUS	CHAMPVA	GROUP HEALTH PLAN	FECA BLK LUNG	OTHER
[X] (Medicare #)	(Medicaid #)	(Sponsor's SSN)	(VA File #)	[X] (SSN or ID)	(SSN)	(ID)

1a. INSURED'S I.D. NUMBER (FOR PROGRAM IN ITEM 1)
419 XX 7272A

2. PATIENT'S NAME (Last Name, First Name, Middle Initial)
BARNES AGUSTA E

3. PATIENT'S BIRTH DATE   MM 08 DD 29 YYYY 1917   SEX M [X] F

4. INSURED'S NAME (Last Name, First Name, Middle Initial)

5. PATIENT'S ADDRESS (No., Street)
356 ENCINA AVENUE

6. PATIENT RELATIONSHIP TO INSURED
Self ☐ Spouse ☐ Child ☐ Other ☐

7. INSURED'S ADDRESS (No., Street)

CITY
WOODLAND HILLS   STATE XY

8. PATIENT STATUS
Single [X] Married ☐ Other ☐
Employed ☐ Full-Time Student ☐ Part-Time Student ☐

CITY   STATE

ZIP CODE 12345 0000   TELEPHONE (include Area Code) (555) 467 2646

ZIP CODE   TELEPHONE (include Area Code) ( )

9. OTHER INSURED'S NAME (Last Name, First Name, Middle Initial)
SAME

10. IS PATIENT'S CONDITION RELATED TO:

11. INSURED'S POLICY GROUP OR FECA NUMBER
NONE

a. OTHER INSURED'S POLICY OR GROUP NUMBER
MEDIGAP 419167272

a. EMPLOYMENT? (CURRENT OR PREVIOUS)
YES ☐ [X] NO

a. INSURED'S DATE OF BIRTH   MM DD YY   SEX M ☐ F ☐

b. OTHER INSURED'S DATE OF BIRTH   MM DD YYYY   SEX M ☐ F ☐

b. AUTO ACCIDENT?   PLACE (State)
YES ☐ [X] NO

b. EMPLOYER'S NAME OR SCHOOL NAME

c. EMPLOYER'S NAME OR SCHOOL NAME

c. OTHER ACCIDENT?
YES ☐ [X] NO

c. INSURANCE PLAN NAME OR PROGRAM NAME

d. INSURANCE PLAN NAME OR PROGRAM NAME
CALFCA002

10d. RESERVED FOR LOCAL USE

d. IS THERE ANOTHER HEALTH BENEFIT PLAN?
YES ☐ NO ☐ *If yes*, return to and complete item 9 a-d.

READ BACK OF FORM BEFORE COMPLETING AND SIGNING THIS FORM.

12. PATIENT'S OR AUTHORIZED PERSON'S SIGNATURE I authorize the release of any medical or other information necessary to process this claim. I also request payment of government benefits either to myself or to the party who accepts assignment below.
SIGNED *Agusta E. Barnes*   DATE *11/21/XX*

13. INSURED'S OR AUTHORIZED PERSON'S SIGNATURE I authorize payment of medical benefits to the undersigned physician or supplier for services described below.
SIGNED *Agusta E. Barnes*

14. DATE OF CURRENT: MM DD YYYY   ◄ ILLNESS (First symptom) OR INJURY (Accident) OR PREGNANCY (LMP)

15. IF PATIENT HAS HAD SAME OR SIMILAR ILLNESS GIVE FIRST DATE   MM DD YYYY

16. DATES PATIENT UNABLE TO WORK IN CURRENT OCCUPATION   MM DD YYYY   FROM   TO   MM DD YYYY

17. NAME OF REFERRING PHYSICIAN OR OTHER SOURCE
GASTON INPUT MD

17a. I.D. NUMBER OF REFERRING PHYSICIAN
32783127XX

18. HOSPITALIZATION DATES RELATED TO CURRENT SERVICES   MM DD YYYY   FROM   TO   MM DD YYYY

19. RESERVED FOR LOCAL USE

20. OUTSIDE LAB?   YES ☐ [X] NO $ CHARGES

21. DIAGNOSIS OR NATURE OF ILLNESS OR INJURY (RELATE ITEMS 1,2,3 OR 4 TO ITEM 24E BY LINE)
1. 78659   3.
2.   4.

22. MEDICAID RESUBMISSION CODE   ORIGINAL REF. NO.

23. PRIOR AUTHORIZATION NUMBER

24. A. DATE(S) OF SERVICE							B. Place of Service	C. Type of Service	D. PROCEDURES, SERVICES, OR SUPPLIES (Explain Unusual Circumstances) CPT/HCPCS	MODIFIER	E. DIAGNOSIS CODE	F. $ CHARGES		G. DAYS OR UNITS	H. EPSDT Family Plan	I. EMG	J. COB	K. RESERVED FOR LOCAL USE
From MM	DD	YYYY	To MM	DD	YYYY													
11	21	20XX					11		93350		1	183	00	1			67	805027XX
11	21	20XX					11		93017		1	68	00	1			67	805027XX

25. FEDERAL TAX I.D. NUMBER   70 64217XX   SSN ☐ EIN [X]

26. PATIENT'S ACCOUNT NO.   060

27. ACCEPT ASSIGNMENT? (For govt. claims, see back)   [X] YES ☐ NO

28. TOTAL CHARGE $ 251 00

29. AMOUNT PAID $

30. BALANCE DUE $

31. SIGNATURE OF PHYSICIAN OR SUPPLIER INCLUDING DEGREES OR CREDENTIALS (I certify that the statements on the reverse apply to this bill and are made a part thereof.)
PERRY CARDI MD
SIGNED *Perry Cardi, MD*   112220XX   DATE

32. NAME AND ADDRESS OF FACILITY WHERE SERVICES WERE RENDERED (if other than home or office)
SAME

33. PHYSICIAN'S, SUPPLIER'S BILLING NAME, ADDRESS, ZIP CODE AND PHONE #
COLLEGE CLINIC
4567 BROAD AVENUE
WOODLAND HILLS XY 12345 0001
555 486 9002
PIN#   GRP# 3664021CC

reference initials

FIGURE 7–11 Example of a completed CMS-1500 Health Insurance Claim Form for a Medicare (primary) and Medigap (secondary) crossover claim. Shaded blocks should not be completed for this type of case.

OTHER INSURANCE/MEDICARE-MSP
(primary)   (secondary)

OTHER INSURANCE COMPANY NAME
MAILING ADDRESS
CITY STATE ZIP CODE

1. MEDICARE	MEDICAID	CHAMPUS	CHAMPVA	GROUP HEALTH PLAN	FECA BLK LUNG	OTHER	1a. INSURED'S I.D. NUMBER (FOR PROGRAM IN ITEM 1)
[X] (Medicare #)	[ ] (Medicaid #)	[ ] (Sponsor's SSN)	[ ] (VA File #)	[X] (SSN or ID)	[ ] (SSN)	[ ] (ID)	609 XX 5523A

2. PATIENT'S NAME (Last Name, First Name, Middle Initial)
BLAIR GWENDOLYN

3. PATIENT'S BIRTH DATE MM 09 DD 01 YYYY 1931 M [ ] SEX F [X]

4. INSURED'S NAME (Last Name, First Name, Middle Initial)
BLAIR GWENDOLYN

5. PATIENT'S ADDRESS (No., Street)
416 RICHMOND STREET

6. PATIENT RELATIONSHIP TO INSURED
Self [X] Spouse [ ] Child [ ] Other [ ]

7. INSURED'S ADDRESS (No., Street)
SAME

CITY WOODLAND HILLS   STATE XY

8. PATIENT STATUS
Single [ ] Married [X] Other [ ]
Employed [X] Full-Time Student [ ] Part-Time Student [ ]

CITY   STATE

ZIP CODE 12345 0000   TELEPHONE (include Area Code) (555) 459 1519

ZIP CODE   TELEPHONE (include Area Code) ( )

9. OTHER INSURED'S NAME (Last Name, First Name, Middle Initial)

10. IS PATIENT'S CONDITION RELATED TO:

11. INSURED'S POLICY GROUP OR FECA NUMBER
7845931Q

a. OTHER INSURED'S POLICY OR GROUP NUMBER

a. EMPLOYMENT? (CURRENT OR PREVIOUS)
[ ] YES [X] NO

a. INSURED'S DATE OF BIRTH MM DD YY   M [ ] SEX F [ ]

b. OTHER INSURED'S DATE OF BIRTH MM DD YYYY M [ ] SEX F [ ]

b. AUTO ACCIDENT?   PLACE (State)
[ ] YES [X] NO

b. EMPLOYER'S NAME OR SCHOOL NAME
CITY LIBRARY

c. EMPLOYER'S NAME OR SCHOOL NAME

c. OTHER ACCIDENT?
[ ] YES [X] NO

c. INSURANCE PLAN NAME OR PROGRAM NAME
ABC INSURANCE COMPANY

d. INSURANCE PLAN NAME OR PROGRAM NAME

10d. RESERVED FOR LOCAL USE

d. IS THERE ANOTHER HEALTH BENEFIT PLAN?
[ ] YES [ ] NO   If yes, return to and complete item 9 a-d.

READ BACK OF FORM BEFORE COMPLETING AND SIGNING THIS FORM.
12. PATIENT'S OR AUTHORIZED PERSON'S SIGNATURE I authorize the release of any medical or other information necessary to process this claim. I also request payment of government benefits either to myself or to the party who accepts assignment below.

SIGNED SOF   DATE

13. INSURED'S OR AUTHORIZED PERSON'S SIGNATURE I authorize payment of medical benefits to the undersigned physician or supplier for services described below.

SIGNED SOF

14. DATE OF CURRENT: MM DD YYYY ◀ ILLNESS (First symptom) OR INJURY (Accident) OR PREGNANCY (LMP)

15. IF PATIENT HAS HAD SAME OR SIMILAR ILLNESS GIVE FIRST DATE MM DD YYYY

16. DATES PATIENT UNABLE TO WORK IN CURRENT OCCUPATION
FROM MM DD YYYY TO MM DD YYYY

17. NAME OF REFERRING PHYSICIAN OR OTHER SOURCE
GERALD PRACTON MD

17a. I.D. NUMBER OF REFERRING PHYSICIAN
46278897XX

18. HOSPITALIZATION DATES RELATED TO CURRENT SERVICES
FROM MM DD YYYY TO MM DD YYYY

19. RESERVED FOR LOCAL USE

20. OUTSIDE LAB? $ CHARGES
[ ] YES [X] NO

21. DIAGNOSIS OR NATURE OF ILLNESS OR INJURY (RELATE ITEMS 1,2,3 OR 4 TO ITEM 24E BY LINE)
1. 110 1   3.
2.   4.

22. MEDICAID RESUBMISSION CODE   ORIGINAL REF. NO.

23. PRIOR AUTHORIZATION NUMBER

24. A DATE(S) OF SERVICE From MM DD YYYY	To MM DD YYYY	B Place of Service	C Type of Service	D PROCEDURES, SERVICES, OR SUPPLIES (Explain Unusual Circumstances) CPT/HCPCS	MODIFIER	E DIAGNOSIS CODE	F $ CHARGES	G DAYS OR UNITS	H EPSDT Family Plan	I EMG	J COB	K RESERVED FOR LOCAL USE
031520XX		11		99243	25	1	103 00	1			54	022287XX
031520XX		11		11750		1	193 00	1			54	022287XX

25. FEDERAL TAX I.D. NUMBER 62 74109XX   SSN [ ] EIN [X]

26. PATIENT'S ACCOUNT NO. 070

27. ACCEPT ASSIGNMENT? (For govt. claims, see back) [X] YES [ ] NO

28. TOTAL CHARGE $ 296 00

29. AMOUNT PAID $ 100 00

30. BALANCE DUE $

31. SIGNATURE OF PHYSICIAN OR SUPPLIER INCLUDING DEGREES OR CREDENTIALS (I certify that the statements on the reverse apply to this bill and are made a part thereof.)
NICK PEDRO DPM   031620XX
SIGNED Nick Pedro, DPM DATE

32. NAME AND ADDRESS OF FACILITY WHERE SERVICES WERE RENDERED (if other than home or office)
SAME

33. PHYSICIAN'S, SUPPLIER'S BILLING NAME, ADDRESS, ZIP CODE AND PHONE #
COLLEGE CLINIC
4567 BROAD AVENUE
WOODLAND HILLS XY 12345 0001
555 486 9002
PIN#   GRP# 3664021CC

reference initials

FIGURE 7–12   Template for a case in which another insurance company is the primary payer and Medicare is the secondary payer (MSP).

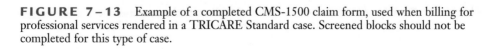

FIGURE 7–13 Example of a completed CMS-1500 claim form, used when billing for professional services rendered in a TRICARE Standard case. Screened blocks should not be completed for this type of case.

CHAMPVA
No secondary coverage

CHAMPVA INSURANCE COMPANY NAME
MAILING ADDRESS
CITY STATE ZIP CODE

1. MEDICARE	MEDICAID	CHAMPUS	CHAMPVA	GROUP HEALTH PLAN	FECA BLK LUNG	OTHER	1a. INSURED'S I.D. NUMBER	(FOR PROGRAM IN ITEM 1)
☐ (Medicare #)	☐ (Medicaid #)	☐ (Sponsor's SSN)	☒ (VA File #)	☐ (SSN or ID)	☐ (SSN)	☐ (ID)	560 XX 4444	

2. PATIENT'S NAME (Last Name, First Name, Middle Initial)	3. PATIENT'S BIRTH DATE	SEX	4. INSURED'S NAME (Last Name, First Name, Middle Initial)
DEXTER BRUCE R	MM 03 DD 13 YYYY 1934	M ☒ F ☐	DEXTER BRUCE R

5. PATIENT'S ADDRESS (No., Street)	6. PATIENT RELATIONSHIP TO INSURED	7. INSURED'S ADDRESS (No., Street)
226 IRWIN ROAD	Self ☒ Spouse ☐ Child ☐ Other ☐	SAME

CITY	STATE	8. PATIENT STATUS	CITY	STATE
WOODLAND HILLS	XY	Single ☒ Married ☐ Other ☐		

ZIP CODE	TELEPHONE (include Area Code)		ZIP CODE	TELEPHONE (include Area Code)
12345 0000	(555) 497 1338	Employed ☐ Full-Time Student ☐ Part-Time Student ☐		( )

9. OTHER INSURED'S NAME (Last Name, First Name, Middle Initial)	10. IS PATIENT'S CONDITION RELATED TO:	11. INSURED'S POLICY GROUP OR FECA NUMBER
		023

a. OTHER INSURED'S POLICY OR GROUP NUMBER	a. EMPLOYMENT? (CURRENT OR PREVIOUS)	a. INSURED'S DATE OF BIRTH	SEX
	☒ YES ☐ NO	MM DD YY	M ☐ F ☐

b. OTHER INSURED'S DATE OF BIRTH	SEX	b. AUTO ACCIDENT? PLACE (State)	b. EMPLOYER'S NAME OR SCHOOL NAME
MM DD YYYY	M ☐ F ☐	☐ YES ☒ NO	USAF

c. EMPLOYER'S NAME OR SCHOOL NAME	c. OTHER ACCIDENT?	c. INSURANCE PLAN NAME OR PROGRAM NAME
	☐ YES ☒ NO	

d. INSURANCE PLAN NAME OR PROGRAM NAME	10d. RESERVED FOR LOCAL USE	d. IS THERE ANOTHER HEALTH BENEFIT PLAN?
		☐ YES ☒ NO If yes, return to and complete item 9 a-d.

READ BACK OF FORM BEFORE COMPLETING AND SIGNING THIS FORM.

12. PATIENT'S OR AUTHORIZED PERSON'S SIGNATURE I authorize the release of any medical or other information necessary to process this claim. I also request payment of government benefits either to myself or to the party who accepts assignment below.

SIGNED ___SOF___ DATE _____

13. INSURED'S OR AUTHORIZED PERSON'S SIGNATURE I authorize payment of medical benefits to the undersigned physician or supplier for services described below.

SIGNED _____

14. DATE OF CURRENT: ILLNESS (First symptom) OR INJURY (Accident) OR PREGNANCY (LMP)	15. IF PATIENT HAS HAD SAME OR SIMILAR ILLNESS GIVE FIRST DATE MM DD YYYY	16. DATES PATIENT UNABLE TO WORK IN CURRENT OCCUPATION
MM DD YYYY		FROM MM DD YYYY TO MM DD YYYY

17. NAME OF REFERRING PHYSICIAN OR OTHER SOURCE	17a. I.D. NUMBER OF REFERRING PHYSICIAN	18. HOSPITALIZATION DATES RELATED TO CURRENT SERVICES
GERALD PRACTON MD	C01402X	FROM MM 07 DD 29 YYYY 20XX TO MM 07 DD 31 YYYY 20XX

19. RESERVED FOR LOCAL USE	20. OUTSIDE LAB?	$ CHARGES
	☐ YES ☒ NO	

21. DIAGNOSIS OR NATURE OF ILLNESS OR INJURY (RELATE ITEMS 1,2,3 OR 4 TO ITEM 24E BY LINE)

1. 600 0   3. |_____
2. |_____   4. |_____

22. MEDICAID RESUBMISSION CODE	ORIGINAL REF. NO.

23. PRIOR AUTHORIZATION NUMBER

24. A. DATE(S) OF SERVICE		B. Place of Service	C. Type of Service	D. PROCEDURES, SERVICES, OR SUPPLIES (Explain Unusual Circumstances)		E. DIAGNOSIS CODE	F. $ CHARGES		G. DAYS OR UNITS	H. EPSDT Family Plan	I. EMG	J. COB	K. RESERVED FOR LOCAL USE
From MM DD YYYY	To MM DD YYYY			CPT/HCPCS	MODIFIER								
072920XX		21	2	52601		1	1193	00	1				C06430X

25. FEDERAL TAX I.D. NUMBER	SSN EIN	26. PATIENT'S ACCOUNT NO.	27. ACCEPT ASSIGNMENT? (For govt. claims, see back)	28. TOTAL CHARGE	29. AMOUNT PAID	30. BALANCE DUE
77 86531XX	☐ ☒	090	☒ YES ☐ NO	$ 1193 00	$	$ 1193 00

31. SIGNATURE OF PHYSICIAN OR SUPPLIER INCLUDING DEGREES OR CREDENTIALS (I certify that the statements on the reverse apply to this bill and are made a part thereof.)	32. NAME AND ADDRESS OF FACILITY WHERE SERVICES WERE RENDERED (if other than home or office)	33. PHYSICIAN'S, SUPPLIER'S BILLING NAME, ADDRESS, ZIP CODE AND PHONE #
GENE ULIBARRI MD 073020XX SIGNED *Gene Ulibarri* DATE	COLLEGE HOSPITAL 4500 BROAD AVENUE WOODLAND HILLS XY 12345 0001 95 0731067	COLLEGE CLINIC 4567 BROAD AVENUE WOODLAND HILLS XY 12345 0001 555 486 9002 PIN# 7786531XX GRP#

reference initials

FIGURE 7–14 An example of a completed CMS-1500 Health Insurance Claim Form for a CHAMPVA case with no secondary coverage. Screened blocks should not be completed for this type of case.

FIGURE 7–15 An example of a completed CMS-1500 Health Insurance Claim Form for a workers' compensation case. Screened blocks should not be completed for this type of case.

CHAPTER OUTLINE

ELECTRONIC DATA INTERCHANGE
ELECTRONIC CLAIMS
ADVANTAGES OF ELECTRONIC CLAIM SUBMISSION
CLEARINGHOUSES
TRANSACTION AND CODE SET REGULATIONS: STREAMLINING ELECTRONIC DATA INTERCHANGE
   Transaction and Code Set Standards
TRANSITION FROM PAPER CMS-1500 TO ELECTRONIC STANDARD HIPAA 837
   Levels of Information for 837P Standard Transaction Format
CLAIMS ATTACHMENTS STANDARDS
   Standard Unique Identifiers

PRACTICE MANAGEMENT SYSTEM
BUILDING THE CLAIM
   Encounter or Multipurpose Billing Forms
   Scannable Encounter Form
   Keying Insurance Data for Claim Transmission
   Encoder
   Clean Electronic Claims Submission
PUTTING HIPAA STANDARD TRANSACTIONS TO WORK
   Interactive Transactions
ELECTRONIC REMITTANCE ADVICE
DRIVING THE DATA
METHODS FOR SENDING CLAIMS

COMPUTER CLAIMS SYSTEMS
   Payer or Carrier-Direct
   Clearinghouse
TRANSMISSION REPORTS
   Electronic Processing Problems
   Billing and Account Management Schedule
   Administrative Simplification Enforcement Tool (ASET)
   The Security Rule: Administrative, Physical, and Technical Safeguards
HIPAA: APPLICATION TO THE PRACTICE SETTING
COMPUTER CONFIDENTIALITY
   Confidentiality Statement
   Prevention Measures
RECORDS MANAGEMENT
   Data Storage
   Electronic Power Protection

KEY TERMS

application service provider (ASP)

Accredited Standards Committee X12 (ASC X12)

back up

batch

business associate agreement

cable modem

clearinghouse

code sets

covered entity

data elements

direct data entry (DDE)

digital subscriber line (DSL)

electronic data interchange (EDI)

electronic funds transfer (EFT)

electronic remittance advice (ERA)

encoder

encryption

HIPAA Transaction and Code Set (TCS)—Rule

National Standard Format (NSF)

password

real time

standard transactions

T-1

taxonomy codes

trading partner agreement

8

Electronic Data Interchange: Transactions and Security

OBJECTIVES*

After reading this chapter, you should be able to:

- Understand HIPAA requirements for electronic claims.

- Identify the transactions and code sets to use for insurance claims transmission.

- Create a successful insurance claim for submission and reimbursement.

- State HIPAA Security Rule compliance guidelines for electronic protected health information.

- Describe necessary components when adopting a practice management system.

- Explain the difference between carrier-direct and clearinghouse electronically transmitted insurance claims.

- State measures used to secure privacy of electronic mail, Internet, and instant messaging.

- Describe the use of patient encounter forms, crib sheets, and scannable encounter forms in electronic claim submission.

- List computer transmission problems that can occur.

- Name some types of interactive computer transactions.

*Performance objectives and exercises for hands-on practical experience for this chapter appear in the *Workbook*.

ELECTRONIC DATA INTERCHANGE

Technology and the use of **electronic data interchange (EDI)** has made the processing of transactions more efficient and reduced administrative overhead costs in other industries. EDI is the exchange of data in a standardized format through computer systems (e.g., health insurance claims). This is a process by which understandable data are sent back and forth via computer linkages between entities that function alternatively as sender and receiver. Electronic transmissions are sent encrypted so that they cannot be opened and read if intercepted (received) by the wrong individual. **Encryption** is used to assign a code to represent data and is done for security purposes. This "secret code" makes data unintelligible to unauthorized parties. In encrypted (encoded) versions, the data look like gibberish to unauthorized users and must be decoded to be used or read. In electronically secure environments, the sending computer system encrypts/encodes the data being sent and the receiving computer decodes the data to make it understandable. Therefore, both computers must speak the same "language." Standardizing transactions and codes sets is required to use EDI effectively, so the industry has witnessed the implementation of standard formats, procedures, and data content through Health Insurance Portability and Accountability Act (HIPAA) regulations.

ELECTRONIC CLAIMS

An electronic claim, like a paper claim, is constructed from data that are used in the reimbursement process (the life cycle of a claim is discussed in Chapter 3). However, the method for submitting an electronic claim is by means of EDI rather than U.S. Postal Service ("snail mail") or paper fax transmission.

In the 1960s and early 1970s, large hospitals began submitting electronic claims for payment to insurance carriers. Today, most health care providers submit electronic claims for reimbursement. As the Medicare program has expanded, thereby increasing the number of covered individuals, the Centers for Medicaid and Medicare Services (CMS) began to emphasize electronic claims submission to reduce the number of paper claims and administrative costs. This system of transmission was practical only for hospitals and large medical practices, because some carriers required 25 or more claims per batch. A **batch** is a group of claims for different patients sent at the same time from one facility.

ADVANTAGES OF ELECTRONIC CLAIM SUBMISSION

Nearly all insurance companies are required under HIPAA to participate in the electronic claim processing standards.

Unlike paper claims, electronic transactions require no signature or stamp, no search for an insurance carrier's address, no postage fees or trips to the post office, and no storage of claim forms in a file cabinet. Electronic transactions build an audit trail, a chronological record of submitted data that can be traced to the source to determine the place of origin. Generally cash flow is improved and less time is spent processing claims, thereby freeing staff for other duties. Information goes from one computer to another, which reduces overhead by decreasing labor costs and human error. After electronic submission of claims, payment can be received in 2 weeks or less. In comparison, when claims are completed manually and sent by mail, payment may take 4 to 6 weeks on average. With EDI, the audit trail offers a proof of receipt and is generated by the carrier, thus eliminating the potential for insurance payers to make the excuse that the claim was never received and therefore not processed.

Another important advantage of electronic claims submission is the online error-edit process that may be incorporated into the software in the physician's office, clearinghouse, or insurance company. This feature alerts the person processing the claim to any errors immediately so a correction can be made before transmission of the claim. Information about problem claims can be telecommunicated immediately, allowing quicker submission of corrected or additional data.

Both paper and electronic claims begin with gathering data before, during, and after the service is rendered. You have learned that the information you need to obtain is crucial when submitting a paper claim for payment; therefore accurate information is key to successful electronic claim submission and timely reimbursement.

CLEARINGHOUSES

For a seamless business process, a **clearinghouse** is an entity that receives the electronic transmission of claims (EDI) from the health care provider's office and translates it into a standard format prescribed in HIPAA regulations. This HIPAA standard is readable by the processing parties (insurance payers) to complete the reimbursement cycle. The clearinghouse's duties include separating the claims by carrier, performing software edits on each claim to check for errors, and transmitting claims electronically to the correct insurance payer (Figure 8–1).

After receiving the claims transmission, a typical clearinghouse process works as follows:

● Claims are checked electronically (scrubbed) for missing or incorrect information using an elaborate editing process. Claims that do not meet all required data for

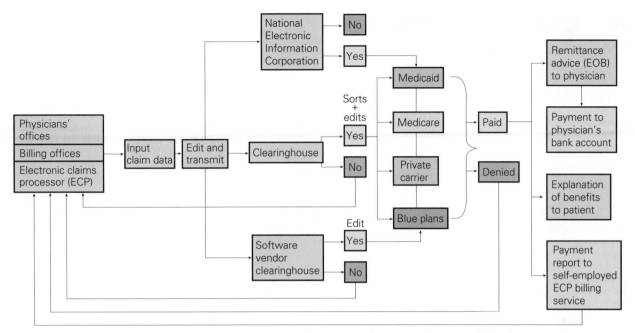

FIGURE 8–1 Flow sheet of electronic transmission systems showing path for claim payment via the National Electronic Information Corporation (NEIC), clearinghouse, and independent software vendor. This system also indicates when payment is made to physician and depicts locations where claims may not pass an edit or are denied.

further processing are rejected and not forwarded to the payer.

● Groups of batches of claims that pass all edits are then sent to each separate insurance payer. Several claims can be submitted to various insurance payers in a single batch electronic transmission.

● Claims that are rejected during the editing process are electronically sent back to the health care provider along with a report that lists needed corrections.

● Once corrections are made, the claims can then be resubmitted for processing and go through the same previous edits to ensure the correct data are present.

Some medical practices have direct links to the insurance companies and do not use the services of a clearinghouse.

CMS has a Medicare Transaction System (MTS) for Part A (hospital services) and Part B (outpatient medical services) claims processing. This system replaces the numerous software programs formerly used by Medicare's claims processing contractors with a national electronic standard program. The system is used for nearly all Medicare transactions, including claims submission, called electronic medical claims (EMC), payment, direct deposit, online eligibility verification, coordination of benefits, and claims status.

Using a clearinghouse offers several advantages:

● Translation of various formats to the HIPAA-compliant standard format

● Reduction in time of claims preparation
● Cost-effective method through loss prevention
● Fewer claim rejections
● Fewer delays in processing and quicker response time
● More accurate coding with claims edits
● Consistent reimbursement

TRANSACTION AND CODE SET REGULATIONS: STREAMLINING ELECTRONIC DATA INTERCHANGE

The **HIPAA Transaction and Code Set (TCS) Rule** was developed to introduce efficiencies into the health care system. The objectives are to achieve a higher quality of care and to reduce administrative costs by streamlining the processing of routine administrative and financial transactions. Department of Health and Human Services (HHS) has estimated that by implementing TCS, almost $30 billion over 10 years would be saved.

TCS regulation required the implementation of specific standards for transactions and code sets by October 16, 2003. The intent of TCS requirements is to achieve a single standard.

For example, in the pre-HIPAA environment, when submitting claims for payment, health care providers had been doing business with insurance payers who required the use of their own version of local code sets (e.g., state

Table 8.1	Recognized Benefits of TCS and EDI
Benefit	**Result**
More reliable and timely processing–quicker reimbursement from payer	Fast eligibility evaluation. Reduced time in claim life cycle. Industry averages for claim turnarounds are 9 to 15 days for electronic vs. 30 to 45 days for paper claims, improving cash flow.
Improved accuracy of data	Decreases processing time, increases data quality, and leads to better reporting.
Easier and more efficient access to information	Improves patient support.
Better tracking of transactions	Facilitates tracking of transactions (i.e., when sent and received), allowing for monitoring (e.g., prompt payments).
Reduction of data entry/manual labor	Electronic transactions facilitate automated processes (e.g., auto payment posting).
Reduction in office expenses	Lowers office supplies, postage, and telephone expenses.

Data from HIPAAdocs Corporation, Columbia, Md.

Medicaid programs) or identifiers and paper forms. More than 400 versions of a **National Standard Format (NSF)** exist to submit a claim for payment. Health care providers' offices will benefit from less paperwork, and standardizing data will result in more accurate information and a more efficient organization.

HIPAA standardization actions are similar to using a bank's automatic teller machine (ATM) or the grocery store's self-checkout. A magnetic strip on a bank card or the bar code on a grocery item can be swiped across a scanning device, allowing customers to process a transaction more quickly than with traditional methods. As these methods are adapted, there are benefits to both the end user and the business providing the technology (Table 8.1).

As learned in Chapter 2, HIPAA governs how a covered entity may handle health information. Whether or not a provider transmits health information in electronic form in connection with a transaction covered by HIPAA will determine whether a provider is considered a covered entity (Figure 8–2). Under HIPAA, the following circumstances would likely make the provider a **covered entity:**

- If the provider submits electronic transactions to any payer.
- Large providers: If the provider submits paper claims to Medicare and has 10 or more employees, the provider

is required to convert to electronic transactions (no later than October 16, 2003) and, therefore, HIPAA compliance is required.

A provider *is not considered a covered entity* under HIPAA in the following circumstances:

- Small providers: If the provider has less than 10 employees and submits claims only on paper to Medicare (not electronic). The provider may continue to submit on paper and therefore is not required to comply with HIPAA guidelines (i.e., not required to submit electronically).
- If the provider only submitted paper claims until and after April 14, 2003, and does not send claims to Medicare, the provider is not required to comply with sending electronic claims.

According to CMS, "After October 16, 2003, (for Medicare claims delayed until July 1, 2004) Electronic Claims will not be processed if they are in a format other than in the HIPAA format. Providers who are not small providers (institutional organizations with fewer than 25 full-time employees or physicians with fewer than 10 full-time employees) must send all claims electronically in the HIPAA format."

Transaction and Code Set Standards

TCS standards have been adopted for health care transactions. HIPAA **standard transactions** are the electronic files in which medical data are compiled to produce a specific format to be used throughout the health care industry.

In general, **code sets** are the allowable set of codes that anyone could use to enter into a specific space (field) on a form. All health care organizations using electronic transactions will have to use and accept (either directly or through a clearinghouse) the code set systems required under HIPAA that document specific health care data elements, including medical diagnoses and procedures, drugs, physician services, and medical suppliers. These codes have already been in common use throughout the industry and should have helped ease the transition to the new transaction requirements. What has been a standard in the health care industry and recognized by most payers has now been *mandated* under HIPAA.

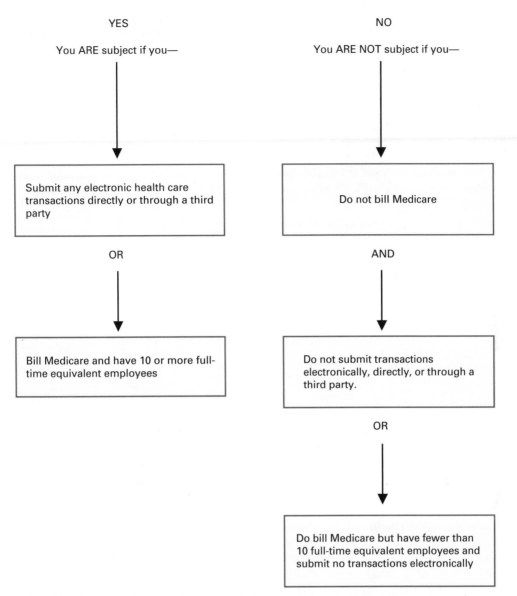

FIGURE 8–2 Decision flow chart of who is subject to the HIPAA Transaction and Code Set (TCS) rule.

HIPAA standard codes are used in conjunction with the standard electronic transactions. It is necessary that the health care industry recognize a standard that eliminates ambiguity when processing transactions. In turn, this will ultimately improve the quality of data and result in improved decision making and reporting in administrative and clinical processes.

Medical codes sets are **data elements** used uniformly to document why patients are seen (diagnosis, ICD-9-CM) and what is done to them during their encounter (procedure, CPT-4 and HCPCS). Each covered entity organization is responsible for implementing the updated codes in a timely manner, using the new HIPAA-mandated TCS codes, and deleting old or obsolete ones (Table 8.2).

When a patient comes into your office and is treated, his or her confidential health information is collected and put into the computerized practice management system. The services rendered are assigned a standard code from the HIPAA-required *code sets* (e.g., CPT), and the diagnosis is selected from another code set (e.g., ICD-9-CM); much the same as pre-HIPAA.

When claims are generated for electronic submission, all data collected are compiled and constructed into an HIPAA *standard transaction*. This EDI is recognized across the health care sector in computer systems maintained by providers, the clearinghouses, and insurance payers. The harmony among the covered entities results in a more efficient claim life cycle.

Data Requirements

Your role as an insurance billing specialist will likely require you to understand what data elements are required to construct an HIPAA standard transaction in comparison to those essential for a paper CMS-1500 form or the old electronic NSF.

The office's practice management software system will produce the required HIPAA standard electronic formats. If the software is not capable of producing such formats, the continued use of clearinghouses will eliminate much of the confusion by translating into the HIPAA standard format. You will be trained on the practice management software system on where to insert or input additionally captured data that have not been collected on the CMS-1500 form or electronic NSF.

Required and Situational

In addition to the major code sets (ICD-9 and CPT/HCPCS), several *supporting code sets* encompass both medical and nonmedical data (Table 8.3) When constructing a claim, the supporting code sets are made up of "Required" and "Situational" data elements, similar to those on the CMS-1500 paper form. These supporting code sets are embedded in the data elements identified by the HIPAA standard electronic formats. You will not need to know all these specific codes, but it will be helpful to know they do exist, especially if you are active in the claims processing procedures. When reviewing reports from the clearinghouse or the insurance payer, you may

Table 8.2	HIPAA Medical Code Sets and Elements	
Standard Code Sets	**Medical Data Elements**
International Classification of Diseases, Ninth Edition, Clinical Modification (ICD-9-CM), Vols 1 and 2 ICD-9-CM replaces DSM-IV.	Diseases Injuries Impairments Other health-related problems and their manifestations Causes of injury, disease, impairment, or other health-related problems
ICD-9-CM, Vol 3	Procedures or other actions taken for diseases, injuries, and impairments on hospital inpatients reported by hospitals, including prevention, diagnosis, treatment, and management
Current Procedural Terminology, Fourth Edition (CPT-4)	Physician services Physician and occupational therapy services Radiologic procedures Clinical laboratory tests Other medical diagnostic procedures Hearing and vision services Transportation services (e.g., helicopter, ambulance) Other services
Code on Dental Procedures and Nomenclature (CDT)	Dental services
National Drug Codes (NDC) for Retail Pharmacy transactions	Pharmaceuticals Biologics
International Classification of Diseases, 10th Edition, Clinical Modification (ICD-10-CM) (diagnosis) ICD-10-PCS (to replace ICD-9-CM, Vol 3 procedural coding system)	Expected to replace ICD-9-CM, possibly by October 2007.

have to correct claims that were rejected for not having correct data elements.

Required refers to data elements that must be used to be in compliance with an HIPAA standard transaction. Conversely, *situational* means that the item depends on the data content or context. For example, a baby's birth weight is obviously "situational" when submitting a claim for the delivery of the infant. Another situational data element would be the last menstrual period (LMP) when a woman is pregnant. Determining the required and situational data elements not currently collected for the CMS-1500 claim or NSF electronic format can be complex; you will learn this process when you are in the office performing claims processing duties. As an insurance billing specialist, you are directly involved in the claims

Table 8.3	HIPAA Transaction Functions and Formats
Standard Transaction Function	**Industry Format Name**
Official title: Health Care Eligibility Benefit Inquiry and Response **Purpose:** Eligibility verification/response when obtaining issues regarding benefits and coverage, this standard is used from a health care provider to a health plan or between two health plans. The 270 is the "inquiry for eligibility verification." The 271 is the "response."	ASC X12N 270/271
Official title: Health Care Claim Status Request and Response **Purpose:** Health claim status inquiry/response. The 276 is the "inquiry" to determine the status of a claim. The 277 is the "response."	ASC X12N 276/277
Official title: Health Care Services Review—Request for Review and Response **Purpose:** Referral certification and authorization for patient health care services.	ASC X12N 278
Official title: Payroll Deducted and Other Group Premium Payment for Insurance Products **Purpose:** Health plan premium payments, including payroll deductions.	ASC X12N 820
Official title: Benefit Enrollment and Maintenance **Purpose:** Used to transmit subscriber enrollment information to a health plan to establish coverage or terminate the policy.	ASC X12N 834
Official title: Payment and Remittance Advice **Purpose:** Transmission indicating the explanation of benefits or remittance advice from a health plan payer to the health care provider. This may also be data sent from a health plan direct to the provider's financial institution (bank) that includes payment and information about the processing of the claim.	ASC X12N 835
Official title: Health Care Claim or Equivalent Encounter **Purpose:** Request to obtain payment for the transmitted health services encounter information. The 837P (Professional) replaces the paper CMS-1500 form and the electronic national standard format (NSF). The 837I (Institutional) replaces the paper UB-92 often used in hospitals. The 837D (Dental) is used for dentistry. Additionally, the Coordination of Benefits for claims and payment will be transmitted through the 837 format.	ASC X12N 837 Includes: 837P - Health Care Claim, Professional 837I - Health Care Claim, Institutional 837D - Health Care Claim, Dental
Proposed official title: First Report of Illness, Injury or Incident **Potential purpose:** Report information on a claim pertaining to factors such as date of onset of illness or date of accident.	PROPOSED— ASC X12N 148
Proposed official title: Health Claims Attachment **Potential purpose:** Transmit additional information to claim. No photocopied attachments stapled to paper claims or additional information mailed after the claim is initially received.	PROPOSED— ASC X12 275 and HL7

processing procedures and will need to know the most important items to look for related to HIPAA requirements and situational data to successfully construct a compliant and payable insurance claim.

In addition to other data elements required under HIPAA TCS, examples include the following:

- **Taxonomy codes.** Taxonomy is defined as the science of classification; thus these are numeric and alpha provider *specialty* codes, which are assigned and classify each health care provider. Common taxonomy codes include "general practice 208D0000X," "family practice 207Q00000X," and "nurse practitioner 363L00000X."
- *Patient account number.* To be assigned to every claim.

- *Relationship to patient.* Expanded to 25 different relationships, including indicators such as "grandson," "adopted child," "mother," and "life partner."
- *Facility code value.* Facility-related element that identifies the place of service, with at least 29 to choose from, including "office," "ambulance air or water," and "end-stage renal disease treatment facility."
- *Patient signature source code.* Indicates how the patient or subscriber signatures were obtained for authorization and how signatures are retained by the provider. Codes include letters such as "B" for "signed signature authorization form or forms for both CMS-1500 claim form block 12 and block 13 are on file" and "P" for "signature generated by provider because the patient was not physically present for services."

Box 8.1 | HIPAA Supporting Code Sets

Adjustment reason code	Disability type code	Place of service code
Agency qualifier code	Discipline type code	Policy compliance code
Amount qualifier code	Employment status code	Product/service procedure code
Ambulatory patient group code	Entity identifier code	Prognosis code
Attachment report type code	Exception code	Provider code
Attachment transmission code	Facility type code	Provider organization code
Claim adjustment group code	Functional status code	Provider specialty certification code
Claim filing indicator code	Hierarchical child code	Provider specialty code
Claim frequency code	Hierarchical level code	Record format code
Claim payment remark code	Hierarchical structure code	Reject reason code
Claim submission reason code	Immunization status code	Related-causes code
Code list qualifier code	Immunization type code	Service type code
Condition codes	Individual relationship code	Ship/delivery or calendar pattern code
Contact function code	Information release code	Ship/delivery pattern time code
Contract code	Insurance type code	Student status code
Contract type code	Measurement reference ID code	Supporting document response code
Credit/debit flag code	Medicare assignment code	Surgical procedure code
Currency code	Nature of condition code	Transaction set identifier code
	Non-visit code	Transaction set purpose code
	Note reference code	Unit or basis measurement code
	Nutrient admin method code	Version identification code
	Nutrient admin technique code	X-ray availability indicator code

TRANSITION FROM PAPER CMS-1500 TO ELECTRONIC STANDARD HIPAA 837P

The American National Standards Institute (ANSI) formed the **Accredited Standards Committee X12 (ASC X12),** which developed the U.S. standards body for the cross-industry development, maintenance, and publication of electronic data exchange standards. In regard to the health care industry, processing administrative functions can be costly and involve many paper forms and communications via telephone, fax, and postal services. Also, the security and privacy of an individual's health information may be jeopardized. So, to address the burden of these high overhead costs, the uniform adoption of HIPAA standards has brought forth electronic formats to complete the following health care related transactions:

- Obtain authorization to refer to a specialist
- Submit a claim for reimbursement
- Request and respond to additional information needed to process a claim
- Health care claims or equivalent encounter information
- Health care payment and remittance advice
- Coordination of benefits
- Health care claim status
- Enrollment and disenrollment in a health plan
- Eligibility for a health insurance plan
- Health plan premium payments
- Referral certification and authorization
- First report of injury
- Health claims attachments
- Other transactions HHS may prescribe by regulation

Each of these standard transactions is identified by a three-digit number preceded by "ASC X12N." The transactions, however, are referred to in the office simply by the three-digit number, for example, 837 or 837P (professional). The 837P replaces the paper CMS-1500 form and the more than 400 versions of the electronic National Standard Format (NSF). HIPAA also provides standards for the complete cycle of administrative transactions and electronic standard formats. Use Box 8.1 to become better acquainted with these HIPAA supporting code sets.

Levels of Information for 837P Standard Transaction Format

Because the 837P is an electronic claims transmittal format, data collected to construct and submit a claim are grouped by levels. It is important for claims processing staff to know the language when following up on claims. You do not need to know exactly how these are grouped. However, if the clearinghouse or payer states that you have an invalid item at the "high level," you will need to understand that it could be incomplete or erroneous information pertaining to the provider, subscriber, or payer (Table 8.4).

A "friendlier" way to understand this new stream-of-data format is to address a "crosswalk" between the legacy CMS-1500 and the 837P (Table 8.5; note that dates on HIPAA transactions will be in the format YYYYMMDD [20030806]). Refer to a paper CMS-1500 Health Insurance Claim Form template as shown in the previous chapter. Use Table 8.6 and compare the block number on the CMS-1500 paper claim with the data element number in the 837 elctronic format.

Table 8.4	Data Grouping in 837P Standard Transaction Format
Level	**Information**
High-level information: Applies to the entire claim and reflects data pertaining to the billing provider, subscriber, and patient.	Billing provider/pay to provider information Subscriber/patient information Payer information
Claim-level information: Applies to the entire claim and all service lines and is applicable to most claims.	Claim information
Specialty claim–level information: Applies to specific claim types.	Specialty
Service line–level information: Applies to specific procedure or service that is rendered and is applicable to most claims.	Service line information
Specialty service line–level information: Applies to specific claim types. Required data are only required for the specific claim type.	Specialty service line information
Other information	Coordination of benefits (COB) Repriced claim/line Credit/debit information Clearinghouse/VAN tracking

CLAIMS ATTACHMENTS STANDARDS

This proposed rule (as of November 2004) is intended to develop an electronic standard for claims attachments as required by HIPAA. Currently, practice management and claims software include a data field that allows you to indicate that a paper claims attachment will be included with the claim. An electronic standard transaction for claims attachment would be used to transmit clinical data, in addition to those data contained in the claims standard, to help establish medical necessity for coverage and eliminate the need for the paper attachment.

Standard Unique Identifiers

Standard Unique Employer Identifier

The employer identification number (EIN) is assigned by the Internal Revenue Service (IRS) and is used to identify employers for tax purposes. HIPAA requires that the EIN be used to identify employers rather than inputting the actual name of the company when submitting claims. The date to comply was July 30, 2004. Employers will use their EINs to identify themselves in transactions involving premium payments to health plans on behalf of their employees or to identify themselves or other employers as the source or receiver of information about eligibility. Employers also will use EINs to identify themselves in

Table 8.5	Comparison of CMS-1500 and 837P			
CMS-1500 Box #	**CMS-1500 Block Name**	**837P Data Element #**	**837P Data Element Name**	**Status**
1	Government program	66	Identification code qualifier	R
1a	Insured ID number	67	Subscriber primary identifier	R
2	Patients name L, F, MI	1035	Patient last name	R
		1036	Patient first name	R
		1037	Patient middle name	R
		1039	Patient name suffix	R
3	Patient date of birth	1251	Patient date of birth	R
3	Sex	1068	Patient gender code	R
4	Insured name L, F, MI	1035	Patient last name	S
		1036	Patient first name	S
		1037	Patient middle name	S
		1039	Patient name suffix	S
5	Patient address	166	Patient address line	R
		166	Patient address line	S
5	City	19	Patient city name	R
5	State	156	Patient state code	R
5	Zip	116	Patient postal zone or zip code	R
5	Telephone		Not used in 837P	
6	Patient relationship to insured, self, spouse	1069	Individual relationship code	S
7	Insured address	166	Subscriber address line	S
		166	Subscriber address line	S
7	City	19	Subscriber city name	S
7	State	156	State code	S
7	Zip code	116	Subscriber postal zone or zip code	S
7	Telephone		Not used in 837P	

Continued

Table 8.5	Comparison of CMS-1500 and 837P—cont'd			
CMS-1500 Box #	**CMS-1500 Block Name**	**837P Data Element #**	**837P Data Element Name**	**Status**
8	Patient status single, married	1069	Individual relationship code	
8	Other	1069	Individual relationship code	
8	Employed		Not used in 837P	
8	Full-time student		Not used in 837P	
8	Part-time student		Not used in 837P	
9	Other insured's name L, F, MI	1035	Other insured last name	S
		1036	Other insured first name	S
		1037	Other insured middle name	S
		1039	Other insured name suffix	S
9a	Other insured policy or group number	93	Other insured group name	S
9b	Other insured date of birth	1251	Other insured birth date	S
9b	Sex	1068	Other insured gender code	S
9c	Employer's name or school name		Not used in 837P	
9d	Insurance plan name or program name	93	Other insured group name	S
10	Is patient's condition related to:		Related causes information:	S
10a	Employment (current or previous)	1362	Related causes code	S
10b	Auto accident	1362	Related causes code	S
10b	Place (state)	156	Auto accident state or province code	S
10c	Other accident	1362	Related causes code	S
11	Insured's policy group or FECA number			S
11a	Insured's date of birth	1251	Subscriber's birth date	S
11a	Sex	1068	Subscriber gender code	S
11b	Employer's name or school name		Not used in 837P	
11c	Insurance plan name or program name	93	Other insured group name	S
11d	Is there another health benefit plan	98	Entity identifier code	
12	Patient's or authorized person's signature (and date)	1363	Release of information code	R
		1351	Patient signature source code	R
13	Insured's or authorized person's signature	1073	Benefits assignment certification indicator	S
14	Date of current: illness, injury, pregnancy (last menstrual period [LMP])	1251	Initial treatment date	S
		1251	Accident date	S
		1251	LMP	S
15	If patient has had same or similar illness, give first date	1251	Similar illness or symptom date	S
16	Dates patient unable to work in current occupation: From	1251	Last worked date	S
16	To	1251	Work return date	S
17	Name of referring physician or other source			S
17a	ID number of referring physician			S
18	Hospitalization dates related to current services: From	1251	Related hospitalization	S
18	To		Related hospitalization discharge date	S
19	Reserved for local use			S
20	Outside lab?			S
20	$ Charges			S
21	Diagnosis or nature of illness or injury, Item 1	1271	Diagnosis code	S
21	Item 2	1271	Diagnosis code	S
21	Item 3	1271	Diagnosis code	S
21	Item 4	1271	Diagnosis code	S
22	Medicaid resubmission code		Not used in 837P	
22	Original reference number	127	Claim original reference number	S
23	Prior authorization number	127	Prior authorization number	S
24a	Dates of service: *from* MM DD YY	1251	Order date	R
24a	*To* MM DD YY	1251	Order date	R
24b	Place of service	1331	Place of service code	S
24c	Type of service		Not required in 837P	
24d	Procedures, services, or supplies CPT/HCPCS	234	Procedure code	R

Table 8.5 Comparison of CMS-1500 and 837P—cont'd

CMS-1500 Box #	CMS-1500 Block Name	837P Data Element #	837P Data Element Name	Status
24d	Modifier	1339	Procedure modifier	S
		1339	Procedure modifier	S
		1339	Procedure modifier	S
24e	Diagnosis code	1328	Diagnosis code pointer	S
			Diagnosis code pointer	S
			Diagnosis code pointer	S
			Diagnosis code pointer	S
24f	$ Charges	782	Line item charge amount	R
24g	Days or units	380	Service unit count	R
24h	EPSDT family plan	1366	Special program indicator	
24i	EMG	1073	Emergency indicator	
24j	COB		Not required for Medicare	
24k	Reserved for local use	127	Rendering provider secondary identifier	S
25	Federal tax ID number	67	Rendering provider identifier	R
25	SSN, EIN	66	Identification code qualifier	R
26	Patient's account number	1028	Patient account number	R
27	Accept assignment?	1359	Medicare assignment code	R
28	Total charge	782	Total claim charge amount	R
29	Amount paid	782	Patient amount paid	S
30	Balance due		Not required for Medicare	
31	Signature of physician or supplier (and date)	1073	Provider or supplier signature indicator	R
32	Name and address of facility where services were rendered	1035	Laboratory or facility name	S
		166	Laboratory or facility address line	S
		166		S
		19	Laboratory or facility city	S
		156	Laboratory facility state or province code	S
		116	Laboratory or facility postal zone or zip code	S
		or		
		1036	Submitter first name	
		1035	Billing provider last or organizational name	R
		1036	Billing provider first name	R
		166	Billing provider address line	R
		166	Billing provider address line	R
		19	Billing provider city name	R
		156	Billing provider state or province code	R
		116	Billing provider postal zone or zip code	R
33	Physicians' suppliers billing name, address, ZIP code, and phone number	1035	Billing provider last or organization name	R
		1036	Billing provider first name	R
		166	Billing provider address line	R
		166	Billing provider address line	R
		19	Billing provider city name	R
		156	Billing provider state or province code	R
		116	Billing provider postal zone or zip code	R
33	PIN	127	Billing provider additional identifier	R
33	Group (GRP) number	67	Billing provider identifier	R

transactions when enrolling or disenrolling employees in a health plan.

Standard Unique Health Care Provider Identifier

Health insurance plans have been assigning an identifying number to each provider with whom they conduct business. Providers have many different identifier numbers when submitting claims to several different payers. HIPAA requires that a National Provider Identifier (NPI) be assigned to each provider to be used in transactions with all health plans. The NPI is all numeric and is 10 characters in length; it is required by May 23, 2007. In April 2005, CMS announced that Fox Systems, Inc., will recieve and process NPI applications. Fox will operate a help desk for providing more information available at www.foxsys.com.

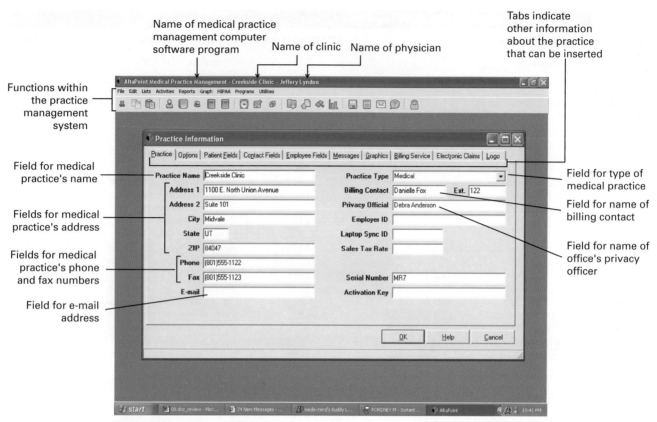

FIGURE 8–3 AltaPoint screen of the Creekside Clinic's medical practice's business information for Dr. Jeffery Lyndon.

According to CMS, NPI is a lasting identifier that would not change based on changes in a health care provider's name, address, ownership or membership in health plans, or Healthcare Provider Taxonomy classification (Taxonomy identifies the specialty). If an NPI is used for fraudulent purposes, an investigation will take place and a different NPI may be assigned.

Standard Unique Health Plan Identifier

This rule is under development and, like the NPI, will assign a standard identifier to identify health plans that process and pay certain electronic health care transactions. As of April 2005, a Notice of Proposed Rulemaking has not been published in the *Federal Register*. Check for updates at www.cms.hhs.gov.

Standard Unique Patient Identifier

The intention to create a standard for a uniform patient identifier prompted protest among public interest groups who saw a universal identifier as a civil liberties threat. Therefore the issue of a universal patient identifier is "on hold."

PRACTICE MANAGEMENT SYSTEM

The most important function of a practice management system (PMS) is accounts receivable. Many offices use features such as scheduling, electronic health record (EHR), and word processing to run an efficient office. However, the goal of maximum value can be attained if the PMS is able to prepare, send, receive and process HIPAA standard electronic transactions. For older PMS versions, a clearinghouse will convert old formats into the HIPAA standard transactions. Keep in mind that HIPAA does not apply to the format of stored data within the PMS databases. Computer systems are free to use any data format when storing data because HIPAA standards apply only to the format in which data is *transmitted* (Figure 8–3).

If your practice is in the market for a new PMS, consider looking for a vendor that understands HIPAA thoroughly–including the Privacy and Security Rules. A PMS can help with the administrative burdens such as tracking the receipt of the Notice of Privacy Practices (NPP), noting a patient's treatment consent or authorization, and mapping disclosures. An HIPAA-ready PMS may allow the following:

● Setting security access to patient files in the software (Figure 8–4)

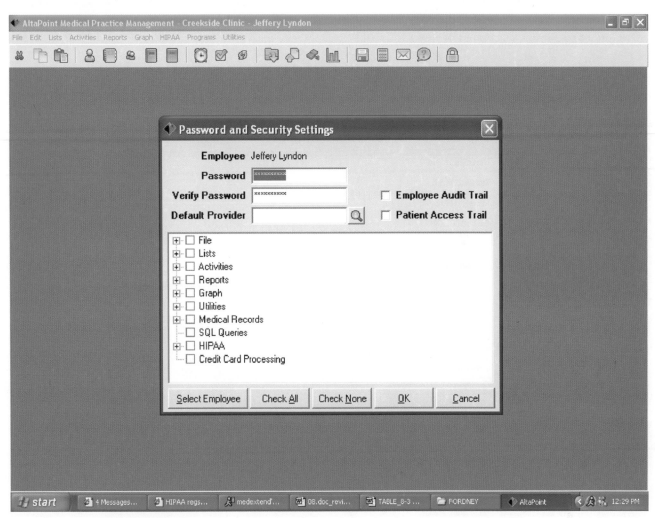

FIGURE 8–4 AltaPoint screen showing password and security settings that allow user access to particular functions of the practice management system.

- Indicating date of receipt and signature of NPP
- Inserting date of patient's authorization
- Maintaining files of practice's authorization and notification forms
- Tracking requests for amendments, request for restrictions on use and disclosure of protected health information (PHI), and indication of whether the physician agreed to the request or denied the request (Figure 8–5)
- Tracking expiration dates

When assessing the PMS's functionality in accounts receivable management, consider the ability to perform the following:
- Set up all practice providers as individuals to bill using correct and appropriate identifiers for each and every health care provider.
- Key in all patient demographics and insurance information.
- Electronic claim batch submission either direct to payer or through clearinghouse. Note that some PMS vendors sell an "add-on" module to go directly to some

carriers such as Medicare, Medicaid, and Blue Cross Blue Shield.

BUILDING THE CLAIM

Encounter or Multipurpose Billing Forms

As mentioned in Chapter 3, an *encounter form* (also known as charge slip, multipurpose billing form, patient service slip, routing form, super bill, or transaction slip) is a document used to record information about the service rendered to a patient. The style and format of the billing form varies because it is customized to meet the needs of each health care office. For easy reference in selecting levels of service and diagnosis, many billing forms include preprinted procedural and diagnostic codes. The list of codes printed on the form are specific to the medical practice's specialty. This aids the health care provider in determining the correct level of evaluation and management service, ensures each component is addressed in the

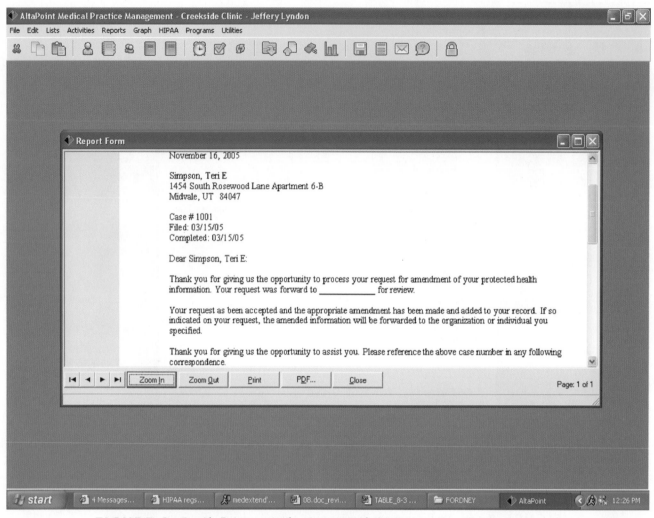

FIGURE 8–5 AltaPoint screen showing a provider's response to a patient's request to amend their protected health information as allowed under HIPAA legislation.

physician's dictation, and expedites data entry of professional services. The provider circles the codes, and the insurance billing specialist takes that information and enters it into the computer system. Billing forms cannot be used in place of documentation in the patient record and may not withstand an external audit.

Scannable Encounter Form

Some encounter forms are designed so that they may be scanned to input charges and diagnoses into the patient's computerized account (see Figure 7–9). Time is saved and fewer errors occur because no keystrokes are involved (Figure 8–6).

Keying Insurance Data for Claim Transmission

Manual claim completion is accomplished by obtaining patient and insurance data, looking up a diagnosis and procedure in an index, referring to medical and financial records, and following block-by-block guidelines for the CMS-1500 insurance claim form. Much of this source information is found on an encounter form that is used to post charges and payments. Additionally, scanning or copying the patient's insurance card and driver's license can assist when obtaining information for a claim or following up on a delinquent account.

When one is operating computer software, the encounter form also may be used to obtain information (Figure 8–7). A screen prompt (question) appears on the monitor, and the data are keyed in reply to the prompt. Reusable data are entered initially in a file and identified by a number. Each treating physician, referring physician, patient, and insurance carrier has an assigned computer code number (Figure 8–8). For example, Dr. Jones might be keyed in as 010; a patient, Jane Doe, might be input as an account number; and the ABC Insurance Company might be 003 (Figure 8–9). This information is stored in the database and is the same as that necessary

CFR

PAT 4140.0   DOCTOR: **2 FRANK CHI, M.D.**   **APPT DATE:**   05/27/XX
                    ROOM: APPT TIME: 2:30 PM
               APPTLOC: APPT LEN: 10 min.
( ) 985-6575   01/22/1936   F63   APPTCD: DEPT/LOC: 0, n/a
PRI: (Y) BLUE SHIELD ENVOY   REASON: OX, F/U visit   DSET/PRT: 1, 12
201-XX-9969   LAST DX: 000.0 No diagnosis applicable   ACCT BAL: 75.00
SEC: SSN/STA: 201-XX-9969, 1 Active   PAT DUE: 0.00
                       OVERLAY: 1 INTERNAL MEDICINE   VOUCHER: 7887

NEW PT OFFICE VISITS
①②③④Ⓟ/L   99203   NP LEVEL THREE
①②③④Ⓟ/L   99204   NP LEVEL FOUR
①②③④Ⓟ/L   99205   NP LEVEL FIVE

EST PT OFFICE VISIT
①②③④Ⓟ/L   99211   EST PT LEVEL ONE
①②③④Ⓟ/L   99212   EST PT LEVEL TWO
①②③④Ⓟ/L   99213   EST PT LEVEL THREE
①②③④Ⓟ/L   99214   EST PT LEVEL FOUR
①②③④Ⓟ/L   99215   EST PT LEVEL FIVE
①②③④Ⓟ/L   00003   GLOBAL VISIT

OTHER PROCEDURES
①②③④Ⓟ/L   99000   COLL & PREP/PAP TEST
①②③④Ⓟ/L   93000   EKG WITH INTERPRETATION
①②③④Ⓟ/L   82270   HEMOCCULT
①②③④Ⓟ/L   81000   URINALYSIS

INJECTIONS
①②③④Ⓟ/L   ~FLU,   FLU INJ/ADMIN/MCR
①②③④Ⓟ/L   ~9065   FLU INJ/NON MCR
①②③④Ⓟ/L   ~PNEU   PNEUMO/ADMIN/MCR
①②③④Ⓟ/L   ~9073   PNEUMO INJ NON MCR

UNLISTED PROCEDURES

_____

STOP FOR VERIFICATION
BREASTS
①②③④Ⓟ/L   610.2   FIBROADENOSIS, BREAST
①②③④Ⓟ/L   611.72   LUMP OR MASS IN BREAST

CARDIOVASCULAR
①②③④Ⓟ/L   441.4   ABDOM AORTIC ANEURYSM
①②③④Ⓟ/L   411.1   ANGINA
①②③④Ⓟ/L   424.1   AORTIC VALVE DISORDER
①②③④Ⓟ/L   427.31   ATRIAL FIBRILLATION
①②③④Ⓟ/L   427.32   ATRIAL FLUTTER
①②③④Ⓟ/L   427.61   ATRIAL PREMATURE BEATS
①②③④Ⓟ/L   426.11   ATRIOVENT BLOCK-1ST DE
①②③④Ⓟ/L   785.2   CARDIAC MURMURS NEC
①②③④Ⓟ/L   429.3   CARDIOMEGALY
①②③④Ⓟ/L   428.0   CONGESTIVE HEART FAILU
①②③④Ⓟ/L   425.1   HYPERTR OBSTR CARDIOMY
①②③④Ⓟ/L   414.01   ISCHEMIC CHR HEART DIS
①②③④Ⓟ/L   426.2   LEFT BB HEMIBLOCK
①②③④Ⓟ/L   424.0   MITRAL VALVE DISORDER
①②③④Ⓟ/L   785.1   PALPITATIONS
①②③④Ⓟ/L   427.0   PAROX ATRIAL TACHYCARD
①②③④Ⓟ/L   427.1   PAROX VENTRIC TACHYCAR

CHEST
①②③④Ⓟ/L   466.0   BRONCHITIS, ACUTE
①②③④Ⓟ/L   491.0   BRONCHITIS, CHRONIC
①②③④Ⓟ/L   493.20   CH OB ASTH W/O STAT AS
①②③④Ⓟ/L   493.00   EXT ASTHMA W/O STAT AS

①②③④Ⓟ/L   491.21   OBS CHR BRNC W ACT EXA
①②③④Ⓟ/L   491.20   OBS CHR BRNC W/O ACT E

ENDOCRINE
①②③④Ⓟ/L   250.61   DMI NEURO CMP CONTROLL
①②③④Ⓟ/L   250.01   DMI WO CMP CONTROLLED
①②③④Ⓟ/L   250.03   DMI UNCONTROLLED
①②③④Ⓟ/L   250.60   DMII NEURO CMP CONTROL
①②③④Ⓟ/L   250.00   DMII WO CMP CONTROLLED
①②③④Ⓟ/L   250.02   DMII UNCONTROLLED
①②③④Ⓟ/L   272.0   HYPERCHOLESTEROLEMIA
①②③④Ⓟ/L   272.1   HYPERGLYCERIDEMIA
①②③④Ⓟ/L   245.2   HYPOTHYROIDISM
①②③④Ⓟ/L   278.01   MORBID OBESITY
①②③④Ⓟ/L   241.0   THYROID NODULE

EXTREMITIES
①②③④Ⓟ/L   782.3   EDEMA
①②③④Ⓟ/L   440.22   LOWER EXT EMBOLISM
①②③④Ⓟ/L   451.0   PHLEBITIS-LEG
①②③④Ⓟ/L   440.21   PVD W/CLAUDICATION
①②③④Ⓟ/L   454.9   VARICOSE VEIN OF LEG

GI
①②③④Ⓟ/L   789.06   ABDMNAL PAIN EPIGASTRI
①②③④Ⓟ/L   789.02   ABDMNAL PAIN LFT UP QU
①②③④Ⓟ/L   789.04   ABDMNAL PAIN LT LWR QU
①②③④Ⓟ/L   789.05   ABDMNAL PAIN PERIUMBIL
①②③④Ⓟ/L   789.03   ABDMNAL PAIN RT LWR QU
①②③④Ⓟ/L   789.01   ABDMNAL PAIN RT UPR QU
①②③④Ⓟ/L   578.1   BLOOD IN STOOL
①②③④Ⓟ/L   575.12   CHOLECYSTITIS, ACUTE
①②③④Ⓟ/L   564.0   CONSTIPATION
①②③④Ⓟ/L   787.91   DIARRHEA
①②③④Ⓟ/L   562.11   DIVERTICULITIS
①②③④Ⓟ/L   562.10   DIVERTICULOSIS
①②③④Ⓟ/L   574.20   GALLSTONE(S), CHRONIC
①②③④Ⓟ/L   535.00   GASTRITIS
①②③④Ⓟ/L   530.81   GERD
①②③④Ⓟ/L   455.3   HEMORRHOID, EXT W/O COM
①②③④Ⓟ/L   455.0   HEMORRHOID, INT W/O COM
①②③④Ⓟ/L   564.1   IRRITABLE COLON
①②③④Ⓟ/L   787.01   NAUSEA WITH VOMITING
①②③④Ⓟ/L   569.3   RECTAL & ANAL HEMORRHA
①②③④Ⓟ/L   530.11   REFLUX ESOPHAGITIS
①②③④Ⓟ/L   V76.41   SCREEN COLORECTAL

GU
①②③④Ⓟ/L   601.0   ACUTE PROSTATITIS
①②③④Ⓟ/L   600   BPH
①②③④Ⓟ/L   592.0   CALCULUS OF KIDNEY
①②③④Ⓟ/L   592.1   CALCULUS OF URETER
①②③④Ⓟ/L   595.0   CYSTITIS, ACUTE
①②③④Ⓟ/L   595.1   CYSTITIS, CHRONIC
①②③④Ⓟ/L   599.7   HEMATURIA
①②③④Ⓟ/L   607.84   IMPOTENCE, ORGANIC ORI
①②③④Ⓟ/L   791.0   PROTEINURIA

HEENT
①②③④Ⓟ/L   380.4   CERUMEN, IMPACTED
①②③④Ⓟ/L   372.02   CONJUNCTIVITIS
①②③④Ⓟ/L   784.7   EPISTAXIS
①②③④Ⓟ/L   784.0   HEADACHE
①②③④Ⓟ/L   464.0   LARYNGITIS/TRACHEITI
①②③④Ⓟ/L   465.0   LARYNGOPHARYNGITIS, A
①②③④Ⓟ/L   780.4   LIGHT-HEADEDNESS
①②③④Ⓟ/L   346.00   MIGRAINE
①②③④Ⓟ/L   460   NASOPHARYNGITIS, ACUT
①②③④Ⓟ/L   381.01   OTITIS MEDIA
①②③④Ⓟ/L   462   PHARYNGITIS, ACUTE
①②③④Ⓟ/L   477.0   RHINITIS ALLERGIC
①②③④Ⓟ/L   461.0   SINUSITIS, ACUTE
①②③④Ⓟ/L   780.2   SYNCOPE/VERTIGO

HEMATOLOGIC
①②③④Ⓟ/L   280.0   CHR BLOOD LOSS ANEMI
①②③④Ⓟ/L   280.1   IRON DEF ANEMIA DIET
①②③④Ⓟ/L   281.0   PERNICIOUS ANEMIA

HYPERTENSION
①②③④Ⓟ/L   404.12   BEN HY HT/REN/CHF
①②③④Ⓟ/L   403.10   BEN HTN REN W/O REN
①②③④Ⓟ/L   403.11   BEN HYP WITH REN FAI
①②③④Ⓟ/L   401.1   BENIGN HYPERTENSION
①②③④Ⓟ/L   401.0   MALIGNANT HYPERTENSI
①②③④Ⓟ/L   458.0   ORTHOSTATIC HYPOTENS

NEURO
①②③④Ⓟ/L   345.10   GEN CNV EPIL W/O INT
①②③④Ⓟ/L   435.3   TIA
①②③④Ⓟ/L   433.10   CAROTID STENOSIS
①②③④Ⓟ/L   437.0   CEREBRAL ATHEREOSCLER

OB GYN
①②③④Ⓟ/L   112.1   CANDIDAL VULVOVAGINI
①②③④Ⓟ/L   627.2   MENOPAUSAL SYMPTOMS
①②③④Ⓟ/L   V76.2   SCREEN MAL NEOP-CERV

RHEUMATOLOGIC
①②③④Ⓟ/L   723.1   CERVICAL PAIN
①②③④Ⓟ/L   274.0   GOUT
①②③④Ⓟ/L   724.2   LUMBAGO/BACK PAIN
①②③④Ⓟ/L   729.5   PAIN IN LIMB
①②③④Ⓟ/L   724.1   PAIN IN THORACIC SPI
①②③④Ⓟ/L   714.0   RHEUMATOID ARTHRITIS
①②③④Ⓟ/L   724.3   SCIATICA
①②③④Ⓟ/L   710.0   SYST LUPUS ERYTHEMAT

MISC
①②③④Ⓟ/L   780.6   FEVER UNKN ORGIN
①②③④Ⓟ/L   054.9   HERPES SIMPLEX NOS
①②③④Ⓟ/L   786.05   SHORTNESS OF BREATH

UNLISTED DIAGNOSIS
①②③④Ⓟ/L   STOP FOR VERIFICATION

①②③④Ⓟ/L   **REFERRALS**   ①②③④Ⓟ/L   **LOCATIONS**   ①②③④Ⓟ/L   **DOCTORS**   ①②③④Ⓟ/L   **NEXT VISIT**
①②③④Ⓟ/L   ①②③④Ⓟ/L   ①②③④Ⓟ/L   ①②③④Ⓟ/L   ____ DAYS
①②③④Ⓟ/L   ①②③④Ⓟ/L   ①②③④Ⓟ/L   F. CHI, MD   ①②③④Ⓟ/L   _1_ WEEKS
①②③④Ⓟ/L   ①②③④Ⓟ/L   ①②③④Ⓟ/L   A. SWERD, MD   ①②③④Ⓟ/L   ____ MONTHS
①②③④Ⓟ/L   ①②③④Ⓟ/L   ①②③④Ⓟ/L   J. STEVEN, MD   ①②③④Ⓟ/L

FIGURE 8–6   Scannable encounter form. Primary service or procedure is marked (with a #2 pencil) in the number 1 location and linked to the primary diagnosis, which also is marked in the number 1 location. The secondary procedures are marked in the number 2 location as is the secondary diagnosis. The primary linkage for all services and procedures is connected to the physician performing the service and the location in which it took place. *(Form template from Pearson NCS, Inc, Bloomington, Minn. Form data are fictitious and not a part of the template.)*

Name and code of
patient file

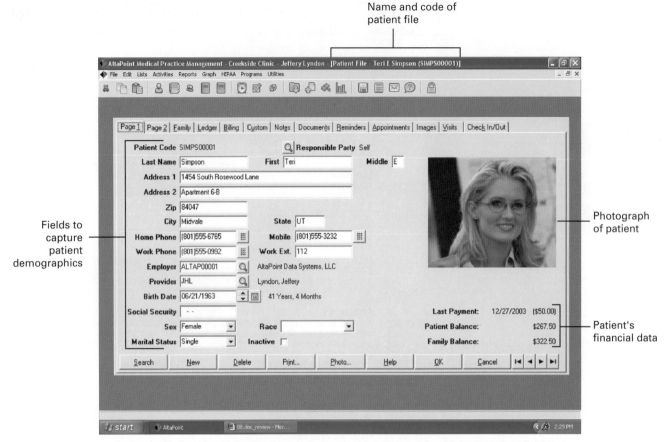

Fields to
capture
patient
demographics

Photograph
of patient

Patient's
financial data

FIGURE 8–7 AltaPoint screen of an open patient account with patient data fields.

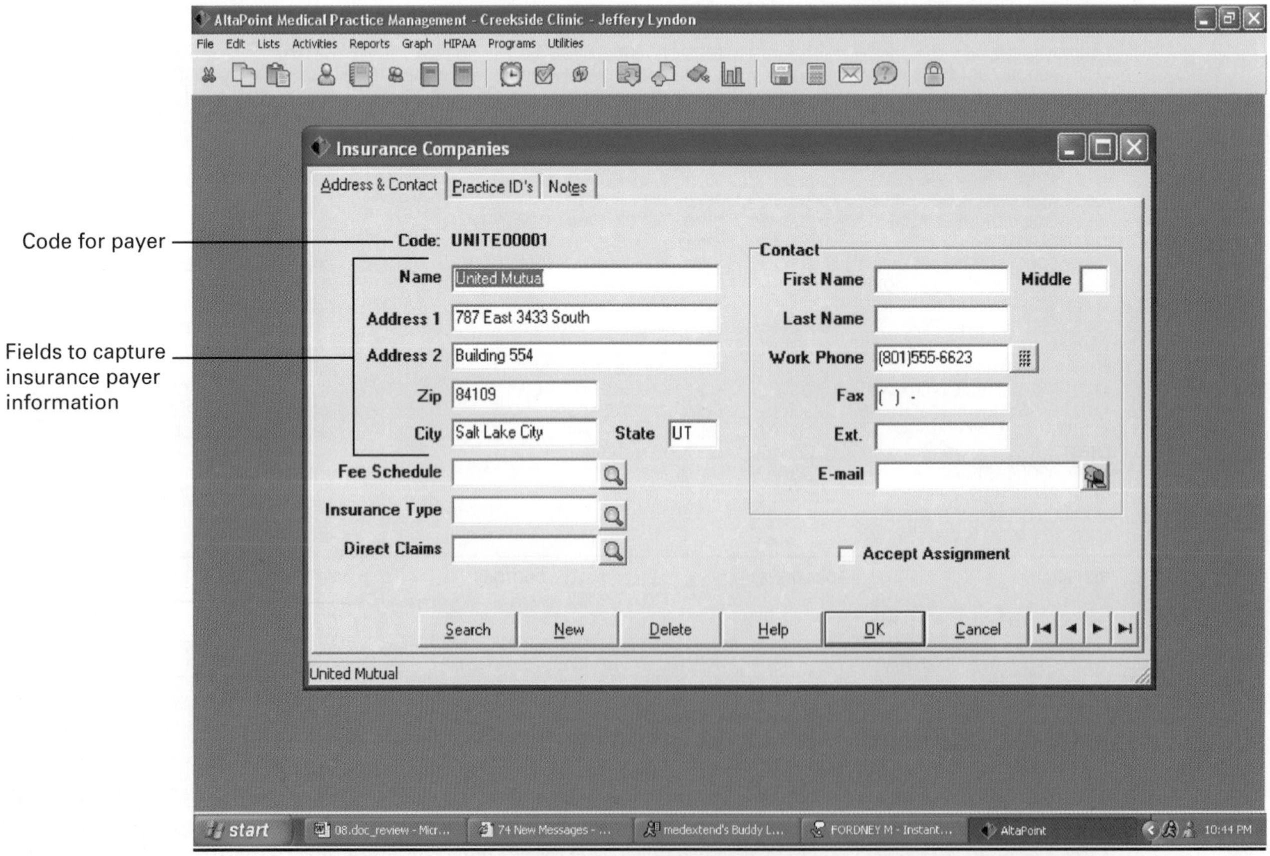

Code for payer

Fields to capture
insurance payer
information

FIGURE 8–8 AltaPoint screen of the payer file showing completed data fields.
Notice that the Code for the Payer is "UNITE00001."

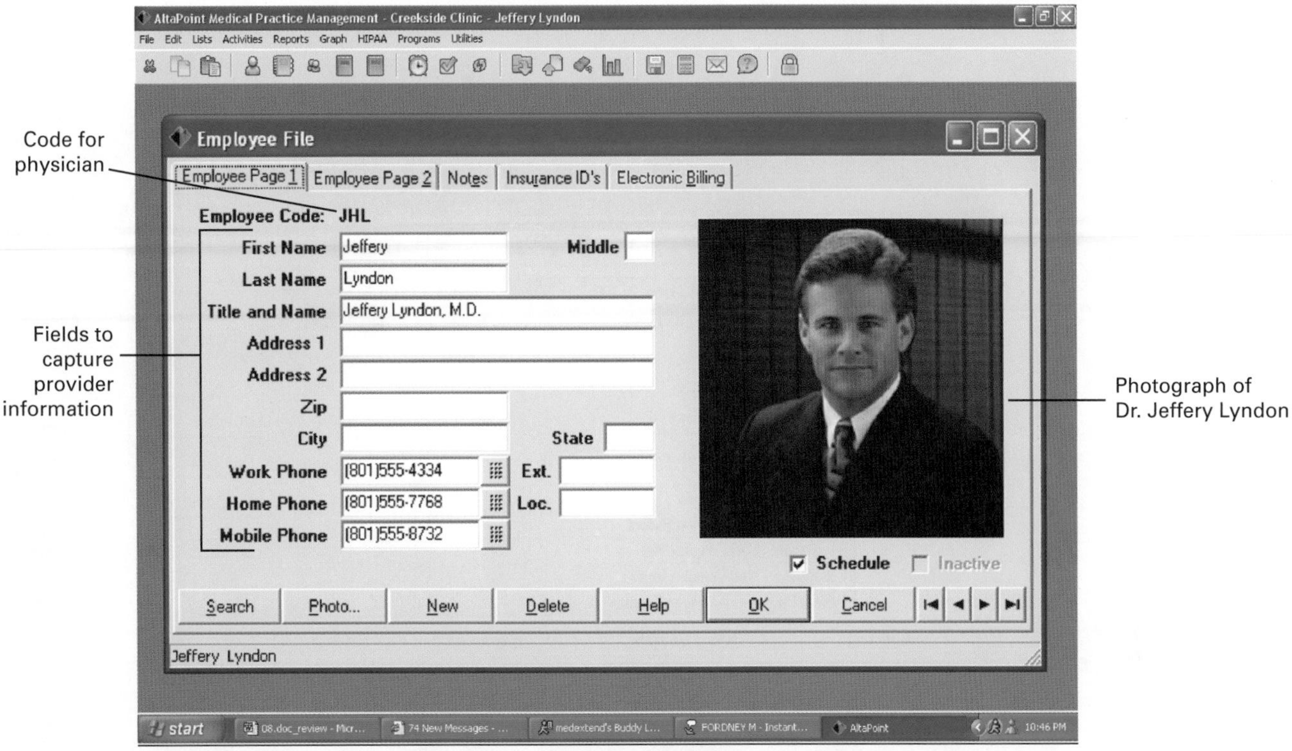

FIGURE 8–9 AltaPoint screen of the provider file of Dr. Jeffery H. Lyndon. Note that he is identified in the PMS as "JHL," so all information keyed into the PMS under "JHL" are assigned as Dr. Lyndon being the responsible physician.

for completing a claim manually. It is automatically retrieved by the system when a computer code number is keyed in and used to generate a computerized claim or electronic claim. Because there are computer code numbers and prompts for each item, there is less chance for error or omitting mandatory information. The program checks to see that data are complete and in proper format. It is important to understand how your particular management system works.

Some entries are made using a "macro." This technique involves a series of menu selections, keystrokes, or commands that have been recorded into memory and assigned a name or key combination. When the macro name is keyed in, the steps or characters in the macro are executed from beginning to end, saving time and key strokes.

Some general do's and don'ts guidelines for keying in data and billing electronic claims follow:

● Do not use special characters (dashes, spaces, or commas)
● Do use the patient account numbers to differentiate between patients with similar names.
● Do use correct numeric locations of service code, current valid CPT, or Healthcare Common Procedure Coding System (HCPCS) procedure codes.
● Do not bill codes using modifiers -21 or -22 electronically unless the carrier receives documents

(called attachments) to justify more payment (Figure 8–10).
● Do print an insurance billing worksheet or perform a front-end edit (online error checking) to look for and correct all errors before the claim is transmitted to the insurance carrier.
● Do request electronic-error reports from the insurance carrier to make corrections to the system.
● Do obtain and cross-check the electronic status report against all claims transmitted.

After input is complete, the information is stored in memory and a claim may be transmitted individually or in batches. Batched claims can be divided according to insurance type or date(s) of service and are ideally sent during low-volume times.

Because the health care provider is responsible for submitting an accurate bill, the insurance billing specialist inputs the codes and claims examiners will not recode (Figure 8–11). Medicare is forbidden to recode a claim. This eliminates transposition of numbers or missing or added digits on transmitted claims. During the edit and error process, software code editors identify invalid codes, age conflicts, gender conflicts, procedural and diagnostic code conflicts, and other data before issuing payment. If certain information is submitted incorrectly (e.g., patient's name or insurance identification number is incorrect,

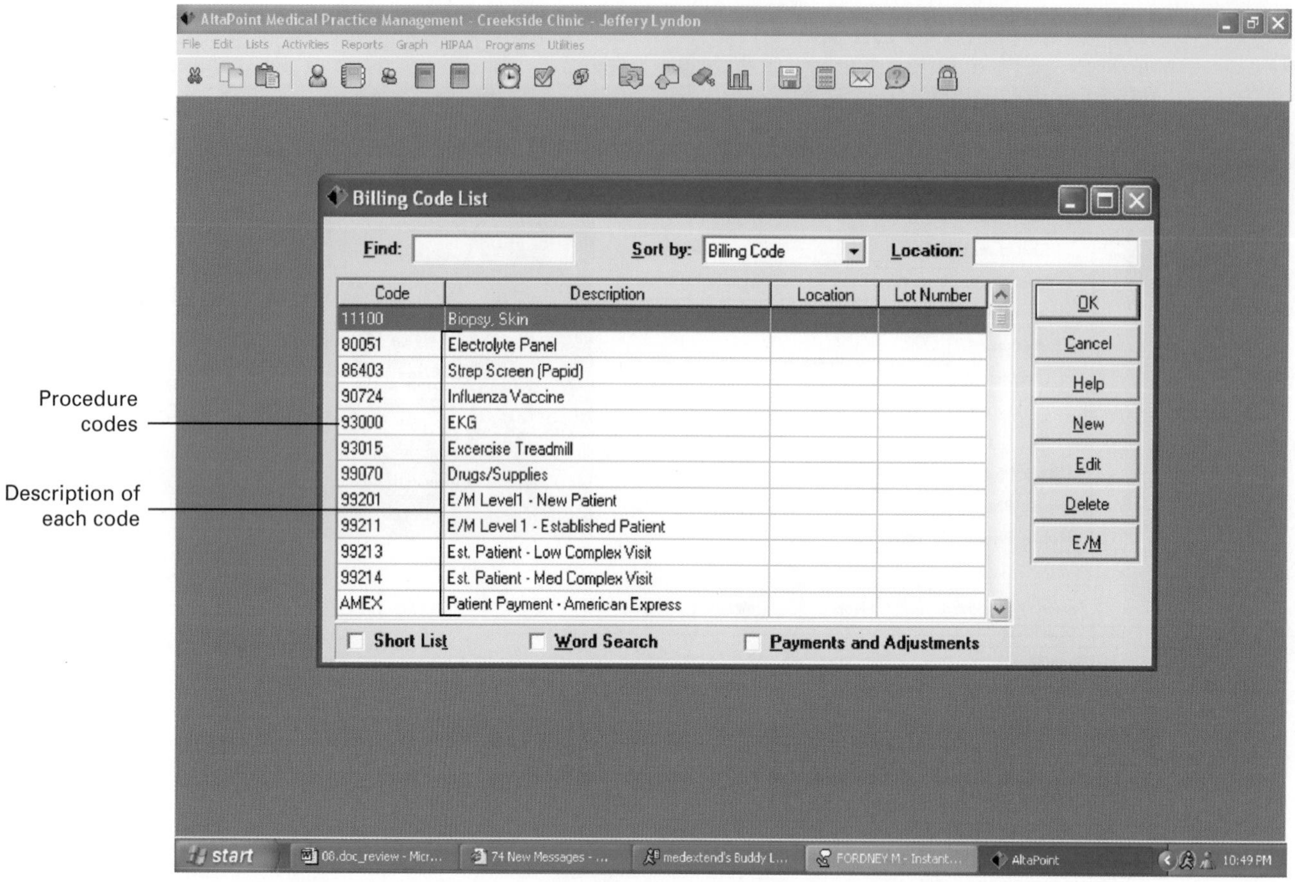

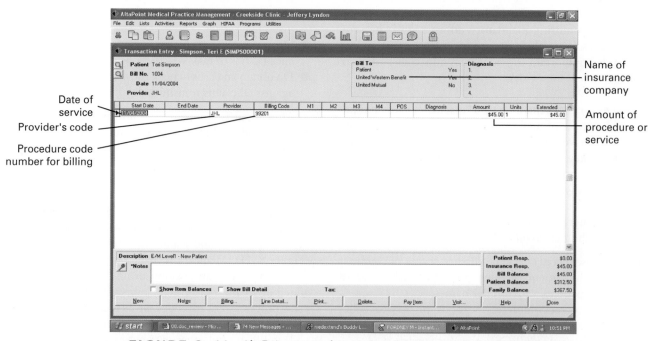

FIGURE 8–10   AltaPoint screen showing billing codes with their descriptions.

FIGURE 8–11   AltaPoint screen showing keyed data necessary for transmitting for payment an insurance claim to the insurance carrier and/or clearinghouse for patient Teri E. Simpson.

a diagnosis code is missing a fifth digit, or a provider's identification number is omitted), the claim is rejected and must be resubmitted with correct data. Incorrect coding may be keying errors, or it may be a deliberate attempt to obtain fraudulent payment. The edit check allows immediate feedback about the status of an electronically transmitted claim.

Medicare requires certain information when submitting paper and electronic claims for some blocks of the CMS-1500 claim form. Carriers may return claims if this information is omitted. A list of mandatory information and conditional requirements is shown in Table 8.6.

The physician or the insurance billing specialist may revise coding on the health record and on the claim to reflect the services more accurately up until the time at which the claim is transmitted for payment.

Encoder

An **encoder** is an add-on software to practice management systems that can greatly reduce the time it takes to build or review a claim before batching. This helps improve overall coding accuracy. The billing specialist or other user is prompted with a series of questions or choices leading to or affecting a specific code assignment by displaying code-specific edits. Using an encoder can enhance a medical practice's compliance program when it comes to accuracy in its billing procedures. Used as an audit tool, the encoder can also be helpful in performance improvement by identifying problem areas in the billing process.

However, there are instances when an encoder does not accurately assign codes; therefore one must never be completely dependent on code-assist software. For example, if a patient has three thorns incised and extracted (removed), the CPT code 10120 "incision and removal

Table 8.6	Medicare Requirements When Submitting Paper and Electronic Claims	
Mandatory Information		
Block No.	**Paper Claims**	**Electronic Claims**
1A.	Insured's ID number	Insured's ID number
2.	Patient's name	Patient's last and first names
11.	Insured's policy group number	Group number/source of payment
13.	Patient's signature source	Patient's signature source/release of information indicator
24a.	Dates of service	Service from/through dates
24b.	Place of service	Place of service
24d.	Procedures, services, and so on	HCPCS procedure code
24f.	$ charges	Line charges
24g.	Days or units of service	Units of service
31.	Provider's signature indicator	Provider's signature indicator
33.	Provider's billing name and address	Provider's last and first names
		Payer organization, name
		Provider 's Medicare number (batch level)
		Provider's pay-to address 1
		Provider's pay-to city
		Provider's pay-to state
		Provider's pay-to ZIP code
		Provider's pay-to telephone number
Conditional Requirements		
4.	Insured's name	Insured's last and first names
6.	Patient's relationship to insured	Patient's relationship to insured
7.	Insured's address	Insured's address-line 1 Insured's city, state, ZIP code, and telephone number
9c.	Employer's or school name	Insured's employer name
9d.	Insurance plan or program name	Group name
14.	Date of current illness and so on	Accident/symptom date
17.	Name of referring/ordering provider	Referring/ordering provider's last name
17a.	ID number of referring/ordering provider	Referring/ordering provider's NPI, referring provider's NPI
19.	Reserved for local use	Date last seen, supervising provider's NPI, date of last x-ray
20.	Outside lab	Laboratory indicator, laboratory charges, purchased service indicator, purchased service charge
21.	Diagnosis	Diagnosis 1, 2, 3, 4
24d.		HCPCS modifier 1, 2, 3, 4
24k.	Reserved for local use	Rendering provider's NPI
32.	Facility name and address	Facility/laboratory name and/or facility/laboratory NPI number, mammography certification number

---

PATIENT'S MEDICARE ELECTRONIC SIGNATURE MONTHLY AUTHORIZATION FORM

I authorize any holder of medical or other information about me to release to the Social Security Administration and Center for Medicare and Medicaid Services or its intermediaries or carriers any information needed for this or a related Medicare claim. I permit a copy of this authorization to be used in place of the original, and request payment of medical insurance benefits either to myself or to the party who accepts assignment.

_____   _____
Signature of Patient   Date

A

PATIENT'S MEDICARE ELECTRONIC SIGNATURE ONE-TIME AUTHORIZATION FORM

I request that payment of authorized Medicare benefits be made either to me or on my behalf to _____ for services furnished me by that physician or supplier. I permit a copy of this authorization to be used in place of the original and authorize any holder of medical information about me to release to the Center for Medicare and Medicaid Services or its agents any information needed to determine these benefits or the benefits payable for related services.

_____   _____
Signature of Patient   Date

B

FIGURE 8–12   Examples of patients' Medicare electronic signature authorization forms. **A,** Monthly form. **B,** One-time form.

of foreign body, subcutaneous tissue; simple (integumentary system)" might be generated by the encoder. But if internally audited, the case may warrant CPT code 27372 "removal of foreign body, deep, thigh region in knee area (musculoskeletal system)." Thus one learns that not all procedures involving the skin are found in the integumentary system and, if deeper skin layers are affected, a code may be found in another system. A *grouper* is software designed for use in a network that serves a group of users working on a related project that allows access to the same data.

Signature Requirements

Physician

The physician's signature on the agreement or contract is a substitute for his or her signature on the claim form.

Patient

For assignment of benefits, each patient's signature must be obtained and retained in the office records, because there are no handwritten signatures on electronic claims (Figure 8–12). Office policy varies on obtaining the patient's signature for release of medical information.

A clause on the patient registration form or an authorization and assignment release document may be designed specifically for obtaining signatures for transmitting electronic claims and acceptance of financial responsibility by the patient. The CMS-1500 Health Insurance Claim form also may be used for this purpose, and the patient should sign in Block 12 or 13 for a specific date of service. Most practice management systems ask a question whether the patient's signature is on file and require a "yes" or "no" answer to populate the required field when the claim is submitted. When a physician sees a patient in the hospital who has never been to the office, the authorizations obtained by the hospital apply to that provider's filing of a claim, for example, as in a consultation process.

Clean Electronic Claims Submission

Because dirty claims cost medical practices, the following is a review of some methods used to ensure clean claims.

● Claim scrubber software (prebill/edit processing)
● Encoder software
● Electronic clearinghouse
● Single and batch claims review

PUTTING HIPAA STANDARD TRANSACTIONS TO WORK

Interactive Transactions

Interactive transaction is back-and-forth communication between two computer systems. One requests information and the other provides information during what is referred to as online **real time.** Real time allows for instant information. An inquiry is made and an answer received within seconds. It can involve eligibility verification, deductible status, claim inquiries, status of claims, and other insurance claim data. Other information also may be accessed, such as limiting charges, fee schedules, allowables, procedure codes, and postoperative days for specific procedures. Many insurance companies, such as Medicare fiscal intermediaries, provide access to information on assigned pending and paid claims. Additional information that may be determined includes whether the individual has other coverage and which insurance carrier should be billed as primary. In addition, some insurance carriers deposit payments into the physician's bank account automatically via **electronic funds transfer (EFT).** EFT is a paperless computerized system that enables funds to be debited, credited, or transferred and eliminates the need for personal handling of checks (Figure 8–13).

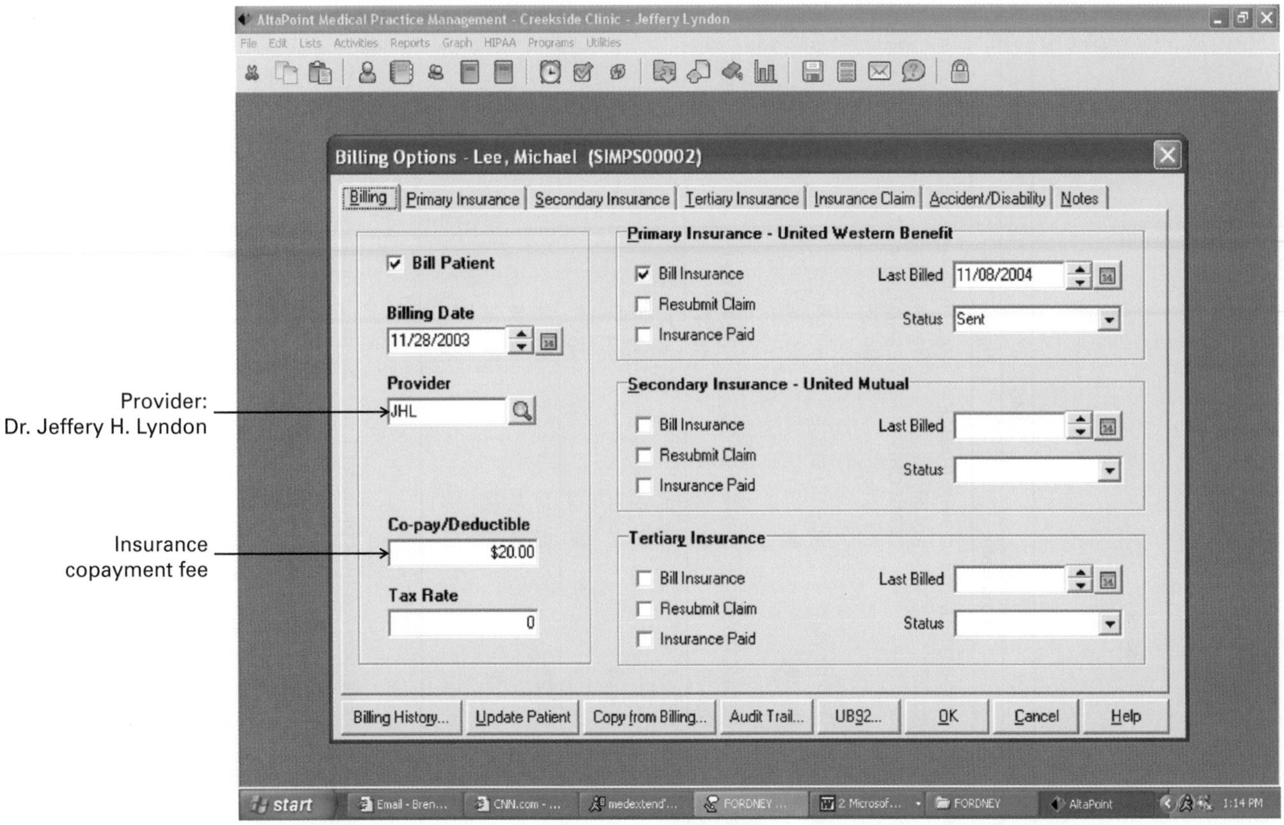

FIGURE 8–13 AltaPoint screen showing the billing options available and set up for patient Michael Lee.

ELECTRONIC REMITTANCE ADVICE

An online transaction about the status of a claim is called an **electronic remittance advice (ERA)**. This gives information on charges paid or denied and automatically posts the information to patients' accounts without data entry if the software has this feature. The computer tests the claims computer data against various guidelines or parameters known as screens. If the services billed on the claim exceed the screens, the claim is denied, returned to the physician for more information, or sent for review. If a claim is denied or rejected, the billing specialist receives a printout stating the reason. The missing, miscoded, or incomplete information should be added or corrected and the claim resubmitted; this process is more efficient than remaining on a telephone on hold or resubmitting a claim via standard mail.

A Medicare ERA, formerly known as explanation of Medicare benefits (EOMB or EOB) is based on the American National Standards Institute (ANSI) Accredited Standards Committee X12 (ASC X12) Health Care Claim Payment/Advice (835), or "ANSI 835" (Figure 8–14). A subcommittee, X12N, has developed standards for a variety of electronic transactions between third-party payers and health care providers.

The use of ANSI 835 Version 4010 generates an electronic Medicare remittance advice instead of the paper RA.

To improve cash flow, ANSI 835 also allows EFT of Medicare payments to the physician's bank account, which is called *direct deposit*.

DRIVING THE DATA

Basic procedures for transmission of a claim electronically:
1. Set up the database.
2. Enter data.
3. Batch or compile a group of claims.
4. Connect the computerized database with the clearinghouse or direct to the payer.
5. Transmit the claims.
6. Review the clearinghouse reports.

METHODS FOR SENDING CLAIMS

The methods for getting claims submitted to either the payer or the clearinghouse vary according to the office system in place. Methods can include the following:
Data transmission via cable modem, DSL, T-1
- **Cable modem.** A modem used to connect a computer to a cable television system that offers online services.
- **Digital subscriber line (DSL).** A high-speed connection through a telephone line jack and usually a means of accessing the Internet.

No. 1 ABC INSURANCE COMPANY	5780 MAIN STREET	WOODLAND HILLS	XY	12345	TEL # 5557639836
No. 2 Prov #	No. 3 Prov Name	No. 4 Part B	No. 5 Paid Date:	No. 6 Remit #	Page:

Row labels (left column):

PATIENT NAME No. 7	PATIENT CNTRL NUMBER No. 12	NACHG Nos. 14	HICHG 15	TOB 16
HIC NUMBER No. 8	ICN NUMBER No. 13	COST Nos. 17	COVDY 18	NCOVDY 19
FROM DT–THRU DT Nos. 9 10				
CLM STATUS No. 11				

Detail field layout (Part B block — each claim cell has four sub-rows):

	RC	REM					
Line 1	No. 20	No. 21	DRG # No. 22	DRG OUT AMT No. 27	COINSURANCE No. 30	PAT REFUND No. 34	CONTRACT ADJ No. 38
Line 2	No. 20	No. 21	OUTCD Nos. 23	CAPCD 24	COVD CHGS No. 31	ESRD NET ADJ No. 35	PER DIEM RTE No. 39
Line 3	No. 20	No. 21	PROF COMP No. 25	MSP PAYMT No. 28	NCOVD CHGS No. 32	INTEREST No. 36	PROC CD AMT No. 40
Line 4	No. 20	No. 21	DRG AMT No. 26	DEDUCTIBLES No. 29	DENIED CHGS No. 33	PRE PAY ADJ No. 37	NET REIMB No. 41

SUBTOTAL FISCAL YEAR

	COST Nos. 17	COVDY 18	NCOVDY 19					
Line 1					No. 27	No. 30	No. 34	No. 38
Line 2						No. 31	No. 35	No. 39
Line 3				No. 25	No. 28	No. 32	No. 36	No. 40
Line 4				No. 26	No. 29	No. 33	No. 37	No. 41

SUBTOTAL PART B

	COST Nos. 17	COVDY 18	NCOVDY 19					
Line 1					No. 27	No. 30	No. 34	No. 38
Line 2						No. 31	No. 35	No. 39
Line 3				No. 25	No. 28	No. 32	No. 36	No. 40
Line 4				No. 26	No. 29	No. 33	No. 37	No. 41

A

FIGURE 8–14 **A,** Example of a computer-generated Medicare Part B Remittance Advice document received by a provider from the payer or fiscal intermediary. For an explanation and to understand each number that appears in this document, refer to Figure 8–14, B. (*From a handout "How to Read a Remittance Advice (RA)" supplied by TrailBlazer Health Enterprises, LLC, Dallas, Texas, a Medicare contractor.*)

Medicare Remittance Advice

No. 1	The payer name, address, city, state, ZIP code, and telephone number	No. 21	Remark codes. These codes are used to return claim-specific information to the provider. Only ANSI codes are used.
No. 2	Medicare provider number	No. 22	*Diagnosis Related Group (DRG) number
No. 3	Provider name	No. 23	*Outlier code 70 = Code is present if a cost outlier is paid
No. 4	Claim type (Part A and Part B claims are listed on separate pages of the remittance advice)	No. 24	*Capital code 22 is present if capital is present
No. 5	Date the claim was paid	No. 25	*Professional fees billed but not payable by the FI
No. 6	Sequential remittance advice assigned code and page number	No. 26	*PPS-DRG operating amount (DSH+OLD+CAP+HSP+FSP)
No. 7	Beneficiary's last name, first initial, and middle initial	No. 27	*PPS-DRG outlier amount
No. 8	Beneficiary's Health Insurance Claim Number (HICN)	No. 28	MSP primary payer amount
No. 9	Statement covers from date (MMDDCCYY)	No. 29	Deductible amounts (Cash deductible and/or blood deductible)
No. 10	Statement covers through date (MMDDCCYY)	No. 30	Coinsurance amounts (including LTR days)
No. 11	Claim Status Code:	No. 31	Covered charges
	1—Paid as primary	No. 32	Noncovered charges
	2—Paid as secondary	No. 33	Denied charges
	3—Paid as tertiary	No. 34	Patient refund amounts
	4—Denied	No. 35	ESRD Network reduction
	5—Pended	No. 36	Interest paid to provider and/or beneficiary for claim. The amount paid by Medicare when there is a delay in processing a clean claim
	10—Received, but not in process	No. 37	Presumptive payment adjustment—forced balancing amount (standard paper remittance only)
		No. 38	Contractual adjustment (amount used to balance claim charges to payment amount). Amount calculated as follows:
	19—Paid as primary and crossed over		Minus the sum of all value codes for MSP
	20—Paid as secondary and crossed over		Minus claim noncovered charges
	21—Paid as tertiary and crossed over		Minus Gramm-Rudman reduction
	22—Reversal of previous payment		Minus ESRD Network reduction
	23—Not our claim and crossed over		Minus claim denied charges
No. 12	Patient control number		Minus the value code amount for professional component
No. 13	Internal control number		Minus blood deductible
No. 14	Patient name change (74 = change in patient name and QC = No change in patient name)		Minus cash deductible
			Minus coinsurance amount
No. 15	HIC number change (C = Change in HIC number and N = No change in HIC number)		Minus net provider reimbursement amount
			Minus patient refund amount
No. 16	Type of bill (three digit code)		*Do not subtract if satisfied by MSP payment
No. 17	*Cost report days	No. 39	Per diem rate
No. 18	*Covered days	No. 40	Fee schedule amount payable amount
No. 19	*Noncovered days	No. 41	Reimbursement amount paid to the provider for this claim
No. 20	Reason codes (up to 4 occurrences—see ANSI code list)		

FIGURE 8-14 cont'd **B,** Explanation of the Medicare Remittance Advice.

B

- **T-1.** A T-carrier channel that can transmit voice or data channels quickly.

Data directly keyed into payer system: DDE via dial-up modem or Internet

- **Direct data entry (DDE).** Keying claim information directly into the payer system by accessing over modem dial-up or DSL. This is a technology to directly enter the information into the payer system via the access whether it is dial-up or DSL.

Practice management system (PMS). In-house shared systems or application service provider (ASP).

- **Application service provider (ASP).** "Renting" a PMS available over the Internet. All data are housed on the server of the ASP but the accounts are managed by the health care provider's staff. Claims are batched and submitted similarly as though the software is stored on the desktop at the provider's office.

COMPUTER CLAIMS SYSTEMS

Payer or Carrier-Direct

For a better understanding of how insurance claims are transmitted, know the types of systems and how they work (e.g., payer or carrier-direct and clearinghouse).

Fiscal agents for Medicaid, Medicare, TRICARE, and many private insurance carriers use the carrier-direct system. With this system, the data are transmitted electronically directly into the payer's system. This eliminates the need for a clearinghouse.

It is necessary to have a signed agreement with each carrier with whom the physician wishes to submit electronic claims.

Clearinghouse

Clearinghouses may charge a flat fee per claim or a monthly charge. Some clearinghouses offer to file claims free of charge to the provider, but recoup the expense from the payer. Most often, a vendor agreement of sorts will be in place between the clearinghouse and the provider submitting the claims. These contracts may be a **business associate agreement,** a **trading partner agreement,** or other contract.

TRANSMISSION REPORTS

Whether claims are submitted carrier-direct or through a clearinghouse, reports are generated and able to be accessed in order to track each function of the claims process. For example:

- *Send and receive files* reports show that a file is received by the clearinghouse and/or payer and also notifies

the billing specialist when a file has been sent to the provider's account for review (Figure 8–15).

- *Scrubber report* indicates the total number of claims, charges, and dollar amounts that were received by the clearinghouse and scrubbed for claim submitted to Massachusetts Insurance Plan (Figure 8–16). The billing specialist reviews the scrubber report for each insurance payer when claims have been transmitted through the clearinghouse.

- *Transaction transmission summary* shows how many claims were originally received by the clearinghouse and/or payer and how many claims were rejected automatically (not included for further processing (Figure 8–17).

- *Rejection analysis* report identifies the most common reasons claims are rejected and indicates what claims were not included for processing (Figure 8–18). Corrections must be made by the billing specialist and the claims need to be refiled.

- *Electronic inquiry or claims status review* lists files received from the provider's office and indicates the progress of the claim. For example, if a claim is sent to a clearinghouse and forwarded to a payer, then the clearinghouse can indicate the status is confirmed received by the payer.

Electronic Processing Problems

Some problems can occur in electronic claims submission. Usually a status report of claims is received electronically from the insurance company. It consists of an acknowledgment report and indicates assigned and not assigned claims, crossed over and not crossed over claims, claims accepted with errors, and rejected claims (see Figure 8–18). Data transmission problems arise periodically because of hardware or software problems.

Billing and Account Management Schedule

Maintaining a schedule will help with EDI transmissions, which will enable a better cash flow. Table 8.7 suggests guidelines and procedures to tailor to the needs of your billing office.

Administrative Simplification Enforcement Tool (ASET)

To address issues of noncompliance in regard to TCS, the federal government has implemented the use of an electronic tool to assist health care providers, payers, clearinghouses, and others to submit complaints regarding the HIPAA TCS rule. This online tool, known as the Administrative Simplification Enforcement Tool, or ASET,

Text continued on p. 296

Raw 837
=========

Electronic Technologies, Inc.
============================

ISA*00* *00*
*ZZ*1234*ZZ*VB6786786*041110*0310*U*00401*123456789*0*P*:~GS*HC*12
34*VB6786786*20041110*0310*123456789*X*004010X098A1~ST*837*0001~B
HT*0019*00*1*20041110*0310*CH~REF*87*004010X098A1~NM1*41*2*GERI
ATRIC ASSOCIATES LLC*****46*1234~PER*IC*JIM
JONES*TE*8005551212~NM1*40*2*MASSACHUSETTS INS
PLAN*****46*XYZ1~HL*1**20*1~NM1*85*2*ALABAMA MEDICAL
ASSOC*****24*54-5555555~N3*PO BOX
123456~N4*BOSTON*MA*12345~REF*1D*123456789~HL*2*1*22*0~SBR*P*1
8*******MC~NM1*IL*1*JONES*DEBRA*K**MI*123456789123~N3*11
JEFFERS POND
ROAD~N4*BOSTON*MA*12345~DMG*D8*19640812*F~NM1*PR*2*VMAP
FHSC FA*****PI*DMAS~N3*PO BOX
123~N4*BOSTON*MA*12345~CLM*123456*150***11::1*Y*A*Y*Y*B~REF*X
4*1242522DD~HI*BK:6110~NM1*DN*1*JACKSON*DONALD~REF*1D*12345
6789~NM1*82*1*ROWLAND*DAVID****24*54-
5555555~PRV*PE*ZZ*207ZP0102X~REF*1D*123456789~NM1*77*2*NORTH
OFFICE*****24*54-5555555~N3*123 LIPPLE
AVENUE~N4*BOSTON*MA*12345~LX*1~SV1*HC:88305:26*150*UN*1***1~
DTP*472*D8*20041028~REF*6R*11265594~
.
.
.
.
SE*160*0001~GE*1*123456789~IEA*1*123456789~

A

Human-Readable 837
===================
Electronic Technologies, Inc.
=============================

==
INTERCHANGE HEADER - Production File
==
Authorization: none   Password: none
SubmitterID: 1234   ReceiverID: VB6786786
Date: 11.10.2004   Time: 0310
Run #: 003   Control #: 123456789
Request Acknowledgement: No Sub-element Separator: :

FUNCTIONAL GROUP HEADER - HC
==
Submitter ID: 1234   ReceiverID: VB6786786
Date: 11.10.2004   Time: 0310 Control #: 123456789
ANSI X10 Version: 004010X098A1

TRANSACTION SET HEADER- 837
==
Control #: 0001
Structure Code: 0019   Purpose Code: 00
Reference ID: 1   Type: CH
Date: 11.10.2004   Time: 0310
Functional Category: 004010X098A1

Submitter - Non-Person

GERIATRIC ASSOCIATES LLC (Electronic Transmitter ID #,1234)
Contact: JIM JONES
Phone Number: 800.555.1212

Receiver - Non-Person

MASSACHUSETTS INS PLAN (Electronic Transmitter ID #,XYZ1)

BATCH #1
==

Billing Provider - Non-Person

ALABAMA MEDICAL ASSOC (Employer ID Number,54-5555555)
PO BOX 123456
BOSTON, MA 12345
Provider Number: 123456789

PATIENT #1
==
Primary Insurance

Patient Relationship: Self

Subscriber - Person

JONES, DEBRA K (Member ID Number,123456789123)
11 JEFFERS POND ROAD
BOSTON, MA 12345

Date of Birth: 19640812 Gender Code: F

Payer - Non-Person

VMAP FHSC FA (Payer ID Number,DMAS)
PO BOX 123
BOSTON, MA 12345

Account Number: 123456
Claim Amount: $150
Facility: Office
This Claim is   ORIGINAL
Provider Signature: On File Assignment Code: Assigned
Assignment of Benefits Indicator: Y
Release of Information: Yes, Provider Has a Signed Statement
Permitting Release of Medical Billing
Data Related to a Claim
CLIA Number: 1242522DD
Principal Diagnosis Code: 6110

Referring Prov. - Person

JACKSON, DONALD
MA Provider Number: 123456789

Rendering Prov. - Person

ROWLAND, DAVID (Employer ID Number,54-5555555)
Provider Taxonomy Code: 207ZP0102X
MA Provider Number: 123456789

Service Location - Non-Person

NORTH OFFICE (Employer ID Number,54-5555555)
123 LIPPLE AVENUE
BOSTON, MA 12345

Service Line # 1

Service Code: 88305
Modifier: 26
Amount: $150 Measurement: Unit Quantity: 1
Diagnosis Pointer: 1
Date of Service: 20041028
Prov. Control #:   11265594

PATIENT #2
==
.
.
.
.
TRANSACTION SET TRAILER
==
Included Segments: 160
Control #: 0001

FUNCTIONAL GROUP TRAILER
==
Transaction Sets Included: 1
Group Control #: 123456789

INTERCHANGE TRAILER
==
Included Functional Groups: 1
Control #: 123456789

B

FIGURE 8–15 **A,** Raw 837 clearinghouse transmission report. If you print the 837 electronic claims transmission file, it looks similar to **A;** however, the report becomes readable after it comes back from the clearinghouse showing the patients' claims that were submitted. **B,** Readable 837 clearinghouse transmission report. *(Reports supplied by Electronic Technologies, Inc., Delmar, New York.)*

Scrubber Report
================

Electronic Technologies, Inc.
=========================

ALIAS : Massachusetts Insurance Plan   Date: November 22, 2004
Trace# : 003   Time: 0310
Filename: 6238   ISA Control #: 1067345273

===

TOTAL CLAIMS   6
TOTAL CHARGES   8
TOTAL DOLLARS $780.16

===

                        END REPORT

         ===================================
           This 837 has been scrubbed at a level two (2)

This Scrubber Report indicates the total number of claims, charges and dollar amount that was received by the clearinghouse and scrubbed for claim submitted to Massachusetts Insurance Plan. The billing specialist will review the Scrubber Report for each insurance payer where claims were transmitted through the clearinghouse.

FIGURE 8–16 Clearinghouse scrubber report. *(Report supplied by Electronic Technologies, Inc, Delmar, New York.)*

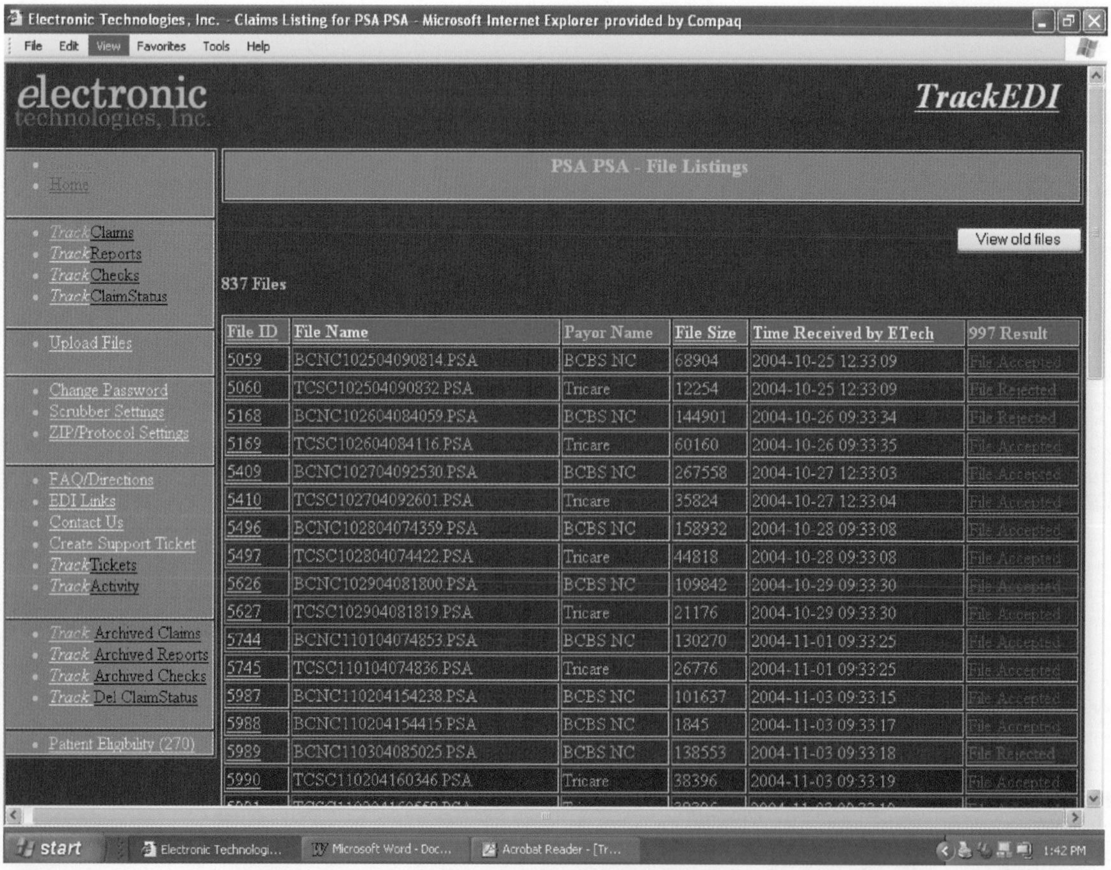

HIPAA Standard Transaction "Functional Acknowledgment" (ASC X12 997)

The 997 indicates whether the claim file was accepted or rejected.

FIGURE 8–17 Clearinghouse 997 report that shows which 837 claim files were accepted and rejected. *(Report supplied by Electronic Technologies, Inc, Delmar, New York.)*

ALIAS: Massachusetts Insurance Plan 997 Report

=======================================

CLAIMS 997 ACKNOWLEDGMENT FILE

Trace#: 941   ID: 114120941
SUBMISSION DATE: 11.22.2004   997 DATE: 11.23.2004
TIME SUBMITTED: 0112   997 TIME: 111346
===============   ===

ERROR CODE	PATIENT ACCT #	LINE# / CHARGE#
251:NM1:9	628263478	2893

DESCRIPTION: Payer Name
Segment Has Data Element Errors
DETAIL: Subscriber Identifier - (Mandatory data element missing)
SUBMITTED:

ERROR CODE	PATIENT ACCT #	LINE# / CHARGE#
251:NM1:10	123456	5454545

DESCRIPTION: Payer Name
Segment Has Data Element Errors
DETAIL: (Invalid character in data element)
SUBMITTED:

ERROR CODE	PATIENT ACCT #	LINE# / CHARGE#
251:NM1:8	4515485	3157654

DESCRIPTION: Payer Name
Segment Has Data Element Errors
DETAIL: Identification Qualifier (Conditional required data element
missing)
SUBMITTED:

This transaction was :   Rejected
Rejection Reason :   One or More Segments in Error
This Functional Group was :   Rejected
Transaction Sets Included :   1
Transaction Sets Received :   1
Transaction Sets Accepted :   0

FIGURE 8–18 Clearinghouse 997 report showing the claims acknowledgment file. This report shows error codes and details the types of errors made. It also shows patient account numbers and names of the payers. *(Report supplied by Electronic Technologies, Inc, Delmar, New York.)*

Table 8.7	Daily, Weekly, and End-of-Month Guidelines and Protocols

Daily	Weekly	End of Month
Post charges in practice management system. Post payments in practice management system. Batch, scrub, edit, and transmit claims (daily or weekly); retrieve transmission reports. Run day sheet. Review clearing-house/payer transmission confirmation reports. Audit claims batched and transmitted with confirmation reports. Correct rejections and resubmit claims.	Batch, scrub, edit, and transmit claims (daily or weekly). Analyze previous week's rejected and resubmitted claims. Note any problematic claims and resolve outstanding files. Research unpaid claims. Make follow-up calls to resolve reasons for rejections, such as incorrect NPI, missing patient ID, incomplete data elements, wrong format, and so on.	Run month-end aging reports. Review all claim rejection reports (clearinghouse and payer) to verify problems are resolved and claims accepted. Update practice management system with payer information, such as EIN, NPI, and so on. Run patient statements in office or through clearinghouse.

enables individuals or organizations to file a complaint online against an entity "whose actions impact the ability of a transaction to be accepted and/or efficiently processed."

The Security Rule: Administrative, Physical, and Technical Safeguards

Security measures encompass all the administrative, physical, and technical safeguards in an information system. The Security Rule addresses only *electronic* protected health information (ePHI), but the concept of protecting PHI that will become ePHI puts emphasis on security for the entire office. The Security Rule is divided into three main sections:

- Administrative safeguards
- Technical safeguards
- Physical safeguards

Administrative safeguards prevent unauthorized use or disclosure of PHI through administrative actions that manage the selection, development, implementation, and maintenance of security measures to protect ePHI. These management controls guard data integrity, confidentiality, and availability and include the following:

- Information access controls authorize each employee's physical access to PHI. This is management of password and access for separate employees that restricts their access to records in accordance with their responsibility in the health care organization. For example, usually the health information records clerk who has authorization to retrieve health records will not have access to billing records located on the computer.
- Internal audits allow the ability to review who has had access to PHI to ensure that there is no intentional or accidental inappropriate access, in both the practice management software system and the paper records or charges.
- Risk analysis and management is a process that assesses the privacy and security risks of various safeguards and the cost in losses if those safeguards are not in place. Each organization must evaluate their vulnerabilities and the associated risks and decide how to lessen those risks. Reasonable safeguards must be implemented to protect against known risks.
- Termination procedures should be formally documented in the office policies and procedures (P&P) manual and include terminating an employee's access to PHI. Other procedures would include changing office security pass codes, deleting user access to computer systems, deleting terminated employees' e-mail accounts, and collecting any access cards or keys.

Technical safeguards are technologic controls in place to protect and control access to information on computers in the health care organization and include the following:

- Access controls consist of user-based access (system set up to place limitations on access to data tailored to each staff member) and role-based access (limitations created for each job category, e.g., receptionist, administrative medical assistant, clinical medical assistant, bookkeeper, insurance billing specialist).
- Audit controls keep track of log-ins to the computer system, administrative activity, and changes to data. This includes changing passwords, deleting user accounts, or creating new user accounts.
- Automatic log-offs prevent unauthorized users from accessing a computer when it is left unattended. The computer system or software program should automatically log-off after a predetermined period of inactivity. Your office's practice management software may have this useful feature; if not, the feature may be temporarily mimicked using a screen-saver and password.
- Each user should have a unique identifier or "username" and an unshared, undisclosed **password** to log into any computer with access to PHI. Identifying each unique user allows the functions of auditing and access controls to be implemented. Other authentication techniques involve more sophisticated devices, such as a magnetic card or fingerprints. Most likely you will be dealing with a password in your office. Passwords for all users should be changed on a regular basis and should never be common names or words.

Physical safeguards also prevent unauthorized access to PHI. These physical measures and P&P protect a covered entity's electronic information systems and related buildings and equipment from natural and environmental hazards and unauthorized intrusion. Appropriate and reasonable physical safeguards should include the following:

- Media and equipment controls are documented in the office P&P manual regarding the management of the PHI. Typical safeguard policies include how the office handles the retention, removal, and disposal of paper records, and recycling of computers and destruction of obsolete data disks or software programs containing PHI.
- Physical access controls limit unauthorized access to areas where equipment is stored as well as medical charts. Locks on doors are the most common type of control.
- Secure workstation locations minimize the possibility of unauthorized viewing of PHI. This includes making sure that password-protected screen savers are in use on computers when unattended and that desk drawers are locked.

HIPAA: APPLICATION TO THE PRACTICE SETTING

Because HIPAA affects all areas of the health care office, from the reception area to the provider, every staff member must be educated about HIPAA and trained in the P&P pertinent to the organization. This is in addition to being trained on job responsibilities.

Reasonable safeguards are measurable solutions based on accepted standards that are implemented and periodically monitored to demonstrate that the office is in compliance. Reasonable efforts must be made to limit the use or disclosure of PHI. If you are the receptionist and you close the privacy glass between your desk and the reception room area when you are making a call to a patient, this is a reasonable safeguard to prevent others in the waiting room from overhearing.

Incidental uses and disclosures are permissible under HIPAA only when reasonable safeguards or precautions have been implemented to prevent misuse or inappropriate disclosure of PHI. When incidental uses and disclosures result from failure to apply reasonable safeguards or adhere to the minimum necessary standard, the Privacy Rule has been violated. If you are in the reception area and you close the privacy glass when having a confidential conversation and are still overheard by an individual in the waiting room, this would be "incidental." You have applied a reasonable safeguard to prevent this from happening.

COMPUTER CONFIDENTIALITY

CONFIDENTIALITY STATEMENT

Most information in patients' medical records and physicians' financial records is considered confidential and sensitive. Employees who have access to such computer data should have integrity and be well chosen because they have a high degree of responsibility and accountability. It is wise to have those handling sensitive computer documents sign an annual confidentiality statement, as recommended by the Alliance of Claims Assistance Professionals (Figure 8–19). In this way the statement can be updated when an individual's responsibilities increase or decrease. The statement should contain the following:

- Written or oral disclosure of information pertaining to patients is prohibited.
- Disclosure of information without consent of the patient results in serious penalty (e.g., immediate dismissal).

An additional example of an employee confidentiality agreement that may be used by an employer when hiring an insurance biller is shown in Figure 2–6.

PREVENTION MEASURES

Employees can take a number of preventive measures to maintain computer security:

1. Obtain a software program that stores files in coded form.
2. Never leave disks or tapes unguarded on desks or anywhere else in sight.
3. Use a privacy filter over the computer monitor so data may be read only when one is directly in front of the computer.

4. Log off the computer terminal before leaving a work station, especially if working in a LAN (local area network) environment, which is used in most hospitals, clinics, or large offices.
5. Check and double-check the credentials of any consultant hired.
6. Read the manuals for the equipment, especially the sections entitled "Security Controls," and follow all directions.
7. Store confidential data on diskettes or "zip" disks rather than only to the computer's hard drive. Diskettes should be stored in a locked, secure location, preferably one that is fireproof and away from magnetic fields.
8. Make sure the computer system has a firewall installed and proper antivirus software. This can keep amateurs, but not professional hackers, from accessing an electronic system. Hackers can access digital copiers, laser printers, fax machines, and other electronic equipment that have internal memories. Some offices leave modems on for transmitting and receiving data during low-cost, low-volume hours.
9. Develop passwords for each individual user and access codes to protect the data. A password is a combination of letters, numbers, or symbols that each individual is assigned to access the system. Passwords should be changed at regular intervals and never written down. A good password is composed of more than five characters and is case sensitive. Case sensitive means that the password must be entered exactly as stored using

Continued

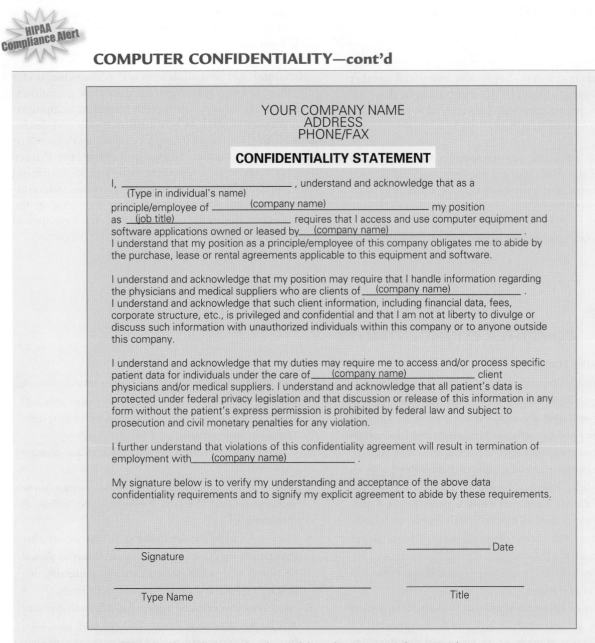

COMPUTER CONFIDENTIALITY—cont'd

YOUR COMPANY NAME
ADDRESS
PHONE/FAX

CONFIDENTIALITY STATEMENT

I, _____ , understand and acknowledge that as a
  (Type in individual's name)
principle/employee of _____(company name)_____ my position
as __(job title)_____ requires that I access and use computer equipment and
software applications owned or leased by___(company name)_____ .
I understand that my position as a principle/employee of this company obligates me to abide by
the purchase, lease or rental agreements applicable to this equipment and software.

I understand and acknowledge that my position may require that I handle information regarding
the physicians and medical suppliers who are clients of___(company name)_____ .
I understand and acknowledge that such client information, including financial data, fees,
corporate structure, etc., is privileged and confidential and that I am not at liberty to divulge or
discuss such information with unauthorized individuals within this company or to anyone outside
this company.

I understand and acknowledge that my duties may require me to access and/or process specific
patient data for individuals under the care of___(company name)_____ client
physicians and/or medical suppliers. I understand and acknowledge that all patient's data is
protected under federal privacy legislation and that discussion or release of this information in any
form without the patient's express permission is prohibited by federal law and subject to
prosecution and civil monetary penalties for any violation.

I further understand that violations of this confidentiality agreement will result in termination of
employment with___(company name)_____ .

My signature below is to verify my understanding and acceptance of the above data
confidentiality requirements and to signify my explicit agreement to abide by these requirements.

_____   _____ Date
  Signature

_____   _____
  Type Name   Title

FIGURE 8–19 Example of a confidentiality statement for an employee using computer equipment and software. (*National Association of Claims Assistance Professionals, Inc, Downers Grove, Ill.*)

upper- or lower-case characters. Delete obsolete pass-words from the system. Change any passwords known by an employee who is fired or resigns. Individuals with their own passwords allow the employer to distinguish work done by each employee. If errors or problems occur, focus may then be directed toward correcting the individual user.

10. Send only an account number (not the patient's name) when e-mailing a colleague with specific questions (e.g., about coding).

RECORDS MANAGEMENT

Data Storage

A paperless office requires an organized and efficient system for keeping files that have been saved to the hard drive against accidental destruction. Keep financial records on disks or tapes and store them in an area that does not have temperature extremes or magnetic fields.

When data is keyboarded, it is wise to **back up** (save data) frequently. Automated backup is possible, and the computer regularly initiates the process. Most financial software programs display a screen prompt instructing the operator to back up before quitting the program. If there is no automated backup, always back up files at the end of the day or several times a week so information is not lost during a power outage (e.g., surge, spike, blackout, brownout, or lightning strike), computer breakdown, or head crash. Head crash occurs when the read-write head on a disk drive strikes the surface of the disk, causing damage at the point of impact.

About once a week, a verification process should be done that compares the original records with the copies. This can take 20% to 30% longer than ordinary backup, but if a comparison is not made, there is no way to ensure that the data have been backed up. Store backup copies away from the office in case of fire, flood, or theft.

Maintain a notebook (log) of the documents on disks or tapes with an index located at the front of the book. The log enables one to keep track of files and should list when the files were backed up last so they can be located quickly. Be sure another employee knows where this notebook is kept and is familiar with how to track down files through this system. Note the code for accessing these documents and date revisions when updating old documents. Do *not* put anything related to personal health information in this log, for example: 31403.DOC, Mrs. Private Patient Positive HIV Report.

Electronic Power Protection

Plug equipment into power surge suppressors or, better yet, receptacles with an uninterruptible power supply (UPS) to prevent computer and data file damage. In addition, the entire office should be protected by a surge suppressor installed near the electric circuit breaker panel. This device is called an *all-office* or *whole-office surge suppressor*.

Selection of an Office Computer System

A medical practice wishing to use an in-office computer or an individual wishing to set up his or her own business should consider the following:

1. What is the cost of the basic equipment and will it be purchased or leased?
2. What accessories will be necessary and what are their costs?
3. How much space will be necessary for the equipment and accessories for the office or home office business?
4. What type of electrical installation should be done to handle electronic transmission of data?
5. Should a computer fax or modem be obtained or should there be a separate fax line installed?
6. How much electrical energy will be used and how much additional cost will be necessary?
7. If the computer is on a time-sharing system with other users, how much will the telephone line cost when communicating online or directly to the computer?
8. What are the hardware maintenance costs and who will do the repair work?
9. What initial software will be necessary and will it be compatible with the operating system?
10. What is the estimated cost of software upgrades and will upgrades require an expanded operating system?
11. What are the software maintenance costs and who will provide technical support?
12. Should a document scanner be obtained?
13. What forms will be used as output from the computer? Also consider their size, design, acquisition, storage, waste, and cost.
14. What other supplies will be necessary and what will their costs be?
15. How many people on the staff will operate the computer? Will recruitment be necessary? Who will train employees? How much training time is necessary?
16. Will there be financing when the equipment is purchased and, if so, what type?
17. Will there be insurance and a warranty on the system?
18. How much will the consulting costs be?
19. What is the backup support and response time when there is a system crash (software or hardware)? Who will respond to software problems and who will respond to hardware problems?
20. How much time will it take to convert the current accounting system to the computerized system, and who will be doing the conversion?

The following are major mistakes that practice administrators and physicians make when selecting an office computer system:

● Practice software process is not structured.
● Specific needs and requirements are not fully addressed.
● Consultant selected for advice is biased.

- Primary users omitted from decision purchasing process.
- Buying more than is required by the practice.
- Allowing vendors to dictate the purchasing process.

- Senior management team finalizes the choice of systems in the process rather than giving end users more input.
- Equating the vendor representative with the product.
- Refusal to use the Request for Proposal concept.

RESOURCES

INTERNET

- Administrative Simplification Enforcement Tool (ASET)
  Web site: **https://htct.hhs.gov/index.jsp**

- American Academy of Professional Coders
  Web site: **www.aapc.com**

- American Health Information Management Association's Clinical Coding Forum
  Web site: **www.ahima.org/coding**

- American Medical Association
  Web site: **www.ama-assn.org**

- Association for Electronic Health Care Transactions (AFEHCT)
  Web site: **http://www.afehct.org/aboutus/index.htm**

- Blue Cross Blue Shield Association
  Web site: **www.bluecares.com**

- *Federal Register*
  Web site: **http://www.gpoaccess.gov/fr/lindex.html**

- Healthcare Information and Management Systems Society
  Web site: **http://www.himss.org/ASP/index.asp**

- Office of Inspector General
  Web site: **www.oig.hhs.gov/**

- Centers for Medicaid and Medicare Services
  Web site: **www.cms.gov**

- Joint Healthcare Information Technology Alliance (JHITA)
  Web site: **http://www.jhita.org**

- Listing of all 50 State Insurance Commissioners
  Web site: **http://www.naic.org/state_contacts/index.htm**

- North Carolina Healthcare Information and Communications Alliance, Inc. (NCHICA)
  Web site: **http://www.nchica.org**

- TRICARE
  Web site: **http://www.tricare.osd.mil/tricareservicecenters/default.cfm**

- TRICARE Support Office
  Web site: **www.tso.osd.mil**

- Workers' Compensation related links
  Web site: **http://www.comp.state.nc.us/ncic/pages/all50.htm**

- Workgroup for Electronic Data Interchange (WEDI)
  Web site: **http://www.wedi.org**

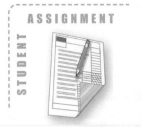

STUDENT ASSIGNMENT

✔ Study Chapter 8.

✔ Answer the review questions in the *Workbook* to reinforce the theory learned in this chapter and to help prepare for a future test.

✔ Complete the assignments in the *Workbook* to edit and correct insurance claims that have been transmitted and rejected with errors.

✔ Turn to the glossary at the end of this textbook for a further understanding of the key terms used in this chapter.

CHAPTER OUTLINE

FOLLOW-UP AFTER CLAIM
  SUBMISSION
CLAIM POLICY PROVISIONS
  Insured
  Payment Time Limits
EXPLANATION OF BENEFITS
  Components of an EOB
  Interpretation of an EOB
  Posting an EOB
CLAIM MANAGEMENT
  TECHNIQUES
  Insurance Claims Register

Tickler File
Insurance Company Payment
  History
CLAIM INQUIRIES
PROBLEM PAPER AND
  ELECTRONIC CLAIMS
  Types of Problems
REBILLING
REVIEW AND APPEAL PROCESS
FILING AN OFFICIAL APPEAL
  Medicare Review and
  Redetermination Process

TRICARE Review and Appeal
  Process
STATE INSURANCE
  COMMISSIONER
  Commission Objectives
  Types of Problems
COMMISSION INQUIRIES
PROCEDURE: TRACE AN UNPAID
  INSURANCE CLAIM
PROCEDURE: FILE AN OFFICIAL
  APPEAL

KEY TERMS

appeal
delinquent claim
denied paper or electronic claim
explanation of benefits (EOB)
inquiry

lost claim
overpayment
peer review
rebill (resubmit)
rejected claim

remittance advice (RA)
review
suspended claim
suspense
tracer

9

Receiving Payments and Insurance Problem Solving

After reading this chapter, you should be able to:

- Identify three health insurance payment policy provisions.

- Name three claim management techniques.

- Identify purposes of an insurance company history reference file.

- Indicate time limits for receiving payment for manually versus electronically submitted claims.

- Explain reasons for claim inquiries.

- Define terminology pertinent to problem paper and electronic claims.

- State solutions for problem paper and electronic claims.

- Identify reasons for rebilling a claim.

- List four objectives of state insurance commissioners.

- Mention seven problems to submit to insurance commissioners.

- Describe situations for filing appeals.

- Name three levels of review under the TRICARE appeal process.

- State the levels of review and redetermination in the Medicare program.

- Determine which forms to use for the Medicare review and redetermination process.

*Performance objectives and exercises for hands-on practical experience for this chapter appear in the *Workbook*.

Service

Assist patients with in-office registration procedures so complete and accurate personal and financial data are obtained initially and during follow-up visits. This may help diminish denied claims.

Verifying insurance coverage is a cost-effective and time-saving habit that benefits the patient and the practice. If a patient does not have active coverage and services are going to be provided, it is helpful for the patient to know that he or she is responsible for all charges.

Improve customer service by implementing an appeals process to help settle any improper patient claim denials. Notify the patient with a telephone call that an appeal letter was sent to the insurance carrier. This satisfies the patient that the practice is investigating. The patient will benefit by knowing why the claim was appealed. Either telephone or send a letter to the patient telling him or her of the insurance carrier's final decision. Give a clear explanation to the patient of the RA or EOB when questions are asked because these documents can lead to confusion or misunderstandings.

If the patient has a complaint about an insurance carrier, prepare a letter or form for the patient's signature and send it to the local insurance commissioner explaining the problem and asking for their help in resolving it.

FOLLOW-UP AFTER CLAIM SUBMISSION

For an overall picture of where and when insurance claim problems occur after submission, all aspects of the insurance picture must be studied from beginning to end. This chapter begins with the provisions for payment in the insurance contract and explains how this affects the timeliness for payment. Then the text demonstrates how to interpret the document that accompanies the payment and how to manage and organize financial records. To improve cash flow, numerous problems that can occur are presented and some solutions are offered. Finally, the review and appeal processes are discussed for various programs.

With the development of proficient skills and experience in following up on claims, one can become a valuable asset to his or her employer and bring in revenue that might otherwise be lost to the business.

CLAIM POLICY PROVISIONS

Insured

Each health insurance policy has provisions relating to insurance claims. There is a provision that the claimant has an obligation to notify the insurance company of a loss (injury, illness, or accident) within a certain period of

time or the insurer has the right to deny benefits for the loss.

In some policies, if the insured is in disagreement with the insurer for settlement of a claim, a suit must begin within 3 years after the claim is submitted. Another provision states that an insured person cannot bring legal action against an insurance company until 60 days after a claim is submitted.

Payment Time Limits

The health insurance policy also has a provision about the insurance company's obligation to pay benefits promptly when a claim is submitted. However, time limits vary in this provision from one insurance carrier or program to another. Specific time limits will be stated either in the insurance contract or the payer's manual outlining claims filing rules. It is reasonable to expect payment within 4 to 12 weeks if claims are submitted on paper or in as little as 7 days when transmitted electronically. If a payment problem develops and the insurance company is slow or ignores, denies, or exceeds time limits to pay a claim, then it is prudent to contact the insurance company. In the letter, the contracted time limit should be stated, the reason the claim has not been paid should be asked, and a copy should be retained for the physician's files. If the problem persists and there is no favorable response, the state insurance commissioner should be contacted to see whether he or she can take action to improve the situation; a copy of the correspondence should also be mailed. Many state insurance commissioners have broad powers to regulate the insurance companies within their state; others have no powers at all. If the carrier is a self-insured plan, a Medicaid or Medicare health maintenance organization (HMO), or an Employee Retirement Income Security Act (ERISA)–based plan, the insurance commissioner will not be able to assist with carrier issues. Claims may be submitted to the insurance company repeatedly with none of them ever being recorded. The one claim that will make it to the insurance company is the one that arrives after the self-determined timely filing deadline. If the provider has no contract with the carrier, the provider is not obligated to the carrier's deadline. Their denial should be appealed and payment demanded.

Managed care plans usually process claims on a daily basis, but some plans release payments quarterly. Some plans withhold a percentage that is reserved in a pool and distributed at the end of the fiscal year. In some states, managed care plans do not come under the jurisdiction of the state insurance commissioner. Read through the contract and if the responsible entity is still unable to find out who is the responsible entity then check with your state medical society. Because managed care plans vary considerably in payment policies and administrative procedures, the next chapter details follow-up procedures and problem-solving techniques.

EXPLANATION OF BENEFITS

An **explanation of benefits (EOB)** may also be referred to as a **remittance advice (RA),** check voucher, or payment voucher. It is a document issued stating the status of the claim, that is, whether it is paid, adjusted, suspended (pending), rejected, or denied. A **suspended claim** is one that is processed by the insurance carrier but is held in an indeterminate (pending) state about payment either because of an error or the need for additional information from the provider of service or the patient. The EOB also states the allowed and disallowed amounts by the insurance carrier. The allowed amount is the maximum dollar value the insurance company assigns to each procedure and service on which payment is based. Insurance carriers pay different percentages (e.g., 80%) of the allowed amount or flat rate based on service depending on the type of contract. If benefits have been assigned, the health care provider receives a copy of the EOB/RA along with a payment check. If benefits have not been assigned, payment goes to the patient and the provider's office personnel should bill the patient.

Components of an EOB

At first glance, the form may seem difficult to understand. Unfortunately, there is no standard format for EOBs from one carrier to the next, but information contained in each one usually is the same. If one line at a time is read, the description and calculations for each patient may be understood easily. The EOB breaks down how payment was determined and contains the following information in categories or columns:

1. Insurance company's name and address
2. Provider of services
3. Dates of services
4. Service or procedure code numbers
5. Amounts billed by the providers
6. Reduction or denial codes. Comment codes (reason, remarks, or notes) indicating reasons payments were denied, asking for more information to determine coverage and benefits, or stating amounts of adjustment because of payments by other insurance companies (coordination of benefits)
7. Claim control number
8. Subscriber's and patient's name and policy numbers
9. Analysis of patient's total payment responsibility (amount not covered, copayment amount, deductible, coinsurance, other insurance payment, and patient's total responsibility)
10. Copayment amount(s) due from the patient
11. Deductible amounts subtracted from billed amounts
12. Total amount paid by the insurance carrier

Figure 9–1 illustrates an EOB for a private insurance carrier and identifies each component mentioned in the preceding list.

Interpretation of an EOB

Reading and interpreting an EOB may be a bit overwhelming initially, so take time to read the document carefully. If several patients' claims are submitted to an insurance carrier, the EOB may reflect the status of all of those claims and one check voucher may be issued. If the provider has signed a contract agreeing to discount fees with a number of insurance carriers and managed care plans, payment amounts may vary along with the percentage of the fee that is adjusted off of the account. In addition, if more than one provider is in the medical practice and the practice is submitting claims using one group tax identification number, more than one physician's patients' claims may appear on a single EOB. The explanation of benefits shown in Figure 9–1 should be read line by line to interpret the meanings under each category or column, and the numbered explanations should be referred to when necessary. A helpful way to separate patients and their corresponding payments is to use a highlighter or ruler to underline the entire row across the EOB. This helps reduce errors when posting payments.

Posting an EOB

When an EOB is received in the physician's office, the claim(s) should be pulled or the patient's computerized account should be referred to, and every payment against the applicable insurance contract should be checked to establish whether the amount paid is correct. Refer to Chapter 3 and see Figure 3–18 for step-by-step directions for posting a patient's financial accounting record.

If services are reimbursed but are not clearly described on an EOB, a telephone call to the payer usually clarifies and resolves the problem so that posting can be completed.

 Claims paid with no errors are put into a file designated for closed claims. An EOB for a single payment may be stapled to the claim form and then filed with the closed claims according to the date the payment was posted. EOBs that have many patients' payments listed may be filed in an EOB file. Some offices prefer to make copies of each multiple EOB, highlight the appropriate patient account, and attach the copy to the individual claim or file it in each patient's financial record.

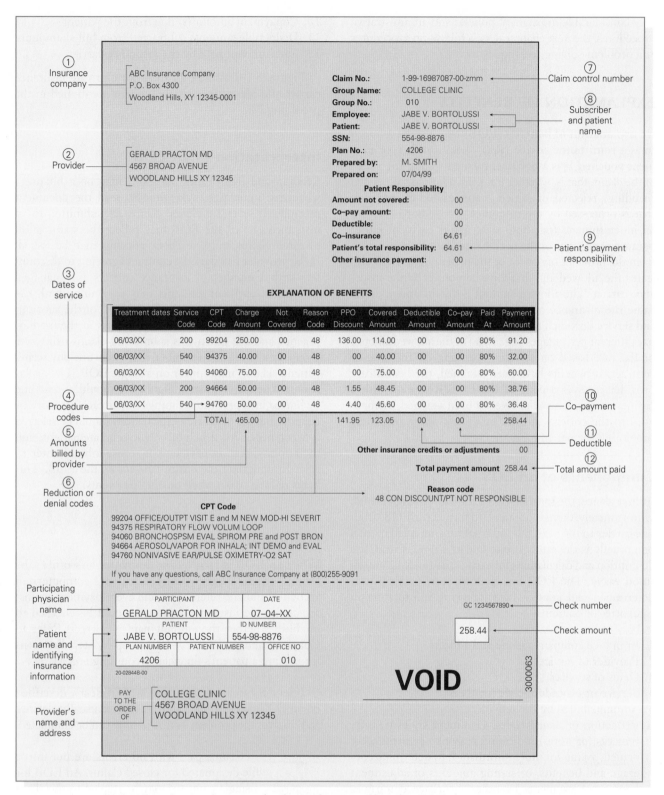

FIGURE 9–1   One example of an explanation of benefits (EOB) document with accompanying check that the provider received from a private insurance company. These payment voucher documents vary among insurance companies.

After posting payments and adjustments to applicable patient accounts, the paper EOB/RA should be filed in a designated area clearly marked in a folder. Some offices may group these remittances by payer, by month received, or by some other method. If your office receives electronic EOBs/RAs and you print them out, file accordingly. Some practice management systems allow for automatic posting of payment by downloading electronic files that work in sync with the format of the remittances.

Additional information and examples of documents may be found in the following chapters: Chapter 11 explains a Statement of Remittance for managed care systems, Chapters 8 and 12 explain both a Medicare electronic RA and a hard copy RA, and Chapter 14 shows a Summary Payment Voucher for the TRICARE program.

CLAIM MANAGEMENT TECHNIQUES

Insurance Claims Register

As discussed in Chapter 3, completed insurance claims are logged onto an insurance claims register (see Figure 3–24). After logging into a register, place a copy of all insurance claims in a pending file labeled for each month of service so that the unpaid claims can be retrieved for easy follow-up. Or, place a copy of the insurance claim in an alphabetic file by insurance company name. This method permits an inquiry on multiple outstanding claims in one letter to the insurance carrier each month rather than many letters covering individual claims. Place the insurance claims register in a loose-leaf notebook indexed according to the various insurance companies. When referring to a claims register, delinquent claims can be quickly located by simply looking through the book under the Date Claim Paid column. If that column is blank, check the Date Claim Submitted column and follow up as needed.

When a payment is received, pull all copies of claims that correspond with the payments and attach the EOB/RA. Post payment received and the contracted adjustment to the patient's financial accounting record and to the day sheet or the computerized financial record. File the EOB/RA and deposit the payment check in the physician's bank account. Use a checkmark or draw a line through the pertinent information in the claim register, but do not obscure data. When all claims on the page have been paid, draw a diagonal line across the page. Some medical practices prefer to date stamp and insert "complete" in the upper right corner of the sheet. Pages may be retained for future reference.

A log like this also could be developed and updated with little effort if using a spreadsheet software program, which would allow statistical data to be retrieved quickly and easily.

Most medical software programs offer practice management reports that can be used to track insurance payments.

Some claims are aged according to date submitted, allowing easy reference for timely follow up. Other offices age by date of service, which is when charges are initiated.

Tickler File

An alternative manual method used to track pending or resubmitted insurance claims is a "tickler file." This file is also called a *suspense* or *follow-up file*. A type of tickler file is also used to remind patients of upcoming or missed appointments (see Figure 3–22). Tickler files also can be set up in computer systems that prompt the insurance billing specialist to telephone or send inquiries about unpaid insurance claims.

To set up a manual reminder system, divide active claims by month and file them in chronologic order by date of service. Subdivisions also can be made by patient name or in numerical order by account number. Maintain the active file (unpaid claims) for the calendar year and put inactive resolved claims (older than 1 year) in storage that is accessible.

To incorporate this manual system into the billing process, start by printing two completed CMS-1500 claim forms or copy completed claim forms. Send the original to the payer and file the copy in the tickler file by date of service. After receiving the payment check and EOB/RA, pull all claims noted on the EOB/RA from the tickler file. Post the payment to the patient's account (financial accounting record) and day sheet or financial record in the computer system. Compare the charges made on each claim to the payments listed on the EOB/RA. If it is a managed care plan, refer to the insurance contract made with the provider, if necessary. If a patient has received many services and the claim was submitted on several forms, determine whether services on all forms were processed for payment. After performing this reconciliation process, attach a copy of the EOB/RA to the claim and put it in a paid file. Each claim should be referenced with the date of payment posted to the patient's account.

Delinquent claims remaining in the tickler file and exceeding the contract time limits should be traced.

Complete the insurance claim tracer form shown in Figure 9–2. If a claim has been denied because of a billing error, send a letter to the appeals division of the insurance company as shown in Figure 9–3. Attach a copy of the tracer or letter to the claim and refile it in the tickler file. It is recommended to send a copy of correspondence marked "For your information" to the patient. Follow-up procedures for claim inquiries are discussed next.

Aging Reports

 Each month a report should be run that will indicate what claims are outstanding. The report can be selected to be aged as "current," "30 days," "60 days," "90 days," "120 days," and so on. After running the report, proper follow-up should be made by inquiry as to why a claim has not yet been paid. The insurance billing specialist can write notes on the aging report documenting calls to the payer or adjustment made. For example, a note indicating the claim is to be corrected and rebilled would be helpful.

After investigating each outstanding item on the aging report, the documentation should be retained properly for future reference. If the office protocol allows notes to be placed directly in the practice management system under the pertinent patient account, then follow the office procedure.

Because time is of the essence, it is wise to be aggressive on claims that are outstanding for more than 60 days, especially when there are issues concerning timely filing.

Insurance Company Payment History

 Manually obtaining information on the payment history of insurance companies can be done by making a file of 3- by 5-inch index cards or 8- by 11-inch three-hole punched sheets in a loose-leaf binder listing the insurance companies or managed care plans that send claim payments directly to the physician. Every time a payment is received, pull out the card or the loose-leaf sheet for that company and update the information. The following information is necessary for tracking:

- Insurance company name and regional office addresses
- Claims filing procedures
- Payment policies (provisions) for each plan
- Time limits to submit claims
- Time limit for receiving payments
- Dollar amount paid for each procedural code number
- Allowable charges for each procedure code number
- Names of patients covered and their policy and group numbers

If the patients' names and group policy numbers are listed, this file is helpful when discussing with the patient what the insurance company may be expected to pay for certain services. Remember that group numbers may change annually as benefits increase or decrease, so keep the policy numbers current.

 Using the practice management system's monthly reporting capabilities is useful when tracking the payment history of insurance companies. This is an easy method to discover which companies pay slowly or pay less on certain services, and it provides excellent reports for tax purposes or to understand trends in the financial operations of the health care office.

An insurance company payment history system can help avoid potential problems and pinpoint requirements that must be met to help secure additional payment on a reduced or denied claim.

CLAIM INQUIRIES

An **inquiry,** most often referred to as a follow-up or **tracer,** is made to an insurance company to learn the status of an insurance claim or inquire about payment determination shown on the EOB/RA. As mentioned, claim status can be accessed electronically or telephonically by digital response systems, thus speeding up response time. Claim status also may be accessed with a telephone call or by mail. The following are reasons for making inquiries:

- There was no response to a submitted claim within 45 days.
- Payment was not received within the time limit for the plan or program.
- Payment is received but the amount is incorrect.
- Payment is received but the amount allowed and the patient's responsibility are not defined.
- Payment received was for a patient not seen by the provider. It is possible to receive a payment check made out to a payee's name that is different from the patient's name. Making a call may quickly clarify for whom the payment is being made.

In addition to nonpayment or reduced payment, there are other reasons for inquiries to an insurance company, including the following:

- EOB/RA shows that a professional or diagnostic code was changed from what was submitted.
- EOB/RA shows that the service was disallowed when it was a benefit.
- The claim should be revised and resubmitted. Check to see whether the procedure codes were correct and that the services listed were described fully enough to justify the maximum allowable benefits. If services were

COLLEGE CLINIC
4567 Broad Avenue
Woodland Hills, XY 12345-0001
Telephone (555) 486-9002
Fax (555) 487-8976

INSURANCE CLAIM TRACER

INSURANCE COMPANY NAME American Insurance   DATE: 09/14/XX   .

ADDRESS P.O. Box 5300, New York, New York 12000   .

Patient name: Marcella Austin

Date of birth: May 25, 1970

Employer: TC Corporation

Insured: Marcella Austin

Policy/certificate No.   9635 402-A

Group name/No.   B0105

Date of initial claim submission: 08/02/XX

Date(s) of service: 07/02/XX to 07/10/XX

Total charges submitted: $536.24

An inordinate amount of time has passed since submission of our original claim. We have not received a request for additional information and still await payment of this assigned claim. Please review the attached duplicate and process for payment within 7 days.

DETAILS OF INQUIRY

Please check the claim status and return this letter to our office. Thank you.

- ☐ No record of claim.
- ☐ Claim received and payment is in process.
- ☐ Claim is in suspense (comment please).
- ☐ Claim is in review (comment please).
- ☐ Additional information needed (comment please).
- ☐ Applied to deductible. Amount: $ _____
- ☐ Patient not eligible for benefits.
- ☐ Determination issued to beneficiary.
- ☐ Claim paid. Date: _____ Amount: $ _____ To whom: _____
- ☐ Claim denied (comment please).

Comments: _____

Thank you for your assistance in this important matter. Please contact the insurance specialist named below if you have any questions regarding this claim.

Insurance Specialist: Katelyn Chang   (555) 486-9002 Ext. 236   .

Treating Physician: Gene Ulibarri, MD   State license number C1480XX   .

Provider Number: 256788831XX   Provider's IRS number 77-86531XX .

FIGURE 9–2   One example of an insurance claim tracer showing how a form may be set up to follow up on a delinquent claim.

ABC MEDICAL GROUP, INC.

123 Main Street
Woodland Hills, XY 12345-0239
Tel. 555/487-4900
Fax. No. 555/486-4834

September 12, 20XX

Ms. Jane Hatfield
Appeals Division
XYZ Managed Care Plan
100 South H Street
Anytown, XY 12345-0001

Dear Ms. Hatfield:

Re: Claim number: A0958
     Patient: Carolyn B. Little
     Dates of service: August 2–10, 20XX

Recently I received a denied claim from your office (see enclosure). A review of the contract I have with your managed care plan shows that these services should have been approved and paid according to your fee schedule.

Enclosed is a photocopy of my chart notes for the professional services rendered to the patient on these dates. I have seen Ms. Little five times in the last nine days and each service was medically necessary by the specific complaints expressed by the patient.

On examination, I found the complaints by the patient were valid.

If after review of this claim you still feel reimbursement is not appropriate, please forward this request to the Peer Review Committee for a final determination.

If you need additional information, please telephone, fax, or write my office.

Sincerely,

John Doe, MD

mtf
Enclosures

FIGURE 9–3 A letter asking for a review about a claim submitted and denied by a managed care plan.

coded correctly and a particular service was disallowed, be sure to meet the requirements of your office in documenting this situation. You may need to talk to your supervisor to better understand how to handle this particular issue.
● There is an error on the EOB/RA.
● The check received was made out to the wrong physician.

Inquire about the claim if any of these situations occurs. If the inquiry is submitted in writing, some programs require special forms be completed with a copy of the claim attached. Figure 9–3 is an example of a letter used when asking for a review about a denied claim that was submitted to a managed care plan. If a claim must be reviewed after payment has been rendered, send in the letter as shown in Figure 9–4. When calling, document the name of the person spoken to, date and time of call, department or extension of the person, and an outline of the conversation.

PROBLEM PAPER AND ELECTRONIC CLAIMS

Types of Problems

There are many types of problem claims (e.g., delinquent, in suspense [pending], lost, rejected, denied, downcoded, partial payment, payment lost in the mail, payment paid

COLLEGE CLINIC
4567 Broad Avenue
Woodland Hills, XY
12345-0001
Telephone 555/486-9002
Fax (555) 487-8976

Committee on Physician's Services

Re: Underpayment	
Identification No.:	M18876782
Patient:	Peaches Melba
Type of Service:	Plastic & Reconstructive Surgery
Date of Service:	1 - 3 - XX
Amount Paid:	$ 75.00
My Fees:	$ 180.00

Dear Sirs:

Herewith a request for a committee review of the above-named case, since I consider the allowance paid very low having in mind the location, the extent, the type, and the necessary surgical procedure performed: The skin graft, one inch in diameter, included the lateral third of eyebrow and was full thickness to preserve hair follicles.

Operative report for the surgery has been sent to you with the claim.

Considering these points I hope that you will authorize additional payment in order to bring the total fee to within reasonable and customary charges.

Sincerely,

Cosmo Graff, M.D.

Cosmo Graff, M.D.

mf
enclosure

FIGURE 9–4 A letter appealing a fee reduction. This letter lists important data and is sent to the insurance carrier after payment has been received that the physician believes should be increased.

to patient, and overpayment). To keep accounting accurate and up to date, these problems require some type of follow-up action. The claim status may be indicated on an EOB; however, sometimes a claim is submitted and no status is reported. As mentioned, sending a claim inquiry form (tracer) is often the quickest way of determining the status of a claim (see Figure 9–2).

To prevent repeated claims errors, if the office manager understands and has a good overview of the insurance claims process, he or she should identify the source of the errors within the medical office. Often a claim may be denied because of an error that occurred when collecting registration information at the front desk or when posting charges to the account. Other errors occur because of wrong procedure or diagnostic codes, incorrect provider numbers, and a variety of situations mentioned in prior chapters. Many claims are denied for wrong gender and wrong year of birth. The more unusual or foreign-sounding a name is, the more denials occur based on gender.

The individual handling the front desk must collect insurance information accurately and update patient demographic information routinely (e.g., insurance identification number and address). The person posting to accounts must be certain to post to the correct account and see that supplemental insurers are billed after the primary insurance carrier has paid. Identified errors should be brought to the attention of the responsible individuals to improve accuracy of outgoing claims and avoid future problems.

Delinquent, Pending, or Suspense

The following are specific claim problems and possible solutions.

PROBLEM: The term **delinquent claim** means payment is overdue from a nonpayer. The nonpayer can be an insurance company, managed care plan, or intermediary for the Medicaid, Medicare, or TRICARE programs. Sometimes nonpayment is caused by a claim in review or in **suspense** because of an error or the need for additional information. The carrier may be investigating a claim because of preexisting conditions or possibly because the patient may have a work-related injury. If a service is not covered, sometimes there is no response; however, a follow-up should be initiated to further investigate.

PAPER CLAIM SOLUTION: Use claim management techniques (e.g., insurance claims register, tickler file, insurance company payment history) to keep on top of delinquent claims, so that follow-up can be accomplished in a timely manner. If the office handles a large volume of claims, divide the unpaid claims into four groups, one for each of the three largest insurers and the fourth for all others. Work on one group each week so the work is spread out over the 4 weeks in the month. Write a follow-up letter to the insurance company asking for payment and enclose a copy of the original claim form or complete the insurance company's claim tracer form or create one as shown in Figure 9–2. If the insurance contract does not bar the provider from billing members for noncovered services and the plan has not responded, send the plan a letter with a copy to the member. In the letter say that you assume its nonresponse means the service is not covered so you will bill the member directly.

ELECTRONIC CLAIM SOLUTION: In-house edit includes trying to resolve the issue as to why the claim is still not paid. Look for evidence of the claim being submitted, this should be identified in the practice management system. If the claim was submitted and confirmed received, then it is wise to look at how the claim was billed (e.g., CPT and ICD-9-CM codes). If this information is correct and the dates are correct on the claim, then contact the payer to find out what other information is holding up the claim or why the claim was denied. If the claim was not successful in being received by the clearinghouse and there is no clear-cut reason on reports or investigating the claim data showing exactly what information was amiss, then perhaps there was a problem with the format. Contacting the clearinghouse gives you more insight as to why the claim was not successfully received or rejected. The insurance billing specialist can contact the payer immediately after finding out that the claim is delinquent or the payer can be contacted after initial steps of investigation take place, such as the in-house edit and contacting the clearinghouse.

Lost Claims

PROBLEM: When an insurance claim is received by the insurance company, the claim is date stamped usually within 24 hours, assigned a claim number, and logged into the payer system. However, if there is a backlog of claims, it may take several days to be logged into the system. If one calls to find out the status of the claim during that time,

one may be told it has not been received or it may be considered a **lost claim.**

PAPER CLAIM SOLUTION: Ask if there is a backlog of claims to resolve the situation. This indicates that the claim probably has not been logged into the system. Always verify that the patient is insured by the insurance carrier and is covered for the basic benefits claimed. If it is determined to be lost, then submit a copy of the original claim referencing it "copy of the original claim submitted on (date)." Before sending it, verify the correct mailing address (e.g., post office box number, ZIP code). There are several ways to track the claim if there have been various problems with the same insurance company. Send it by certified mail with return receipt or fax the claim and ask for a confirmation. Another method available to show proof that a special communication was sent by a deadline is to obtain and complete a Certificate of Mailing form from the post office. The form is initialed and postmarked at the post office and returned to the insurance biller for office file records. Because the post office does not keep a record of the mailing, this certificate costs less than certified mail. If there is verifiable information of a lost claim, call or write to the provider relations department or member services and explain the problem. If a managed care plan, possibly check the time limit in the contract with the payer in question. Some contracts have a clause that specifies any claims not paid within a certain number of days (e.g., 30 days) after receipt will be paid at an increased rate or in full. If there is a possibility that claims have been mishandled, gather documentation and send a letter to the state insurance commission with a letter to the insurance carrier about the action taken.

ELECTRONIC CLAIM SOLUTION: Always retain the electronic response or confirmation from the carrier saying it received the specific claim. Keep all clearinghouse reports that confirm received transmission and relay information back regarding claim status. Practice management software programs show the date of every claim submitted. This is tamper-proof data recorded by the computer and may be used as a legal form of proof that the claim was submitted to the insurance carrier. Unfortunately this does not "prove" the payer received the claim, so some payers do not always accept this. Send a printed copy of the electronic proof of timely filing to the insurance carrier. Or you may send a letter with the proof of filing, a copy of the claim, and a copy of the denial if you received one for exceeding the timely filing limit.

Rejected Claims

Chapter 7 discusses some common reasons why paper claims are rejected or delayed. A **rejected claim** is a claim submitted that does not follow specific insurance carrier instructions or contains a technical error. Such claims may be disproved or discarded by the system and returned to the biller. Technical errors consist of missing or incorrect information and are found through computer edits, screening processes for benefit provisions, and proofreading. Medicare-mandated prepayment screens are discussed in Chapter 12.

PROBLEM: Paper or electronic claim rejections may occur due to one or more of the following:

- Transposed numbers
- Missing required Health Insurance Portability and Accountability Act (HIPAA) transaction code sets
- Missing subscriber date of birth
- Missing, invalid, or incorrect procedure codes and modifiers
- Missing or invalid place of service
- Mismatch of place of service to type of service
- Missing referring physician when billing tests
- Missing or invalid provider number when the patient was referred
- Incorrect, invalid, nonspecific, or missing diagnostic code numbers
- Incorrect dates of service
- Incorrect year of service
- Incorrect number of days in the month (e.g., February)
- Code description does not match services rendered
- Duplicate dates of service
- Duplicate charges

PAPER CLAIM SOLUTION: If a claim is rejected and returned, add the missing or incomplete information and resubmit a corrected claim for regular claims processing. Never send a corrected claim for review or appeal because this type of claim should always be resubmitted.

ELECTRONIC CLAIM SOLUTION: Likely, an electronic claim will not make it in a batch to be transmitted to the payer if a series of computer edits have been performed before batching (grouping claims together). The system will flag this particular claim as needing edits and will not batch it in with the rest. Correct the data in the appropriate fields and rebatch the claim.

If the claim does go through to the payer and is reported as being rejected, review the rejection reason code and correct the field. Then, rebatch the claim and submit again.

PROBLEM: A claim is submitted for several services. One service is rejected for incomplete information but the other services are paid.

PAPER CLAIM SOLUTION: Complete a new CMS-1500 claim form including all information and resubmit

for the rejected services only. Note in Block 19 that it is a resubmission.

ELECTRONIC CLAIM SOLUTION: As with a paper claim, add the required information and retransmit only the claim that was rejected, not all the claims that were originally batched and transmitted. Because this was rejected, it will likely be in the payer system for processing.

PROBLEM: Insurance carrier requests further information or information about another carrier.

PAPER CLAIM SOLUTION: Verify primary and secondary insurance information with the patient and call or mail the information to the insurance company. Identify the subscriber, subscriber number, and date of service on all correspondence.

ELECTRONIC CLAIM SOLUTION: As with a paper claim, verify all insurance information and provide accurate payer information in all applicable fields and resubmit.

PROBLEM: Resubmitted claim is returned a second time.

PAPER CLAIM SOLUTION: Review the EOB/RA statement to see if there is a denial code or narrative explanation. Examine the claim for missing, incomplete, or incorrect information and, if found, correct it. Evaluate the claim to determine if it is a candidate for the appeal process. Determine if a specific appeal form must be submitted. Submit chart notes, a detailed summary, or a copy of the operative or pathology report, as applicable, to clearly identify the procedure or service. Enclose a cover letter with the resubmitted data. The letter must specifically say what course of action is being requested (i.e., review) and it must have the name and signature of the person requesting the review.

ELECTRONIC CLAIM SOLUTION: Verify all data required for processing the claim at the payer end. Determine whether an appeal process is warranted and follow steps as outlined by the payer.

Denied Claims

A **denied paper or electronic claim** is one that may be denied because of benefits coverage policy issues or program issues. It stands to reason that insurance companies save money when a claim is denied, and only a small percentage of individuals pursue appeals. State laws require insurance companies to notify the insured of a denial and state why the claim was denied. It is possible that payment can be received even after a claim has been denied in whole or in part.

When a claim is denied and the responsible party is the patient, then transfer the balance to the patient's financial account record. If the patient has not been contacted by the insurance company, notify the patient by telephone or mail as soon as possible to keep him or her informed. Always retain the correspondence from the insurance company so it can be quickly retrieved in the event a patient inquires and has additional questions. The recourse to a denied claim is to appeal and request a review in writing. The appeals process varies between insurance carriers. A Medicare claim may be redetermined (appealed) by requesting a review in writing, and federal laws require that an explanation be given for each denied service. In Medicare Part B redetermination cases, carriers have been instructed to pay an appealed claim if the cost of the hearing process is more than the amount of the claim.

Some reasons why paper or electronic claims are not paid because of denial include the following:

● Selected diagnoses not covered.
● Frequency limitations or restrictions per benefit period
● Procedure performed by ineligible specialty provider (e.g., podiatrist would not be paid for neurosurgery)
● Bundled with other services
● Payable only in certain locations (e.g., outpatient only)
● Prior approval needed and not obtained
● Service or procedure not justified by diagnosis
● Missing or incorrect place of service code

Because denials usually involved policy coverage issues, electronic claims may be denied for the same reasons as a paper claim.

In either case of paper or electronic claim denial, simply changing information on the claim and resubmitting will not resolve the problem. Additional examples with suggested solutions are as follows:

PROBLEM: Service was not a policy or program benefit (e.g., routine physical examination, routine tests, routine foot care, routine dental care, cosmetic surgery, custodial care, eye or hearing examinations for glasses or hearing aids, and some immunizations). Plastic surgery is considered a general exclusion in many insurance policies.

PAPER AND ELECTRONIC CLAIM SOLUTION: Send the patient a statement with a notation of the response from the insurance company. Before providing services, always verify coverage for routine physical examinations or tests and services that are in question as to whether they will be paid by the insurance policy. Discuss this with the patient before service is provided and advise of the likelihood of no coverage. It may be appropriate to request payment at the time of service. In a Medicare case before service is given, have the patient sign an advanced beneficiary notice (see Figure 12–11).

PROBLEM: Treatment is given for a preexisting condition. (Currently some policies do not include this exclusion.)

PAPER AND ELECTRONIC CLAIM SOLUTION: When a patient is referred, ask the referring physician to forward information on all preexisting conditions that may be relevant to the surgery or procedure to be performed. Under HIPAA policies, physicians may treat patients, seek payment, and conduct routine health care operations without having to obtain a patient's written consent. Request verification of insurance coverage from the insurer for the surgery or procedure with regard to preexisting conditions. Request authorization for the surgical procedure or diagnostic tests. If authorization is denied, have the physician discuss other treatment or payment options with the patient. If the physician believes that the patient's condition is not preexisting, send an appeal to the insurance company. Otherwise bill the patient, noting the insurance company's response on the statement.

PROBLEM: Insurance coverage is canceled before service.

PAPER AND ELECTRONIC CLAIM SOLUTION: Send the patient a statement with notation of the insurance determination on the bill.

PROBLEM: Insurance coverage lapsed before service is rendered.

PAPER AND ELECTRONIC CLAIM SOLUTION: Send the patient a statement with notation of the response from the insurance company on the bill.

PROBLEM: Service is provided before coverage is in effect.

PAPER AND ELECTRONIC CLAIM SOLUTION: Send the patient a statement with notation of the response from the insurance company on the bill.

PROBLEM: Insurance company indicates provided service was not medically necessary.

PAPER AND ELECTRONIC CLAIM SOLUTION: Determine under what circumstances the insurance carrier considers the service to be medically necessary. The problem may be that the diagnostic code does not properly support the procedural codes being reported. It is vital that the physician's documentation be specific enough to support the necessity of the services provided. If the physician believes the patient's condition supported the medical necessity for the service, send an appeal for review to the insurance company, explaining in detail the reasons why. Keep a list of codes that have been denied for medical necessity and what further determinations were made in the insurance company payment history. Check the insurance contract to determine whether the patient may be billed. Consider asking patients to sign an Advanced Beneficiary Notice or Waiver of Liability form before treatment. Beware that you do not have every patient sign such documents because then such documents would be considered a blanket waiver. Bill the patient if payment may be denied.

PROBLEM: Service was for an injury that is considered as payable or covered under workers' compensation. Create a workers' compensation information sheet asking the employee and employer to fill out separate sections with space for the following: explanation of the injury, insurance information, adjuster's name and telephone number, and claim or case number.

PAPER AND ELECTRONIC CLAIM SOLUTION: Locate the carrier for the industrial injury, request permission to treat, and send the carrier a report of the case with a bill. Notify the patient's health insurance carrier monthly about the status of the case.

PROBLEM: Service was not precertified for a surgery, hospitalization, or diagnostic procedure.

PAPER AND ELECTRONIC CLAIM SOLUTION: Telephone the insurance company and ask whether precertification was necessary for the service or if any sanctions were imposed. The office may want to institute a policy that all surgical procedures and durable medical equipment/supplies be called in to insurance companies before rendering the service. Document the contact name, date, and time of the call. If there were problems or difficulties about the case leading to the reason precertification was not obtained, write a letter of appeal noting the history. Insurance payers can change their policies on certain procedure codes throughout the year.

PROBLEM: Patient or employer did not pay premium.

PAPER AND ELECTRONIC CLAIM SOLUTION: Verify insurance coverage before treatment begins, especially for procedures and surgery. Change patient's account to "cash" if insurance is not in force and discuss this with the patient.

PROBLEM: Service or procedure is experimental.

PAPER AND ELECTRONIC CLAIM SOLUTION: Verify whether the procedure is approved by the insurance company before the procedure is done.

PROBLEM: Deductible was not met.

PAPER AND ELECTRONIC CLAIM SOLUTION: Ask the patient when he or she arrives at the office about the status of the deductible. Or telephone the payer to find out this information, which often may be obtained from an automated system. Collect the deductible from the patient if it has not been paid. Consider holding the claim if several services are performed during the same time period and the patient paid the deductible at another office but the deductible has not been recorded by the insurance company.

PROBLEM: Services are considered cosmetic.

PAPER AND ELECTRONIC CLAIM SOLUTION: Appeal the claim if the problem was treated because of a medical condition, not for cosmetic reasons. Otherwise, collect from the patient before services are provided.

PROBLEM: Claim duplicates an existing claim.

PAPER AND ELECTRONIC CLAIM SOLUTION: Verify the services or charges have not been previously submitted and processed.

PROBLEM: Claim is missing a modifier or has an incomplete or invalid modifier.

PAPER AND ELECTRONIC CLAIM SOLUTION: Become familiar with the modifier descriptions and their appropriate use, and verify that the payer recognizes them.

Measures to Prevent Denied Claims

Prevention measures to avoid denied claims are as follows:

1. Be proactive and verify insurance coverage at the first visit—this saves time and surprises for everyone. Make sure demographic information is current at each visit.
2. Include progress notes and orders for tests for extended hospital services.
3. Submit a letter from the prescribing physician documenting necessity when ambulance transportation is used.
4. Clarify the type of service (e.g., primary surgical services versus assist-at-surgery services).
5. Use modifiers to further describe and identify the exact service rendered.
6. Keep abreast of the latest policies for all contracted payers as well as the federal programs by going to the Centers for Medicare and Medicaid Services (CMS) Web site to read currently posted Medicare Transmittals (formerly called Program Memorandums) and reading news releases from the Blue Plans, Medicaid, TRICARE, workers' compensation insurance carriers, and managed care plans.
7. Obtain current provider manuals for all contracted managed care payers as well as the Blue Plans, Medicaid, Medicare, and TRICARE for quick reference. When bulletins or pages are received from these programs during the year, keep the manuals up-to-date by inserting the current material.

Downcoding

Lowered reimbursement is the result of downcoding. As mentioned in Chapter 6, downcoding occurs for the following problems:

PROBLEM: There is insufficient diagnostic information on a claim.

PAPER CLAIM SOLUTION: Be sure each procedure listed on the paper claim form is linked to an appropriate diagnosis. Refer to the health record if necessary. A code link book is an excellent resource and is available from Ingenix. See Appendix A.

PROBLEM: Unspecified diagnoses are listed on the claim form. Routine use of too many nonspecific diagnostic codes (ICD-9-CM codes that have number "9" as the fourth or fifth digit) result in denials, especially if extensive or specific surgery is involved.

PAPER CLAIM SOLUTION: Make sure the physician dictates specific diagnoses and does not circle nonspecific diagnoses on an encounter form. Always code to the highest level of specificity. Refer to the patient's health record when necessary.

Payment Paid to Patient

PROBLEM: Sometimes an insurance payment may be sent in error to the patient after an assignment of benefits has been signed and sent in with the insurance claim. In some cases, a clause may be in the insurance policy that payment may be made only to the insured. In another instance this might happen when a patient uses the services of a provider who is outside of his or her preferred provider organization.

PAPER AND ELECTRONIC CLAIM SOLUTION: Call the insurance company to verify whether the payment was made and to whom. If the provider has a participating agreement, then the insurance company is obligated to pay the provider and must proceed by correcting the error. If the account is substantially overdue, ask for a copy of the endorsed check or EOB/RA statement that indicates where payment was sent. If the carrier refuses, ask for help from the supervisor of the provider or customer relations department. There are two different courses of action to take after this has been verified.

1. Call the patient explaining that the insurance company sent payment to him or her in error and ask when full payment can be expected. Document the commitment in the patient's financial record. If the patient cannot be reached by telephone, send a letter by certified mail to the patient. Discuss with the physician whether he or she wishes to discharge the patient from the practice.
2. Send a letter to the insurance company including a copy of the claim with EOB/RA indicating payment was made to the patient and a copy of the assignment of benefits. Demand payment from the insurance company, stating the need to honor the assignment and the signed participation agreement. The insurance company must recover the payment from the patient. If a

dead-end is reached after pursuing reimbursement from the insurance company, then file a complaint with the state insurance commissioner. After receiving the physician's complaint, the commissioner will write to the insurance company and request a review of the claim. If the insurance company admits that there is an assignment of benefits and that it inadvertently paid the patient, the insurance company must pay the physician within 2 to 3 weeks and honor the assignment even before it recovers its money from the patient. The insurance company then files for payment from the patient.

Two-Party Check

PROBLEM: A check is received made out to both the physician and the hospital and only part of the sum is the physician's payment. This might occur when the provider is contracted with the hospital.

SOLUTION: If you do not receive an EOB containing the breakdown of both party's payments, then call the insurance company and ask how much should be retained by the physician. Request the allocation be sent in writing. Ask whose tax identification number will be used on the 1099 form for reporting income to the Internal Revenue Service. The hospital's income should not be reflected on the physician's 1099 form. To avoid another problem like this, inquire why the insurance company paid in this manner. Sometimes a participating agreement may exist that the physician did not know about.

Overpayment

An **overpayment** is a sum of money paid by the insurance carrier or patient to the provider of service that is more than the bill or more than the allowed amount. Overpayments may be discovered immediately, called to one's attention by the patient or insurance carrier, or not discovered for several months or years. The Office of Inspector General strongly advises to return overpayment promptly. Not doing so can lead to severe fines and implicate fraudulent activity.

Some states have laws or court decisions barring or restricting managed care plans and other insurers from recovering mistaken payments from providers. Some states bar insurers from collecting any mistaken payment from an innocent provider. Some states will not let insurers recover if the provider "changed its position" in reliance on the payment (i.e., the provider spent the money to pay its bills). First determine whether an overpayment exists by reviewing the available financial documents on the case in question. Then decide how to handle the overpayment. Be sure to get the physician's attorney's advice on the extent to which you can challenge a plan's demand for repayment based on state law or court decisions.

It is wise to develop an overpayment policy and procedure for each type of insurer, program, or managed care plan and for every type of overpayment situation that may occur.

PROBLEM: Overpayment scenarios that may occur are as follows:

● Receiving more than one's fee from an insurance carrier
● Receiving more than the contract rate from a managed care plan
● Receiving payments that should have been paid to the patient
● Receiving duplicate payments from two or more insurance carriers or from the patient and one or more third-party payers
● Receiving payment made for someone who is not the provider's patient

SOLUTION: When an overpayment occurs, post the activity to the appropriate patient account with additional notation that it was received in error and a refund was made. Creation of an account specifically for overpayments is advisable to track all funds in this category. In any type of overpayment situation, cash the third-party payer's check and make out a refund check payable to the originator of the overpayment. The refund check should always be sent to the attention of a specific person at the insurance company. In case of an audit, this establishes documentation showing the problem has been resolved. Usually insurance companies process a credit of the overpayment amount to the next check voucher.

Refund checks should be given top priority and written as soon as reasonably possible. Make sure this office policy is clearly stated and adhered to in all cases. If the patient pays and a third-party pays and the overpayment must be refunded to the patient, always write a check—never refund in cash. If the patient pays by credit card, wait until the charges have cleared to draft a check.

If the patient cannot be located to return the money, send a check by registered mail to the patient's last known address. When it comes back marked "undeliverable," retain the document as legal proof that an honest effort was made to return the overpayment. The money should be listed as taxable income and put in the bank.

Commercial Carriers

PROBLEM: Usually an overpayment mistake made by a commercial carrier is the insurer's problem.

SOLUTION: First call and notify the patient; then proceed cautiously before refunding money by doing the following:

● Investigate the refund request by sending a letter to the insurance payer disputing the recoupment. Include documentation as proof (e.g., operative report, health record, bundling guidelines).
● Obtain documentation from the insurance payer to prove why the refund is legitimate.
● The general rule is to not pay old recoupments dating back more than 4 or 5 years.
● If two or more insurance carriers send duplicate payments, write a letter to each explaining the situation and let them straighten it out. Then send a refund to the correct insurance carrier to the attention of a specific person after receiving a letter explaining to whom the money should be sent.

Managed Care Plan

PROBLEM: An overpayment from a managed care plan is discovered.

SOLUTION: Review the payer's policy about overpayments and be sure it is clearly documented in the provider's contract. Address this issue if it is not defined by the payer. Follow your office protocol for documenting overpayments.

Medicare

PROBLEM: An overpayment is made from Medicare, Medicaid, or a Blue Plan.

SOLUTION: Check the billing and health records to determine whether the provider made any mistakes. If an error has been made by the insurance carrier, send a letter with documentation to appeal and prove the provider's case. Medicare, Medicaid, and the Blue Plans usually process a credit of the overpayment on the next payment voucher.

REBILLING

If a claim has not been paid, do not automatically **rebill (resubmit)** the insurance carrier without researching the reason why it is still outstanding. Simply rebilling claims can be considered duplicate claims, and the insurance company may audit the physician's practice for trying to collect duplicate payment unless you mark it "Possible duplicate." Instead, follow up on the claim as indicated in the previous section. If it is discovered that an error has been made in billing a case, then send in a corrected claim or use a claim correction form (Figure 9–5). This form was developed by a special committee convened

Claim Correction Form

Physician offices are encouraged to submit claims electronically. This form should be used in situations where the provider cannot submit corrected claims electronically or where electronic submissions would not adequately address the issue.

Submitted To:

Plan/Payer Name:_____ Date Submitted:_____

Plan/Payer Address: _____

City:_____ State_____ Zip_____

Telephone: (_____) _____ Fax: (_____) _____ E-mail:_____

Patient Name: ___Susan_____ D.O.B.:_____
  First   M.I.   Last

Subscriber Name: _____ Date of Service:_____

Policy #:_____ Group #: _____ Original Claim #:_____

Submitted From:

Provider Name:_____ TIN or ID#: _____

Contact: _____ Telephone: (_____) _____ Ext._____

Fax:(_____) _____ E-mail _____

THE FOLLOWING WAS CORRECTED ON THIS CLAIM:

❑ The patient's policy/group number was incorrect. The correct number(s) are shown above.

❑ The correct CPT code is _____ instead of _____

❑ Wrong date of service was filed. The correct date is _____

❑ Visits were denied based on the diagnosis given. Proper diagnosis code is _____ instead of _____

❑ Visit: ❑ Procedure: denied as over carrier's utilization limits. Please see attached letter to justify extensions of these limits.

❑ Carrier indicated that the patient is covered by another plan that is Primary. This is incorrect. Patient indicates you are Primary.

❑ The secondary carrier is: _____   ❑ There is no secondary carrier.

❑ The procedure was denied as medically not necessary. Documentation to support the medical necessity of this service is attached.

❑ Our clerk: ❑ Carrier's clerk: failed to enter correct number of times (units) procedure was performed. Correct units are as follows:

   D.O.S.: _____   Code: _____   Units: _____   Charge Total $: _____

❑ Multiple Surgical Procedures:
   ❑ Carrier failed to approve any procedure at 100%.   ❑ Carrier approved incorrect procedure at 100%.
   Carrier should have approved code _____ @ ❑ 100% or ❑ 50% instead of _____
   Carrier should have approved code _____ @ ❑ 100% or ❑ 50% instead of _____
   Carrier should have approved code _____ @ ❑ 100% or ❑ 50% instead of _____

❑ Modifiers should be attached to code(s)

Code	Code		Code	Code
❑ -50 _____ _____			❑ -51 _____ _____	
❑ -58 _____ _____			❑ -59 _____ _____	
❑ -79 _____ _____			❑ -GA _____ _____	
❑ ___ _____ _____			❑ _____ _____	

❑ The following E/M visit was denied as included in the global surgical fee. In fact, the service was a significant separately identifiable service provided above and beyond the procedure and submitted with appropriate E/M modifier. Please reconsider with attached documentation:

   Code: _____   with modifier(s); ❑ -24 ❑ -25   Charge $ _____

❑ UPIN information for code _____ was omitted. Physician Name: _____ UPIN: _____

❑ Plan specific provider I.D. omitted. The I.D. # is _____

❑ CLIA number was omitted. The CLIA number is _____

❑ The place of service was incorrect. The place of service should be _____

❑ The service was rendered at the physician's physical location listed in Box 32 of the claim form.

❑ Failed to attach EOB from Primary carrier. The EOB is attached to this form.

❑ Failed to enter correct information on indicated line of claim form.

   Line #:_____   Correct Information: _____

❑ Other reason for claim correction: _____

❑ Comment: _____

June 2003

FIGURE 9–5 One example of a claim correction form that may be adapted or photocopied for use by medical practices that was developed by a special committee convened by the American Association of Health Plans, the Healthcare Financial Management Association, and the Specialty Society Coalition, June 2003. These data may not always apply to all third-party insurers because each has its own procedures.

by the American Association of Health Plans, the Healthcare Financial Management Association, and the Specialty Society Coalition, which included representatives of the American Academy of Family Physicians, the American College of Obstetricians and Gynecologists, and the American Academy of Dermatology, among others. Medical practices may adapt it or photocopy it for use.

Generally if a bill has not been paid, the provider's office personnel have a strategy to automatically rebill the claim or the patient every 30 days. Bill patients on a monthly basis, even when insurance payment is expected so that they understand what has been submitted and what is pending. The statement should clearly identify the claim that has been submitted and what action is expected from the patient. If collection becomes a problem, action can be referenced to the date of service if the patient has been billed consistently. See Chapter 10 for the wording of notations on statements and in the collection process.

In December 2004 the Centers for Medicare and Medicaid Services (CMS) implemented a process that allows providers to resubmit corrected claims that have been rejected for minor errors or omissions rather than appealing those claims. For example, claims with missing or incorrect provider numbers, incorrect modifiers, or claims with keying errors (incorrect date or place of service) can be rebilled.

REVIEW AND APPEAL PROCESS

An **appeal** is a request for payment by asking for a review of an insurance claim that has been inadequately or incorrectly paid or denied by an insurance company. In the Medicare program, appeals are referred to as *redeterminations*. Usually there is a time limit for appealing a claim. Always check every private insurance carrier, Medicare, TRICARE, managed care, and workers' compensation payment against the appropriate fee schedule or customary profile to determine whether the benefits were allowed correctly. To find out this information, read the payment voucher document or refer to provider manuals for the various programs.

An appeal on a claim should be based not only on billing guidelines but also on state and federal insurance laws and regulations.

There may be a discrepancy in the way the physician or physician's staff and insurance company interpret a coding guideline. The decision to appeal a claim should be based on several factors. The provider should determine that there is sufficient information to back up his or her claim, and the amount of money in question should be sufficient in the physician's opinion. Ultimately the

decision to appeal rests in the physician's hands, not the insurance billing specialist. It takes a team effort to appeal a claim successfully. To proceed, make a telephone call to the insurance company. It may save time and money and an expert who is able to solve the problem may be reached. The following are basic guidelines:

- Assemble all documents needed (e.g., patient's medical record, copy of the insurance claim form, and EOB/RA).
- Remain courteous at all times.
- Obtain the name and extension number of the insurance claims representative or adjuster and keep this with the telephone records. After developing rapport, one may wish to call on him or her in the future for help. Ask for any toll-free numbers that the company may have, and keep these for future reference.
- Listen carefully. Jot down the date and take notes of how to solve the problem. This may be of help if another problem of the same type occurs.

An appeal is filed in the following circumstances:

- Payment is denied and the reason for denial is not known.
- Payment is received but the amount is incorrect. Verify that initially the correct amount was billed. Perhaps there was an excessive reduction in the allowed payment.
- The physician disagrees with the decision by the insurance carrier about a preexisting condition.
- Unusual circumstances warranted medical treatments that are not reflected in payment.
- Precertification was not obtained within contract provisions because of extenuating circumstances, and the claim was denied.
- Inadequate payment was received for a complicated procedure.
- "Not medically necessary" is stated as the reason for denial and the physician disagrees.

FILING AN OFFICIAL APPEAL

Refer to the end of this chapter for carrying out the procedure when filing an official appeal.

If the appeal is won but copies of the same documents must be submitted each time this issue arises, ask the insurance carrier how future claims with the same issue may be handled. Keep track of this information in a file.

Appeals must be in writing, but some programs require completion of special forms. Always send a copy of the original claim, EOB/RA, and any other documents to justify the appeal.

It is always important to keep track of the status after inquiry or appeal until payment for the case is resolved.

Use the insurance claims register shown in Chapter 3 or a separate active file labeled "Appeals Pending."

If an appeal is not successful, the physician may want to proceed to the next step, which is a peer review. A **peer review** is an evaluation done by a group of unbiased practicing physicians to judge the effectiveness and efficiency of professional care rendered. This group determines the medical necessity and subsequent payment for the case in question. Some insurance companies send a claim for peer review routinely for certain procedures that have been done for particular diagnoses.

Additional information on tracing delinquent claims, appealing or reviewing a claim, or submitting a claim for a deceased patient can be found in the chapters on Medicaid, Medicare, TRICARE, and workers' compensation.

Medicare Review and Redetermination Process

A physician or beneficiary has the right to appeal a claim after payment or denial. The Medicare program has five levels of redetermination and special guidelines to follow. They are as follows:

1. Redetermination (telephone, letter, or CMS-20027 Form)
2. Hearing officer (HO) hearing (reconsideration)
3. Administrative law judge (ALJ) hearing
4. Departmental Appeal Board review
5. Judicial review in U.S. District Court

Telephone Review

Most Medicare carriers have a telephone appeals phone (TAP) service. This may save you from filing a formal paper "Post Payment Review." When requesting a telephone appeal, gather information, such as the beneficiary's name, date of birth, Medicare health insurance claim number, name and address of provider of service, telephone and group tax identification number, date of initial determination, date of service for which the initial determination was issued, and which items are at issue in the appeal (progress notes, operative report).

Table 9.1 illustrates the Medicare Part B appeals process.

Redetermination (Level 1)

On October 1, 2004, the redetermination step became effective. If the claim was denied because of a simple error made by the insurance biller, such as omission of the National Provider Identifier (NPI) or Unique Provider Identification Number (UPIN) of the referring physician or failure to code a diagnosis, then resubmit a corrected claim. Include only the denied services and indicate in Block 19 "resubmission, corrected claim." In the event the insurance carrier made an error—for example, a procedure code was different from what was submitted or the date of service was entered incorrectly from the paper claim into the carrier's computer—then resubmit the claim with an attachment explaining the error. If response to the resubmission indicates that the claim has been "processed" previously, then go to the next appeal level.

A notice must be mailed by the Medicare intermediary within 60 days of receipt of a request from a beneficiary or provider. It must include reasons for the decision, a summary of clinical or scientific evidence used in making the redetermination, a description of how to obtain additional information, a notification of the right to appeal, and instructions on how to appeal the decision to the next level. If requested, the Medicare intermediary must provide information about the policy, manual, or regulation used in making the redetermination decision. The decision must be written in language the beneficiary can understand.

Table 9.1	**Medicare Part B Redetermination Process**				
Step	**Time Limit for Request**	**Amount in Controversy**	**Jurisdiction**	**Form**
Redetermination (telephone, letter, or CMS-20027 Form)	120 days from initial claim determination	None	Carrier	CMS-20027 (possibly fax) CMS-1500 corrected claim resubmitted
Hearing officer (HO) hearing (reconsideration)	180 days from date of initial determination	$100 or more	Carrier/qualified independent contractors	CMS-1964
Administrative law judge (ALJ) hearing	60 days from receipt of the HO determination	$100 or more	Carrier/Social Security Bureau of Hearings and Appeals	CMS-1965
Departmental Appeal Board (DAB) review	60 days from receipt of hearing decision		U.S. District Court	HA-520
Judicial review in U.S. District Court	60 days of receipt of the DAB's decision	$1050 or more		

Reconsideration (Level 2)

The physician may ask for a **review** when a claim is assigned. The request must be within 6 months from the date of the original determination shown on the RA. Figure 9–6 shows Form CMS-1964, which may be used in requesting a review of Medicare Part B claims. However, some carriers have developed their own request forms. Contact the carrier to find out the necessary form to use. Review the RA for the denial code or narrative stating why the claim has been denied. Check the claim for accuracy of diagnostic, procedural, or Healthcare Common Procedure

---

DEPARTMENT OF HEALTH AND HUMAN SERVICES
HEALTH CARE FINANCING ADMINISTRATION

FORM APPROVED
OMB No. 0938-0033

REQUEST FOR REVIEW OF PART B MEDICARE CLAIM
Medical Insurance Benefits – Social Security Act

NOTICE—Anyone who misrepresents or falsifies essential information requested by this form may upon conviction be subject to fine and imprisonment under Federal Law.

1 Carrier's Name and Address

Medicare Blue Cross and
Blue Shield of Texas, Inc.
P.O. Box 660031
Dallas, TX 75266-0031

2 Name of Patient

Jose F. Perez

3 Health Insurance Claim Number

032-XX-6619

4 I do not agree with the determination you made on my claim as described on my Explanation of Medicare Benefits dated:
3-2-20XX

5 MY REASONS ARE: (Attach a copy of the Explanation of Medicare Benefits, or describe the service, date of service, and physician's name—NOTE.—If the date on the Notice of Benefits mentioned in item 3 is more than six months ago, include your reason for not making this request earlier.)

01-21-20XX Electrocardiographic monitoring; 24 hours (93224)

Physician: Gerald Practon, MD

6 Describe Illness or Injury: Heart palpitations, tachycardia, & light headedness (near syncopal episode). Although patient

had a previous Holter monitor within the 6 mo time limitation, it did not provide any clinical evidence of disease.

Patient underwent recent monitoring after experiencing additional symptoms that were more severe than the initial

symptoms.

7 [X]   I have additional evidence to submit. (Attach such evidence to this form.)

[ ]   I do not have additional evidence.

COMPLETE ALL OF THE INFORMATION REQUESTED. SIGN AND RETURN THE FIRST COPY AND ANY ATTACHMENTS TO THE CARRIER NAMED ABOVE. IF YOU NEED HELP, TAKE THIS AND YOUR NOTICE FROM THE CARRIER TO A SOCIAL SECURITY OFFICE, OR TO THE CARRIER. KEEP THE DUPLICATE COPY OF THIS FORM FOR YOUR RECORDS.

8   SIGNATURE OF *EITHER* THE CLAIMANT *OR* HIS REPRESENTATIVE

Claimant	Representative
	Gerald Practon, MD
Address	Address 4567 Broad Avenue
City, State, and ZIP Code	City, State, and ZIP Code Woodland Hills, XY 12345

Telephone Number	Date	Telephone Number	Date
		555-486-9002	6-5-20XX

FORM CMS-1964 (9/91)

CARRIER'S COPY

FIGURE 9–6   Request for Review of Part B Medicare Claim Form CMS-1964. This form can be used by the Medicare beneficiary or physician when requesting a review of a submitted claim.

Coding System (HCPCS) codes or missing modifiers, as well as any other item that might be incorrect or missing.

A request on the physician's letterhead must include the following information:

1. Current date
2. Medicare provider number
3. RA number or claim number
4. Date of RA
5. Patient's name
6. Patient's health insurance claim number (HICN)
7. Date of service
8. Place of service
9. Procedure code(s)
10. Amount billed
11. Amount approved
12. Amount paid
13. Denial reason (action code description from the RA)
14. Brief statement of why service should be reviewed

Attach the following with the review request:

1. Copy of the original insurance claim
2. Copy of the RA showing the denial
3. Photocopy of other documents such as operative or pathology report or detailed summary about the procedure with appropriate words highlighted to help the reviewer
4. Cover letter explaining the procedure indicating justification for the services and the reason the provider should receive more reimbursement. Include the physician's NPI and signature in the letter (Figure 9–7).

Mail the documents by certified mail with return receipt requested and retain copies of all documents sent to the carrier in the provider's pending file.

If a claim is unassigned, the beneficiary (patient) can pursue the review or appoint the physician as an

---

PHYSICIAN'S LETTERHEAD

January 2, 20XX

Committee on Physician's Services
Medicare
Street address of fiscal intermediary
City, State, ZIP Code

Dear Madam or Sir:

Re: Underpayment

Identification No.:	1910-2192283-101
Patient:	Mrs. Sarah C. Nile
Type of Service:	Exploratory laparotomy
Date of Service:	December 1, 20XX
Amount Paid:	$000.00
My Fees:	$0000.00

Herewith a request for a committee review of the above-named case, since I consider the allowance paid very low having in mind the patient's condition prior to surgery, the location, the extent, the type, and the necessary surgical procedure performed.

Enclosed are photocopies of the history and physical showing the grave status of the patient prior to surgery, operative report, pathology report, and discharge summary. The Medicare Remittance Advice and the Medicare CMS-1500 claim originally submitted are also enclosed.

Considering these points, I hope that you will authorize additional payment in order to bring the total fee to a more reasonable amount.

Sincerely,

Hugh R. Aged, MD
NPI# 73542109XX

mf

Enclosures (6)

FIGURE 9–7   A cover letter for a Medicare review request to be sent with photocopies of documents pertinent to a claim.

authorized representative. The patient completes forms CMS-1964 and SSA-1696 (Figures 9–6 and 9–8) and obtains the physician's acceptance signature. Decisions on unassigned claims are sent to the patient.

Send all requests to the review department. Most insurance carriers have an address or post office box for review requests that is different from initial claim submissions, so be sure to send it to a correct current address. A review usually is completed by the insurance carrier within 30 to 45 days. Make a follow-up inquiry if no response is received in that time frame.

If certain procedures are consistently denied, ask the carrier what information is necessary to process the claim. If the provider is not satisfied with the results of the review, move to the next level.

Administrative Law Judge Hearing

A request for a hearing before an administrative law judge (ALJ) may be made if the amount still in question is $100 or more (usually in combined claims). The request must be made within 60 days of receiving the reconsideration officer's decision (Figure 9–9). It may take 18 months to receive an ALJ assignment. Proof that the claim represents an unusual case and warrants special consideration may lead to a successful conclusion. However, the decision might be reversed, allow partial adjustment of the carrier's payment, or deny payment. If the final judgment is not satisfactory, then proceed to the next level.

Judicial Review

The Appeals Council is part of the Office of Hearings and Appeals of the Social Security Administration. A request must be made within 60 days of the ALJ decision; if there is a question that the final judgment was not made in accordance with the law, the council by its own election may review the ALJ decision. If the council denies a review, the provider may file a civil action for a federal district court hearing.

The amount in controversy must be $1000 or more, and an attorney must be hired to represent the provider and manage the case. The case may be filed where the physician's business is located. Contact the local medical society for suggestions of names of attorneys experienced at this level of the appeals process.

CMS Regional Offices

One final suggestion (and this can be done with steps for a hearing or a review) is to write or telephone the medical director at one of the CMS regional offices. Sometimes a regional officer intercedes or takes steps to correct problems or inequities. CMS regional offices may be located by accessing the Medicare Web site; see Internet Resources at the end of this chapter.

Medigap

Insurance companies that sell Medigap policies must be certified before being allowed to sell in each state. The certification can be lifted from any insurer that does not honor its contract agreements. Only the state insurance commissioner can exert pressure on Medigap insurance companies. If payment is slow in coming or is not received from a Medigap insurer, tell the insurer "If I do not receive payment, I will have no alternative but to contact the state insurance commissioner."

Document complete follow-up information on each Medigap insurer (firm name, address, telephone number, and policy numbers) of every patient seen.

TRICARE Review and Appeal Process

 A provider who treats a TRICARE patient but is out of network is not able to obtain information from TRICARE. Contact the patient for their assistance. Also, out-of-network providers who wish to treat an obstetric case may need a nonavailability request form completed and processed before a patient can receive care. There must be a reason the patient cannot go to a providing facility and TRICARE determines whether or not it will approve the request. Otherwise claims will be denied.

Before appealing a TRICARE claim, an inquiry should be sent to verify claim status and attempt to resolve the problem. Figure 9–10 shows an example of a form that may be used for inquiring about a TRICARE Standard claim. TRICARE appeals procedures applicable to the routine processing of TRICARE Standard claims are described here. However, TRICARE managed care contracts have been adopted throughout the United States and the appeals procedures that TRICARE contractors use in these areas may vary. For information on how to file reviews and appeals for those contracts, ask the contracting insurance carrier for instructions and forms.

Three levels for review under TRICARE Standard appeal procedures exist:

1. *Reconsideration* (conducted by the claims processor or other TRICARE contractor responsible for the decision in a particular case)
2. *Formal review* (conducted by TRICARE headquarters)
3. *Hearing* administered by TRICARE headquarters but conducted by an independent hearing officer

DEPARTMENT OF
HEALTH AND HUMAN SERVICES
CENTERS FOR MEDICARE & MEDICAID SERVICES

NAME (Print of Type)	H.I. CLAIM NUMBER
Carol T. Usner	432-XX-9821
WAGE EARNER (if different)	SOCIAL SECURITY NUMBER

Section I   **APPOINTMENT OF REPRESENTATIVE**

I appoint this individual Gene Ulibarri, MD 4567 Broad Ave., Woodland Hills, XY 12345
(Print or type name and address of individual you want to represent you)

to act as my representative in connection with my claim or asserted right under Titles XI, or XVIII of the Social Security Act. I authorize this individual to make or give any request or notice; to present or to elicit evidence; to obtain information; and to receive any notice in connection with my claim wholly in my stead.

SIGNATURE (Beneficiary) *Carol T. Usner*	ADDRESS 530 Hutch Street, Woodland Hills, XY 12345
TELEPHONE NUMBER (555) 386-0122 (Area Code)	DATE August 3, 20XX

Section II   **ACCEPTANCE OF APPOINTMENT**

I,   Gene Ulibarri, MD   , hereby accept the above appointment. I certify that I have not been suspended or prohibited from practice before the Social Security Administration; that I am not, as a current or former officer or employee of the United States, disqualified from acting as the claimant's representative; and that I will not charge or receive any fee for the representation unless it has been authorized in accordance with the laws and regulations referred to on the reverse side hereof. In the event that I decide not to charge or collect a fee for the repesentation, I will notify the Social Security Administration. (Completion of Section III satisfies this requirement.)

I am a/an medical doctor
(Attorney, union representative, relative, law student, etc.)

SIGNATURE (Representative)	ADDRESS 4567 Broad Ave., Woodland Hills, XY 12345
TELEPHONE NUMBER (555)-486-9002 (Area code)	DATE August 3, 20XX

Section III (Optional)   **WAIVER OF FEE OR DIRECT PAYMENT**
(Note to Representative: You may use this portion of the form to waive a fee or to waive direct payment of the fee from withheld past-due benefits.)

I waive my right to charge and collect a fee for representing _____
_____ before the Social Security Administraion or the Centers for Medicare & Medicaid Services.

SIGNATURE	DATE

(See important information on reverse)
Form SSA-1696-U4 (3-88)

FIGURE 9–8   Form SSA-1696-U4 completed by a Medicare patient appointing the physician as his or her authorized representative.

HOW TO COMPLETE THIS FORM

Print or type your full name and your Social Security Number.

Section I—APPOINTMENT OF REPRESENTATIVE

You may appoint as your representative an attorney or any other qualified individual. You may appoint more than one person, but see "The Fee You Owe The Representative(s)." You may NOT appoint as your representative an organization, the law firm, a group, etc. For example, if you go to a law firm or legal aid group for help with your claim, you may appoint any attorney or other qualified individual from that firm or group, but NOT the firm or group itself.

Check the block(s) for the program in which you have a claim. Title II, check if your claim concerns disability or retirement benefits, etc. Title XVI, check if the claim concerns Supplemental Security Income (SSI) payments. Title IV FMSHS (Federal Mine Safety and Health Act), check if the claim is for black lung benefits. Title XVIII, check only in connection with a proceeding before the Social Security Administration involving entitlement to medicare coverage or enrollment in the supplementary medical insurance plan (SMIP). More than one block may be checked.

Section II—ACCEPTANCE OF APPOINTMENT

The individual whom you appoint in Section I above completes this part. Completion of this section is desirable in all cases, but it is mandatory only if the appointed individual is not an attorney.

Section III—WAIVER OF FEE

This section may be completed by your representative if he/she will not charge any fee for services performed in this claim. If you had appointed a co-counsel (second representative) in Section I and he/she will also not charge you a fee, then the co-counsel should also sign this section or give a separate waiver statement.

GENERAL INFORMATION

1. When you have representative:

   We will deal directly with your representative on all matters that affect your claim. Occasionally, with the permission of your representative, we may deal directly with you on the specific issues. We will rely on your representative to keep you informed on the status of your claim, but you may contact us directly for any information about your claim.

2. The authority of your representative:

   Your representative has the authority to act totally your on behalf. This means he/she can (1) obtain information about your claim the same as you; (2) submit evidence; (3) make statements about facts and provisions of the law; and (4) make any request (including a fee request). It is important, therefore, that you are represented by a qualified individual.

3. When will the representative stop:

   We will stop recognizing or dealing with your representative when (1) you tell us that he/she is no longer your representative; (2) your representative does any one of the following; (a) submits a fee petition, or (b) tells us that he/she is withdrawing from the claim, or (c) he/she violates any of our rules and regulations, and a hearing is held before an administrative law judge (designated as hearing officer) who orders your representative disqualified or suspended as representative of any Social Security claimant.

4. The fee you owe the representative(s):

   Every representative you appoint has a right to petition for a fee. To charge you a fee, a representative must first file a fee petition with us. Irrespective of your fee agreement, you never owe more than the fee we have authorized in a written notice to you and representative(s). (Out-of-pocket expenses are not included). If your claim went to court, you may owe an additional fee for your representative's service before the court.

5. How we determine the fee:

   We use the criteria on the back of the fee petition (Form SSA 1560-U4), a copy of which your representative must send you.

6. Review of the fee authorization:

   If you or your representative disagrees with the fee authorization, either of you may request a review. Instructions for filing this review are on the fee authorization notice.

7. Payment of fees:

   If past-due benefits are payable in your claim, we generally withhold 25 percent of the past-due benefits toward possible attorney fees. If no past-due benefits are payable or this is an SSI claim, then payment of the fee we have authorized is your responsibility.

8. Penalty for charging an unauthorized fee:

   If your representative wants to charge and collect from you a fee that is greater than what we had authorized, then he/she is in violation of the law and regulations. Promptly report this to your nearest Social Security office.

Form SSA-1696-U4 (3-88)

FIGURE 9–8 cont'd Form SSA-1696-U4 completed by a Medicare patient appointing the physician as his or her authorized representative.

DEPARTMENT OF HEALTH AND HUMAN SERVICES
CENTERS FOR MEDICAIRE & MEDICAID SERVICES

Form Approved
OMB No. 0938-0034

REQUEST FOR HEARING
PART B MEDICARE CLAIM
Medical Insurance Benefits–Social Security Act

NOTICE—Anyone who misrepresents or falsifies essential information requested by this form may upon conviction be subject to fine and imprisonment under Federal Law.

CARRIER'S NAME AND ADDRESS

Medicare Blue Cross
Blue Shield of North Dakota
4510 13th Avenue, S.W.
Fargo, ND 58121-0001

1 NAME OF PATIENT

Deborah P. Sawyer

2 HEALTH INSURANCE CLAIM NUMBER

481-XX-6491

3 I disagree with the review determination on my claim and request a hearing before a hearing officer of the insurance carrier named above.
    MY REASONS ARE: *(Attach a copy of the Review Notice. NOTE.—If the review decision was made more than 6 months ago include your reason for not making this request earlier.)*

Complications arose during the surgical procedure requiring additional procedures performed. See attached chart notes and medical reports.

4 CHECK ONE OF THE FOLLOWING:

[X] I have additional evidence to submit.
(Attach such evidence to this form or forward it to the carrier within 10 days.)

[ ] I do not have additional evidence.

CHECK ONLY ONE OF THE STATEMENTS BELOW

[ ] I wish to appear in person before the Hearing Officer.

[X] I do not wish to appear and hereby request a decision on the evidence before the Hearing Officer.

5 **EITHER THE CLAIMANT OR REPRESENTATIVE SHOULD SIGN IN THE APPROPRIATE SPACE BELOW**

SIGNATURE OR NAME OF CLAIMANT'S REPRESENTATIVE		CLAIMANT'S SIGNATURE	
Gaston Input, MD		*Deborah P. Sawyer*	
ADDRESS		ADDRESS	
4567 Broad Avenue		1065 Evans Road	
CITY, STATE, AND ZIP CODE		CITY, STATE, AND ZIP CODE	
Woodland Hills, XY 12345		Woodland Hills, XY 12345	
TELEPHONE NUMBER 555-486-9002	Date 10-11-20XX	TELEPHONE NUMBER 555-742-1821	DATE 10-11-20XX

(Claimant should not write below this line)

ACKNOWLEDGEMENT OF REQUEST FOR HEARING

Your request for a hearing was received on _____. You will be notified of the time and place of the hearing at least 10 days before the date of the hearing.

SIGNED   DATE

FORM CMS-1965 (8-79)

FIGURE 9–9 Request for Hearing: Part B Medicare Claim Form CMS-1965.

Reconsideration

Participating providers may appeal certain decisions made by TRICARE and request reconsideration. Providers who do not participate may not appeal, but TRICARE Standard patients and parents or guardians of patients younger than 18 years of age who seek care from nonparticipating providers may file appeals. Providers who do not participate may not receive any information about a particular claim without the signed authorization of the patient or the patient's parent or guardian.

TRICARE CLAIM INQUIRY

Date: _____

TO: TRICARE
                    Address of fiscal intermediary
                    City, State, Zip Code

FROM: Provider's name   Telephone number
               Address   Fax number
               City, State, Zip Code

RE: Sponsor's Social Security Number _____

       Sponsor's Name _____

       Patient's Name _____

       Patient's Mailing Address:

       _____

       Street   City   State   Zip Code

       Dates of service claim: _____

       Total charges billed on claim: _____

       Claim number that appears on TRICARE Explanation of Benefits
       (leave blank if the claim has not been paid and information is not available)

       _____

A. _____   I have submitted a claim, but have not received any payment
                    or other notification from you.

B. _____   I have received notification or payment concerning the claim,
                    but feel it may have been processed incorrectly.

C. _____   Deductible Status. Please confirm that individual and family
                    deductibles have been applied correctly.

D. _____   Coverage for this patient is under

                   _____ **TRICARE**   _____ **CHAMPVA**

E. _____   Additional information or explanation that will assist
                    reviewing or processing the claim is attached to this letter or
                    written in this area.

FIGURE 9–10 A TRICARE Standard claim inquiry form that may be completed to obtain a quick reply. Mail to the TRICARE fiscal intermediary for your region.

Matters that can be appealed include the following:

1. Medical necessity disagreements (inappropriate care, level of care, investigational procedures)
2. Factual determinations (hospice care, foreign claims, provider sanction cases)
   a. Denials or partial denials of requests for preauthorization for certain services or supplies
   b. Coverage issues—notification that TRICARE will not pay for services before or after a certain date

Matters that cannot be appealed include the following:

1. Denial of services received from a provider not authorized to provide care under TRI CARE
2. A specific exclusion of law or regulation
3. Allowable charges for particular services

4. Issues relating to the establishment and application of diagnosis-related groups
5. Decisions by the claims processor to ask for additional information on a particular case
6. A determination of a person's eligibility as a TRICARE beneficiary

The TRICARE department that handles appeals collects and organizes all information necessary to review the case effectively. Usually a determination decision is made within 60 days from receipt of the appeal. Disagreements about the amount allowed for a particular claim may be reviewed by the claims processor to determine whether it was calculated correctly. However, an individual cannot appeal the amount that the TRICARE contractor determines to be the allowable charge for a certain medical service.

Requests must be sent to the claims processor of the state in which services were provided and must be postmarked within 90 days of the date the provider receives the Summary Payment Voucher (formerly referred to as an EOB). Include photocopies of the claim, Summary Payment Voucher, and other supporting documents with the request form or letter. The claim identification number assigned by the claims processor should be included in any inquiry concerning payment of the claim. If TRICARE denies the initial request, then the other two levels of review, formal review and hearing, may be pursued.

Formal Review

A formal review must be done within 60 days from the date on the reconsideration decision notice. Include photocopies of the notice as well as any other information or documents to support why there is a disagreement in the TRICARE decision. The case is reviewed again and a formal review decision is issued. The formal review decision is final if the amount in dispute is less than $300.

Hearing

An independent hearing may be pursued if the amount in dispute is $300 or more. The request must be postmarked or received within 60 days from the date of the formal review decision. A hearing is conducted by an independent hearing officer at a location convenient to both the requesting party and the government.

STATE INSURANCE COMMISSIONER

Commission Objectives

The insurance industry is protected by a special exemption from the Federal Trade Commission (FTC) under the McCarran Act (named for the late Senator Pat McCarran of Nevada). Under the exemption, the FTC cannot attack unfair or deceptive practices if there is any state law about such practices. The regulations vary widely from state to state, and by no means are all 50 states equally strict. If a complaint arises about an insurance policy, medical claim, or insurance agent or broker, the insurance department of the state of residence or the state where the insurance company's corporate office is headquartered should be contacted. Sometimes this department is referred to as the insurance commission of the state. State insurance departments usually have various objectives, including the following:

- To make certain that the financial strength of insurance companies is not unduly diminished
- To monitor the activities of insurance companies to make sure the interests of the policyholders are protected
- To verify that all contracts are carried out in good faith
- To make sure that all organizations authorized to transact insurance, including agents and brokers, are in compliance with the insurance laws of that state
- To release information on how many complaints have been filed against a specific insurance company in a year
- To help explain correspondence related to insurance company bankruptcies and other financial difficulties
- To assist if a company funds its own insurance plan
- To help resolve insurance conflicts

The insurance commissioner can hold a hearing to determine whether licensed insurers, agents, or brokers are in compliance with the insurance laws of the state, but the commissioner does not have the authority vested in a court of law to order an insurance company to make payment on a specific claim.

The insurance commissioner reviews the policy to see whether the denial of a claim by the insurance company was based on legal provisions of the insurance contract and advises the patient if there is an infraction of the law. If there is an infraction, the patient should consult an attorney to determine whether the claim should be submitted to a court of law.

Types of Problems

The types of problems that should be submitted to the insurance commissioner are as follows:

1. Improper denial of a claim or settlement for an amount less than that indicated by the policy, after proper appeal has been made
2. Delay in settlement of a claim, after proper appeal has been made
3. Illegal cancellation or termination of an insurance policy
4. Misrepresentation by an insurance agent or broker
5. Misappropriation of premiums paid to an insurance agent or broker
6. Problems about insurance premium rates
7. Two companies that cannot determine which is primary

COMMISSION INQUIRIES

An insurance billing specialist may not be in a position to know the particulars about a case and should never assume or accuse unless he or she is certain or has concrete evidence. Remember "Jump to conclusions, suffer contusions."

Requests to the insurance commissioner must be submitted in writing. An example of an insurance complaint form showing pertinent necessary information when making a request for assistance from the state insurance commissioner is shown in Figure 9–11. In some states, the insurance commissioner requires that the complaint come from the patient even if an assignment of benefits form has been signed. In such a case, a letter or form should be prepared for the patient to sign and then submit. Depending on the circumstances of the case, one may wish to send copies to the state medical association or an attorney. Mail may be sent certified, return receipt requested. The request should contain the following information:

1. The inquiring person's (patient) or policyholder's name, because the commissioner's responsibility is to the patient (the consumer), not the physician
2. The policyholder's address
3. The policyholder's telephone number
4. The insured's name
5. Name, address, and title of the insurance agent or official of the insurance company
6. A statement of the complaint including, if possible, a copy of the policy, medical bills, unpaid medical insurance claim, canceled checks, and any correspondence from the company pertaining to the claim
7. The patient's signature
8. The name and address of the insurance company, agent, or broker, or name and address of the finance company if the premium was financed
9. The policy or claim number
10. The date of loss
11. The date the patient signed the complaint form

FIGURE 9–11 Insurance complaint form, showing pertinent necessary information when stating a complaint and making a request for assistance from the state insurance commissioner.

If an insurance company is continually a slow payer, a method to speed up payments is to include a note to the carrier that reads "Unless this claim is paid or denied within 30 days, a formal written complaint will be filed with the state insurance commissioner."

Another method is to send a letter to the insurance commissioner with a copy notation inserted at the end to the insurance company. It might read, "The attached claim has been submitted to the XYZ Insurance Company. It has not been paid or denied. Please accept this letter as a formal written complaint against the XYZ Insurance Company."

Insurance companies are rated according to the number of complaints received about them, so they do not want the insurance commissioner to be alerted to any problems. Some states have information available to the public on how many claims have been submitted against a company if this information is needed. Refer to Internet Resources at the end of this chapter to contact the state insurance commissioner in your state for assistance or information about state laws.

PROCEDURE

TRACE AN UNPAID INSURANCE CLAIM

OBJECTIVE: To complete an insurance claim tracer and attach to this document a photocopy of the claim submitted.

EQUIPMENT/SUPPLIES: Typewriter or computer, insurance claims register (tracing or log file), insurance Claim Tracer Form, a previously submitted insurance claim form, and pen or pencil.

DIRECTIONS: Follow these basic step-by-step procedures, which include rationales, to learn this skill and practice it by completing the *Workbook* assignment.

1. Review the insurance claims register (tracing or log file) to learn and verify which claims are overdue for payment and have not been paid by the insurance carrier.
2. Obtain a copy of the previously submitted insurance claim that has not been paid.
3. Abstract data from the insurance claim and insert it on the insurance claim tracer form.
4. Make a photocopy of the unpaid insurance claim form.
5. Have the physician, office manager, or insurance biller sign the form.
6. Post an entry to either the patient's accounting financial record or insurance claims register (tracing or log file) indicating a tracer was submitted to the insurance carrier.

PROCEDURE

FILE AN OFFICIAL APPEAL

OBJECTIVE: To compose, format, key, proofread, and print a letter of appeal and attach to this document photocopies of information to substantiate reimbursement requested.

EQUIPMENT/SUPPLIES: Typewriter or computer, printer, letterhead paper, envelope, attachments (if necessary), thesaurus, English dictionary, medical dictionary, and pen or pencil.

DIRECTIONS: Follow these basic step-by-step procedures, which include rationales, to learn this skill and practice it by completing the *Workbook* assignment.

1. Refer to the end of Chapter 4 and follow the procedure to compose, format, key, proofread, and print a letter.
2. Include the beneficiary's name, health insurance claim number, date of initial determination, dates of service in question, items or services in question, name and address of the provider, and signature of appellant.
3. Compose a letter with an introduction that stresses the medical practice's qualifications, the physician's commitment to complying with regulations and providing appropriate services, and the importance of the practice to the payer's panel of physicians or specialists.
4. Provide a detailed account of the necessity of the treatment given and its relationship to the patient's problems and chief complaint. You might cross reference the medical record and emphasize parts of it that the reviewer may have missed.
5. Explain the reason why the provider does not agree with the claim denial listed on the EOB/RA.
6. Abstract excerpts from the coding resource book and attach a photocopy of the article or pertinent information showing the name of the article, coding resource, and date of publication.
7. Send copies of similar cases with increased reimbursement from the same insurance company, if available from the insurance company payment history file.
8. Call the insurance company and speak to the individual responsible for appeals, explaining what the resubmission is trying to accomplish. Direct the correspondence to this person.
9. Retain copies of all data sent for the physician's files.
10. Use a method that confirms the payer received the letter, such as a certified return receipt or signature using Federal Express or Airborne Express services.

RESOURCES

INTERNET

- Medicare forms may be downloaded and printed and regional offices may be located at:
  Web site: **www.medicare.gov**

- A bimonthly newsletter that links to regulatory information online is located at:
  Web site: **www.integsoft.com/appeals/tal**

- Subscription repository of appeal letters and comments that assists the health care community in sharing successful appeal information may be found at:
  Web site: **www.integsoft.com/appeals/tal**

- State insurance commissioners may be found at:
  Web site: **www.naic.org/state contacts/sid websites.htm**

ASSIGNMENT

STUDENT

✔ Study Chapter 9.

✔ Answer the review questions in the *Workbook* to reinforce the theory learned in this chapter and to help prepare you for a future test.

✔ Complete the assignments in the *Workbook* to fill in a form for tracing a delinquent claim, locate errors on a returned claim, and complete a form to appeal a Medicare case.

✔ Turn to the glossary at the end of this textbook for a further understanding of the key terms used in this chapter.

RESOURCE

VIDEO

Medical Assistant Video Series, Tape 6: "The CMS Files: A Case for Medical Billing Accuracy." This video is an interesting and entertaining presentation about what happens to rejected claim forms. It gives reasons why claims are denied and ways to avoid such problems. It gives excellent reinforcement of material learned in this chapter, especially when viewed after the chapter has been read. An assignment is presented in the *Workbook* for completion after viewing this video.

CHAPTER OUTLINE

CASH FLOW CYCLE
  Accounts Receivable
  Patient Education
  Patient Registration Form
FEES
  Fee Schedule
  Fee Adjustments
  Communicating Fees
  Collecting Fees
CREDIT ARRANGEMENTS
  Payment Options
CREDIT AND COLLECTIONS LAWS
  Statute of Limitations
  Equal Credit Opportunity Act
  Fair Credit Reporting Act

Fair Credit Billing Act
Truth in Lending Act
Truth in Lending Consumer
  Credit Cost Disclosure
Fair Debt Collection
  Practices Act
THE COLLECTION PROCESS
  Office Collection Techniques
  Insurance Collection
  Collection Agencies
  Credit Bureaus
  Credit Counseling
  Small Claims Court
  Tracing a Skip
  Special Collection Issues

PROCEDURE: SEVEN-STEP
  BILLING AND COLLECTION
  GUIDELINES
PROCEDURE: TELEPHONE
  COLLECTION PLAN
PROCEDURE: CREATE A
  FINANCIAL AGREEMENT WITH
  A PATIENT
PROCEDURE: FILE A CLAIM IN
  SMALL CLAIMS
PROCEDURE: FILE AN ESTATE
  CLAIM

KEY TERMS

accounts receivable (A/R)

age analysis

AMA Code of Medical Ethics

automatic stay

balance

bankruptcy

bonding

cash flow

Code of Medical Ethics

collateral

collection ratio

credit

credit card

creditor

cycle billing

debit card

debt

debtor

discount

dun messages

embezzlement

estate administrator

estate executor

fee schedule

financial accounting record

garnishment

insurance balance billing

itemized statement

lien

manual billing

netback

no charge (NC)

nonexempt assets

professional courtesy

reimbursement

secured debt

skip

statute of limitations

unsecured debt

write-off

10

Office and Insurance Collection Strategies

OBJECTIVES*

After reading this chapter, you should be able to:

- Define credit and collection terminology.

- Translate collection abbreviations.

- Describe office billing procedures.

- Define aging analysis.

- Discuss ways to determine fees and describe an office's fee policies.

- Summarize credit laws applicable to a physician office setting.

- Define accounts receivable and explain how it is handled.

- Recite types of fee adjustments available to patients.

- Name credit options available to patients.

- Perform oral and written communication collection techniques.

- State the role of a billing service, collection agency, and credit bureau in the collection process.

- List possible solutions to collection problems.

- Explain the purpose of small claims court in the collection process.

- Name basic actions in tracing a debtor who has moved and left no forwarding address.

*Performance objectives and exercises for hands-on practical experience for this chapter appear in the *Workbook*.

CASH FLOW CYCLE

The practice of medicine is both a profession and a business. Although the physician decides what type of medicine he or she will practice, it is often the practice manager or administrator who is responsible for the business portion of the practice. It is extremely important for the physician and insurance specialist to work together to provide all patients the best possible medical care and ensure that the physician is paid fairly for services rendered.

Today this process has become increasingly difficult. Physician office and billing practices have evolved from the barter system of days past, and since the Great Depression, the availability of credit and credit cards have become a common feature of the financial marketplace. The word **credit** comes from the Latin *credere*, which means "to believe" or "to trust." This trust is in an individual's business integrity and his or her financial ability to meet obligations when they become due. For many, the idea of credit has changed and may simply mean to put off paying today what one can pay tomorrow.

A large percentage of **reimbursement** to physicians' offices is generated from third-party payers (private insurance, government plans, managed care contracts, and workers' compensation). The physician, the practice administrator responsible for financial affairs, and the patient must understand these insurance contracts, which list reimbursement provisions, medical services not covered, the portion of the bill the patient is responsible for, and the process for reimbursing the office.

Accounts Receivable

Accounts receivable (A/R) include the unpaid balances due from patients for services that have been rendered. Each medical practice has a policy about handling A/R. The effectiveness of this policy and its enforcement are reflected in the practice's **cash flow.** The cash flow is the ongoing availability of cash in the medical practice. When charges are collected at the time of service, the A/R is zero. In an ideal situation, all outstanding balances are paid within 60 days; however, this is not possible for the following reasons:

1. Health care expenses have increased and exceed the expenses the patient pays for everyday living.

2. The public feels it is a right, rather than a privilege, to receive the best possible health care. Therefore care of the indigent becomes an unreimbursable expense in the medical office.
3. Legal proceedings often delay the payment of medical expenses.
4. Insurance carriers do not pay claims in a timely manner, resulting in further delays in the collection of patient copayments.

By monitoring the A/R, the insurance billing specialist is able to evaluate the effectiveness of the collection process. The formula for finding out the A/R ratio is to divide the month-end A/R balance by the monthly average charges for the prior 12-month period. An average total A/R (all monies not collected at the time of service) should be one and a half to two times the charges for 1 month of services (Examples 10.1 and 10.2).

Example 10.1 Formula

Physician's Charges Monthly Total	$50,000 × 1.5 = $75,000	Total Outstanding Accounts Receivable

or

$50,000 × 2.0 = $100,000

Total outstanding A/R should range from $75,000 to $100,000.

Example 10.2 Calculation of Accounts Receivable Ratio

Annual gross charges	$150,000
Average monthly gross charges (150,000 ÷ 12 months)	12,500
Current Accounts Receivable Balance	20,000
Accounts Receivable Ratio: 20,000 ÷ 12,500 = 1.60 months	

Accounts that are 90 days or older should not exceed 15% to 18% of the total A/R. To calculate this figure, divide the total amount of A/R by the amount of accounts that are 90 days old and older (Example 10.3).

Example 10.3 Formula for Determining Percentage of Accounts Over 90 Days

Amount of A/R over 90 days	A/R Total	Percentage of A/R over 90 days
$12,000 ÷ $75,000 = 16%		

Practice management systems should calculate this automatically when an aging report is needed.

The best way to keep the A/R down is to verify insurance benefits before sending claims, collect copays and deductibles at the time of service, obtain authorizations for noncontracted health maintenance organization (HMO) patients, and monitor the A/R on a weekly basis. Electronic claims that have not been paid within 30 days and paper claims unpaid within 45 days of submission have problems that can range from the carrier asking for additional information from the patient to the patient not being one of the carrier's insured.

The **collection ratio** is the relationship of the amount of money owed to a physician and the amount of money collected on the physician's A/R. A collection rate of 100% is obviously desirable, although unrealistic, and should always be sought as a goal for the person managing collections in the physician's office. To calculate

the collection rate for a 1-month period, divide the amount of monies collected during the current month by the total amount of the A/R.

Patient Education

Information should be provided about office fees and payment policies during the initial contact with the patient. This decreases the number of billing statements sent and increases collections. Never allow a patient to believe that he or she is not responsible for the bill. Discuss copayment requirements (see Chapter 3) with patients who are enrolled in managed care plans, and convey the office policy of collecting this amount when registering the patient for the office visit. A new patient information pamphlet or brochure and confirmation letter (Figure 10–1) may be sent to welcome the new patient to the practice. This letter informs the patient about the practice, clearly outlines payment expectations,

COLLEGE CLINIC
4567 Broad Avenue
Woodland Hills, XY 12345-0001
Tel. (555) 486-9002
FAX (555) 487-8976

February 3, 20XX

Mrs. Mary M. McLean
4919 Dolphin Way
Woodland Hills, XY 12345-0001

Dear Mrs. McLean:

Thank you for making an appointment with Dr. Ulibarri and entrusting us with your personal health care. Your appointment has been scheduled on ———— (date) at ——o'clock (time). Please arrive 15 minutes early and bring the completed patient registration and history form.

The fee for your physical examination is approximately $——— (charge). If laboratory tests, an electrocardiogram, or any procedures are necessary, there will be additional charges. For patients covered by insurance, our office policy requires a payment of 20% of all charges at the time of service. Please expect to pay this on the day of your visit. For your convenience, we accept cash, checks, and credit cards (Visa, American Express, and MasterCard).

Enclosed is a brochure with information regarding our medical practice and a map on the back for your convenience. We look forward to your visit. Please call me at (555) 486-9002 if you have any questions.

Sincerely,

Fran Staple, CMA
Office Manager

Enc: brochure, patient registration, history form

1. State with which doctor the patient has the appointment.

2. Confirm the date and time.

3. State the approximate fee for services ahead of time.

4. Alert the patient that additional charges may be added for additional services.

5. Offer payment options.

6. Enclose patient brochure, patient registration, and history form.

7. Establish a contact person and invite questions.

FIGURE 10–1 New patient confirmation letter emphasizing information to incorporate when writing to a new patient.

provides collection policies and procedures in printed form, establishes a contact person, invites questions, and confirms all specific details discussed.

Patient Registration Form

There is no substitution for good information-gathering techniques at the time of initial patient registration. Always obtain complete and accurate information from the patient on the first visit and confirm the accuracy of that information on each subsequent visit. Chapter 3 describes what data should be obtained from the patient; Figure 3–7 is an example of a patient registration information form, also called a patient information sheet. Have the guarantor agree in writing to pay for all medical treatment. By obtaining the guarantor's signature, he or she is then bound by contract to pay the bill.

Learn as much as possible about the patient before any services are provided. This is when the patient is likely to be the most cooperative. Information provided on the patient information sheet will prove critical to any billing and collection efforts. The patient should be instructed to answer all questions and indicate any spaces on the form that do not apply by marking "N/A" (not applicable). Review of the completed patient information sheet ensures that all blanks have been addressed and accurate information has been collected. It also alerts office staff of an account that may be a future problem. Items often overlooked are the street address, when a post office box is given; an apartment or mobile home number; and a business telephone number with department and extension. These help to trace a patient who has moved. If a patient refuses to divulge any information, invoking the privacy laws, it should be policy to require payment for services at the time care is rendered. A potential nonpaying patient may be recognized at this time. Some indications to look for follow:

● Incomplete information on the registration form
● Multiple changes of residence
● Questionable employment record
● No business or home telephone
● Post office box listed with no street address
● Motel address
● Incomplete insurance information or no insurance coverage
● No referral information or authorization from a primary care physician for patients enrolled in a managed care plan

Employers are changing health plans with increasing frequency and patients are more transient than ever, so update this form each time the patient is seen or every 6 months. This can be done by printing out a data sheet or having the patient review a copy of his or her registration form and inserting changes or corrections with a red pen. New information also can be obtained using an updated or abbreviated form (see Figure 3–9).

FEES

Fee Schedule

Most medical practices operate with a set of fees that must be applied to all patients in the practice uniformly. As discussed in Chapter 6, a **fee schedule** is a listing of accepted charges or established allowances for specific medical procedures. Always quote fees and state policies about the collection of fees to the patient at the initial visit. Under federal regulations, a list of the most common services the physician offers, including procedure code numbers, with a description of each service and its price, must be available to all patients, and a sign must be posted in the office advising patients of this.

Occasionally a physician assigns a fee for a service that is not on the fee schedule and not reimbursed by insurance, such as an uncanceled appointment (referred to as a "no show"), completion of an insurance form, a long-distance telephone consultation, a narrative medical report for an insurance company, or interest assessed on a delinquent account. It is advisable to inform patients before billing for any such services to preserve the patient–physician relationship. If such charges are imposed or the fee schedule is increased at a later date, a notice should be placed in the reception room and communicated to patients via their monthly billing statements. This information should be included in the medical practice's information brochure that is given to patients.

Fee Adjustments

Discounted Fees

A physician may choose to discount his or her fees for various reasons, but it is ill-advised and may be illegal in some circumstances. A **discount** is a reduction of the normal fee based on a specific amount of money or a percentage of the charge. When a physician offers a discount, it must apply to the total bill, not just the portion that is paid by the patient (copayment or coinsurance amount). By following this rule, the physician is giving a discount to the patient and the insurance company, but the same discount must be given to each member of the insurance plan. This practice could reduce the physician's profile with the insurance company and trigger a reduction in the physician's allowable reimbursement schedule; therefore the physician should consider the outcome of discounting fees. All discounts must be noted on the patient's **financial accounting record**/ledger card (Figure 10–2), and any financial reasons or special circumstances should be documented in the patient's medical record. This ensures

STATEMENT

College Clinic
4567 Broad Avenue
Woodland Hills, XY 12345-0001
Telephone: (555) 486-9002
Fax: (555) 487-8976

Jake Herron
439 Zinfendale Lane
Woodland Hills, XY 12345

Phone No. (H) ___555/862-4193___ (W) _555/862-5900_ Birthdate: _02/12/79_

Insurance Co. ____None____ Policy No. _____

DATE	REFERENCE	PROFESSIONAL SERVICE DESCRIPTION	CHARGE	CREDITS		CURRENT BALANCE	
				PAYMENTS	ADJUSTMENTS		
3-3-XX	99203	OV Level 3, NP	70 92			70	92
3-6-XX	81000	UA	8 00			78	92
3-6-XX	93000	ECG Hosp admit, C Hx PX	34 26			113	18
4-6-XX		Billed pt. **We can clear this account on MasterCard, VISA, or Discover.** Please authorize this by giving us your account number, expiration date, type of card, and the amount you would like to charge.					
4-26-XX	Ck #602	ROA Pt		50 00		63	18
5-6-XX		Billed pt. **PLEASE NOTE**—This account is Past Due. Your prompt attention is courteously requested.				63	18
6-6-XX		Billed pt. **FINAL NOTICE**—If we do not hear from you within 10 days this account will be turned over to our collection agency				63	18
6-29-XX	Ck #639	ROA Pt		50 00		13	18
6-29-XX		Courtesy Adjustment			13 18		0
8-14-XX	99213	OV Level 3	40 20			40	20
8-14-XX	Cash	ROA Pt (20% Cash discount)		32 18	8 02		0

1. First dun message
2. Second dun message
3. Third dun message
4. Courtesy adjustment (write-off)
5. Cash discount

Due and payable within 10 days.   **Pay last amount in balance column**

Key: PF: Problem-focused
EPF: Expanded problem-focused
D: Detailed
C: Comprehensive

SF: Straightforward
L: Low complexity
M: Moderate complexity
H: High complexity

CON: Consultation
HX: History
PX: Phys Exam

ED: Emergency Dept.
HCD: House call
HV: Hospital visit
OV: Office visit

FIGURE 10–2 Financial accounting record (ledger card) showing dun messages, courtesy adjustment (write-off), and cash discount.

complete record keeping and safeguards any questions that may be brought up during a financial audit.

Cash Discounts

Cash discounts may be offered (5% to 20%) to patients who pay the entire fee, in cash, at the time of service. If a cash discount system is offered, this policy should be posted in the office and every active patient sent notification.

Research your state laws because some states do not allow cash discounts. Also, refer to your office's compliance protocol to be sure any such discounts do not implicate fraud.

Financial Hardship

Financial hardship cases are the most difficult for the physician to determine. The insurance billing specialist should never assume anything about a patient's financial

2005 GUIDELINES ON POVERTY INCOME			
Size of family unit	48 contiguous states and D.C.	Alaska	Hawaii
1	$ 9570	$11,950	$11,010
2	$12,830	$16,030	$14,760
3	$16,090	$20,110	$18,510
4	$19,350	$24,190	$22,260
5	$22,610	$28,270	$26,010
6	$25,870	$32,350	$29,760
7	$29,130	$36,430	$33,510
8	$32,390	$40,510	$37,260
For each additional person add:	$ 3260	$ 4080	$ 3660

FIGURE 10–3   Department of Health and Human Services 2004 guidelines on poverty income, published in the *Federal Register*.

status, nor judge a patient's ability to pay by his or her appearance. The Department of Health and Human Services has published a 2004 guideline on poverty income (Figure 10–3), which is used to determine eligibility for uncompensated services under the Hill-Burton program, the Community Services Block Grant program, and the Head Start program. Physicians may choose to follow these guidelines to direct patients to government-sponsored programs, obtain public assistance, and determine who is eligible for a hardship waiver. A hardship waiver can vary from 25% to 100% of the bill. Various financial forms are available to obtain this information; a copy of the patient's wage and tax statement (W2) or income tax return should be examined to make a reliable decision. The patient also should sign a written explanation to verify true financial hardship. This helps in the collection process and allows the physician to accept the insurance as payment in full, in certain circumstances, without being suspected of insurance fraud. The reason for a fee reduction must be documented in the patient's medical record.

Be very careful about giving a discount because it can be construed as discriminatory if not given to other patients consistently. To avoid problems, develop a written policy about what qualifies a patient for a financial hardship discount.

Write-off or Courtesy Adjustment

A **write-off** or *courtesy adjustment* (preferred term) is an asset or debt that has been determined to be uncollectable and is taken off (subtracted/credited) the accounting books. It is considered lost income but may not be claimed as a loss for tax purposes. The insurance specialist should obtain financial information on all patients who request a write-off. Office policies about adjustments and all discounts

should be in writing, and all staff members should be informed. The physician must approve the portion of the charge to be credited to the financial record before the debt is forgiven. There are three circumstances when a write-off can be performed. The first is as stated in the preceding discussion, when the patient has proved a financial hardship. The second is when it will cost more to bill the balance than what is owed. For example, the balance may be $1.05. It will cost the practice more to collect this than what it is worth. This type of write-off is known as a *small balance write-off*. The last situation is when the provider has made a good faith effort to collect the balance with no success. In this case, the balance is written off and the account is sent to a professional collection agency for collection.

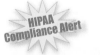

The Office of the Inspector General issued guidance to providers that he or she is free to use whatever policy they want on charity care, discounts, write-offs, and collections, as long as it is done consistently and the reasons for granting these are documented. Make sure that these deviations from standard collection procedures are not tied to or conditioned on referrals or use of the provider's services. Be sure office policy states the minimum effort in collection of debts, such as one or more letters or telephone calls. The provider that uses minimum collection efforts can waive the obligations of patients in financial need in accordance with office policy and try to collect more aggressively from other patients who are not financially needy.

Professional Courtesy

Professional courtesy is a concept attributed to Hippocrates, but the foundations actually are derived from Thomas Percival's *Code of Medical Ethics* written in 1803. The *American Medical Association Code of Ethics,* formulated and adopted in 1847, closely mirrored Percival's code. The practice of professional courtesy served to build bonds between physicians and reduce the incentive for physicians to treat their own families. Most physicians agree that one of the greatest honors and privileges in the practice of medicine is to be asked to care for a physician and his or her family members. The practice of professional courtesy often was extended to others in the health care profession and members of the clergy. Most hospitals and many surgeons have given up the practice of free care today because most physicians now have insurance coverage for medical expenses.

Professional courtesy means making no charge to anyone, patient or insurance, for medical care.

An interim rule from Centers for Medicare and Medicaid Services (CMS) effective July 24, 2004, identifies proper ways to offer professional courtesy:

1. The professional courtesy is offered to all physicians on the entity's bona fide medical staff or in the entity's local community or service area without regard to volume or value of referrals or other business generated between the parties.
2. The health care items and services provided are of a type routinely provided by the entity.
3. The entity's professional courtesy policy is written and approved in advance by the entity's governing body.
4. The professional courtesy is not offered to a physician (or immediate family member) who is a federal health care program beneficiary unless there has been a good faith showing of financial need.
5. If the professional courtesy involves any whole or partial reduction of any coinsurance obligation, the insurer is informed in writing of the reduction.
6. The arrangement does not violate the anti-kickback statute (section 1128b[b] of the act), or any federal or state law or regulation governing billing or claims submission.

Physicians must examine their policies on professional courtesy to ensure that they do not violate the contractual terms in private or managed care insurance policies or Medicare/Medicaid laws and regulations. If the treating physician does not bill the physician-patient for services rendered, the third-party payer is relieved of its contractual obligation. If the treating physician waives the deductible and copayment, the physician may be accused of not treating others with the same insurance coverage in an equal manner. Although there may be some situations in which it is defensible to not charge for services to health care professionals, the physician should ensure that this professional courtesy is not linked to patients who have been referred to the practice. There are laws that prohibit any inducement or kickbacks from physicians (or others) that could influence the decision of a physician (or other) to refer patients or that may affect a patient's decision to seek care.

Professional courtesy may violate fraud and abuse laws depending on how the recipients of the professional courtesy are selected and how the courtesy is extended. If selection depends on referral of individuals, then it may implicate the anti-kickback statute. An insurance claim submitted as a result of such a professional courtesy may also be affected by the False Claims Act.

Copayment Waiver

Waiving copayments is another way physicians have reduced the cost of medical care for patients in the past. In doing so, the physician accepts the insurance payment only. In most situations, both private insurers and the federal government ban waiving the copayment; therefore it is not suggested or recommended. Waiving copayments could violate the contract between the patient and insurance company. Some insurance companies look at this as a means of recouping its losses by undergoing litigation against the provider or demanding the return of all payments made to the provider.

No Charge

No charge (NC) means waiving the entire fee for professional care. This is permitted as long as it is not part of a fraudulent scheme and is offered to all patients. All NC visits must be fully documented in the clinical portion of the patient's medical record and the financial record. A physician or insurance specialist cannot assess a fee for services for which the insurance company does not approve as a way of trying to satisfy a patient's deductible.

Another instance when "no charge" occurs on a patient's account is when follow-up visits are posted after a patient undergoes surgery considered under a surgical package or Medicare global fee structure. When posting such charges in a computer system, Current Procedural

Terminology (CPT) procedure code 99024 (postoperative follow-up visit included in global fee) may be used.

Reduced Fee

Precautions should be taken before reducing the fee of a patient who dies. The doctor's sympathy in this case could be misinterpreted and result in a malpractice suit. A fee reduction should never be based on a poor result in the treatment of a patient.

If a patient disputes a fee and the physician agrees to settle for a reduced fee, the agreement should be in writing with a definite time limit for payment and the words "without prejudice" inserted. By doing this, the physician protects the right to collect the original sum if the patient fails to pay the reduced fee. The physician and patient should sign the agreement and each should receive a copy.

Because the patient's financial history is personal, in-the-office conversations about fees must be private so other individuals cannot overhear. The patient should be made to feel comfortable so he or she feels free to discuss any financial problems. Be firm. Use tact. Always use a courteous but businesslike approach when discussing financial matters.

Communicating Fees

People have a difficult time asking each other for money and talking about financial obligations. Financial arrangements should be discussed up front and in great detail before any services are provided (Figure 10–4). Many medical practices create their own collection problems by not being clear about how and when they expect to be paid. If patients are not told that payment is due at the time of service, most assume they can pay at a later time. Following are some guidelines to help communicate effectively about money:

1. Be courteous at all times but express a firm, businesslike approach that will not offend the patient.
2. Never badger or intimidate a patient into paying; merely state the payment policy and educate the patient.
3. Inform the patient of the fee and any deductible and balance due in a clear manner.
4. Verify the patient's copayment listed on his or her insurance card and collect this amount before the patient's office visit.

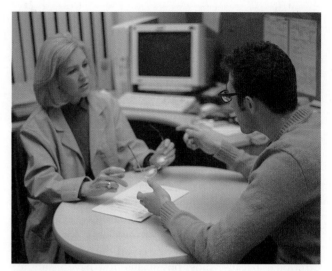

FIGURE 10–4   Insurance billing specialist discussing fees with the patient.

5. Make it easier for the patient to pay rather than leave without making payment.
6. Do not give the patient an option by asking if he or she would like to pay now or have a bill sent.
7. Motivate the patient to pay by appealing to his or her honesty, integrity, and pride.

The following are examples of communicating in a positive manner and letting the patient know exactly what is expected:

- "The office visit is $62, Mrs. Smith. Would you like to pay by cash, check, credit card, or debit card?"
- "Your copayment is $10, Mr. Jones. I will collect it before your office visit."
- "Your insurance policy shows a $100 deductible that is your responsibility and currently has not been met, Miss Rodriguez. You must pay the full fee today, which is $75."
- "Mrs. Merryweather, I must collect $4.77 today for your vitamin B_{12} injection. The injection is not covered by your insurance policy."
- "We look forward to seeing you on Tuesday, March 3, at 10 AM., Mr. Gillespie. The consultation fee will be approximately $150 and payment is expected at the time of service. We accept cash, check, credit cards, or debit cards for your convenience."

Collecting Fees

Payment at the Time of Service

Collecting applicable copayments and other amounts due from the patient upon each office visit is strongly recommended. To avoid difficulties in collecting at a future date, ask for fixed copayments before the patient is seen by the provider. This will alleviate billing for small amounts or possible problems with collection if statements are sent

FINANCIAL AGREEMENT

1. Total amount of the debt; wording "cash price" must be used according to Regulation Z
2. Amount of down payment
3. Finance charge; must be in capital letters and stand out
4. Interest rate expressed as an annual percentage; must be in capital letters and stand out
5. Amount of each payment
6. Date each payment is due
7. Date final payment is due; itemized payment record allows tracking of payments and balance owed
8. Signature of patient and physician with copies retained by both; narrative must be included

For professional SERVICES rendered or to be rendered to:

Patient Keenan Kellog Daytime phone 555-486-0132

Parent if patient is a minor ______

1. Cash price for services.................... $ 5000.-
2. Cash down payment.................... $ 300.-
3. Charges covered by insurance service plan.................... $ 4000.-
4. Unpaid balance of cash price.................... $ 700.-
5. Amount financed (the amount of credit provided to you).................... $ 700.-
6. **FINANCE CHARGE** (the dollar amount the credit will cost you).................... $ -0-
7. **ANNUAL PERCENTAGE RATE** (the cost of credit as a yearly rate).................... $ 0%
8. Total of payments (5 + 6 above – the amount you will have paid when you have made all scheduled payments).................... $ 700.-
9. Total sales price (1 + 6 above – sum of cash price, financing charge and any other amounts financed by the creditor, not part of the finance charge).................... $ 5000.-

You have the right at anytime to pay the unpaid balance due under this agreement without penalty. You have the right at this time to receive an itemization of the amount financed.

☒ I want an itemization ☐ I do not want an itemization

Total of payments (#8 above) is payable to Dr. Astro Parkinson in 7 monthly installments of $100. each and -0- installments of $-0- each. The first installment being payable on Feb. 15 20 XX and subsequent installments on the same day of each consecutive month until paid in full.

NOTICE TO PATIENT

Do not sign this agreement if it contains any blank spaces. You are entitled to an exact copy of any agreement you sign. You have the right at any time to pay the unpaid balance due under this agreement.

The patient (parent or guardian) agrees to be and is fully responsible for total payment of services performed in this office including any amounts not covered by any health insurance or prepayment program the responsible party may have. See your contract documents for any additional information about nonpayment, default, any required prepayment in full before the scheduled date and prepayment refunds and penalties.

Signature of patient or one parent if patient is a minor:

X Keenan Kellog

Doctor's Signature Astro Parkinson, MD

SCHEDULE OF PAYMENT

No.	Date due	Amount of installment		Date paid		Amount paid		Balance owed	
Total amount								700	–
D.P				Ck #					
1	2/15	100	–	572	2/10	100	–	600	–
2	3/15	100	–	598	3/13	100	–	500	–
3	4/15	100	–						
4	5/15	100	–						
5	6/15	100	–						
6	7/15	100	–						
7	8/15	100	–						
8									
9									
10									
11									
12									
13									
14									
15									
16									
17									
18									
19									
20									
21									
22									
23									

FIGURE 10–5 Financial Agreement Form (#1826) used for financial payment plans. By completing this form the physician provides full disclosure of all information required by the Truth in Lending Act, Regulation Z. *(From SYCOM, A Division of New England Business Service, Inc., Groton, Mass.)*

by mail after the visit. The importance of collecting outstanding bills, coinsurance amounts, and money from cash-paying patients up front should be communicated to office staff. One-on-one communication is the best way to motivate a **debtor.** Each patient's account **balance** (amount due) should be reviewed before his or her appointment. If the appointment schedule is on a computer system, print the account balance by each patient's name. If an appointment book is used, make a copy of the page showing the day's schedule. Write overdue balances by the patient's name after obtaining overdue amounts from each patient's financial accounting record card. This information also should be recorded on the transaction slip for that day's visit and may be "flagged" when the transaction slips are printed or written. Treat this information confidentially and keep it out of view of other patients. When a patient arrives whose name is "flagged," alert the patient accounts manager.

To do effective preappointment collection counseling, the patient should be taken to a quiet area away from the general activity of the office. Sit down with the patient and discuss the situation. Use an understanding attitude and helpful nature while verbalizing phrases such as "I understand" and "I can help." Ask direct questions to learn exactly what problems the patient is facing. Answers to questions such as, "When do you expect your next paycheck?" and, "How much are you able to pay today?" help determine the strategy. The goal should be to try and collect the full amount. If that is not possible, try to collect a portion of the balance. Get a promise to pay for the remaining balance by a specific date. If the patient is unable to comply, set up a payment plan. The chances of reaching a mutually satisfactory resolution are greatly improved when the two parties are face to face.

A personal interview is better than a telephone interview because a financial agreement can be signed when the debtor is present (Figure 10–5), resulting in a better follow-up response. Let the patient know that the practice is willing to help and that the debtor should inform the insurance specialist if he or she runs into further

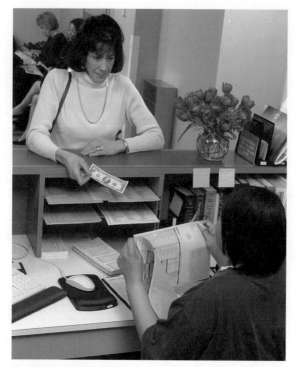

FIGURE 10–6   Receptionist collecting copayment from the patient.

problems making the payment. This personal contact helps if a renegotiation of the agreement is needed. A medical practice cannot refuse to let an established patient see the doctor because of a **debt,** but the office staff has every right to ask for payment while the patient is in the office (Figure 10–6). Some practices are placing automated teller machines (ATMs) in their waiting rooms. ATMs are almost everywhere today and they help generate a small income for having the ATMs in place. Putting an ATM machine in the waiting room gives the reluctant patient a means of obtaining funds to pay the medical bill while in the office.

Encounter Forms

Multipurpose billing forms (see Chapter 3) are known by many names, including *encounter form.* They are helpful when collecting fees at the time of service. Encounter forms can be given to patients to bill their insurance companies, used to inform patients of current charges and outstanding balances, and used as receipts for payment (Figure 10–7).

Patient Excuses for Nonpayments

Nonpayers show a tendency to dismiss financial arrangements with curt remarks. Look directly at the patient, confidently expecting payment. Demonstrate to the patient the right to request payment. Be ready if excuses are offered. Table 10.1 shows examples of patients' excuses and possible responses.

When a patient chatters nervously, it may be a way of setting up reasons to rationalize not paying. Do not let this be distracting. Pause after asking for payment and do not say another word until the patient responds. Many people feel uncomfortable with silence, but pauses may work to advantage and help complete a transaction. The cash flow and collection ratio are increased by taking this approach, while decreasing billing chores and collection costs. The quick identification of nonpayers may be obtained and the person responsible for collections notified.

Payment by Check

Check Verification

Check verification requires the insurance specialist to become familiar with the appearance of a good check. A personal check is the most common method of payment in most medical offices, but it is not a personal guarantee of payment. A driver's license and one other form of identification always should be required. Check these against existing records. Call the bank to verify all out-of-state and suspicious checks. A verification service (which is a private company with resources to quickly identify patient information over the telephone) or a check authorization system may be worthy of consideration for clinics and larger group practices.

Check Forgery

Forgery is false writing or alteration of a document to injure another person or with intent to deceive (e.g., signing another person's name on a check to obtain money or pay off a debt without permission). To guard against forgery, always check to be sure the endorsement on the back of the check matches the name on the front. Be suspicious if the beneficiary or provider states that he or she did not receive the check but the insurance company shows it as being cashed, or if the payee of the check claims that the signature is not his or hers.

Payment Disputes

Problem checks appear in many forms. One is the check for partial payment when the debtor (the patient) writes "payment in full" on the check. If the **creditor** (the physician) cashes the check, it may be argued that the debt is paid in full. A legal theory called "accord and satisfaction" may apply to this situation if the debt is truly disputed by the debtor. If the check is retained (and cashed) by the physician, it can be considered "accord and satisfaction," and the physician cannot procure the balance from the patient. The operative words are "truly disputed." If there is a legitimate, genuine dispute over the amount of the bill, and an amount less than the full amount of the bill is accepted, the physician could be

TAX ID #3664021CC
Medicaid #HSC12345F
Medicare DME #34007

COLLEGE CLINIC
4567 Broad Avenue
Woodland Hills, XY 12345-0001
Tel. (555) 486-9002
FAX (555) 487-8976

CO-PAY: $10.00
CO. NAME: Quality Care
IPA:

1. Insurance identifying data

☐ PRIVATE ☐ BLUE CROSS ☐ MEDI-CAL ☐ MEDICARE ☒ HMO ☐ PPO

ACCOUNT #	PATIENT'S LAST NAME	FIRST	INITIAL	TODAY'S DATE
3794	McDonald	Lydia	P.	5/6/ XX

ASSIGNMENT: I hereby assign payment directly to College Clinic of the surgical and/or medical benefits, if any, otherwise payable to me for his/her services as described below.
SIGNED (Patient, or Parent, if Minor) *Lydia McDonald*   DATE: 5/6/ XX

2. Assignment of medical benefits

ICD-9	DESCRIPTION							
789.0	Abdominal pain	433.1 ✓	Coronary A dis.	401.	Hypertension	353.2	Radiculopathy, cervical	
995.3	Allergic reaction	733.	Costochondritis	242.90	Hyperthyroidism	353.4	Lumbar	
290.10	Alzheimer's	430.	CVA	790.6	Hyperuricemia	592.0	Renal stone	
285.	Anemia	595.0	Cystitis	276.8	Hypokalemia	714.0	Rheumatoid arthritis	
413.9	Angina	311.	Depression	244.	Hypothyroid	724.3	Sciatica	
300.4	Anxiety reaction	692.	Dermatitis	244.	Hypothyroidism	461.	Sinusitis	
414.0	ASHD	250.0	Diabetes mell	564.1	Irritable bowel synd.	V45.0	Stat post pacemaker	
493.	Asthma bronchial	562.11	Diverticulitis	386.	Labyrinthitis	780.2	Syncope	
491.2 ✓	Asth broncho-chr.	427.9	Ectopy or VPC's	724.5	Low back pain	727.	Tendonitis	
781.2	Ataxia	782.3	Edema	780.7	Malaise and fatigue	531.	Ulcer	
427.31	Atrial fib	610.1	Fibrocystic breast	424.0	Mitral valve prolapse	465.	URI	
586	Azotemia	535.	Gastritis	728.85	Muscle spasm	599.	Urin. tract inf.	
600	BPH	558.	Gastroenteritis	410.	Myocardial infar.	616.10	Vaginitis	
466.0	Bronchitis acute	274.	Gout	715.80	Osteoarthritis	079.	Viral syndrome	
490.	Bronchitis chr.	784.0	Headache	733.	Osteoporosis			
426.50	Bundle BR block	389.9	Hearing loss	382.	Otitis media			
786.50	Chest pain	578.1	Hematochezia	785.1	Palpitations			
428.0	CHF	599.7	Hematuria	462	Pharyngitis			
575.1	Cholecystitis	455.6	Hemorrhoids	486	Pneumonitis			
564.1	Colitis	553.3	Hernia hiatal	511.	Pleurisy			
416.	COPD	550.	Hernia inguinal	601.	Prostatitis			
		274.4	Hyperlipidemia	696.1	Psoriasis			

3. Additional diagnostic codes

4. Additional procedure codes

✓	DESCRIPTION	CPT-4/MD	FEE	✓	DESCRIPTION	CPT-4/MD	FEE	✓	DESCRIPTION	CPT-4/MD	FEE
	OFFICE VISIT–NEW PATIENT				OFFICE PROCEDURES				X-RAY		
	Intermediate	99203	60.00	✓	EKG 12 lead	93000	55.00		Chest	71020	55.00
	Extended	99204	95.00		2DM mode echo	99307	500.00				
✓	Compreh.	99205	195.		Doppler	93320	250.00				
	Consultation	99245	250.00		Color doppler	93325	200.00				
	OFFICE VISIT–ESTAB. PATIENT				Treadmill	93015	295.00				
	Intermediate	99213	55.00		Stress echo	93350-YB			IMMUNIZATIONS/INJECTIONS		
	Extended	99214	65.00		Oximetry w/Exercise	94761	75.00	✓	Flu	90724	20.00
	Compreh.	99215	195.00		Aspiration major jt.	20610	60.00		Pneumococcal	90732	20.00
					Intermediate jt.	20605	45.00		Injection	907	
	MISCELLANEOUS				Trigger point/ten. inj.	20550	45.00		LABORATORY: See attached requisition sheet		
					Sigmoidoscopy-flex.	45330	145.00		Collection and handling	36415	9.00
					Slow flow loop	94375	35.00		Urinalysis	81000	10.00
					Spirometry	94010	50.00				
					w/Bronchodilator	94060	65.00				
					Cerumen removal	69210	40.00				

RETURN APPOINTMENT INFORMATION
____ WEEKS 3 MONTH(S)

SET UP FOLLOWING TESTS

DOCTOR'S SIGNATURE: *PCardi MD*

PLEASE REMEMBER THAT PAYMENT IS YOUR OBLIGATION REGARDLESS OF INSURANCE OR OTHER THIRD PARTY INVOLVEMENT.

REC'D BY:
☐ BANK CARD
☑ CASH
☐ CHECK
_____

PREVIOUS BALANCE	-0-
TODAY'S FEE	270.00
AMOUNT REC'D/CO-PAY	10.00
BALANCE	260.00

5. Patient's previous balance

6. Total charges and payments received

FIGURE 10–7 Encounter form; diagnostic codes from *International Classification of Diseases, Ninth Revision, Clinical Modification* (ICD-9-CM), and procedural codes for professional services from Current Procedural Terminology (CPT). *(Courtesy Bibbero Systems, Inc., Petaluma, Calif. Phone: 800-242-2376; Fax: 800-242-9330;* ***www.bibbero.com.****)*

precluded from seeking the balance. However, acceptance of payment does not necessarily mean acceptance of the "paid in full" remark. A good safeguard is to read the state's accord and satisfaction laws; the Uniform Commercial Code, Articles 3, 4, and 9; and the Retail Installment Sales Act and Escheats Law. Even if a check marked "paid in full" is accidentally cashed, 90 days may be available to rectify the situation by returning the fund to the patient and informing him or her that the accord and satisfaction is not acceptable.

Table 10.1 | **Possible Responses to Patients' Excuses for Avoiding Payment**

Excuse	Response
"Just bill me."	"As we explained when we made your appointment, Mr. Barkley, our practice bills for charges more than $50. Amounts under $50 are to be paid at the time of the visit. That will be $25 for today's visit, please."
"I have insurance to cover this."	"We will be billing your insurance for you, Miss Butler, but your policy shows a deductible in the amount of $300 that still must be met. We must collect the full fee for today's visit, which is $150 to meet that deductible responsibility."
"I get paid on Friday; you know how it is."	"I understand. Why don't you write the check today and postdate it for Saturday. We will hold the check and deposit it on the next business day" (depending on office policy).
"If I pay for this, I won't be able to pay for the prescription."	"Our payment policy is very much like the pharmacy; we expect payment at the time of service. Let me check and see if the doctor can dispense some medication samples to last until you can get your prescription filled."
"I don't have that much with me."	"How much can you pay, Mrs. Fish? I can accept $10 now and give you an envelope to send us the balance within the week, or I can put it on your credit or debit card." (Get a commitment and write the balance due under the sealing flap of the envelope. Also write the date on a tickler calendar or the patient's financial accounting record while the patient is watching.)
"I'll take care of it."	"I know you will, Mr. Stone; I just need to know when that will be so I can document your intentions for our bookkeeper." (Get a commitment and write down the date on a tickler calendar or on the patient's financial accounting record card while in view of the patient. Hand him an envelope with the amount due written under the sealing flap.)
"I forgot my checkbook."	"We take Visa, MasterCard, and American Express, Mr. Storz." (If the patient still does not pay, provide him with a self-addressed envelope and write the patient's name, account number, date of service, amount due, and expected payment date under the sealing flap. Restate the expected payment date as you hand the patient the envelope. Note the date on a tickler calendar or on the patient's financial accounting record card while the patient is watching.)

Unsigned Checks

Another problem is unsigned checks. First ask the patient to come to the office and sign the check or send a new one. If unable to reach the patient or if there is a transportation or time limitation problem, write the word "over" or "see reverse" on the signature line on the front of the check. On the back of the check, where the endorsement should appear, write "lack of signature guaranteed," the practice's name, and one's own name and title. This endorsement in effect is a guarantee that the practice will absorb the loss if the patient's bank or the patient does not honor the check.

Returned Checks

When the physician's office receives notice that a check was not honored, the reason should be stated on the back of the check. The most common reason is nonsufficient funds (NSF). Call the bank to find out if there are adequate funds in the account to cover the check and take the NSF check to the bank immediately. Friday afternoon is a good time to do this. You might telephone the patient to see if they suggest redepositing it. It may be an oversight or miscalculation by the patient. If it is not worth redepositing or if a second NSF notice is received, call the patient immediately. Be courteous but straight to the point. Check the state laws about NSF checks. There is a time limit for making the check good, and there are additional charges (up to 10% of the value of the check) that the patient must make to restore the check. If the patient does not respond, the matter may be turned over

to the State Attorney or satisfaction may be obtained through small claims court. Send an NSF demand letter (Figure 10–8) by certified mail with return receipt requested and include the following:

1. Check date
2. Check number
3. Name of the bank where the check is drawn
4. Name of person the check was payable to
5. Check amount
6. Any allowable service charge
7. Total amount due
8. Number of days the check writer has to take action

Once a patient has been informed of the returned check, explain that the facility will no longer be able to accept checks as payment. Future payments should be in the form of cash, money order, or a cashier's check. If the patient wishes the check returned, be sure to photocopy it and keep it in the financial record because it serves as an acknowledgment of the debt. The bad check may be returned to the patient after it has been replaced with a valid payment. Place a notation on the patient's record to this effect.

Larger facilities may consider a check authorization system to guard against bad checks. With such a system the company supplies a terminal that gives an approval number for each check that is taken in and guarantees payment on the checks authorized. If no approval is given, another form of payment is necessary. The check guarantee service receives a percentage for the checks that it

COLLEGE CLINIC
4567 Broad Avenue
Woodland Hills, XY 12345-0001
Tel. (555) 486-9002
FAX (555) 487-8976

August 15, 20XX

Mrs. Maxine Holt
444 Labina Lane
Woodland Hills, XY 12345-0001

Dear Mrs. Holt:

The following check has been dishonored by the bank and returned without payment:

Date: 08/04/20XX
Check No.:   755
Amount: $106.11
Payable to: Perry Cardi, MD
Bank: Woodland Hills National Bank
Reason: Nonsufficient funds

This is a formal notice demanding payment in the amount of $106.11 within 15 days from today's date or your account will be considered for legal action.

Please make payment immediately by cash, cashier's check, or money order at the above address. Your immediate attention will be appreciated.

Sincerely,

Delores Yee, CMA-A

Patient Accounts Manager
for Perry Cardi, MD

FIGURE 10–8 Demand letter for returned check. This letter serves as a formal notice to collect payment and notifies a patient of impending legal action.

approves and collects all bad check charges from the patient. One way to help discourage bad checks is to charge a penalty for returned checks. This information should be included in the new patient brochures and posted in the office for all patients to view. Perhaps make reference to the particular section of the state Civil Code's provisions about checks for nonsufficient funds if it is desired to collect more than the face value of the check.

If notified that the checking account is closed, do not waste time trying to contact the patient. Send a demand letter immediately. In most states, legal action can be taken if the patient does not respond in 30 days. Consider filing a claim in small claims court. Most states have written codes or statutes pertaining to bad checks. Often legislation allows the creditor to add punitive damages to the amount of the debt being collected, sometimes up to three times the amount of the check.

When a patient stops payment on a check, it is usually done to resolve a good faith dispute. In this case, the patient believes that he or she has legal entitlement to withhold payment. The physician may want to contact a

lawyer to discuss his or her legal rights and responsibilities before sending a demand letter and trying to collect.

Itemized Patient Statements

Every patient receives an **itemized statement** (Figure 10–9) of his or her account showing the dates of service, a list of detailed charges, copayments and deductibles paid, the date insurance claim was filed (if appropriate), applicable adjustments, and the account balance. These items also are listed on the patient's account or financial accounting record card (see Figure 3–17 and Figure 10–2). Timeliness, accuracy, and consistency have a significant effect on the cash flow and collection process when sending itemized statements. A credit card option should be printed on the statement to encourage easier and faster payment.

Professional bills are a reflection of the medical practice. The billing statement should be patient oriented and easy to read and understand. Avoid technical terms and abbreviations that might lead to misunderstandings

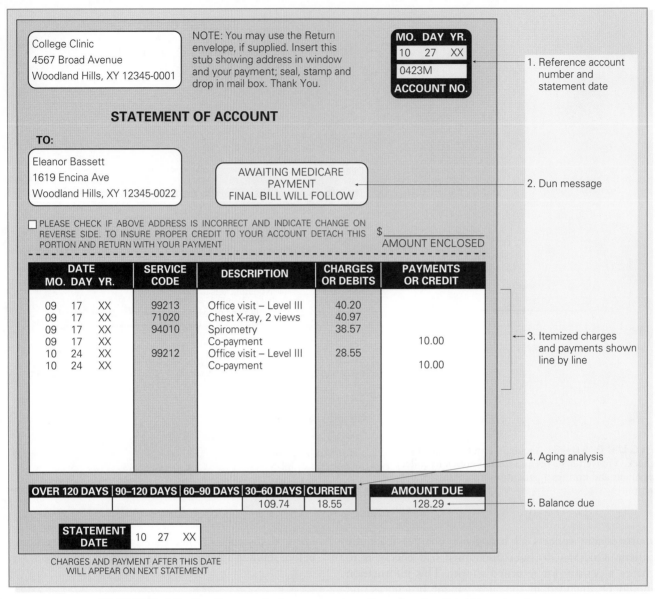

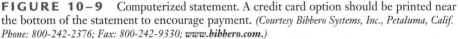

FIGURE 10–9   Computerized statement. A credit card option should be printed near the bottom of the statement to encourage payment. *(Courtesy Bibbero Systems, Inc., Petaluma, Calif. Phone: 800-242-2376; Fax: 800-242-9330; **www.bibbero.com**.)*

and confusion. Enclose a return envelope. Addressed envelopes should contain the statement "Forwarding Service Requested" so the postal service can forward the mail and provide the physician's office with a notice of the patient's new address. When this notice is received in the physician's office, it should be circulated to all necessary departments to record the new information.

Patients can be oriented to the billing process by having the insurance specialist generate a printed statement when they are ready to leave the office and explain pertinent information, such as account number, dates of service, payments, procedures, interest fees, copayments, and deductibles. Patient information pamphlets about common health concerns such as blood pressure,

cholesterol, or back pain can be sent along with the bill to convey a caring attitude.

The office is likely to experience an increase in telephone calls from inquiring patients when statements go out in the mail. One person or one department should handle all billing questions, ensuring a consistent response.

Age Analysis by Aging Report

Age analysis is a term used for the procedure of systematically arranging the A/R by age from the date of service. Accounts are usually aged in time periods of 30, 60, 90, and 120 days and older, as shown at the bottom

Collection Decision Tree

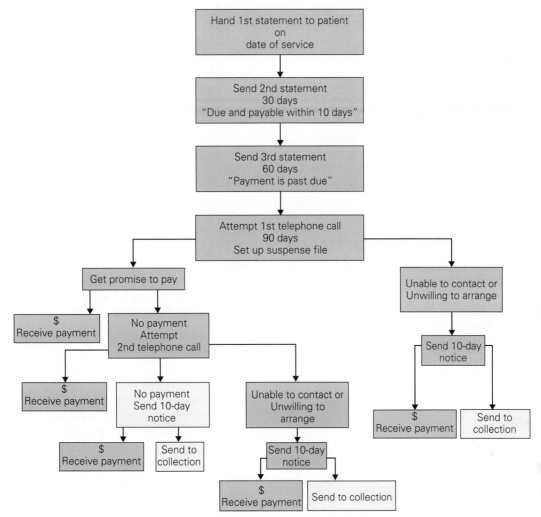

FIGURE 10–10 Collection decision tree. This is a quick reference used to help determine when to send statements, make telephone calls, and send accounts to a collection agency.

of Figure 10–9. An aging report can be generated by the practice management system or by use of other software in a computer system. This helps collection follow-up by providing easy recognition of overdue accounts and allows the insurance specialist to determine which accounts need action in addition to a regular statement. A decision tree showing time frames for sending statements and telephone calls is presented in this chapter in Figure 10–10.

Dun Messages

Dun messages are used on statements to promote payment (see Figures 10–2 and 10–9). The best and most effective collection statements include a handwritten note; however, this is seldom possible. Dun messages also can be printed by the computer system or applied with brightly colored labels. Examples of dun messages follow:

● "If there is a problem with your account, please call me at (555) 486-0000—Marlayn."

● "This bill is now 30 days past due. Please remit payment."

● "This bill is now 60 days past due. Please send payment immediately."

● "Your account is 90 days past due. Please remit payment now to avoid collection action."

● "FINAL NOTICE: If we do not hear from you within 10 days, this account will be turned over to our collection agency."

Do not send intimidating, impatient, or threatening statements. These only serve to antagonize patients. Dun messages should be printed in different languages and sent to patients who speak English as a second language. Examples follow.

● "No payment yet; your payment by return mail will be appreciated."

● "No hemos recibido pago. Agracieramos remita por correo."

● "Payment needed now. No further credit will be extended."
● "Se requiere pago hoy. No se le estendera mas credito."

Manual Billing

Manual billing is usually done by photocopying the patient's financial accounting record and placing it in a window envelope. The financial accounting record becomes the statement and should be clear and readable with no crossouts or misspellings. Typewritten statements may be used by small offices and generally are typed on continuous form paper. The completed statements are separated, folded, and placed into billing envelopes.

A coding system with metal clip-on tabs or peel-off labels that are placed on the financial accounting record card can be used with a manual system. Each time the account is billed, a different color tab or label is placed on the financial accounting record card, which shows at a glance how many times the account has been billed. It also provides aging of accounts, although if a report is desired it must be done manually in addition to this process.

Computer Billing

Computerized patient statements can be generated by the practice management software. All charges, payments, and adjustments will be reflected on hardcopy and made readily available to mail to the patient (see Figure 10–9). The computer program usually offers choices of billing types, including patient billing, **insurance balance billing,** discounted billing, and no bill. The insurance specialist can instruct the computer to print all bills of a specific type. The computer also can be instructed to print bills according to specific accounts, dates, and insurance types. Accounts are automatically aged, and standard messages can be printed on the statements for each of the aged dates (30, 60, 90, or 120 days). Some systems allow personalized messages to be inserted that override the standard messages.

Billing Services

Billing services are employed by many medical practices to reduce administrative paperwork by taking over the task of preparing and mailing patient statements. These services also may be employed to prepare and mail insurance claim forms or send them electronically. They may provide data entry of patients' demographic and billing information, charges, receipts, and adjustments; tracking of payments from patients and third-party payers; production of management reports, purging of inactive accounts, and collection of accounts.

Some advantages of billing services are advanced technology, professional and understandable bills, experts answering all billing-related telephone inquiries, and no downtime caused by vacations, or medical or personal leave. This service allows the medical office to have fewer disruptions and the freedom from worry about financial matters when trying to provide medical care.

The physician's office sends billing and receipt information into the system daily. This may be done in writing or through a computer system. The billing service then prepares the bills, mails them, and may also receive payments. Regular reports, whether weekly or monthly, are sent to the physician summarizing the transactions. Billing services may offer full account management services and in many cases customize a service that meets the needs of the provider. Using a billing service company is most commonly referred to as *outsourcing*. When choosing a billing service, make a list of important questions and visit the facility. Also ask for references so that you may obtain valuable feedback from other provider offices that have used the same billing service.

Billing Guidelines

Billing procedures are determined by the size of the practice, the number of accounts, and the number of staff members assigned to the collection process. Adopt a specific method of handling accounts and decide which billing routine best fits the practice. Check insurance and managed care contracts carefully to determine which circumstances allow for patients to be billed. Be sure to conform to federal guidelines if there is a need to bill managed care patients. Refer to the end of this chapter for the seven-step billing and collection procedures and guidelines.

CREDIT ARRANGEMENTS

Although payment at the time of service is ideal, many patients do not have funds available to pay at the time of the office visit. Alternative payment methods may be offered to help continuous cash flow and reduce collection costs.

Payment Options

Credit Card Billing

Credit card payment is an option that provides patients with an alternative to clear their account balances. Credit cards are issued by organizations that entitle the cardholder to credit at their establishments. This method of payment may be most useful as a downpayment on uninsured or elective procedures. According to a survey by American Express, 33% of patients said they would use a credit card to pay for health care–related expenses if the option is given. Credit cards can help manage the A/R by improving cash flow, reducing billing costs, lowering overhead, and reducing the risk of bad debts. If a practice accepts credit cards, advise all patients in the following ways: display a credit card acceptance sign, include an insignia or message on the statement, include the credit card policy in the new patient brochure, and have staff members verbalize to patients that this option is available. Patients may prefer to clear a debt immediately and make monthly payments to the credit card company instead of owing money to their doctor.

Verifying Credit Cards

A one- or two-physician office may have a simple credit card imprinter in the office. The insurance specialist should check credit card warning bulletins to make sure that the card has not been canceled or stolen. Large practices may have an electronic credit card machine that allows the insurance specialist to swipe the card through the machine that is linked to the credit card company. Transactions then are approved, processed, and deposited into a bank account, usually in 2 working days. These machines may be rented or purchased.

Verifone terminals also are used for credit card authorization. They are small computers with built-in software and modems for communicating with other computers over telephone lines. They have a small alphanumeric keypad and a small display screen that can show a line or two of data. This device reads the information off the magnetic card as it is swiped through the machine, dials a telephone number, connects with another computer, verifies the patient's credit, and displays a message.

Verifying Credit Card Holders

Always verify the cardholder by asking for photo identification such as a driver's license. Examine the card carefully and observe the following guidelines:

- Accept a credit card only from the person whose name is on the card.
- Match the name on the card with the patient's other identification and make sure the expiration date has not passed.
- Look on the back of the card for the word "void." This is an alert that the card has been heated, which is a method used to forge a signature.
- Check the "hot list" for problem cards.
- Verify all charges regardless of the amount and get approval from the credit card company.
- Complete the credit card voucher (Figure 10–11) before asking for a signature.
- Compare the signature on the credit card voucher against the signature on the card.

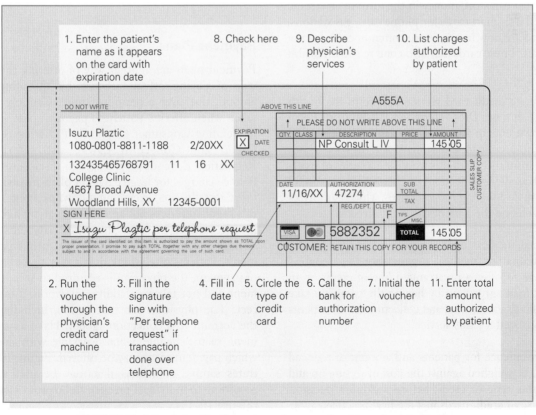

FIGURE 10–11 Credit card voucher completed in a physician's office.

● Record the credit card number in the patient's financial file for future use if the patient's account has to be traced or transferred to a collection agency.

Credit Card Fees

Most banks directly deposit the credit card voucher and subtract the monthly fees from the practice's bank account. A statement from the bank indicates how much has been credited to the account. The fees can be negotiated based on volume, but usually range from 2% to 10% on each transaction. Some medical practices charge patients a service fee for using credit cards. Do not issue cash or check refunds for any payments made by credit card. Credit vouchers (see Figure 10–11) used for crediting a credit card account are available at local banks. Patients who want to make payments may have their credit cards charged for each scheduled payment.

Credit Card Options

Other cards also are used for credit in a physician's office. ATM cards sometimes are accepted for medical care if the practice has a credit card scanner. Private-label cards are credit vehicles that can be used only to pay for health care. Some large practices offer their own private-label health cards. Smart cards also are used in some locations. They are small credit or debit cards that contain a computer chip that can store money in the form of electronic data. Special use smart cards for phone calls, gas stations, and fast food are now in use, as are common cards having multiple uses. These cards may also contain patient health care data.

Visa offers a credit card service unique to the health care market. It has a Pre-Authorized Health Care Form that allows patients to authorize the medical office to bill their account directly for copayments and the balance not covered by insurance. Patients who need a series of treatments, such as allergy injections or chemotherapy, can fill out one form designating these services, which authorizes the staff to charge the patient's account directly.

A national medical card is now available for use by any professional or medical organization and enables the physician to offer a prearranged line of credit or an installment loan agreement by having the company take over the billing, accounting, and collecting for all patients who are approved for this service.

The convenience for patients and amount of reduced A/R should be weighed against the cost of setting up and operating this type of credit before making a decision about the use of credit cards in a medical practice.

Debit Cards

A **debit card** is a card permitting bank customers to withdraw cash at any hour from any affiliated ATM in the country. The holder also may make cashless purchases from funds on deposit without incurring revolving finance charges for credit. A small fee is charged to the customer's checking account when the card is used; however, this fee is usually applied only once a month (if the debit card is used), regardless of how many times the card is used during the month. Medical practices offering credit card payment may use the same electronic credit card machine to swipe the debit card for verification and approval. Separate debit card machines are also available for businesses that do not accept credit cards. Debit cards take the place of check writing; however, once the debit card is approved for a certain amount, the bank that issued the debit card is responsible for paying the funds that were approved. There are no returned checks for nonsufficient funds with this method of payment.

E-Checks

Another payment option that is becoming popular is payment by e-check. With an e-check, the patient gives his or her checking account information, such as account number and bank routing number. No signature is necessary, and the check is deposited as though it were sent by the patient.

Payment Plans

Payment plans are another way of offering the patient a way of paying off an account by spreading out the amount due over a period of time. Caution should be taken when offering patients a payment plan. The Truth in Lending Consumer Credit Cost Disclosure Law (see Credit and Collection Laws), also referred to as Regulation Z, requires full written disclosure about the finance charges for large payment plans involving four or more installments, excluding a downpayment. However, this regulation does not apply if the patient agrees to pay in one sum or in fewer than four payments and then decides independently to make drawn-out partial payments. Patients often think that if they make any amount of payment, the physician is required to accept that payment and not take any additional action. This is incorrect. The physician can take action, including sending the account to a collection agency. Have a written payment plan schedule when working with accounts in which payment plans may be offered. Figure 10–12 illustrates sample guidelines that may be used or revised according to individual practice and management policies (Figure 10–13).

PAYMENT PLAN SCHEDULE

Balance due amount	Minimum monthly payment	Time frame for full payment
$0 – $200	$35	6 months
$201 – $500	$50	1 year
$500 – $1000	$100	1 year
$1001 – $3000	$125	2 years
$3001 – $5000	$150	2 years
>$5001*	$200	5 years

*Accounts over $5,000 must complete credit card application to certify minimum required payment and are subject to approval by office manager.

FIGURE 10–12 Payment plan schedule used in the physician's office to negotiate monthly payments shows balance due amounts, minimum monthly payment, and payment time frames.

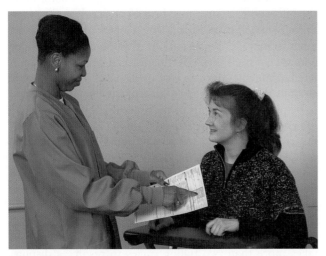

FIGURE 10–13 Insurance billing specialist setting up a payment plan with a patient.

CREDIT AND COLLECTION LAWS

The following laws are important because they provide the legal framework within which the insurance specialist must execute the physician's collection policy. In addition, each state may have specific collection laws that are necessary to research and obey.

The Fair and Accurate Credit Transactions (FACT) Act of December 4, 2003 (Public Law 108-159), establishes medical privacy provisions as part of consumer credit law. The bill amends the Fair Credit Reporting Act (FCRA) to include improved medical privacy protections and protections against identity theft. Credit bureaus and creditors must comply with a number of medical privacy restrictions that ban the sharing of medical information. Title IV of the FACT Act limits the use and sharing of medical information in the financial system and provides an expanded definition of medical information. For additional information at the Web site, see Internet Resources at the end of this chapter.

Statute of Limitations

A formal regulation or law setting time limits on legal action is known as a **statute of limitations.** In regard to collections, the statute of limitations is the maximum time during which a legal collection suit may be rendered against a debtor. However, for a lawsuit to be successful, a concerted effort should be made to collect on an account from the time services are rendered. The patient should receive regular statements indicating that if the insurer does not pay the patient will be held responsible.

Statutes vary according to three kinds of accounts:

1. *Open book accounts* (also called open accounts): Accounts that are open to charges made from time to time. Payment is expected within a specific period but credit has been extended without a formal written contract. Physicians' patient accounts usually are open book accounts.
2. *Written contract accounts:* Accounts having a formal written agreement in which a patient signs to pay his or her bill in more than four installments (see Truth in Lending Act).
3. *Single-entry accounts:* Accounts having only one entry or charge; usually these are for a small amount.

Equal Credit Opportunity Act

The Equal Credit Opportunity Act (which is a federal law) prohibits discrimination in all areas of granting credit. If credit is offered, credit must be available fairly and impartially to all patients who request it. Obtaining detailed credit information before performing services will prevent accusations of credit discrimination. New patients can be informed that payment is due at the time of service, and they should arrive 20 minutes early to fill out a credit application if they would like to establish credit for possible future treatment. Check all information with a credit bureau that will verify data such as the patient's address, previous addresses, length of residence, employment history, and approximate wage. The report will also contain the patient's name changes, the patient's bill-paying history, and any history of bankruptcy. If the patient has a poor credit rating, credit may be denied and the patient then has 60 days to request the reason in writing.

The law prohibits discrimination against any applicant for credit for the following reasons:

● Age, color, marital status, national origin, race, religion, or sex
● He or she has exercised rights under consumer credit laws
● An applicant is receiving income from any public assistance program

Fair Credit Reporting Act

Agencies that either issue or use reports on consumers (patients) in connection with the approval of credit are regulated by the Fair Credit Reporting Act. The act states that credit reporting agencies can only provide reports when:

● A court order is issued.
● The report is requested by the consumer (patient) or instructions are given by the patient to provide the report.
● There is a legitimate business need for the information.

If credit is refused, the physician must provide the patient with a reason credit was denied. Specific information about what the report contains is not necessary and should not be given. The provider also must give the name and address of the agency from which the report came. The patient must have an opportunity to correct any inaccuracies if they occur.

Fair Credit Billing Act

Per the Federal Trade Commission, the Fair Credit Billing Act (FCBA) applies to "open end" credit accounts, such as credit cards, and revolving charge accounts for department store accounts. It does not cover installment contracts such as loans or extensions of credit you repay on a fixed schedule. Consumers often buy cars, furniture, and major appliances on an installment basis, and they repay personal loans in installments as well. The FCBA settlement procedures apply only to disputes about "billing errors," such as unauthorized charges. Federal law limits the consumer's responsibility for unauthorized charges to $50; charges that list the wrong date or amount; charges for goods and services that the consumer did not accept or were not delivered as agreed; math errors; failure to post payments and other credits, such as returns; failure to send bills to the current address—provided the creditor receives the change of address, in writing, at least 20 days before the billing period ends; and charges for which an explanation or written proof of purchase along with a claimed error or request for clarification are requested.

To take advantage of the law's consumer protections, write to the creditor at the address given for "billing inquiries," not the address for sending payments, and include one's name, address, account number, and a description of the billing error. Send the letter so that it reaches the creditor within 60 days after the first bill was mailed that contained the error. Send the letter by certified mail, return receipt requested, for proof of what the creditor received. Include copies (not originals) of sales slips or other documents that support the position. Keep a copy of the dispute letter. The creditor must acknowledge the complaint in writing within 30 days after receiving it, unless the problem has been resolved. The creditor must resolve the dispute within two billing cycles (but not more than 90 days) after receiving the letter. Payment may be withheld on the disputed amount (and related charges) during the investigation. Any part of the bill not in question must be paid, including finance charges on the undisputed amount. The creditor may not take any legal or other action to collect the disputed amount and related charges (including finance charges) during the investigation. Although the account cannot be closed or restricted, the disputed amount may be applied against the credit limit. If the creditor's investigation determines the bill is correct, one must be told promptly and in writing how much is owed and why. Copies of relevant documents may be requested. At this point the disputed amount is owed plus any finance charges that accumulated while the amount was in dispute. The minimum amount that was missed because of the dispute may have to be paid. If the results of the investigation are disputed, the creditor may be written to within 10 days after receiving the explanation, and the disputed amount may be refused. At this point, the creditor may begin collection procedures. Any creditor who fails to follow the settlement procedure may not collect the amount in dispute, or any related finance charges, up to $50, even if the bill turns out to be correct. For example, if a creditor acknowledges the complaint in 45 days—15 days too late—or takes more than two billing cycles to resolve a dispute, the penalty applies. The penalty also applies if a creditor threatens to report, or improperly reports, one's failure to pay to anyone during the dispute period.

Truth in Lending Act

The federal Truth in Lending Act (TILA) of 1969 is a consumer protection act that applies to anyone who charges interest or agrees on payment of a bill in more than four installments, excluding a downpayment. When a specific agreement is reached between patient and physician, Regulation Z of this act requires that a written disclosure of all pertinent information be made, regardless of the existence of a finance charge (see Figure 10–5). This full disclosure must be discussed at the time the agreement is first reached between patient and physician and credit is extended. It is essential to include the following items:

1. Total amount of the debt
2. Amount of down payment
3. Finance charge
4. Interest rate expressed as an annual percentage

5. Amount of each payment
6. Date each payment is due
7. Date final payment is due
8. Signature of patient and physician with copies retained by both

In addition, it might be wise to also include the account balance with the total interest and total amount paid by the patient at the end of the contract.

According to the Federal Trade Commission (FTC), the Truth in Lending provision is not applicable and no disclosures are necessary if a patient decides on his or her own to pay in installments or whenever convenient.

Late Payment Charges

Medical practices that implement late payment charges that meet the criteria defined in the TILA as a finance charge must comply with a host of requirements that revolve around proper disclosure to patients.

Charges must meet the following criteria to qualify as late payment charges:

1. The account balance must be paid in full at the time of initial billing.
2. The account is treated as delinquent when unpaid.
3. The charge is assessed to a patient's account only because of his or her failure to make timely payments.
4. Installments are limited to no more than three.
5. The creditor (physician or insurance specialist) makes a "commercially reasonable" effort to collect these accounts.

When a physician continues to treat a patient with an overdue account, the courts have viewed this as continuation of care and an extension of credit. Patients who fall into this delinquent status should be referred elsewhere. See Chapter 4 for instructions on sending a discharge letter. After the patient has paid the overdue amount, the patient can be taken back and treated on a cash-only basis.

Truth in Lending Consumer Credit Cost Disclosure

The Truth in Lending Consumer Credit Cost Disclosure is similar to the Federal Truth in Lending Act. It requires businesses to disclose all direct and indirect costs and conditions related to the granting of credit. All interest charges, late charges, collection fees, finance charges, and so forth must be explained up front, before the time of service. Include the following on all statements to charge interest and bill the patient monthly:

● Amount of each payment
● Due date

● Unpaid balance at the beginning of the billing period
● Finance charges
● Date balance is due

Fair Debt Collection Practices Act

The Fair Debt Collection Practices Act (FDCPA) was designed to address the collection practices of third-party debt collectors and attorneys who regularly collect debts for others. Although this act does not apply directly to physician practices collecting for themselves, a professional health care collector must avoid the actions that are prohibited for collection agencies. The main intent of the act is to protect consumers from unfair, harassing, or deceptive collection practices. Refer to the guidelines in Box 10.1, which are taken from the FDCPA, to help avoid illegalities, enhance collections, and maintain positive patient relations. For more information about

---

Box 10.1 | **Fair Debt Collection Practices Act Guidelines**

1. Contact debtors only once a day; in some states, repeated calls in 1 day or the same week could be considered harassment.
2. Place calls after 8 AM and before 9 PM.
3. Do not contact debtors on Sunday or any other day that the debtor recognizes as a Sabbath.
4. Identify yourself and the medical practice represented; do not mislead the patient.
5. Contact the debtor at work *only* if unable to contact the debtor elsewhere; no contact should be made if the employer or debtor disapproves.
6. Contact the attorney if an attorney represents the debtor; contact the debtor only if the attorney does not respond.
7. Do not threaten or use obscene language.
8. Do not send postcards for collection purposes; keep all correspondence strictly private.
9. Do not call collect or cause additional expense to the patient.
10. Do not leave a message on an answering machine indicating that you are calling about a bill.
11. Do not contact a third party more than once unless requested to do so by the party or the response was erroneous or incomplete.
12. Do not convey to a third party that the call is about a debt.
13. Do not contact the debtor when notified in writing that a debtor refuses to pay and would like contact to stop, except to notify the debtor in writing that there will be no further contact or that there will be legal action.
14. Stick to the facts; do not use false statements.
15. Do not prepare a list of "bad debtors" or "credit risks" to share with other health care providers.
16. Take action immediately when stating that a certain action will be taken (e.g., filing a claim in small claims court or sending the patient's case to a collection agency).
17. Send the patient written verification of the name of the creditor and the amount of debt within 5 days of the initial contact.

collection laws in your state, contact your state attorney general's office. The stricter law prevails if there is a conflict between state and federal laws.

THE COLLECTION PROCESS

For collections to be handled effectively, staff members should be trained in collection techniques. Most insurance specialists can be trained to be efficient collectors when given the correct tools. New collectors need time to gain confidence, which is an important aspect of being a good collector.

Office Collection Techniques

Telephone Debt Collection

Telephone collections are made easier if the insurance billing specialist is convinced that he or she can collect before trying to convince the patient to pay. Two important factors to consider are the insurance specialist's ability to contact the patient and the patient's ability to pay the bill. Contact the patient in a timely manner at the first sign of payment delay. Prepare before making a telephone collection call by reviewing the account and noting anything unusual. Locate information as to where the patient is employed (or if unemployed) by reviewing the patient registration form. Decide what amount will be settled for if payment cannot be made in full. Make the first call count. Act in a calm, businesslike manner and combine empathy with diligence. Be positive and persuasive. Listen to what the patient has to say, even if he or she gets angry and raises his or her voice. Lower the volume of your own voice and respond in a composed manner. Try to pick up clues from what the patient is saying; he or she may be giving the real reason for nonpayment. Ask questions, show interest, and let the patient know that he or she is being listened to. Respond in a respectful manner and carefully word the reply; when patients are distressed they do not always make sense. The goal is to encourage the patient to pay, not agitate the patient. Use all resources and learn to negotiate.

Use an organized approach to determine which collection calls to make first. Print out the A/R by age and target the accounts that are in the 60- to 90-day category. The most effective results come from this group. If financial accounting record cards are used, pull all the cards with tabs or labels that indicate the patient has received two or three statements, depending on office protocol. Start with the largest amount owed and work the accounts in decreasing amounts owed. After this category has been completed, move on to the 90- to 120-day accounts. Finally, go after accounts that are more than 120 days old.

Most state collection laws allow telephone calls to the debtor between 8 AM and 9 PM. Never call between 9 PM and 8 AM because to do so may be considered harassment. However, according to collection experts, the best time to telephone is between 5:30 PM and 8:30 PM on Tuesdays and Thursdays and 9 AM to 1 PM on Saturdays. However, regardless of when the call is made, track the times when the most patients are contacted and adjust the calling schedule accordingly. Perhaps the physician's office hours should be increased to include one evening a week or Saturday mornings to make collection calls. Another option is the use of flex time in which the employee can choose his or her own working hours from within a broad range of hours approved by management. Use a private phone away from the busy operations of the office to eliminate interruptions. Patients may be embarrassed about not being able to pay their bills, and patient confidentiality must be maintained. Follow the rules stated in the Fair Debt Collection Practices Act.

Be alert for new ideas or approaches to collection by watching how banks and other retailers implement sophisticated collection skills. Decide if any of these could be used to the medical practice's advantage and present the techniques to the office manager. Keep abreast of improvements made to collection software that improve collection results and allow more collectors to work from their homes. Other advances (e.g., call block, which is an expanded telephone service) have made it more difficult to make collection calls. This service was originally intended to screen out unwanted telemarketing calls by intercepting blocked, unlisted, or unknown numbers. Standard numbers are usually allowed to go through. The key to averting a block is to make sure the number the call is being placed from is listed and within the patient's area. Telephone companies' services vary, so research to discover all expanded services used in your area.

For step-by-step procedures on making telephone collection calls, refer to the end of this chapter.

Telephone "Don'ts"

Communication is very important, especially when trying to work with a patient through difficulties in making payments. Remain professional at all times and treat the patient with respect. The following is a list of *do nots* for telephone collections:

- Do not raise your voice and antagonize the patient.
- Do not accuse the patient of dishonesty or lying.
- Do not act like a "tough guy" or threaten a patient.
- Do not consent to partial payments until payment in full has been asked for and do not agree to a long string of small partial payments.
- Do not engage in a debate.

● Do not report a disputed account to a collection agency or bureau until the patient's dispute is disclosed as part of the record.

Telephone collection calls also are effective the day before patients are due for their appointments. State the date and time of the appointment and then remind the patient of the balance owed and ask whether he or she would please bring payment to the appointment.

Telephone Collection Scenarios

The most difficult part of one-on-one collections is preparing for the many situations that may be encountered and the various responses the patient may make. Following are some statements patients make for not paying an account and examples of responses the insurance specialist can make:

Statement: "I can't pay anything now."
Response: "Are you employed? Are you receiving unemployment compensation, welfare, or Social Security benefits?"

You are determining the patient's ability to pay.

"Are you paying some of your bills?"

You are uncovering the fact that the patient is paying certain bills. You can then tell the patient that the bill must be taken care of, also, even if only a small amount at a time.

Statement: "I can't pay the whole bill now."
Response: "How long will it take you to pay this bill?"

Ask this question instead of "How much can you pay?"

Statement: "I can pay, but not until next month."
Response: "When do you get paid?"

Ask for payment the day after payday.

"Do you have a checking account?"

Ask for a postdated check.

Statement: "I have other bills."
Response: "This is also one of your bills that should be paid now. Let's talk about exactly how you plan payment."

Statement: "How about $10 a month (on a $350 bill)?"
Response: "I'd like to accept that, but our accountant does not allow us to stretch out payments beyond 90 days, which would be $105 a month."

This adheres to (Truth in Lending Law) regulations for collecting payment in installments without a written agreement. If the patient tries to cooperate, then compromise. If not, turn the account over to a collection agency.

Statement: "I sent in the payment."

Response: "When was the payment sent? To what address was it sent? Was it a check? On what bank was it drawn and for what amount? What is the canceled check number?"

Investigate to determine whether the check was posted to a wrong account. If not, call the patient back and ask if he or she would call his or her bank to see if it cleared; if it has not, the patient should stop payment. Ask the patient to call back and verify the status of the check. If the patient is lying, he or she will not follow through. Ask for a new check and tell the patient that a refund will be made if the other one shows up.

Statement: "I cannot make a payment this month."
Response: "The collection agency picks up all our delinquent accounts next Monday. I don't want to include yours, but I need a check today."

Statement: "The check's in the mail."
Response: "May I have the check number and date it was mailed?"

Call back in 3 days if not received.

Statement: "I'm not going to pay the bill because the doctor didn't spend any time with me."
Response: "May I confirm the doctor you saw, the date, and time? For what reason did you see the doctor? Do you still have the problem for which you saw the doctor?"

Get as much information as possible and research the office schedule the day the patient was seen. Let the doctor know about the patient's complaint and inquire how he or she would like to handle the complaint.

Statement: "I thought the insurance company was paying this."
Response: "Your insurance paid most of the bill; now the balance is your responsibility. Please send your check before Friday to keep your account current."

Explain why (deductible, copayment benefit) the service is not covered under the insurance plan.

Collection Letters

Collection letters are another method of reaching patients and reminding them of their debt. Knowledge of the patient base and of individual patients may help determine the effectiveness of collection letters. Every facility is unique, and the number of accounts, the geographic spread of patients, the staff size, and the amount of time collectors have to spend on individual accounts helps determine which collection method best suits the practice.

COLLEGE CLINIC
4567 Broad Avenue
Woodland Hills, XY 12345-0001
Tel. (555) 486-9002
FAX (555) 487-8976

November 13, 20XX

Miss Melanie Markham
1001 Swallow Lane
Woodland Hills, XY 12345-0001

Dear Miss Markham:

It is the office policy of College Clinic to contact patients who have
received two billing statements but have not responded. We realize this
could be an oversight on your part, not a willful disregard of an assumed
obligation. If you have a financial problem or a question about your
account, please call me at (555) 486-9002 extension 443 or stop by
our office.

We would like to thank you in advance for your cooperation in attending
to this matter.

Sincerely,

Shirley Summer, CMA
Clarence Cutler, MD

FIGURE 10–14   Collection form letter sent to all patients who have not responded after two billing cycles.

The positive aspect of collection letters is that they can reach a large number of patients rapidly and the cost is relatively low (especially if form letters are used; Figure 10–14).

Collection letters have some negative aspects:

● Letters usually take 2 or 3 days to reach the patient and may lie unopened for a week or more.
● Letters are one-way communication, thus lacking the ability to provide the reason for nonpayment.
● The response and recovery through letters are relatively poor.
● Manual preparation takes time (especially if a decision must be made before sending each letter).

The insurance specialist is often the one to compose collection letters and devise a plan for collection follow-up. A series of collection letters may be written using varying degrees of forcefulness, starting with a gentle reminder. When a collection letter is written, use a friendly tone and ask why payment has not been made. Imply that the patient has good intentions to pay. This may be done by suggesting that the patient has overlooked a previous statement. Communicate the doctor's sincere interest in the patient. Always invite the patient to explain the reason for nonpayment in a letter, telephone call, or office visit. It should sound as though the patient is anxious to clear the debt.

When collection letters are sent toward the end of the year, include a statement letting the patient know that if the account is paid in full by the end of the year, the medical expense may be used as an income tax deduction. Another tactic is to send a notice advising the patient that he or she may skip December's payment because of increased expenses during the holidays. This tactic may be used as an opportunity to build patient relationships, but the collector must be firm and clear when offering such leeway. Collection letters sent after the first of the year can suggest that the patient clear the debt by using an income tax refund check.

Types of Collection Letters

A form letter saves time and can go out automatically at specific times during the billing cycle (see Figure 10–14). Letters with checklists are a type of form letter (Figure 10–15) that makes it easier for the patient to choose a payment option. Personally typed letters can be individualized to suit any situation. Collection letters should contain the following information:

● Full amount owed
● Services performed
● What action the patient should take
● Time frame in which the patient should respond
● How the patient should take care of the bill

COLLEGE CLINIC
4567 Broad Avenue
Woodland Hills, XY 12345-0001
Tel. (555) 486-9002
FAX (555) 487-8976

March 16, 20XX

Mr. Frank Lincoln
3397 Westminster Avenue
Woodland Hills, XY 12345-0001

Account No.   593287
Amount Due: $ _____

Dear Mr. Lincoln:

The care of our patients is more important than writing letters about overdue accounts. Yet, as you must realize, the expense of furnishing care can only be met by payments from appreciative patients.

Your account is seriously past due and has been removed from our current files because of its delinquent status. Our office policy indicates that your account should be placed with a collection agency. However, we would prefer to hear from you regarding your preference in this matter.

Enclosed is a current statement of your account. Please indicate your payment choice.

- ☐ I would prefer to settle this account immediately. Please find payment in full enclosed.

- ☐ I would prefer to make monthly payments (up to six months). To exercise this option please call and make arrangements to come into our office to sign a financial agreement.

- ☐ Please charge the full amount to my credit card. (We accept American Express, MasterCard, and Visa). To exercise this option, please telephone our office or fill in the enclosed form and return it with the envelope provided.

_____   _____
Signature   Date

Please select one of the three options above, sign the form, and return this notice within 10 days from the date indicated in the letter. A postmarked return envelope is provided. Failure to respond will result in an automatic referral to our collection agency. Please do not hesitate to call if you have any questions regarding this matter.

Sincerely,

Gil Steinberg
Office Manager

Enc. Envelope, Credit Card Agreement Form

FIGURE 10–15 Multipurpose collection letter with checklist. This advises patient of a seriously past due account, offers the patient three payment options, and warns the patient that failure to respond will result in a referral to a collection agency.

- Why the patient should take care of the bill
- Address to which patients send payment
- Telephone number to contact the office
- Contact person's name
- Signature, which can be listed as "Financial Secretary," "Insurance Specialist," "Assistant to Doctor _____," or one's name and title with the physician's name below.

When pursuing collection, the insurance specialist should stay within the authorization of the physician.

All letters should be noted on the back of the financial accounting record, in the collection log, or in the computer comment area. Abbreviations can be used to indicate which letter was sent (Table 10.2) along with the date the letter was mailed. Letters can be sent in brightly colored envelopes to attract attention. The envelope should include "Address Service Requested" or "Forwarding Service Requested" on the outside to ensure the letter is forwarded if the patient has moved so that the office will be notified of the patient's new address. Always include a self-addressed stamped envelope.

Table 10.2 | **Collection Abbreviations**

ATTY	Attorney	NSN	No such number
B	Bankrupt	OFC	Office
Bal	Balance	OOT	Out of town
Bk*	Bank	OOW	Out of work
BLG	Belligerent	PA	Payment arrangement
BTTR	Best time to reach	PH or PH'D	Phoned
CB	Call back	Ph/Dsc*	Phone disconnected
CLM	Claim	PIF	Payment in full
DA*	Directory assistance	PIM	Payment in mail
DFB	Demand for balance	PMT	Payment
DNK	Did not know	POE	Place of employment
DSC	Disconnected	POLK†	Polk directory
EMP	Employment	POW	Payment on way
EOM	End of month	PP	Promise to pay or partial payment
EOW	End of week	PT	Patient
FA	Further action	RCD	Received
FN	Final notice	R/D*	Reverse directory
H	He (or husband)	RE	About
HHCO	Have husband call office	RES	Residence
HSB	Husband	S	She (or wife)
HTO	He telephoned office	SEP	Separated
HU	Hung up	SK*	Skip or skipped
INS	Insurance	SOS	Same old story
L1, L2	Letter one, letter two (sent)	SP/DEL*	Special delivery
LB	Line busy	STO	She telephoned office
LD	Long distance	T	Telephoned
LM	Left message	TB	Telephoned business
LMCO	Left message, call office	TR	Telephoned residence
LMVM	Left message, voice mail	TT	Talked to
LTR	Letter	TTA	Turned to agency
MR	Mail return	UE	Unemployed
N1, N2	Note one, note two (sent)	U/Emp	Unemployed
NA	No answer	UTC	Unable to contact
N/B*	Nearby or neighbors (no phone listing)	VFD	Verified
NFA*	No forwarding address	Vfd/E	Verified employment
NHD*	Never heard of debtor	Vfd/I	Verified insurance
NI	Not in	W/	Will
NLE	No longer employed	WCO	Will call office
NPL	No phone listed	WCIO	Will come in office
NPN	Nonpublished number	W/I	Walk-in
NR	No record	WVO	Will visit office
NSF	Not sufficient funds	X	By

*Used in skip tracing.
†Directories used to locate patients by street address or telephone number.

Collection Abbreviations

Collection abbreviations can be used to save time and space while documenting efforts to collect and patients' responses. A few of the most common abbreviations are listed in Table 10.2. Always use standard abbreviations so anyone working on the account will know exactly what attempts have been made to collect and what action has been taken. Figure 10–16 illustrates some abbreviated collection entries, with interpretations, on the back of a financial accounting record.

Insurance Collection

Most patients carry some form of insurance; however, filing an insurance claim is only the first step in collecting fees owed. Good follow-up techniques (see Chapter 9) are necessary to ensure payment from the insurance carrier and copayment or coinsurance payment from the patient.

First, affirm that a clean insurance claim was sent with all necessary precertification, preauthorization, and documentation for services. Next, follow up in a timely manner with telephone calls and written tracers. Track all denials to learn what services are being denied and which insurance companies are denying payment. It is worth investing money and staff resources to identify the cause of claim denials. Send all high-dollar claims by certified mail to alleviate the problem of the insurance company saying that "it was never received." This saves time and is cost effective.

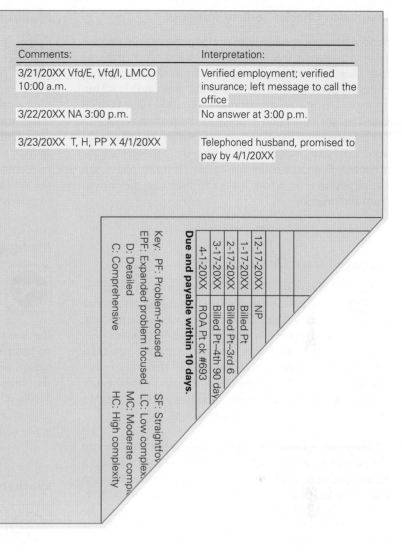

Comments:	Interpretation:
3/21/20XX Vfd/E, Vfd/I, LMCO 10:00 a.m.	Verified employment; verified insurance; left message to call the office
3/22/20XX NA 3:00 p.m.	No answer at 3:00 p.m.
3/23/20XX T, H, PP X 4/1/20XX	Telephoned husband, promised to pay by 4/1/20XX

Due and payable within 10 days.	
12-17-20XX	NP
1-17-20XX	Billed Pt
2-17-20XX	Billed Pt
3-17-20XX	Billed Pt-3rd 6
4-1-20XX	Billed Pt-4th 90 day
	ROA Pt ck #693

Key: PF: Problem-focused SF: Straightfo[rward]
EPF: Expanded problem focused LC: Low complex[ity]
D: Detailed MC: Moderate compl[exity]
C: Comprehensive HC: High complexity

FIGURE 10–16 The back of a financial accounting record (ledger card) that shows examples of abbreviated collection entries with interpretation.

History of Accounts

If the insurance company seems to be ignoring all efforts to trace the claim, an exact history of the account may be the best weapon with which to proceed. A history of the account is a chronologic record of all events that have occurred. Keep all communications received from the insurance company, note all telephone calls, and keep copies of all documents sent. Send a copy of the history of the account directly to the insurance company and demand a reply. This may also be done in the case of an insurance company dispute or a refusal to pay.

Coinsurance Payments

Use a letter or statement to collect from patients who have insurance coverage. Clearly indicate to the patient that the insurance biller has submitted an insurance claim and advise the patient what action is expected. The status of the insurance claim should be noted on all statements. Notify patients promptly when insurance payment has been received. Ask patients to get involved in the insurance process or to pay the bill within 10 days if a problem exists. Following are examples of notations on statements for patients with insurance coverage:

● "We have received payment from your insurance company. The balance of $_____ is now your responsibility."
● "Your insurance company has paid its share of your bill. This statement is for the amount payable directly by you."
● "Your insurance company has paid $_____ for the above services. The remaining portion of $_____ is now your responsibility."
● "The balance of this account is your share of the cost. Please remit today. For questions, call 486-9002."
● "Your insurance company has not responded. The account is due and payable. Please contact your insurance company about payment. Thank you for your assistance."

Insurance Checks Sent to Patients

Send a letter immediately to notify patients who receive insurance checks (see Chapter 9). Advise such patients that they have received payment from their insurance company and that their account is due and payable within 10 days. Do not send continuous monthly bills; instead speed up the collection process. If the patient refuses to pay and the physician does not want the patient to return, send a 10-day notification advising the patient that the account will go to a collection agency; if no response, ask the physician if he or she wishes to discharge the patient from the practice.

Managed Care Organizations

 When a medical practice deals with several managed care organizations, trying to remember all the contract information can be confusing. A managed care desk reference (see Chapter 11) can help staff members find information quickly. "Promised payment date" along with all the other information on the desk reference grid or matrix can be easily referred to by the insurance specialist when trying to collect from managed care organizations.

Make sure all referral authorizations are in place before the patient is to be seen. If a patient shows up without a referral, offer to reschedule or inform the patient that the visit must be paid for in cash before leaving the office. If the patient has no money, a promissory note may be executed, but this action is not preferred and would be carried out as a last option.

When dealing with managed care contracts, do not sign any contract that holds a third party "harmless." The "hold harmless" clause is a way for one party to shift financial responsibilities to another party. Such "hold harmless" clauses often include phrases that state that the third party is "held harmless" to pay claims, liabilities, costs, expenses, judgments, or damages awarded by any court to all patients who bring any legal action against the medical practice. If the third party goes out of business or goes bankrupt before the contract is honored, the physician cannot collect any money from the patient that the third party was to have paid. To avoid such possibilities, make sure payments from all managed care organizations are current.

Check to see that all third-party payers are insured by a federal agency. Such insurance would pay the physician in the event the managed care organization could not. Managed care bankruptcy is discussed in Chapter 11.

Medicare

 A provider must make genuine collection efforts to collect the unpaid deductible and coinsurance amounts from all Medicare patients. Reasonable efforts must include subsequent billings, telephone calls, and in-person collection efforts done in the same manner as with all patients. Accounts may not be written off until sequential statements (spaced 15 to 30 days apart) have been sent with an increasing intensity in the collection message. A telephone call should be placed to the debtor asking for payment, as well as requesting payment when the patient is seen in person.

Medigap Insurance

 When a patient has Medigap insurance, make sure the patient's signature appears in Block 13 of the CMS-1500 insurance claim form. Do not routinely enter "signature on file" unless the insured has signed an insurance-specific statement authorizing assignment of benefits to the physician named on the claim form. A signed statement allowing the physician to bill for and receive payment for Medigap-covered services until the beneficiary revokes authorization is preferred. A Medicare "signature on file" is not sufficient.

Workers' Compensation

Verify the validity of work-related injury and illness through the patient's employer and obtain accurate billing information. Send timely bills and reports using the correct coding system and fee schedule. Always keep the adjuster assigned to the case informed of ongoing treatment. The patient and employer should both be notified if a problem exists. Document all correspondence, including telephone authorizations for treatment and any tracing efforts. Any disputed or unresolved workers' compensation cases may be revised to self-pay, or be referred to a Financial Service Representative or the proper state-level authority. The physician may file for mediation on behalf of the patient if proper authorization was obtained and a claim form sent at the time of the patient's treatment. A claim also may be filed with the state labor board naming the patient's employer and workers' compensation carrier whenever there is difficulty getting full payment. The industrial board has the employer pressure the carrier to resolve the matter. If an insurance company has not paid or has sent a written notice of nonpayment, the provider may file a request for default judgment from the state authority. If the judgment is in the provider's favor, the payer is ordered to pay in full. See Chapter 15 for more information on delinquent workers' compensation claims.

Suing an Insurance Carrier

As stated under Statute of Limitations, there are time periods during which an insured person may sue the insurance company to collect the amount the claimant believes is owed. An insured person may not initiate a legal action against the insurer until 60 days after the initial claim has been submitted. A lawsuit against the insurer must be filed within 3 years of the date the initial claim was submitted for payment.

When the insurance company does not respond to reason or negotiation after the physician's office has tried to collect from an insurance plan, the only alternatives are surrender or litigation. A lawsuit may be worthwhile if a high-dollar claim is in question. Insurance carriers may be sued for payment under two circumstances: claim for plan benefits or breach of contract and claim for damages.

Claim for plan benefits is used when the claim is governed by the Employee Retirement Income Security Act (ERISA), a Federal Employee Health Benefit Act (FEHBA). ERISA governs health insurance that is provided as a benefit of employment. FEHBA governs all health insurance provided as a benefit to federal employees. An insured person is entitled to appeal a denied claim under these two federal laws. A timely request must be filed to sue for payment. The time limit for ERISA is within 60 days of denial; for FEHBA the time limit is within 6 months. Federal laws apply across the country and overrule all state laws. Suits based on claims for plan benefits may be made when denial is based on the following:

● Medical necessity
● Preexisting condition
● Usual and customary rate issues
● Providers or facilities that are not covered
● Services that fall within an exclusion to coverage
● Failure to offer Consolidated Omnibus Budget Reconciliation Act (COBRA) coverage by a plan administrator

When the claim falls outside of the scope of these federal laws, it is possible to sue if the conduct of the payer constitutes a violation of state laws relating to unfair insurance practices.

Suing based on claim for damages falls entirely under state law. This is most likely to occur if the patient has no plan benefit but the patient or physician's office is led to believe so by the insurer or plan administrator. Examples may include the following:

● Insurer misquoting benefits during a verification of those benefits
● Denial of payment because of lack of medical necessity when preauthorization of treatment was obtained

Collection Agencies

Delinquent accounts should be turned over to a collection agency only after all reasonable attempts have been made to collect by the physician's office. Knowing when to turn accounts over helps determine the success of the collection agency. The longer the unpaid balance remains in the physician's office, the less chance the agency has to collect the account, so the determination that an account is uncollectable should be made quickly. Some guidelines follow:

● When a patient states that he or she will not pay or there is a denial of responsibility
● When a patient breaks a promise to pay
● When a patient makes partial payments and 60 days have lapsed without payment
● When a patient fails to respond to the physician's letters or telephone calls
● When payment terms fail for no valid reason
● When a check is returned by the bank because of insufficient funds and the patient does not make an effort to rectify the situation within 1 week of notification
● When delinquency coexists with marital problems, divorce proceedings, or child support agreements
● When a patient is paid by the insurance company and does not forward the payment to the physician (this constitutes fraud and may be pursued with legal action)
● When a patient gives false information
● When a patient moves and the office has used all resources to locate the patient

Not all accounts should go to a collection agency. Such accounts include those of personal friends, elderly widows or widowers living on pensions, and accounts with balances under $25. Many physicians prefer to adjust small bad debts off of the books rather than increase administrative costs. All disputed accounts should be reviewed and approved by the physician before they are sent to collection. There should be a systematized approach for turning accounts over to a collection agency that still allows room for exceptions.

Choosing an Agency

A collection agency should be chosen with great care because it is a reflection of the medical practice.

Choose a reputable agency that is considerate and efficient with a high standard of ethics. The agency should specialize in physician accounts and have an attitude toward debtors with which the physician agrees. Find out how long the agency has been in business and request a list of at least 10 references and statistics on their collection effectiveness. The average collection rate varies greatly but falls between 20% and 60% on assigned accounts. Be sure the report rate includes all accounts more than 1 year old and does not exclude accounts with small balances.

An agency's performance can be evaluated by the amount collected, less the agency's fees, which is called the **"netback."** For instance, if the collector recovered 25% of $5000 ($1250) and takes a 50% commission, the physician's netback is $625. If the collector recovered 25% of the $5000 ($1250) and charged a 30% commission, the netback is $375. Although the second agency collected less, its lower commission afforded the physician more money.

When choosing a collection agency, make sure (1) to set up a separate P.O. Box or Lock Box for the collection project; (2) to set up a separate bank account for the collection project; (3) that the contract stipulates that all correspondence is sent to the P.O. Box. (no correspondence is to be sent to the collection agency's physical or payment address); (4) that all e-checks and credit card receipts are deposited into the physician's bank account; and (5) that under no circumstance is the collection agency to receive any payments. If money goes to the collection agency (whether insured, bonded, registered, or licensed), there is nothing to stop the collection agency from stealing the physician's money. The collection agency also could have a hidden lawsuit against it or an income tax lien, and the physician may lose all of his or her money if the money goes to the agency's bank account. Do not put "hold harmless" clauses in contracts. Hold the collection agency responsible for its actions. Many states do not regulate collection agencies. Many simply require the collection agency to be registered. In addition to checking references, check with the state's Department of Corporations to determine whose name is on the collection agency's registration, if the tax identification number is correct and current, and if the address listed is different than the one the agency gave. Contact the circuit court to determine whether there are any lawsuits or judgments against the collection agency. Find out how many of the collection agency's employees will be assigned to the account, then monitor them once the contract is signed. They may have the best credentials and references and belong to all the correct organizations, but if they acquire an increasing number of accounts and the amount of recoupment remains constant each month or is less than the national average, they may be picking and choosing

the accounts. This is especially true when they are over-anxious to receive a new file. If this happens, consider looking for another collection agency. Make sure an account can be recalled without a penalty. The patient may have coverage with a carrier already contracted with, so find out if the collection agency has the ability to resend a claim or if the billing company or office staff handle this. If so, does the contract have provisions for this, and does the collection agency receive recoupment for obtaining insurance information?

The biggest key to the agency's effectiveness is the doctor's own credit and collection policy. A comprehensive patient registration form, along with verifying employment, turning accounts over quickly when they qualify, and giving the agency all the available information, helps the agency pick up the paper trail and secure payment. A good collection agency has membership in a national collection society and the approval of the local medical society. Review the agency's financial statement and make sure the agency is licensed, bonded, and carries "hold harmless clause" insurance. If a patient should sue because of harassment, this insurance will protect the physician from being sued as well. The local bar association and state licensing bureaus can be contacted to determine whether any complaints have been lodged against the agency or law firm. Find out if the agency reports uncollectable debtors ("deadbeats") to a credit bureau and investigate which one is used.

Types of Agencies

There are local, regional, and national agencies. National agencies and ones that use the Internet may have better results tracing skips (patients who owe balances on their accounts and move without leaving a forwarding address). Local agencies are more aware of the socioeconomic status of patients. Some agencies pay their staff commissions and bonuses for high productivity, and others are low-key and more customer-oriented. Find out the experience level of the staff and make sure the agency values the physician's business.

Another option is to use a collection service such as CollectNet, which gives small and mid-sized facilities with limited budgets the collection capabilities of large collection systems by connecting to databases. The medical practice is able to make calling lists, print collection letters, search for telephone numbers and addresses, access patient credit reports, write and format reports, monitor collection progress, and set automatic callback reminders. Optional features include BankruptcyNet, SkipNet, LetterNet, and BureauNet. Collection agencies use this service, but it is also available to large groups and clinics.

Agency Operating Techniques

Collection agencies must follow all the laws stated in the Fair Debt Collection Practices Act. They may not "harass" the debtor or make false threats, and they may not use letters that appear to be legal documents. A provision should be included for the agency to seek permission from the physician's office before suing a debtor in municipal court and charging a percent of the judgment. A progress report should be provided to the physician's office on a regular basis at least monthly. The agency also should return any uncollectable accounts to the physician's office within a reasonable time and not charge for these accounts. If a debtor moves, ask if the account is forwarded to another collection office. All procedures used to make collections should be shown to the physician's office, including collection letters and telephone script. The physician's office should be aware if the agency uses a personalized or standard approach. A personal visit to the premises of the collection agency can provide a first-hand view of its operating techniques.

Agency Charges

Agencies may be paid a flat rate on all accounts according to volume. Some agencies may leave the accounts in the control of the physician's office where the staff speaks with the patient and posts all delinquent incoming monies. Other agencies charge a commission based on a percentage of an account, and the physician's office refers all calls to the agency once the account is turned over to it. A standard rate for most agencies to break even is one third of all monies collected, and an average rate charged is 50%. Make sure the commission is based on how much is collected on the overdue accounts and not the total amount of overdue accounts turned over to the agency.

Agency Assigned Accounts

Patients' accounts turned over to a collection agency should have a letter of withdrawal sent by certified mail (see Figure 4–20). Place a note on all financial accounting records indicating the date the account was assigned. Once an account has been given to a collection agency, it is illegal to send the patient a monthly statement. Financial management consultants usually recommend that the patient's balances be written off of the A/R at the time the account is assigned. A portion of the account balance can be written back on if and when the agency collects on the debt. Accounts also should be listed in a separate journal to help track the effectiveness of the agency. Allow enough columns to show the future date, amount, and percentage of an account collected by the agency, as well as the total account balance.

Flag or insert a full sheet of brightly colored paper in the patient's chart noting the date the account was assigned to collection. This will alert all medical staff of the situation if the patient calls on short notice or walks in to be seen. If the patient sends payment to the physician's office after the account has been turned over to an agency, notify the collection agency immediately. Any calls about accounts that have gone to collection should be referred to the agency.

Credit Bureaus

Collection agencies also can offer the services of a credit bureau. Credit bureaus gather credit information from many sources and make it available for a fee to members of a credit bureau service. Credit reports can be issued on new patients enabling the physician's office to verify credit. The information may consist of the patient's residence and moving habits (a measure of permanency), number of dependents, verification of employment and approximate salary, the patient's payment history on other merchant accounts, and any history of bankruptcy or use of an alias. This report can be obtained over the telephone or provided in written form.

The Fair Credit Reporting Act of 1971 allows a person to see and correct his or her credit report. The credit report can be checked for negative credit information, disputed information, mistakes, and out-of-date information. If credit is denied based in whole or in part on an adverse credit report, a letter should be sent advising the patient the name and address of the agency and stating that credit has been denied because credit requirements have not been met. The insurance specialist need not reveal data or specify the exact nature of the information obtained from the credit bureau but must name the bureau. A copy of the letter should be kept in the patient's file.

Credit Counseling

A consumer credit counseling service is a nonprofit agency that assists people in paying off their debts. The insurance specialist may have to refer patients for this service if continued medical care is being provided and the patient becomes overwhelmed by the cost. The patient may also contact his or her own bank or credit union, which may provide counseling at no charge. Care must be given with such referrals; use only legitimate agencies and warn patients that many private commercial debt consolidators may charge high fees. Dissatisfied patients may blame the physician or the insurance specialist if satisfactory financial arrangements are not made.

A patient seeking medical care who is unable to pay for services and is ineligible for state aid should be directed to the local hospital that services recipients under the Hill-Burton Act of 1946. These hospitals obtained federal construction grants to enlarge their facilities in exchange for their provision of health care for needy patients. The Department of Health and Human Services will furnish the names of local hospitals that participate in this service. Patients must complete financial applications to determine eligibility before care is rendered.

Small Claims Court

Small claims court is a part of our legal system that allows lay people to have access to a court system without the use of an attorney. Some advantages are a modest filing fee, minimal paperwork, exclusion of costly lawyers, and a short time frame from filing the action to trial date. Incorporated physicians usually must be represented by an attorney, and the agency must file in a municipal or justice court if an account has already been sent to a collection agency.

Most states have small claims courts (also called conciliation, common pleas, general sessions, justice courts, or people's court). Each state has monetary limits on the amount that can be handled in small claims court, and accounts should be reviewed for eligibility. The dollar amount varies from state to state and sometimes from one county to another. The national median small claims jurisdiction is $5000. There are several legislative bills being considered by U.S. Senate and House committees that address raising the dollar limit. Several states already have had such bills signed into law. The new limits in these states vary from $3000 to $25,000. There also may be limits on the number of claims filed per year that are more than a specific dollar amount.

When filing a claim, the person filing the petition (the physician's office) is referred to as the plaintiff and the party being brought to suit (the patient) is called the defendant. It is generally recommended that the plaintiff send a written demand to the defendant before filing a lawsuit to give the defendant a last opportunity to resolve the claim.

For step-by-step procedures on filing a claim, refer to the procedure at the end of this chapter.

After filing a claim, a trial date will be set, and both plaintiff and defendant will be ordered to appear before the judge. Often a postcard is sent notifying the plaintiff when the defendant has been served. If the amount of delinquent debt is more than the monetary limit for the small claims court, consider "cutting the claim to fit" the limit. For example, if the amount of a debt is $2757 and the state limit is $2500, consider waiving (giving up) the $257 (difference) to bring the amount down to the limit. The claim cannot be divided into two different suits of $1378.50, and one cannot sue twice on the same claim.

Claim Resolutions

The plaintiff has four options after he or she is served:

1. Pay the claim. The court clerk will receive the money and forward it to the physician's office, but the filing fee or service charges will not be refunded.
2. Ignore the claim. The judge may ask the physician's representative to state the physician's side, but the physician will win by default and the judgment will be awarded in the physician's favor, usually including court costs.
3. Answer the petition. A contested court hearing will be held. The plaintiff (physician) has the burden of proving his or her claim to the court. A counterclaim may be filed by the patient at this time.
4. Demand a jury trial. The case will be taken out of small claims court and the physician will be notified by the county clerk to file a formal complaint in a higher court. An attorney must represent the physician if this occurs.

Trial Preparation

The plaintiff and defendant must both appear on the trial date or the claim will be dismissed and cannot be refiled. Instead of attending the trial in person, the doctor may send a representative, such as his or her assistant or bookkeeper. If the claim is settled before trial, a dismissal form should be dated, signed, and filed with the clerk.

Preparation for the trial is essential and can mean the difference between success and failure. Decide what the judge should hear to conclude in the physician's favor. Although one cannot be represented in court by a lawyer, a lawyer can be asked for advice before going to court. Following are recommendations to help prepare for trial:

1. Be on time; otherwise the court may give a judgment in the defendant's favor.
2. Be ready to submit the basic data required by the court: the physician's name, address, and telephone number; the patient's name and address; the delinquent amount being claimed; and a brief summary of the claim.
3. Show all dates of service and amounts owed, the date the physician's bill was due (if a series of treatments is involved), the date of the last visit, the date of the last payment (if any payment was made), and the amount still unpaid.
4. Include all attempts to collect the debt and organize all exhibits in chronologic order. Include documentation

such as copies of statements, letters, notes, receipts, contracts, dishonored checks, telephone calls, other discussions with the patient, and other evidence to present to the court. A timeline showing the sequence of events may be useful.

5. Speak slowly and clearly, present the case in a concise manner, and use a businesslike approach. Answer all questions accurately but briefly.
6. Present a witness if live testimony is relevant. A notarized statement from a witness is admissible but not as effective.
7. Try to anticipate the opposing party's evidence and arguments so a rebuttal may be prepared. Keep in mind that a third party will be making the decision.

The judge will question the physician or representative and the patient, review the evidence, and then make a ruling. Winning the case gives the physician the right to attach a debtor's bank assets, salary, car, personal assets, or real property. The small claims office can show the assistant how to execute a judgment. Judgments usually are effective for many years. There is a small charge if the physician decides to execute against the patient's assets, but the charge is recoverable from the defendant.

A losing defendant may appeal and request a new trial in superior court. The defendant may ask the judge to make small installment payments, but not all judges will order this alternative. If the defendant fails to pay, a writ of execution may be obtained from the clerk's office to enforce judgment. This writ of execution permits the marshal to obtain funds from a losing party's bank account or take items of the losing party's property to satisfy the judgment.

Federal Wage Garnishment Laws

Federal wage garnishment laws provide a limit on the amount of employee earnings withheld in a work week or pay period when a debtor's future wage is seized to pay off a debt. It also protects the employee from being dismissed if his or her pay is garnished for only one debt regardless of the number of levies that must be made to collect. This law is enforced by the compliance officers of the Wage and Hour Office of the U.S. Department of Labor. The law does not apply to federal government employees, court-ordered support of any person, court orders in personal bankruptcy cases, or state or federal tax levies. The patient's employer becomes involved as the "trustee" because the employer owes money to the debtor for wages earned.

Once a **garnishment** has been ordered by the court, an employer has to honor it by satisfying the terms of garnishment before wages can be paid to the debtor.

Only a percentage of the wage (usually 25%) is garnished and paid to the creditor. This amount is determined from the employee's disposable earnings. Disposable earnings is the amount left after Social Security and federal, state, and local taxes are deducted. The statute resulting in the smaller garnishment applies when state garnishment laws conflict with federal laws. This method of collection should be considered a last resort for the medical office and used only with large bills.

Tracing a Skip

A patient who owes a balance on his or her account and moves but leaves no forwarding address is called a **skip.** In these cases an unopened envelope is returned to the office marked "Returned to Sender, Addressee Unknown." Instead, place the words "Forwarding Service Requested" below the doctor's return address on the envelope, and the post office will make a search and forward the mail to the new address. The physician's office will be informed of this new address for a nominal fee. Complete a Freedom of Information Act Form at the post office if the address is a rural delivery box number, and the United States Postal Service will provide the physical location of a person's residence. When patients send payments by mail, precautions must be taken to avoid discarding envelopes with a change of address. Always match the address on the envelope, along with the check, against the patient's account. One staff person should have the responsibility of updating all patients' addresses in all locations to prevent this problem.

Skip Tracing Techniques

Once it is determined that a patient is a skip, tracing should begin immediately. Office policies should be established stating how the skip should be traced, whether he or she is to be traced in the office, or at what point the account should be sent to a collection agency. Some offices choose to make only one attempt, whereas others prefer to do most of the detective work themselves. Box 10.2 lists techniques that can be used to initiate the search for the debtor.

Never state one's business with the patient when trying to make any of these contacts. Keep all information confidential. A good skip tracer must be patient and have the ability to pursue all necessary steps with tenacity and tact. A good imagination, a detective's instincts, and the ability to get along with people help in this tedious job.

Skip Tracing Services

There are several outside services from which to choose. Some agencies offer customized service with several levels

Box 10.2 Search Techniques Used to Trace a Debtor

1. Cross-check the address on the returned envelope with the patient registration form and account to ensure it was mailed correctly.
2. Check the ZIP code directory to determine whether the ZIP code corresponds with the patient's street address or post office box.
3. File a request with the local post office to obtain a new or corrected address.
4. Look in the local telephone directory. Call people with names that are spelled the same. Check directory assistance for a new or current listing.
5. Call the primary care physician for updated information when investigating for a physician specialist or any referring practice.
6. Determine whether the patient has been seen at the hospital; if so, speak to someone in the accounts department.
7. Inquire at the patient's place of employment. If the patient is no longer employed, ask to speak to the personnel department in an effort to locate the patient. Do not divulge the reason for the call.
8. Contact persons listed on the patient registration form, including personal referrals.
9. Request information from the Department of Motor Vehicles if a driver's license number is available.
10. Obtain information from street directories, city directories, and cross-index directories (available at many public libraries) for a new address or the names and telephone numbers of neighbors, relatives, or landlords.
11. Telephone the local moving company or moving rental service and ask for the patient's new address.
12. Request information from utility companies.
13. Inquire at the patient's bank to determine whether he or she is still a customer.
14. Obtain the services of a local credit bureau to check reports and receive notification if the patient's Social Security number shows up under a different name or at a new address.
15. Contact the Board of Education when the patient has children or is a student to find out the patient's school district and the school closest to his or her former residence. Request a forwarding address.
16. Call the police department if it is suspected that the patient may have a criminal record.
17. Check public records such as tax records, voter registration, court records, death and probate records, hunting and fishing licenses, and marriage licenses.

of skip tracing available. Each level is more extensive and costly. The physician's office decides at which level it would like the search conducted. The first level usually involves verifying the patient's information and checking for typographical errors. The highest level uses every resource available to find the patient. The age of the account, the account balance, and the cost of the level of skip tracing service are all considerations when deciding which level to choose. A collection agency or credit bureau (as mentioned) also may offer the services of skip tracing.

Search via Computer

Another method of skip tracing is to use electronic databases or online services. "Information wholesalers" also exist that cater to bill collectors and similar interested parties. Currently there are a number of bills pending in Congress aimed at restricting the flow of personal data in cyberspace. Perhaps in the future this information will not be so easy to obtain; however, conducting a successful electronic search is relatively easy at present. Following are several methods used to search electronic databases to locate a debtor's address and home telephone number.

- Surname scan. This can be done locally, regionally, or nationally based on data banks that have been compiled from public source documents.
- Address search. This provides property search and any change of address from all suppliers of data to the database, including the U.S. Postal Service. Names of other adults in the household also may be included who may have the debtor's telephone number listed under their name.
- Electronic directory. This allows access to the regional telephone operating company's screen of information.
- Credit holder search. This is used to establish occupation.
- Phone number search. This permits access to the names of other adults within the same household who have a telephone number.
- Neighbor search. This displays the names, addresses, and telephone numbers of the debtor's former neighbors.
- ZIP code search. This provides the names, addresses, and telephone numbers of everyone within that ZIP code who has the same last name as the debtor.
- City search. This locates everyone with the same last and first name within a given city, as well as all people who live in that city.
- State search. This finds all people with the same last name or same last and first name within the state and lists their addresses and telephone numbers.
- National search. This operates the same way as the state search. It is recommended for people with unusual last names.
- Business search. This lists all the names of the businesses in the neighborhood of the patient's last known residence. This search may help find where the patient has relocated or verify the patient's place of employment.

Refer to the end of the chapter for a listing of some of the larger directories used on the Internet and explore several directories to cross-check results because of frequent data change. Information is not secure when using the Internet. The patient's right to privacy must never be violated.

Special Collection Issues

Bankruptcy

Bankruptcy laws are federal laws applicable in all states that ensure equal distribution of the assets of an individual among the individual's creditors. There are two kinds of bankruptcy petitions: voluntary and involuntary. A voluntary petition is one filed by a person asking for relief under the Bankruptcy Reform Act (the Code). An involuntary petition is one filed against a person by his or her creditors requesting that a person obtain relief under the Code.

When a patient files for bankruptcy, he or she becomes a ward of the court and has its protection. The patient is granted an **automatic stay** against creditors, which means that the physician may contact patients only for the name, address, and telephone number of their attorney. The insurance specialist should no longer send statements, make telephone calls, or attempt to collect the account. A creditor can be fined for contempt of court if he or she continues to proceed against the debtor. If a collection agency has the account and has been notified of the bankruptcy, the situation is the same as if the physician has been notified. If the physician is notified first, the collection agency should be called and informed of the fact. Notification of bankruptcy does not have to be in writing; verbal communication is valid (e.g., if a patient telephones the doctor's office to inform him or her of the bankruptcy). Bankruptcy remains part of the debtor's permanent credit record for 10 years.

After a patient informs the physician's office of the bankruptcy, determine what type of bankruptcy the debtor has filed. Refer to Table 10.3 for a listing of the five types of bankruptcy cases.

Bankruptcy Rules

Under the bankruptcy rules, an unsecured creditor must file proof of claim in Chapter 7 or Chapter 13 bankruptcies within 90 days after the first date set for the meeting of creditors. When filing a claim, the proper form may be obtained from a stationery store or by writing to the presiding judge of the bankruptcy court. If a creditor fails to file a claim, the creditor will lose his or her right to any proceeds from the bankruptcy. A plan for payment will be approved by the court. The trustee may be contacted from time to time to check the status of the claim and the payments that should be expected. Once a patient has filed for bankruptcy there must be a time lapse of 6 years

Table 10.3	Types of Bankruptcy Cases
Chapter 7 Case	

This is sometimes called a *straight petition in bankruptcy* or *absolute bankruptcy*. In this case, all of the **nonexempt assets** of the bankrupt person are liquidated and are distributed according to the law to the creditors. Secured creditors are first in line for payment of all **secured debt.** Unsecured creditors are last. A person declares those to whom he or she owes money and is not required to make payment, thus eliminating all of the debtor's outstanding legal obligations for **unsecured debt.** Most medical bills are considered unsecured debt because they are not backed by any form of **collateral.** The only debt that is discharged in Chapter 7 bankruptcy is the debt that had been incurred up to the point of filing for protection	under Chapter 7. So, if a patient files before services are rendered, the bankruptcy laws do not apply for the treatment provided. A Chapter 7 bankruptcy does not necessarily result in the discharge of all debts. If the patient lies about his or her financial status, the debt may not be dischargeable. If the debt incurred was for a luxury service (e.g., facelift), immediately preceding the filing, it is possible that it may not be discharged. Consult the practice's attorney before adjusting the debt off the books in such a situation. All creditors are notified by the Administrator in Bankruptcy as to the proceedings and may choose either to attend the proceedings or make a claim against whatever assets remain.

Chapter 9 Case	**Chapter 12 Case**
This case is used for reorganization proceedings when a city or town is insolvent or unable to meet its debts. A plan is put into effect to adjust such debts.	This case is used for reorganization when a farmer is unable to meet his or her debts.

Chapter 11 Case	**Chapter 13 Case**
This case is used for reorganization of a business enterprise when the company is unable to meet its debts but would like to continue business and would be unable to do so if creditors took away its assets. A plan of arrangement is confirmed by the court, and each class of creditor must accept the plan or receive at least that which it would receive on liquidation of the company.	This is sometimes called a wage earner's bankruptcy. It is designed to protect the wage earner from creditors while allowing the wage earner to make arrangements to repay a portion of his or her bills (about 70%) over a 3- or 5-year period. The debtor pays a fixed amount agreed upon by the court to the trustee in bankruptcy. A claim needs to be filed as directed by the debtor's attorney.

before he or she can file again. The only exception to this is Chapter 13 bankruptcy.

Terminally Ill Patients

Although it may be difficult to collect from patients who are terminally ill, it is usually harder to collect from the estate after they have died. When a patient is too sick or scared to communicate necessary information, speak to family members and stress the need for help. Usually, terminally ill patients want to do the right thing. Call the patient before he or she comes in to receive service. Make sure the patient is aware of the existing balance and try to work with the patient to eliminate at least a portion of the balance before the next appointment. Estimate costs and prepare a plan that is agreeable to both the physician and the patient.

Estate Claims

Great care and sensitivity should be taken when trying to collect on a deceased patient's account. The entire probate system was set up to help protect families from painful involvement in estate settlements. Do not offend the deceased's family by making contact during the time of bereavement. However, a claim should be filed after the first or second week so the physician's name can be added to the list of creditors.

Refer to the procedure at the end of this chapter for filing an estate claim.

After filing, the claim is then denied or accepted. If accepted, an acknowledgment of the debt is sent to the physician's office. Many delays arise because of the legal complications of settling an estate, but the debts are paid according to a priority system when the estate is settled. Usually funeral expenses are paid first; following in order are estate administration expenses, claims due for the deceased person's last illness, and taxes and other debts. Any amounts left are divided among family members. A lien or lawsuit may be filed against the estate in the rare case of a rejection of the claim.

Various state time limits and statutes govern the filing of a claim against an estate. Check with the county court in your state to obtain filing deadlines. Deadlines may range from 2 months to 3 years but must be adhered to for successful collection from an estate.

Litigation

A difficult question arises when the physician is advised that a patient is involved in a pending litigation related to the services provided to the patient. It may not be necessary to wait until the litigation is resolved to pursue payment. Assess whether the patient has the ability to pay before possibly receiving a settlement in a lawsuit. Before withholding collection activity, the medical practice should get a guarantee that the physician will be paid in full before the patient (debtor) receives money out of a settlement. The agreement must be guaranteed by the lawyer representing the patient. If the patient is working, regular payments should be required pending the settlement of the patient's litigation. It is always advisable to contact a malpractice attorney in such cases.

Liens

A **lien** is a claim on the property of another as security for a debt. This may include a claim on a future settlement of a lawsuit. The physician may be asked to accept a lien by a patient or the patient's attorney when the patient has been involved in an automobile accident and is awaiting a settlement (Figure 10–17). In litigation cases, a lien is a legal promise to satisfy a debt owed by the patient to the physician out of any proceeds received on the case. See Chapter 15 for further details about industrial cases.

Patient Complaints

It is generally in the physician's best interest to resolve patient complaints and billing disputes quickly, accurately, and amicably. Always address collection complaints seriously. Listen to the patient with an open mind. Note specifically what the patient is saying and what the patient wants to do. Look beyond the complaint to determine what caused the problem. The source of the problem should be resolved, not just the result of the problem. A patient complaint form may be adapted to prompt staff to pay close attention to positive customer relations. This form may help screen poor collection techniques by staff members, pinpoint billing department problems, and identify policies and procedures that need improvement.

The patient may refuse to pay the physician if the patient's complaint is not addressed. Following are some guidelines to follow when a patient calls or writes a letter complaining about the physician or the medical practice:

1. Listen carefully (or read the letter carefully) and establish exactly what the patient complaint is and what the patient wants done about it.
2. Thank the person for calling (or writing); demonstrate appreciation of his or her input into the situation.
3. Apologize, regardless of whether the patient is right or wrong.

**REQUEST FOR ALLOWANCE OF LIEN
ASSIGNMENT AND AUTHORIZATION**

WHEREAS, I have a right or cause of action out of personal injury, to wit:

I, _____ hereby authorize _____ ,
    patient's name   physician's name

to furnish upon request, to my attorney, _____ , any and all medical records, or reports of examination, diagnosis, treatment, or prognosis but not necessarily limited to those items as set forth herein, in addition to an itemized statement of accounts for services rendered therefore or in connection therewith, which my attorney may from time to time request in connection with the injuries described above and sustained by me on the _____ day of _____ , 20XX.

I hereby irrevocably authorize and direct my said attorney set forth herein to pay to _____ all charges for attendance in court,
      patient's name

if required as an expert witness whether he testifies or not; reports or other data supplied by him; depositions given by said doctor; medical services rendered or drugs supplied; and any other responsible and customary charges incurred by my attorney as submitted by _____ and in
                                    physician's name

connection with said injury. Said payment or payments are to be made from any money or monies received by my attorney whether by judgment, decree, or settlement of this case, prior to disbursement to me and payment of the amount as herein directed shall be the same as if paid by me. This authorization to pay the aforementioned doctor shall constitute and be deemed as assignment of so much of my recovery I receive. It is agreed that nothing herein relieves me of the primary responsibility and obligation of paying my doctor for services rendered, and I shall at all times remain personally liable for such indebtedness unless released by the aforementioned doctor or by payment disbursed by my attorney. I accept the above assignment:

Dated: _____ Patient: _____

As the attorney of record for the above-named, I hereby agree to observe the terms of this agreement, and to withhold from any award in this case such sums as are required for the adequate protection of Dr. _____

Date: _____ Attorney: _____

FIGURE 10–17 A patient's authorization to release information to an attorney and grant lien to the physician against proceeds of settlement in connection with accident, industrial, or third-party litigation cases.

4. Answer the complaint. Explain what happened, if applicable, and state what is being done about it.
5. Use a professional and sincere approach. If the patient is wrong, state that the complaint is unjustified, but first explain your estimation of the situation and its resolution. Otherwise, he or she is likely to become quite upset. Do not be sarcastic, condescending, or insulting.
6. Take all complaints seriously. Do not respond in a lighthearted manner or use humor; it will only serve to upset the patient.
7. Respond in letter form. Whether the complaint has been received by telephone or by letter, take the time to write to answer the complaint. This indicates that the matter is not being taken lightly.
8. Be cordial and sincere. Express to the patient the hope of continuing a friendly relationship, but that payment is needed. Treat the patient with respect, good will, and sincere appreciation. Often kindness can turn a negative into a positive. The complaint can be turned into a payment.
9. Follow up after the complaint has been resolved by looking at the root of the problem and taking the necessary time to communicate this to the office manager. This will allow for a plan of action that will help prevent the same type of problem from recurring.

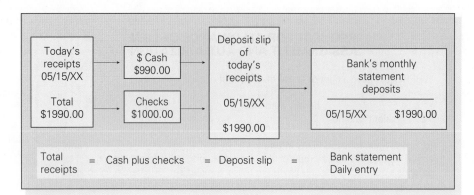

FIGURE 10–18   Explanation of an audit trail to review monies received by a medical practice and monies deposited into a bank account.

Collection Controls

All collections should be carefully controlled to prevent lost checks and embezzlement.

Embezzlement

Embezzlement means stealing money that has been entrusted in one's care. In many cases of insurance claims embezzlement, the physician is held as the guilty party and has to pay huge sums of money to the insurance carrier when false claims are submitted by an employee. If an undiscovered embezzler leaves the employer and you are hired to replace that person, you could be accused some months down the line of doing something that you did not do. Take precautions as an employee and to protect the medical practice.

Precautions for Financial Protection

To prevent the temptation to steal from a medical practice, these office policies should be routinely practiced. Ask the physician or supervisor to initial all entries about adjustments, discounts, and write-offs on either the ledger cards or day sheets. If a patient owes money to the physician that is uncollectable and adjusted off, be sure the physician dates and initials the ledger that shows the closed account. Ask the physician, an auditor, or an outside consultant to occasionally check an entire day's records (the patient sign-in log and appointment schedule) with the day sheet, ledger cards, encounter forms, and cash receipt slips. A daily trail balance of accounts receivable including daily deposit of checks and cash can assist in reviewing monthly income and aid in discovering embezzlement. Review the monthly bank statement to verify that all deposits tally with the receipts for each business day (Figure 10–18). If poor bookkeeping and record keeping are noticed, bring this to your employer's attention.

All insurance payment checks should be immediately stamped within the endorsement area on the back "For Deposit Only," called a *restrictive endorsement*. The bank should be given instructions never to cash a check made payable to the physician.

Encounter forms, transaction slips, and cash receipts should be prenumbered. If a mistake is made when completing one, void it and keep the slip as part of the financial records. It is especially imperative to have prenumbered insurance forms if the physician's practice allows the use of a signature stamp when submitting claims. Thus, filing of fictitious insurance claims can be totally eliminated.

As a precautionary measure, always type your initials at the bottom left or top right corner of the insurance claim forms that you submit. This will indicate to office personnel who did the work. Always retain the Explanation of Benefits or Remittance Advice documents that accompany checks from insurance companies.

Only a few of the many precautions for protection are mentioned here; embezzlement can occur in accounts receivable, accounts payable, with petty cash, use of computers, and in various other aspects of a medical practice.

Bonding

Insurance billers, claims assistance professionals, or anyone who handles checks or cash should be bonded or insured. A practice that carries a fidelity or *honesty bond* means that an insurance company will prosecute any guilty employees. **Bonding** is an insurance contract by which a bonding agency guarantees payment of a certain sum to a physician in case of a financial loss caused by an employee or some contingency over which the payee has no control. Bonding methods for a practice with three or more office employees follow:

- *Position-schedule bond* covers a designated job, such as a bookkeeper or nurse, rather than a named individual. If one employee in a category leaves, the replacement is automatically covered.

- *Blanket-position bond* provides coverage for all employees regardless of job title.
- *Personal bond* provides coverage for those who handle large sums of money. A thorough background investigation is required.

Such bonding contracts may be obtained from a casualty insurance agent or broker. Bond coverage should be reviewed periodically with the insurance agent to ensure that coverage is keeping pace with the expansion of the business.

PROCEDURE

SEVEN-STEP BILLING AND COLLECTION GUIDELINES

OBJECTIVE: To properly bill and collect payments for professional services rendered to patients.

EQUIPMENT/SUPPLIES: Patients' financial accounting statements, envelopes, calendar, and telephone.

DIRECTIONS: Follow these step-by-step procedures and guidelines, which include rationales, to learn this job skill.

1. Present the first statement at the time of service. This can be a formal statement or an encounter form (multipurpose billing form).
2. Mail the second itemized statement within 30 days of treatment. The phrase "due and payable within 10 days" should be printed on each statement. Local paycheck issuing patterns should be considered before selecting a date for statements to be mailed. Choose which billing routine the office will use:
   a. Monthly billing. Using the monthly billing system, all statements are mailed at the same time during the month. Choose a mail-out day at the beginning of the month so the patient will receive the bill near the 15th, or send statements near the end of the month, so the patient receives the bill on the 1st.
   b. Cycle billing. **Cycle billing** is a system of billing accounts at spaced intervals during the month based on a breakdown of accounts by alphabet, account number, insurance type, or date of first service. This relieves the pressure of having to get all the statements out at one time and allows collection at a faster, more organized rate than accounts collected at random. It also allows continuous cash flow throughout the month and distributes the influx of incoming calls from patients about problem accounts. The number of cycles may be determined

by how the collector wishes to divide the workload. Using two cycles per month, statements would be sent on the 25th to arrive by the 1st, and on the 10th to arrive by the 15th of the month. Using four cycles per month, statements should be sent every Tuesday or Wednesday to arrive at the end of the week. If a cycle that was established by the first date of service is used, and the patient was first seen on the 11th of the month, then every month on the 11th he or she should receive a bill.

3. Send the third statement 30 days after the second statement was sent. Indicate that the payment is past due.
4. If there is no response to the third statement, place the first telephone call to the patient depending on office policy (7 to 14 days). Ask if there is a problem. Ask for a payment commitment and set up a suspense file. Accounts are put in a suspense file for active follow-up. Action must be taken within the time frame mentioned, after the patient has been so advised.
5. Check for payment as promised. Allow 1 day for mail delay. Place the second telephone call to the patient and ask for payment. Set up a new payment date. Allow 5 days.
6. Check for payment as promised. Send a 10-day notice advising the patient that unless payment is received in 10 days, the account will be turned over for legal action.
7. Check for payment. Promptly surrender the account for collection or legal action. Figure 10-10 shows a collection decision tree to be used when determining when to send statements, 10-day notices, and accounts to a collection agency and when to make telephone calls.

PROCEDURE

TELEPHONE COLLECTION PLAN

OBJECTIVE: To obtain payment of a delinquent account balance due by making the first collection telephone call.

EQUIPMENT/SUPPLIES: Telephone, pen or pencil, patient's financial accounting record, computerized account, or collection telephone log.

DIRECTIONS: Follow these step-by-step procedures and guidelines, which include rationales, to learn this job skill.

1. Set the mood of the call by the manner of speech and tone of voice. The first 30 seconds of the call set the scene for the relationship with the patient. Follow the Fair Debt Collection Practices Act when making a telephone call.

2. State the name of the caller, the practice represented, and identify the patient. Be certain the debtor is being spoken to before revealing the nature of the call.

3. Identify oneself and the facility.

4. Verify the debtor's address and any telephone numbers.

5. State the reason for the call by asking for full payment and stating the total amount owed. Ask for payment courteously but firmly.

6. Take control of the conversation and establish urgency by asking for full payment now. Speak slowly in a low voice; staying calm and polite prevents quarreling.

7. Ask when payment will be made, how it will be made, and if it will be sent by mail or in person.

8. Pause for effect. This turns the conversation back to the patient to respond to the demand or explain why payment has not been made. Never assume that if a patient does not respond, it means no.

9. Find out if the patient needs clarification of the bill.

10. Inquire if the patient has a problem. Ask if the practice can be of assistance, especially when the patient is unable to give a reason for nonpayment.

11. If the patient is reluctant to agree to an amount, question him or her by asking one of the following: "How much are you willing to pay?" "Do you have a regular paycheck?" "Will payment be made through a checking account?"

12. Obtain a promise to pay with an agreeable amount and a due date; be clear how and when payment is

---

COLLEGE CLINIC
4567 Broad Avenue
Woodland Hills, XY 12345-0001
Tel. (555) 486-9002
FAX (555) 487-8976

October 2, 20XX

Mr. Leonard Blabalot
981 McCort Circle
Woodland Hills, XY 12345-0001

Dear Mr. Blabalot:

I am glad we had an opportunity to discuss your outstanding balance with our practice during our phone conversation on October 1, 20XX. This will confirm and remind you that you agreed to pay $100 on your account on or before October 15, 20XX.

A return envelope is enclosed for your convenience.

Sincerely,

Charlotte Rose Routingham
Business Office

Enc. envelope

FIGURE 10–19 Telephone confirmation letter sent to remind patient of the payment terms agreed to in a telephone conversation.

PROCEDURE—CONT'D

expected, but give the patient a choice of action. Set immediate deadlines for payment.

13. Ask for half of the amount if full payment is not possible.

14. Discuss a payment plan if the patient is not able to pay half of the balance owed. Be realistic and reasonable. It is self-defeating to set up payment arrangements the patient cannot afford. Advise the patient that the entire balance will become due and payable if the payment is even 1 day late. Ask the patient to please call before the due date with an explanation if any problems arise to prevent payment.

15. Restate the importance of the agreement.

16. Tell the patient to write down the amount and due date.

17. Document the agreement on the patient's financial accounting record by inserting the date of the call and abbreviated notations, in the computer system, or in a collection telephone log. Note the time the patient was spoken to.

18. Send confirmation of the agreement (Figure 10–19) as a follow-up to the telephone call.

19. Check the account the day after the payment was due; allow 1 day for mail delay. If the patient fails to make payment as promised, make another telephone call and ask the patient if there is still a problem. Get a new commitment to pay and confirm again. If the patient continues to avoid payment, advise the patient that the account will be turned over to a collection agency and follow through as stated.

PROCEDURE

CREATE A FINANCIAL AGREEMENT WITH A PATIENT

OBJECTIVE: To assist the patient in making credit arrangements by completing and signing a Truth in Lending form.

EQUIPMENT/SUPPLIES: Patient's financial accounting record (ledger), calendar, Truth in Lending form, typewriter or computer, calculator, and quiet private room.

DIRECTIONS: Follow the step-by-step procedures that include rationale to learn this job skill. An assignment is presented in the *Workbook* to practice this skill.

1. Explain the patient's balance due and answer questions about credit.

2. Inform the patient of the medical practice's office policy about extending credit payments.

3. Discuss an installment plan concerning the amount of the total debt, the downpayment, amount and date of each installment, and the date of final payment.

4. Subtract the down payment from the total debt. Decide the remaining amount by the number of months the debt is being carried to determine the monthly installment amounts and date of final payment.

5. Complete a Truth in Lending form after mutually agreeing on the terms if the payments require more than four installments. This procedure complies with Regulation Z.

6. Review the completed Truth in Lending form with the patient.

7. Ask the patient to sign the Truth in Lending form.

8. Make a photocopy of the form for the patient to retain.

9. File the original Truth in Lending form in the patient's financial files in the office.

PROCEDURE

FILE A CLAIM IN SMALL CLAIMS

OBJECTIVE: To file a claim to obtain payment for a delinquent or uncollectable financial account in small claims court.

EQUIPMENT/SUPPLIES: Small claims court filing form, photocopy of the patient's financial accounting record, computer or typewriter, pen or pencil, envelope, and check for filing fee.

DIRECTIONS: Follow these step-by-step procedures and guidelines, which include rationales, to learn this job skill.

1. Obtain a Claim of Plaintiff or Plaintiffs Original Petition form to notify the patient that action is being filed. This can be obtained from the clerk's office located at the municipal or justice court. Obtain booklets and material to help guide the claimant through the process.

2. Complete and file the papers with the small claims court; make sure to have the patient's correct name and street address.

3. Make a photocopy of the small claims court form for the office files.

Continued

PROCEDURE—CONT'D

FILE A CLAIM IN SMALL CLAIMS

4. Pay the clerk the small filing fee. Filing fees vary by state, by county within some states, and by the amount of the claim.

5. Make arrangements to serve the defendant. The summons or citation can be served on the patient by a sheriff or court-appointed officer by paying a small fee plus mileage for the constable who serves it. The person serving the defendant must fill out a proof of service form.

6. After being served, a patient has one of four options:
   a. *Pay the claim*—to the court clerk. This will be forwarded to the physician but the filing fee or service charge will not be refunded.
   b. *Ignore the claim*—the physician will win by default. In some states, a judgment may be requested in writing, but in other states the physician or the medical assistant must appear on a specified date. If the patient does not appear, the judgment is granted in the physician's favor and usually court costs are included in the judgment.
   c. *Request a small claims hearing*—the court clerk will let both parties know when to appear. The patient may file a counterclaim against the physician at this time.
   d. *Demand a jury trial*—the case will be taken out of small claims court. The physician will be notified by the court clerk to file a formal complaint in a higher court, and an attorney must represent the physician.

7. Appear in court (physician or the medical assistant) on the specified date; claim will be dismissed and cannot be refiled.

8. Basic information required by the court follows:
   a. Physician's name, address, and telephone number
   b. Patient's name and address
   c. Delinquent amount
   d. Summary of the claim including the date the physician's bill was due, date of the last visit, date of the last payment, unpaid amount, and all records of telephone contacts and letters sent.

9. Determine what the judge needs to hear to decide a favorable case. Good preparation for the trial can make the difference between success or failure.

10. Organize all the exhibits in a notebook, in chronologic order. A time-line showing the sequence of events can be useful.

11. Take a businesslike professional approach at the hearing by giving concise and accurate answers to the judge's questions, speaking slowly and clearly. The physician or assistant must bring any witnesses, statements, receipts, contracts, notes, dishonored checks, or other evidence to court. The judge will question the medical assistant or physician and the patient, review the evidence, and then make a ruling.

12. Put a lien on the debtor's wages, automobile, bank or personal assets, or real property if the judgment, which is usually effective for many years, is in the physician's favor. This is the physician's legal right. The small claims office will show the medical assistant or physician how to execute a judgment.

13. Pay a small fee if the physician decides to execute against the patient's assets. It is recoverable from the patient.

PROCEDURE

FILE AN ESTATE CLAIM

OBJECTIVE: To file a claim on an estate for a deceased patient who has an outstanding balance on his or her financial accounting record.

EQUIPMENT/SUPPLIES: Statement of Claim form, computer or typewriter, pen or pencil, photocopy machine, patient's financial accounting record, USPS certified mail forms, and envelope.

DIRECTIONS: Follow these step-by-step procedures and guidelines, which include rationales, to learn this job skill.

1. Confirm the date and place of death with the hospital, nursing home, or funeral home.

2. Pursue payment from all third-party payers first.

3. Contact the Register of Wills' office in the county where the patient lived or the probate department of the superior court, County Recorder's Office. Request a Statement of Claim form or the county's proper document to formally register a claim against an estate.

4. File the claim according to the instructions received with the claim form. When probate is filed, a notification will be sent advising the court of probate, the attorney representing the estate, and the **estate executor** or **estate administrator.** Perhaps a small fee should be included for court costs.

5. Send a photocopy of the patient's financial accounting record (itemized statement) by certified mail, return receipt, to the attorney and copies to the executor and the court. If the physician treated the deceased patient's last illness, that fact should be clearly indicated on the statement.

6. Allow the legal system to take its course. A call to the executor can be made periodically to check on the status of the estate.

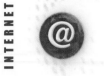

RESOURCES

INTERNET

Web sites to help you search for a debtor:

- Anywho
  Web site: **www.anywho.com**

- Bigfoot
  Web site: **www.bigfoot.com/**

- InfoSpace
  Web site: **www.infospace.com**

- Info USA
  Web site: **www.infousa.com**

- SearchBug
  Web site: **www.searchbug.com**

- Switchboard
  Web site: **www.switchboard.com**

- WhoWhere?
  Web site: **www.whowhere.com/**

- Yahoo People Search
  Web site: **www.yahoo.com/search/people/**

- 411Locate
  Web site: **www.411locate.com**

- Web site for small claims court
  Web site: **http://www.small-claims-courts.com**

- Fair and Accurate Credit Transactions (FACT) Act
  Web site: **www.hipaadvisory.com/news/2004/0216fact.htm**

- State statutes that correspond to Articles of the Uniform Commercial Code.
  Web site: **http://www.law.cornell.edu/uniform/ucc.html**

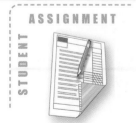

ASSIGNMENT

STUDENT

✓ Study Chapter 10.

✓ Answer the review questions in the *Workbook* to reinforce the theory learned in this chapter and to help prepare you for a future test.

✓ Complete the assignment in the *Workbook* to give you hands-on experience in selecting a dun message, posting a courtesy adjustment and insurance or patient payment, composing a collection letter, and completing a credit card voucher and a financial agreement.

✓ Turn to the glossary at the end of this textbook for a further understanding of the key terms used in the chapter.

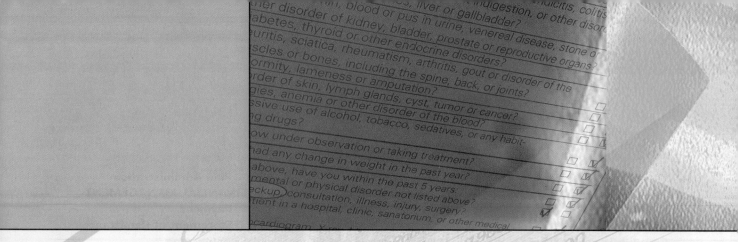

Health Care Payers

CHAPTER OUTLINE

PRIVATE INSURANCE
  Blue Cross and Blue Shield
    Plans
MANAGED CARE
  Prepaid Group Practice Health
    Plans
  Benefits
  Health Care Reform
MANAGED CARE SYSTEMS
  Health Maintenance
    Organizations
  Exclusive Provider
    Organizations
  Foundations for Medical Care
  Independent Practice
    Associations

  Preferred Provider
    Organizations
  Physician Provider Groups
  Point-of-Service Plans
  Triple-Option Health Plans
MEDICAL REVIEW
  Quality Improvement
    Organization
  Utilization Review of
    Management
MANAGEMENT OF PLANS
  Contracts
  Preauthorization of Prior
    Approval
  Diagnostic Tests
  Managed Care Guide

  Plan Administration
FINANCIAL MANAGEMENT
  Payment
  Statement of Remittance
  Accounting
  Fee-for-Service
  Year-End Evaluation
  Bankruptcy
CONCLUSION

KEY TERMS

ancillary services

buffing

capitation

carve outs

churning

claims-review type of foundation

closed panel program

comprehensive type of foundation

copayment (copay)

deductible

direct referral

disenrollment

exclusive provider organization
  (EPO)

fee-for-service

formal referral

foundation for medical care
  (FMC)

gatekeeper

health maintenance organization
  (HMO)

in-area

independent (or individual)
  practice association (IPA)

managed care organizations
  (MCOs)

participating physician

per capita

physician provider group (PPG)

point-of-service (POS) plan

preferred provider organization
  (PPO)

prepaid group practice model

primary care physician (PCP)

self-referral

service area

staff model

stop loss

tertiary care

turfing

utilization review (UR)

verbal referral

withhold

11

The Blue Plans, Private Insurance, and Managed Care Plans

OBJECTIVES*

After reading this chapter, you should be able to:

- Define a prepaid health plan (PHP).
- Identify types of managed care health plans.
- List two types and two different functions of foundations.
- State the provisions of the Health Maintenance Organization Act of 1973.
- Explain health maintenance organization (HMO) benefits and eligibility requirements.
- State reasons for a quality improvement organization.
- Define independent practice associations.
- Name the elements of preferred provider organizations (PPOs).
- Identify four types of authorizations for medical services, tests, and procedures.

*Performance objectives and exercises for hands-on practical experience for this chapter appear in the *Workbook*.

Service

Carefully follow guidelines for each managed care contract in regard to preauthorization for certain tests and services, hospital admissions, inpatient or outpatient surgeries, elective procedures, or when the patient must be seen by someone other than the primary care physician. If authorization is obtained in a timely manner, the patient's health care will not be delayed and payment will be forthcoming.

PRIVATE INSURANCE

Numerous private insurance companies across the United States offer health insurance to individuals and groups. Most offer a variety of managed care plans. This chapter describes the difference between private insurance and managed care. Fee-for-service reimbursement was discussed in previous chapters. This chapter explains managed care capitation as a form of reimbursement.

Blue Cross and Blue Shield Plans

Blue Cross/Blue Shield plans are pioneers in private insurance and had a nonprofit status that made them unique among all private insurance carriers for many years. Blue Cross/Blue Shield is the largest insurance company in the United States. Each plan is independently owned and operated in each state but work together in a network similar to a spider web. Originally, Blue Cross plans were developed to cover hospital expenses and Blue Shield plans were primarily established to cover physician services. Today different plans have been developed that allow members to seek treatment from Blue Cross/Blue Shield providers anywhere in the United States. There are so many different plans that it is difficult for the medical biller to know which type the member is enrolled in. However, the patient's identification card is important and very helpful in obtaining the correct information needed for billing purposes. The patient may have a traditional plan or a managed care plan (e.g., preferred provider organization [PPO], point-of-service [POS plan], independent [or individual] practice association [IPA], health maintenance organization [HMO], or Medicare HMO). Plans are different and may have diverse names in each state (e.g., Premera in Alaska and Washington state; Care First in Maryland, northern Virginia, Washington, D.C., and Delaware; and Horizon in New Jersey). This chapter describes these managed care systems.

Nationally the Blue Cross/Blue Shield Association is a single corporation administering the rules and regulations for the regional plans to follow. The regional plans process claims for members who have plan coverage for hospital expenses, outpatient care, other institutional services, home care, dental benefits, and vision care. Most of the affiliated organizations have converted to for-profit status and operate in much the same way as other private insurance carriers. In some areas, Blue Cross and Blue Shield are separate organizations, and in some situations they may compete against each other. They have plans that are similar to other private insurance companies and they do not have standardized claim form guidelines. In addition, Blue Cross/Blue Shield may act as a Medicare fiscal intermediary in certain regions. An experienced medical biller should be aware of the many problems these circumstances cause. For example, the policy number may require the claim to be sent to the home plan, or the policy number may require the claim to be sent through the provider's state carrier. Blue Cross/Blue Shield realizes this is a problem, so the organization is developing a product called Blue Plan that incorporates all products. The intent is to help the patient avoid making payments.

There are other unique situations with Blue Cross/Blue Shield in regard to contracts. Blue Cross/Blue Shield would like to have contracts with both medical groups and the providers that work for the group. This poses unique problems when the group and provider are contracted, when the group is contracted and the provider is not, and when there is no contract with either the provider or group. Each situation has a different effect on claims processing and payment. A provider must be individually contracted with Blue Cross/Blue Shield to receive reimbursement as a member physician. Deductibles and copayments vary according to the patient's plan.

Because Blue Cross/Blue Shield contracts are like other types of private and managed care plans, in this textbook the organization is not listed separately in the description of types of fee structures, network physicians, managed care plans, and guidelines for completing the CMS-1500 insurance claim form or electronic claims processing. A medical practice should have available for reference, current provider manual for their state's Blue Cross/Blue Shield plans.

MANAGED CARE

Until the early 1970s, most health insurance was delivered through traditional fee-for-service plans. This scenario has changed from indemnity plans to managed health care plans, such as HMOs. In this chapter, the health care reforms of the past and present are defined and explained. In addition to HMOs, other types of prepaid group practice models that use a managed care approach and are operated by **managed care organizations (MCOs)** are discussed.

In prepaid group plans, patients join the plan and pay monthly medical insurance premiums individually or through their employer. The physician renders service to the patient, and the patient usually pays a small copayment and occasionally a deductible as required by the plan. Providers that join the plan are paid using the capitation method. **Capitation** is a system of payment used by managed care plans in which physicians and hospitals are paid a fixed per capita amount for each patient enrolled over a stated period of time, regardless of the type and number of services provided.

Prepaid Group Practice Health Plans

The *Ross-Loos Medical Group* in Los Angeles was America's oldest privately owned prepaid medical group. It was founded in 1929 by Drs. Donald E. Ross and H. Clifford Loos and existed only in southern California, where it expanded to 17 medical group locations. In 1975 the Ross-Loos Medical Group formed a corporation and received a federal grant to develop a health care system under the federal Health Maintenance Organization Act of 1973. In 1980, INA Healthplan, Inc., of Philadelphia merged with Ross-Loos. Ross-Loos is now known as *CIGNA Healthplans of California*.

Most CIGNA patients are served under a prepayment group plan by which they pay a monthly premium and receive hospital, surgical, and professional benefits from a CIGNA staff physician or CIGNA Health Care Center. Several thousand other CIGNA patients are private and are treated on a fee-for-service basis. In the case of an emergency when the patient is outside the area of a CIGNA Health Care Center, he or she may seek professional or hospital care in other facilities, but CIGNA must be notified as soon as possible. A dental plan and Medicare supplemental plan also are available through CIGNA.

Another pioneer of the prepaid group practice concept is the *Kaiser Permanente Medical Care Program*. It began in 1933 when Dr. Sidney R. Garfield and a few physicians working for him gave combined industrial accident and personal medical care to approximately 5000 workers building a fresh-water aqueduct across the California desert to Los Angeles. Dr. Garfield charged the insurance carriers $1.50 per man per month and the workers 5 cents a day. In return he provided comprehensive health care. Then in 1938, Henry J. Kaiser and his son Edgar started a joint venture to complete the Grand Coulee Dam in Washington and invited Dr. Garfield to form a medical group to furnish care to the workers for 7 cents a day prepaid by the employer. The group expanded to include the workers' wives and children.

Kaiser Permanente now has centers in 12 regions covering 16 states. Patients are served under a prepayment group plan and receive hospital, surgical, and professional benefits from physicians located at the Kaiser Permanente Medical Care Centers. In most regions, the Kaiser Permanente Medical Plan is a **closed panel program** composed of multispecialty physicians, and the plan limits the patient's choice of personal physicians to those practicing in one of the 12 geographic regions.

In January 1994, Kaiser Permanente announced a venture with Pacific Mutual Life Insurance Company to give Kaiser's 4.6 million California patients a less cost-effective option of using physicians and medical facilities outside the vast Kaiser network. This was the first time that Kaiser allowed certain member groups of its two California health maintenance organizations to seek medical help from non-Kaiser physicians and is termed a POS option (see discussion later in this chapter). In this option, Kaiser pays up to a specified amount and the patient pays the rest, depending on the contract. Kaiser does not provide care on a fee-for-service or cost reimbursement basis.

In emergency situations when patients cannot reach a Kaiser Center, they may seek the services of outside facilities or physicians. They are transferred to a Kaiser facility when their condition stabilizes.

Health Maintenance Organization Act of 1973

An HMO is a prepaid group practice that can be sponsored and operated by the government, medical schools, clinics, foundations, hospitals, employers, labor unions, community or consumer groups, insurance companies, hospital medical plans, or the Veterans Administration.

In 1973, Congress passed the Health Maintenance Organization Act of 1973 (Public Law 93-222), creating authority for the federal government to assist HMO development in a number of ways, including (1) providing grants, loans, and loan guarantees to offset the initial operating deficits of new HMOs that meet federal standards (e.g., are federally qualified) and (2) requiring most employers to offer an HMO to their employees as an alternative to traditional health insurance.

Accreditation

The National Committee for Quality Assurance (NCQA) is a not-for-profit organization that accredits HMOs, including traditional staff and group model HMOs, network and IPA model HMOs, mixed models, and open-ended HMOs. NCQA developed HEDIS (Health Plan Employer Data Information Set), which is a set of data reporting standards that compares performance between plans. For further information, go to the Web site listed in Internet Resources at the end of this chapter.

Eligibility

Those who have voluntarily enrolled in an HMO plan from a specific geographic area (**in-area** or **service area**) or who are covered by an employer who has paid an established sum per person to be covered by the plan are eligible. The law states that an employer employing 25 or more persons may offer the services of an HMO as an alternative health treatment plan for employees. Medicare and Medicaid beneficiaries also may become members of managed care plans whether retired or employed. The federal government reimburses the HMOs on a **per capita** basis, depending on the size of the enrollment. This means that the HMO is paid a fixed per capita amount (also known as capitation) for each patient served without considering the actual number or nature of services provided to each person.

To qualify as an HMO, an organization must present proof of its ability to provide comprehensive health care. To retain eligibility, an HMO must render periodic performance reports to the offices of the Department of Health and Human Services. Thus accurate and complete medical records are imperative to the survival and cost control of an HMO.

Primary Care Physician

Most managed care plans use a **primary care physician (PCP)** as a gatekeeper. A **gatekeeper** is a physician who controls patient access to specialists and diagnostic testing services. PCPs usually are physicians who practice in the fields of internal medicine, family practice, general practice, or pediatrics. Although obstetrics/gynecology is considered specialty care, the obstetrician/gynecologist may be contracted as a PCP, and when not, it is common for MCOs to allow self-referral by members to obstetricians/gynecologists for certain services (e.g., Pap smears).

Identification Card

Each enrollee of a managed care plan is given an identification card as shown in Figure 3–11. The card usually lists the patient's name, member number, group number, and primary care physician's name. The name of the MCO and type of plan with the amount of copayment for various outpatient services (e.g., office visit, emergency department, urgent care center, and pharmacy) may be included by some plans.

Both sides of the patient's card should be photocopied because the insurance address, telephone numbers used for inquiries and authorizations, or other important information may be listed on the front or back of the card.

Benefits

Benefits under the HMO Act fall under two categories: basic and supplemental health service, which are listed in Box 11.1.

Box 11.1 | **Health Maintenance Organization Act Benefits of 1973**

BASIC HEALTH SERVICES

Alcohol, drug abuse, and addiction medical treatment
Dental services (preventive) for children younger than age 12 years
Diagnostic laboratory, x-ray, and therapeutic radiology services
Emergency health services in or out of the HMO service area
Family planning and infertility services
Health education and medical social services
Home health services
Hospital services (inpatient and outpatient)
Mental health services on an outpatient basis, short-term (not to exceed 20 visits) ambulatory, evaluative, and crisis intervention
Physicians' services and consultant or referral services without time or cost limits
Preventive health services (e.g., physical examinations for adults, vision and hearing tests for children through age 17 years, well-baby care, immunizations, health education)

SUPPLEMENTAL HEALTH SERVICES

Dental care not included in basic benefits
Extended mental health services not included in basic benefits
Eye examinations for adults
Intermediate and long-term care (nursing facilities and nursing homes)
Prescription drugs
Rehabilitative services and long-term physical medicine (e.g., physical therapy)

Health Care Reform

Over the past 70 years, leaders of the United States, from President Roosevelt to President Bush, have announced reforms of the health care system. Medical practices have made transitions from rural to urban, generalist to specialist, solo to group practice, and fee-for-service to capitation, and have expanded to a number of health care delivery systems that try to manage the cost of health care. Before capitation, **fee-for-service** was the usual method of billing by physicians in private practice. A professional service was rendered by the physician to the patient, and the physician made a separate charge for each service and expected to receive a fee for each service provided. Early insurance contracts were indemnity plans. They paid a flat fee for covered services and the patient paid the full balance. There were no participating agreements with physicians or hospitals.

A major restructuring of the United States health care system was needed during the 1990s for the following reasons:

● A growing percentage of Americans were not covered by private or government insurance.

- Employers had to pay escalating health care premiums and did not want to cut wages to cover these costs.
- Government needed to reduce the deficit by keeping down increases in the Medicare and Medicaid programs.
- Physicians and hospital costs soared with no end in sight because of inflation, high-tech equipment, expensive medications, and so on.
- Patients spent more and more money for less and less care and coped with a system riddled with inefficiency and fraud.
- Services were being overused by patients.

Integrated health care delivery systems have been formed in many states in the past decade to reduce costs. These have included MCOs, physician–hospital organizations, and group practices accepting a variety of MCOs and fee-for-service patients. These systems allow for better negotiations for contracts with large employers and managed care plans, as well as with medical and office suppliers for discounts. Each type of organization differs in ownership, purpose, governance, management, and type of services provided. Even before the government released its health care reform proposal, some states began establishing laws implementing managed care for the general populations, as well as for Medicaid patients and those injured on the job (workers' compensation cases). Hawaii has had a statewide universal health insurance plan since 1974. Many regions have large groups of Medicare-eligible people who have opted to belong to an HMO or other prepaid plans.

In 1994, California put together the first working alliance in the nation, followed by Florida's voluntary purchasing group, the Community Health Purchasing Alliances. In California the alliance is formally known as the Health Insurance Plan of California. This allows firms with 5 to 50 workers to offer their employees a wide choice of different insurance programs. All plans must offer the same benefits, but some physicians and hospitals are more desirable than others. The company must pay an amount equal to at least half of the cost of the lowest priced plan; the worker pays the remainder.

In the future, those on Medicaid, younger than age 65 years and not receiving either Temporary Assistance to Needy Families (TANF), formerly known as Aid to Families with Dependent Children (AFDC), or Supplemental Security Income (SSI) may no longer be part of Medicaid. They might obtain their health benefits like everyone else. TANF and SSI recipients would be covered under a Medicaid plan, but Medicaid would pay a capitated premium (payment per capita) to the alliance. The recipient would pick a low-cost plan from the state alliance. Some states have pilot projects in certain communities to determine whether this is feasible for the entire state.

MANAGED CARE SYSTEMS

Health Maintenance Organizations

The oldest of all the prepaid health plans is the **health maintenance organization (HMO).** An HMO is a plan or program by which specified health services are rendered by participating physicians to an enrolled group of persons. Fixed periodic payments are made in advance to providers of services **(participating physicians)** by or on behalf of each person or family. If a health insurance carrier administers and manages the HMO, it contracts to pay in advance for the full range of health services to which the insured is entitled under the terms of the health insurance contract.

HMO Models

There are important differences in the structure of various HMOs that influence the way physicians practice and, perhaps, the quality of medical care delivered. Following are several types of HMO models.

Prepaid Group Practice Model

The **prepaid group practice model** delivers services at one or more locations through a group of physicians who contract with the HMO to provide care or through its own physicians who are employees of the HMO. For example, Kaiser Permanente is a prepaid group practice model wherein physicians form an independent group (Permanente) and contract with a health plan (Kaiser) to provide medical treatment to members enrolled by the plan. Although the physicians work for a salary, it is paid by their own independent group, not by the administrators of the health plan. This is designed to permit the physicians to concentrate on medicine.

Staff Model

The **staff model** is a type of HMO in which the health plan hires physicians directly and pays them a salary instead of contracting with a medical group.

Network HMO

A *network HMO* contracts with two or more group practices to provide health services. It is common for those physicians to see patients in their own offices, seeing both HMO and non-HMO patients. Network physicians are typically paid a capitation amount for the care of each HMO patient in their panel of patients, regardless of whether or not the patient is actually seen by the physician in any given month.

Direct Contract Model

A common type of model in open-panel HMOs is the *direct contract model*. This type of managed care health plan contracts directly with private practice physicians in the community rather than through an intermediary such as an IPA or a medical group. Contracted health care services are delivered to subscribers by individual physicians in the community.

Write to the Office of Health Maintenance Organizations for further information on HMOs.*

Exclusive Provider Organizations

An **exclusive provider organization (EPO)** is a type of managed care plan that combines features of HMOs (e.g., enrolled population, limited provider panel, gatekeepers, utilization management, capitated provider reimbursement, authorization system) and PPOs (e.g., flexible benefit design, negotiated fees, and fee-for-service payments). It is referred to as exclusive because employers agree not to contract with any other plan. The member must choose medical care from network providers with certain exceptions for emergency or out-of-area services. If a patient decides to seek care outside the network, generally he or she is not reimbursed for the cost of the treatment. Technically, many HMOs can be considered EPOs. However, EPOs are regulated under insurance statutes rather than federal and state HMO regulations.

Foundations for Medical Care

A **foundation for medical care (FMC)** is an organization of physicians sponsored by a state or local medical association concerned with the development and delivery of medical services and the cost of health care. The first foundation for medical care was established in 1954 in Stockton, California. Foundations have sprung up across the United States, and some comprehensive foundations have assumed a portion of the underwriting risk for a defined population. Foundations deal primarily with various groups—employer groups, government groups, and county and city employees. Some plans are open to individual subscribers, but these instances usually represent a small percentage of the foundation activity.

There are basically two types of foundations for medical care operations and each functions differently: (1) a **comprehensive type of foundation,** which designs and sponsors prepaid health programs or sets minimum benefits of coverage, and (2) a **claims-review type of foundation,** which provides evaluation of the quality and efficiency of services by a panel of physicians to the numerous fiscal agents or carriers involved in its area, including the ones processing Medicare and Medicaid. Reviews are done for services or fees that exceed local community guidelines.

A key feature of the foundation is its dedication to an incentive reimbursement system. For a participating physician, income is received in direct proportion to the number of medical services delivered (e.g., fee-for-service) rather than payment through capitation. The FMC offers a managed care plan fee schedule to be used by member physicians. In some areas, foundation physicians agree to accept the foundation allowance as payment in full for covered services. The patient is *not* billed for the balance. However, the patient is billed for nonbenefit items, a deductible, and coinsurance.

The patient may select any member or nonmember physician he or she wishes. Member physicians agree to bill the foundation directly, and a nonmember physician may wish to collect directly from the patient. Many foundations submit claims on the CMS-1500 form, and others transmit data electronically. The foundation movement has a national society, the American Managed Care and Review Association (AMCRA),* which can provide further information on AMCRA or foundations in an individual state.

Independent Practice Associations

Another type of MCO is the **independent (or individual) practice association (IPA),** in which the physicians are not employees and are not paid salaries. Instead they are paid for their services on a capitation or fee-for-service basis out of a fund drawn from the premiums collected from the subscriber, union, or corporation by an organization that markets the health plan. A discount of up to 30% is withheld to cover costs of operating the IPA. IPA physicians make contractual arrangements to treat HMO members out of their own offices. A participating physician may also treat non-HMO patients.

Preferred Provider Organizations

A **PPO** is another type of managed care plan. A PPO contracts with a group of providers (designated as "preferred") to deliver care to members. PPO members have the freedom to choose any physician or hospital for services, but they receive a high level of benefits if the preferred providers are used. There are usually coinsurance requirements and deductibles, and claims have to be filed. Occasionally the PPOs pay 100% of the cost of care but most do not. As with major medical policies,

---

*Centers for Medicaid and Medicare Services, Room 4350, Cohen Building, 330 Independence Ave, SW, Washington, DC 20201.

*1227 25th St., NW, #610, Washington, DC 20037 (formerly known as the American Association of Foundations for Medical Care).

coinsurance requires the patient to pay 20% to 25% of the allowed amount up to a certain point and then the PPO pays 80% to 100% of the balance. Predetermination of benefits may be required, as well as fee limits, quality control, and utilization review. Some hospital indemnity plans pay fixed fees for various services. The patient pays the difference if the charges are higher.

Silent Preferred Provider Organizations

Sometimes preferred provider payers and plan administrators purchase existing preferred provider networks without talking to those providers who have signed contracts. These may be referred to as either silent, blind, or phantom PPOs, discounted indemnity plans, nondirected PPOs, or wraparound PPOs. They gain the ability to limit reimbursement (lower or discount payments) without the provider's knowledge or consent. Providers that are taken in by silent PPOs are unable to get paid out-of-network, which reduces their income. Silent PPOs complicate the appeal process because it may be difficult to contact another payer directly and may lose claims because of timely filing laws. Silent PPOs are considered legitimate in most states. Whenever you see "network discount applied" on an explanation of benefits document, investigate further into the claim to determine whether a silent PPO is operating. To discover silent PPOs, always precertify procedures and look at patients' insurance cards even if the patients are established.

Physician Provider Groups

A **physician provider group (PPG)** is a physician-owned business entity that has the flexibility to deal with all forms of contract medicine and still offer its own packages to business groups, unions, and the general public. One division may function as an IPA under contract to an HMO. Another section may act as the broker or provider in a PPO that contracts with hospitals, as well as other physicians, to market services or medical supplies to employers and other third parties. Still another portion might participate in joint ventures with hospitals, freestanding imaging centers and laboratories, purchase of diagnostic equipment, retail medical equipment as a corporate subsidiary, and so on. The sideline businesses do not pay dividends but provide income to make future assessments to participating physicians unnecessary. The difference between an IPA and a PPG is that an IPA may not be owned by its member physicians, whereas a PPG is physician owned.

The ability of the PPGs to combine services (joint purchasing, marketing, billing, collections, attorneys, and accountant fees) is an advantage because it cuts down on the cost of running a business and allows each physician to retain his or her own practice in addition to these joint ventures. The physicians turn over a small percentage of their income to the PPG for expenses. Patients call one telephone number to make appointments, and the billing is done in one location.

Point-of-Service Plans

The typical **point-of-service (POS) plan** combines elements of an HMO and a PPO while offering some unique features. It is basically an HMO consisting of a network of physicians and hospitals that provides an insurance company or an employer with discounts on its services. In a POS program, members choose a primary care physician who manages specialty care and referrals. A POS plan allows the covered individual to choose service from a participating or nonparticipating provider, with different benefit levels. The POS program pays members a higher level of benefits when they use program (network) providers. The member may use providers outside the network, but higher deductibles and coinsurance percentages for out-of-network services give members incentives to stay within the network.

The POS plan may also provide nonparticipating benefits through a supplemental major medical policy. The key advantage of POS programs is the combination of HMO-style cost management and PPO-style freedom of choice.

Triple-Option Health Plans

This type of plan allows members to select from three choices: HMOs, PPOs, or "traditional" indemnity insurance. Some of these plans allow the employee to change plans more often than traditional arrangements. They incorporate cost containment measures, such as precertification for hospital admission, hospital stays, and second surgical opinions.

Table 11.1 gives an overview or summary of five of the most common types of managed care plans.

MEDICAL REVIEW

Quality Improvement Organization

A *Quality Improvement Organization (QIO)* program (formerly known as *professional* or *peer review organization*), contracts with CMS to review medical necessity, reasonableness, appropriateness, and completeness and adequacy of inpatient hospital care for which additional payment is sought under the outlier provisions of the Prospective Payment System. Generally it operates at the

Table 11.1 Managed Care Plans

Plan	Network		Copay Deductible	Payment Method	Authorization Required
	In	Out			
HMO (health maintenance organization)	X		Fixed copay	Capitated Fee-for-service (carve outs)	X
PPO (preferred provider organization)	75/25% 80/20% 90/10%	60/40% 70/30%	Fixed copay Deductible	Fee-for-service	X
IPA (independent practice association)	Limit Large group		Fixed copay	Capitated Fee-for-service (carve outs)	X
EPO (exclusive provider organization)	X		Fixed copay	Fee-for-service Capitated	X
POS (point-of-service)	X	X	Fixed copay Deductible	Fee-for-service Capitated	X

state level. A review addresses whether the services met professionally recognized standards of health care and may include whether the appropriate services were provided in appropriate settings. The QIO's professional medical staff performs these reviews. The results of the reviews are submitted to CMS. A review is an evaluation of the quality and efficiency of services rendered by a practicing physician or physicians within the specialty group. Practitioners in a managed care program may come under peer review by a QIO. A review may be used to examine evidence for admission and discharge of a hospital patient and to settle disputes over fees (see Figure 9–4 and Chapter 17). QIOs are not restricted to MCO programs but also play a role in Medicare inpatient cases.

Quality Improvement System for Managed Care

Quality Improvement System for Managed Care (QISMC) is a CMS initiative to strengthen managed care organization efforts to protect and improve the health and satisfaction of Medicare and Medicaid beneficiaries. QISMC adopts a very broad definition of "quality" to include the "measurement of health outcomes, consumer satisfaction, accountability of managed care organizations for achieving ongoing quality improvement, the need for intervention to achieve this improvement, and the importance of data collection, analysis, and reporting."

Utilization Review of Management

A management system called **utilization review (UR)** is necessary to control costs in a managed care setting. UR is a formal assessment of the cost and use of components of the health care system. The utilization review committee reviews individual cases to determine medical necessity for medical tests and procedures. It also watches over how providers use medical care resources. If medical care, tests, or procedures are denied, the patient must be informed of the need for the denied service and the risks of not having it. The written reasons for denial let the patient know his or her rights to receive the service and obligation to pay before obtaining such services.

Emphasis is placed on seeing a high volume of patients in a performance-based reimbursement system. **Churning** is when a physician sees a patient more than medically necessary and is done to increase revenue through an increased number of services. Churning may be seen in fee-for-service as well as some managed care environments. **Turfing** is to transfer the sickest, high-cost patients to other physicians so the provider appears to be a low utilizer. **Buffing** is to make this practice look justifiable to the plan. All of these situations may affect utilization review.

MANAGEMENT OF PLANS

Contracts

Obtain nationwide data from Medirisk, Inc.,* to make a knowledgeable financial decision on how a managed care plan will impact an existing medical practice. Data supplied by this company can be used to evaluate existing fees, negotiate with managed care firms, and weigh practice expansions (e.g., add partners or a satellite office). A physician should have the contract reviewed by an attorney before signing a contract with a managed care plan.

_____

*5901 Peachtree Dunwoody Rd, NE, Suite 455, Building B, Atlanta, GA 30328.

Carve Outs

When an MCO contracts with a physician group, several important considerations are as follows:

1. How many patients will the MCO provide?
2. What is the per capita rate (capitation amount per patient)?
3. What services are included in the capitated amount?

Medical services not included in the contract benefits are called **carve outs** (not included within the capitation rate) and may be contracted for separately. For example, if an internist contracts with an MCO, all evaluation and management services, as well as electrocardiograms, spirometries, hematocrits, fasting blood sugar tests, and urinalyses, might be included in the capitation amount that is received per person, per month, regardless of whether any of these services were rendered. However, sigmoidoscopies and hospital visits might be "carved out" of the contract and paid on a fee-for-service basis. Generally physicians prefer carve outs for expensive procedures when contracting with MCOs.

Preauthorization or Prior Approval

Some managed care plans require preauthorization for certain services or referral of a patient to see a specialist. The following are several types of referrals that a plan may use.

1. **Formal referral.** An authorization request is required by the MCO contract to determine medical necessity. This may be obtained via telephone or a completed authorization form mailed or transmitted via fax (Figure 11–1) or email.
2. **Direct referral.** An authorization request form is completed and signed by the physician and handed to the patient. Certain services may not require completion of a form and may be directly referred (e.g., obstetric care, dermatology).
3. **Verbal referral.** Primary care physician informs the patient and telephones the referring physician that the patient is being referred for an appointment.
4. **Self-referral.** The patient refers himself or herself to a specialist. The patient may be required to inform the primary care physician.

Patients may be unaware of preapproval requirements. A good precaution is to ask the patient about insurance coverage at the time the appointment is made. If the patient is a member of a managed care plan, carefully review the patient's preauthorization requirements. If approval is necessary for certain situations, inform the patient of this before he or she sees the physician. If a patient has obtained the written authorization approval, remind him or her to bring the form at the time of the scheduled visit. Even if preapproved, *the treatment must be medically*

necessary or payment may be denied after submission of a claim. If an authorization is delayed and the patient comes in for the appointment, the plan should be called to obtain a verbal authorization. The date, time, and name of the authorizing person should be documented; otherwise the patient's appointment may have to be rescheduled. A referral recommendation must be documented in the patient's record and, if applicable, sent to the referring physician.

A tracking system such as a referral tracking log should be in place for pending referrals so care may be rendered in a timely manner and patients do not get "lost" in the system (Figure 11–2). This log should include the date the authorization is requested, patient's name, procedure or consultant requested, insurance plan, dates of follow-up, name of person who approved or denied the request, and appointment date for consult or procedure. Sometimes authorization approvals are sent to the primary care physician and not to the referring or ordering physician. In these cases, follow-up must be made with the primary care physician. A maximum 2-week turnaround time should be allowed and all authorization requests should be tracked.

If a managed care plan refuses to authorize payment for a recommended treatment, tests, or procedures, have the primary care physician send a letter to the plan that is worded similarly to that shown in Figure 11–3. Then send a letter such as that shown in Figure 11–4 to the patient informing him or her of this fact and asking the patient to appeal the denial of benefits.

In some managed care plans, when a primary care physician sends a patient to a specialist for consultation who is not in the managed care plan, the specialist bills the primary care physician. This is done because the primary care physician receives a monthly capitation check from the plan and any care for the patient must come from the capitation pool. This type of plan encourages primary care physicians not to refer patients so he or she can retain profits.

If a specialist recommends referral to another specialist **(tertiary care),** be sure the recommendation is in writing. Call the specialist at a later date to determine whether the recommendation was acted upon. If the patient refuses to be referred, be sure this is documented. If a referral form is necessary, *do not* telephone or write a letter. The managed care plan may refuse payment if the proper form is not completed.

When a referral authorization form is received, make a copy of the form for each approved office visit, laboratory test, or series of treatments. Then use the form as a reference to bill for the service. All copies being used

College Clinic
4567 Broad Avenue, WH
Telephone No.: (555) 486-9002
Fax No.: (555) 487-8976

MANAGED CARE PLAN AUTHORIZATION REQUEST

☐ Health Net   ☐ Met Life
☒ Pacificare   ☐ Travelers
☐ Secure Horizons   ☐ Pru Care
☐ Other

Member/Group No.: 54098XX

**TO BE COMPLETED BY PRIMARY CARE PHYSICIAN
OR OUTSIDE PROVIDER**

Patient Name: Louann Campbell   Date: 7-14-20XX

☐ Male   ☐ Female   Birthdate: 4-7-1952   Home Telephone Number: (555) 450-1666

Address: 2516 Encina Avenue, Woodland Hills, XY 12345-0439

Primary Care Physician: Gerald Practon, MD   Provider ID #: TC 14021

Referring Physician: Gerald Practon, MD   Provider ID #: TC 14021

Referred to: Raymond Skeleton, MD   Office Telephone number: (555) 486-9002

Address: 4567 Broad Avenue, Woodland Hills, XY 12345

Diagnosis Code: 724.2   Diagnosis Low back pain

Diagnosis Code: 722.10   Diagnosis Sciatica

Treatment Plan: Orthopedic consultation and evaluation of lumbar spine; R/O herniated disc L4-5

Authorization requested for: ☐ Consult only   ☐ Treatment only   ☐ Consult/Treatment

☐ Consult/Procedure/Surgery   ☐ Diagnostic Tests

Procedure Code: 99244   Description: New patient consultation

Procedure Code: _____   Description: _____

Place of service: ☒ Office ☐ Outpatient ☐ Inpatient ☐ Other   Number of Visits: 1

Facility: _____   Length of Stay: _____

List of potential future consultants (i.e., anesthetists, surgical assistants, or medical/surgical):

Physician's Signature: *Gerald Practon, MD*

TO BE COMPLETED BY PRIMARY CARE PHYSICIAN

PCP Recommendations: See above   PCP Initials: *GP*

Date eligibility checked: 7-14-20XX   Effective Date: 1-15-20XX

TO BE COMPLETED BY UTILIZATION MANAGEMENT

Authorized: _____ Auth. No. _____ Not Authorized _____

Deferred: _____   Modified: _____

Comments: _____

FIGURE 11–1 A managed care plan treatment authorization request form completed by a primary care physician for preauthorization of a professional service.

AUTHORIZATION REQUEST LOG

Date requested	Patient name	Procedure/ consult	Insurance plan	1st F/U	2nd F/U	3rd F/U	Approved	Scheduled date
2/8/XX	Juan Percy	Bone scan- full body	Health Net	2/20			J. Smith	2/23/XX
2/8/XX	Nathan Takai	MRI-L-knee	Pru-Care	2/20	3/3			
2/9/XX	Lori Smythe	Consult Neuro G. Frankel MD	FHP	2/22			T. Hope	2/26/XX
2/10/XX	Bob Mason	Cervical collar	Secure Horizons	2/22	3/5	3/19		

FIGURE 11–2 An authorization request log to be used as a system for tracing referral of patients for diagnostic testing, procedures, and consultations.

Ms. Jane Smith
Chairperson
Utilization Review Committee
ABC Managed Care Plan
111 Main Street
Anytown, XY 12345-0122

Dear Ms. Smith:

On _____ I prescribed_____ for_____ .
     Date   List treatment, test, procedure   Patient's name

On _____ you refused to authorize for that treatment. I find that I
     Date
must take issue with your determination for the following reasons:

In my medical judgment, the treatment is a very important part of my overall care of_____
_____ . This patient suffers from _____ . The treatment is
Patient's name   Describe condition
necessary to _____ . Failure to perform the treatment could
       Describe why necessary
result in the following problem(s):

For these reasons, I urge you to reconsider your refusal to authorize payment for the
procedure I have prescribed.

By copy of this letter to_____ I am reiterating my suggestion that
           Patient's name
he/she obtain the treatment despite your refusal to authorize payment, for the reasons I
have set forth in this letter and in prior discussions with _____ .
                     Patient's name
Yours truly,

John Doe, MD

cc: (Name of patient)

FIGURE 11–3 A letter to a managed care plan when there is a refusal to authorize payment for a recommended treatment, test, or procedure.

Mr. Avery Johnson
130 Sylvia Street
Anytown, XY 12345-0022

Dear Mr. Johnson:

On _____ I prescribed _____ for you. On _____ ,
     Date   Treatment, test, procedure   Date

_____ refused to authorize for same. On that basis,
   Name of Managed Care Plan
you have informed me of your decision to forego the treatment I have prescribed. I
expressed my concerns regarding your decision during our discussion on _____ about
                                                               Date

the potential ramifications of your refusal to undergo the treatment.

The purpose of this letter is to recommend that you appeal_____
                                           Name of Managed Care Plan's
denial of benefits and reconsider your decision to forego the treatment in light of the
potential consequences of your refusal.

Should you wish to discuss this further, please do not hesitate to contact me.

Sincerely yours,

John Doe, MD

FIGURE 11–4 A letter to inform the patient about refusal of payment for treatment, test, or procedure by the managed care plan.

indicates that all the services that the patient's plan has approved are completed. Ask the primary care physician or the managed care plan for a new authorization to continue treatment on the patient. The request should be generated in a timely manner so that treatment is not delayed.

Diagnostic Tests

Many managed care plans require that patients have laboratory and radiology tests performed at plan-specified facilities. These are referred to as *network facilities*. Obtain the necessary authorizations for such services and allow sufficient time to receive the test or x-ray results before the patient's return appointment.

Inform the patient ahead of time when there is doubt about coverage for a test or the managed care plan indicates a test is not covered. Disclose the cost and have the patient sign a waiver agreement to pay for the service, thus enabling the billing of the patient for the service. If an authorization is denied because a test is deemed "medically unnecessary" and the physician wishes to appeal, the physician can present clinical reasons to the MCO's medical director to receive approval and bring attention to possible expansion of benefits for future patients.

Managed Care Guide

To help you keep up with the growth of local managed care plans and remember which physician belongs to which plan in the practice, create a grid or matrix of all MCOs with which the practice has contracts. Use a sheet of paper and list each plan with billing address vertically in a column to the left; then list significant data horizontally across the top. Suggested titles for column categories are as follows: eligibility telephone numbers, copayment amounts, preauthorization requirements, restrictions on tests frequently ordered, participating laboratories, participating hospitals, and the contract's time limit for promised payment. Referring to this grid will provide specifics at a glance about each plan's coverage and copayment amounts (Figure 11–5).

Plan Administration

Patient Information Letter

Inform managed care subscribers in writing what is expected from them and what they can expect in turn. The patient information letter should outline possible restrictions, noncovered items, expectations for copayment, and names of the managed care plans in which the physician is currently participating. Note if the patient

MANAGED CARE PLAN REFERENCE GUIDE

Plan name/address	Telephone eligibility	Copay	Preauthorization requirements	Test restrictions	Contracted lab(s) radiology	Contracted hospital(s)	Promised payment
Aetna PPO POB 43 WH XY 12345	555-239-0067	$5	hosp/surg/all dx tests	PE 1/yr	ABC Labs	College Hosp	30 days
Blue PPO POB 24335 WH XY 12345	555-245-0899	$8	referral specialist	PE 1/yr	Main St. Lab	St. John MC	30 days
Health Net POB 54000 WH XY 12345	555-408-5466	$5	hosp/surg see check list referrals	Mammo- gram 1/yr	Valley Lab	St. Joseph MC	45 days
Travelers MCO POB 1200 WH XY 12345	555-435-9877	$10	surg/hosp admit referrals	Pap >50 q3yr <50 q1yr	College Hosp. Metro Lab	College Hosp	30 days

FIGURE 11–5 Managed care plan quick reference guide to help keep track of specifics for each managed care plan in which the physician participates.

neglects to notify the office of any change about eligibility status in the plan, such as **disenrollment;** the patient is then held personally responsible for the bill. Also mention that the managed care patient must inform the office if hospitalization, surgery, or referral to a specialist is necessary. State that because of restrictions, failure to do so will make the patient liable for denied services. This letter may be referred to as a waiver of liability and in the Medicare program is called an advance beneficiary notice (ABN). Post a sign in the waiting room advising managed care patients to check with the receptionist about participating plans.

Figure 11–6 is a sample letter of appropriate wording and content. File a copy of the letter given to the patient in the patient's medical record. Document in the medical record if the patient refuses to agree with managed care policy. Reimbursement may depend on the documentation.

RIGHT TO AUDIT RECORDS

When the patient is a member of a managed care organization (MCO) and the physician has signed a contract with the MCO that has a clause that states "for quality care purposes, the MCO has a right to access the medical records of their patients, and for utilization management purposes," the MCO has a right to audit those patients' financial records.

Medical Records

Medical record management may differ when handling multiple managed care contracts. Place colored adhesive dots on patient file folder labels or color-code managed care files by using a different colored chart for each EPO, HMO, IPA, and PPO patient. This decreases confusion and saves time in identifying individual plans so that coverage, copayment, billing, and authorization requirements are met.

Scheduling Appointments

Screen patients when they call for appointments to determine whether they belong to the same prepaid health plan as the physician. Ask the patient to read from the insurance card to determine whether the physician's name is listed as the patient's primary care physician. Keep on hand an alphabetical list and profile of all plans with which the practice has a signed contract. It might also be useful to have a list of plans to which the practice does not belong. If the patient is not in a participating plan and still wishes to schedule a visit, inform him or her that payment at the time of the appointment is necessary and the amount is determined by the private fee schedule. This is an excellent idea if the patient is not a member of an HMO. In some states, Florida for example, an HMO patient cannot be billed for services that are covered. The provider must obtain authorization to treat the patient if the person is an HMO patient and the provider is not a participating provider because collecting from the HMO patient could "backfire" on the provider. The patient will pay for the visit, then send a copy of the receipt to his or her HMO. The HMO could file a complaint with the appropriate HMO regulatory agency because the provider

XYZ MEDICAL GROUP, INC.
1400 Avon Road, Suite 200
Woodland Hills, XY 12345

January 1, 20XX

TO: OUR PATIENTS

RE: PREFERRED PROVIDER ORGANIZATIONS

The following is a list of the PPOs and health insurance plans that we are members of and, therefore, will bill for you:

1. Georgia County Foundation
2. VIP Health Plan
3. Blue Cross Prudent Buyer Plan
4. Georgia County PPO
5. Northwest PPO
6. Blue Shield PPO

We are participating providers in several different PPOs. In order that we may maintain proper records for referrals and/or hospitalization, we request that each patient who is enrolled in a specific PPO keep our office currently informed regarding his or her eligibility status in that plan. Each time you are in the office for a visit, please verify with the receptionist that we have the correct coverage information.

If you have not informed us of changes in the status of your eligibility within the plan, you will be held responsible for any outstanding balance on your account due to that change.

Additionally, when your physician feels it is necessary to either hospitalize you or refer you to another physician outside this group, it is your responsibility to inform your physician that you belong to a specific PPO, as there may be restrictions imposed by that PPO regarding admission and referrals. If you fail to inform your physician at the time of referral or admission, our group may not be held responsible for noncoverage charges due to these restrictions.

If you have any questions regarding the above, please ask to speak to our insurance specialist.

I have read and understand the above text.

Signed: _____ Date: _____
Patient (subscriber)

FIGURE 11–6 Letter to preferred provider organization subscribers outlining restrictions and noncovered services.

treated their client without authorization and billed their client for the balance. The HMO could request a claim form from the provider and the provider would enter his or her private fee, which is more than the provider billed the HMO for another patient. This would open the door to possible fraud and abuse charges. The HMO could contact the patient, stating it should not have had to pay for the visit because the patient was in an HMO. Finally, the patient could demand a refund, and the provider would have no choice but to refund the money because the patient could turn the provider over to the HMO regulatory agency. The assignment of benefits must be checked on the claim form either to the provider or the patient.

Encounter Form

Many managed care plans use an internal document on which the services rendered to the patient are checked off (charge ticket, encounter form, routing slip). It also may be used as a billing statement. The original is forwarded to the health plan's administrative office, and a copy is retained in the physician's files. Some plans require such documentation on a CMS-1500 Health Insurance Claim form. Examples of encounter forms are shown in Figures 3–15, 8–9, and 10–7.

FINANCIAL MANAGEMENT

Payment

Deductibles

Usually there is no **deductible** for a managed care plan. However, if there is one, be sure to ask patients if they have met their deductibles and collect them in the early months of the year (January through April).

Copayments

In a managed care plan, a **copayment** is a predetermined fee paid by the patient to the provider at the time service is rendered. It is commonly referred to as a *copay* and is a form of cost sharing because the managed care plan or insurance company pays the remaining cost. Always collect the copay at the time of the patient's office visit. Billing for small amounts is not cost effective. Copays are commonly made for office visits, prescription drugs, inpatient mental health services, urgent care visits, and emergency department visits. However, the amount may vary according to the type of service.

Payment Mechanisms

Payment mechanisms in managed care plans vary and can range from fee for service and capitation to salaried physicians. Following are some details about other payment mechanisms.

Contact Capitation

Contact capitation is based on the concept of paying physicians for actual patient visits or "contacts." A scenario under this payment method is when a patient is referred to a specialist for care. A "contact" occurs when the patient visits the specialist for treatment. The patient is assigned to the specialist for a defined period of time called the contact period. The length of the contact period is set in advance for each type of specialty by the participating specialty physician panel and MCO and may be tailored to the demographic and practice needs of the group. Each new patient visit during a contact period initiates a "contact point." Contact points determine how much to pay each physician. The average contact point value is determined by dividing the net specialty capitation pool or total amount of money set aside to be used for a particular specialty by the number of contacts in a certain time period. The average contact value is used to determine the amount paid to each specialist during each month in the contact period.

Case Rate Pricing

For specialists, another payment method is *case rate pricing*. This means the specialist contracts with the managed care plan for an entire episode of care. This may be done for certain high-volume, expensive surgical procedures (e.g., knee surgery, cataracts, and bypass surgery).

Stop-Loss Limit

Some contracts have a **"stop-loss"** section, which means that if the patient's services are more than a certain amount, the physician can begin asking the patient to pay (fee for service). Monitor each patient's financial accounting record in those instances.

Contract Payment Time Limits

Usually state laws dictate the time limit within which a managed care plan must pay. The contract may or may not state the terms of payment, time limits, and late payment penalties, all of which can vary from one plan to another. Prompt payment laws require payment within 30, 45, 55, or 60 days. To diminish late payment of claims, a contract can specify that late claims accrue interest (e.g., 5% interest for claims paid after the payment time limit has elapsed). Some states have enacted laws enforcing interest penalties for late payment for either or both private payers as well as managed care plans. Therefore know the laws for the pertinent state. A time limit payment provision is an important factor to consider when reviewing a contract before a medical practice participates.

Monitoring Payment

Monitor payments made from all managed care plans and note whether the payment received is less than the agreed amount as stated in the contract. If payment has been reduced, send a letter to the plan citing, "As per contract, see page xx about the fee for the consultation."

Sometimes a procedure (e.g., angioplasty with an assistant) may be done and the plan will not pay for an assistant, stating that it is not usual practice. However, perhaps the standard practice in a specific region is to always use an assistant for an angioplasty. When this is emphasized, the plan may remit additional payment.

Some states may have screening fees for emergency services and may or may not require prior approval for such services as defined by the Consolidated Omnibus Budget Reconciliation Act of 1985 (COBRA). Some states have adjudication laws with penalties if the managed care plan does not pay promptly. Take the following steps if claims are not paid in a timely manner (30 days):

1. Write to the plan representative and list the unpaid claims, claims paid after the payment time limit, and claims paid in error.
2. Send a statement to the director of the managed care plan notifying him or her that if the bill is not paid, the employer's benefits manager or patient will be contacted and alerted to outstanding, slow-paying accounts. Say that this will prevent the physician from renewing the plan's contract, and ask the recipient to contact the plan's representative. The consumer has a choice of managed care plans; if the present plan does not fulfill his or her expectations, then the managed care plan loses members because of dissatisfaction.
3. Take examples and statistics to the next renegotiating session when the physician's contract is expiring.

Chapters 9 and 10 present information on how to handle slow or delinquent managed care plan payers.

Statement of Remittance

Managed care plans pay by either a capitation system (monthly check for the number of patients in the plan) or based on the services given to the patient (monthly check with a statement of remittance or explanation of benefits [EOB]).

In the capitation system a monthly check arrives written out for the total amount of monthly capitation. The accompanying paperwork lists all eligible patients being paid for on a per capita basis divided into two groups, commercial and senior. Patients categorized as commercial are usually younger than age 65 and are paid at a lesser rate because their risk is lower (e.g., they do not need to see the doctor frequently). The senior patient category includes those older than 65 years of age; these are paid at a higher rate because of the increased risk. Always verify the individual capitated amounts listed by each name on the accompanying paperwork against the monthly eligibility list to balance the amount of the check. Contact the MCO if an error appears. If a specialist is capitated, there may be thousands of patients on the capitation plan and a list of patients will not be provided. The capitation amount for a specialist may be only a few cents per month calculated according to the risk of the patient needing specialty services.

In the system when payment is based on services rendered and an EOB is generated, such statements itemize services that have been rendered to patients and usually indicate the amount billed, amount allowed, amount paid, and any copayment to be made by the patient (Figure 11–7). Generally patients under managed care plans do not receive an EOB. Payments are checked against the managed care contract for verification and then posted to the patients' accounts. An error should be brought to the attention of the plan's administrator and, depending on the circumstances, appealed.

Accounting

Managed care plans vary in their financial reimbursement structure, and careful accounting procedures are required. Accounting can become a confusing issue because of mixture of private and managed care patients with copayment requirements, coinsurance amounts, deductibles, and withholds.

Fee-for-Service

Some medical practices handle managed care patient accounts the same as fee-for-service patient accounts. If coinsurance payment is necessary at the time of service,

STATEMENT OF REMITTANCE

PATIENT NAME (ID NUMBER)	SERVICE DATE MO. DAY YR	POS	NO SVC	PROCEDURE NUMBER AND DESCRIPTION	AMOUNT BILLED	AMOUNT ALLOWED	RISK WITHHELD	CO PAY	AMOUNT PAID	ADJ. CODE
380224171-01 ALAN E.				CLAIM NO. 62730406 ACCOUNT NO.						
	092620XX	03	1	81000 URINALYSIS-ROUTINE	1000	1000	100	0	900	
	092620XX	03	1	82270 OCCULT BLOOD ANY S	1200	1200	120	0	1080	
	092620XX	03	1	99243 COMPRE RE-EXAM OR	6500	6500	650	0	5850	
	092620XX	03	1	36415 VENIPUNCTURE W/CEN	1700	1700	170	0	1530	
				CLAIM TOTALS =10400	10400	1040	0	9360		
558700321-01 RONALD B.				CLAIM NO. 62730407 ACCOUNT NO.						
	092520XX	03	1	90050 LIM EXAM EVAL A/O	3000	3000	300	300	2400	
				CLAIM TOTALS = 3000	3000	300	300	2400		
473760096-01 DORMA L.				CLAIM NO. 62730408 ACCOUNT NO.						
	092520XX	03	1	90050 LIM EXAM EVAL A/O	3000	3000	300	300	2400	
				CLAIM TOTALS = 3800	3000	300	380	3120		

VENDOR SUMMARY: TOTAL AMOUNT PAID $1,638.96   TOTAL WITHHELD $194.39

             AMOUNT PAID YEAR-TO-DATE: $42,411.95   AMOUNT WITHHELD YEAR-TO-DATE $5,109.94

Adjustment Code Legend
A = Adjusted: Billed amount exceeds VIP allowed.
O = Claim for service denied. Charges for this service included in other benefit payment. No patient liability.

FIGURE 11–7 Statement of remittance or explanation of benefits for noncapitated patients or contracted fee for service indicating the amount billed, amount allowed, amount paid, and any copayment that is to be made by the patient.

post first the charge and then the coinsurance prepayment, either calculated based on the percentage of the charge the plan allows or the flat copayment amount, for example, $15 for each office visit. Finally, post an adjustment entry of the disallowed amount, which is calculated on a percentage of the MCO's allowable charge to balance the account (Figure 11–8). An overpayment should be shown as a refund or credit to the account.

Year-End Evaluation

Withhold

Depending on the contract, a managed care plan may retain a percentage of the monthly capitation payment or a percentage of the allowable charges to physicians until the end of the year to cover operating expenses. This is known as **withhold.** A statement of remittance from the MCO shows the risk amounts withheld for each patient's

visit in Column 8 of Figure 11–7. The withhold plus interest is returned to the physician at the end of the plan-year if the budgeted services for the plan are not overused. However, the withhold or a portion of it is retained by the plan if services are overutilized. Thus the physicians share in any surplus or pay part of any deficit at year's end. This risk sharing creates an incentive for limiting care by the gatekeeper and limiting referrals to specialists, thereby keeping medical costs down. The withhold can cover all services or be specific to hospital care, **ancillary services** (laboratory/x-ray use), or specialty referrals.

A managed care plan that withholds a percentage of the allowable charge must be tracked in the physician's accounts receivable so it is not prematurely written off as a bad debt. To do this, develop a capitation accounting worksheet listing the dates of service, patients' names, CPT code for the service rendered, fee-for-service

STATEMENT

College Clinic
4567 Broad Avenue
Woodland Hills, XY 12345-0001
Telephone: 555-486-9002
Fax: 555-487-8976

Account No. 78650
Brian Wu
8700 Mason Drive
Woodland Hills, XY 12345

DATE	PROFESSIONAL SERVICE DESCRIPTION	CHARGE	CREDITS		CURRENT BALANCE	
			PAYMENTS	ADJUSTMENTS		
4-7-XX	Surgery	4000 00		600 00	3400 00	Disallowed amount
4-7-XX	Coinsurance payment (required)		680 00		2720 00	Patient's copay
4-7-XX	Adj.				2720 00	
5-15-XX	Plan payment ck #2408		2720 00		-0-	MCO payment

Due and payable within 10 days.   **Pay last amount in balance column** ⇧

Key: PF: Problem-focused   SF: Straightforward   CON: Consultation   HCD: House Call (Day)
EPF: Expanded problem-focused LC: Low complexity CPX: Complete Phys Exam HCN: House Call (Night)
D: Detailed   MC: Moderate complexity E: Emergency   HV: Hospital Visit
C: Comprehensive   HC: High complexity   ER: Emergency Dept.   OV: Office Visit

FIGURE 11–8 Posting to a patient's financial accounting record (ledger card) showing charge of $4000. The plan allows $3400; therefore the patient's prepaid coinsurance amount is $680 (20% of $3400). The managed care plan sent a check for $2720 (80% of $3400) and the disallowed amount ($600) is adjusted off of the account, which brings the account balance to zero.

charges, withheld amounts, and disallowed amounts (Figure 11–9). Then total all columns. The total of the withheld column is a debit entry that indicates what the managed care plan owes to the medical practice pending its year-end reconciliation. If and when the withheld amount arrives, the accounting worksheet can be compared with the amount withheld during the year. The amount of withholds that are not returned to the physician is adjusted once withholds are settled. The total of the column for disallowed amounts shows the amount written off by the medical practice. Combine the withheld returned amount with the managed care payment for the year to determine whether it is worthwhile for the practice to participate in the plan. Some practices can use the information to renegotiate increased fees when the managed care contract is to be renewed.

Capitation versus Fee-for-Service

Financial management reports are generated via computer and are the responsibility of the manager or accountant in most medical practices. However, it can be an asset for an insurance biller to have some knowledge of the content of these reports. Most medical practices monitor plan payments for profit or loss by comparing actual income from managed care patients with what would have been received from fee-for-service plans. To do this one designs a capitation accounting sheet for each capitated plan. This sheet shows a listing of dates of service and professional service descriptions (procedures, injections, and laboratory work), as well as charges and payments (Figure 11–10). As managed care plan patients receive services, actual service fees are posted in a charge column from the office fee schedule as if the patient were a private payer. In a payment column, office visit, copayments, and the monthly capitation payment are posted. Then all columns are totaled. It is necessary to apply a discount to the total charged amount for a realistic comparison because the physician usually is paid on an allowed amount rather than an actual charge. Calculate the difference between the actual charge and the average allowed amount to do this.

Compare the capitated payment amounts plus copayment amounts with the total discounted charges at the end of the year. This gives an accurate idea of whether the capitated payment received is adequate for the services the physician performed. Compiling monthly records and reviewing them at the end of the year helps a medical practice assess the gain or loss of each capitation plan.

Bankruptcy

If an MCO declares bankruptcy, such as a Chapter 11 filing, it is obligated to pay all bills incurred after the filing. If the patient had treatment before the filing, a delay in getting reimbursed may occur because the MCO cannot repay debts incurred before its filing until it has worked out a reorganization plan. Physicians under contract with the MCO are obligated to honor their contractual commitments. If their contracts expire or if they have escape clauses, they may be required to continue accepting patients depending on the contract provisions.

Some clauses allow a physician to withdraw from seeing managed care patients or leave if the MCO is in bankruptcy proceedings for more than 4 months. However, bankruptcy courts have broad powers to prevent physicians from leaving MCOs in bankruptcy proceedings if the court deems such actions to be detrimental to the rehabilitation of the debtor.

In some states, laws such as California's Knox-Keene Health Care Service Plan Act of 1975 prohibit hospitals and physicians under contract to an MCO from billing patients. Other states do not have such protection but may have emergency insurance funds to limit the financial liability of enrollees in bankruptcy MCOs. If the insurance commissioner is contacted by letter, he or she will refer the letter to the MCO. However, letters make insurance commissioners aware of problems that have developed.

Chapter 10 contains information on the topic of bankruptcy.

CONCLUSION

In summary, the medical biller should be aware that no matter what the type of plan, coverage is either purchased by an individual or paid by an employer. This is extremely important to know because if the plan is paid by the employer it is regulated by the Employee Retirement Income Security Act, also known as ERISA. This law regulates all managed care insurance paid by the employer or supplemented by the employee for the employee's spouse or children, which today is about 85% of the claims that are non–Medicare/Medicaid/workers' compensation. ERISA is regulated by the Department of Labor, and if the plan is an ERISA plan, the State Insurance Commissioners have no power to help with insurance carrier issues. Consequently, if the managed care organization is "related to" an employee benefit plan (EBP), the requirements of ERISA and its regulations are of overriding importance and severely restrict patient rights.

No employer is obligated to establish an EBP. To encourage them to do so, Congress has given them, their plans, their HMOs and insurers, and their administrators

DEBIT

Date	Patient	Service	Charge	Withhold	Disallow	
5/15/20XX	Mason	99204	106.11	5.94	21.22	← Disallowed amounts
5/15/20XX	Mason	93000	34.26	1.92	3.43	
5/15/20XX	Mason	81000	8.00	.38	2.40	
5/15/20XX	Self	93501	1500.00	240.00	300.00	
Total			1648.38	248.24	327.05	← Total withheld amount owed by MCO

FIGURE 11–9 A managed care plan when payment is on a fee-for-service basis. Note the disallowed portion of the charge, which is based on the plan's allowable charge. A portion of the allowable charge is withheld.

CAPITATION ACCOUNTING WORKSHEET

NAME OF PLAN ABC Managed Care Plan

DATE OF SERVICE	PROFESSIONAL SERVICE DESCRIPTION	CHARGES	PAYMENTS		
		Services Fees	Capitation	Copay	
20XX 1/15	Capitation (105 members) @ $8 ea		840.00		← Capitation payment
2/15	Capitation (115 members)		920.00		
2/20	Sanchez OV/Copay	35.00		5.00	← Copayment amount
2/22	Jones OV/Copay	35.00		5.00	
2/23	Davis OV/Copay	35.00		5.00	← Actual fee-for-service charge
3/6	Evans OV/Copay	35.00		5.00	
3/15	Capitation (130 members)		1040.00		
4/10	Wu OV/Copay	35.00		5.00	
4/15	Capitation (135 members)		1080.00		
	May through December are not shown				
END OF YEAR TOTALS		3500.00	6880.00	500.00	

FIGURE 11–10 An accounting sheet for a capitation plan from January through April showing dates of service, professional service descriptions, members' charges, and capitation payments and copayments received by the medical practice. Charges and payments columns may be totaled at the end of the year to compare capitation with fee-for-service earnings.

substantial immunities from liability. State regulation of HMOs administered by self-insured EBPs is preempted by ERISA; therefore employees cannot be protected by those state laws that limit the excesses of other HMOs not subject to ERISA.

Any case "relating to" an EBP falls under federal jurisdiction and is always removed from state to federal court when a lawsuit is initiated. There the patient and provider will find that the usual state law tort claims also are preempted by ERISA; therefore any claims against the HMO or EBP for medical malpractice, wrongful death, fraud, nonpayment or incorrect payment of claims, and so on will be summarily dismissed if filed in state courts. As of January 1, 2003, new changes were made to ERISA about time limitations on claims processing and the appeals process. Therefore know if the policy is paid for by the patient or employer. Refer to the resources at the end of this chapter for more information on ERISA.

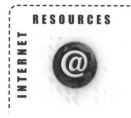

RESOURCES

INTERNET

- American Association of Health Plans (AAHP) (formerly known as American Managed Care and Review Association and American Association of Foundations for Medical Care) Web site: **www.aahp.org**

- Employee Retirement Income Security Act (ERISA) Web site: **http://www.dol.gov/ebsa/compliance_assistance.html** Then do a search and select "E." ERISA is listed as a selection.

- Federal Register Web site: **http://www.gpoaccess.gov/fr/index.html**

- National Committee for Quality Assurance Web site: **http://hprc.ncqa.org**

✔ Study Chapter 11.

✔ Answer the review questions in the *Workbook* to reinforce the theory learned in this chapter and to help prepare you for a future test.

✔ Complete the assignments in the *Workbook* to give you hands-on experience in abstracting information from a medical record to complete treatment authorization forms for prepaid health insurance cases.

✔ Turn to the glossary at the end of this textbook for a further understanding of the key terms used in this chapter.

CHAPTER OUTLINE

BACKGROUND
POLICIES AND REGULATIONS
  Eligibility Requirements
  Health Insurance Card
  Enrollment Status
  Benefits and Nonbenefits
ADDITIONAL INSURANCE
  PROGRAM
  Medicare/Medicaid
  Medicare/Medigap
  Medicare Secondary Payer
  Automobile or Liability
    Insurance Coverage
MEDICARE MANAGED CARE
  PLANS
  Health Maintenance
    Organizations
  Carrier Dealing Prepayment
    Organization
UTILIZATION AND QUALITY
  CONTROL
  Quality Improvement
    Organizations
  Federal False Claims
    Amendment Act
MEDICARE BILLING
  COMPLIANCE ISSUES

  Clinical Laboratory
    Improvement Amendment
PAYMENT FUNDAMENTALS
  Provider
  Prior Authorization
  Waiver of Liability Provision
  Elective Surgery Estimate
  Prepayment Screens
  Correct Coding Initiative
MEDICARE REIMBURSEMENT
  Chronology of Payment
  Reasonable Fee
  Resource-Based Relative
    Value Scale
  Healthcare Common Procedure
    Coding System (HCPCS)
CLAIM SUBMISSION
  Local Coverage Determination
  Fiscal Intermediaries and Fiscal
    Agents
  Provider Identification
    Numbers
  Patient's Signature
    Authorization
  Time Limit
  Paper Claims
  Electronic Claims

  Medicare/Medicaid Claims
  Medicare/Medigap Claims
  Medicare/Employer
    Supplemental Insurance
    Claims
  Medicare/Supplemental and
    MSP Claims
  Deceased Patients Claims
  Physician Substitute Coverage
AFTER CLAIM SUBMISSION
  Remittance Advice
  Medicare Summary Notice
BENEFICIARY REPRESENTATIVE/
  REPRESENTATIVE PAYEE
  Posting Payments
  Review and Redetermination
    Process
PROCEDURE: DETERMINE
  WHETHER MEDICARE IS
  PRIMARY OR SECONDARY
  AND DETERMINE
  ADDITIONAL BENEFITS
PROCEDURE: COMPLETE AN
  ADVANCE BENEFICIARY
  NOTICE (ABN) FORM

KEY TERMS

advance beneficiary notice (ABN)

approved charges

assignment

benefit period

Centers for Medicare and
  Medicaid Services (CMS)

Correct Coding Initiative (CCI)

crossover claim

diagnostic cost groups (DCGs)

disabled

end-stage renal disease (ESRD)

fiscal intermediary (FI)

hospice

hospital insurance

intermediate care facilities (ICFs)

limiting charge

medical necessity

Medicare

Medicare Part A

Medicare Part B

Medicare Part C

Medicare/Medicaid (Medi-Medi)

Medicare Secondary Payer (MSP)

Medicare summary notice (MSN)

Medigap (MG)

national alphanumeric codes

nonparticipating physician
  (nonpar)

nursing facility (NF)

participating physician (par)

peer review organization (PRO)

premium

prospective payment system (PPS)

qui tam action

reasonable fee

relative value unit (RVU)

remittance advice (RA)

resource-based relative value
  scale (RBRVS)

respite care

Supplemental Security
  Income (SSI)

supplementary medical
  insurance (SMI)

volume performance standard
  (VPS)

whistleblowers

12

Medicare

OBJECTIVES*

After reading this chapter, you should be able to:

- Explain eligibility criteria for Medicare.

- Name important information to abstract from a patient's Medicare card.

- Identify the benefits and nonbenefits of Medicare.

- List the federal laws adopted to increase health benefits for employed workers and the elderly.

- Name the conditions when an HMO-Medicare patient can be seen by a nonmember HMO physician.

- Differentiate between an HMO Risk Plan and an HMO Cost Plan.

- Name the federal laws that relate to cost containment of health services and to reduction of fraud and abuse issues.

- Explain when to obtain a patient's signature on an advance beneficiary notice or waiver of liability agreement.

- Define a Medicare-mandated prepayment screen.

- State the benefits for a participating versus nonparticipating physician.

- Calculate a payment for a procedure using the current conversion factor.

- List situations for using a lifetime beneficiary claim authorization and information release document.

- Determine the time limit for submitting a Medicare claim.

- Explain claims submission for individuals who have Medicare with other insurance.

- List CMS-1500 block numbers that require Medigap information when submitting a Medicare/Medigap claim.

- Post information on the patient's financial accounting record after a Medicare payment has been received.

*Performance objectives and exercises for hands-on practical experience for this chapter appear in the *Workbook*.

Service

Remind the patient to bring in his or her insurance identification card or cards. Give assistance to patients who may be visually impaired or have hearing impairment and need to complete registration forms for filing insurance claims. Work closely with caregivers and be aware of each patient's limitations, caring for each one with dignity.

Answer the patient's questions about Medicare Summary Notice documents because these can be confusing to elderly patients and can lead to misunderstandings about payments for services rendered.

BACKGROUND

Although Social Security is one of the United States' most important domestic programs, this system is by no means the first. There were a number of social insurance programs throughout Europe and Latin America before the Social Security Act was signed into law in 1935. Before the United States had Social Security, 20 other nations already had similar systems in operation. Another 30 countries had different social insurance programs in place, such as workers' compensation.

POLICIES AND REGULATIONS

Medicare is administered by the **Centers for Medicare and Medicaid Services (CMS),** formerly known as the Health Care Financing Administration (HCFA). CMS is subdivided into three divisions with the following responsibilities:

1. The Center for Medicare Management oversees traditional fee-for-service Medicare, including development of payment policy and management of fee-for-service contractors.
2. The Center for Beneficiary Choices provides beneficiaries with information on Medicare, Medicare Select, and Medicare Plus (+) Choice programs and Medigap options. It also manages the Medicare + Choice plans, consumer research, and grievance and appeals functions.
3. The Center for Medicaid and State Operations focuses on federal–state programs, such as Medicaid, the State Children's Health Insurance Program, insurance regulations, and the Clinical Laboratory Improvements Act (CLIA).
4. CMS also enforces the insurance portability and transaction and code set requirements of the Health Insurance Portability and Accountability Act.

Eligibility Requirements

The Social Security Administration (SSA) offices take applications for Social Security, controls the eligibility process, and provides information about the Medicare program. If an individual already receives Social Security or Railroad Retirement benefits, he or she is automatically enrolled in Medicare Parts A and B starting the first day of the month that the individual turns 65 years of age. In the year 2000, the retirement age gradually increased for people born in the year 1938 or later. By 2027, full-time retirement age will be 67 for people born after 1959. Benefits may increase if retirement is delayed beyond full-retirement age. As of this edition, Medicare still may begin at age 65. Those who apply for Social Security early (at age 62 years) do not receive Medicare but receive monthly reduced Social Security benefits. If an individual is younger than 65 years of age and disabled, he or she will automatically get Medicare Parts A and B after they get Social Security disability or Railroad Retirement benefits for 24 months. An individual does not have to be retired to receive Medicare benefits.

Medicare is a federal health insurance program for the following categories of people:

1. People 65 years of age or older who are on Social Security
2. People 65 years of age or older who are retired from the railroad or Civil Service
3. **Disabled** individuals who are eligible for Social Security disability benefits* and who are in the following categories:
   a. Disabled workers of any age
   b. Disabled widows of workers who are fully or currently insured through the federal government, Civil Service, SSA, **Supplemental Security Income (SSI),** or the Railroad Retirement Act and whose husbands qualified for benefits under one of these programs
   c. Adults disabled before age 18 years whose parents are eligible for or retired on Social Security benefits
4. Children and adults who have chronic kidney disease requiring dialysis or **end-stage renal disease (ESRD)** requiring a kidney transplant
5. Kidney donors (all expenses related to the kidney transplantation are covered)

All persons who meet one of the previously stated eligibility requirements determined by SSA are eligible for **Medicare Part A** (hospital coverage) at no charge. Those who qualify for full Medicare benefits may also elect to take **Medicare Part B** (outpatient coverage). Medicare Part B recipients pay annually increasing basic premiums to the SSA, and some pay a Medicare surtax on federal income tax payments. This premium may be deducted automatically from the patient's monthly Social

---

*In the disabled categories, a person must be disabled for not less than 12 months to apply for disability benefits. A disabled beneficiary must receive disability benefits for 24 months before Medicare benefits begin. See Chapter 16 for further information on this topic.

This is the patient's health insurance claim number. It must be shown on all Medicare claims exactly as it is shown on the card — including the letter at the end.

This shows hospital insurance coverage.

This shows medical insurance coverage.

MEDICARE   HEALTH INSURANCE

SOCIAL SECURITY ACT

NAME OF BENEFICIARY
JANE DOE

MEDICARE CLAIM NUMBER   SEX
      123-XX-6789A   FEMALE

IS ENTITLED TO   EFFECTIVE DATE
HOSPITAL INSURANCE (PART A)   01/01/20XX
MEDICAL INSURANCE (PART B)   01/01/20XX

SIGN ➡ _Jane Doe_
HERE

Special code indicating patient status

The date the insurance starts is shown here.

FIGURE 12–1   Medicare health insurance identification card.

Security check if he or she wishes. Those individuals not eligible for Medicare Part A (hospital insurance) at 65 years of age may purchase Part B from the SSA.

Aliens

An alien on Medicare may be eligible for Part A or B coverage. To be eligible, the applicant must have lived in the United States as a permanent resident for 5 consecutive years. It is usually not necessary to state on the CMS-1500 form that the patient is an alien when billing Medicare.

Health Insurance Card

The patient should present his or her Medicare health insurance card indicating the patient's insurance claim number (Figures 12–1 and 12–2). The claim number is the Social Security number of the wage earner with an alpha suffix. However, a spouse's card might have the husband's claim number if she has never worked and has no SSA work credits. The card indicates hospital and medical coverage, effective date, and patient status. When a husband and wife both have Medicare, they receive separate cards and claim numbers. Medicare cards are red, white, and blue, and cards issued after 1990 are plastic.

The letters after the Medicare number on the patient's identification card indicate the patient's status as follows (this is only a partial listing):

A = wage earner (shown in Figure 12–1)
B = husband's number (wife 62 years or older)
D = widow

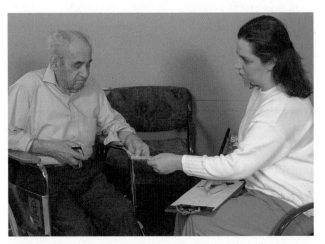

FIGURE 12–2   Insurance billing specialist obtaining the identification card from a disabled Medicare patient.

HAD = disabled adult
C = disabled child
J, Kl, or Jl = special monthly benefits, never worked under Social Security
M = Part B benefits only
T = uninsured and entitled only to health insurance benefits

A patient whose Medicare card claim number ends in "A" has the same Social Security and claim numbers. A patient whose Medicare card claim number ends in "B" or "D" has *different* Social Security and claim numbers. A quick check between Social Security and card claim numbers may identify a submission error and forestall a claims rejection.

The letters preceding the Medicare number on the patient's identification card indicate *railroad retirees:*

A = retired railroad employee
Examples: A 000000 (6 digits); A 000-00-0000 (9 digits)
MA = spouse of a retired railroad employee
WA/WD = widow or widower of deceased employee (age or disability)
Examples: WA000000 (6 digits); WA000-00-0000 (9 digits)
CA = child or student
WCA/WCD = widow of retiree with child in her care or disabled child of deceased employee
PA/PD = parent of deceased employee (male or female)
H = railroad retirement board pensioner before 1937
MH = wife of railroad retirement board pensioner before 1937
WH = widowed wife of railroad retirement board pensioner before 1937
WCH = widow of railroad retirement board pensioner with child in her care
PH = parent of railroad retirement board pensioner before 1937
JA = widow receiving a joint and survivor annuity
X = divorced spouse's annuity, for use on forms AA-3 and AA-7 only
Example: CA 123-45-6789C

Enrollment Status

If an individual receiving Social Security or Railroad Retirement benefits did not sign up for Medicare at the time of eligibility, then an individual is eligible to enroll in Medicare 3 months before his or her 65th birthday. The enrollment period ends 3 months after the month in which the person turns 65. If the enrollment period is missed, the individual must wait until the next general enrollment period, January 1 through March 31, of the following year.

A telephone hotline or, in some states, a modem connection is available to verify the enrollment status. This is useful because patients can switch coverage to a senior managed care plan on a month-to-month basis. Most carriers also allow information on deductible status. The patient's numeric information (Medicare number and date of birth) is entered into the telephone system, and the digital response indicates how much of the deductible has been satisfied. Contact the Medicare local fiscal agent for information about this service.

Benefits and Nonbenefits

Medicare Part A: Hospital Benefits

Part A of Medicare is **hospital insurance** benefits for people 65 years of age or older, for people younger than age 65 with certain disabilities, or for people with end-stage renal disease. Funds for this health service come from special contributions from employees and self-employed persons, with employers matching contributions. These contributions are collected along with regular Social Security contributions from wages and self-employment income earned during a person's working years.

A **benefit period** begins the day a patient enters a hospital and ends when the patient has not been a bed patient in any hospital or **nursing facility (NF)** (formerly called skilled nursing facility) for 60 consecutive days. It also ends if a patient has been in a nursing facility but has not received skilled nursing care for 60 consecutive days. A nursing facility offers nursing or rehabilitation services that are medically necessary to a patient's recovery. Services provided are not custodial. Custodial services are those that assist the patient with personal needs (e.g., dressing, eating, bathing, and getting in and out of bed). Hospital insurance protection is renewed every time the patient begins a new benefit period. There is no limit to the number of benefit periods a patient can have for hospital or nursing facility care. However, special limited benefit periods apply to hospice care.

Medicare Part A provides benefits to applicants in any of the following situations:

1. A bed patient in a hospital (up to 90 hospital days for each benefit period)
2. A bed patient in a nursing facility receiving skilled nursing care (up to 100 extended-care days for each benefit period)
3. A patient receiving home health care services
4. A patient who needs care in a psychiatric hospital (up to 190 days in a lifetime)
5. A terminally ill patient diagnosed as having 6 months or less to live who needs hospice care. A **hospice** is a public agency or private organization that is primarily engaged in providing pain relief, symptom management, and supportive services to terminally ill people and their families.
6. A terminally ill patient who needs respite care. **Respite care** is a short-term inpatient stay that may be necessary for the terminally ill patient to give temporary relief to the person who regularly assists with home care. Inpatient respite care is limited to stays of no more than 5 consecutive days for each respite period.

Figure 12–3 contains information on five major classifications of inpatient hospital cost-sharing benefits for Medicare Part A. Miscellaneous hospital services and supplies might consist of intensive care unit (ICU) costs, blood transfusions, drugs, x-ray and laboratory tests, medical supplies (casts, surgical dressings, splints), use of wheelchair, operating room (OR) and recovery room costs, and therapy (physical, occupational, and speech language). There are no benefits for personal convenience items

MEDICARE (PART A): HOSPITAL INSURANCE–COVERED SERVICES FOR 2005

Services	Benefit	Medicare Pays	Patient Pays
HOSPITALIZATION Semiprivate room and board, general nursing and miscellaneous hospital services and supplies. (Medicare payments based on benefit periods.)	First 60 days	All but $912	$912 deductible
	61st to 90th day 91st to 150th day[1]	All but $228 a day	$228 a day
	60-reserve-days benefit	All but $456 a day	$456 a day
	Beyond 150 days	Nothing	All costs
NURSING FACILITY CARE Patient must have been in a hospital for at least 3 days and enter a Medicare-approved facility generally within 30 days after hospital discharge.[2] (Medicare payments based on benefit periods.)	First 20 days	100% of approved amount	Nothing
	21st to 100th day	All but $114 a day	Up to $114 a day
	Beyond 100 days	Nothing	All costs
HOME HEALTH CARE Part-time or intermittent skilled care, home health aide services, durable medical equipment and supplies, and other services.	Unlimited as long as Medicare conditions are met and services are declared "medically necessary."	100% of approved amount; 80% of approved amount for durable medical equipment.	Nothing for services; 20% of approved amount for durable medical equipment.
HOSPICE CARE Pain relief, symptom management, and support services for the terminally ill.	If patient elects the hospice option and as long as doctor certifies need.	All but limited costs for outpatient drugs and inpatient respite care.	Limited cost sharing for outpatient drugs and inpatient respite care.
BLOOD	Unlimited if medically necessary.	All but first 3 pints per calendar year.	For first 3 pints.[3]

[1] This 60-reserve-days benefit may be used only once in a lifetime.
[2] Neither Medicare nor private Medigap insurance will pay for most long-term nursing home care.
[3] To the extent the blood deductible is met under Part B of Medicare during the calendar year, it does not have to be met under Part A.

FIGURE 12–3 Five major classifications of Medicare Part A benefits. *(Updated from Medicare and You 2005, U.S. Government Printing Office.)*

(television, radio, and telephone), private duty nurses, or a private room unless the private room is determined medically necessary. Similar benefits also relate to nursing facilities.

Benefits for hospice and respite care consist of nursing and physicians' services, drugs, therapy (physical, occupational, and speech-language pathology), home health aide, homemaker services, medical social services, medical supplies and appliances, short-term inpatient care, and counseling.

Medicare Part B: Medical Benefits

Part B of Medicare is **supplementary medical insurance (SMI)** benefits for the aged and disabled. Funds for this program come equally from those who sign up for it and the federal government. A medical insurance **premium** is automatically deducted from monthly checks for those who receive Social Security benefits, Railroad Retirement benefits, or a Civil Service annuity. Others pay the premium directly to the SSA. In some states, when a person is eligible for Medicare Part B and Medicaid, Medicaid pays for the monthly Part B premiums.

Figure 12–4 contains information on five major classifications of medical benefits for Medicare Part B. In addition to medical and surgical services by a doctor of medicine (MD), doctor of osteopathy (DO or MD), or a doctor of dental medicine or dental surgery (DDS), certain services by a doctor of podiatric medicine (DPM), and limited services by a doctor of chiropractic (DC) are paid for. Dental care is covered only for fractures or surgery of the jaw. Optometric examinations are provided if a person has aphakia (absence of the natural lens of the eye).

Preventive Care Benefits

Medicare's preventive care benefits are listed in Table 12.1. Other benefits are ambulance service, meeting medical necessity requirements rental or purchase of durable medical equipment for home use, prosthetic devices for internal body organs, artificial limbs and eyes, and braces or supports (leg, arm, back, and neck).

MEDICARE (PART B): MEDICAL INSURANCE-COVERED SERVICES FOR 2004

Services	Benefit	Medicare Pays	Patient Pays
MEDICAL EXPENSES Doctor's services (not routine physical exams), outpatient medical and surgical services and supplies, diagnostic tests, ambulatory surgery center facility fees for approved procedures, and durable medical equipment (such as wheelchairs, hospital beds, oxygen, and walkers). Also covers second surgical opinions, outpatient mental health care, and outpatient physical and occupational therapy, including speech-language therapy	Unlimited if medically necessary	80% of approved amount (after $100 deductible); reduced to 50% for most outpatient mental health services	$100 deductible,[1] plus 20% of approved amount or limited charges[2]
CLINICAL LABORATORY SERVICES Blood tests, urinalyses, and more	Unlimited if medically necessary	100% of approved amount	Nothing for services
HOME HEALTH CARE Part-time skilled nursing care, physical therapy, occupational therapy, speech-language therapy, home health aide services, medical social services, durable medical equipment (such as wheelchairs, hospital beds, oxygen, and walkers), medical supplies, and other services	Unlimited as long as patient meets conditions and benefits are declared medically necessary	100% of approved amount; 80% of approved amount for durable medical equipment	Nothing for services; 20% of approved amount for durable medical equipment
OUTPATIENT HOSPITAL TREATMENT Services for the diagnosis or treatment of illness or injury	Unlimited if medically necessary	Medicare payment to hospital based on hospital cost	$100 deductible, plus 20% of whatever the hospital charges
BLOOD	Unlimited if medically	80% of approved amount	First 3 pints plus 20% of approved amounts for additional pints (after $100 deductible)[3]

[1]Once the patient has had $100 of expenses for covered services in the year, the Part B deductible does not apply to any further covered services received for the rest of the year. The Part B deductible in 2005 will rise to $110.

[2]See Figure 12–8 for an explanation of approved amount for participating physicians and limited charges for nonparticipating physicians.

[3]To the extent the blood deductible is met under Part A of Medicare during the calendar year, it does not have to be met under Part B.

FIGURE 12–4 Five major classifications of Medicare Part B benefits. *(Updated from Medicare and You 2005, U.S. Government Printing Office.)*

On December 8, 2003, the Medicare Prescription Drug Improvement and Modernization Act of 2003 (MMA) became effective. This legislation provides seniors and people living with disabilities with a prescription drug benefit. Because the new drug benefit does not go into operation until 2006 (Medicare Part D), there is an interim plan, which is as follows:

● Interim discount card. From spring 2004 through 2005, beneficiaries could purchase a card that is estimated to save 10% to 15% off drug prices.
● Interim low-income assistance. Individuals with incomes less than $12,390 ($16,720 for couples) in 2004 would each get $600 a year on the card.

● Coverage choice. From January 2006 beneficiaries can choose the following:
  ● To remain in standard Medicare, current Medicare HMO, or retiree plan without signing up for a drug benefit
  ● To stay in standard Medicare and enroll in a stand-alone drug plan
  ● To enroll in a private health plan offering drug coverage and Medicare benefits
● Drug benefit. Enrollees' annual deductible is $250 with an estimated premium of $35 a month (varies depending on plan) and a 25% copayment of drug costs up to $2250 in a year. After that, enrollees pay all drug costs until they have spent $3600 out of pocket (equal to

Table 12.1 Medicare Preventive Services

Covered Service	Who is Covered	Patient Liability
Bone mass measurements: Once every 24 mo for qualified individuals and more frequently if medically necessary	Certain people with Medicare who are at risk for losing bone mass	20% of the Medicare approved amount (or a set coinsurance amount) after the yearly Part B deductible
Cardiovascular screening (blood)	All people	20% of the Medicare-approved amount after the yearly Part B deductible
Colorectal cancer screening *Fecal occult blood test:* Once every 12 mo **Flexible sigmoidoscopy:** Once every 48 mo **Colonoscopy:** Once every 24 mo if at high risk for colon cancer; otherwise once every 10 yr, but not within 48 mo of a screening flexible sigmoidoscopy **Barium enema:** May be used instead of a sigmoidoscopy or colonoscopy	All people with Medicare age 50 and older, except colonoscopy for which there is no minimum age requirement	Nothing for fecal occult blood test For all other tests, 20% of the Medicare-approved amount after the yearly Part B For flexible sigmoidoscopy or colonoscopy, patient pays 20% of the Medicare-approved amount after the yearly Part B deductible if the test is done in a hospital outpatient department
Diabetes: Coverage for glucose monitors, tests strips, and lancets Diabetes Self-management training Diabetes screening tests twice a year	All people with Medicare who have diabetes (insulin and noninsulin dependent) Certain people with Medicare who are at risk for complications from diabetes must be ordered by a physician	20% of the Medicare-approved amount after the yearly Part B deductible
Glaucoma screening: Once every 12 mo	People with Medicare who are at high risk for glaucoma, including people with diabetes, a family history of glaucoma, or African-Americans who are age 50 and older	20% of the Medicare-approved amount after the yearly Part B deductible
Mammogram screening: Once every 12 mo Medicare also covers digital technologies for mammogram screenings	All women with Medicare age 40 and older. A baseline mammogram is recommended for women between ages 35 and 39	20% of the Medicare-approved amount with no Part B deductible
Papanicolaou (Pap) test/pelvic examination (includes clinical breast examination): Once every 24 mo Once every 12 mo if at high risk for cervical or vaginal cancer, or if childbearing age and have an abnormal Pap test in the past 36 mo	All women with Medicare	Nothing for the Pap laboratory test. For Pap test collection and pelvic and breast examinations, 20% of the Medicare-approved amount (or a set coinsurance amount) with no Part B deductible
Prostate cancer screening **Digital rectal examination:** Once every 12 mo **Prostate specific antigen (PSA) test:** Once every 12 mo	All men with Medicare age 50 and older (coverage begins the day after the 50th birthday)	Generally, 20% of the Medicare-approved amount for the digital rectal examination after the yearly Part B deductible. No coinsurance and no Part B deductible for the PSA test
Vaccinations **Influenza (flu) vaccine:** Annually **Pneumococcal pneumonia vaccine (PPV):** Once in a lifetime **Hepatitis B vaccine:** Physician recommendation only	All people with Medicare	Nothing for flu and PPV if the physician accepts assignment For hepatitis B vaccine, 20% of the Medicare-approved amount after the yearly Part B deductible
Wellness physical examination: Within 6 mo of the day patient enrolled in Medicare Part B	All people with Medicare	20% of the Medicare-approved amount after the yearly Part B deductible

$5100 in annual costs for those with no other drug insurance). At that point, catastrophic coverage takes effect and enrollees pay 5% of prescriptions or copays of $2 for generics and $5 for brand names (whichever is greater).

● Dual eligible subsidies. People eligible for Medicaid and Medicare will pay no premium or deductible and have no gap in coverage. They will pay $1 per prescription for generics and $3 for brand names. Copays are waived for those in nursing homes.

● Other low-income subsidies. Individuals with incomes less than about $13,000 ($17,600 for couples) in 2006 and assets of less than $6000 ($9000 for couples) will pay no premium or deductible and have no gap in coverage. They will pay $2 for generics, $5 for brand names, and nothing above the catastrophic limit.

People with incomes between $13,000 and $14,400 ($17,600 and $19,500 for couples) in 2006 and assets less than $10,000 ($20,000 for couples) will pay premiums on a sliding scale, a $50 deductible and 15% of drug costs with no gap in coverage. After spending $3600 out of pocket in a year, copays will be $2 for generics, $5 for brand names.

Nonbenefits

Nonbenefits, also referred to as *noncovered services*, consist of routine physical examination, routine foot care, eye or hearing examinations, and cosmetic surgery unless caused by injury or performed to improve functioning of a malformed part. A physician may bill a patient separately for noncovered services.

The numerous other benefits and nonbenefits are too numerous to list here. Refer to Medicare newsletters or contact the Medicare carrier to find out whether a particular procedure qualifies for payment.

Medicare Part C: Medicare Plus (+) Choice Program

The Balanced Budget Act of 1997 created **Medicare Part C,** called Medicare + Choice. This program increased the number of health care options in addition to those that are available under Part A and Part B. Medicare + Choice plans receive a fixed amount of money from Medicare to spend on their Medicare members. Some plans may require members to pay a premium similar to the Medicare Part B premium. The Medicare Advantage (MA) program introduced in 2004 will eventually replace Medicare + Choice in 2006.

Plans available under this program may include the following: health maintenance organization (HMO), point-of-service (POS) plan, preferred provider organization (PPO), private fee-for-service (PFFS) plan, provider-sponsored

organization (PSO), religious fraternal benefit society (RFBS), and a pilot program, Medicare medical savings account (MSA). Most of these (except for PSO and RFBS) are discussed in Chapters 3 and 11.

A PSO is a managed care plan that is owned and operated by a hospital and provider group instead of an insurance company. An RFBS is a managed care option that is associated with a church, group of churches, or convention. Membership is restricted to church members and is allowed regardless of the person's health status. In an MSA plan, the patient chooses an insurance policy approved by Medicare that has a high annual deductible. Medicare pays the premiums for this policy and deposits the dollar amount difference between what it pays for the average beneficiary in the patient's area and the cost of the premium into the patient's MSA. The patient uses the MSA money to pay medical expenses until the high deductible is reached. If the MSA money becomes depleted, the patient pays out of pocket until the deductible is reached. Unused funds roll over for use the next year.

Railroad Retirement Benefits

Railroad Retirement Board offices maintain eligibility records for Medicare and provide information about the program for railroad workers and their beneficiaries. Medical insurance premiums are automatically deducted from the monthly checks of people who receive Railroad Retirement benefits. Those who do not receive a monthly check pay their premiums directly or, in some cases, have premiums paid on their behalf under a state assistance program. If the allowed fees differ from those allowed by the regular Medicare carrier, write or fax the Medicare railroad retiree carrier, asking that fees be based on fee data from the local carrier.

Railroad Retirement beneficiaries generally are entitled to benefits for covered services received from a qualified American facility. However, under certain circumstances, a Medicare beneficiary may receive care in Canada or Mexico. Benefits and deductibles under Parts A and B are the same as for other Medicare recipients.

Some railroad retirees are members of a railroad hospital association or a prepayment plan. These members pay regular premiums to the plan and then can receive health services that the plan provides without additional charges. In some plans, small charges are made for certain services, such as drugs or home visits. Many prepayment plans make arrangements with Medicare to receive direct payments for services they furnish that are covered under Medicare Part B. Some prepayment plans have contracts with Medicare as HMOs or competitive medical plans and can receive direct payment for services covered by either hospital or medical insurance. After a claim is submitted to the Medicare railroad retiree carrier, a remittance advice (RA) document is generated explaining the decision made on the claim and what services Medicare paid for.

Employed Elderly Benefits

To understand various types of scenarios that may be encountered when submitting claims for elderly individuals, one must know about several powerful federal laws that regulate health care coverage of those age 65 and older who are employed. Such individuals may have group insurance or a Medigap (MG) policy and may fall under billing categories of Medicare first payer or Medicare secondary payer (all are presented in detail later in this chapter).

Omnibus Budget Reconciliation Act

The Omnibus Budget Reconciliation Act (OBRA) of 1981 required that, in the case of a current or former employee or dependent younger than age 65 years and eligible for Medicare solely because of ESRD, the employer's group coverage is primary for up to 30 months. The Balanced Budget Act of 1997 mandated this change in the length of the coordination period. OBRA applies to all employers regardless of the number of employees. OBRA of 1986, effective in 1987, required that, if an employee or dependent younger than age 65 years has Medicare coverage because of a disability other than ESRD, the group coverage is primary and Medicare is secondary. This act applies only to large group health plans having at least 100 full- or part-time employees.

Tax Equity and Fiscal Responsibility Act

The Tax Equity and Fiscal Responsibility Act (TEFRA) of 1982 established that an employee or spouse age 65 to 69 years is entitled to the same health insurance benefits offered under the same conditions to younger employees and their spouses. The group insurance is primary and Medicare is secondary. TEFRA applies to employers with at least 20 full- or part-time employees.

Deficit Reduction Act

The Deficit Reduction Act (DEFRA) of 1984, effective 1985, was an amendment to TEFRA and stated that a spouse age 65 to 69 years or an employee of any age is entitled to the same group health plan offered to younger employees and their spouses. The group's coverage is primary and Medicare is secondary. DEFRA applies to employers with at least 20 full- or part-time employees.

Consolidated Omnibus Budget Reconciliation Act

The Consolidated Omnibus Budget Reconciliation Act (COBRA) of 1985, effective 1986, is another amendment to TEFRA eliminating the age ceiling of 69 years. An employee or spouse age 65 or older is entitled to the same group health plan offered to younger employees and their spouses. COBRA requires that third-party payers reimburse for certain care rendered in government-run veteran and military hospitals. The group's coverage is primary and Medicare is secondary. COBRA applies to employers with at least 20 full- or part-time employees.

Tax Reform Act

The Tax Reform Act was passed in 1986; it clarified certain aspects of COBRA. A spouse and dependents may elect to receive continued coverage even if the employee does not wish insurance coverage and terminates the plan. However, the spouse and dependents must have been covered under the plan before the covered employee terminates it. Spouses who are widowed or divorced while receiving continued coverage must report such changes to the benefit plan administrator within 60 days of the employee's death to determine how many additional months of coverage are available.

ADDITIONAL INSURANCE PROGRAMS

Many Medicare recipients have Medicare in combination with other insurance plans. This section explains various coverage combinations. Guidelines for processing claims for these plans are presented later in this chapter.

Medicare/Medicaid

Patients designated as **Medicare/Medicaid (Medi-Medi)** are on both Medicare and Medicaid (in California Medi-Cal) simultaneously. These patients qualify for Old Age, Survivors, and Disability Insurance (OASDI) assistance benefits (older than age 65), are severely disabled, or are blind.

Medicare/Medigap

A specialized insurance policy devised for the Medicare beneficiary is called **Medigap** or *Medifill*. This type of policy is designed to supplement coverage under a fee-for-service Medicare plan. It may cover prescription costs and the deductible and copayment (e.g., 20% of the Medicare allowed amount) that are typically the patient's responsibility under Medicare. These plans are offered by private third-party payers to Medicare beneficiaries who pay the monthly premiums for this supplemental insurance.

The federal government in conjunction with the insurance industry established predefined minimum benefits for 10 Medigap policies categorized by alpha letters A through J (Figure 12–5). Basic benefits are found in policy A. Each subsequent letter represents basic benefits

TEN MEDIGAP STANDARDIZED POLICIES

(Not all may be available in all states.)

A	B	C	D	E	F	G	H	I	J
Basic Benefit	Basic Benefit	Basic Benefit	Basic Benefit	Basic Benefit	Basic Benefit	Basic Benefit	Basic Benefit	Basic Benefit	Basic Benefit
		Skilled Nursing Coinsurance	Skilled Nursing Coinsurance	Skilled Nursing Coinsurance	Skilled Nursing Coinsurance	Skilled Nursing Coinsurance	Skilled Nursing Coinsurance	Skilled Nursing Coinsurance	Skilled Nursing Coinsurance
	Part A Deductible	Part A Deductible	Part A Deductible	Part A Deductible	Part A Deductible	Part A Deductible	Part A Deductible	Part A Deductible	Part A Deductible
		Part B Deductible			Part B Deductible				Part B Deductible
					Part B Excess 100%	Part B Excess 100%		Part B Excess 100%	Part B Excess 100%
		Foreign Travel Emergency	Foreign Travel Emergency	Foreign Travel Emergency	Foreign Travel Emergency	Foreign Travel Emergency	Foreign Travel Emergency	Foreign Travel Emergency	Foreign Travel Emergency
		At-Home Recovery			At-Home Recovery		At-Home Recovery	At-Home Recovery	
							Basic Drug Benefit ($1250 Limit)	Basic Drug Benefit ($1250 Limit)	Extended Drug Benefit ($3000 Limit)
			Preventive Care						Preventive Care

FIGURE 12–5   Ten Medigap standardized policies.

plus other coverage, with the most comprehensive benefits in policy J. Sale of all policies are not available in all states, so individuals in some states have fewer options than others.

A slightly different variation of a Medigap policy is *Medicare Select*. This policy has the same coverage as regular Medigap policies, but there is a restriction in that the beneficiary must obtain medical care from a list of specified network doctors and providers.

Medicare Secondary Payer

In some instances, Medicare is considered secondary and classifies the situation as **Medicare Secondary Payer (MSP)**. Follow the suggested steps in the procedure at the end of the chapter to identify whether Medicare is primary or secondary and to determine what additional benefits the patient might have.

Managed Care and Medicare

When a patient's primary insurance is a managed care plan that requires fixed copayments, it is possible to obtain reimbursement from Medicare for those amounts. An assigned MSP claim must be filed with Medicare after the managed care organization (MCO) has paid. When Medicare's copayment reimbursement has been received, the provider must refund to the patient the copayment amount previously collected.

The practice is paid a capitated amount and there is no explanation of benefits (EOB) document. Have the patient sign a statement that explains the situation. Attach the statement and the copayment receipts to the claim. The statement may read as shown in the following box:

Patient Name _____
Medicare Number _____
There is no Explanation of Benefits documentation available for the attached billed services. I am currently enrolled with _____ managed care plan for my health care. My physician, _____ MD, is paid on a capitated basis, and the copayment that I pay is $ _____ for each service or visit.

Patient's signature _____
Date _____

A nonparticipating physician (nonpar) must file an unassigned MSP claim. The patient is directly reimbursed by Medicare and no refund is necessary.

Automobile or Liability Insurance Coverage

Liability insurance is not secondary to Medicare because there is no contractual relationship between the injured party and third-party payer. A physician who treats a Medicare patient who has filed a liability claim must bill the liability insurer first *unless* the insurer will not pay promptly (e.g., within 120 days after the liability insurance claim is filed). After 120 days have gone by without a payment from the liability insurer and if the services performed are covered Medicare benefits, a participating (par) or nonpar physician may seek conditional payment from Medicare. However, if a claim is filed with Medicare, the provider must drop the claim against the liability insurer.

If the payment made by the liability insurer is less than the physician's full charge, the physician may file an assigned claim and must accept as full payment the greater of either the Medicare-approved charge or sum of the liability insurance primary payment and the Medicare secondary payment.

A nonpar physician may file an unassigned claim for Medicare secondary payment only if the payment by the liability insurer is less than the Medicare limiting charge. If the payment equals or exceeds the limiting charge, the physician must accept the disbursement as full payment.

If Medicare payments have been made but should not have been because the services are excluded under this provision, or if the payments were made on a conditional basis, they are subject to recovery. A copy of the notice of payment or denial form from the other insurer should be included when sending in the CMS-1500 claim form. Medicare is secondary even if a state law or a private contract of insurance states that Medicare is primary. The physician must bill the other insurer first. A claim for secondary benefits may be submitted to Medicare only after payment or denial has been made by the primary coverage. Liability insurance is not considered an MSP.

MEDICARE MANAGED CARE PLANS

Health Maintenance Organizations

During the spring of 1984, the Department of Health and Human Services published regulations giving Medicare enrollees the right to join and assign their Medicare benefits to HMOs. HMOs had been in operation for nearly

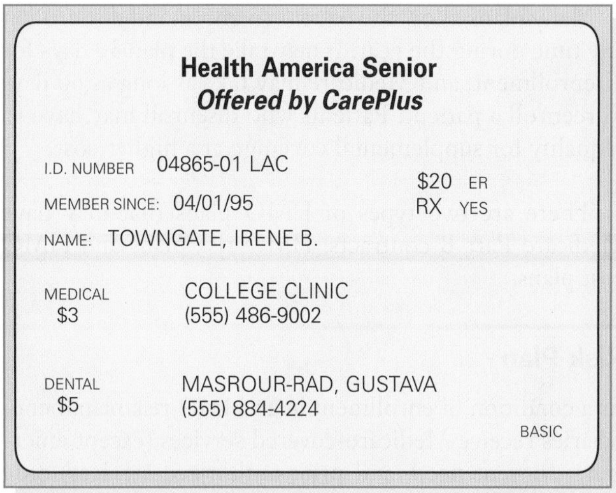

Health America Senior
Offered by CarePlus

I.D. NUMBER 04865-01 LAC
MEMBER SINCE: 04/01/95
NAME: TOWNGATE, IRENE B.

$20 ER
RX YES

MEDICAL COLLEGE CLINIC
$3 (555) 486-9002

DENTAL MASROUR-RAD, GUSTAVA
$5 (555) 884-4224

BASIC

FIGURE 12–6 A senior managed care plan card.

50 years when they became available as an option for Medicare enrollees. With a Medicare HMO (also known as a senior HMO or senior plan), the patient does not need a Medicare supplemental insurance plan. Upon enrollment, the Medicare beneficiary is sent an insurance card from the managed care plan (Figure 12–6). However, Medicare cards are not forfeited and an elderly patient may show two cards, leading to confusion about what the coverage is and who to bill.

Medicare makes payments directly to the HMO on a monthly basis for Medicare enrollees who use the HMO option. Enrollees pay the HMO a monthly premium, which is an estimate of the coinsurance amounts for which the enrollee would be responsible plus the Medicare deductible. It appears that HMOs contracting to provide services for Medicare patients will be converted to a Medicare + Choice plan as their contract renewal dates occur.

Some HMOs provide services not usually covered by Medicare, such as eyeglasses, prescription drugs, and routine physical examinations. Once a person has converted from Medicare to an HMO, he or she cannot go back to a former physician of personal choice and expect Medicare to pay the bill. The patient should receive services from a physician and hospital facility that are contracted with the HMO plan.

If a Medicare patient has switched over to a managed care plan and wishes to disenroll, the patient must do the following:

1. Notify the plan in writing of disenrollment.
2. Complete Medicare form Medicare Managed Care Disenrollment CMS-566, attach a copy of the disenrollment letter, and take it to the Social Security office.

Many plans allow the patient to enroll and disenroll at any time during the year. It may take the plan 30 days for disenrollment, and Medicare may take as long as 60 days to reenroll a patient. Patients who disenroll may have to requalify for supplemental coverage at a higher cost.

There are two types of HMO plans that may have Medicare Part B contracts: HMO risk plans and HMO cost plans.

Risk Plan

As a condition of enrollment in an HMO risk plan, beneficiaries receive Medicare-covered services (except emergency, urgent need, and prior authorized services) only from providers who are contracted members of the HMO network. Enrollees of HMO risk plans are referred to as "restricted" beneficiaries. Usually services rendered by "out-of-plan" physicians are not covered when the same services are available through the organization unless a referral or prior authorization is obtained. The only exception is for emergency care. Claims for HMO risk plan beneficiaries must be sent directly to the organization.

A system of Medicare reimbursement for HMOs with risk contracts is called **diagnostic cost groups (DCGs).** The HMO enrollees are classified into various DCGs on the basis of each beneficiary's prior 12-month history of hospitalization, and payments are adjusted accordingly. This payment system does not apply to disabled and hospice patients, those on renal dialysis, or those enrolled only in Medicare Part B. Patients are reclassified each year according to their previous year's use of hospital service.

Cost Plan

Under an HMO cost plan, beneficiaries receive Medicare-covered services from sources in or outside of the HMO network. Enrollees are referred to as "unrestricted" beneficiaries. Claims for cost plan beneficiaries may be sent to the HMO plan or the regular Medicare carrier.

Noncontract Physician

If a noncontract physician treats a Medicare HMO patient, the services are considered "out-of-plan" services. The claim must be submitted to the managed care plan, which determines whether it is responsible to pay for the services. Conditions that must be met follow:

1. The service was an emergency and the patient was not able to get to an HMO facility or member physician (patient was out of the HMO area).

2. The service was covered by Medicare.
3. The service was medically necessary.
4. The service was authorized previously or was an approved referral.

The patient is responsible for the fee if the HMO determines there was no emergency and denies payment. The HMO reimburses according to the Medicare Fee Schedule Allowable Amount, so the physician cannot bill the patient for the balance. If the physician does not receive 100% of the allowable, steps must be taken through the HMO's appeals process. If this fails, contact the Medicare Managed Care Department at the Medicare Regional CMS Operations Office. Denied services can be billed to the patient (no more than the Medicare fee schedule or limiting charge) after the HMO EOB is received.

Carrier Dealing Prepayment Organization

A Carrier Dealing Prepayment Organization may be set up by a medical practice under contract to the government. Such plans are considered a service contract rather than insurance. In the past, such plans were run by HMOs, but now practices of 12 to 15 physicians are opting to run their own plans. These organizations must be incorporated and have their own Medicare provider number. The organization must furnish physicians' services through employees and partners or under formal arrangement with medical groups, independent practice associations, or individual physicians. Part B services must be provided through qualified hospitals or physicians. When operating this type of organization, the physician accepts Medicare assignment and agrees to deal with the Medicare carrier instead of CMS. Patients sign a contract agreeing to pay a monthly fee (usually $20 to $25). This is supposed to cover all Medicare copayments, deductibles, and nonreimbursable expenses (annual physical examinations and preventive care). The patient is not responsible to pay for noncovered services.

UTILIZATION AND QUALITY CONTROL

Quality Improvement Organizations

As explained in detail in Chapter 11, a *Quality Improvement Organization (OIO)* program (formerly known as *professional* or *peer review organization*), contracts with CMS to review medical necessity, reasonableness, appropriateness, and completeness and adequacy of inpatient hospital care for which additional payment is sought under the outlier provisions of the Prospective Payment System (PPS).

CMS has assigned a point system for medical documentation as discussed in Chapter 3. If sufficient points are lacking, penalties can lead to fines or forfeiture of the physician's license. Therefore it is extremely important that each patient's care be well documented from the treatment standpoint, as well as for justifying maximum reimbursement. A physician who receives a letter from a QIO about quality of care should consult his or her attorney before responding by letter or personal appeal. A photocopy of the patient's health record can be used to substantiate the claim if there is detailed clinical documentation.

Federal False Claims Amendment Act

Another federal law to prevent overuse of services and to spot Medicare fraud is the Federal Claims Amendment Act of 1986. This act offers financial incentives of 15% to 25% of any judgment to informants **(whistleblowers)** who report physicians suspected of defrauding the federal government. This is called a *qui tam action.* The laws are intended to help catch Medicare and Medicaid cheaters. The health insurance companies that process Medicare claims have a Medicare fraud unit whose job is to catch people who steal from Medicare. The Office of the Inspector General (OIG), Department of Health and Human Services, is the law enforcement agency that investigates and prosecutes people who steal from Medicare. The OIG works closely with Medicare insurance companies, the Federal Bureau of Investigation (FBI), the Postal Inspection Service, and other federal law enforcement agencies. If the physician is on an optical disk retrieval (ODR) A-1000 system, it is possible for the OIG to obtain procedure codes that show comparison billing with peers in the area. The Centers for Medicaid and Medicare Services alerts the OIG of offices to investigate.

For information on fraud and abuse, see Boxes 2–9 and 2–10. See Chapter 15 for information about fraud in the workers' compensation program.

Clinical Laboratory Improvement Amendment

The CLIA of 1988 established federal standards, quality control, and safety measures for all freestanding laboratories, including physician office laboratories (POLs). Various laboratory procedures fall within CLIA categories depending on the complexity of each test. If a physician performs only tests that pose no risk to the patient, the laboratory may be eligible for a certificate of waiver that exempts it from CLIA regulations' quality control and personnel standards; however, a registration fee must still be paid for the waived category. The other two categories are moderate or high-complexity laboratory services. Each category level requires a yearly licensing fee to be paid by the physician. A certificate is then issued and must be posted in the laboratory. Various levels of quality control measures are necessary for each CLIA level and must be performed in a timely manner (e.g., daily or weekly). Fines may be levied if federal standards are not maintained. This has had an impact on office laboratories; because of the strict requirements, many physicians send patients to independent laboratories for tests (e.g., blood cell counts, cytology specimens, and cultures). However, some physicians prefer to draw blood from a patient, particularly if the patient has a history of difficult venous access.

When claims to Medicare fiscal intermediaries are submitted for laboratory services performed in the physician's office, the 10-digit CLIA certificate number should be entered in Block 23 of the CMS-1500 claim

---

HIPAA Compliance Alert

MEDICARE BILLING COMPLIANCE ISSUES

Because Medicare is a federal program, legislation sets down the policies that must be followed. Therefore whoever participates in the program must comply with all the regulations. Billing issues about which medical practices should be aware may include but are not limited to the following:

- Release of medical information
- Reassignment of payment
- Limiting charges for nonparticipating providers
- Correct procedural code assignment and service utilization
- Accurate diagnostic code assignment
- Medical necessity of services performed

- Billing for ancillary employees (physician assistants and nurse practitioners) called "incident to" billing
- Documentation related to selection of procedural codes for services performed
- Ancillary orders and supervision requirements
- Teaching physician and resident billing
- Routine waiver of copayments, deductibles, or professional courtesy discounts
- Stark I and II antireferral and compensation regulations
- Credit balance refunds
- Correct coding initiative edits

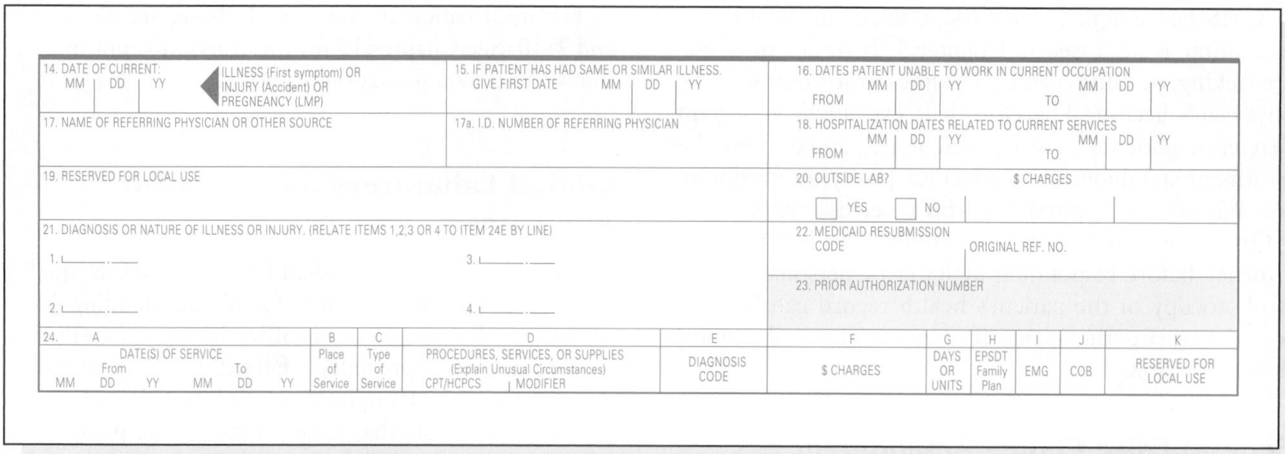
14. DATE OF CURRENT: MM | DD | YY ◀ ILLNESS (First symptom) OR INJURY (Accident) OR PREGNEANCY (LMP)
15. IF PATIENT HAS HAD SAME OR SIMILAR ILLNESS. GIVE FIRST DATE MM | DD | YY
16. DATES PATIENT UNABLE TO WORK IN CURRENT OCCUPATION MM | DD | YY FROM MM | DD | YY TO
17. NAME OF REFERRING PHYSICIAN OR OTHER SOURCE
17a. I.D. NUMBER OF REFERRING PHYSICIAN
18. HOSPITALIZATION DATES RELATED TO CURRENT SERVICES MM | DD | YY FROM MM | DD | YY TO
19. RESERVED FOR LOCAL USE
20. OUTSIDE LAB? YES NO $ CHARGES
21. DIAGNOSIS OR NATURE OF ILLNESS OR INJURY. (RELATE ITEMS 1,2,3 OR 4 TO ITEM 24E BY LINE)
1. 3.
2. 4.
22. MEDICAID RESUBMISSION CODE ORIGINAL REF. NO.
23. PRIOR AUTHORIZATION NUMBER
24. A DATE(S) OF SERVICE From MM DD YY To MM DD YY | B Place of Service | C Type of Service | D PROCEDURES, SERVICES, OR SUPPLIES (Explain Unusual Circumstances) CPT/HCPCS MODIFIER | E DIAGNOSIS CODE | F $ CHARGES | G DAYS OR UNITS | H EPSDT Family Plan | I EMG | J COB | K RESERVED FOR LOCAL USE

FIGURE 12–7 Section of the CMS-1500 claim form with Block 23 emphasized indicating where to insert a certificate number for laboratory services (CLIA No.) or a prior authorization number for a procedure when permission has been granted.

form (Figure 12–7). Physicians billing patients for outside laboratory work are not held to these standards but may charge the patient only what the laboratory charges (based on a fee schedule), plus any additional services the physician provides (e.g., drawing, handling, shipping, and interpretation of the blood or office visit).

PAYMENT FUNDAMENTALS

Provider

Participating Physician

In a **participating physician (par)** agreement, a physician agrees to accept payment from Medicare (80% of the **approved charges**) plus payment from the patient (20% of approved charge) after the $110 deductible has been met (Figure 12–8). The Medicare annual deductible is based on the calendar year, January 1 through December 31. This agreement is referred to as accepting **assignment.** The physician must complete and submit the CMS-1500 claim form to the fiscal intermediary. The assignment of benefits, Block 12, is signed by the patient, the physician indicates that assignment is being accepted by checking "Yes" in Block 27, and the payment goes directly to the physician (Figure 12–9). Physicians, practitioners, and suppliers who fail to submit claims are subject to civil monetary penalties up to $2500 for each claim.

Nonparticipating Physician

A **nonparticipating physician (nonpar)** does not have a signed agreement with Medicare and has an option about assignment. The physician may decline assignment for all services or accept assignment for some services and collect from the patient for other services performed at the same time and place. An exception to this policy is mandatory assignment for clinical laboratory tests and services by physician assistants. Unassigned electronic claims that are denied have no appeal rights.

Nonpar physicians receive only 95% of the Medicare-approved amount. Nonpar physicians may decide on a case-by-case basis whether to accept assignment. If the nonpar physician accepts assignment for a claim, Medicare pays 80% of the nonpar Medicare-approved amount directly to the physician and the physician collects the remaining 20% from the patient. If the nonpar physician does not take assignment on a particular claim, he or she may balance bill the patient 115% of the nonpar rate because Medicare will send the payment to the patient. For example, if the nonpar rate is $100, the provider can balance bill the patient for $115. However, in this case, even though the physician is required to submit the claim to Medicare, the carrier pays the patient directly and the physician therefore must collect his or her entire fee from the patient; thus physicians must "chase the money." Consequently, physicians should evaluate whether the ability to balance bill and collect a higher fee from the patient is worth the potential extra billing and collection costs. Furthermore, some hospitals and states—including Minnesota, Pennsylvania, Vermont, and New York—prohibit or limit balance billing, so physicians must ascertain whether or not these restrictions apply before making a Medicare participation or nonparticipation decision.

Limiting charge is a percentage limit on fees, specified by legislation, that nonpar physicians may bill Medicare beneficiaries above the allowed amount. Nonpar physicians may submit usual and customary fees for assigned claims. Because of these two situations, nonpar physicians usually have a fee schedule that lists

PAYMENT EXAMPLES

	Actual charge	Medicare approved amount*	Deductible	Medicare pays	Beneficiary responsible for	Medicare courtesy adjustment†
Doctor A accepts assignment	$480	$400	$110 already satisfied	$320 (80% of approved amount)	$80 (20% of approved amount)	$80 (difference between actual charge and approved amount)
Doctor B does not accept assignment and charges the limiting amount	$437	$380	$110 already satisfied	$304 (80% of approved amount)	$133 (20% of approved amount [$76] plus difference between limiting charge [actual charge] and approved amount [$57] = $133)	None
Doctor C accepts assignment; however, the patient has not met the deductible amount	$480	$300 ($400 minus the deductible)	$110 has not been met	$240 (80% of approved amount determined after subtracting the deductible)	$160 (deductible plus 20% of approved amount)	$80 (difference between actual charge and approved amount)

*The Medicare approved amount is less for nonparticipating physicians than for participating physicians.
†The courtesy adjustment is the amount credited to the patient's account in the adjustment column. The word "courtesy" implies that Medicare patients are treated well and is preferred to phrases like "not allowed."

FIGURE 12–8 Payment examples for three physicians showing a physician accepting assignment versus not accepting assignment, and the amounts the patient is responsible for paying with deductible satisfied and not met.

both usual fees and limiting charges. Some states have set limiting charges that are more restrictive than Medicare policies. These states are Connecticut, Massachusetts, New York, Ohio, Pennsylvania, Rhode Island, and Vermont. Inquire from the fiscal intermediary of those states for guidelines.

Prior Authorization

For Medicare patients who have additional insurance, many insurance carrier group plans and MCO senior plans require prior authorization for surgical procedures, diagnostic testing, and referrals to specialists. Some of these procedures requiring authorization are on a mandatory list, whereas others are chosen by the regional carrier. The mandatory list is composed of procedures such as:

● Bunionectomy
● Carotid endarterectomy
● Cataract extractions
● Cholecystectomy
● Complex peripheral revascularization
● Coronary artery bypass graft surgery
● Hysterectomy
● Inguinal hernia repair
● Joint replacements (hip, shoulder, or knee)
● Transurethral prostatectomy

Carriers may have a toll-free line to call for authorization, require the completion of a preauthorization form, or require a letter only if there is a dispute over claims payment. Check with the local carrier on its policy for preauthorization.

The prior authorization number is used when billing the Medicare carrier and is entered on the CMS-1500 claim form in Block 23 (see Figure 12–7). If the procedure is not approved, the carrier sends a denial to the physician, patient, and hospital, if applicable. If the procedure is done as an emergency, notify the carrier within the time frame designated by the insurance plan so an authorization can be arranged.

ADVANCE BENEFICIARY NOTICES

Medicare considers the appropriate use of advance beneficiary notices (ABNs) as a compliance issue. Ask the patient to sign an ABN document if you know the service is not covered or if there is a possibility that a service may be denied for medical necessity or limitation of Medicare benefits. A step-by-step procedure of how to complete an ABN form is presented at the end of this chapter.

PLEASE
DO NOT
STAPLE
IN THIS
AREA

APPROVED OMB-0938-008

CARRIER

☐☐☐ PICA

HEALTH INSURANCE CLAIM FORM

PICA ☐☐☐

| 1. MEDICARE | MEDICAID | CHAMPUS | CHAMPVA | GROUP HEALTH PLAN | FECA BLK LUNG | OTHER | 1a. INSURED'S I.D. NUMBER (FOR PROGRAM IN ITEM 1) |
| ☐ (Medicare #) | ☐ (Medicaid #) | ☐ (Sponsor's SSN) | ☐ (VA File #) | ☐ (SSN or ID) | ☐ (SSN) | ☐ (ID) | |

2. PATIENT'S NAME (Last Name, First Name, Middle Inital)

3. PATIENT'S BIRTH DATE MM DD YY   SEX M ☐ F ☐

4. INSURED'S NAME (Last Name, First Name, Middle Initial)

5. PATIENT'S ADDRESS

6. PATIENT RELATIONSHIP TO INSURED
Self ☐ Spouse ☐ Child ☐ Other ☐

7. INSURED'S ADDRESS (No., Street)

CITY   STATE

8. PATIENT STATUS
Single ☐ Married ☐ Other ☐
Employed ☐ Full-Time Student ☐ Part-Time Student ☐

CITY   STATE

ZIP CODE   TELEPHONE (Include Area Code) ( )

ZIP CODE   TELEPHONE (Include Area Code) ( )

9. OTHER INSURED'S NAME (Last Name, First Name, Middle Initial)

10. IS PATIENT'S CONDITION RELATED TO:

11. INSURED'S POLICY GROUP OR FECA NUMBER

a. OTHER INSURED'S POLICY OR GROUP NUMBER

a. EMPLOYMENT? (CURRENT OR PREVIOUS)
☐ YES ☐ NO

a. INSURED'S DATE OF BIRTH MM DD YY   SEX M ☐ F ☐

b. OTHER INSURED'S DATE OF BIRTH MM DD YY   SEX M ☐ F ☐

b. AUTO ACCIDENT?   PLACE (State)
☐ YES ☐ NO

b. EMPLOYER'S NAME OR SCHOOL NAME

c. EMPLOYER'S NAME OR SCHOOL NAME

c. OTHER ACCIDENT?
☐ YES ☐ NO

c. INSURANCE PLAN NAME OR PROGRAM NAME

d. INSURANCE PLAN NAME OR PROGRAM NAME

10d. RESERVED FOR LOCAL USE

d. IS THERE ANOTHER HEALTH BENEFIT PLAN?
☐ YES ☐ NO   If yes, return to and complete item 9 a-d.

READ BACK OF FORM BEFORE COMPLETING & SIGNING THIS FORM.
12. PATIENT'S OR AUTHORIZED PERSON'S SIGNATURE I authorize the release of any medical or other information necessary to process this claim. I also request payment of government benefits either to myself or to the party who accepts assignment below.

SIGNED *SOF*   DATE

13. INSURED'S OR AUTHORIZED PERSON'S SIGNATURE I authorize payment of medical benefits to the undersigned physician or supplier for services described below.

SIGNED

PATIENT AND INSURED INFORMATION

14. DATE OF CURRENT: MM DD YY ILLNESS (First symptom) OR INJURY (Accident) OR PREGNANCY (LMP)

15. IF PATIENT HAS HAD SAME OR SIMILAR ILLNESS. GIVE FIRST DATE MM DD YY

16. DATES PATIENT UNABLE TO WORK IN CURRENT OCCUPATION MM DD YY FROM TO MM DD YY

17. NAME OF REFERRING PHYSICIAN OR OTHER SOURCE

17a. I.D. NUMBER OF REFERRING PHYSICIAN

18. HOSPITALIZATION DATES RELATED TO CURRENT SERVICES MM DD YY FROM TO MM DD YY

19. RESERVED FOR LOCAL USE

20. OUTSIDE LAB? ☐ YES ☐ NO $ CHARGES

21. DIAGNOSIS OR NATURE OF ILLNESS OR INJURY. (RELATE ITEMS 1,2,3 OR 4 TO ITEM 24E BY LINE)
1.   3.
2.   4.

22. MEDICAID RESUBMISSION CODE   ORIGINAL REF. NO.

23. PRIOR AUTHORIZATION NUMBER

24. A DATE(S) OF SERVICE From MM DD YY To MM DD YY	B Place of Service	C Type of Service	D PROCEDURES, SERVICES, OR SUPPLIES (Explain Unusual Circumstances) CPT/HCPCS	MODIFIER	E DIAGNOSIS CODE	F $ CHARGES	G DAYS OR UNITS	H EPSDT Family Plan	I EMG	J COB	K RESERVED FOR LOCAL USE
1											
2											
3											
4											
5											
6											

PHYSICIAN OR SUPPLIER INFORMATION

25. FEDERAL TAX I.D. NUMBER ☐ SSN ☐ EIN

26. PATIENT'S ACCOUNT NO.

27. ACCEPT ASSIGNMENT? (For govt. claims, see back) ☒ YES ☐ NO

28. TOTAL CHARGE $

29. AMOUNT PAID $

30. BALANCE DUE $

31. SIGNATURE OF PHYSICIAN OR SUPPLIER INCLUDING DEGREES OR CREDENTIALS (I certify that the statements on the reverse apply to this bill and are made a part thereof.)

SIGNED   DATE

32. NAME AND ADDRESS OF FACILITY WHERE SERVICES WERE RENDERED (If other than home or office)

33. PHYSICIAN'S, SUPPLIER'S BILLING NAME, ADDRESS, ZIP CODE & PHONE #

PIN#   GRP#

(APPROVED BY AMA COUNCIL ON MEDICAL SERVICE 8/88)

FORM HCFA-1500 (12-90)
FORM OWCP-1500   FORM RRB-1500

FIGURE 12–9 Block 12 of the CMS-1500 claim form where the patient signs authorizing payment to be sent to the physician and Block 27 marked with an X showing that the physician accepts Medicare assignment of benefits.

Waiver of Liability Provision

Limited Liability

When a patient is to receive a service from a participating physician that might be denied for **medical necessity** or because of *limitation of liability* by Medicare, inform the patient and have him or her agree to pay for the denied service in advance. If the Medicare guidelines or parameters are not known for a certain procedure or service, refer to *Medicare transmittals* (formerly called program memorandums) or call the Medicare carrier and ask. Some medical practices use a computerized method to screen for the medical necessity of a service but must have access to national coverage determinations (NCDs) and local coverage decisions (formerly called local medical review policies, or LMRPs) to find out if there is limited coverage.

If you expect Medicare to deny payment (entirely or in part) instruct the patient to sign an **advance beneficiary notice (ABN),** also known as a waiver of liability agreement or responsibility statement, as shown in Figures 12–10 and 12–11. This form should not be given to someone

---

Patient Name: *Mary Judd*   Medicare # (HICN): 432XX1234

ADVANCE BENEFICIARY NOTICE (ABN)

Note: You need to make a choice about receiving these health care items or services.

We expect that Medicare will not pay for the item(s) or service(s) that are described below. Medicare does not pay for all of your health care costs. Medicare only pays for covered items and services when Medicare rules are met. The fact that Medicare may not pay for a particular item or service does not mean that you should not receive it. There may be a good reason your doctor recommended it. Right now, in your case, **Medicare probably will not pay for –**

Items or Services: *B12 injections*

Because: *Medicare does not usually pay for this injection or this many injections.*

The purpose of this form is to help you make an informed choice about whether or not you want to receive these items or services, knowing that you might have to pay for them yourself.
Before you make a decision about your options, you should **read this entire notice carefully.**
- Ask us to explain, if you don't understand why Medicare probably won't pay.
- Ask us how much these items or services will cost you (**Estimated Cost**: $35.00), in case you have to pay for them yourself or through other insurance.

PLEASE CHOOSE **ONE** OPTION. CHECK **ONE** BOX. **SIGN & DATE** YOUR CHOICE.

☒ **Option 1. YES.** **I want to receive these items or services.**
I understand that Medicare will not decide whether to pay unless I receive these items or services. Please submit my claim to Medicare. I understand that you may bill me for items or services and that I may have to pay the bill while Medicare is making its decision.
If Medicare does pay, you will refund to me any payments I made to you that are due to me.
If Medicare denies payment, I agree to be personally and fully responsible for payment.
That is, I will pay personally, either out of pocket or through any other insurance that I have.
I understand I can appeal Medicare's decison.

☐ **Option 2. NO.** **I have decided not to receive these items or services.**
I will not receive these items or services. I understand that you will not be able to submit a claim to Medicare and that I will not be able to appeal your opinion that Medicare will not pay.

March 20, 20XX
Date

Mary Judd
Signature of patient or person acting on patient's behalf

NOTE: Your health information will be kept confidential. Any information that we collect about you on this form will be kept confidential in our offices. If a claim is submitted to Medicare, your health information on this form may be shared with Medicare. Your health information, which Medicare sees, will be kept confidential by Medicare.

OMB Approval No. 0938-0566   Form No. CMS-R-131-G   (June 2002)

FIGURE 12–10 Advance beneficiary notice, which is also known as a responsibility statement or waiver of liability agreement.

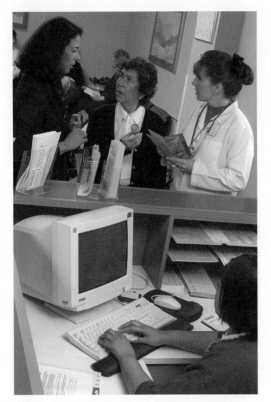

FIGURE 12–11 Insurance billing specialist instructing an elderly patient to sign an Advance Notice Medicare Beneficiary Waiver of Liability Agreement for services not covered.

who is in a medical emergency, confused, legally incompetent, or otherwise under great duress. It cannot be signed after a patient has received the service and must specifically state what service or procedure is being waived. Write the specific time frequency limitation for a particular service, such as screening colonoscopy once every 10 years. Each space on the ABN must be completed before providing the ABN to the patient. Blank or partially completed ABNs, even with the patient's signature, are not acceptable. An ABN may be mailed to a patient when presenting it face-to-face is not possible, but the patient must have an opportunity to ask questions. When the ABN is mailed, it should be sent with a cover letter explaining that the procedure will be denied by Medicare and include contact information so the patient can ask questions before the procedure.

To determine which services require an ABN, refer to the National Coverage Determinations and the Local Coverage Decisions (LCDs), formerly known as Local Medical Review Policies (LMRPs) from the insurance carrier. An office policy should be in place for handling patients who refuse to sign an ABN. When sending in a claim, the Healthcare Common Procedure Coding System (HCPCS) level II modifier -GA (waiver of liability on file)

must be added to pertinent codes to indicate a patient has signed the waiver. The Medicare carrier then informs the patient that he or she is responsible for the fee. Keep this signed waiver with other patient financial documents and not with the patient's health record.

If the service was not reasonable because of Medicare guidelines but the patient thought it was covered and there is no advance notice given with signed waiver of liability agreement, then:

● Neither Medicare nor the patient can be collected from.
● The patient does not have to pay the deductible or coinsurance.
● The patient is refunded any amount paid to the provider on the item or service.

If assignment is accepted and the physician and patient thought the service was covered under reasonable assumptions, then:

● Medicare is billed to pay for the service.
● The patient must pay the deductible and coinsurance.
● Medicare will not seek a refund of money already paid to the physician.

Nonparticipating providers must refund any amount collected from the beneficiary when services are later found to be not reasonable and necessary.

Noncovered Services

Do not get confused with the issue of *noncovered* Medicare services because these may always be billed to the patient. Do not give a patient an ABN when a service is never covered by Medicare. Instead give those patients a different form, the Notice of Exclusions of Medicare Benefits (NEMB) (Figure 12–12). This form clearly states that the service is never covered by Medicare and the patient is responsible for payment. It is not a requirement to give the patient an NEMB for a never-covered service in order to bill the patient but use of the form makes it clear before the procedure is done that he or she must pay for it. Services denied as inclusive of another service (a payment already made for the other service) are not considered a noncovered item and may not be billed to the patient. If a formal denial is necessary to bill the patient or another insurer, a claim should be sent with a letter attached stating the need for the denial to bill another payer; otherwise to bill for a noncovered service is inappropriate and may be viewed as fraud.

Elective Surgery Estimate

Effective October 1, 1987, under the Tax Reform Act, a nonparticipating physician who does not accept assignment for an *elective surgery* for which the actual charge

NOTICE OF EXCLUSIONS FROM MEDICARE BENEFITS (NEMB)

There are items and services for which Medicare <u>will not pay</u>.

- Medicare does **not** pay for all of your health care costs. Medicare only pays for covered benefits. **Some items and services are not Medicare benefits and Medicare will not pay for them.**

- When you receive an item or service that is **not** a Medicare benefit, **you are responsible to pay for it,** personally or through any other insurance that you may have.

> The purpose of this notice is to help you make an informed choice about whether or not you want to receive these items or services, knowing that you will have to pay for them yourself. **Before you make a decision, you should read this entire notice carefully.**
> Ask us to explain, if you don't understand why Medicare won't pay.
> Ask us how much these items or services will cost you (**Estimated Cost: $_____**).

Medicare will not pay for: _____

_____ ;

☐ **1.** **Because it does not meet the definition of any Medicare benefit.**

☐ **2.** **Because of the following exclusion * from Medicare benefits:**

☐ Personal comfort items.	☐ Routine physicals and most tests for screening.
☐ Most shots (vaccinations).	☐ Routine eye care, eyeglasses and examinations.
☐ Hearing aids and hearing examinations.	☐ Cosmetic surgery.
☐ Most outpatient prescription drugs.	☐ Dental care and dentures (in most cases).
☐ Orthopedic shoes and foot supports (orthotics).	☐ Routine foot care and flat foot care.
☐ Health care received outside of the USA.	☐ Services by immediate relatives.
☐ Services required as a result of war.	☐ Services under a physician's private contract.

- ☐ Services paid for by a governmental entity that is not Medicare.
- ☐ Services for which the patient has no legal obligation to pay.
- ☐ Home health services furnished under a plan of care, if the agency does not submit the claim.
- ☐ Items and services excluded under the Assisted Suicide Funding Restriction Act of 1997.
- ☐ Items or services furnished in a competitive acquisition area by any entity that does not have a contract with the Department of Health and Human Services (except in a case of urgent need).
- ☐ Physicians' services performed by a physician assistant, midwife, psychologist, or nurse anesthetist, when furnished to an inpatient, unless they are furnished under arrangements by the hospital.
- ☐ Items and services furnished to an individual who is a resident of a skilled nursing facility (a SNF) or of a part of a facility that includes a SNF, unless they are furnished under arrangements by the SNF.
- ☐ Services of an assistant at surgery without prior approval from the peer review organization.
- ☐ Outpatient occupational and physical therapy services furnished incident to a physician's services.

* This is only a general summary of exclusions from Medicare benefits. It is not a legal document. The official Medicare program provisions are contained in relevant laws, regulations, and rulings.

FIGURE 12–12 Notice of Exclusions from Medicare Benefits (NEMB) form.

will be $500 or more must provide the beneficiary with the following in writing: (1) the estimated fee for the procedure, (2) the estimated Medicare-approved allowance for the procedure, and (3) the difference in the physician's actual charge (limiting charge and the allowed amount) (Figure 12–13). *Elective surgery* means a surgical procedure that can be scheduled in advance, is not an emergency, and is discretionary on the part of the physician and the patient. Failure to undergo elective surgery does

not pose a mortality threat. Give a copy of the estimation letter to the Medicare patient and keep the original for the files. Document the patient's acknowledgment by obtaining his or her signature at the bottom of the letter.

Prepayment Screens

On some procedures, Medicare limits the number of times a given procedure can be billed during 1 year (e.g., four

**WORKSHEET FOR
ESTIMATED MEDICARE PAYMENT FOR ELECTIVE SURGERY**

Worksheet

1. Physician's actual fee (limiting charge) .... $ 1248.03
2. Medicare approved or allowed amount .... $ 1085.24
3. Difference between physician's actual fee and
   Medicare approved or allowed amount .... – 162.79
   (1 – 2 = 0)
4. Twenty percent coinsurance (0.20 × 2 = 0) .... + 217.05
5. Beneficiary's out-of-pocket expense (3 + 4 + 0) .... $ 379.84
   Assume the $110 deductible has been met

Items 1, 2, and 5 must be included in the letter to the beneficiary

A

Beneficiary Letter

Dear Patient:

Because I do not accept assignment for elective surgery, Medicare requires that I give you certain information before surgery when my charges are $500 or more.

The following information concerns the surgery we have discussed. These estimates assume that you have already met the $110 deductible.

Type of surgery ...... Osteotomy, proximal left tibia
Limiting charge $ 1248.03
Medicare estimated payment $ 868.19
Patient's estimated payment $ 379.84

This estimate is based upon our present expectations of what surgical procedure(s) will be required. Please remember that this is only an estimate of charges; we cannot be sure that additional procedures will or will not be necessary.

Sincerely,

John Doe, M.D.
Medicare Provider Number 126XX5479

I understand the foregoing physician charges and my financial responsibility with respect to those estimated charges.

Patient's Signature .... *Jane Doe* .... Date 5-18-20XX
                                Jane Doe

B

FIGURE 12–13 **A,** Worksheet. **B,** sample beneficiary letter for estimated Medicare payment for elective surgery.

office visits per month or one treatment every 60 days for routine foot care). This is known as a Medicare Prepayment Screen. The screens or flags are computer triggers that suspend processing. These screens are used to identify and review claims for medical necessity and determine compliance with other appropriate criteria. The suspended claim is checked by a reviewer who decides whether the services are medically necessary. If the patient previously submitted a claim for the procedure performed in the same year by another physician and has met the limit for the year, the claim will be downcoded or denied. Refer to the local Medicare fiscal agent's transmittals (formerly known as program memorandums) or contact them for a complete list of the Medicare prepayment screens, which are applicable locally.

To avoid problems, use good procedure code guidelines discussed in Chapter 6 and adhere to the following criteria:

● The level of service is appropriate to documentation.
● The procedure is accurate to the gender of the patient.
● The frequency is appropriate.
● The diagnosis and procedure match.
● The provider has certification for performing services (e.g., laboratories).
● The fee is within the Medicare-approved charge.

Correct Coding Initiative

Medicare's **Correct Coding Initiative (CCI)** is implemented by CMS in an attempt to eliminate unbundling or other inappropriate reporting of Current Procedural Terminology (CPT) codes. As you may recall, *unbundling* is coding and billing numerous CPT codes to identify procedures that usually are described by a single code. Coding conflicts are picked up and claims are reviewed, suspended, or denied when conflicts occur. Software is available to give physicians, private insurance companies, and billing services access to the same government database used in auditing physicians for improper use of CPT codes. It is currently available on the CMS Web site at no charge. Refer to the Internet Resources at the end of this chapter.

MEDICARE REIMBURSEMENT

Chronology of Payment

For many years, Medicare payments were based on reasonable fees (e.g., the amounts approved by the Medicare carrier [fiscal agents]). Medicare paid 80% of the approved charge. On October 1, 1983, an important development in the Medicare Part A program, the **prospective payment system (PPS),** became effective. Under the regulations enacted by the Social Security Amendments of 1983, hospitals treating Medicare patients are reimbursed according to preestablished rates for each type of illness treated based on diagnosis. Payments to hospitals for Medicare services are classified according to more than 500 diagnosis-related group (DRG) numbers. Beneficiaries (patients) cannot be billed beyond the preestablished DRG rate except for normal deductible and copayment amounts. (See Chapter 17 for an in-depth discussion of DRGs.)

In 1984, the Deficit Reduction Act established a participating physician program that offered incentives to participating physicians and froze the fees of nonparticipating physicians. The 1987 Omnibus Budget Reconciliation Act (OBRA) introduced the maximum allowable actual charge (MAAC) formula, which developed the maximum fee (limiting charge) that a nonpar physician could charge Medicare patients for each service.

Reasonable Fee

Reasonable fee is the amount that Medicare participating providers agree to accept. It is listed on the RA, formerly known as the EOB, as an allowed (approved) charge for a procedure. This charge may be higher or lower than the fee the physician lists on the claim. When a physician accepts assignment, he or she may bill the patient only 20% of the Medicare-allowed charge. Charging for completion and submission of a claim form on an assignment claim violates the terms of the assignment. Interest fees cannot be assessed to Medicare patients.

It is permissible to collect the deductible at the time of service if you know how much of the deductible has already been paid; but the Medicare copayment should not be collected until Medicare pays.

Mandatory assignment laws have been adopted in several states, and legislation is under consideration and pending in many more states. These state laws would require physicians to accept the approved charge for their Medicare patients as a condition for being licensed to practice medicine in the state. Arkansas, Florida, Illinois, Maryland, Montana, and New Hampshire have rejected mandatory assignment proposals.

Resource-Based Relative Value Scale

As mentioned in Chapter 6, a **resource-based relative value scale (RBRVS)** is the system Medicare uses for establishing fees. This system takes into account work, overhead expense, and malpractice values for all CPT codes that are published in the *Federal Register* each November. These are adjusted for each Medicare local carrier by geographic practice cost indices (GPCI) by using a formula that gives the total value for a code.

The formula for obtaining the allowed amount of a given service or procedure is to choose an HCPCS/CPT code and use the **relative value unit (RVU)** amounts listed in the *Federal Register* for work value, practice expense, and malpractice value and multiply each of those by the GPCI. Then to obtain the total adjusted RVU, add the three amounts together. Finally, to discover the allowed amount for this code, multiply the annual Medicare conversion factor (CF) by the HCPCS/CPT code's total adjusted RVU amount. For a graphic illustration of this formula, see Figure 6–2. To give you experience in using this formula, do the assignments relating to RBRVS for this chapter in the *Workbook.*

Healthcare Common Procedure Coding System (HCPCS)

As mentioned in Chapter 6, the federal government developed the Healthcare Common Procedure Coding System (HCPCS) for the Medicare program. To obtain correct payment for a procedure or service, a code number must be selected from level I or II of HCPCS coding system. When submitting a claim, be sure to use the level II HCPCS **national alphanumeric codes** and modifiers rather than CPT procedure codes for certain appliances and procedures when indicated. When billing CPT modifiers, a good reference is presented in Table 6–4, as helpful hints in italics entitled "Medicare Payment Rule."

CLAIM SUBMISSION

Local Coverage Determination

Local Coverage Determination (LCD), formerly known as Local Medical Review Policy (LMRP), is a decision by a fiscal intermediary or carrier whether to cover a particular service on a contractor-wide basis in accordance with the Social Security Act (SSA) (i.e., a determination as to whether the service is reasonable and necessary). LCD is an educational and administrative tool to assist physicians, providers, and suppliers in submitting correct claims for payment. Contractor medical directors and staff develop LCDs with input from the public. LCDs list covered and noncovered codes for a given Medicare policy but do not include any of the coding guidance that were found in LMRPs. LCDs outline how contractors will review claims to determine whether Medicare coverage requirements have been met. CMS requires that local policies be consistent with national guidance. Use of LCDs helps avoid situations in which claims are paid or denied without a full understanding of the basis for payment and denial. LCDs may be obtained from the Medicare carrier Web site at www.cms.hhs.gov/mcd.

Fiscal Intermediaries and Fiscal Agents

An organization handling claims from hospitals, NFs, **intermediate care facilities (ICFs),** long-term care facilities (LTCFs), and home health agencies is called a **fiscal intermediary (FI).** The National Blue Cross Association holds the fiscal intermediary contract for Medicare Part A; in turn, it subcontracts it out to member agencies.

Organizations handling claims from physicians and other suppliers of services covered under Medicare Part B are called *carriers* or *fiscal agents.* Medicare Part B payments are handled by private insurance organizations under contract with the government. Since January 1, 1992, the rule for where to send a Medicare claim is to bill the carrier who covers the area where the service occurred or was furnished, not the carrier who services the physician's office.

See Internet Resources at the end of this chapter to go to the Web site for the names and addresses for claims submission in each state and to obtain further information about this program.

Provider Identification Numbers

Another requirement of the Tax Reform Act was the establishment of several types of identification numbers for each physician and nonphysician practitioner providing services paid by Medicare. Because there are so many numbers, they are easily confused and end up being the source of many errors when completing blocks on the CMS-1500 claim form. The numbers defined and shown in template examples with correct placement in Chapter 7 follow:

- Provider identification numbers (PINs), group and individual. With the implementation of the National Provider Identifier on May 23, 2007, PINs will no longer be used.
- Unique physician identification numbers (UPINs). With the implementation of the National Provider Identifier on May 23, 2007, UPINs will no longer be used.
- National provider identifier (NPI) scheduled to be implemented on May 23, 2007.
- Durable Medical Equipment (DME) supplier number.

Patient's Signature Authorization

A Medicare patient's signature authorization for release of medical information and assignment of benefits to the insurance carrier is obtained in Block 12 of the CMS-1500 claim form. This block should be signed regardless of whether the physician is a participating or nonparticipating physician. The signed authorization should be kept on file in the patient's health record for an episode of care or for a designated time frame (e.g., 1 year or lifetime). Subsequent claims may then indicate "Signature on file" or "SOF" in Block 12 of the claim form. The lifetime beneficiary claim authorization and information release form shown in Figure 12–14 is an example that can be used for assigned and nonassigned Medicare claims and kept in the patient's health record. An original copy of a CMS-1500 claim form may be used to obtain a lifetime signature authorization. Write across the top of the form "Lifetime Signature Authorization" and file as just described. Further information on this topic may be found in Chapters 4 and 7.

Signature on file situations that may occur in a medical practice are follow:

- Illiterate or physically handicapped. When an illiterate or physically handicapped enrollee signs by mark (X), a witness should sign his or her name and address next to the mark. If the claim is filed for the patient by another person, that person should enter the patient's name and write "By," sign his or her own name and address, indicate relationship to the patient, and state why the patient cannot sign.
- Confinement in a facility. Sometimes it is not possible to obtain the signature of a Medicare patient because of confinement in a nursing facility, hospital, or home. In such cases, physicians should obtain a lifetime signature authorization from the patient.

College Clinic
4567 Broad Avenue
Woodland Hills, XY 12345-0001
Tel (555) 486-9002
Fax (555) 487-8976

LIFETIME BENEFICIARY CLAIM AUTHORIZATION AND INFORMATION RELEASE

Patient's
Name _____ Jane Doe _____ Medicare I.D. number _____ 540-XX-8755A

I request that payment of authorized Medicare benefits be made either to me or on my behalf to (name of physician/supplier) for any services furnished me by that physician/supplier. I authorize any holder of medical information about me to release to the Center for Medicare and Medicaid Services and its agents any information needed to determine these benefits or the benefits payable to related services.

I understand my signature requests that payment be made, and I consent to the release of medical information necessary to pay the claim. If other health insurance is indicated in Item 9 of the CMS-1500 claim form or elsewhere on other approved claim forms or electronically submitted claims, my signature authorizes release of the information to the insurer or agency shown. In Medicare assigned cases, the physician or supplier agrees to accept the allowed amount of the Medicare carrier as the full charge, and the patient is responsible only for the deductible, coinsurance, and noncovered services. Coinsurance is based upon the allowed amount of the Medicare carrier.

_____ Jane Doe _____   _____ January 3, 20XX _____
Patient's Signature   Date

FIGURE 12–14 Lifetime Assignment of Benefits and Information Release.

- Medigap claim. When submitting a crossover claim to a Medigap carrier, obtain a lifetime signature authorization for the Medigap carrier.
- Deceased patient. Refer to Deceased Patient Claims later in this chapter for signature requirements.
- Medicare/Medicaid (Medi-Medi) claim. These crossover claims do not require the patient's signature.

Time Limit

The *time limit* for sending in claims is the end of the calendar year after the fiscal year in which services were furnished. The fiscal year for claims begins October 1 and ends September 30 (see the following box).

For services furnished on:	The time limit for filing is:
October 1, 2004, to September 30, 2005	December 31, 2006
October 1, 2005, to September 30, 2006	December 31, 2007

On assigned claims, the provider may file without penalty up to 27 months after providing service if reasonable cause for the delay is shown to the insurance carrier. Otherwise there is a 10% reduction in the reimbursement. On unassigned claims, the provider may be fined up to $2000 for delinquent claim submission or be dropped from Medicare. When submitting a late claim, ask the fiscal intermediary for the guidelines that CMS considers reasonable cause for delay.

Paper Claims

The form that physicians use to submit paper claims to Medicare is the CMS-1500. Refer to Chapter 7 for instructions on how to complete the CMS-1500 claim form for the Medicare program. The reference templates for Medicare and supplemental coverage shown at the end of that chapter are as follows:

- Medicare, no secondary coverage: Figure 7–9
- Medicare/Medicaid, crossover: Figure 7–10
- Medicare/Medigap, crossover: Figure 7–11
- Other insurance/Medicare MSP: Figure 7–12

Patients are not allowed to submit claims to Medicare (with four exceptions). Situations when a patient may file a claim are the following:

- Services covered by Medicare for which the patient has other insurance that should pay first; called MSP
- Services provided by a physician who refuses to submit the claim
- Services provided outside the United States
- Situations where durable medical equipment is purchased from a private source

Medicare claim status is also explained in detail in Chapter 7 (e.g., clean, incomplete, rejected, dirty, and other claims). To obtain the mailing address for sending Medicare claim forms for your state or county, go to the Internet Web site http://www.cms.hhs.gov/contacts/incardir.asp. For further information and booklets, pamphlets, and the annual *Medicare Handbook*, contact the nearest Social Security office.

Electronic Claims

Medicare requests that all providers submit claims electronically. All electronic transmission formats are scheduled to be standardized by the use of ANSI ASC X12N (837) Version 4010. Refer to Chapter 8 on how to transmit claims electronically to the Medicare carrier.

Medicare/Medicaid Claims

Medi-Medi patients qualify for the benefits of Medicare and Medicaid. Use the CMS-1500 claim form and check "Yes" for the assignment in Block 27. If the physician does not accept assignment, then payment goes to the patient and Medicaid (in California Medi-Cal) will not pick up the residual. The CMS-1500 claim form will be crossed over and processed automatically by Medicaid after processing is completed by Medicare. The fiscal intermediary may refer to this as a **crossover claim,** or *claims transfer*. It is not necessary to submit another form. Claims should be sent according to the time limit designated by the Medicaid program in the state. Generally the Medicare payment exceeds the Medicaid fee schedule, and little or no payment is received except when the patient has not met his or her annual Medicare deductible.

In some states, the fiscal intermediary for a crossover claim may have a different address from that used for the processing of a patient who is on Medicare only. Write or call the nearest Medicare fiscal intermediary for the guidelines pertinent to the state.

Medicare/Medigap Claims

Medicare has streamlined the processing of Medicare/Medigap claims in most states. Medicare carriers transmit Medigap claims electronically for participating physicians, thus eliminating the need to file an additional claim. This is also called a *crossover claim*. Medigap payments go directly to the participating physicians, and a Medicare Summary Notice is sent to the patient that states "This claim has been referred to your supplemental carrier for any additional benefits."

To assure the crossover of the Medicare/Medigap claim, complete Blocks 9 through 9d of the CMS-1500 claim form and list the PAYRID number of the Medigap plan in Block 9d. The PAYRID for Medigap plans is referred to as the Other Carrier Name and Address (OCNA) number, and a list of all OCNAs is published in the Medicare newsletter.

If automatic crossover capabilities are not offered in one's state, attach the Medicare RA to the claim form and submit a claim to the Medigap plan separately.

Refer to Figure 7–11 for submitting claims when Medicare is primary and the patient has a Medigap (supplemental) policy.

Medicare/Employer Supplemental Insurance Claims

Some individuals have supplemental coverage with complementary benefits by employment plans even after retirement. In some cases, this coverage may be paid by a former employer after retirement. Usually crossover relationships exist with many insurance carriers who insure Medicare beneficiaries.

Medicare/Supplemental and MSP Claims

Completing the CMS-1500 claim form for a Medicare patient who has supplemental insurance can be confusing. First, decide whether the case is Medicare primary or secondary payer. If Medicare is primary and the secondary payer is a Medigap policy, follow Medicare/Medigap processing guidelines. After determining who is primary, follow the directions on what should be entered in each block of the CMS-1500 claim form, depending on the primary payer, or follow MSP guidelines.

Templates shown at the end of Chapter 7 make it easier to learn which blocks to complete and which to ignore, depending on the primary and secondary payer. Figure 7–12 is for billing other insurance primary and Medicare secondary (MSP). A copy of the front and back sides of the primary insurance's EOB document must be attached to the claim when billing Medicare.

See Chapter 7 for general instructions for completing claims in Medicare and Medicare secondary payer cases.

Deceased Patients Claims

There are two ways in which to submit billing for a patient who has died:

1. Participating physician accepts assignment on the claim form. This results in the quickest payment. No signature by a family member is needed on the CMS-1500 claim form. Type "Patient died on

(indicate date)" in Block 12 where the patient's signature is necessary.

2. The nonparticipating physician does not accept assignment, bills Medicare, and submits the following:
   a. A CMS-1500 claim form signed by the estate representative who is responsible for the bill
   b. A statement or claim for all services provided
   c. Name and address of the responsible party
   d. Provider's statement, signed and dated, refusing to accept assignment

Nothing can be done about the open balance on the account until the estate is settled, and then Medicare will pay.

Physician Substitute Coverage

Many times special substitute coverage arrangements are made between physicians (e.g., on-call, vacation, or unavailable because of another commitment). These arrangements are referred to as either reciprocal for on-call situations or *locum tenens* for a vacation situation. Specific modifiers are used to distinguish these situations, and special billing guidelines are stated as follows:

● *Reciprocal arrangement.* When submitting Medicare claims, the regular physician must identify the service provided by the *substitute* doctor by listing the -Q5 modifier after the procedure code.
● *Locum tenens arrangement.* When submitting Medicare claims, the *regular* physician must identify the service provided by the *substitute* doctor by listing the -Q6 modifier after the procedure code.

AFTER CLAIM SUBMISSION

Remittance Advice

Medicare sends a payment check and a nationally standardized document to participating physicians called a Medicare **remittance advice (RA),** formerly known as an explanation of Medicare benefits (EOMB). On the front side of the RA are status codes that are the same nationwide, representing the reason a claim may not have been paid in full or was denied, and so forth. These codes are defined on the reverse side of the RA. If the patient has Medigap, supplementary, or complementary crossover coverage, the "other payer" statement will say whether the claim has been transferred to the supplemental insurer.

Nonparticipating physicians also receive an RA with payment information about unassigned claims. The RA will separate payment information about assigned claims from unassigned claims to avoid posting errors by the practice. Check the payment against the fee schedule to determine whether the benefits are for the correct amount. On each claim form, note the date the payment is posted for reference. Optional items to document are amount of payment, RA processing data, and batch number.

Offices transmitting claims electronically receive an electronic remittance advice (ERA) showing payment data, and this may be automatically uploaded into the office computer system. The ERA electronically posts payments, and the provider does not have to manually post them. Paper and electronic remittance notices have the same format.

Medicare Summary Notice

A patient is mailed a similar document called a **Medicare summary notice (MSN).** This document is designed to be easier for the patient to understand, but because many patients do not know what is meant by *amount charged, Medicare approved, deductible,* and *coinsurance,* it often becomes necessary for the insurance billing specialist to educate the patient. First, photocopy an RA to be used as an example, deleting the patient's name to ensure confidentiality. Then use the RA to illustrate to future patients what various terms mean. This will increase patient understanding and save time.

When a claim is denied the MSN will identify the number of the Local Medical Review Policy (LMRP), Local Coverage Decision (LCD), or National Coverage Decision (NCD) used in denial of the claim.

BENEFICIARY REPRESENTATIVE/REPRESENTATIVE PAYEE

Medicare beneficiaries may have memory impairment or may be confined to a wheelchair or bed so they have a legal right to appoint an individual to serve as their representative.

Claims assistance professionals (CAPs) act as client representatives. They have some legal standing and are recognized by Medicare to act on the beneficiary's behalf if the beneficiary completes a Beneficiary Representative Form SSA-1696. This form is available from the Social Security district office. Copies of the completed form should be sent to the Medicare intermediary or carrier when appropriate.

In contrast, a representative payee is an individual or organization chosen by the SSA to receive and administer SSA benefit funds on behalf of the beneficiary. Other duties consist of assisting the beneficiary with check writing for financial obligations, such as personal care and maintenance, housing, medical service expenses, and investing any surplus monies for the beneficiary's benefit. A representative payee is responsible for using payments received only for the benefit of the beneficiary, accounting for the benefits received on request, and contacting SSA when anything affects eligibility for SSA benefits or prevents the representative payee's ability to perform these responsibilities. Additional information on CAPs is found in Chapters 1 and 18.

Posting Payments

Usually a physician's charge is higher than the charge approved by the Medicare carrier or fiscal agent. This does not mean that his or her charges are unreasonable. As mentioned, payments are established using a fee schedule based on an RBRVS, a **volume performance standard (VPS)** for expenditure increases, and a *limiting charge* for nonparticipating physicians. *Volume performance standard* is the desired growth rate for spending on Medicare Part B physician services that is set each year by Congress.

Because some services may be disallowed or the payments on them may be lower than those charged by the physician, know how to post payments to the patient's financial accounting record card or computerized account. Figure 12–15 illustrates how payments and courtesy adjustments are posted. The word "courtesy" implies that Medicare patients are treated well and is preferred to phrases like "not allowed" or "write-off."

Medicare does not allow for the standardized waiving of copayments. Medicare regulations require that a patient be billed for the copayment at least three times before the balance is adjusted off as uncollectable. Document this as further justification if the patient is suffering financial hardship.

When an RA is received, it may list many patients (Figure 12–16). Do not post the entire payment made in a lump sum to the daysheet. Individually post each line item paid to the patient's financial accounting record card or computerized account and to the daysheet (Figure 12–17). To prevent funds from going astray, some offices prefer to post Medicare payments to a separate daysheet and deposit each multiple reimbursement check separately. The daysheet totals will then agree with the deposit slip totals and not get confused with other monies collected.

Figure 12–18, *A*, illustrates an example of a Medicare/Medicaid case after payment by Medicare. Medicare applied the patient's full $110 deductible amount to the Medicare allowed amount, reducing payment to $4. The Medicaid RA (see Figure 12–18, *B*) shows reimbursement of the coinsurance and deductible amounts dual-billed to Medicaid.

Calculations are shown in the following box:

Medicare		Medicaid	
$115	Allowed amount	$115	Medicare allowed
−110	Deductible		amount
$ 5	Balance on which	−32	Medicaid cutback
	payment is	$ 83	Medicaid allowed
× .80	calculated		
$ 4	Medicare paid 80%	−4	Medicare paid
		$ 79	Medicaid payment

When referring to the Medicaid program, a *cutback* means a reduction, that is, reducing Medicare's allowable charges to Medicaid's allowable charges. This would require an adjustment entry on the patient's financial accounting record. Cutbacks are common on Medicaid claims.

Medicare overpayments can occur in the following situations:

● The carrier processes the charge more than once.
● The physician receives duplicate payments from Medicare and a secondary payer.
● The physician is paid directly on an unassigned claim.
● The item is not covered but is paid.
● The payment is made on erroneous information.

If an overpayment check is received, deposit the check and then write to Medicare notifying them of the overpayment. Include a copy of the check and the RA. This overpayment will be deducted from the next Medicare payment and will be shown on the RA. If the physician wishes to repay a Medicare overpayment on the installment plan, Financial Statement of Debtor CMS-379 form may be used. This form is sent to the physician when the carrier notifies the physician that money is due back.

Refer to Chapter 9 for additional information about EOB documents from private insurance carriers.

Review and Redetermination Process

Chapter 9 outlines in detail the steps to take for having a claim reviewed and the process of appealing a claim in the Medicare program.

STATEMENT

College Clinic
4567 Broad Avenue
Woodland Hills, XY 12345-0001
Telephone: 555-486-9002
Fax: 555-487-8976

Account No. 946
John Smith
100 James Street
Woodland Hills, XY 12345-0001

DATE	PROFESSIONAL SERVICE DESCRIPTION	CHARGE		CREDITS		CURRENT BALANCE	
				PAYMENTS	ADJUSTMENTS		
2-15-xx	Surgery	800	00			800	00
2-17-xx	Medicare/Medigap billed (2-15-xx)					800	00
4-2-xx	Medicare payment voucher #12498 (2-15-xx)			440 00		360	00
4-12-xx	Medigap payment voucher #45500 (2-15-xx)			110 00		250	00
4-12-xx	Medicare courtesy (adjustment 2-15-xx)				250 00	-0-	

Due and payable within 10 days   **Pay last amount in balance column** ⇧

Key: PF: Problem-focused   SF: Straightforward   CON: Consultation   HCD: House Call (Day)
   EPF: Expanded problem-focused   LC: Low complexity   CPX: Complete Phys Exam   HCN: House Call (Night)
      D: Detailed   MC: Moderate complexity   E: Emergency   HV: Hospital visit
      C: Comprehensive   HC: High complexity   ER: Emergency Dept.   OV: Office Visit

FIGURE 12–15 Financial accounting record (ledger card) illustrating how payments and courtesy adjustments should be posted. The Medicare allowed amount is $550 in the case illustrated.

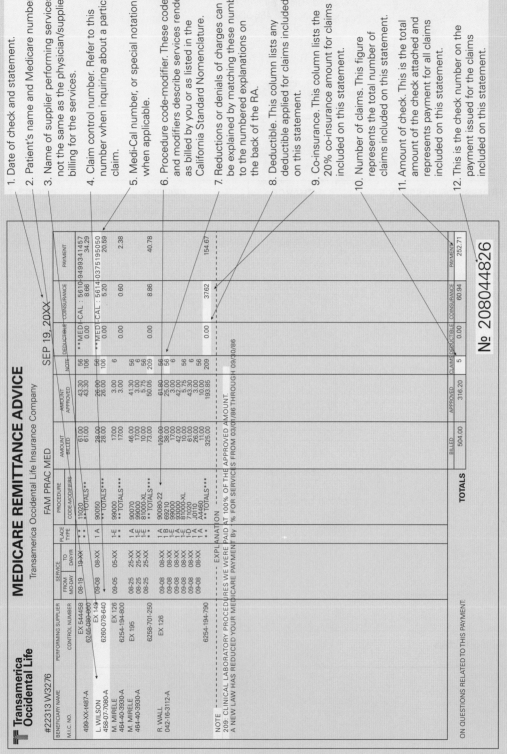

FIGURE 12–16   Medicare remittance advice (RA) document. A, Front. Insurance carriers are required to use Center for Medicare and Medicaid Services messages for Medicare RA, but each carrier has its own code numbers to denote the messages.

EXPLANATION OF NOTES
Additional notes may be listed on the front of this form.

1 – See enclosed letter.

2 – Claim was filed after the time limit.

4 – These bills are handled by a special intermediary.

5 – This payment is for an adjustment of a previous claim.

6 – Charges over the maximum Medicare allowance are not covered.

7 – Services before Medicare entitlement are not covered.

8 – Services after Medicare entitlement ended are not covered.

10 – Other charges submitted with this claim may be on a separate statement which you have received or will receive soon.

12 – Routine examinations and related services are not covered.

13 – Immunizations or other routine and preventative services are not covered.

16 – We need an itemization of this charge. Please resubmit your claim with this information.

17 – Prescription drugs are not covered.

18 – Charges for this physician/supplier are not covered.

19 – We need a full description of the service or supply to consider this charge. Please resubmit your claim with this information.

23 – We need a written report for this service. Please resubmit your claim with this information.

26 – More than $312.50 annual psychiatric expense is not covered.

27 – We need from the prescribing physician the specific length of time this medical equipment is needed. Please resubmit your claim with this information.

30 – This charge was previously considered.

37 – Claims for these services will be made by a home health agency or hospital.

39 – Equipment that is not medically necessary is not covered. (See Note 89)

42 – These supplies or services are not covered.

45 – Over 62½% of psychiatric expenses is not covered.

46 – Routine foot care is not covered.

47 – Routine eye examinations or eye refractions are not covered.

48 – Partial payment of this claim was made to the beneficiary.

49 – This service cannot be considered until the hospital makes the necessary arrangement with the carrier for its processing.

50 – The beneficiary is not responsible for this reduction/denial under the assignment agreement.

54 – Care before and/or after surgery is included in the surgery benefit. (See Note 50)

56 – This is the full charge allowed based upon the prevailing or usual and customary rate.

62 – Payment has been reduced because this test is commonly part of an automated test group. (See Note 50)

66 – This service is not covered when done by this laboratory.

70 – There were no charges or bills with your claim form. Please resubmit your claim with this information.

72 – We need a signed and dated prescription showing medical necessity and specific length of time needed. Please resubmit your claim with this information.

73 – Before another month's payment can be made, we need a new signed and dated prescription showing further necessity of the medical equipment and specific length of time needed.

80 – We need to know the place of service to consider this charge. Please resubmit your claim with this information.

83 – SSA advises us that they are unable to verify the patient's eligibility for Part B Medical Insurance Plan. For this reason, no payment can be made on this claim.

84 – The patient's HIC number shown on this claim was incorrect. Please use the correct HIC number on all future claims.

85 – The patient's name shown on this claim was incorrect. Please use the correct name on all future claims.

86 – Over 62½% of the allowable charges for psychiatric services is not covered.

89 – If you did not know that Medicare does not pay for this medical service, you may request a review of this decision. See below paragraph entitled "Your right to review of a case."

90 – This service by a chiropractor is not covered.

93 – Over $500.00 annual expense billed by a physical therapist is not covered.

95 – These specific services by this supplier are not covered.

96 – Please verify the date of this service. Resubmit your claim with this information.

99 – We need a complete diagnosis before the claim can be considered. Please resubmit your claim with this information.

106 – The Medicare covered services on this claim have been forwarded for additional processing under Medi-Cal.

107 – This claim was not forwarded for Medi-Cal processing. Please bill Medi-Cal directly and attach a copy of this statement.

108 – The bills for these services have been transferred to Blue Shield of California Medicare Claims, Chico, CA 95976. You will hear from them.

129 – Payment for services prior to July 1 is based on the previous year's payment rate.

131 – Payment for this physician service in a hospital department is reduced since this service is commonly performed in the physician's office. (See Note 50)

138 – This amount is more than Medicare pays for maintenance treatment of renal disease.

147 – This charge is not covered because an allowance for purchase of the same equipment was previously made.

151 – Your claim was transferred to a Health Maintenance Organization for processing.

153 – These are more visits (treatments) for this diagnosis than Medicare covers unless there were unusual circumstances. (See Note 89)

154 – This service is not covered for your patient's reported condition. (See Note 89)

155 – Only one visit per month to a nursing home is covered unless special need is indicated. (See Note 89)

156 – This laboratory test for the reported condition and/or illness is not covered. (See Note 89)

158 – Procedures whose effectiveness has not been proven are not covered. (See Note 89)

161 – The frequency of services for this condition are not covered. (See Note 89)

162 – More than one visit per day for this condition are not covered. (See Note 89)

172 – This type of services billed by a psychologist are not covered.

179 – The amount for this service is included in the approved amount for the consultation/office/hospital visit.

181 – Payment for this service is included in the major surgical fee.

187 – We need the name and address of the individual doctor who performed this service. Please resubmit your claim with this information.

192 – Medicare benefits have been reduced because the patient's employer group health plan has paid some of these expenses.

198 – A claim must be sent to the patient's employer group health plan first. After the claim has been processed by that plan, resubmit this claim with the bills and the notice the other insurance company sent you.

203 – Clinical laboratory services. Blood Gas Studies and Rhythm Strips (1–3 leads) furnished in a hospital setting are reimbursed through the hospital.

205 – The date of this service is after the patient's expiration date provided to us by SSA. If service was rendered to this patient on this date, have the patient's estate contact the local Social Security Office for assistance.

206 – For payment, these services must be billed by the performing laboratory with the assignment accepted.

213 – We did not send this claim to Medicaid. Please send this statement and a copy of the claim to the agency that handles Medicaid in your area.

216 – This service or item cannot be processed until your application for a Medicare provider identification number is received and approved.

218 – Since you are Medicare participating, we have processed this claim as assigned. Future claims must be billed on assignment. If the bill was paid in full, you must immediately refund the amount due to the beneficiary.

219 – We need this charge submitted on your letterhead bill. Please resubmit your claim with this information.

221 – The name and Medicare number submitted on this claim do not match. Please verify for whom these services were rendered and provide the correct name and number on the claim and resubmit.

223 – We did not consider this for payment because you did not send the extra information we asked for. Payment can be requested again by sending us another claim form and all the information.

226 – Medicare will pay rent for the prescribed number of months or until the equipment is no longer needed, whichever occurs first. This is the first monthly rental payment.

227 – You will receive a notice each month when additional rental payments are paid.

231 – Medicare will no longer pay for rental on this item since the purchase price has been paid.

237 – The amount of this payment is the difference between the approved purchase allowance and the rental payments you have received.

YOUR RIGHT TO REVIEW OF A CASE

If you have a problem or question about the way a claim was handled or about the amount paid, please write Transamerica Occidental Life, Box 54905, Terminal Annex, Los Angeles, California 90054, within 6 months of the date of this notice. We will give your request full consideration.

Your Social Security office will help you file a request for review of a claim if it is more convenient for you.

WHERE TO SEND REFUNDS

When refunding a payment you should send a check with a letter of explanation. The letter should include your Transamerica Occidental/Medicare check number, beneficiary name and Medicare identification number (HIC No.), control number to which the payment relates and any other information which may be pertinent to the refund. Send this information to:

Transamerica Occidental Life
C/O Check and Payment Control
Box 54905, Terminal Annex
Los Angeles, CA 90054-0905

KEY TO CODES FOR PLACE AND TYPE OF SERVICE

Place of service	Type of service
1. Office	A. Medical care
2. Home	B. Surgery (includes treatment of fractures)
3. Inpatient hospital	C. Consultation
4. Skilled nursing facility	D. Diagnostic X-ray
5. Outpatient hospital	E. Diagnostic laboratory
6. Independent laboratory	F. Radiation therapy
7. Other	G. Anesthesia
8. Independent kidney disease treatment center	H. Assistance at surgery
	I. Other medical service
	J. Whole blood or packed red cells

B

FIGURE 12–16, cont'd **B,** Back of Medicare RA document.

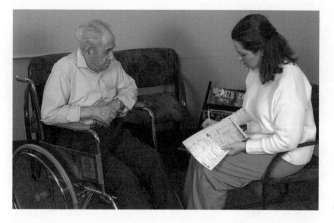

FIGURE 12–17   Insurance billing specialist explaining a Medicare remittance advice document that the physician's office has received.

MEDICARE REMITTANCE ADVICE

XYZ Insurance Company

Physician or supplier name	Dates of service From To MMDD MMDDYY	See back serv typl	Sub code (alwcode)	Billed amount	Amount allowed	See ** act cde	Beneficiary obligation Deductible Co-ins		Medicare payment to Beneficiary provider

BENEFICIARY: BILL HUTCH   HIC NUMBER: 5432-112-34
CONTROL NO.: 92106-30810-00   DE/MI: 2121D52

John Doe MD 0310	031094	D 03	120101	145.00	105.00	101	110.00	1.00	0.00	4.00
CLAIM TOTALS:				145.00	105.00	101	110.00	1.00	0.00	4.00

A

MEDICAID REMITTANCE ADVICE

RECIPIENT NAME	RECIPIENT MEDICAID ID NO.	CLAIM CONTROL NUMBER	SERVICE DATE MO DAY YR	PROCEDURE CODE	PATIENT ACCT. NO.	QTY.	MEDICARE ALLOWED	MEDICAID ALLOWED	PATIENT LIABILITY	COMPUTED MCR AMT.	MEDICAID PAID	EOB MESSAGE
BILL HUTCH	521345678	4006984891200	03 10 XX	49555–80		001	105.00	73.00		4.00	.00	
		4006984891200	00 00 XX			000	105.00	73.00		4.00	69.00	
BLOOD DEDUCT	00 DEDUCTIBLE	110.00 COINSUR	1.00 CUTBACK 32.00									CUTBACK 443

B

FIGURE 12–18   **A,** A Medicare/Medicaid case after payment by Medicare. **B,** The Medicaid remittance advice shows reimbursement of the coinsurance and deductible amounts dual billed to Medicaid.

PROCEDURE

DETERMINE WHETHER MEDICARE IS PRIMARY OR SECONDARY AND DETERMINE ADDITIONAL BENEFITS

1. Inquire whether the patient is covered under one or more of the following plans or situations:

   Automobile liability insurance, no-fault insurance, and self-insured liability insurance. An individual injured or ill because of an automobile accident may be covered by liability insurance or no-fault insurance.

   Disability insurance. Disability insurance coverage offered through an employer-sponsored large group health plan (LGHP).

   Employee group health plan (EGHP). Insurance policies for individuals 65 years of age or older who are still employed. Employers with 20 or more employees are required to offer workers and their spouses ages 65 through 69 years the same health benefits offered to younger workers. Workers may accept or reject the employer's health insurance plan. If they accept it, Medicare becomes the secondary insurance carrier.

   Employer supplemental insurance. A Medicare beneficiary has this plan through a former employer. Some people are covered by employment plans even after retirement, as long as the plan allows it and the insured informs the insurance company that he or she wishes to maintain coverage. These are known as *conversion policies.* Complementary benefits can vary in these supplemental plans, and these policies are not considered "Medigap" as defined by federal law. Note: When an employee retires and Medicare becomes the primary coverage, the company's group health plan coordinates benefits with Medicare.

   Federal Black Lung Act. An act was formed to cover employees or former coal miner employees who have illness related to black lung disorder and have acceptable diagnoses that occur on the Department of Labor's list.

   Veterans Affairs (VA). A Medicare beneficiary is also receiving benefits from the Department of Veterans Affairs. In this situation, there must be a decision made as to where to send the claim. Medicare is not secondary to the VA and the VA is not secondary to Medicare.

   The claim is sent where specified by the patient. The claim can be sent to Medicare, where, if the claim is processed, the patient must satisfy his or her contractual requirement to pay any deductible and copayment amounts. If the patient asks that the claim be sent to the VA instead of Medicare, the claim is processed and any payments issued are considered as payment in full. Many veterans want the claim sent to the VA.

   Workers' compensation. An individual suffers a disease or injury connected with employment.

   These plans are billed as primary (first) payer and Medicare second. Payments for these types of policies may not necessarily go to the physician but may go to the insured.

2. Ask to see the Medicare card, as well as any other insurance cards, and make photocopies of both sides of each card.
3. Inquire of the patient whether the supplemental coverage was carried over (conversion policy) from his or her employer.
4. Call the carrier if the type of plan is not clearly identified.
5. Bill the correct insurance plan.

   For Medigap cases, nonparticipating physicians may collect copayments and deductibles up to their limiting charge (unless the state forbids collection of more than the allowed amount) from patients at the time of service. Participating physicians may not collect copayments/deductibles from patients covered by Medigap if the patient requests the physician to submit the claim to the Medigap insurer. Collect copayments after receiving the Medicare/Medigap RA document.

   For other secondary insurance, write the patient's group and policy (or certificate) numbers on the Medicare RA, attach it to a copy of the original Health Insurance Claim Form CMS-1500, and submit it to the secondary carrier. Then copy the physician's billing statement shows date of treatment, description of service(s) rendered, fees, and diagnosis.

PROCEDURE

COMPLETE AN ADVANCE BENEFICIARY NOTICE (ABN) FORM

1. Complete an ABN form by inserting the patient's name and health insurance claim number as it appears on the Medicare card.
2. Include the service or treatment that Medicare will likely deny in the appropriate block.
3. State the reason for anticipated denial in the appropriate block.
4. Insert the estimated cost for the service or procedure. However, not including an amount does not invalidate an ABN.
5. The patient must select one of the following options on the ABN form:
   a. Receive the services affected by coverage limitations
   b. Decline the service or procedure
6. Date the form and have the patient or the patient's representative sign it.

RESOURCES

INTERNET

@

For current information or to download Medicare publications, visit the Medicare Web site.

- Centers for Medicare and Medicaid Services
  Forms, Publications, Regulations, Transmittals (formerly called Program Memorandums)
  Web site: **http://www.CMS.gov**

- CMS Manual System
  Web site: **http://www.cms.hhs.gov/manuals**

- Education and training
  Web site: **http://www.cms.hhs.gov/medlearn**
  www.cms.hhs.gov/medlearn/matters

- CLIA waived tests
  Web site: **http://www.CMS.gov/clia/waivetbl.pdf**

- key term "CLIA"
  Federal Register
  Web site: **www.archives.gov/federal_register/index.html**

- For the mailing address for sending Medicare claim forms for your state or county
  Web site: **http://www.cms.hhs.gov/contacts/incardir.asp**

- Social Security Online
  Web site: **http://www.ssa.gov**

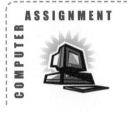

STUDENT ASSIGNMENT

✔ Study Chapter 12.

✔ Answer the review questions in the *Workbook* to reinforce the theory learned in this chapter and to help prepare you for a future test.

✔ Complete the assignments in the *Workbook* to give you experience in computing Medicare in mathematic calculations, selecting HCPCS code numbers, abstracting from patients' health records, preparing financial accounting record cards, and completing forms pertinent to the Medicare program.

✔ Turn to the glossary at the end of this textbook for a further understanding of the key terms used in this chapter.

COMPUTER ASSIGNMENT

Do the exercises for cases 8, 9, and 10 on the CD Rom to review concepts you have learned for this chapter.

CHAPTER OUTLINE

HISTORY

MEDICAID PROGRAMS

   Maternal and Child Health
      Program

   Low-Income Medicare
      Recipients

MEDICAID ELIGIBILITY

   Verifying Eligibility

   Categorically Needy

   Medically Needy

MATERNAL AND CHILD HEALTH
PROGRAM ELIGIBILITY

Accepting Medicaid Patients

   Identification Card

   Point-of-Service Machine

   Retroactive Eligibility

MEDICAID BENEFITS

   Covered Services

   Disallowed Services

MEDICAID MANAGED CARE

CLAIM PROCEDURE

   Copayment

   Prior Approval

   Time Limit

Reciprocity

Claim Form

AFTER CLAIM SUBMISSION

   Remittance Advice

   Appeals

MEDICAID FRAUD CONTROL

KEY TERMS

categorically needy

covered services

Early and Periodic Screening,
Diagnosis, and Treatment
(EPSDT)

fiscal agent

Maternal and Child Health
Program (MCHP)

Medicaid (MCD)

Medi-Cal

medically needy (MN)

prior approval

recipient

share of cost

State Children's Health Insurance
Program (SCHIP)

Supplemental Security Income
(SSI)

13

Medicaid and Other State Programs

OBJECTIVES*

After reading this chapter, you should be able to:

- Understand the benefits and nonbenefits of Medicaid.

- Define terminology relating to Medicaid.

- Interpret Medicaid abbreviations.

- Name the two Medicaid eligibility classifications.

- List important information to abstract from the patient's Medicaid card.

- State eligibility requirements and claims procedures for the Maternal and Child Health Program.

- Identify those eligible for the Medicaid Qualified Medicare Beneficiaries program.

- Explain basic operations of a Medicaid-managed care system.

- Describe basic Medicaid claim procedure guidelines.

- File claims for patients who have Medicaid and other coverage.

- Minimize the number of insurance forms rejected because of improper completion

*Performance objectives and exercises for hands-on practical experience for this chapter appear in the *Workbook*.

Service

Avoid stereotyping patients. Provide the same quality of service regardless of the patient's age, sex, race, nationality, economic level, education, occupation, religion, or diagnosis. Signs of discrimination and prejudice have no place in the health care field.

HISTORY

Federal participation in providing medical care to needy persons began between 1933 and 1935 when the Federal Emergency Relief Administration made funds available to pay the medical expenses of the needy unemployed. The Social Security Act of 1935 set up the public assistance programs. Although no special provision was made for medical assistance, the federal government paid a share of the monthly assistance payments, which could be used to meet the costs of medical care. However, the payment was made to the assistance recipient rather than the provider of medical care.

In 1950, Congress passed a law mandating that all states set up a health care program of assistance, which meant that the states had to meet minimum requirements. As a result of this mandate, the states set up **Medicaid (MCD)** programs. Congress authorized vendor payments for medical care—payments from the welfare agency directly to physicians, health care institutions, and other providers of medical services. By 1960, four fifths of the states had made provisions for medical vendor payments.

A new category of assistance recipient was established for the medically needy aged population. The incomes of these individuals were too high to qualify them for cash assistance payments, but they needed help in meeting the costs of medical care. The federal government financially supports the minimum assistance level, and the states must wholly support any part of the program that goes beyond the federal minimum. This is referred to as *state share*.

In 1965, Title XIX of the Social Security Act became federal law, and Medicaid legally came into being. To a large extent it was the result of various attempts during the previous 30 years to provide medical care to the needy. The program has always had somewhat of a split personality. On one hand, it is viewed as an attempt on the part of the government to provide comprehensive quality health care to those unable to afford it. On the other hand, Medicaid has been seen as merely a bill-paying mechanism that uses the most efficient and economic system possible to administer the provision of health care.

Since 1983, the trend in many states has been to expand Medicaid eligibility requirements and services. Changes in Medicaid eligibility allowing more people into the program were made by many states after the passage by the federal government of the Deficit Reduction Act of 1984 (DEFRA) and the Child Health Assurance Program (CHAP).

In 1982, the Tax Equity and Fiscal Responsibility Act (TEFRA) set down laws affecting those under the Medicare program, as well as Medicaid medically needy recipients and those in certain other categories. See Chapter 12 for information about how this act affects Medicare recipients.

In 2002 and 2003, states across the nation faced steep budget shortfalls. A vast majority of them made cuts of some kind in their Medicaid programs by either instituting or boosting copayments for certain types of services or eliminating some services.

MEDICAID PROGRAMS

Title XIX of the Social Security Act provides for a program of medical assistance for certain low-income individuals and families. The program is known as Medicaid in 48 states and **Medi-Cal** in California. Arizona is the only state without a Medicaid program similar to those existing in other states. Since 1982, Arizona has received federal funds under a demonstration waiver for an alternative medical assistance program (prepaid care) for low-income persons called the Arizona Health Care Cost Containment System (AHCCCS).

Medicaid is administered by state governments with partial federal funding. Coverage and benefits vary widely from state to state because the federal government sets minimum requirements and the states are free to enact more benefits. Thus each state designs its own Medicaid program within federal guidelines. The Centers for Medicaid and Medicare Services (CMS) of the Bureau of Program Operations of the United States Department of Health and Human Services is responsible for the federal aspects of Medicaid. Medicaid is not so much an insurance program as it is an assistance program.

Maternal and Child Health Program

 Each state and certain other jurisdictions, including territories and the District of Columbia (56 programs total), operate a **State Children's Health Insurance Program (SCHIP)** with federal grant support under Title V of the Social Security Act. In some states this program may be known as **Maternal and Child Health Program**

(MCHP) or Children's Special Health Care Services (CSHCS). Although Title V has been amended on a number of occasions, notably between 1981 and 1987, no changes have been as sweeping as those in the Omnibus Budget Reconciliation Act (OBRA) of 1989. SCHIP insures children from families with slightly higher incomes than the federal poverty level. Because Medicaid's income requirements change with the age of the child, a family may have children enrolled in both programs.

Federal funds are granted to states, enabling them to:

● Provide low-income mothers and children access to quality maternal and child health services.
● Reduce infant mortality and the incidence of preventable diseases and handicapping conditions among children.
● Increase the number of children immunized against disease and the number of low-income children receiving health assessments and follow-up diagnostic and treatment services.
● Promote the health of mothers and infants by providing prenatal, delivery, and postpartum care for low-income, at-risk pregnant women.
● Provide preventive and primary care services for low-income children.
● Provide rehabilitation services for the blind and disabled younger than age 16 years.
● Provide, promote, and develop family-centered, community-based, coordinated care for children with special health care needs.

The state agency tries to locate mothers, infants, and children younger than 21 years of age who may have conditions eligible for treatment under the MCHP. The conditions are diagnosed, and the necessary medical and other health-related care, any hospitalization, and any continuing follow-up care are given.

After a child is examined at an MCHP clinic and a diagnosis is made, the parents are advised about the treatment that will benefit the child. The state agency then helps them locate this care. If the parents cannot afford this care, the agency assists them with financial planning and may assume part or all of the cost of treatment, depending on the child's condition and the family's resources.

Low-Income Medicare Recipients

There are three aid programs for Medicare patients who have low incomes and have difficulty paying Medicare premiums, copayments, and deductibles. Each program addresses a different financial category, and the monthly income figures are adjusted each year. The titles of the three programs follow:

● Medicaid Qualified Medicare Beneficiary Program

● Specified Low-Income Medicare Beneficiary Program
● Qualifying Individuals Program

The programs usually are administered through county social services departments, the same ones that administer Medicaid. One application is completed that pertains to all three programs, and an individual is placed in one of the programs depending on how he or she qualifies financially.

Medicaid Qualified Medicare Beneficiary Program

The Medicaid Qualified Medicare Beneficiary (MQMB) program was introduced in the Medicare Catastrophic Act of 1988 as an amendment to the Social Security Act. In 1990, the Omnibus Budget Reconciliation Act allowed for assistance to qualified Medicare beneficiaries (QMBs, pronounced "kwim-bees") who are aged and disabled and are receiving Medicare and have annual incomes below the federal poverty level. Eligibility also depends on what other financial resources an individual might have.

Under this act, states must provide limited Medicaid coverage for QMBs. They must pay Medicare Part B premiums (and Part A premiums if applicable), along with necessary Medicare deductibles and coinsurance amounts. Coverage is restricted to Medicare cost sharing unless the beneficiary qualifies for Medicaid in some other way. Medicaid will not pay for the service if Medicare does not cover the service to the patient.

States also are required to pay Part A premiums, but no other expenses, for qualified disabled and working individuals. It is optional for states to provide full Medicaid benefits to QMBs who meet a state-established income standard.

Specified Low-Income Medicare Beneficiary Program

The Specified Low-Income Medicare Beneficiary (SLMB, pronounced "slim-bee") program was established in 1993 for elderly individuals whose income is 20% above the federal poverty level. It pays the entire Medicare Part B premium. The patient must pay the deductible and copay, and for noncovered items.

Qualifying Individuals Program

The Qualifying Individuals (QI) program was created in 1997 for qualifying individuals whose income is at least 135% but less than 175% of the federal poverty level (FPL). It also pays for the Medicare Part B premium.

MEDICAID ELIGIBILITY

Medicaid is available to certain needy and low-income people, such as the elderly (65 years or older), blind, disabled, and members of families with dependent children deprived of the support of at least one parent and financially eligible on the basis of income and resources. If a person may be eligible for Medicaid, he or she goes to the local public service welfare office, human service, or family independence agency and applies for benefits.

Verifying Eligibility

After acceptance into the program, the patient brings a form or card to the physician's office that verifies acceptance into the program (Figure 13–1), but this does not indicate proof of eligibility. It is the provider's responsibility to verify that the person to receive care is eligible on the date the service is rendered and is the individual to whom the card was issued.

Each state decides which services are covered and what the payments are for each service. There are two classifications that contain several basic groups of needy and low-income individuals.

Categorically Needy

The first classification, the **categorically needy** group, includes all cash recipients of the Temporary Assistance to Needy Families (TANF) (formerly known as Aid to Families with Dependent Children [AFDC]) program, certain other TANF-related groups, most cash recipients of the **Supplemental Security Income (SSI)** program, other SSI-related groups, QMBs, and institutional and

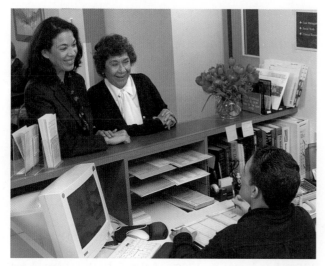

FIGURE 13–1 Medicaid patient checking in with the receptionist.

long-term care and intermediate-care facility patients (Box 13–1).

Medically Needy

The second classification involves state general assistance programs for low-income people, the medically indigent, and individuals losing employer health insurance. This classification is sometimes referred to as the **medically needy (MN)** class. A Medicaid **recipient** in this category may or may not pay coinsurance or a deductible, which

---

Box 13.1   Groups Eligible for Medicaid Benefits

MANDATORY ELIGIBILITY GROUPS

Families, pregnant women, and children
- Temporary Assistance to Needy Families (TANF)-related groups
- Non-TANF pregnant women and children
- Infants born to Medicaid-eligible pregnant women
- Children under age 6 and pregnant women whose family income is at or below 135% of the federal poverty level (FPL)
- Recipients of adoption assistance or foster care assistance under Title IV-E of the Social Security Act

Aged and disabled
- Supplemental Security Income (SSI)-related groups
- Qualified Medicare Beneficiaries (QMBs)

Persons who receive institutional or other long-term care in nursing facilities (NFs) and intermediate care facilities (ICFs)
- Certain Medicaid beneficiaries
- Medicare-Medicaid beneficiaries

OPTIONAL ELIGIBILITY GROUPS

Low-income persons losing employer health insurance coverage (Medicaid purchase if COBRA coverage)

Infants up to age 1 and pregnant women not covered under the mandatory roles whose family income is not more than 185% of the FPL (note that percent may be modified by each state)

Children under age 21 who meet TANF income and resource requirements buy who otherwise are not eligible for TANF

Persons who would be eligible if institutionalized, but receive care under home- and community-based service waivers

Persons infected with tuberculosis who would be financially eligible for Medicaid at the SSI income level if they were within a Medicaid-covered category (limited coverage)

Low-income children with the State Children's Health Insurance Program (SCHIP)

Low-income, uninsured women and diagnosed through the Centers for Disease Control and Prevention's National Breast and Cervical Cancer Early Detection program and in need of treatment for breast or cervical cancer

MEDICALLY NEEDY ELIGIBILITY GROUP

Medically indigent low-income individuals and families who have too much income to qualify under mandatory or optional eligibility Medicaid groups

must be met within the eligibility month or other specified time frame before he or she can receive state benefits (also known as **share of cost**). Emergency care and pregnancy services are exempt by law from copayment requirements. This may be a component of a state's general assistance program for low-income people. Another method to meet Medicaid eligibility requirements is to *spend down* to or below the state's medically needy income level by incurring medical expenses that reduce excess income. This then makes it low enough to make him or her eligible for the program.

For those individuals who may become medically indigent as a result of high medical care expenses and inadequate health insurance coverage, a number of states have adopted a State Program of Assistance for the Medically Indigent. Box 13–1 lists the classes and basic groups for Medicaid eligibility.

MATERNAL AND CHILD HEALTH PROGRAM ELIGIBILITY

 Specific conditions qualify a child for benefits under the MCHP. The state law under which each agency operates either defines the conditions to be included or directs the children's agency to define them. All state laws include children who have some kind of handicap that requires orthopedic treatment or plastic surgery; a few states add other conditions. A list of both types of conditions that qualify children for MCHP follows:

- Cerebral palsy
- Chronic conditions affecting bones and joints
- Cleft lip
- Cleft palate
- Clubfoot
- Cystic fibrosis*
- Epilepsy*
- Hearing problems*
- Mental retardation*
- Multiple handicaps*
- Paralyzed muscles
- Rheumatic and congenital heart disease*
- Vision problems requiring surgery*

Accepting Medicaid Patients

Program Participation

A provider must enroll for participation in the Medicaid program by signing a written provider agreement, depending on state guidelines, with the fiscal agent, local public service welfare office, human service agency, or family independence agency.

Individual physicians have their own office procedures for handling Medicaid patients. A patient can be on Medicaid one month and then off the following month, or the patient could be on the program for several months or years; each case is different. The physician may accept or refuse to treat Medicaid patients but must make the decision on the basis of the entire Medicaid program, not an individual patient's personality, medical situation, or other discriminating factor. The patient must receive quality care and be treated the same as the paying patient. If the physician decides to take Medicaid patients, he or she must accept the Medicaid allowance as payment in full (Figure 13–2). The Medicaid allowance is the maximum dollar amount to be considered for payment for a service or procedure by the program.

When obtaining personal information from the patient at the time of the first visit or a follow-up visit, always check the patient's name, address, and telephone number in a reverse address directory to verify that it is correct. Another type of directory, such as City Directory, is one that lists everyone on a given block or even in an apartment building who has a telephone. These easy reference guides cut verification time in half. However, they may be too expensive for a small office but the information

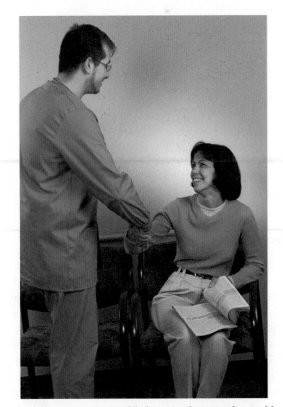

FIGURE 13–2 Disabled patient being welcomed by an insurance biller who is asking for her Medicaid card.

---

*Only some states include this item in their Maternal and Child Health Program.

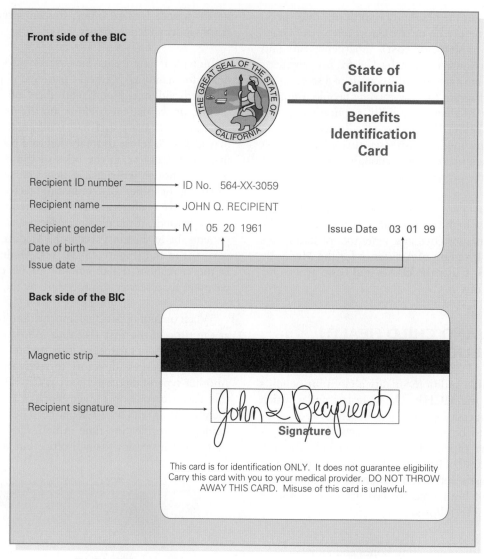

Front side of the BIC

THE GREAT SEAL OF THE STATE OF CALIFORNIA

State of California

Benefits Identification Card

Recipient ID number ⟶ ID No.   564-XX-3059

Recipient name ⟶ JOHN Q. RECIPIENT

Recipient gender ⟶ M   05 20 1961   Issue Date   03 01 99

Date of birth

Issue date

Back side of the BIC

Magnetic strip ⟶

Recipient signature ⟶ *John Q Recipient*
Signature

This card is for identification ONLY. It does not guarantee eligibility
Carry this card with you to your medical provider. DO NOT THROW
AWAY THIS CARD. Misuse of this card is unlawful.

FIGURE 13–3   Plastic Medi-Cal benefits identification card.

may be accessible via the Internet or through a local library or hospital library if there is an online service. Some Medicaid individuals are homeless and may list fake addresses, which makes locating them difficult.

Identification Card

A plastic or paper Medicaid identification card (or coupons in some states) usually is issued monthly (Figure 13–3). Under certain classifications of eligibility, identification cards are issued in some states on the 1st and 15th of each month, every 2 months, every 3 months, or every 6 months. Sometimes an unborn child can be issued an identification card that is used for services promoting the life and health of the fetus. Obtain a photocopy of the front and back of the card. Carefully check the expiration date of the card each time the patient visits the physician's office to see whether eligibility is indicated for the month of service.

Note whether the patient has other insurance, copayment requirements, or restrictions, such as being eligible for only certain types of medical services.

Point-of-Service Machine

When professional services are rendered, eligibility for that month must be verified, which may be done in a number of ways. The Potomac Group, Inc., in Nashville, Tennessee, has developed MediFAX for some states. This is a machine that allows the user to verify coverage in seconds and is available for several states. There are some states that provide their own electronic system for Medicaid verification via touch-tone telephone, modem, or specialized Medicaid terminal equipment such as a point-of-service (POS) machine (Figure 13–4). Some states issue cards that contain adhesive labels listing the month of eligibility that must be used on the billing claim form.

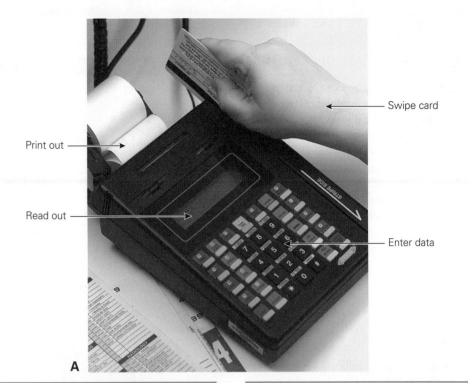

A

POS Device: Medi-Service Printout

EDS BROAD AVENUE TERMINAL T309006
XX-02-15
17:16:36

PROVIDER NUMBER:
12345F

TRANSACTION TYPE: MEDI-SERVICES

RECIPIENT ID:
5077534XX

YEAR & MONTH OF BIRTH:
1975-12

DATE OF ISSUE:
XX-02-15

DATE OF SERVICE:
XX-02-15

PROCEDURE CODE:
45339

LAST NAME: MORRISON MEDI SVC
RESERVATION APPLIED

B

POS Device: Share of Cost Printout

EDS BROAD AVENUE TERMINAL T309006
XX-02-15
17:16:36

PROVIDER NUMBER:
12345F

TRANSACTION TYPE: SHARE OF COST

RECIPIENT ID:
5077534XX

YEAR & MONTH OF BIRTH:
1984-10

DATE OF ISSUE:
XX-02-15

DATE OF SERVICE:
XX-02-15

CASE NUMBER:

PROCEDURE CODE:
90945

PATIENT APPLIED AMOUNT:
$50.00

TOTAL BILLED AMOUNT:
$100.00

LAST NAME: ADAMS
AMOUNT DEDUCTED: $50.00
SHARE OF COST HAS BEEN MET

C

FIGURE 13–4 **A,** Insurance biller using a point-of-service (POS) device machine to check a patient's Medicaid eligibility. **B,** Printout from a POS device for Medi-Service. **C,** Printout from a POS device for share of cost.

Retroactive Eligibility

Retroactive eligibility may be granted to a patient in some cases. When patients are seeking medical care who are in hope of qualifying for Medicaid but have not done so at the time of service, the account must be set up as a cash account until retroactive eligibility has been established. If the patient has documentation or a retroactive card confirming this and has paid for any services during the retroactive period, a refund must be made and Medicaid billed. As described and shown in the previous chapter, a waiver of liability agreement rewritten to the Medicaid program and signed by the patient might be used in such cases.

MEDICAID BENEFITS

Covered Services

Under federal guidelines, the state Medicaid basic benefits offered to eligible recipients include the types of **covered services** shown in Box 13–2; consult state regulations for additional benefits.

Early and Periodic Screening, Diagnosis, and Treatment

Another benefit of the Medicaid program is the **Early and Periodic Screening, Diagnosis, and Treatment (EPSDT)** service. This is a program of prevention, early detection, and treatment of welfare children (younger than age 21). In California (Medi-Cal), it is known as the Child Health and Disability Prevention (CHDP) program and in Ohio as Healthcheck. Because many states are changing the name of EPSDT and the services offered under the program, check with the state Medicaid vendor.

The EPSDT guidelines include a medical history and physical examination; immunization status assessment; dental, hearing, and vision screening; developmental assessment; and screening for anemia and lead absorption, tuberculosis, bacteriuria, and sickle cell disease and trait. States are required to provide necessary health care, diagnostic services, treatment, and other services to correct physical or mental defects found.

Disallowed Services

If a service is totally disallowed by Medicaid (denied claim), a physician is within legal rights in many states to bill the patient; consult state regulations before deciding to bill. However, it is wise to have the patient sign a waiver of liability agreement if the service to be provided may be a denied service from known past claim submission experience. An example of a waiver of liability agreement is shown in Figure 12–10. Write or telephone the state agency (see Internet Resources at the end of this chapter)

Box 13.2 | Medicaid Basic Benefits

Family planning
Home health care
Immunizations
Inpatient hospital care
Laboratory and x-ray
Outpatient hospital care
Physicians' care
Screening, diagnosis, and treatment of children younger than 21 years of age
Skilled nursing care
Transportation to and from health care providers
In some states additional services included might be the following:
  Allergy care
  Ambulance services
  Certain medical cosmetic procedures
  Chiropractic care
  Clinic care
  Dental care
  Dermatologic care
  Diagnostic, screening, preventive, and rehabilitative services (e.g., physical therapy)
  Emergency department care
  Eyeglasses and eye refractions
  Hospice care
  Intermediate care
  Occupational therapy
  Optometric services
  Podiatric care
  Prescription drugs
  Private duty nursing
  Prosthetic devices
  Psychiatric care
  Respiratory care
  Speech therapy

---

to obtain up-to-date information and details on the Medicaid program in a particular state.

MEDICAID MANAGED CARE

As early as 1967, some states began bringing managed care to their Medicaid programs. In the past decade, many states have adopted pilot projects to see whether a managed care system will work and what benefits might be received. Mainly this has been done as an effort to control escalating health care costs by curbing unnecessary emergency department visits and emphasizing preventive care.

When the last state, Arizona, joined Medicaid, it began with prepaid care rather than adhering to the way most states have structured their programs. By then most states had been struggling with Medicaid for nearly 20 years. In these systems, the Medicaid recipient enrolls either in an existing or specifically formed plan similar to a health maintenance organization (HMO). Some plans are run by independent commissions appointed by county boards of supervisors. Usually the patient can either choose or be assigned a gatekeeper (primary care physician) who must approve all specialty care and inpatient or outpatient hospital treatment. Patients must use physicians, clinics, and hospitals participating in their assigned plan.

Patients can be cared for side by side with private-paying patients. Some states have adopted capitated (a flat fee per patient) rather than fee-for-service reimbursement. There may be a small copayment for services. In programs run for a number of years, it has been found that there is better access to primary health care and savings of monies in delivering the care if the programs are well managed.

CLAIM PROCEDURE

Medicaid policies and claim procedures about identification cards, prior approval regulations, claim forms, and time limits vary from state to state. General guidelines for submitting claims are stated here.

For specific state guidelines, consult the current *Medicaid Handbook* online at the state fiscal agent's Web site. See Internet Resources at the end of this chapter for the Web site address.

Claim procedures and information on the Medi-Cal program are presented in Appendix B to assist those working as an insurance billing specialist for a clinic or physician's practice in California.

Copayment

There are two types of copayment requirements that may apply to a state. Some states require a small fixed copayment paid to the provider at the time services are rendered. This policy was instituted to help pay some of the administrative costs of physicians participating in the Medicaid program.

Another requirement is the **share of cost** or *spend down* copayment. Some Medicaid recipients must meet this copayment requirement each month before Medicaid benefits can be claimed. The amount may change from month to month so be sure to verify the copayment each time it is collected. Obtain this copay amount when the patient comes in for medical care and report on the claim form that it has been collected.

Prior Approval

Many times **prior approval** is necessary for various services, except in a bona fide emergency. Some of these services are the following:

- Durable medical equipment
- Hearing aids

- Hemodialysis
- Home health care
- Inpatient hospital care
- Long-term care facility services
- Medical supplies
- Medications
- Prosthetic or orthotic appliances
- Surgical procedures
- Transportation
- Some vision care

Usually prior authorization forms are completed to obtain permission for a specific service or hospitalization (Figure 13–5) and mailed or faxed to the Department of Health or a certain office in a region for approval. In some cases, time does not allow for a written request to be sent for prior approval, so an immediate authorization can be obtained via a telephone call to the proper department in any locale. Note the date and time the authorization was given, the name of the person who gave authorization, and any verbal number given by the field office. Usually a treatment authorization form indicating that the service was already authorized must be sent in as follow-up to the telephone call.

Time Limit

Each state has its own time limit for the submission of a claim. The time limit can vary from 2 months to 12 or 18 months from the date that the service was rendered. A bill can be rejected if it is submitted after the time limit unless the state recognizes some valid justification. Some states have separate procedures for billing over-one-year (OOY) claims. A percent of the claim may be reduced according to the date of a delinquent submission. Prescription drugs and dental services are often billed to a different intermediary than are services performed by a physician, depending on the state guidelines.

Reciprocity

Most states have reciprocity for Medicaid payments if a patient requires medical care while out of state. Contact the Medicaid intermediary in the patient's home state and ask for the appropriate forms. If the case was an emergency, state this on the form. File the papers with Medicaid in the patient's home state. Reimbursement will be at that state's rate.

Claim Form

As of October 1, 1986, federal law has mandated that the CMS-1500 Insurance Claim Form be adopted for the processing of Medicaid claims in all states.

Physicians either submit a claim form to a **fiscal agent,** which might be an insurance company, or the bill

STATE USE ONLY

SERVICE CATEGORY

3

TYPEWRITER ALIGNMENT
Elite Pica

CONFIDENTIAL PATIENT INFORMATION
FOR F.I. USE ONLY

CCN

TREATMENT AUTHORIZATION REQUEST
STATE OF CALIFORNIA DEPARTMENT OF HEALTH SERVICES

F.I. USE ONLY
40 ☐   41 ☐
42 ☐   43 ☐

TYPEWRITER ALIGNMENT
Elite Pica

(PLEASE TYPE)   FOR PROVIDER USE   (PLEASE TYPE)

VERBAL CONTROL NO.

TYPE OF SERVICE REQUESTED
☐ DRUG   ☒ OTHER

REQUEST IS RETROACTIVATE?
☐ YES   ☒ NO

IS PATIENT MEDICARE ELIGIBLE?
☐ YES   ☒ NO

PROVIDER PHONE NO.
(555) 555-1111
AREA

PATIENT'S AUTHORIZED REPRESENTATIVE (IF ANY)
ENTER NAME AND ADDRESS
•
•
•

PROVIDER NAME AND ADDRESS

PLEASE TYPE YOUR NAME AND ADDRESS HERE

SMITH, SUSAN MD
727 ELM BLVD
ANYTOWN, CA 90101

PROVIDER NO.
HSC12345F

30 83

FOR STATE USE

33   PROVIDER; YOUR REQUEST IS:

1 ☒ APPROVED AS REQUESTED   ☐   ☐ DEFERRED

2 ☐ APPROVED AS MODIFIED (ITEMS MARKED BELOW AS AUTHORIZED, MAY BE CLAIMED)   ☐ JACKSON VS RANK PARAGRAPH CODE

BY   *John Doe*
MEDICAL CONSULTANT

REVIEW COMMENTS INDICATOR

I.D. #   DATE
34 0 1   35 0 8 2 0 X X   44 ☐

NAME AND ADDRESS OF PATIENT

PATIENT NAME (LAST, FIRST, M. I.)
APPLEGATE, NANCY

STREET ADDRESS
1515 RIVER ROAD

CITY, STATE, ZIP CODE
SACRAMENTO, CA 95822

PHONE NUMBER
(555) 545-1123

MEDICAL IDENTIFICATION NO.
253971060   CHECK DIGIT

SEX AGE   DATE OF BIRTH
F   32   06 18 70

PATIENT STATUS:
☒ HOME   ☐ BOARD AND CARE
☐ SNF/ICF   ☐ ACUTE HOSPITAL

COMMENTS/ EXPLANATION

DIAGNOSIS DESCRIPTION:
ENDOMETRIOSIS

ICD-9-CM DIAGNOSIS CODE
617.9

MEDICAL JUSTIFICATION:
VISTA HOSPITAL - 1200 MAPLE ST., ANYTOWN, CA

UNCONTROLLABLE ENDOMETRIOSIS

RETROACTIVE AUTHORIZATION GRANTED IN ACCORDANCE WITH SECTION 51003 (B)

36 ☐ 1 ☐ 2 ☐ 3 ☐ 4 ☐ 5 ☐ 6

	AUTHORIZED YES	NO	APPROVED UNITS	SPECIFIC SERVICES REQUESTED	UNITS OF SERVICE	PROCEDURE OR DRUG CODE	QUANTITY	CHARGES
1	9 ☒	☐	10 *3*	DAYS: 3 HOSPITAL DAYS REQUESTED	11		12	$
2	13 ☒	☐	14 *1*	HYSTERECTOMY	1	15 5815070	16 1	$ $1300.00
3	17 ☐	☐	18			19	20	$
4	21 ☐	☐	22			23	24	$
5	25 ☐	☐	26			27	28	$
6	29 ☐	☐	30			31	32	$

TO THE BEST OF MY KNOWLEDGE, THE ABOVE INFORMATION IS TRUE, ACCURATE AND COMPLETE AND THE REQUESTED SERVICES ARE MEDICALLY INDICATED AND NECESSARY TO THE HEALTH OF THE PATIENT.

Susan Smith   MD   8-10-XX
SIGNATURE OF PHYSICIAN OR PROVIDER   TITLE   DATE

AUTHORIZATION IS VALID FOR SERVICES PROVIDED

37 FROM   DATE   38 TO   DATE
0 9 0 1 X X   0 9 3 0 X X

TAR CONTROL NUMBER

36 OFFICE   12   SEQUENCE NUMBER   61240229   PI 0

NOTE: AUTHORIZATION DOES NOT GUARANTEE PAYMENT. PAYMENT IS SUBJECT TO PATIENT'S ELIGIBILITY. BE SURE THE IDENTIFICATION CARD IS CURRENT BEFORE RENDERING SERVICE.   SEND TO FIELD SERVICES (F.I. COPY)

SEE YOUR PROVIDER MANUAL FOR ASSISTANCE REGARDING THE COMPLETION OF THIS FORM.   50-1 12/87

FIGURE 13–5 Completed treatment authorization request form used in California for the Medi-Cal program.

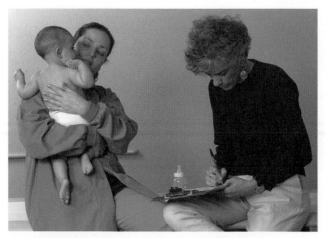

FIGURE 13–6 Physician holding a child and interacting with an insurance biller.

is sent directly to the local public service welfare office, human service, or family independence agency (Figure 13–6). These agencies have different names in each state. Refer to Internet Resources at the end of this chapter to locate the Web site for your local Medicaid fiscal agent.

In Chapter 7 there are general instructions for block-by-block entries on how to complete the CMS-1500 claim form for the Medicaid program. Because guidelines for completing the form vary among all Medicaid intermediaries, refer to the local Medicaid intermediary for their directions. Figure 7–8 is a template emphasizing placement of basic elements on the claim form and shaded blocks that do not require completion.

To keep up-to-date, always read the current bulletins or program memos on the Medicaid or Medi-Cal program at the state fiscal agent's Web site. Read and implement the rule changes and updates to avoid rejected claims.

Medicaid Managed Care

When filing a claim for a Medicaid managed care patient, send the bill to the managed care organization (MCO) and not the Medicaid fiscal agent. The MCO receives payment for services rendered to eligible members via the capitation method.

Maternal and Child Health Program

Each jurisdiction operates its own MCHP with its own unique administrative characteristics. Thus each has its own system and forms for billing and related procedures. The official plans and documents are retained in the individual state offices and are not available on either a regional or national office basis. For specific information

about a state's policies, contact your local Department of Health to locate the office near you or go to Internet Resources at the end of this chapter for the Web site address.

Medicaid and Other Plans

When Medicaid and a third-party payer cover the patient, Medicaid is always considered the payer of last resort. The third-party payer (other insurance) is billed first.

Government Programs and Medicaid

When a Medicaid patient has Medicare (sometimes referred to as a crossover case), TRICARE, or CHAMPVA, always send the insurance claim first to the federal program fiscal agent servicing the region. Then bill Medicaid second and attach to the claim form the remittance advice/explanation of benefits (RA/EOB) or check voucher that has been received from the federal program. Only send in a claim if the other coverage denies payment or pays less than the Medicaid fee schedule, or if Medicaid covers services not covered by the other policy.

Electronic claims may be automatically crossed over from primary government programs. Chapter 12 gives additional information on crossover claim submission. Figure 7–10 is a template emphasizing placement of basic elements on the claim form and shaded blocks that do not require completion for a crossover claim. Chapter 14 gives further information on patients who receive benefits from TRICARE and CHAMPVA.

Group Health Insurance and Medicaid

It is possible that a person can be eligible for Medicaid and also have group health insurance coverage through an employer. Third-party liability occurs if any entity is liable to pay all or part of the medical cost of injury, disease, or disability. In these cases, the primary carrier is the other program or insurance carrier, and it is sent the claim first. After an RA/EOB or check voucher is received from the primary carrier, Medicaid (the secondary carrier) is billed; a copy of the RA/EOB or check voucher is enclosed.

Medicaid and Aliens

Some aliens may have Medicare Part A or Part B or both (see Chapter 12). If an alien is older than 65 years and on Medicaid (Medi-Cal in California) and not eligible for Medicare benefits, bill the Medicaid processing agent and use the proper Medicaid claim form for the region. On the CMS-1500 claim form in Block 19, indicate "Alien is older than 65 years and not eligible for Medicare benefits." Your *Medicaid Handbook* should provide specifics for your region or state.

MEDICAID REMITTANCE ADVICE					TO: ANYBODY, FERNANDO G. 1000 ELM STREET ANYTOWN, XY 12345-0001							

REFER TO PROVIDER MANUAL FOR DEFINITION OF RAD CODES

PROVIDER NUMBER 00AX65800		CLAIM TYPE MEDICAL		WARRANT NO 39248026		EDS SEQ NO 20000617		DATE 06/01/20XX		PAGE 1 of 1 pages		
RECIPIENT NAME	RECIPIENT MEDICAID I.D. NO.	CLAIM CONTROL NUMBER	SERVICE DATES FROM MMDDYY	TO MMDDYY	PROCED CODE MODIFIER	PATIENT ACCOUNT NUMBER	QTY	BILLED AMT	PAYABLE AMT		PAID AMT	RAD CODE
APPROVES (RECONCILE TO FINANCIAL SUMMARY)												
TORRES R	559978557	5079350917901	030720XX	030720XX	Z4802		0001	20.00	16.22		16.22	0401
		5079350917901	030720XX	030720XX	Z4802		0001	20.00	16.22		16.22	0401
						TOTAL		40.00	32.44		32.44	
CHAN B	561198435	5044351314501	020320XX	020320XX	Z4800		0001	30.00	27.03		27.03	0401
		5044351314501	020320XX	020320XX	Z4800		0001	20.00	16.22		16.22	0401
						TOTAL		50.00	43.25		43.25	
		TOTALS FOR APPROVES						90.00	75.69		75.69	
											75.69	AMT PAID
DENIES (DO NOT RECONCILE TO FINANCIAL SUMMARY)												
GOMEZ M	624163192	501134031900	122720XX	122720XX	Z4800		0001	30.00				0036
		TOTAL NUMBER OF DENIES					0001					
SUSPENDS (DO NOT RECONCILE TO FINANCIAL SUMMARY)												
HERN D	562416373	5034270703001	010520XX	010520XX	Z4800		0001	20.00				0602
MART E	623105478	5034270712305	010520XX	010520XX	Z4800		0001	20.00				0602
		5034270712305	010520XX	010520XX	Z4800		0001	20.00				0602
						TOTAL		40.00				0602
LOPEZ C	560291467	5034270712502	012420XX	012420XX	Z4800		0001	20.00				0602
		PAT LIAB 932.00 OTH COVG		0.00		SALES TX		0.00				
		TOTAL NUMBER OF SUSPENDS					0004	80.00				

EXPLANATION OF DENIAL/ADJUSTMENT CODES
0401 PAYMENT ADJUSTED TO MAXIMUM ALLOWABLE
0036 RESUBMISSION TURNAROUND DOCUMENT WAS EITHER NOT RETURNED OR WAS RETURNED UNCORRECTED, THEREFOR YOUR CLAIM IS FORMALLY DENIED
0602 PENDING ADJUDICATION
        OHC CARRIER NAME AND ADDRESS
N049 NORTHWESTERN NATIONAL LIFE   111 WASHINGTON AVE. FL 3   MINNEAPOLIS MN 55401

FIGURE 13–7 Medicaid remittance advice form showing adjustments, cutbacks, denied claims, and claims in suspense.

AFTER CLAIM SUBMISSION

Remittance Advice

A remittance advice (RA) or check voucher, accompanies all Medicaid payment checks sent to the physician. Sometimes five categories of adjudicated claims appear on an RA—adjustments, approvals, denials, suspends,

and audit/refund (A/R) transactions—although this terminology may vary from one fiscal agent to another (Figure 13–7).

Adjustments occur from overpayments or underpayments. Approval is when an original claim or a previously denied claim is approved for payment. Denied claims are listed with a reason code on the RA. Claims in suspense for a certain period of time may be listed on the RA. A/R transactions are miscellaneous transactions as a result of cost settlements, state audits, or refund checks received. An RA for a Medicare or Medicaid case is illustrated in Figure 12–18.

Appeals

The time limit to appeal a claim varies from state to state, but it is usually 30 to 60 days. Most Medicaid offices consider an appeal filed when they receive it, not when it is sent. Usually appeals are sent on a special form or with a cover letter along with photocopies of documents applicable to the appeal (e.g., claim form, RA, and preauthorization forms). Appeals go first to either the regional fiscal agent or Medicaid bureau, next to the Department of Social Welfare or Human Services, and then to an appellate court that evaluates decisions by local and government agencies. At each level, an examiner looks at the case and makes a decision. If not satisfied, the physician may ask for further review at the next level.

MEDICAID FRAUD CONTROL

Each state has a Medicaid Fraud Control Unit (MFCU), which is a federally funded state law enforcement entity usually located in the state Attorney General's office. The MFCU investigates and prosecutes cases of fraud and other violations, including complaints of mistreatment in long-term care facilities. The state Medicaid agency must cooperate and ensure access to records by the MFCU and agree to refer suspected cases of provider fraud to this division of the Attorney General's office for investigation.

RESOURCES

INTERNET

- Many states have Medicaid Web sites. Get the Internet address for the state by contacting the local Medicaid office. To compare state-to-state Medicaid programs and obtain general data, contact the Centers for Medicaid and Medicare Service.
  Web site: **http://www.CMS.gov/Medicaid**

- To obtain information about State Children's Health Insurance program (SCHIP), which in some states is known as Maternal and Child Health Program or Children's Special Health Care Services, go to:
  Web site: **www.cms.hhs.gov/schip**

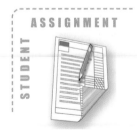

ASSIGNMENT

STUDENT

✔ Study Chapter 13.

✔ Answer the review questions in the *Workbook* to reinforce the theory learned in this chapter and to help prepare you for a future test.

✔ Complete the assignments in the *Workbook* to give you hands-on experience in abstracting from case histories, posting to financial accounting record cards, and completing forms pertinent to the Medicaid program in your state. Note: For students in California, study Appendix B, Medi-Cal. Complete the assignments in the *Workbook* for Chapter 12 and apply the knowledge learned from Appendix B.

✔ Turn to the glossary at the end of this textbook for a further understanding of the key terms used in this chapter.

CHAPTER OUTLINE

HISTORY OF TRICARE

TRICARE PROGRAMS
  Eligibility
  Nonavailability
    Statement

TRICARE STANDARD
  Enrollment
  Identification Card
  Benefits
  Fiscal Year
  Authorized Providers
    of Health Care
  Preauthorization
  Payment

TRICARE EXTRA
  Enrollment
  Identification Card
  Benefits
  Network Provider
  Preauthorization
  Payments

TRICARE PRIME
  Enrollment
  Identification Card
  Benefits
  Primary Care Manager
  Preauthorization
  Payments

TRICARE FOR LIFE
  Enrollment

  Identification Card
  Benefits
  Referral and
    Preauthorization
  Payment

TRICARE PLUS
  Enrollment
  Identification Card
  Benefits
  Payment

**TRICARE PRIME
  REMOTE PROGRAM**
  Enrollment
  Identification Card
  Benefits
  Referral and
    Preauthorization
  Payments

**SUPPLEMENTAL HEALTH
  CARE PROGRAM**
  Enrollment
  Identification Card
  Benefits
  Referral and
    Preauthorization
  Payments

**TRICARE HOSPICE
  PROGRAM**

**TRICARE AND HMO
  COVERAGE**

CHAMPVA PROGRAM
  Eligibility
  Enrollment
  Identification Card
  Benefits
  Provider
  Preauthorization

**MEDICAL RECORD
  ACCESS**
  Privacy Act of 1974
  Computer Matching
    and Privacy
    Protection Act of
    1988

CLAIMS PROCEDURE
  Fiscal Intermediary
  TRICARE Standard
    and CHAMPVA
  TRICARE Extra and
    TRICARE Prime
  Prime Remote and
    Supplemental
    Health Care
    Program
  TRICARE for Life
  TRICARE/CHAMPVA
    and Other
    Insurance
  Medicaid and
    TRICARE/CHAMPVA

  Medicare and
    TRICARE
  Medicare and
    CHAMPVA
  Dual or Double
    Coverage
  Third-Party Liability
  Workers'
    Compensation

**AFTER CLAIM
  SUBMISSION**
  TRICARE Summary
    Payment Voucher
  CHAMPVA
    Explanation of
    Benefits Document
  Quality Assurance
  Claims Inquiries and
    Appeals

**PROCEDURE:
  COMPLETING A
  CHAMPVA CLAIM
  FORM**

KEY TERMS

active duty service
  member (ADSM)

allowable charge

authorized provider

beneficiary

catastrophic cap

catchment area

cooperative care

coordination of benefits

cost-share

Defense Enrollment
  Eligibility Reporting
  System (DEERS)

emergency

fiscal intermediary (FI)

health benefits advisor
  (HBA)

health care finder (HCF)

medically (or
  psychologically)
  necessary

military treatment facility
  (MTF)

nonparticipating
  provider (nonpar)

other health insurance
  (OHI)

participating provider
  (par)

partnership program

point-of-service (POS)
  option

preauthorization

primary care manager
  (PCM)

quality assurance
  program

service benefit program

service-connected injury

service retiree (military
  retiree)

sponsor

summary payment
  voucher

The Civilian Health and
  Medical Program of
  the Department of
  Veterans Affairs
  (CHAMPVA)

total, permanent service-
  connected disability

TRICARE Extra

TRICARE for Life (TFL)

TRICARE Prime

TRICARE service center
  (TSC)

urgent care

veteran

14

TRICARE and CHAMPVA

OBJECTIVES*

After reading this chapter, you should be able to:

- State who is eligible for TRICARE and CHAMPVA.

- Define pertinent TRICARE and CHAMPVA terminology and abbreviations.

- Enumerate the differences between TRICARE Prime and Extra and the TRICARE Standard programs.

- Identify the difference between the TRICARE program and CHAMPVA.

- Explain the benefits and nonbenefits of these government programs.

- Name various forms used with these federal health care programs.

- List the circumstances when a nonavailability statement is necessary.

- Describe how to process claims for individuals who are covered by TRICARE and CHAMPVA.

*Performance objectives and exercises for hands-on practical experience for this chapter appear in the *Workbook*.

HISTORY OF TRICARE

The U.S. Congress created CHAMPUS in 1966 under Public Law 89-614 because individuals in the military were finding it increasingly difficult to pay for the medical care required by their families. CHAMPUS (Civilian Health and Medical Program of the Uniformed Services) is a congressionally funded comprehensive health benefits program. Beginning in 1988, CHAMPUS beneficiaries had a choice of retaining their benefits under CHAMPUS or enrolling in a managed care plan called CHAMPUS Prime, a plan to control escalating medical costs and standardize benefits for active duty families, military retirees, and their dependents. In January 1994, TRICARE became the new title for CHAMPUS. Individuals have three choices to obtain health care under TRICARE:

- TRICARE Standard (fee-for-service cost-sharing type of option)
- TRICARE Extra (preferred provider organization type of option)
- TRICARE Prime (health maintenance organization type of option)

In 2005, the former 11 TRICARE regions in the United States consolidated and merged to form the following: Region West, Region North, and Region South. In addition, there is TRICARE Europe, Canada/Latin America, and Puerto Rico/Virgin Islands. Figure 14–1 shows the locations of the states merged into these regions.

TRICARE PROGRAMS

Eligibility

The following individuals are entitled to medical benefits under TRICARE:

- Active duty uniformed service members in a program called TRICARE Prime Remote for members of Army, Navy, Air Force, Marines, U.S. Coast Guard, Public Health Service, and National Oceanic and Atmospheric Administration.
- Eligible family members of active duty service members
- Military retirees and their eligible family members
- Surviving eligible family members of deceased active or retired service members
- Wards and preadoptive children
- Former spouses of active or retired service members who meet certain length-of-marriage rules and other requirements
- Family members of active duty service members who were court-martialed and separated from their families for spouse or child abuse
- Abused spouses, former spouses, or dependent children of service members who were eligible for retirement but lost that eligibility as a result of abuse of the spouse or child

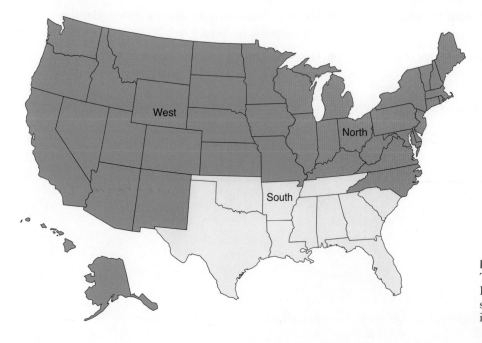

FIGURE 14–1 Map of TRICARE West Region, North Region, and South Region, which shows states that have been merged into each of the regions.

- Spouses and children of North Atlantic Treaty Organization (NATO) nation representatives, under certain circumstances
- Families of activated Reserve and National Guard members if military sponsor's active duty orders are for 30 consecutive days or an indefinite period
- Disabled beneficiaries younger than 65 years of age who have Medicare parts A and B and who qualify under one of the aforementioned categories
- Medicare-eligible beneficiaries in a program called TRICARE for Life

An individual who qualifies for TRICARE is known as a **beneficiary;** the active duty service member is called the **sponsor.** A person who is retired from a career in the armed forces is known as a **service retiree** or **military retiree** and remains in a TRICARE program until age 65, at which time the individual becomes eligible for the Medicare program. No further family benefits are provided in the event that an active duty military person served from 4 to 6 years and then chose to leave the armed services, thereby giving up a military career. CHAMPVA beneficiaries are not eligible for TRICARE.

Defense Enrollment Eligibility Reporting System

All TRICARE-eligible persons must be enrolled in the **Defense Enrollment Eligibility Reporting System (DEERS)** computerized database. TRICARE claims processors check DEERS before processing claims to verify beneficiary eligibility. A TRICARE beneficiary may check his or her status by contacting the nearest personnel office of any branch of the service or by calling the toll-free number of the DEERS center.

Nonavailability Statement

A Nonavailability Statement (NAS) is a certification from a military hospital stating that it cannot provide the care needed. As of December 2003, this type of certification is no longer necessary for TRICARE and CHAMPVA beneficiaries for outpatient procedures or for those who wish to receive treatment as inpatients at a civilian hospital and who live within a catchment area surrounding a **military treatment facility (MTF).** An MTF is a uniformed services hospital sometimes referred to as a military hospital, formerly called a U.S. Public Health Service (USPHS) hospital. The only exception is that an NAS is still required for nonemergency inpatient mental health care services.

Catchment Area

The **catchment area** is defined by ZIP codes and is based on an area of approximately 40 miles in radius

surrounding each U.S. MTF. Individuals whose home address ZIP code falls outside the local military hospital's service area do not need an NAS before seeking civilian health care under TRICARE.

TRICARE STANDARD

Enrollment

Those entitled to medical benefits under TRICARE are automatically enrolled in the TRICARE Standard program.

Identification Card

All dependents 10 years of age or older are required to have a Uniformed Services (military) identification and privilege card for TRICARE Standard. Dependents and survivors of active duty personnel and retirees carry a military identification card DD Form 1173 (Figure 14–2). Dependents younger than 10 years of age are not normally issued Uniformed Services identification cards; information for their claims should be provided from either parent's card. Refer to the back of the card under "medical" to ensure that the card authorizes civilian medical benefits. Essential information must be abstracted from the front and back of the card; therefore photocopy both sides to retain in the patient's medical record.

Benefits

In the TRICARE Standard program, beneficiaries may receive a wide range of civilian health care services, with a significant portion of the cost paid by the federal government. Patients are not limited to using network providers, and benefits include medical or psychological services or supplies that are considered appropriate care. Such services generally are accepted by qualified professionals to be reasonable and adequate for the diagnosis and treatment of illness, injury, pregnancy, and mental disorders, or are reasonable and adequate for well-baby care. These services are referred to as **medically (or psychologically) necessary.**

Beneficiaries also may receive urgent care and emergency care services. **Urgent care** is medically necessary treatment needed for an immediate illness or injury that would not result in further disability or death if not treated immediately. Treatment should not be delayed but should occur within 24 hours to avoid development of further complications. An **emergency** is a sudden and unexpected medical condition, or the worsening of a condition, which poses a threat to life, losing a limb, or sight and requires immediate treatment to alleviate suffering (e.g., shortness of breath, chest pain, and

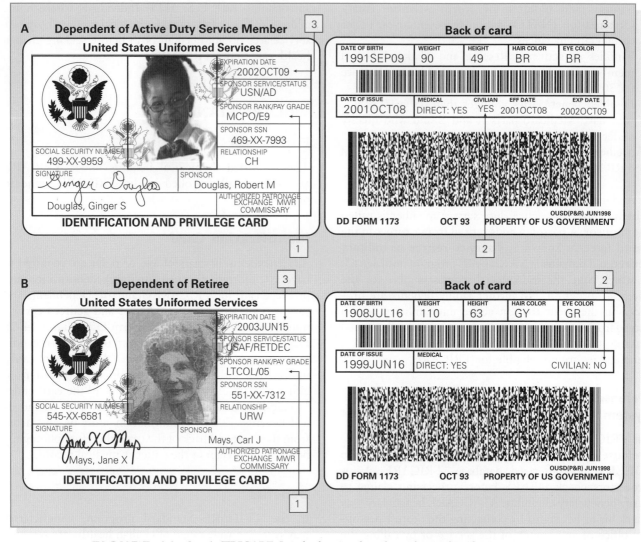

FIGURE 14–2 **A,** TRICARE Standard active duty dependent's identification card (DD Form 1173) from which essential information must be abstracted. **B,** Sample identification card (DD Form 1173) for a retiree's widowed spouse. Cards indicate *1,* sponsor's status and rank; *2,* authorization status for treatment by a civilian provider; and *3,* expiration date.

drug overdose). Usually it is obtained at a hospital emergency department.

TRICARE Standard patients usually seek care from a military hospital near their home. The military physician may refer the patient to a civilian source if the service hospital that is managing the TRICARE Standard patient cannot provide a particular service or medical supplies. **Cooperative care** consists of services or supplies that may be cost-shared by TRICARE Standard under certain conditions.

A **partnership program** is another option that lets TRICARE Standard–eligible persons receive inpatient or outpatient treatment from civilian providers of care in a military hospital, or from uniformed services providers of care in civilian facilities. Whether a partnership program is instituted at a particular military hospital is up to the facility's commander, who makes the decision based on economics.

In addition, there are times when there is no service hospital in the area and a TRICARE Standard beneficiary may seek care through a private physician's office or hospital. Delivery of care through the private physician is emphasized in this chapter.

Read carefully through Figures 14–3 and 14–4 to see the overall picture of TRICARE benefits, which includes cost-sharing (deductibles and copayments).

Fiscal Year

The TRICARE fiscal year begins October 1 and ends September 30. It is different from most programs;

ADFM = active duty family members RFMS = retirees, family members, and survivors	Benefit and Coverage Chart					
Inpatient Services	**Programs and Beneficiary Costs**					
Program and Classification	**TRICARE Prime**		**TRICARE Extra**		**TRICARE Standard**	
	ADFM	RFMS	ADFM	RFMS	ADFM	RFMS
Hospitalization* including **Maternity Benefits***	No copayment	$11.45/day; civilian care $11/day or $25 min charge per/admission, whichever is greater	$11.45/day; civilian care $11/day or $25 min charge per/admission, whichever is greater	$11.45/day; civilian care $250/day or 25% cost-share (contracted fee) whichever is less, plus 20% cost-share for separately billed professional charges	$11.45/day; civilian care $11/day or $25 min charge per/admission, whichever is greater	$11.45/day; civilian care $512/day or 25% cost-share (contracted fee) whichever is less, plus 25% cost-share (maximum allowable charge) for separately billed professional charges
Skilled Nursing Care					$25/admission, or $11.45/day, whichever is greater	25% cost-share (billed charges), plus 25% cost-share (maximum allowable charge) for separately billed professional charges
Mental Illness Hospitalization* and **Substance Use Treatment*** (inpatient, partial hospital program)	None	$40/day (no copayment or cost-share for separately billed professional charges)	$20/day	20% cost-share (contracted fee), plus 20% cost-share (contracted fee) for separately billed professional charges	$20/day	25% cost-share (max allowable charge), for separately billed professional charges plus: 25% of (1) per diem, (2) fixed daily amount or billed charges, or (3) 25% of allowed amount (RTC & partial hospitalization)
Partial Hospitalization* (mental illness)	None	$40/day or $25/admission, whichever is greater	$20/day	20% cost-share (contracted fee), plus 20% cost-share for separately billed professional charges	$20/day	25% of allowed amount, plus 25% maximum allowable charge for separately billed professional charges
Hospice Care	Available in lieu of other TRICARE benefits (provided by Medicare approved program).					
*Preauthorization required.						

FIGURE 14–3 TRICARE Prime, Extra, and Standard inpatient services benefits and coverage chart.

therefore office staff should be alert when collecting deductibles.

Authorized Providers of Health Care

An **authorized provider** may treat a TRICARE Standard patient. This means the provider can be reimbursed by TRICARE for its share of costs for medical benefits and the provider is qualified to provide certain health benefits to TRICARE beneficiaries. Only "certified" providers, those who have passed a credentialing process, can be authorized by TRICARE. Beneficiaries who use nonauthorized providers may be responsible for their entire bill, and there are no legal limits on the amounts these providers can bill beneficiaries. Examples of nonauthorized providers are most chiropractors and acupuncturists and those physicians who do not meet state licensing or training requirements or were rejected

ADFM = active duty family members
RFMS = retirees, family members and survivors

Benefit and Coverage Chart

Outpatient Services	Programs and Beneficiary Costs					
Program and Classification	TRICARE Prime		TRICARE Extra		TRICARE Standard	
	ADFM	RFMS	ADFM	RFMS	ADFM	RFMS
Annual Enrollment Fee* (per fiscal year)	None	$230/person $460/family	None ──────────────▶		None ──────────────▶	
Annual Deductible (per fiscal year 10/1 to 9/30) (applied to outpatient services before cost-share is determined)	None (except when using Point-of-Service option)		E-4 and below $50/person $100/family E-5 and above $150/person $300/family	$150/person $300/family	E-4 and below $50/person $100/family E-5 and above $150/person $300/family	$150/person $300/family
Physician Services	None	$12	15% of contracted fee	20% of contracted fee	20% of maximum allowable charge	25% of maximum allowable charge
Ancillary Services (certain radiology, laboratory, & cardiac services)	None ──────────────▶ (RFMS may have $12 copay if test provided independent of office visit)					
Ambulance Services	None	$20				
Home Health Services	None	$12				
Family Health Services	None	$12				
Durable Medical Equipment (greater than $100)	None	20% cost-share				
Emergency Services (network and non-network)	None	$30 copayment				
Outpatient Behavioral Health (limitations apply)	None	$25 copayment $17 group visits				
Immunizations (for required overseas travel)	None	Not covered		Not covered		Not covered
Ambulatory Surgery (same day)	None	$25 copayment (applied to facility charges only)	$25 copayment for hospital charges	20% of contracted fee	$25 copayment for hospital charges	*Professional:* 25% of maximum allowable charge *Facility:* 25% of maximum allowable charge OR billed charges, whichever is less
Eye Examinations (limitations apply)	None	Clinical Preventive Service	15% of contracted fee	Not covered	20% of maximum allowable charge	Not covered
Prescription Drugs– Network Pharmacy	$3 copayment for each 30-day supply of **generic** medication $9 copayment for each 30-day supply of **brand name** medication					
Prescription Drugs– National Mail Order Pharmacy	$3 copayment for each 90-day supply of **generic** medication $9 copayment for each 90-day supply of **brand name** medication (Note: if the beneficiary has primary insurance that covers presciption medication, the beneficiary is not eligible for the mail order pharmacy benefit)					
Prescription Drugs– Non-network Pharmacy	$9 or 20% of total cost (whichever is greater) plus deductible					

*No enrollment fee for those who are eligible for Medicare (enrolled in Part B) on the basis of disability or end-stage renal disease.

NOTE: TRICARE Prime Remote–benefits are similar to TRICARE Prime program; however, ADSMs have no copayment costs-share or deductible

Program for Persons with Disabilities–no deductible; monthly cost-share varies from $25 to $250, depending on sponsor's rank

FIGURE 14–4   TRICARE Prime, Extra, and Standard outpatient services benefits and coverage chart.

for authorization by TRICARE. Authorized providers include the following:

- Doctor of medicine (MD)
- Doctor of osteopathy (DO or MD)
- Doctor of dental surgery (DDS)
- Doctor of dental medicine (DDM)
- Doctor of podiatric medicine or surgical chiropody (DPM or DSC)
- Doctor of optometry (DO)
- Psychologist (PhD)

Other authorized nonphysician providers include audiologists, certified nurse midwives, clinical social workers, licensed practical nurses, licensed vocational nurses, nurse practitioners, physician assistants, psychiatric social workers, registered nurses, registered physical therapists, and speech therapists.

Preauthorization

There are certain referral and **preauthorization** requirements for TRICARE Standard patients. When specialty care or hospitalization is necessary, the MTF must be used if services are available. If services are not available, the **health care finder (HCF)** will assist with the referral or preauthorization process. An HCF is a health care professional, usually a registered nurse, who helps the patient work with his or her primary care physician to locate a specialist or obtain a preauthorization for care. HCFs are found at a **TRICARE service center (TSC),** which is an office staffed by HCFs and beneficiary service representatives. All admissions, ambulatory surgical procedures, and other selected procedures require preauthorization. Certain types of health care services requiring prior approval from the TRICARE health contractor follow:

- Arthroscopy
- Breast mass or tumor removal
- Cardiac catheterization
- Cataract removal
- Cystoscopy
- Dental care
- Dilatation and curettage
- Durable medical equipment purchases
- Gastrointestinal endoscopy
- Gynecologic laparoscopy
- Hernia repairs
- Laparoscopic cholecystectomy
- Ligation or transection of fallopian tubes
- Magnetic resonance imaging (MRI)
- Mental health care
- Myringotomy or tympanostomy
- Neuroplasty
- Nose repair (rhinoplasty and septoplasty)
- Strabismus repair
- Tonsillectomy or adenoidectomy

Payment

Deductible and Copayment

Deductibles and copayments are determined according to two groups: (1) active duty family members and (2) retirees, their family members, and survivors.

Spouses and Children of Active Duty Members

For inpatient (hospitalized) care, the beneficiary pays the first $25 of the hospital charge or a small fee for each day, whichever is greater, and TRICARE pays the remainder of the allowable charges for authorized care.

For outpatient (nonhospitalized) care, the beneficiary pays the first $150 (deductible) plus 20% of the charges more than the $150 deductible. A family with two or more eligible beneficiaries pays a maximum of $300 (deductible) plus 20% of the charges in excess of $300. TRICARE pays the remainder of the allowable charges, which is 80%.

All Other Eligible Beneficiaries

This category includes retired members, dependents of retired members, dependents of deceased members who died in active duty, and so forth.

For inpatient (hospitalized) care, the beneficiary pays 25% of the hospital charges and fees of professional personnel. TRICARE pays the remaining allowable charges for authorized care, or 75%.

For outpatient (nonhospitalized) care, the beneficiary pays $150 (deductible) plus 25% of the charges more than the $150 deductible. A family with two or more eligible beneficiaries pays a maximum of $300 plus 25% of the charges in excess of $300. TRICARE pays the remainder of the allowable charges for authorized care, which is 75%.

Refer to Figures 14–3 and 14–4 for further clarification and to see the differences in benefits between the three TRICARE program options.

Participating Provider

If the physician agrees to accept assignment a TRICARE Standard case, the **participating provider (par)** agrees to accept the TRICARE-determined **allowable charge** as payment in full. Providers may choose to accept TRICARE assignment on a case-by-case basis. Assignment should always be accepted when the service member is transferring within 6 months because this avoids collection problems. The provider may bill the patient for his or her **cost-share** or coinsurance (20% to 25% of the allowable charge after the deductible has been met) and for any noncovered services or supplies. The provider may not bill for the difference between the provider's usual charge and the allowable charge.

Beneficiaries pay only a certain amount each year for the cost-share and annual deductible. This amount is known as the **catastrophic cap.** After this cap is reached, TRICARE pays 100% of the allowable charges for the rest of the year. A note should be attached to the claim when the patient has met the catastrophic cap; this may help expedite claims processing and payment. After the claim is completed and sent to the fiscal intermediary, the payment goes directly to the physician.

Nonparticipating Provider

A health care provider who chooses not to participate in TRICARE is called a **nonparticipating provider (nonpar)** and, as of November 1, 1993, may not bill the patient more than 115% of the TRICARE allowable charge. For example, if the TRICARE allowable charge for a procedure is $100, providers who decide not to participate in TRICARE may charge TRICARE patients no more than $115 for that procedure. The patient pays the deductible (20% or 25% of the charges determined to be allowable) and any amount more than the allowable charge up to 115% when the physician does not accept assignment.

TRICARE EXTRA

Enrollment

TRICARE Extra is a preferred provider organization type of option in which the individual does not have to enroll or pay an annual fee. On a visit-by-visit basis, the individual may seek care from an authorized network provider and receive a discount on services and reduced cost-share (copayment). A nonenrolled beneficiary automatically becomes a TRICARE Extra beneficiary when care is rendered by a network provider. If a nonenrolled beneficiary receives care from a non-network provider, the services received are covered under TRICARE Standard. Providers receive a contract rate for giving care.

Identification Card

A TRICARE Extra beneficiary must present the military identification card when receiving care as proof of eligibility. The military identification card indicates a "Yes" in Box 15B (back of card) if the beneficiary is eligible. Children younger than 10 years of age may use the sponsor's identification card (attach a copy of the child's card to the claim). Individuals older than 10 years must have their own identification card. Contact the local HCF to verify eligibility. Active duty and retiree dependents and survivors carry an orange or brown military identification

card (see Figure 14–2). Retirees carry a blue-gray military identification card.

Benefits

See Figures 14–3 and 14–4 for outpatient and inpatient benefits and deductible and copayment amounts.

Network Provider

The network provider is the physician who provides medical care to TRICARE beneficiaries under the TRICARE Extra program at contracted rates. They have discount agreements with the TRICARE program.

Preauthorization

Referrals from other network providers are coordinated through the HCF. The network provider refers the beneficiary for additional services, when necessary, after precertification requirements and completing a referral form.

Payments

Deductible and Copayment

Deductibles and copayments are determined by group: (1) active duty family members and (2) retirees, their family members, and survivors.

Spouses and Children of Active Duty Members

No copayment is required for inpatient (hospitalized) care.

For outpatient (nonhospitalized) care, the beneficiary pays the first $150 (deductible) plus 15% of the charges more than the $150 deductible. A family with two or more eligible beneficiaries pays a maximum of $300 (deductible) plus 15% of the charges in excess of $300. TRICARE pays the remainder of the allowable charges (85%).

All Other Eligible Beneficiaries

For inpatient (hospitalized) care, the copayment is $250 per day or 25% of the plan's allowable charges, whichever is less, plus 20% of separately billed professional charges at the plan's allowable rate.

For outpatient (nonhospitalized) care, the beneficiary pays $150 (deductible) plus 20% of the charges more than the $150 deductible. A family with two or more eligible beneficiaries pays a maximum of $300 plus 20% of the charges in excess of $300. TRICARE pays the remainder of the allowable charges for authorized care (80%).

See Figures 14–3 and 14–4 for further clarification of deductibles and copayments.

TRICARE PRIME

TRICARE Prime is a voluntary health maintenance organization (HMO)–type option. Participation in TRICARE Prime is optional. Beneficiaries who are not enrolled as members in TRICARE Prime may continue to receive services through TRICARE Extra from network providers or through TRICARE Standard using non-network providers. The beneficiary may no longer use the TRICARE Standard program once enrolled in TRICARE Prime.

Enrollment

An individual must complete an application and enroll for a minimum of 12 months to become a TRICARE Prime member. There is an annual enrollment fee charged per person or family except for active duty families, who may enroll free. Active duty service members are enrolled automatically in TRICARE Prime and are not eligible for benefits under TRICARE Standard or TRICARE Extra. These members are able to use the local military and civilian provider network with necessary authorization.

Enrollees normally receive care from within the Prime network of civilian and military providers. The beneficiary has the option of choosing or being assigned a **primary care manager (PCM)** for each family member. The PCM manages all aspects of the patient's health care (except emergencies) including referrals to specialists. Enrolled beneficiaries may not use a non-network provider, except in emergencies or for pharmaceuticals, without a specific referral from an HCF.

Identification Card

Individuals who enroll are issued a TRICARE Prime identification card, as shown in Figure 14–5. This card does not guarantee TRICARE eligibility; therefore providers must check the TRICARE Uniformed Services military identification card for the effective and expiration dates or call the local HCF. Copies of the military identification card and the TRICARE Prime card should always be made and retained in the patient's file. For TRICARE Prime patients, both cards should be checked at every visit.

Benefits

Covered services are the same as those for TRICARE Standard patients plus additional preventive and primary care services. For example, periodic physical examinations are covered at no charge under TRICARE Prime but are not covered under TRICARE Extra or TRICARE Standard. Prime also covers certain immunizations and annual eye examinations for dependent children of retirees that are not a benefit under Extra or Standard. A dental plan is available for an additional monthly premium. An NAS is necessary for certain inpatient services if the beneficiary resides within the designated MTF catchment area. See Figures 13–3 and 13–4 for outpatient and inpatient benefits and deductible and copayment amounts.

Primary Care Manager

The PCM is a physician who is responsible for coordinating and managing the entire beneficiary's health care unless there is an emergency. A provider who decides to participate in a managed care program goes through a credentialing process. This is done approximately every 2 years for all physicians who participate as providers. The PCM may refer the beneficiary for additional services, when necessary, but specific referral and preauthorization requirements must be carried out. Referral patterns are evaluated to determine excessive or inappropriate referrals to specialists. A pattern of such referrals could result in termination of participation in TRICARE Prime.

Preauthorization

All admissions, ambulatory surgical procedures, and other selected procedures require preauthorization. Outpatient or ambulatory surgery must be on the approved procedure list before it is performed. The list is in the *TRICARE Handbook* available on the Web site: http://www.tricare.osd.mil.

The **health benefits advisor (HBA)** at the nearest military medical facility should be called to determine whether an NAS statement is needed for the procedure before the surgery is scheduled in the approved facility. An HBA is a person at a military hospital or clinic who is there to help beneficiaries obtain medical care needed through the military and TRICARE. A **point-of-service (POS) option** is available if no authorization is obtained. This means that the individual can choose to get TRICARE-covered nonemergency services outside the Prime network of providers without a referral from the PCM and without authorization from the HCF. There is an annual deductible and 50% cost-share if the POS option is used.

Payments

Copayment

TRICARE Prime copayments for inpatient hospital services vary for active duty family members and for retirees and their family members and survivors. For outpatient services, copayments are the same for active duty family members and for retirees and their family members and survivors but vary in amounts depending on the type of service received. Copayments should be collected at the time services are rendered. Refer to Figures 13–3 and 13–4 for further clarification of copayments.

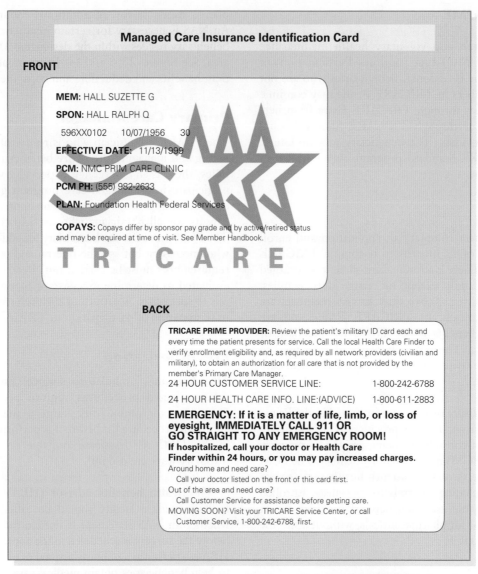

Managed Care Insurance Identification Card

FRONT

MEM: HALL SUZETTE G

SPON: HALL RALPH Q

596XX0102   10/07/1956   30

EFFECTIVE DATE: 11/13/1999

PCM: NMC PRIM CARE CLINIC

PCM PH: (555) 982-2633

PLAN: Foundation Health Federal Services

COPAYS: Copays differ by sponsor pay grade and by active/retired status and may be required at time of visit. See Member Handbook.

T R I C A R E

BACK

TRICARE PRIME PROVIDER: Review the patient's military ID card each and every time the patient presents for service. Call the local Health Care Finder to verify enrollment eligibility and, as required by all network providers (civilian and military), to obtain an authorization for all care that is not provided by the member's Primary Care Manager.

24 HOUR CUSTOMER SERVICE LINE: 1-800-242-6788

24 HOUR HEALTH CARE INFO. LINE:(ADVICE)   1-800-611-2883

EMERGENCY: If it is a matter of life, limb, or loss of eyesight, IMMEDIATELY CALL 911 OR GO STRAIGHT TO ANY EMERGENCY ROOM!
If hospitalized, call your doctor or Health Care Finder within 24 hours, or you may pay increased charges.

Around home and need care?
    Call your doctor listed on the front of this card first.
Out of the area and need care?
    Call Customer Service for assistance before getting care.
MOVING SOON? Visit your TRICARE Service Center, or call
    Customer Service, 1-800-242-6788, first.

FIGURE 14–5   TRICARE Prime identification card. A new TRICARE Prime identification card has been redesigned to incorporate essential contact information to help enrollees access health care. This card will be introduced gradually.

TRICARE FOR LIFE

In October 2001, **TRICARE for Life (TFL)** was enacted and offered additional TRICARE benefits as a supplementary payer to Medicare for uniformed service retirees, their spouses, and survivors age 65 or older. When beneficiaries become entitled to receive Medicare Part A and Medicare Part B upon attaining the age of 65, they experience no break in TRICARE coverage. The only change is that TRICARE will pay secondary to Medicare beginning on the first day of the month they turn 65.

TRICARE for Life is provided to the following beneficiaries:
- Medicare-eligible uniformed service retirees, including retired guard and reservists

- Medicare-eligible family members, including widows and widowers
- Certain former spouses if they were eligible for TRICARE before age 65

Dependent parents and parents-in-law are not eligible for TRICARE benefits. They may continue to receive services within a MTF on a space-available basis.

Enrollment

Most beneficiaries must be eligible for Medicare Part A and enrolled in Medicare Part B to qualify for TFL. An exception is Uniformed Services Family Health Plan (USFHP) members. Prospective TFL beneficiaries do not have to sign up or enroll for the program; however, they should be enrolled in DEERS. There are no enrollment fees for TFL. The member is required to enroll in Medicare Part B but without surcharge.

The DEERS notifies a beneficiary within 90 days before his or her 65th birthday that the medical benefits are about to change. They ask the beneficiary to contact the nearest Social Security Administration office about enrollment in Medicare. The beneficiary must elect to enroll in Medicare Part B to be eligible for TFL benefits. If the beneficiary is age 65 or older and only has Medicare Part A, he or she can enroll in Medicare Part B during the annual general enrollment period, which runs from January 1st to March 31st every year. Medicare Part B coverage then begins on July 1st of the year in which the beneficiary enrolls.

Refer to Internet Resources at the end of this chapter for more information about enrolling in Medicare Part B and monthly fees that apply.

Identification Card

Beneficiaries who qualify for TFL do not need a TRICARE enrollment card.

Benefits

Each beneficiary receives a matrix comparing Medicare benefits to TRICARE benefits. Refer to Internet Resources at the end of this chapter for the TRICARE Management Activity Web site address to download this information. Certain benefits (e.g., prescription medications) are covered under the TRICARE Senior Pharmacy Program. Pharmacy benefits provide Medicare-eligible retirees of the uniformed service, their family members, and survivors the same pharmacy benefit as retirees who are younger than age 65. This includes access to prescription drugs at MTFs, retail pharmacies, and through the National Mail Order Pharmacy. Medicare Part B enrollment is not mandatory to receive TRICARE Senior Pharmacy Program benefits.

Referral and Preauthorization

There are no preauthorization requirements for the TFL program. All services and supplies must be benefits of the Medicare or TRICARE programs to be covered.

Payment

The following four scenarios represent most cases and explain the payment mechanism:

1. Services covered under both Medicare and TRICARE. Medicare pays first at the Medicare rate and the remaining is paid by TRICARE, which covers the beneficiary's cost-share and deductible. No copayment, cost-share, or deductible is paid by the TFL beneficiary.
2. Services covered under Medicare but not TRICARE. Medicare pays the Medicare rate and the beneficiary pays the Medicare cost-share and deductible amounts. TRICARE pays nothing.
3. Services covered under TRICARE but not Medicare. TRICARE pays the allowed amount and Medicare pays nothing. The beneficiary is responsible for the TRICARE cost-share and the deductible amounts.
4. Services not payable by TRICARE or Medicare. The beneficiary is entirely responsible for the medical bill.

TRICARE PLUS

Enrollment

TRICARE Plus is open to persons eligible for care in military facilities and not enrolled in TRICARE Prime or a commercial HMO. TRICARE Plus allows some Military Health System (MHS) beneficiaries to enroll with a military primary care provider. There is no enrollment fee.

Identification Card

Persons enrolled in TRICARE Plus are issued an identification card and identified in the DEERS.

Benefits

The TRICARE Plus program is designed to function in the following ways:

- Enrollees use the MTF as their source of primary care; it is not a comprehensive health plan.
- Enrollees may seek care from a civilian provider but are discouraged from obtaining nonemergency primary care from sources outside the MTF.
- Enrollees are not guaranteed access to specialty providers at the MTF.
- Enrollees may not use their enrollment at another facility.

The MTF's commander determines the enrollment capacity at each MTF.

Payment

TRICARE Plus offers the same benefits as TRICARE Prime when using an MTF. It has no effect on the enrollees' use or payment of civilian health care benefits; therefore TRICARE Standard, TRICARE Extra, or Medicare may pay for civilian health care services obtained by a TRICARE Plus enrollee.

ARMED FORCES OF THE UNITED STATES

Active Duty

PHOTO PLACED HERE

U.S. NAVY ACTIVE

RANK/PAY GRADE
LT/03

EXPIRATION DATE
2005 AUG 23

SIGNATURE
John B. Davis

SOCIAL SECURITY NUMBER
654-XX-4567

DAVIS JOHN B.

GENEVA CONVENTIONS IDENTIFICATION CARD

Back of Card

DATE OF BIRTH	WEIGHT	HEIGHT	HAIR COLOR	EYE COLOR
1960JUN20	190	70	BR	BR

DATE OF ISSUE	BLOOD TYPE	GENEVA CONV CATEGORY
1999AUG23	O+	IV

DD FORM 2 (ACTIVE)   OCT 93   PROPERTY OF US GOVERNMENT

FIGURE 14–6 Military identification card for an active duty individual in the Armed Forces. It is used as the identification card for the TRICARE Prime Remote Program and is considered a sponsor identification card.

	TRICARE Prime Remote (TPR)	Supplemental Health Care Program (SHCP)
Plan description	TPR is a program for Active Duty Service Members (ADSMs) who live and work more than 50 miles or one hour from a military treatment facility (MTF). ADSMs must enroll.	SHCP is a program for • Active Duty Service Members (ADSMs) • Inpatients at military treatment facilities who are not TRICARE eligible (e.g., eligible parents, parents-in-law) referred by an MTF to a civilian provider for care (usually for a specific test, procedure or consultation). • Non-MTF referred ADSMs (e.g., ROTC students, cadets/midshipmen, eligible foreign military).
Provider type	Any civilian provider.	Any civilian provider.
Beneficiary access to care	TPR ADSMs receive from any civilian provider, or from a military treatment facility when available. Under TPR, ADSMs will have the same priority to care as other ADSMs at the MTF.	The beneficiary may receive services from any civilian provider, in accordance with referral and preauthorization requirements, below.
Beneficiary responsibility	TPR ADSMs have no annual deductible, cost-shares, or copayments. The TPR ADSM must present his/her Military ID card at the time care is received.	ADSMs and others eligible for SHCP referred to civilian providers have no copayment, deductible, or cost share. Beneficiary must present his/her Military ID card at the time care is recieved.
Point-of-Service (POS)	Point-of-Service does not apply. If the ADSM receives care without a referral or preauthorization, the claim will be processed if it meets all other TRICARE requirements on a case-by-case basis.	The Point-of-Service option does not apply.
Program benefits	Offers benefits similar to TRICARE Prime. Some benefits (including all behavioral health care) require preauthorization.	Offers benefits similar to TRICARE Prime. Some benefits (including all behavioral health care) require preauthorization.
Referrals and preauthorizations	Primary care – ADSMs can receive primary care from a provider without a referral or preauthorization. ADSMs with an assigned PCM will receive primary care from their PCM. ADSMs with no PCM can use any TRICARE-certified provider. Or, he/she can contact a HCF for assistance in locating a provider. Specialty and inpatient care – The SPOC will review requests for specialty and inpatient care.	Specialty and inpatient care – The MTF will review all requests for specialty and inpatient care for ADSMs. **The MTF Commander or designee signature on a DD Form 2161** is required for designated patients **referred** for civilian care. Preauthorization for **non-referred** Active Duty Service Members for specialty, inpatient, and behavioral health care must be **obtained from the SPOC or the Health Care Finder.**

FIGURE 14–7 Summary of unique aspects of TRICARE Prime Remote Program and Supplemental Health Care Program.

TRICARE PRIME REMOTE PROGRAM

Enrollment

TRICARE Prime Remote (TPR) is a program designed for **active duty service members** who work and live more than 50 miles or 1 hour from military treatment facilities (military hospitals and clinics). Active duty service members must enroll for this program, which enables them to receive care from any civilian provider. TRICARE Prime Remote for Active Duty Family Members (TPRADFM) is the TPR benefit for family members with similar benefits and program requirements. TPR/TPRADFM is offered in the 50 United States only, and both require enrollment.

Identification Card

Active duty service members must present their military identification card to receive care from providers (Figure 14–6). Photocopy front and reverse sides of the card so information is available for reference when completing the insurance claim form.

Benefits

TPR program benefits are similar to TRICARE Prime. Services may be received from an MTF when available or from any civilian provider. Primary routine care does not require prior authorization (e.g., office visits and preventive health care). The HCF must be contacted to receive authorization for referrals, inpatient admissions, maternity, physical therapy, orthotics, hearing appliances, family planning (tubal ligation or vasectomy), outpatient and inpatient behavioral health services, and transplants. Figure 14–7 is a summary of the unique aspects of TPR.

Referral and Preauthorization

Routine primary care does not require prior authorization (e.g., office visits and preventive health care). The PCM must initiate all specialty referrals and coordinate requests through the HBA for certain outpatient services, all inpatient surgical or medical services, maternity services, physical therapy, orthotics, hearing appliances, family planning, transplants, and inpatient or outpatient behavioral health services. The HBA is a government employee who is responsible for helping all MHS beneficiaries to obtain medical care.

Payments

Those persons covered and receiving benefits under TPR are not responsible for any out-of-pocket costs. Active duty service member claims for services provided by a TRICARE network provider are paid at the same contracted rate as other TRICARE beneficiary claims.

SUPPLEMENTAL HEALTH CARE PROGRAM

Enrollment

The Supplemental Health Care Program (SHCP) covers both military treatment facility–referred care as well as civilian health care provided to active duty service members. The MTF always administers routine care (e.g., routine office visits and preventive health care).

Identification Card

Active duty service members must present their military identification card to receive care from providers (see Figure 14–6). The front and reverse sides of the card should be photocopied so information is available for reference when the insurance claim form is completed.

Benefits

See Figure 14–7 for a summary of the unique aspects of SHCP.

SHCP enables beneficiaries to be referred to a civilian provider for care. The MTF must initiate all referrals to civilian providers and use a DD Form 2161 signed by the facility commander. There is no deductible, copayment, or cost-share for services provided by a civilian provider.

Referral and Preauthorization

The MTF initiates all referrals for active duty service members and other designated patients to civilian specialists when needed.

Payments

Those covered and receiving benefits under SHCP are not responsible for any out-of-pocket costs. Active duty service member claims for services provided by a TRICARE network provider are paid at the same contracted rate as other TRICARE beneficiary claims.

TRICARE HOSPICE PROGRAM

The TRICARE hospice program is based on Medicare's hospice program. It is designed to provide care and comfort to patients who are expected to live less than 6 months if the terminal illness runs its normal course. Those persons who receive care under the hospice program cannot receive other services under the TRI-CARE basic programs (treatments aimed at a cure) unless the hospice care has been formally revoked. There are a number of additional rules and limits to the hospice program; therefore HBA at the nearest military medical facility should be called and a copy of the guidelines requested.

TRICARE AND HMO COVERAGE

TRICARE considers HMO coverage to be the same as any other primary health insurance coverage. TRICARE shares the cost of covered care received from an HMO (including the HMO's user fees), after the HMO has paid all it is going to pay, under the following conditions:

● The provider must meet TRICARE provider certification standards.
● The type of care must be a TRICARE benefit and medically necessary.
● TRICARE does not pay for emergency services received outside the HMO's normal service area.

TRICARE does not cost-share services an individual obtains outside the HMO if the services are available through the HMO. For example, if an HMO provides psychiatric services but the patient does not like the HMO's psychiatrist and obtains services outside the HMO, TRICARE will not pay anything on the claim.

CHAMPVA PROGRAM

The Veterans Health Care Expansion Act of 1973 (PL93-82) authorized a CHAMPUS–like program called **CHAMPVA** (Civilian Health and Medical Program of the Veterans Administration; now known as the Department of Veterans Affairs), which became effective on September 1, 1973. CHAMPVA is not an insurance program in that it does not involve a contract guaranteeing the indemnification of an insured party against a specified loss in return for a premium paid. It is considered a **service benefit program;** therefore there are no premiums.

This program is for the spouse and children of a veteran with a **total, permanent service-connected disability** or for the surviving spouse and children of a veteran who died as a result of a service-connected disability. A **veteran** is any person who has served in the armed forces of the United States, is no longer in the service, and has received an honorable discharge. Just as in the TRICARE program, individuals who qualify for CHAMPVA are known as beneficiaries and the veteran is called the sponsor.

Examples of service-connected total, permanent disabilities include an injury with paraplegic results, a bullet wound with neurologic damage, and loss of a limb. This contrasts with a chronic or temporary service-connected disability, which might exist if an individual improperly lifts a heavy object while in the Navy, suffers a back injury with ongoing sporadic symptoms, and requires continuing medical care after leaving the service. Both scenarios present service-connected disabilities; however, the first example illustrates a person permanently disabled, whereas the second illustrates what may be a chronic or temporary disability.

Eligibility

The following persons are eligible for CHAMPVA benefits as long as they are not eligible for TRICARE Standard and not eligible for Medicare Part A as a result of reaching age 65:

● The husband, wife, or unmarried child of a veteran with a total disability, permanent in nature, resulting from a **service-connected injury**
● The husband, wife, or unmarried child of a veteran who died as the result of a service-connected disability or who, at the time of death, had a total disability, permanent in nature, resulting from a service-connected injury
● The husband, wife, or unmarried child of an individual who died in the line of duty while in active service

Qualifying children are those unmarried and younger than age 18, regardless of whether dependent or not, or those up to age 23 who are enrolled in a course of instruction at an approved educational institution.

Determination of eligibility is the responsibility of the Department of Veterans Affairs (VA). The prospective beneficiary visits the nearest VA medical center and receives a VA identification card if eligible.

Enrollment

Dependents of veterans must have a Social Security number and have contacted the local VA regional office to establish dependency on the veteran sponsor. The individual obtains and completes an application by telephone, fax, or downloading from the VA's Web site (see Internet Resources at the end of this chapter).

Identification Card

The issuing station's number appears on the identification card to identify the home station where the

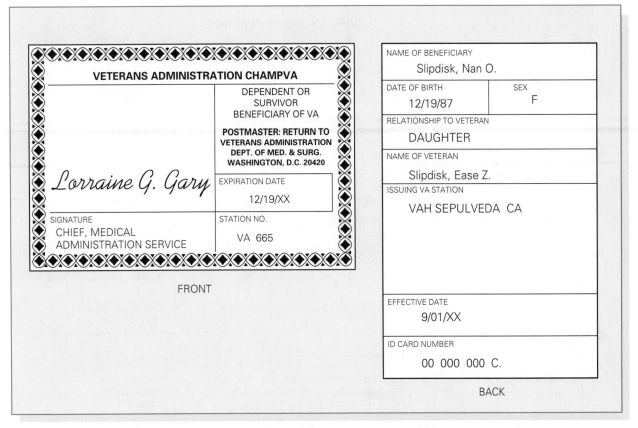

FIGURE 14–8 CHAMPVA card.

beneficiary's case file is kept. The identification card number is the veteran's VA file number with an alpha suffix. The suffix is different for each beneficiary of a sponsor. All dependents 10 years of age or older are required to have a uniformed services (military) identification and privilege card for CHAMPVA, as shown in Figure 14–8.

Benefits

The Department of Veterans Affairs elected to provide these beneficiaries with benefits and cost-sharing plans similar to those received by dependents of retired and deceased uniformed services personnel under TRICARE Standard. An overall picture of CHAMPVA benefits, which includes cost-sharing (deductibles and copayments), can be seen in Figure 14–9.

Provider

The beneficiaries of the CHAMPVA program have complete freedom of choice in selecting their civilian health care providers.

Preauthorization

Preauthorization is necessary for organ and bone marrow transplants, hospice services, most mental health or substance abuse services, all dental care, and all durable medical equipment with a purchase price or total rental cost of $300 or more. Preauthorization for mental health and substance abuse care must be requested from Health Management Strategies (HMS) International, Inc., at 800-240-4068 or mailed to CVAC-MHP, P.O. Box 26128, Alexandria, VA 22313. All other preauthorization requests are made directly to CHAMPVA at 303-331-7599, by fax at 303-331-7804, or by mail to VA Health Administration Center, CHAMPVA, Attn: Preauthorization, P.O. Box 65023, Denver, CO 80206-9023.

CLAIMS PROCEDURE

Fiscal Intermediary

TRICARE Standard is governed by the DoD. As such, it is not subject to those state regulatory bodies or agencies that control the insurance business. The DoD and the VA have agreed to use the Office of the Assistant

CHAMPVA Cost Share Summary

| Benefit (Covered Services) | Beneficiary Pays [1,2] | | CHAMPVA Pays |
	Deductible ($50/individual or $100/family per calendar year)	Cost Share	
Outpatient services			
Ambulatory surgery *Family services*	No	25% of allowable	75% of allowable
Professional services	Yes	25% of allowable	75% of allowable
Pharmacy services	Yes	25% of allowable	75% of allowable
Durable Medical Equipment (DME)			
Non–VA source VA source	Yes No	25% of allowable NONE	75% of allowable 100% of VA cost
Inpatient services			
Facility services DRG based	No	Lesser of: 1) per day amt x number of inpatient days; 2) 25% of billed amount; or 3) DRG rate	DRG rate less beneficiary cost share
Non–DRG based	No	25% of allowable	75% of allowable
Mental health High volume/RTC	No	25% of allowable	75% of allowable
Low volume	No	Lesser of: 1) per day amt x number of inpatient days; 2) 25% of billed amount.	Balance of allowable AFTER beneficiary cost share
Professional services	No	25% of allowable	75% of allowable

[1] Services received at VA health care facilities under the CHAMPVA Inhouse treatment Intiative (CITI) program are exempt from beneficiary cost sharing.
[2] Under catastrophic protection plan (Cat Cap), annual beneficiary cost sharing is limited to $7500.

FIGURE 14–9 CHAMPVA service benefits and cost-share summary chart.

Secretary of Defense and the TRICARE Standard system of fiscal intermediaries and hospital contractors to receive, process, and pay CHAMPVA claims, following the same procedures currently used for TRICARE Standard.

A **fiscal intermediary (FI)** (also known as a contractor or claims processor) is an organization under contract to the government that handles insurance claims for care received under the TRICARE Standard or CHAMPVA program.

TRICARE Standard and CHAMPVA

TRICARE Standard and CHAMPVA claims must be billed on the CMS-1500 claim form and submitted to the claims processor (fiscal intermediary). Remember to abstract the correct information from front and back sides of the patient's identification card. Refer to Chapter 6 and follow the TRICARE or CHAMPVA instructions for completing the CMS-1500 claim form. Refer to Figure 7–13 for an example of a completed TRICARE case with no other insurance and Figure 7–14 for an example of a completed CHAMPVA case. If electing to complete the

HIPAA Compliance Alert

MEDICAL RECORD ACCESS

Privacy Act of 1974

The Privacy Act of 1974 became effective on September 27, 1975, and establishes an individual's right to review his or her medical records maintained by a federal medical care facility, such as a VA medical center or U.S. Public Health Service facility, and to contest inaccuracies in such records. The act directs each agency to make its own rules establishing access procedures. Agencies are allowed to adopt special procedures when it is believed that direct access could be harmful to a person. The act requires that an individual from whom personal information is requested be informed of (1) the authority for the request, (2) the principal purpose of the information requested, (3) routine use of the information, and (4) the effect on an individual who does not provide the information.

Some federal agencies or federally funded institutions may be regulated by both the Privacy Act and the HIPAA standards. Such entities are required to comply with both sets of regulations. While the HIPAA standards generally provide more restrictive regulations, entities are advised to revise their policies and procedures to comply with both the HIPAA standards and the privacy act. Under certain situations, HIPAA standards are likely to prevail and require regulated entities to obtain individual authorization for some disclosures that they now make without authorization under the "routine uses" exception. HIPAA compliance managers should make a determination of the effects of the interplay between the federal laws and the HIPAA standards, consult with legal counsel, and plan an entity's compliance initiatives accordingly.

Computer Matching and Privacy Protection Act of 1988

The Computer Matching and Privacy Protection Act of 1988 was established and is specific to TRICARE. It permits the government to verify information by way of computer matches. By law, the provider must tell a TRICARE member that he or she is calling TRICARE, which is governed by the Department of Defense (DoD), and only information to determine eligibility and to learn what services are covered is to be obtained.

Both of these acts are mentioned on the back of the CMS-1500 claim form. TRICARE patients must be made aware of this information by physicians who treat them, so that they are knowledgeable about routine use and disclosure of medical data. Providers must follow both HIPAA and the Computer Matching and Privacy Protection Act of 1988. Patients may make a Privacy Protection Act request in writing, in person, or by telephone. Individuals should call the facility to determine the required procedures to obtain access to the records and what to include in making a written request.

VA Form 10-1759A for a CHAMPVA case, refer to the instructions presented later in this chapter.

If the physician is nonparticipating and does not accept assignment, the patient completes the top portion of the CMS-1500 claim form, attaches the physician's itemized statement, and submits the claim. Alternatively, the patient may submit on the white TRICARE claim DD Form 2642 Patient's Request for Medical Payment. Patients and providers of care for health services in foreign countries must use DD Form 2520. The Uniform Bill (UB-92) form is used for inpatient hospital billing.

Time Limit

Effective January 1, 1993, claims must be filed within 1 year from the date a service is provided or (for inpatient care) within 1 year from the patient's date of discharge from the inpatient facility.

Claims Office

The TRICARE program is administered by the Department of Defense, TRICARE Management Activity, 16401 East Centretech Parkway, Aurora, CO 80011-9043, but claims are not processed in Colorado. The medical biller must understand that when sending the claim to TRICARE, the claim is sent to the TRICARE claims office nearest to the residence of the military sponsor. For example, if the patient is a child who was treated in California, but the sponsor is an active duty service member stationed in Florida, the claim should be sent to the TRICARE claims office in Camden, SC, and not to the claims office in Surfside Beach, SC. Refer to the Internet Resources at the end of this chapter for the Web site to locate the address of the regional claims processor for submitting a TRICARE Standard claim in each state. Write to the TRICARE Support Office or contact the HBA at the nearest MTF to obtain a current

TRICARE Standard Handbook or for answers to any questions about the name of the regional claims processor, benefits, nonbenefits, when an NAS is necessary, and so on.

Because of the September 11, 2001, attack in New York City and the activation of the United States National Guard and Reserve components to the Middle East, the provider's office may come into contact with members of the National Guard or Reserve Component. The members of these two organizations normally join a unit located near their place of residence. The National Guard and Reserve are only called to active duty in certain circumstances. Otherwise they are required to perform their duties once in "drill status" and to participate in "annual training." Drill status occurs on a Saturday and a Sunday. Annual training occurs for 2 weeks, normally during the summer months. While these service members are on drill status or in annual training, they are entitled to medical care at government expense. The government will pay for an illness or injury incurred while on the way to drill status, during drill status, and on the way home from drill status. If the service member stops anywhere on the way to or from drill (e.g., to put gas in the car), any injury received is not paid for by the government. Sometimes when a service member is injured or becomes ill, he or she may have medical personnel available within the unit to provide medical care. If not, the service member is sent to a clinic or hospital near the drill center. This injury or illness is not covered by workers' compensation. The military unit must be contacted to be compensated for the medical care. Each unit has a staff member called a full-time manager (FTM). This person is assigned to the unit and works full-time during the week and attends drills with the unit on weekends. He or she processes all medical claims for unit members. Medical records must accompany the claim for it to be paid. The unit also may require the physician to prepare additional forms that must accompany the claim. The payment is not paid by the unit. The claim is sent to a higher command where the illness or injury is investigated. This is a very time-consuming procedure, and it could take months for the claim to be paid. It is better to bill the service member for payment if payment is not received with 60 to 90 days.

The CHAMPVA program is administered by the Department of Veterans Affairs, Health Administration Center, P.O. Box 65023, Denver, CO 80206-9023.

TRICARE Extra and TRICARE Prime

The beneficiary does not file any claim forms under TRICARE Extra or TRICARE Prime programs when using network providers. Providers must submit claims on CMS-1500 claim forms to TRICARE subcontractors for services given to beneficiaries. Referral and preauthorization numbers are required on claim forms when applicable.

Time Limit

For outpatient care a claim must be received by the state's or region's TRICARE contractor within 1 year of the date the provider rendered the service to the patient. For inpatient care, a claim must be received by the contractor within 1 year from the date the patient was discharged from the facility. If a claim covers several different medical services or supplies that were provided at different times, the 1-year deadline applies to each item on the claim.

When a claim is submitted on time but the contractor returns it for more information, the claim should be resubmitted with the requested information so it is received by the contractor no later than 1 year after the medical services or supplies were provided or 90 days from the date the claim was returned to the provider, whichever is later.

A contractor may grant exemptions from the filing deadlines for several reasons. A request that includes a complete explanation of the circumstances of the late filing, all available documentation supporting the request, and the claim denied for late filing should be submitted to the contractor.

Claims Office

See the Internet Resources for the Web site to find the name and address to which claims should be submitted and to obtain more information about this program.

TRICARE Prime Remote and Supplemental Health Care Program

Outpatient professional services are submitted using a CMS-1500 claim form. Primary care service claims are processed and paid without a referral or preauthorization from a network or non-network provider. A referral number provided by the HCF must be included on the claim form for specialty medical or surgical care and for behavioral health counseling and therapy sessions. The POS option and NAS requirements do not apply to TPR and SHCP claims.

Time Limit

A claim must be filed within 1 year from the date a service is provided or (for inpatient care) within 1 year from the patient's date of discharge from the inpatient facility.

Claims Office

Do not file claims of active duty armed service patients to TRICARE. Claims for patients on active duty must be sent to the specific branch of service (e.g., Army, Navy, Air Force, or Marines). Claims are submitted to Palmetto Government Benefits Administrators (PGBAs) for processing and payment (see Internet Resources at the end of this chapter to locate the address).

TRICARE for Life

If the beneficiary receives care from a civilian provider, the provider submits claims to Medicare. Medicare pays its portion and then automatically forwards the claim to TRICARE for the remaining amount. TRICARE sends its payment directly to the provider. The beneficiary receives a TRICARE summary payment voucher that indicates the amount paid to the provider.

TRICARE/CHAMPVA and Other Insurance

By law TRICARE/CHAMPVA is usually the second payer when a beneficiary is enrolled in **other health insurance (OHI),** a civilian health plan, or belongs to an HMO or preferred provider organization. However, there are two exceptions:

● When a plan is administered under Title XIX of the Social Security Act (Medicaid)
● When coverage is specifically designed to supplement TRICARE benefits (e.g., Medigap health plan)

When the patient has other health insurance that is primary (meaning that it pays before TRICARE Standard or CHAMPVA does), submit the claim using the CMS-1500 insurance claim form. Attach the explanation of benefits from the primary carrier. If the patient is submitting his or her claim to the other insurance, take these steps:

1. Bill the other insurance carrier with the form it has supplied.
2. Bill TRICARE or CHAMPVA by completing the top section of the CMS-1500 after receiving payment and an explanation of benefits from the other insurance company. Submit the physician's itemized statement, which must contain the following:
   a. Provider's name
   b. Date the services or supplies were provided
   c. Description of each service or supply
   d. Place of treatment
   e. Number or frequency of each service
   f. Fee for each item of service or supply
   g. Procedure code numbers
   h. Diagnostic code number or description of condition for which treatment is being received
   i. Billing statements showing only total charges, canceled checks, or cash register receipts (or similar-type receipts) are not acceptable as itemized statements
3. Attach a photocopy of the explanation of benefits from the other insurance company.
4. Send the TRICARE or CHAMPVA claim to the local claims processor (fiscal intermediary).

Medicaid and TRICARE/CHAMPVA

File TRICARE or CHAMPVA claims first if the beneficiary is a recipient of the Medicaid program.

Medicare and TRICARE

TRICARE is considered secondary to Medicare for persons younger than age 65 who have Medicare Part A as a result of a disability and who have enrolled in Medicare Part B. Those eligible for Medicare Part A are not covered by TRICARE unless disabled. Claims should be submitted to Medicare, then to TRICARE with a copy of the Medicare remittance advice. Services covered by TRICARE but not covered by Medicare (e.g., prescriptions) are paid by TRICARE. Participating providers may obtain a TRICARE fee schedule by contacting their fiscal intermediary.

Medicare and CHAMPVA

Effective December 5, 1991, CHAMPVA became secondary payer to Medicare for persons younger than age 65 who are enrolled in Medicare Parts A and B and who are otherwise eligible for CHAMPVA. Claims first must be submitted to Medicare because CHAMPVA is a secondary payer.

Dual or Double Coverage

A claim must be filed if a patient has additional insurance that provides double coverage. Refusal by the beneficiary to claim benefits from other health insurance coverage results in a denial of TRICARE benefits. In double coverage situations, TRICARE pays the lower of the following:

● The amount of TRICARE-allowable charges remaining after the double coverage plan has paid its benefits
● The amount TRICARE would have paid as primary payer

There must be **coordination of benefits** so that there is no duplication of benefits paid between the double coverage plan and TRICARE.

Third-Party Liability

If the patient is in an automobile accident or receives an injury that may have third-party involvement, the following two options are available for reimbursement:

Option 1: TRICARE Form DD 2527 (Statement of Personal Injury, Possible Third-Party Liability) must be sent in with the regular claim form for cost-sharing of the civilian medical care. All five sections of the form should be completed by the patient. This form allows TRICARE to evaluate the circumstances of the accident and the possibility that the government may recover money for the medical care from the person who injured the patient. If a CMS-1500 claim form is submitted without TRICARE Form DD 2527, a request is made to complete it. This form must be returned within 35 days of the request, or the claims processor will deny the original and all related claims. Then the fiscal intermediary submits a claim to the third party for reimbursement or files a lien for reimbursement with the liability insurance carrier, the liable party, or the attorneys or court involved.

Option 2: The provider can submit claims exclusively to the third-party liability carrier for reimbursement. Claims submitted with ICD-9-CM diagnostic codes between 800 and 999 (Injury and Poisoning) trigger the fact that there might be third-party litigation, and the claims processor may request the completion of DD Form 2527.

Workers' Compensation

If a TRICARE or CHAMPVA beneficiary is injured on the job or becomes ill because of his or her work, a workers' compensation claim must be filed with the compensation insurance carrier. TRICARE or CHAMPVA can be billed when all workers' compensation benefits have been exhausted.

In some situations, it must be decided whether a case that involves an accident or illness is work-related, and the claim might be sent to the TRICARE or CHAMPVA claims fiscal intermediary. In those instances, the claims processor files a lien with the workers' compensation carrier for recovery when the case is settled.

AFTER CLAIM SUBMISSION

TRICARE Summary Payment Voucher

For each TRICARE claim the claims processor issues a **summary payment voucher** (Figure 14–10) that details

the payment of the claim. When the provider participates (accepts assignment), the voucher is sent to him or her with the check. The patient always receives a copy of the voucher, even if the provider receives payment directly from the fiscal intermediary.

CHAMPVA Explanation of Benefits Document

Upon completion of the processing of a claim, a payment check is generated and an explanation of benefits document is sent to the beneficiary (including the provider if the claim is filed by the provider). The explanation of benefits summarizes the action taken on the claim and contains information as graphically illustrated and explained in Figure 14–11. Beneficiaries who receive durable medical equipment or VA services from a CHAMPVA In-house Treatment Initiative (CITI, pronounced "city") do not receive an explanation of benefits.

Quality Assurance

A **quality assurance program** continually assesses the effectiveness of inpatient and outpatient care. The quality assurance department reviews providers' outpatient records on a random basis for clinical and administrative quality. Grievance procedures have been established for members and providers if any complaint arises from an administrative process, a service provided by a physician, or an issue involving quality of care.

TRICARE-managed care programs have a quality assurance program to continually assess the effectiveness of care and services rendered by providers. This includes inpatient and outpatient hospital care, mental health services, long-term care, home health care, and programs for people with disabilities. Providers are notified in writing when a potential quality issue has been confirmed as a breach of quality standards. Recommended corrective action plans are given, and noncompliance may lead to suspension or termination of a provider.

Claims Inquiries and Appeals

Through the appeal process, providers may request reconsideration of a denial of certification for coverage or of the amount paid for a submitted claim. See Chapter 9 for inquiring about the status of a claim and to learn the procedures on how to file reviews and appeals.

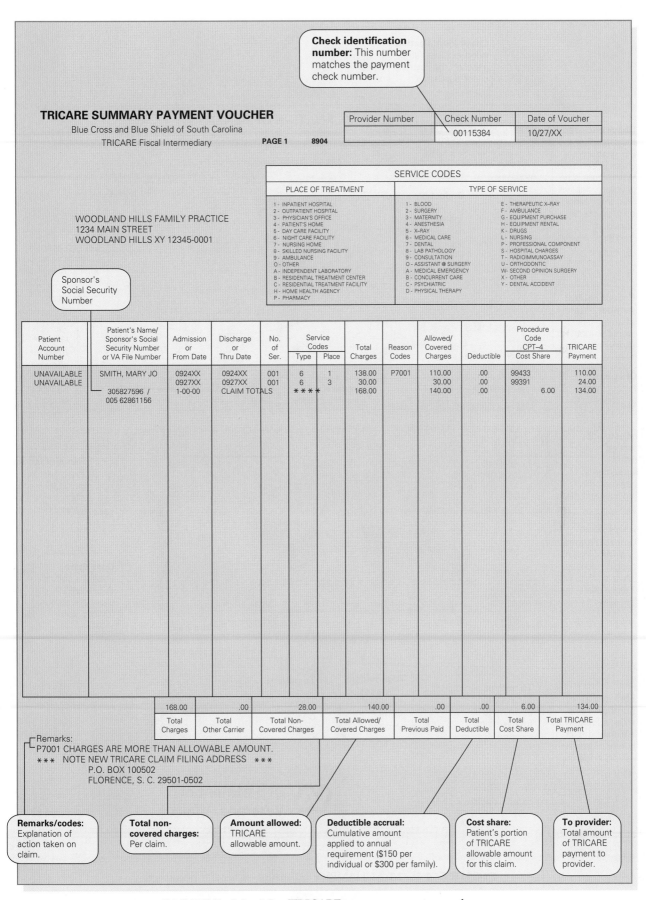

Check identification number: This number matches the payment check number.

TRICARE SUMMARY PAYMENT VOUCHER
Blue Cross and Blue Shield of South Carolina
TRICARE Fiscal Intermediary **PAGE 1** **8904**

Provider Number	Check Number	Date of Voucher
	00115384	10/27/XX

WOODLAND HILLS FAMILY PRACTICE
1234 MAIN STREET
WOODLAND HILLS XY 12345-0001

Sponsor's Social Security Number

SERVICE CODES

PLACE OF TREATMENT	TYPE OF SERVICE
1 - INPATIENT HOSPITAL 2 - OUTPATIENT HOSPITAL 3 - PHYSICIAN'S OFFICE 4 - PATIENT'S HOME 5 - DAY CARE FACILITY 6 - NIGHT CARE FACILITY 7 - NURSING HOME 8 - SKILLED NURSING FACILITY 9 - AMBULANCE 0 - OTHER A - INDEPENDENT LABORATORY B - RESIDENTIAL TREATMENT CENTER C - RESIDENTIAL TREATMENT FACILITY H - HOME HEALTH AGENCY P - PHARMACY	1 - BLOOD E - THERAPEUTIC X–RAY 2 - SURGERY F - AMBULANCE 3 - MATERNITY G - EQUIPMENT PURCHASE 4 - ANESTHESIA H - EQUIPMENT RENTAL 5 - X-RAY K - DRUGS 6 - MEDICAL CARE L - NURSING 7 - DENTAL P - PROFESSIONAL COMPONENT 8 - LAB PATHOLOGY S - HOSPITAL CHARGES 9 - CONSULTATION T - RADIOIMMUNOASSAY O - ASSISTANT @ SURGERY U - ORTHODONTIC A - MEDICAL EMERGENCY W - SECOND OPINION SURGERY B - CONCURRENT CARE X - OTHER C - PSYCHIATRIC Y - DENTAL ACCIDENT D - PHYSICAL THERAPY

Patient Account Number	Patient's Name/ Sponsor's Social Security Number or VA File Number	Admission or From Date	Discharge or Thru Date	No. of Ser.	Service Codes Type	Service Codes Place	Total Charges	Reason Codes	Allowed/ Covered Charges	Deductible	Procedure Code CPT–4	Cost Share	TRICARE Payment
UNAVAILABLE UNAVAILABLE	SMITH, MARY JO 305827596 / 005 62861156	0924XX 0927XX 1-00-00	0924XX 0927XX CLAIM TOTALS	001 001	6 6 ****	1 3	138.00 30.00 168.00	P7001	110.00 30.00 140.00	.00 .00 .00	99433 99391	6.00	110.00 24.00 134.00

168.00	.00	28.00	140.00	.00	.00	6.00	134.00
Total Charges	Total Other Carrier	Total Non-Covered Charges	Total Allowed/ Covered Charges	Total Previous Paid	Total Deductible	Total Cost Share	Total TRICARE Payment

Remarks:
P7001 CHARGES ARE MORE THAN ALLOWABLE AMOUNT.
*** NOTE NEW TRICARE CLAIM FILING ADDRESS ***
P.O. BOX 100502
FLORENCE, S. C. 29501-0502

Remarks/codes: Explanation of action taken on claim.

Total non-covered charges: Per claim.

Amount allowed: TRICARE allowable amount.

Deductible accrual: Cumulative amount applied to annual requirement ($150 per individual or $300 per family).

Cost share: Patient's portion of TRICARE allowable amount for this claim.

To provider: Total amount of TRICARE payment to provider.

FIGURE 14–10 TRICARE summary payment voucher.

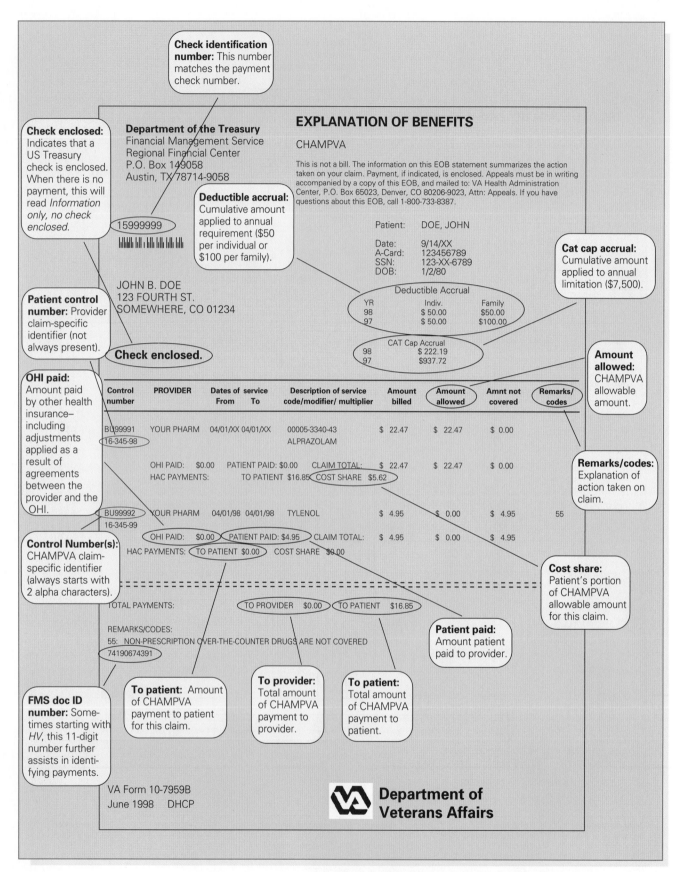

FIGURE 14–11   CHAMPVA explanation of benefits document.

PROCEDURE

COMPLETING A CHAMPVA CLAIM FORM

An example of a completed CHAMPVA claim form is provided in Figure 14-12.

1. Enter the patient's last name, first name, and middle initial (do not use nicknames or abbreviations).
2. Enter the patient's Social Security number exactly as it appears on the Social Security card. If the patient does not have a Social Security number, print "None."
3. Enter the patient's complete address. If the patient's address has changed, place an "X" in the box.
4. Enter the patient's home telephone number. Include the area code.
5A. Enter the number from Item 6 of the patient's current CHAMPVA Authorization Card.
5B. Enter the date from Item 4 of the patient's current CHAMPVA Authorization Card.
5C. Enter the date from Item 5 of the patient's current CHAMPVA Authorization Card.
6. Enter the patient's date of birth.
7. Enter the patient's relationship to the sponsor.
8. Enter the patient's gender.
9. Enter the sponsor's last name, first name, and middle initial (do not use nicknames or abbreviations).
10. Enter the sponsor's VA Claim or File Number.
11. Enter the sponsor's complete address (if different from the patient's).
12A. Place an "X" in the appropriate box if the patient is covered under any other medical benefits plan or health insurance coverage. CHAMPVA does not duplicate benefits of any other health insurance plan or program.
12B. Place an "X" beside all applicable types of medical plans or other health insurance to which the patient is entitled.
12C. Enter the name and address of the other insurance carrier.
12D. Enter the name and address of the employer if other health insurance is provided by the patient's employer.
12E. Enter the policy identification number of the other health insurance carrier.
12F. Enter the insurance agent's name. If this information is not known, enter "Unknown."
12G. Enter the insurance agent's telephone number. If this information is not known, enter "Unknown."
13. Check the appropriate box according to the type of medical care the patient received.
    Inpatient: Check the Inpatient box for admission to a civilian hospital.
    Outpatient: Check the Outpatient box for all eligible CHAMPVA beneficiaries provided medical care from civilian facilities unless otherwise authorized by the VA.
    Pharmacy: Check the Pharmacy box for claims for payment of drugs and medicines requiring a prescription by law.
    Travel: Check the Travel box for claims for ambulance travel to, from, or between hospitals for inpatient care.
    Dental: Check the Dental box for dental care for which the patient has an approved preauthorization.
    Durable Medical Equipment (DME): Check the DME box for payment of durable medical equipment costing more than $100.
    College Infirmary: Check the Other box for College Infirmary.
    Other Inpatient Care: Check the Inpatient box for admissions to an approved nursing facility (including a Christian Science sanatorium).
14. If the patient needs treatment for any kind of an injury (e.g., broken toe, sprained knee, lacerated forehead, or back injury), check "YES" and briefly describe the injury and circumstances of how the patient was injured.
15. Be sure to read the release of medical record information contained in this item and complete the blanks, if appropriate.
16. CHAMPVA is a benefit program. As such, the patient (or sponsor) must assign the benefit to the provider of care if he or she wishes the payment to be made to the provider. Otherwise payment will be made to the patient.
17A. Every CHAMPVA claim must be signed by a patient 18 years of age or older. If the beneficiary is unable to sign on his or her own behalf, the sponsor (or other parent) may sign. In the absence of either parent, a guardian or fiduciary may sign. (NOTE: For privacy reasons a patient younger than 18 years of age may sign his or her own claim form.)
17B. Insert date of signature.
17C. Enter the claimant's relationship to sponsor.
    Part V: To be completed by physician or other provider.
    Top of page II: Enter patient and sponsor's last name, first name, and middle initial.
18. Enter provider's (physician's) name and title.
19. Enter provider's tax identification number.
20. Enter the name of the referring physician or agency.
21. Enter the admission and discharge dates if the patient is hospitalized.
22. Enter the name and address of the facility where services were rendered if other than home or office.

Continued

COMPLETING A CHAMPVA CLAIM FORM

OMB NC: 2900-
Estimated burden: 30 min

VA Department of Veterans Affairs

CHAMPVA CLAIM FORM

CHAMPVA CENTER, 4500 Cherry Creek Drive South, Box 300, Denver CO 80222

WARNING: IF YOU KNOWINGLY MAKE A FALSE STATEMENT OF ANY MATERIAL FACT IN OR IN CONNECTION WITH THIS CLAIM, YOU ARE SUBJECT TO PROSECUTION IN A U.S. COURT

PART 1 - PATIENT INFORMATION (To be completed by the beneficiary, patient or sponsor)

1. PATIENT'S NAME
CHIEU, MARION W.

2. PATIENT'S SOCIAL SECURITY NUMBER
742-XX-0491

3. PATIENT'S ADDRESS (Street, City, State, ZIP)   (Check if new address)
321 OAK STREET,   WOODLAND HILLS, XY 12345

4. TELEPHONE NUMBER (Include area code)
(555)492-7800

5A. CHAMPVA IDENTIFICATION CARD/AUTHORIZATION NUMBER
49-467-081C

	5B. EFFECTIVE DATE			5C. EXPIRATION DATE		
	MONTH	DAY	YEAR	MONTH	DAY	YEAR
	09	01	XX	12	19	XX

6. PATIENT'S DATE OF BIRTH (Month, day, year)
12-01-77

7. PATIENT'S RELATIONSHIP TO SPONSOR (Check one)
☒ SPOUSE   ☐ CHILD

8. PATIENT'S SEX (Check one)
☐ MALE ☒ FEMALE

PART II - SPONSOR INFORMATION (To be completed by the beneficiary, patient or sponsor)

9. SPONSOR'S NAME (Last, first, middle initial)
CHIEU, FRANK T.

10. VA CLAIM/FILE NUMBER
421-05-0129

11. SPONSOR'S ADDRESS IF DIFFERENT FROM PATIENT'S (Street, City, State, Zip)

PART III - PATIENT INSURANCE INFORMATION (To be completed by the beneficiary, patient or sponsor)

12A. IS PATIENT'S TREATMENT COVERED BY OTHER HEALTH INSURANCE
☐ YES   ☒ NO   IF YES, PLEASE COMPLETE ITEMS 12B THROUGH 12G BELOW

12B. TYPE OF COVERAGE
☐ GROUP HEALTH   ☐ PRIVATE (NON–GROUP)
☐ MEDICARE   ☐ CHAMPVA SUPPLEMENTAL
☐ MEDICAID   ☐ WORKERS COMPENSATION
☐ OTHER   ☐ NONE

12C. NAME AND ADDRESS OF INSURANCE CARRIER

12D. IF COVERAGE IS THROUGH WORK, NAME AND ADDRESS OF EMPLOYER

12E. POLICY IDENTIFICATION NUMBER

12F. INSURANCE AGENT'S NAME

12G. AGENT'S TELEPHONE NUMBER

PART IV - TREATMENT INFORMATION (To be completed by the beneficiary, patient or sponsor)

13. TYPE OF CLAIM (Check one)
☐ INPATIENT   ☐ DENTAL
☒ OUTPATIENT   ☐ DME
☐ PHARMACY   ☐ OTHER
☐ TRAVEL

14. WAS NEED OF TREATMENT DUE TO A PHYSICAL INJURY?   YES☐ NO☒
(If "Yes", briefly describe injuries and give a statement of circumstances)

15. I authorize the identified provider of service to disclose to CHAMPVA medical record information that pertains to the medical services described on this form. Unless limitations are shown below, this consent pertains to all of my medical records, including records related to treatment for medical or dental conditions, psychological or psychiatric impairments, drug or alcohol abuse, acquired immune deficiency syndrome (AIDS) or infection with the human immunodeficiency virus (HIV), and sickle cell disease.
The information will be used to process my CHAMPVA claim and determine my (or the patient identified above) eligibility for medical benefits. I also authorize the release of or obtaining of medical and/or other coverage information to and from another organization with which I have other medical benefits plan or health insurance coverage. I understand that I may revoke this authorization at any time, except to the extent that action has already been taken to comply with it. Without my express revocation, this consent will automatically expire: (1) upon satisfaction of the need for disclosure; (2) on February 2, 20XX (date supplied by the beneficiary); or (3) under the following conditions:

LIMITATIONS:

16. I assign payment to the provider(s) of these claim services   ☐ YES   ☒ NO

17. I CERTIFY THAT THE ABOVE STATEMENTS AND ATTACHMENTS ARE CORRECT AND REPRESENT ACTUAL SERVICES, DATES AND FEES CHARGED TO ME OR MY ELIGIBLE DEPENDENTS.

17A. CLAIMANT'S SIGNATURE

17B. DATE
2-2-XX

17C. RELATIONSHIP TO SPONSOR
WIFE

FIGURE 14–12 Completed CHAMPVA claim form VA Form 10-7959A, used when billing for professional services.

PATIENT'S NAME (Last, first, middle initial) CHIEU, MARION W.		SPONSOR'S NAME (Last, first, middle initial) CHIEU, FRANK T.

PART V - PHYSICIAN/OTHER PROVIDER (To be completed by physician or other provider)

18. PROVIDER'S NAME DOE, JOHN M.D.	19. PROVIDER'S TAX I.D. NUMBER 93-4267890	20. NAME OF REFERRING PHYSICIAN OR OTHER SOURCE (e.g. public health agency)

21. WHEN SERVICES ARE RELATED TO A PERIOD OF HOSPITALIZATION, GIVE DATES		22. NAME AND ADDRESS OF FACILITY WHERE SERVICES RENDERED (if other than home office)
ADMITTED	DISCHARGED	

23. DIAGNOSIS OR NATURE OF ILLNESS OR INJURY. RELATE DIAGNOSIS TO PROCEDURE BY USING PROCEDURE NUMBER IN COLUMN 24E BELOW.

A. Dysfunctional uterine bleeding.

B.

C.

24A DATE OF SERVICE	24B * PLACE OF SERVICE	24C PROCEDURE CODE	24D DESCRIBE UNUSUAL SERVICE OR CIRCUMSTANCES	24E DIAGNOSIS CODE	24F CHARGES		24G DAYS OR UNITS	24H TYPE OF SERVICE
02-02-XX	0	99213	Ofc visit Eval & Mgmt Level 3	626.8	45	00	1	1

25. I certify that the statements on the reverse of this bill apply and are made a part hereto. *John Doe, MD* 02-02-XX SIGNATURE OF PROVIDER DATE	26. PROVIDER'S SOCIAL SECURITY NO 272-XX-5731	27. TOTAL CHARGES	45.00	▮▮▮▮

28. PROVIDER'S ADDRESS, ZIP CODE AND TELEPHONE NUMBER
123 MAIN STREET, WOODLAND HILLS, XY 12345   013/486-9002

* PLACE OF SERVICE CODE FOR ITEM 24B IN -INPATIENT HOSPITAL OH -OUTPATIENT HOSPITAL O -DOCTOR'S OFFICE H -PATIENT'S HOME DCF -DAY CARE FACILITY (PSY)	NCF -NIGHT CARE FACILITY (PSY) NH -NURSING HOME SNF -SKILLD NURSING FACILITY AMB -AMBULANCE OL -OTHER LOCATIONS	IL -INDEPENDENT LABORATORY OF -OTHER MEDICAL/SURGICAL FACILITY RTC -RESIDENTIAL TREATMENT CENTER STF - SPECIALIZED TREATMENT FACILITY

PART VI- PHARMACY INFORMATION (To be completed by pharmacist)				PATIENT'S NAME	
29A. NATIONAL DRUG CODE	29B. RX NUMBER	29C. PHARMACY NAME	29D. FILL DATE (Month, day, year)	29E. PHYSICIAN NAME	29F. CHARGES

30. TOTAL CHARGES – $

VA FORM 10-7959A
DEC 1990

reference initials

Pg II

FIGURE 14-12, cont'd For legend see opposite page.

Continued

PROCEDURE—CONT'D

COMPLETING A CHAMPVA CLAIM FORM

23. Enter diagnostic description or nature of illness or injury.
24A. Enter the date of service.
24B. Enter the place of service using one of the codes shown midway down on this page of the form.
24C. Enter the CPT procedure code number with modifier.
24D. Insert a description of the service or procedure.
24E. Enter the ICD-9-CM diagnostic code number for each diagnosis as described in Item 23.
24F. Enter the fee for each service, procedure, or test described in 24D.
24G. Enter the number of days or units. This block is commonly used for multiple visits, number of miles, units of supplies including drugs, anesthesia minutes, or oxygen volume.
24H. Enter the type of service code from the following list:
   1 Medical care
   2 Surgery
   3 Consultation
   4 Diagnostic x-ray
   5 Diagnostic laboratory dialysis
   6 Radiation therapy
   7 Anesthesia
   8 Assistance at surgery
   9 Other medical service
   0 Blood or packed red cells
   A Used DME
   F Ambulatory surgical center
   H Hospice
   L Renal supply in home
   M Alternate payment for maintenance
   N Kidney donor
   V Pneumococcal vaccine
   Y Second opinion on elective surgery
   Z Third opinion on elective surgery
25. Show the signature of the physician, or his or her representative, and the date the form was signed.
26. Enter the provider's Social Security number.
27. Enter the total of all charges.
28. Enter the provider's street address, city, state, ZIP code, and telephone number, including area code.

Items 29A through 30 may be completed if the patient is receiving prescription drugs.

RESOURCES

INTERNET

- CHAMPVA
  Web site: **http://www.va.gov/hac/champva**

- Medicare
  Web site: **http://www.medicare.gov**

- Social Security Administration (for information about enrolling in Medicare Part B)
  Web site: **http://www.ssa.gov**

- TRICARE (for download of a TRICARE manual)
  Web site: **http://www.tricare.osd.mil/tricaremanuals/**

- TRICARE fiscal intermediary directory
  Web site: **http://www.tricare.osd.mil**

Click on Your TRICARE Benefit, click on Claims from the pop-up menu, then click on your state on the map for the name and address of the fiscal intermediary.

- TRICARE military health care beneficiary
  Web site: **http://www.TRICAREOnline.com**

- TRICARE University (basic student course)
  Web site: **http://199.211.83.208/public/index.html**

- VA government forms
  Web site: **http://www.va.gov/forms/medical**

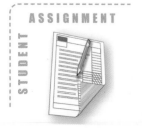

✔ Study Chapter 14.

✔ Answer the review questions in the *Workbook* to reinforce the theory learned in this chapter and help prepare you for a future test.

✔ Complete the assignments in the *Workbook* for computing mathematical calculations and giving you hands-on experience in completing TRICARE and CHAMPVA insurance claim forms and proficiency in procedural and diagnostic coding.

✔ Turn to the glossary at the end of this textbook for a further understanding of the key terms used in this chapter.

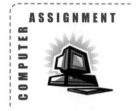

Complete *Workbook* assignment 14–7 on the CD-ROM to transmit a TRICARE electronic insurance claim and review concepts you have learned for this chapter.

CHAPTER OUTLINE

HISTORY
  Workers' Compensation
    Statutes
  Workers' Compensation
    Reform
**WORKERS' COMPENSATION
  LAWS AND INSURANCE**
  Purposes of Workers'
    Compensation Laws
  Self-Insurance
  Managed Care
ELIGIBILITY
  Industrial Accident
  Occupational Illness
COVERAGE
  Federal Laws
  State Laws
  State Disability and Workers'
    Compensation
BENEFITS
TYPES OF STATE CLAIMS
  Nondisability Claim

  Temporary Disability Claim
  Permanent Disability Claim
FRAUD AND ABUSE
**OCCUPATIONAL SAFETY AND
  HEALTH ADMINISTRATION
  ACT OF 1970**
  Background
  Coverage
  Regulations
  Filing a Complaint
  Inspection
  Record Keeping and
    Reporting
LEGAL SITUATIONS
  Medical Evaluator
  Depositions
  Medical Testimony
  Liens
  Third-Party Subrogation
MEDICAL REPORTS
  Privacy and Confidentiality
  Documentation

  Health Information Record
    Keeping
  Terminology
REPORTING REQUIREMENTS
  Employer's Report
  Medical Service Order
  Physician's First Report
  Progress or Supplemental
    Report
  Final Report
CLAIM SUBMISSION
  Financial Responsibility
  Fee Schedules
  Helpful Billing Tips
  Billing Claims
  Out-of-State Claims
  Delinquent or Slow Pay
    Claims
**PROCEDURE: COMPLETING THE
  DOCTOR'S FIRST REPORT OF
  OCCUPATIONAL INJURY OR
  ILLNESS**

KEY TERMS

accident

adjudication

by report (BR)

claims examiner

compromise and release
  (C and R)

deposition

ergonomic

extraterritorial

Federal Employees' Compensation
  Act (FECA)

fee schedule

injury

insurance adjuster

lien

medical service order

nondisability (ND) claim

occupational illness (or disease)

Occupational Safety and Health
  Administration (OSHA)

permanent and stationary
  (P and S)

permanent disability (PD)

petition

second-injury fund

sequelae

sub rosa films

subsequent-injury fund (SIF)

temporary disability (TD)

third-party liability

third-party subrogation

waiting period (WP)

work hardening

Workers' Compensation Appeals
  Board (WCAB)

workers' compensation (WC)
  insurance

15

Workers' Compensation

OBJECTIVES*

After reading this chapter, you should be able to:

- State the purpose of workers' compensation laws.

- Enumerate who is covered under federal workers' compensation laws.

- Name who is covered under state workers' compensation laws.

- Differentiate between workers' compensation insurance and employers' liability insurance.

- Determine the waiting period in each state before benefits begin.

- Describe the types of compensation benefits.

- Define nondisability, temporary disability, and permanent disability claims.

- Explain OSHA's role in protecting employees.

- Define third-party subrogation.

- Define second-injury fund.

- Name the contents of a medical report.

- Complete workers' compensation forms properly.

- Explain how to handle out-of-state claims.

- Define terminology and abbreviations pertinent to workers' compensation cases.

- Explain the advantages of filing a lien.

- List signs of fraud and abuse involving employees, employers, insurers, medical providers, and lawyers.

- State when to report fraud or abuse involving a workers' compensation claim.

- Describe workers' compensation record-keeping methods.

- Explain two ways in which depositions are used.

- Describe actions to take in following up on delinquent workers' compensation claims.

*Performance objectives and exercises for hands-on practical experience for this chapter appear in the *Workbook*.

Service

If a patient arrives for an appointment who has a work-related injury or illness without the employer's signed permission for treatment, telephone the employer and ask to have an official person fax the authorization. This will expedite the medical care and necessary documents and/or forms that must be completed for the patient in a workers' compensation case.

Always educate the patient with regard to the medical practice's billing policies for workers' compensation cases by having him or her complete a patient agreement form to pay the physician's fees if the case is declared not work related or an illness is discovered that is not work related.

HISTORY

Before the establishment of a workers' compensation program in the United States, the employer was responsible for any injury or death to his or her employees resulting from administrative negligence. *Employees* are individuals employed by another, generally for wages, in exchange for labor or services. A physician who is incorporated also is considered an employee under workers' compensation laws.

Originally the worker had to prove legally that injury was caused by negligence on the part of the employer. By the close of the nineteenth century, the number of accidents had increased and legal processes were uncertain; therefore federal and state legal provisions were required. In the early 1900s, employers' liability laws were adopted by many states, but there was still a great need for improvement. In 1911, the first workers' compensation laws were enacted that allowed injured employees to receive medical care without first taking employers to court. All states currently have workers' compensation laws.

Workers' compensation insurance is the most important coverage written to insure industrial accidents. Previously this form of insurance was known as "workmen's compensation." The term *workmen* was changed to *workers* for a more generic title and to avoid sexual bias in language. Employers use employers' liability coverage occasionally to protect themselves when their employees do not come within the scope of a compensation law.

Workers' Compensation Statutes

There are two kinds of statutes under workers' compensation: federal compensation laws and state compensation laws. Federal laws apply to miners, maritime workers, and those who work for the government; they do not apply to state and private business employees. State compensation laws apply to employers and employees within each state, but the laws vary for each state.

The workers' compensation statutes relieve the employer of liability for injury received or illness contracted by an employee in a work situation, except in gross negligence cases. They also enable the employee to be more easily and quickly compensated for loss of wages, medical expenses, and permanent disability. Before these statutes were passed, the employer could be found legally responsible for his or her employees' injuries or illnesses, and frequently there were delays in the employee's attempt to recover damages.

HIPAA Compliance Alert

WORKERS' COMPENSATION AND HIPAA COMPLIANCE

It is important to note that workers' compensation programs are not included under the definition of a "health plan" as identified in the HIPAA statutes. Therefore, workers' compensation programs are not required to comply with HIPAA standards; however, it is beneficial to workers' compensation insurance payers and health care providers to use the adopted HIPAA *Transaction and Code Set* (TCS) to work harmoniously within the claims processing activities used throughout the industry.

Workers' Compensation Reform

By 1994, dysfunctional workers' compensation systems were costing companies more than $65 billion annually in many U.S. cities, driving insurers to deny insurance to businesses and causing companies to close their doors. Some employers began moving their businesses to states requiring lower premiums. Widespread legal and medical corruption and abuse had evolved throughout the system in the form of record-high medical treatment and legal expenses. Reforms of the compensation of health care workers became necessary because of these problems. Reform laws have been introduced in a number of states that deal with the following issues:

- Antifraud legislation and increased penalties for workers' compensation fraud
- Antireferral provisions (e.g., restrictions of physicians referring patients for diagnostic studies to sites where the physician has a financial interest)
- Proof of the medical necessity for treatment (or tests), as well as appropriate documentation. If guidelines are not adhered to, the carrier may refuse to pay the entire fee (e.g., utilization review of inpatient and outpatient claims and treatment plans)

● Preauthorization for major operations and expensive tests (e.g., computed tomography and magnetic resonance imaging)
● Caps on vocational rehabilitation
● Utilization of a disabled worker in another division of the company where he or she was employed so that the worker may be gainfully employed while not using the injured part of the body
● Increase in occupational safety measures
● Employers offering a variety of managed care plans from which employees can choose, with some of these restricting their choice of provider (e.g., health maintenance organizations [HMOs] and preferred provider organizations [PPOs])
● Development of fee schedules
● Medical bill review (mandatory review by law or payers' voluntary review identifying duplicate claims and billing errors)
● Use of mediators instead of lawyers to reach agreement between employers and the injured employee
● Prosecuting physicians, lawyers, and employees who abuse the system

Although the system is far from perfect or complete, much progress has been made toward reducing high costs by trimming reimbursement for medical services and minimizing abuses of the system.

WORKERS' COMPENSATION LAWS AND INSURANCE

Purposes of Workers' Compensation Laws

Workers' compensation laws have been developed for a variety of reasons and accomplish much, including the following:

1. Provide the best available medical care necessary to ensure a prompt return to work of any injured or ill employee, as well as the achievement of maximum recovery.
2. Provide income to the injured or ill worker or to his or her dependents, regardless of fault.
3. Provide a single remedy and reduce court delays, costs, and workloads arising out of personal injury litigation.
4. Relieve public and private charities of financial drains resulting from uncompensated industrial accidents.
5. Eliminate payment of fees to attorneys and witnesses, as well as time-consuming trials and appeals.
6. Encourage maximum employer interest in safety and rehabilitation through an appropriate experience-rating mechanism.

7. Promote the study of causes of accidents and reduce preventable accidents and human suffering rather than concealing fault.

Self-Insurance

Self-insurance is another way that employers can fight high medical costs after an accident. A very large employer can save money by self-insuring employees for a predetermined amount of money and then purchasing policies with large deductibles to cover catastrophic problems. A self-insuring company pays for medical expenses instead of insurance premiums. Benefits are variable from plan to plan, and precertification for certain services may be required.

Self-insured employers are covered by the Employee Retirement Income Security Act (ERISA). This federal law mandates reporting and disclosure requirements for group life and health plans, with guidelines for administration, servicing of plans, some claims processing, and appeals; therefore the state insurance commissioner does not have jurisdiction over such plans. Because they are not state regulated, they often overlook timely payment. ERISA regulations state that a claim must be paid or denied within 90 days of receipt or submission; however, this regulation is not helpful because there is no penalty for violation of the 90-day deadline. Thus physicians who care for individuals under such plans may wish to negotiate payment terms to be 60 days or less.

Sometimes a self-insured plan may have stop-loss or reinsurance that becomes active on large claims, or a set dollar limit per policy year or employee, depending on how it is structured. Such provisions give them an excuse to delay claims until the reinsurer decides to fund the claim. In such cases it may be necessary to become aggressive and ask for the name, address, and telephone number of the reinsurer to learn the claim status. Prompt processing and payment should be demanded because delaying claims is a violation of federal laws and ERISA regulations. Read the conclusion at the end of Chapter 11 for additional information on ERISA.

A form of self-insurance designed to serve a small manufacturing company is known as *captive insurance*. This is best for companies that have good safety records and those willing to implement worker safety programs to keep claims to a minimum. Members of captive self-insurance programs may hire an outside firm to process claims and purchase extra insurance for major claims. They share overhead expenses and investment income if any remains after paying expenses and claims. Most captive programs are based in Bermuda or the Cayman Islands to take advantage of favorable tax benefits.

Managed Care

Increasing numbers of employers are seeking managed care contracts with PPOs and HMOs. Some states have adopted laws authorizing managed care programs, and other states are conducting pilot programs to test the effectiveness of managed care networks. Managed care contracts are not uniform and may limit the choice of providers, use fee schedule–based payments, require pre-certification for certain procedures, implement hospital and medical bill review, and incorporate utilization review of medical services.

ELIGIBILITY

Individuals entitled to workers' compensation insurance coverage are private business employees, state employees, and federal employees (e.g., postal workers, Internal Revenue Service [IRS] employees, coal miners, and maritime workers). **Workers' compensation (WC) insurance** coverage provides benefits to employees and their dependents if employees suffer work-related injury, illness, or death.

Industrial Accident

An **accident** is an unplanned and unexpected happening traceable to a definite time and place and causing **injury** (damage or loss).

Workers' compensation (industrial) accidents do not necessarily occur at the customary work site. For example, an individual may be asked to obtain cash for the petty cash reserve during the lunch hour. He or she may misstep off the curb while walking to the bank and suffer a fractured ankle. This person is considered to be working, although not at the customary work site, and the injury is covered under workers' compensation insurance.

Occupational Illness

Occupational illness or **disease** is any abnormal condition or disorder caused by exposure to environmental factors associated with employment, including acute and chronic illnesses or diseases that may be caused by inhalation, absorption, ingestion, or direct contact. Occupational diseases usually become apparent soon after exposure. However, some diseases may be latent for a considerable amount of time. Therefore some states have extended periods during which claims may be filed for certain slowly developing occupational diseases. These diseases include silicosis, asbestosis, pneumoconiosis, berylliosis, anthracosilicosis, radiation disability, loss of hearing, cumulative trauma, or repetitive motion illnesses (e.g., carpal tunnel syndrome).

COVERAGE

Federal Laws

Employees who work for federal agencies are covered by a number of federal workers' compensation laws:

● Workmen's Compensation Law of the District of Columbia. This law became effective on May 17, 1928, and provides benefits for those working in Washington, DC.
● Federal Coal Mine Health and Safety Act. This act, also referred to as the Black Lung Benefits Act, became effective on May 7, 1941. The act provides benefits to coal miners and is administered through the national headquarters in Washington, DC.
● Federal Employees' Compensation Act. The **Federal Employees' Compensation Act (FECA)** was instituted on May 30, 1908, to provide benefits for on-the-job injuries to all federal employees. The insurance is provided through an exclusive fund system. Many different claim forms are used depending on the type of injury. Payment is based on a schedule of maximum allowable charges. The time limit for submitting a bill is by December 31 of the year after the year in which services were rendered (or by December 31 of the year after the year the condition was accepted as work compensable, whichever is later). For further information locate your regional office of the FECA by going to the Web site listed in Internet Resources at the end of this chapter.
● Longshoremen's and Harbor Workers' Compensation Act (LHWCA). This act became effective on March 4, 1927, and provides benefits for private or public employees engaged in maritime work nationwide. It is administered through regional offices in Boston, Chicago, Cleveland, Denver, Honolulu, Jacksonville, Kansas City, New Orleans, New York City, Philadelphia, San Francisco, Seattle, and Washington, DC. This type of insurance corresponds to that available through the private insurance system. Locate the nearest district office by going to the Web site listed in Internet Resources at the end of this chapter.

State Laws

State compensation laws cover those workers not protected by the previously mentioned federal statutes. Federal law mandates that states set up laws to meet minimum requirements. If an employer does not purchase workers' compensation insurance from a private insurance company, the employer must self-insure and have enough cash in reserve to cover the cost of medical care for all workers who suffer work-related injuries. An employer may be reluctant to file a workers' compensation report with the state in some instances, preferring to pay medical expenses out of pocket rather than have premium rates increase. It is illegal for an employer to fail to report a work-related accident when reporting is required by state law, and some states consider it a misdemeanor. Different penalties can be imposed, depending on state law, such as imprisonment or assessment of fines of from $50 to $2500 or more.

Statutes require that employers have employers' liability insurance in addition to workers' compensation protection. The difference between workers' compensation insurance and employers' liability insurance is that the latter is coverage that protects against claims arising out of bodily injury to others (nonemployees) or damage to their property when someone is on business premises. It is not considered insurance coverage for someone who is working at a business site.

State compensation laws are compulsory or elective, which may be defined as follows:

1. *Compulsory law.* Each employer is required to accept its provisions and provide for specified benefits.
2. *Elective law.* The employer may accept or reject the law. If the statute of the law is rejected, the employer loses the three common-law defenses, which are the following:
   a. Assumption of risk
   b. Negligence of fellow employees
   c. Contributory negligence

Coverage is elective in only two states, New Jersey and Texas. This means that, in effect, all laws are "compulsory."

Minors

Minors are covered by workers' compensation; in some states, double compensation or added penalties are provided. Minors also receive special legal benefit provisions in many states.

Interstate Laws

Questions may arise as to which state's law determines payment of compensation benefits if a worker's occupation takes him or her into another state (e.g., truck drivers). Most compensation laws are **extraterritorial** (effective outside of the state) by either specific provisions or court decision. When billing, follow the rules and fee schedule of the state in which the workers' compensation claim was originally filed. This may or may not be the same as the patient's current state of residence. The only exception is workers' compensation for federal employees, which has nationwide rules. For railroad workers, most states abide by nationwide rules but some states have their own. Claims submission for out-of-state claims is discussed later in this chapter.

Volunteer Workers

Several states have laws to compensate civil defense and other volunteer workers, such as firefighters who are injured in the line of duty.

Funding

Six states (Nevada, North Dakota, Ohio, Washington, West Virginia, and Wyoming), two U.S. territories, and most provinces require employers to insure through a *monopolistic state* or *provincial fund.* Puerto Rico and the Virgin Islands require employers to insure through a *territorial fund.* Employers may qualify as self-insurers in 48 states and territories. A number of states permit employers to purchase insurance from either a competitive state fund or a private insurance company.

The employer pays the premiums for workers' compensation insurance, the amount depending on the employee's job and the risk involved in job performance. The physician usually must supply comprehensive information, and the reporting requirements vary from state to state (Table 15.1). The state bureau or individual insurance carrier should be contacted to obtain instructions and proper forms. State bureaus may be found by going to the Web site listed in Internet Resources at the end of this chapter.

Second-Injury Fund (Subsequent-Injury Fund)

The **second-injury fund,** also known as the **subsequent-injury fund (SIF),** was established to meet problems arising when an employee has a preexisting injury or condition and is subsequently injured at work. The preexisting injury combines with the second injury to produce disability that is greater than that caused by the latter alone.

Two functions of the fund are (1) to encourage hiring of the physically handicapped and (2) to allocate more equitably the costs of providing benefits to such employees. Second-injury employers pay compensation related

Scenario: Second-Injury Fund

Bob Evans loses his left thumb while working a lathe. Then, 2 years later, Bob loses his left index finger in a second work-related accident. A question could arise of whether the second injury added to a preexisting condition or was related to the prior injury. This case illustrates that the existence of the former injury or disability substantially increased (added to) the disability caused by the latter injury. The employer would pay compensation related to the second injury, and funds would come from a second-injury fund to pay for the difference between the first and second injuries.

Table 15.1 | **Employers' or Physicians' Report of Accident[1]**

Jurisdiction	Time Limit	Injuries Covered
Alabama	Within 15 days	Death or disability exceeding 3 days
Alaska	Within 10 days	Death, injury, disease, or infection
Arizona	Within 10 days	All injuries
Arkansas	10 days from notice of injury	Indemnity, injuries, or death. Medical claims reported monthly[2]
California	Immediately[3] (employer)	Death or serious injuries
	As prescribed	1-day disability or more than first aid
	Within 5 days	Occupational diseases or pesticide poisoning
Colorado	Immediately[4]	Death
	Within 10 days[4]	Injuries causing lost time of 3 days or more[4(b)]
	Immediately	Any accident in which three or more employees are injured
	10 days[4]	Occupational disease cases
	10 days[4]	Cases of permanent physical impairment
Connecticut	7 days or as directed	Disability of 1 day or more
Delaware	Within 48 hours[5]	Death or injuries requiring hospitalization
	Within 10 days	Other injuries
District of Columbia	Within 10 days	All injuries
Florida	Within 24 hours[6]	Death
	Within 7 days of carrier receipt of notice	All injuries
Georgia	Within 21 days[7]	All injuries requiring medical or surgical treatment or causing over 7 days of absence
Guam	Within 10 days[8]	Injury, illness, or death
Hawaii	Within 48 hours	Death
	Within 7 working days	All injuries
Idaho	As soon as practicable but not later than 10 days after the accident[9]	All injuries requiring medical treatment or causing 1 day's absence
Illinois	Within 2 working days	Death or serious injuries
	Between 15th and 25th of month	Disability of over 3 days
	As soon as determinable	Permanent disability
Indiana	Within 7 working days[10]	Disability of more than 1 day
Iowa	Within 4 days	Disability of more than 3 days, permanent partial disability, death
Kansas	Within 28 days[11]	Death
	Within 28 days	Disability of more than remainder of day or shift
Kentucky	Within 7 days[12]	Disability of more than 1 day
Louisiana	Within 10 days of employer's actual knowledge of injury[13]	Lost time over 1 week or death
Maine	Within 7 days[14]	Only injuries causing 1 day or more of lost time[14]
Maryland	Within 10 days	Disability of more than 3 days
Massachusetts	Within 7 days, except Sundays and holidays	Disability of 5 or more calendar days
Michigan	Immediately	Death, disability of 7 days or more, and specific losses
Minnesota	Within 48 hours	Death or serious injury
	Within 14 days	Disability of 3 days or more
Mississippi	Within 10 days	Death or disability of more than 5 days[15]
Missouri	Within 10 days[16]	Death or injury
Montana	Within 6 days	All injuries
Nebraska	Within 48 hours[17]	Death
	Within 7 days	All injuries
Nevada	Within 6 working days after report from physician[18]	All injuries requiring medical treatment
New Hampshire	Within 5 calendar days	All injuries involving lost time or medical expenses
New Jersey	Immediately[19]	All injuries
New Mexico	Within 10 days of employer notification	Any injury or illness resulting in 7 or more days of lost time
New York	Within 10 days	Disability of 1 day beyond working day or shift on which accident occurred or requiring medical care beyond 2 first aid treatments
North Carolina	Within 5 days[20]	Disability of more than 1 day or charges for medical compensation exceeding the amount set by the disability commission

Table 15.1 | Employers' or Physicians' Report of Accident—cont'd

Jurisdiction	Time Limit	Injuries Covered
North Dakota	Within 7 days	All injuries
Ohio	Within 1 week	Injuries causing total disability of 7 days or more
Oklahoma	Within 10 days or a reasonable time	Fatalities; all injuries causing lost time or requiring treatment away from worksite
Oregon	Within 5 days[21]	All claims or injuries that may result in compensable inquiry claims injuries
Pennsylvania	Within 48 hours	Death
	After 7 days but not later than 10 days	Disability of 1 day or more
Puerto Rico	Within 5 days	All injuries
Rhode Island	Within 48 hours	Death
	Within 10 days	Disability of 3 days of more and all injuries requiring medical treatment
	Within 3 years of injury	Any claim resulting in medical expense to be reported within 10 days
South Carolina	Within 10 days[22]	All injuries requiring medical attention costing more than $500, more than 1 day disability or permanency
South Dakota	Within 7 days	All injuries[23]
Tennessee	Within 14 days	All injuries requiring medical attention
Texas	Within 8 days[22]	Disability of more than 1 day, or occupational disease
Utah	Within 7 days	All injuries requiring medical attention
Vermont	Within 72 hours[22]	Disability of 1 day or more requiring medical care
Virgin Islands	Within 8 days	Injury or disease
Virginia	Within 10 days[22]	All injuries
Washington	Immediately	Death and accidents resulting in workers' hospitalizations or inability to work
West Virginia	Within 5 days	All injuries
Wisconsin	Within 14 days	Disability beyond 3-day waiting period
Wyoming	Within 10 days	All injuries
FECA	Immediately	All injuries involving medical expenses, disability, or death
LHWCA	10 days	Injuries that cause loss of 1 or more shifts of work or death

[1]Federal Occupational Safety and Health Act of 1970 established uniform requirements and forms to meet its criteria for all businesses affecting interstate commerce to be used for statistical purposes and compliance with the Act. 12 U.S.C. §651.

[2]Arkansas. Medical only claims reported monthly.

[3]California. To Division of Occupational Safety and Health. Within 5 days of employer's notice or knowledge of employee death, employer must report death to the Department of Industrial Relations.

[4]Colorado. (a) Failure to report tolls time limit for claims. (b) Disability of less than 3 days must be reported to insurer.

[5]Delaware. Supplemental report upon termination of disability.

[6]Florida. Death cases—by phone to workers' compensation division within 24 hours. All injuries—carrier to send first report form to division, if injury involved lost time.

[7]Georgia. Supplemental report on first payment and suspension of payment and within 30 days after final payment.

[8]Guam. Failure to report tolls limits for claims.

[9]Supplemental report required after 60 days (for Rhode Island and South Carolina every 6 months), or upon termination of disability.

[10]Indiana. Supplemental report within 10 days after termination of compensation period.

[11]Kansas. Failure to report tolls time limit for claims. Childress v. Childress Painting Co., 1979.

[12]Kentucky. Supplemental report required after 80 days or upon termination of disability

[13]Louisiana. Employers with more than 10 employees must also report, within 90 days, death, any nonfatal occupational illness or injury causing loss of consciousness, restriction of work or motion, job transfer, or medical treatment other than first aid. Violation of confidentiality of any record, subject to $500 fine.

[14]Maine. Must report asbestosis, mesothelioma, silicosis, and exposure to heavy metals no later than 30 days from date of diagnosis.

[15]Mississippi. Permanent disability, serious head or facial disfigurement also covered. $100 may be added to any award and $100 may be ordered payable to the workers' compensation commission.

[16]Missouri. Supplemental report within 1 month after original notice to workers' compensation division.

[17]Nebraska. Report may be made by insurance carrier or employer. Failure to report tolls time limits.

[18]Nevada. For minor injuries not requiring medical treatment, the employee may file a "Notice of Injury," which must be retained by the employer for 3 years.

[19]New Jersey. Uninsured employers are required to report compensable injuries only. If insured, carrier is also required to make report.

[20]North Carolina. Supplemental report required after 60 days or upon termination of disability.

[21]Oregon. Insurers to send initial disabling claims acceptance, aggravation claim acceptance, and claim denial to WC Division within 14 days.

[22]South Carolina, Texas, Vermont, and Virginia. Supplemental report required after 60 days or upon termination of disability.

[23]South Dakota. Any injury that requires treatment other than first aid or that incapacitates employee for at least 7 calendar days.

Table 15.2 | **Minimum Number of Employees for State Workers' Compensation Laws**

		Number Of Employees		
	1	**3**	**4**	**5**
Alaska	Nebraska	American	Florida	Alabama
Arizona	Nevada	Samoa	South Carolina	Mississippi
California	New Hampshire	Arkansas		Missouri
Colorado	New Jersey	Georgia		Tennessee
Connecticut	New York	Michigan		
Delaware	North Dakota	New Mexico		
District of Columbia	Ohio	North Carolina		
Guam	Oklahoma	Virginia		
Hawaii	Oregon			
Idaho	Pennsylvania			
Illinois	Puerto Rico			
Indiana	Rhode Island			
Iowa	South Dakota			
Kansas	Texas			
Kentucky	Utah			
Louisiana	Vermont			
Maine	Virgin Islands			
Maryland	Washington			
Massachusetts	West Virginia			
Minnesota	Wisconsin			
Montana	Wyoming			

primarily to the disability caused by the second injury, even though the employee receives benefits relating to the combined disability. The difference is made up from the subsequent-injury fund.

Minimum Number of Employees

Table 15.2 shows the minimum number of employees at one business required by each state before the state workers' compensation law comes into effect. There are exemptions in many states for certain occupations such as domestic or casual employees, laborers, babysitters, newspaper vendors or distributors, charity workers, and gardeners. Some states do not require compensation insurance for farm laborers or may specify a larger number of farm employees than the number shown in the table.

Waiting Periods

The laws state that a **waiting period (WP)** must elapse before income benefits are payable. This waiting period affects only wage compensation because medical and hospital care are provided immediately. See Table 15.3 to find the waiting period of each state.

State Disability and Workers' Compensation

Five states and one U.S. territory have state disability insurance (also known as unemployment compensation disability insurance): California, Hawaii, New Jersey, New York, Rhode Island, and Puerto Rico. If a recipient is collecting benefits from a workers' compensation insurance carrier and the amount that the compensation carrier pays is less than that allowed by the state disability insurance program, then the latter pays the balance. See Chapter 16 for further information on state disability insurance.

BENEFITS

Five principal types of state compensation benefits that may apply in ordinary cases are the following:

1. *Medical treatment.* This includes hospital, medical and surgical services, medications, and prosthetic devices. Treatment may be rendered by a licensed physician, osteopath, dentist, or chiropractor.
2. *Temporary disability indemnity.* This is in the form of weekly cash payments made directly to the injured or ill person.
3. *Permanent disability indemnity.* This may consist of either weekly or monthly cash payments based on a rating system that determines the percentage of permanent disability or a lump sum award. California has a unique system of permanent disability evaluation that requires a separate determination by the disability rating bureau in San Francisco. No other state has this system.
4. *Death benefits for survivors.* This consists of cash payments to dependents of employees who are fatally injured. A burial allowance also is given in some states.

Table 15.3 Waiting Period for Income and Medical Benefits*

Jurisdiction	Waiting Period (Days)	Jurisdiction	Waiting Period (Days)
Alabama	3	Nebraska	7
Alaska	3	Nevada	5
Arizona	7	New Hampshire	3
Arkansas	7	New Jersey	7
California	3	New Mexico	7
Colorado	3	New York	7
Connecticut	3	North Carolina	7
Delaware	3	North Dakota	5
District of Columbia	3	Ohio	7
Florida	7	Oklahoma	3
Georgia	7	Oregon	3
Guam	3	Pennsylvania	7
Hawaii	3	Puerto Rico	3
Idaho	5	Rhode Island	3
Indiana	7	South Dakota	7
Illinois	3	South Carolina	7
Iowa	3	Tennessee	7
Kansas	7	Texas	7
Kentucky	7	Utah	3
Louisiana	7	Vermont	3
Maine	7	Virgin Islands	0
Maryland	3	Virginia	7
Massachusetts	5	Washington	3
Michigan	7	West Virginia	3
Minnesota	3	Wisconsin	3
Mississippi	5	Wyoming	3
Missouri	3	FECA	3
Montana	4 days or 32 hours, whichever is less	LHWCA	3

*These are statutory provisions for waiting periods. Statutes provide that a waiting period must elapse during which income benefits are not payable. This waiting period affects only compensation, because medical and hospital care are provided immediately.
FECA, Federal Employees Compensation Act; LHWCA, Longshoremen's and Harbor Workers' Compensation Act.

5. *Rehabilitation benefits.* This can be medical or vocational rehabilitation in cases of severe disabilities.

TYPES OF STATE CLAIMS

There are three types of state workers' compensation claims: nondisability (ND) claims, temporary disability claims, and permanent disability claims. Each type is discussed in detail for a clear definition and understanding of the determination process.

Nondisability Claim

This is the simplest type of claim. Generally a **nondisability (ND)** claim involves a minor injury in which the patient is seen by the physician but is able to continue working (Figure 15–1). This type of case does not require weekly temporary disability payments.

Temporary Disability Claim

Temporary disability (TD) occurs when a worker has a work-related injury or illness and is unable to perform the duties of his or her occupation for a specific time or range of time. The time period of temporary disability can extend from the date of injury until the worker either returns to full duty without residual ratable disability (discussed later), returns to modified work, or has ratable residual disability that the physician states is permanent and stationary.

An **insurance adjuster** is the person at the workers' compensation insurance carrier who oversees the industrial case. He or she is responsible for keeping in contact with the physician's office about the patient's ongoing progress. The insurance adjuster's most important function is *adjusting an industrial claim*. This means that the insurance adjuster must evaluate the injury or illness, predict in advance the amount of money reserves needed to cover medical expenses, and calculate as accurate a reserve as possible for weekly TD payments to the injured. This is frequently a difficult task because a seemingly minor back strain ultimately may require fusion, or a small cut may become gangrenous and lead to an amputation. The insurance carrier wants to provide the best possible medical care for the patient. The patient is immediately referred to the specialist if a specialist is necessary.

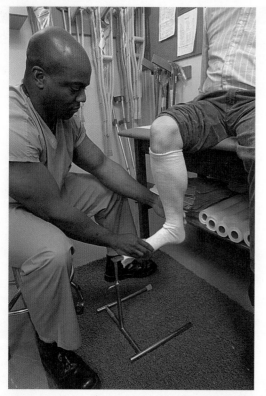

FIGURE 15–1 Physician interacting with an injured worker in the examination room.

Usually workers' compensation weekly TD payments are based on the employee's earnings at the time of the injury. Compensation benefits are not subject to income tax.

Sometimes a patient is released to modified work to effect a transition between the period of inactivity caused by disability and a return to full duty, especially when heavy work is involved. Other times an employee is returned to the company and placed in a different department or division so that he or she is gainfully employed while not using the injured body part. This topic is further detailed in the next section.

Vocational Rehabilitation

Many states provide rehabilitation in the form of retraining, education, job guidance, and placement, to assist an injured individual in finding work before temporary disability compensation benefits expire. In any successful rehabilitation program, insurance carrier, physician, physical therapist, employer supervisor, and personnel department must act as a team with the common goal of getting an injured employee back to light duty or regular work as soon as possible. It is believed that the longer a person remains out of work, the less chance there is that he or she will return to the workplace. The employer and insurance adjuster must remain in communication with rehabilitation center therapists to determine when the injured person will be able to resume some form of work. The physician may suggest a rehabilitation center that provides good care, or the employer may have an in-house program.

Work Hardening

Sports medicine therapy and physical medicine rehabilitation often are used to strengthen the injured worker. Physical medicine/therapy CPT codes 97001 to 97542 are used to report these services. Another type of therapy, called **work hardening,** is an individualized program using simulated or real work tasks to build up strength and improve the worker's endurance toward a full day's work. Common Procedure Terminology (CPT) codes 97545 and 97546 are used to report work hardening conditioning.

Ergonomics

In some cases, an **ergonomic** evaluation of the work site is performed and modifications may be instituted to the job or work site to lessen the possibility of future injury and to get the employee back to gainful employment. CPT code 97537 may be used to report a work site modification analysis. Injured individuals also may be retrained into another career field if their disability prevents them from returning to their former occupation.

Permanent Disability Claim

In this type of claim, the patient or injured party is usually on TD benefits for a time and then concludes that he or she is unable to return to his or her former occupation. The physician states in the report that the patient has residual disability that will hamper his or her opportunity to compete in the open job market. Examples of residual disability include loss of a hand, an eye, or a leg, or neurologic problems. Each patient who has **permanent disability (PD)** is rated according to the severity of the injury, the age of the injured person, and the patient's occupation at the time of the injury. The older the person, the greater the PD benefit. One might think that a younger person deserves higher compensation because he or she will be disabled for a longer portion of his or her working career. However, the workers' compensation laws assume that a young person has a better chance of being rehabilitated into another occupation.

In a PD claim, the physician's final report must include the words **"permanent and stationary" (P and S).** This phrase means that damage from the injury or illness is permanent, the patient has recovered to the fullest extent possible, the physician is unable to do anything more for the patient, and the patient will be hampered by the disability to some extent for the rest of his or her life. The P and S examination usually is comprehensive, and a level 5 CPT code may be appropriate. Depending on the fee schedule, a modifier indicating that the evaluation and management service is a P and S examination also may be used. The case is rated for PD, and a settlement, called a **compromise and release (C and R),** is made. This is an agreement between the injured party and insurance company on a total sum. The case can then be closed.

Reasons that may delay closing a workers' compensation case include the following:

1. Unanswered questions or incomplete answers to data required on workers' compensation forms by the employee, employer, or physician
2. Vague terminology used by the physician in medical reports
3. Omitted signatures on forms or written reports by the employee, employer, or physician
4. Incorrect billing by the physician's office
5. Inadequate progress reports (e.g., the physician fails to send in a medical report routinely to update the insurance carrier when the injured employee is seen in subsequent visits)

Rating

Final determination of the issues involving settlement of an industrial accident is known as **adjudication,** or the rating of a case. A physician does not rate disability but renders a professional opinion on whether the injured individual has temporary or permanent disability that prevents him or her from gainful employment. Rating itself is carried out by the state's industrial accident commission or workers' compensation board. Wage loss, earning capacity, and physical impairment are three categories that may be taken into consideration to rate temporary partial, permanent partial, or total disabilities.

In addition, permanent partial disabilities may be rated by using a scheduled or nonscheduled injury award system. This system is based on a set number of weeks of compensation for a specific loss, such as 288 weeks for the loss of a leg. Scheduled injuries may include loss of a body part, disfigurement, permanent hearing loss, and so on. Nonscheduled injuries are more general, such as disability caused by injury to the back or neck.

If an injured person is dissatisfied with the rating after the case has been declared P and S, he or she may appeal the case (by **petition**—formal written request) to the **Workers' Compensation Appeals Board (WCAB)** or the Industrial Accident Commission.

Surveillance

Sub rosa films sometimes are provided when rating a case to document the extent of a patient's permanent disability. *Sub rosa* means under the rose. In ancient times, the rose was a symbol of silence or secrecy. Videotapes are made over a period of 2 to 3 days without the patient's knowledge. This surveillance is expensive and is used as a last resort, especially in a case in which a person receiving workers' compensation benefits is suspected of making exaggerated complaints. It is also used in cases when a worker has been off work for a long time and supposedly is unable to perform any work activity, even light duty.

Investigators have been known to carry a camera in a gym bag and videotape a supposedly disabled claimant bench pressing at the gym. Patients also have been videotaped going into the physician's office for an appointment wearing a neck brace and removing the brace after returning to their car.

FRAUD AND ABUSE

Increases in the number of fraudulent workers' compensation claims were noted throughout many large metropolitan cities in the 1990s. These problems involved employers, employees, insurers, medical providers, and lawyers. An increasing number of states have enacted some kind of antifraud legislation and stiffened penalties for workers' compensation fraud, making it a felony. Some states require reporting suspected insurance fraud and have forms to incorporate wording in regard to fraudulent statements. An example is shown in Figure 15–2.

Physicians are responsible for determining the legitimacy of work injuries and reporting findings accurately. If a report is prepared with the intent to use it in support of a fraudulent claim, or if a fraudulent claim is knowingly submitted for payment under an insurance contract, the physician may be subject to fines or imprisonment and the revocation or suspension of his or her medical license. Some physicians sign and send a disclosure statement with the medical report certifying that they personally performed an evaluation. The physician may list the total time spent in reviewing records, face-to-face time with the patient, preparation of a report, and other relevant activities.

State of California
Department of Industrial Relations
DIVISION OF WORKERS' COMPENSATION

EMPLOYEE'S CLAIM FOR
WORKERS' COMPENSATION BENEFITS

Estado de California
Departmento de Relaciones Industriales
DIVISION DE COMPENSACIÓN AL TRABAJADOR

PETICION DEL EMPLEADO PARA BENEFICIOS
DE COMPENSACIÓN DEL TRABAJADOR

If you are injured or become ill because of your job, you may be entitled to workers' compensation benefits.

Complete the **"Employee"** section and give the form to your employer. Keep the copy marked **"Employee's Temporary Receipt"** until you receive the dated copy from your employer. You may call the Division of Workers' Compensation at **1-800-736-7401** if you need help in filling out this form or in obtaining your benefits. An explanation of workers' compensation benefits is included on the back of this form.

You should also have received a pamphlet from your employer describing workers' compensation benefits and the procedures to obtain them.

Si Ud. se ha lesionado o se ha enfermado a causa de su trabajo, Ud. tiene derecho a recibir beneficios de compensación al trabajador.
Complete la sección "Empleado" y entregue la forma a su empleador. Quédese con la copia designada "Recibo Temporal del Empleado" hasta que Ud. reciba la copia fechada de su empleador. Si Ud. necesita ayuda para completar esta forma o para obtener sus beneficios, Ud. puede hablar con la Division de Compensación al Trabajador llamando al 1-800-736-7401. En la parte de atrás de esta forma se encuentra una explicación de los beneficios de la compensación al trabajador.

Ud. también debería haber recibido de su empleador un folleto describiendo los beneficios de compensación al trabajador lesionado y los procedimientos para obtenerlos.

Any person who makes or causes to be made any knowingly false or fraudulent material statement or material representation for the purpose of obtaining or denying workers' compensation benefits or payments is guilty of a felony.

Toda aquella persona que a propósito haga o cause que se produzca cualquier declaración o representación material falsa o fraudulenta con el fin de obtener o negar beneficios o pagos de compensación a trabajadores lesionados es culpable de un crimen mayor "felonía".

Employee: *Empleado*

1. Name. *Nombre.* __Ima B. Hurt__ Today's date. *Fecha de hoy.* __4-3-20XX__

2. Home address. *Dirección residencial.* __300 East Central Avenue__

3. City. *Ciudad.* __Woodland Hills__ State. *Estado.* __XY__ Zip. *Código postal* __12345-0001__

4. Date of injury. *Fecha de la lesión (accidente).* __4-3-XX__ Time of injury. *Hora en que ocurrió.* _____ a.m. __2:00__ p.m.

5. Address and description of where injury happened. *Dirección/lugar dónde occurió el accidente.* __The Conk Out Company__ __45 South Gorman Street, Woodland Hills, XY 12345__ injured in stock room

6. Describe injury and part of body affected. *Describa la lesión y parte dél cuerpo afectada.* __Fell off ladder in stock room.__ Injured left ankle.

7. Social Security Number. *Número de Seguro Social del Empleado.* __120 XX 6542__

8. Signature of employees. *Firma del empleado.* __Ima B. Hurt__

Employer–complete this section and give the employee a copy immediately as a receipt.
Empleador–complete esta sección y déle inmediatamente una copia al empleado como recibo.

9. Name of employer. *Nombre del empleador.* __The Conk Out Company__

10. Address. *Dirección.* __45 South Gorman Street, Woodland Hills, XY 12345__

11. Date employer first knew of injury. *Fecha en que el empleador supo por primera vez de la lesión o accidente.* __4-3-20XX__

12. Date claim form was provided to employee. *Fecha en que se le entregó al empleado la petición.* __4-3-20XX__

13. Date employer received claim form. *Fecha en que el empleado devolvió la petición al empleador.* __4-3-20XX__

14. Name and address of insurance carrier or adjusting agency. *Nombre y dirección de la compañía de seguros o agencia administradora de seguros.* __XYZ Insurance Company, P.O. Box 5, Woodland Hills, XY 12345__

15. Insurance policy number. *El número de la poliza del Seguro.* __B 12345__

16. Signature of employer representative. *Firma del representante del empleador.* __J. D. Hawkins__

17. Title. *Título.* __Owner__ 18. Telephone. *Teléfono.* __555-430-3488__

Employer: You are required to date this form and provide copies to your insurer or claims administrator and to the employee, dependent or representative who filed the claim within **one working day** of receipt of the form from the employee.

SIGNING THIS FORM IS NOT AN ADMISSION OF LIABILITY

Empleador: Se requiere que Ud. feche esta forma y que provéa copias a su compañía de seguros, administrador de reclamos, o dependiente/répresentante de reclamos y al empleado que hayan presentado esta petición dentro del plazo de **un día hábil** desde el momento de haber sido recibida la forma del empleado.

EL FIRMAR ESTA FORMA NO SIGNIFICA ADMISION DE RESPONSABILIDAD

Original (Employer's Copy)
DWC Form 1 (REV. 1/94)

ORIGINAL (Copia del Empleador)
DWC Forma 1 (REV. 1/94)

FIGURE 15–2 Employee's Claim for Workers' Compensation Benefits. Notice the insert about fraudulent material.

It is the responsibility of all individuals who deal with workers' compensation cases to notify the insurance carrier of any suspicious situation. By doing so, action can be taken to have the case investigated further by personnel from the fraud divisions or referred to the district attorney's office. Perpetrators and signs of workers' compensation fraud and abuse are listed in Box 15.1.

See Chapters 2, 12, and 13 for further information on fraud and abuse in the medical setting.

OCCUPATIONAL SAFETY AND HEALTH ADMINISTRATION ACT OF 1970

Background

Congress has established an office known as the **Occupational Safety and Health Administration (OSHA)** to protect employees against on-the-job health and safety hazards. This program includes strict health and safety standards and a sensible complaint procedure enabling individual workers to trigger enforcement measures.

Box 15.1 | Perpetrators and Signs of Workers' Compensation Fraud and Abuse

EMPLOYEE

- Symptoms are all subjective.
- Misses the first physician's visit, or cancels or repeatedly reschedules appointments
- Cannot describe the pain or is overly dramatic, such as an employee who comes into the physician's office limping on the left leg, suddenly starts limping on the right leg, and then goes back to limping on the left leg
- Delays in reporting the injury
- Does not report Friday's injury until Monday morning
- First reports an injury to a legal or regulatory agency
- Reports an injury after missing several days of work
- Changes physicians frequently
- Is a short-term worker
- Has a curious claim history
- Fabricates an injury
- Exaggerates a work-related injury to obtain larger benefits, such as an injured employee who has a back pain and claims inability to bend over or lift. Surveillance cameras capture the individual at work on weekends repairing cars in the driveway at home—a task he is supposedly unable to perform
- Blames an injury that occurred off the job on the employer
- Adds symptoms in response to efforts to return the person to work

EMPLOYER

- Misrepresents the annual payroll to get lower premium rates
- Misrepresents the number of workers employed
- Gives a false address with the least expensive premium rates
- Falsely classifies the job duties of workers (as not hazardous), such as stating the job title as a clerical worker when, in fact, the employee is using a lathe every day

INSURER

- Refuses to pay valid medical claims
- Forces the injured worker to settle by using unethical tactics. An insurance agent told an employee that he had a back sprain. Relying on that information, the worker settled the case. Later, a myelogram revealed a herniated intervertebral disk. The patient was left with a permanent partial disability.

MEDICAL PROVIDER

- Makes immediate referral for psychiatric care despite the worker's report of a trauma injury
- Orders or performs unnecessary tests
- Treatment dates fall on weekends and holidays
- Renders unnecessary treatment
- Lists a diagnosis that is not consistent with the course of treatment
- Charges the insurance carrier for services never rendered
- Prolongs treatment for what appears a minor injury
- Participates in a provider mill scheme (see explanation under "Lawyer")
- Makes multiple referrals from a clinic practice regardless of type of injury
- Sends medical reports that look photocopied with the same information typed in (e.g., employer's address, description of injury) or that read almost identical to other reports
- Sends in many claims in which injuries are of a subjective nature, such as stress, emotional distress, headaches, inability to sleep
- Sends in claims from one employer showing several employees with similar injuries, using the same physicians and/or attorneys
- Bills both the workers' compensation carrier and the health insurer for the same service

Continued

Box 15.1   **Perpetrators and Signs of Workers' Compensation Fraud and Abuse—cont'd**

LAWYER

- Overbills clients
- Participates in a medical provider mill scheme. An individual is solicited while in the unemployment line by a recruiter known as a "capper." The capper tells the worker it is possible to obtain more money on disability than through unemployment. The worker is referred to an attorney and a "provider mill" clinic, which help the individual fabricate a claim by claiming stress or an on-the-job injury. In some states, such acts may be considered a public offense and punishable as a misdemeanor or felony.

Work standards are designed to minimize exposure to on-the-job hazards such as faulty machinery, noise, dust, and toxic chemical fumes. Employers are required by law to meet these health and safety standards. Failure to do so can result in fines against the employer that could run into thousands of dollars.

Coverage

The act provides that if a state submits an OSHA plan and it is approved by the government, the state may assume responsibility for carrying out OSHA policies and procedures and is excluded from federal jurisdiction.

The act applies to almost all businesses, large or small. It applies to heavy, light, and service industries, nonprofit and charitable institutions, churches' secular activities in hospitals, farmers, and retailers. Employees of state and local governments are also covered. Federal employees, a farmer's immediate family, church employees engaged in religious activities, independent contractors, and household domestic workers are *not* covered.

Regulations

Specific regulations that affect the medical setting are those aimed at minimizing exposure to hepatitis B virus (HBV), human immunodeficiency virus (HIV), and other bloodborne pathogens. Any worker who comes in contact with human blood and infectious materials must receive proper information and training and use universal precautions to avoid infection. Vaccinations must be provided for those who are at risk for exposure to hepatitis B, and comprehensive records must be maintained. For fact sheets, booklets, and guidelines on bloodborne pathogens, contact the nearest OSHA office or write to OSHA Publications Office, 200 Constitution Avenue, NW, Room N3101, Washington, DC 20210.

Chemicals and hazardous substances are used that impose dangers in many work settings. Businesses are required to obtain material safety data sheets (MSDS) for each hazardous chemical used on site. Employers that produce a hazardous chemical must develop MSDSs. A compliance kit is available from the Superintendent of Documents, U.S. Government Printing Office, Washington, DC 20402.

Filing a Complaint

To file a complaint, the proper form is obtained from the federal Division of Industrial Safety or a state OSHA office and completed by the employee. It is against the law for an employer to take any adverse action against an employee who files such a complaint.

Inspection

A compliance officer (inspector) may call for an appointment or may be sent unannounced to the place of employment. If an officer arrives unannounced, the office manager must be notified so an appointment may be arranged for the inspection to take place. A court warrant may be required to search a company's premises if the employer does not consent to OSHA entry. A business may be cited and, depending on the violation, fines or criminal penalties may be imposed.

Record Keeping and Reporting

Employers must keep records of their employees' work-related injuries and illnesses on OSHA Form No. 200. Forms may be obtained from the OSHA office or from any office of the U.S. Department of Labor. This document must be on file at the workplace and available to employees and OSHA compliance officers on request. Form 200 must be retained in the file for 5 years. After 6 days, a case recorded on Form 200 must have a supplementary record (OSHA Form 101) completed and kept in the files. Some states have modified their workers' compensation forms so they may be used as substitutes for Form 101. Certain low-hazard industries are exempt from having to complete and retain Forms 200 and 101.

Companies with fewer than 11 employees must complete safety survey OSHA Form 200-S. Companies also are required to display OSHA posters to inform employees of their job safety rights. Federal law states that an accident that results in the death or hospitalization of five or more employees must be reported to OSHA.

LEGAL SITUATIONS

Medical Evaluator

Physicians who conduct medicolegal evaluations of injured workers must pass a complex medical examination. They are then certified by the Industrial Medical Council (IMC) and may be referred to under one of the following titles:

- Agreed medical evaluator (AME)
- Independent medical evaluator (IME)
- Qualified medical evaluator (QME)

The medical evaluator is hired by the insurance company or appointed by the referee or appeals board to examine an individual, independent from the attending physician, and render an unbiased opinion about the degree of disability of an injured worker. When the physician performs an evaluation on an injured worker, the workers' compensation fee schedule may have specific procedure codes to bill for the examination. Evaluation and management consultation codes or the CPT code for work-related evaluation by "other" physician (99456) may be used. Some state fee schedules may have specific medical-legal (ML) procedure codes to bill for various levels of examination. When a case involves a medical evaluation, a deposition may be taken of his or her testimony.

Depositions

A **deposition** is a proceeding in which an attorney asks a witness questions about a case, and the witness answers under oath but not in open court. It may take place in the attorney's office or often in the physician's office. In permanent disability workers' compensation cases, depositions usually are taken from the physician and the injured party by the attorney representing the workers' compensation insurance company. The injured party's attorney is also present if the witness is the defendant. Direct questioning and cross-examination may be done by both attorneys.

The session may be recorded on a stenotype machine, in shorthand, or by audiotape or videotape. Video depositions are used in several instances. For example, if a plaintiff in a case is terminally ill and the plaintiff's attorney wishes to preserve the plaintiff's testimony, a video deposition may be used as substantive (essential) evidence. A video deposition also may be taken if a witness cannot be present at the trial. In a case in which a witness may be in Arizona and cannot appear in Pennsylvania, the attorney takes the deposition in Arizona and proves to the court that the witness is beyond its jurisdiction. The same is true for a physician defendant who is not available for some reason.

Exhibits may be entered into evidence. The witness is allowed to read the transcript and make corrections or changes. The witness may be asked to sign the transcript but can waive signature if his or her attorney recommends against signing it. The deposition is used when the case comes to trial.

Depositions may be taken to find out additional information, the physician's version of the facts, the patient's version of the facts, what kind of witnesses the physician and patient will be, and so on. Another use for a deposition is to impeach (challenge the credibility or validity of) a witness on cross-examination. If the witness takes the stand and the testimony is inconsistent with the deposition, the attorney will make this known to the jury.

Medical Testimony

In the instance of an accident case with third-party liability, the physician may have to testify as an expert witness, take time to give a deposition, or attend a pretrial conference. There should be a clear understanding of the terms of testimony and payment to eliminate future misunderstandings. A written agreement from the patient's lawyer should be obtained stating exactly what compensation the physician will receive for research (preparation), time spent waiting to testify (if appointments must be canceled), and actual testimony time (Figure 15–3). In some cases, the physician may want to ask for partial payment in advance. If the physician is subpoenaed, he or she must appear in court regardless of whether an agreement exists. The correct CPT code for medical testimony is 99075. This agreement should be signed by the physician and sent to the attorney. The attorney should return the original to the physician, retaining a copy for his or her files.

Liens

The word **lien** derives from the same origin as the word *liable*, and the right of lien expresses legal claim on the property of another for the payment of a debt (Figure 15–4). Liens sometimes are called *encumbrances* and may be filed for a number of reasons.

The advantages of filing a lien are as follows:

- It is a written agreement and is recognized in court.
- It is a source of protection in the event of litigation.
- It ensures that payment for previously rendered medical services will be received when the attorney and patient have reached a settlement with the insurance company in an accident case.
- It is an inexpensive method of collecting the fee. The physician can file suit and try to get a judgment

---

MEDICAL TESTIMONY AGREEMENT

AGREEMENT made this _____day of _____20XX, between_____
herein referred to as attorney, and _____,
of_____ , _____ , _____ _____ , a licensed _____ .
    (street address)   (city)   (state)   (ZIP code)

In consideration of their mutual covenants set forth herein, the parties agree as follows:

1. The doctor will give medical testimony in the case of:

_____

as a treating physician or as an expert witness (delete the unwanted phrase).

2. The doctor agrees to appear promptly when called and to present his or her medical testimony in a well-prepared professional manner.

3. The doctor will be compensated for time away from the practice of his or her medical duties in accordance with the following:
   (a) $_____ per hour for reports and preparation of medical testimony.
   (b) $_____ per hour for pretrial conferences.
   (c) $_____ per hour for court appearance, including travel time to and from the office.
   (d) $_____ per hour for deposition.
   (e) $_____ per hour for being on call with cancellation of appointments but not appearing in court.

4. The doctor will appear in court on_____ hour's notice from the attorney, unless prior arrangements have been made for the exact time of appearance.

5. The doctor will be compensated on completion of his or her medical testimony, and payment will not be contingent upon the outcome of the case. However, if the case is settled before reaching the court, the doctor will be compensated for being on call as noted above.

This contract shall be binding upon the parties.

IN WITNESS WHEREOF, the said parties hereto have subscribed their respective signatures.

_____
     (physician)

_____
     (attorney)

Date:_____

FIGURE 15–3 Example of a medical testimony agreement between physician and attorney. This is signed by the physician and sent to the attorney for signature. A copy is retained by the attorney and the original is kept by the physician.

---

against the patient, but this is relatively expensive in comparison with filing a lien.

● The physician will collect the full fee. If the physician assigns such a delinquent account to a collection agency, he or she may lose as much as 50% of the fee when it is collected.
● If the physician wishes to bill more than what is allowed for a given service or services, a lien can be filed and the judge will determine whether it is reasonable.
● It avoids harassment in trying to collect the bill.

The chief disadvantage of not filing a lien is that there is no legal documentation should the case go to court as far as collecting monies owed to the physician. A case could be settled, the attorney would get his or her fee, and the physician's fee may be placed last on the list for payment or remain unpaid.

A time limit should be specified when a lien form is completed; reaching a settlement may involve several years of litigation. Some patients may be persuaded to pay before a legal settlement is made or at least make

Scenario: Filing a Lien

Problem 1. Suppose Attorney Blake advises client Roger Reed not to pay the physician until after the trial. Or, what happens if payment is not made for Dr. Practon's courtroom testimony and the case is lost? Suppose medical reports are ordered and Attorney Blake neglects to pay for them. What happens if Roger Reed forgets about the physician's bill?

Solution. If a lien had been signed, then once the case has been settled, the money would be paid to the physician; otherwise, the settlement would belong to the patient, Roger Reed, and he could take any action with the money that he wanted.

Problem 2. Suppose Dr. Practon had an oral agreement covering his fee. The patient, Katie Crest, was unable to pay for medical treatment except on legal monetary recovery. When Katie Crest settled her case, the proceeds went almost entirely to welfare agencies because she received retroactive Medicaid. Dr. Practon sued the patient's attorney and lost.

Solution. If Dr. Practon had gotten a written assignment of the proceeds, the lawyer could have been held liable for the fee.

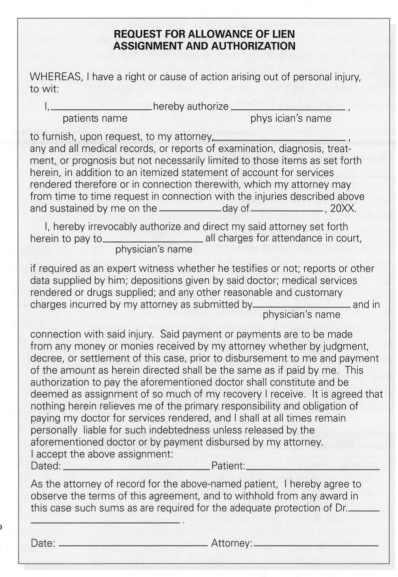

**REQUEST FOR ALLOWANCE OF LIEN
ASSIGNMENT AND AUTHORIZATION**

WHEREAS, I have a right or cause of action arising out of personal injury, to wit:

I,_____hereby authorize_____ ,
   patients name   phys ician's name

to furnish, upon request, to my attorney,_____ , any and all medical records, or reports of examination, diagnosis, treatment, or prognosis but not necessarily limited to those items as set forth herein, in addition to an itemized statement of account for services rendered therefore or in connection therewith, which my attorney may from time to time request in connection with the injuries described above and sustained by me on the _____ day of _____ , 20XX.

I, hereby irrevocably authorize and direct my said attorney set forth herein to pay to_____ all charges for attendance in court,
             physician's name

if required as an expert witness whether he testifies or not; reports or other data supplied by him; depositions given by said doctor; medical services rendered or drugs supplied; and any other reasonable and customary charges incurred by my attorney as submitted by_____ and in
                physician's name

connection with said injury. Said payment or payments are to be made from any money or monies received by my attorney whether by judgment, decree, or settlement of this case, prior to disbursement to me and payment of the amount as herein directed shall be the same as if paid by me. This authorization to pay the aforementioned doctor shall constitute and be deemed as assignment of so much of my recovery I receive. It is agreed that nothing herein relieves me of the primary responsibility and obligation of paying my doctor for services rendered, and I shall at all times remain personally liable for such indebtedness unless released by the aforementioned doctor or by payment disbursed by my attorney.
I accept the above assignment:
Dated:_____ Patient:_____

As the attorney of record for the above-named patient, I hereby agree to observe the terms of this agreement, and to withhold from any award in this case such sums as are required for the adequate protection of Dr._____
_____ .

Date: _____ Attorney:_____

FIGURE 15–4 Patient's authorization to release information to an attorney and grant lien to the physician against proceeds of settlement in connection with accident, industrial, or third-party litigation cases.

payments until a settlement is reached. The lien becomes null and void at the end of the time limit. If the patient's financial status has changed, one might be able to collect because the patient can then be billed. If not, an amended or subsequent lien should be filed that states the actual balance of the patient's account. The word "amended" should be typed on the new lien below the Workers' Compensation Appeals Board case number.

The physician's fee should be protected by having the attorney sign the lien, thereby indicating that he or she will pay the physician directly from any money received in a settlement. This makes the attorney responsible for the fee. The patient's file must be placed in a Hold for Settlement category until the case comes up in court. In some states, the physician's fee owed by the patient constitutes a first lien against any such money settlement, and the attorney must first satisfy the lien of the physician before the patient or attorney receives any

money from the settlement. State laws should be checked. The office of the patient's attorney should be called at least quarterly for an update.

If there is a third-party litigation involved in an industrial case or a decision has not been reached as to whether an accident is caused by industrial or nonindustrial causes, both a regular lien and a workers' compensation lien should be filed. In most states, a special lien form for workers' compensation filing is available and should be used. A copy of the lien should be completed and sent to all concerned parties:

● Appeals board
● Employer of the patient
● Employee (the patient)
● Insurance carrier
● Physician's files (lien claimant or one who is filing for the lien)

The patient/employee consents to the lien by his or her signature. Do not accept a lien form unless it is also signed by the patient's attorney. Check with the local Division of Industrial Accidents for forms pertinent to filing a lien and instructions on the formalities, number of copies required, and where they are to be sent.

Third-Party Subrogation

The legal term *subrogation* is the process of initiating a legal claim against another individual, an individual's insurer, or, in the case of a car accident, one's own automobile insurance company to pay health insurance bills. **Third-party subrogation** means "to substitute" one person for another. When applied to workers' compensation cases, it means a transfer of the claims and rights from the original creditor (workers' compensation insurance carrier) to the **third-party liability** carrier. In a compensation case, the insurance carrier that is "subrogated" to the legal claims has a right to reimbursement of all of the monies paid for the injuries. That reimbursement is obtained from any money the injured collects from a legal claim, directly from the individual who caused the injury, or from another insurer.

Scenario: Third-Party Subrogation

Problem. Monica Valdez, a secretary, goes to the bank to deposit some money for her employer. While on the errand, Monica's car is rear-ended by another automobile and she is injured.

Solution. In such a case there is no question of fault and no question of cause. Monica was hurt during the performance of her work, and the workers' compensation insurance carrier is liable. The carrier must adjust the claim, provide all medical treatment, and pay all TD and PD benefits.

However, the insurance carrier does have legal recourse. It may send a representative to visit with Monica, explain to her that she has a good subrogation case, encourage her to seek the advice of an attorney, and sue the third party (other automobile driver) in civil court. This is sometimes referred to as litigation, which is the process of carrying on a lawsuit. If Monica agrees to sue, the insurance carrier files a demand with the court for repayment of all the money that it has paid out. This is called a lien, which was discussed earlier in the chapter. When the case is settled, if an award is made to Monica, the insurance carrier is reimbursed for all that it has paid and Monica receives the balance. In some states, such as California, the patient is legally prevented from collecting twice.

If the patient's attorney should call the physician's office for information, it is only ethical and legal to get a signed authorization from the patient and to ask permission from the insurance carrier before giving out any medical information. The contract exists between the physician and insurance carrier, not the physician and patient.

MEDICAL REPORTS

Privacy and Confidentiality

The HIPAA Privacy Rule allows for the disclosure of personal health information (PHI) to workers' compensation insurers, state administrators, and employers to the extent necessary to comply with laws relating to workers' compensation. The HIPAA Privacy Rule recognizes the legitimate need of insurers and other entities involved in the workers' compensation systems to have access to individuals' health information as authorized by state or other law. Because of the significant variability among such laws, the HIPAA Privacy Rule permits disclosures of health information for workers' compensation purposes in a number of different ways:

1. *Disclosures without Individual Authorization.* The HIPAA Privacy Rule permits covered entities to disclose protected health information to workers' compensation insurers, state administrators, employers, and other persons or entities involved in workers' compensation systems, without the individual's authorization. This relates to workers' compensation injuries or illnesses and federal programs such as Black Lung Benefits Act, Federal Employees' Compensation Act, the Longshore and Harbor Workers' Compensation Act, and Energy Employees' Occupational Illness Compensation Program Act. The disclosure must comply with and be limited to what the state law requires. Disclosure is allowed for purposes of obtaining payment for any health care provided to the injured or ill worker.

2. *Disclosures with Individual Authorization.* Covered entities may disclose PHI to workers' compensation insurers and others involved in workers' compensation systems to which the individual has provided his or her authorization for the release of the information to the entity.

3. *Minimum Necessary.* Covered entities are required to limit the amount of PHI disclosed to the minimum necessary to accomplish the workers' compensation purpose. Under this requirement, PHI may be shared for such purposes to the full extent authorized by state or other law.

It is preferable that a patient not be scheduled to see a physician for a workers' compensation follow-up examination and an unrelated complaint during the same appointment time. Separate appointments (back to back, if necessary) should be arranged. This allows for separate dictation without intermixing the required documentation for each chart.

Terminology

Most workers' compensation cases involve accidents causing bodily injuries. Therefore one should become familiar with anatomic terms, directional and range-of-motion words, types of fractures, body activity terms, and words that describe pain and symptoms. This terminology appears in progress chart notes and industrial injury reports. The more knowledgeable one becomes about the meaning of the documentation, the more proficient he or she will be in knowing whether the procedure and diagnostic codes assigned are substantiated or if code selection is deficient and should be enhanced for better payment. Figures 15–5 through 15–9, Table 15.4, and Box 15.2 should be studied carefully. One should learn how to spell the words and find the definitions of the words in the dictionary.

Directional Terms

Directional terms are commonly used in workers' compensation reports. Figure 15–5 illustrates positional and directional terms referring to movements and planes of the body. The subject is standing upright, facing forward, arms at the sides with palms forward, and feet parallel. Imaginary lines divide the body in half, forming body planes (e.g., frontal plane dividing right and left sides and coronal plane dividing front and back).

If you get the patient's authorization to disclose the information, then you do not need to include it or track it for accounting, because the disclosures that are made following somebody's authorization do not need to be accounted for.

Documentation

Documentation must show the necessity for the procedures performed. If there is no accurate diagnostic code to explain the patient's condition, a report should be sent that describes the details of the diagnosis.

As learned in Chapter 5, the ICD-9-CM code book has a section that lists E codes, which are categorized by external causes of injuries, poisonings, and adverse effects. E codes describe how injuries occur. In workers' compensation cases, it is important to use E codes because they indicate the external cause of injury, such as E849.3 (Place of occurrence; industrial place and premises). Some cases may need two E codes, one for the circumstance of the event and one for its location. E codes are never used as a primary diagnosis but they give supplemental information to the insurance carrier. This may help the insurance carrier to differentiate between the claims and get a claim paid quicker.

CPT code 99080 may be used to bill for workers' compensation reports. The monetary value assigned to the code usually is determined by the number of pages in the report. If health records are reviewed before consulting or treating a workers' compensation patient, a bill should be submitted for this service. Refer to Chapter 4 for comprehensive information on this topic.

Health Information Record Keeping

If a private patient comes to the office with an industrial injury, a separate health record (chart) and financial record (ledger) should be set up for the work-related injury. A private health record should never be combined with an industrial case record because separate disclosure laws apply to each, and the workers' compensation case may go to court. Some medical practices use a colored file folder or tabs for the industrial health record, which makes filing of all private and workers' compensation documents easier for the insurance billing specialist. If two charts are maintained, it is easy to pull the industrial health record and financial accounting record quickly without having to go through the patient's previously unrelated private health records.

Box 15.2 **Terms That Describe Intensity of Pain and Frequency of Occurrence of Symptoms**

Definitions that describe intensity of pain and frequency of symptoms were developed to assist the physician when documenting subjective complaints.

A **severe** pain would preclude the activity causing the pain.

A **moderate** pain could be tolerated but would cause marked handicap in the performance of the activity precipitating the pain.

A **slight** pain could be tolerated but would cause some handicap in the performance of the activity precipitating the pain.

A **minimal** (mild) pain would constitute an annoyance but would cause no handicap in the performance of the particular activity. It would be considered a nonrateable permanent disability.

Occasional means approximately 25% of the time.

Intermittent means approximately 50% of the time.

Frequent means approximately 75% of the time.

Constant means 90% to 100% of the time.

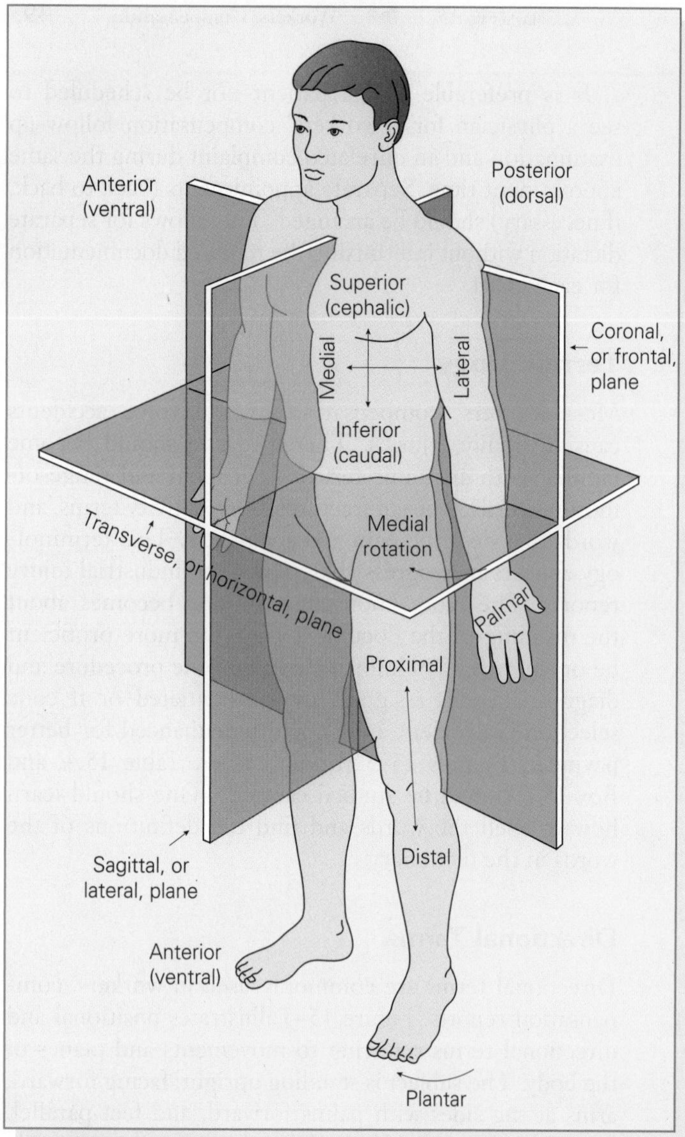
Anterior
(ventral)
Posterior
(dorsal)
Superior
(cephalic)
Medial
Lateral
Inferior
(caudal)
Coronal,
or frontal,
plane
Transverse, or horizontal, plane
Medial
rotation
Palmar
Proximal
Distal
Sagittal, or
lateral, plane
Anterior
(ventral)
Plantar

FIGURE 15–5 Directional terminology. *(From Chabner D-E: Medical Terminology: A Short Course, 2nd ed. Philadelphia, Saunders, 1999.)*

Table 15.4 Body Activity Terms

Body activity terms are used when the physician describes activities that the patient is able to perform and restrictions when a patient returns to work before full recovery.

Balancing	Maintaining body equilibrium to prevent falling when walking, standing, crouching, or running on narrow, slippery, or erratically moving surfaces, or maintaining body equilibrium when performing gymnastic feats.
Bending	Angulation from neutral-straight position about joint (e.g., elbow) or spine (e.g., forward or lateral spine flexion).
Carrying	Transporting an object usually holding it in the hands or arms or on the shoulder.
Climbing	Ascending or descending ladders, stairs, scaffolding, ramps, and poles using feet and legs and/or hands or arms. For climbing, the emphasis is placed on body agility; for balancing, it is placed on body equilibrium.
Crawling	Moving about on hands and knees or hands and feet.
Crouching	Bending body downward and forward by bending legs and spine.
Feeling	Perceiving attributes of objects such as size, shape, temperature, or texture by means of receptors in skin like those of fingertips.
Fingering	Picking, pinching, or working with fingers primarily.
Handling	Seizing, holding, grasping, turning with hands; fingering not involved.
Kneeling	Bending legs at knees to come to rest on knees.
Lifting	Raising or lowering an object from one level to another.
Pulling	Exerting force on an object so the object moves toward the force (includes jerking).
Pushing	Exerting force on an object so the object moves away from the force (includes slapping, striking, kicking, and treadle action).
Reaching	Extending the arm(s) in any direction.
Sitting	Remaining in the normal seated position.
Standing	Remaining on one's feet in the upright position at a work station without moving about.
Stooping	Bending body downward and forward by bending spine and waist.

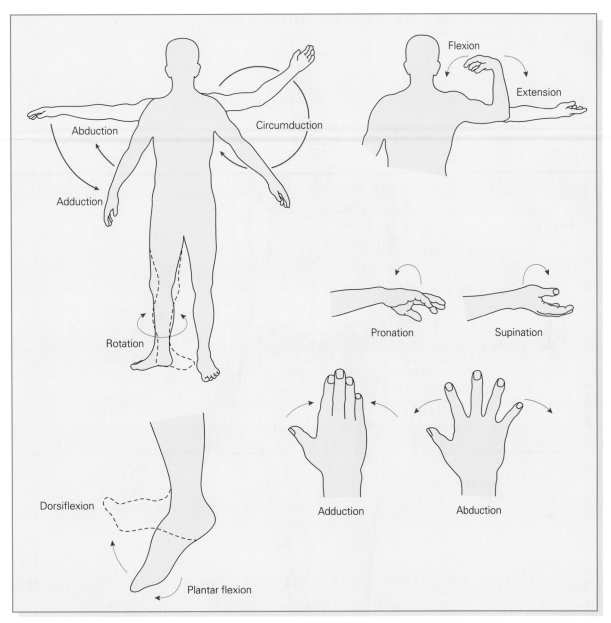

FIGURE 15-6 Range of motion for upper and lower extremities. *(From Sloane S, Fordney MT: Saunders Manual of Medical Transcription. Philadelphia, Saunders, 1994.)*

The positional and directional terms indicate the location or direction of the body part with respect to each other (e.g., medial, toward the midline of the body, and lateral, toward the sides of the body).

Range of Motion of Upper and Lower Extremities

Figure 15–6 shows commonly dictated terms for range of motion (ROM) of upper and lower extremities. ROM tests determine whether the body part is able to move to the full extent possible. Often after an injury to an extremity or joint there is restriction of motion and loss of strength (e.g., grip). ROM can be improved with activity and therapy and is measured with special measurement devices and documented each time a patient is examined.

Types of Fractures

A fracture is a break in the continuity of a bone. Figures 15–7 and 15–8 illustrate the many bones of the body and Figure 15–9 explains each type of fracture. Such injuries can occur from falling, blows, impact hits, a disease process, or direct violence, such as in an automobile accident. Healing may take months and depends on the location and severity of the injured part, associated injury, and complications or infections.

THE SKELETON (ANTERIOR VIEW)

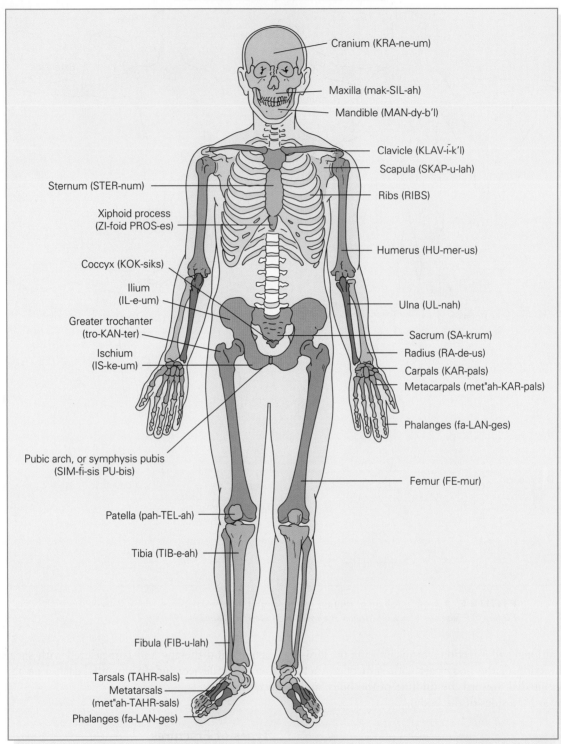

FIGURE 15–7   Terminology pertinent to the skeletal anatomy commonly used in reports on injury cases. *(From Chabner D-E: The Language of Medicine, 6th ed. Philadelphia, Saunders, 1999.)*

THE SKELETON (POSTERIOR VIEW)

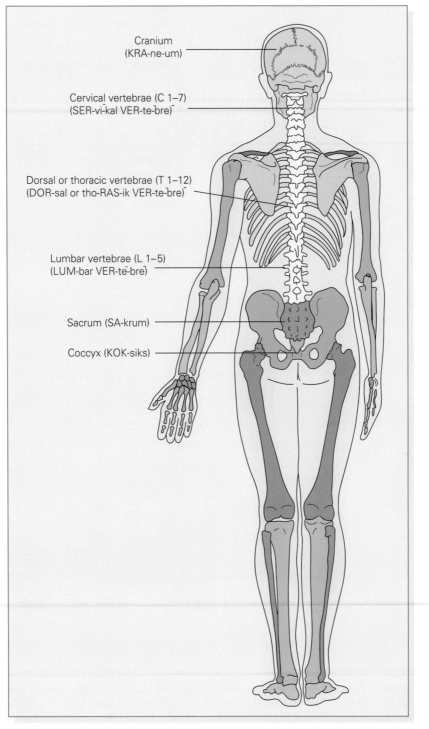

Cranium
(KRA-ne-um)

Cervical vertebrae (C 1–7)
(SER-vi-kal VER-te-bre)

Dorsal or thoracic vertebrae (T 1–12)
(DOR-sal or tho-RAS-ik VER-te-bre)

Lumbar vertebrae (L 1–5)
(LUM-bar VER-te-bre)

Sacrum (SA-krum)

Coccyx (KOK-siks)

FIGURE 15–7, cont'd   Terminology pertinent to the skeletal anatomy commonly used in reports on injury cases. *(From Chabner D-E: The Language of Medicine, 6th ed. Philadelphia, Saunders, 1999.)*

BONES OF THE HAND AND FOOT

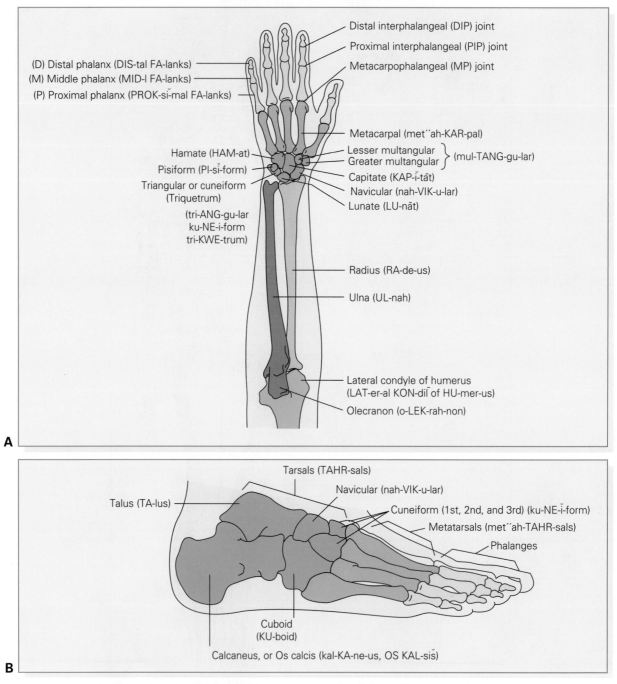

FIGURE 15–8 Terminology pertinent to the hand **(A)** and foot **(B),** indicating the common medical terms seen in reports on injury cases. *(A, Redrawn from Marble HC: The Hand: A Manual and Atlas for the General Surgeon. Philadelphia, Saunders, 1960. B, Redrawn from Chabner D-E: The Language of Medicine, 6th ed. Philadelphia, Saunders, 1999.)*

REPORTING REQUIREMENTS

Employer's Report

The laws clearly state that the injured person must promptly report the industrial injury or illness to his or her employer or immediate supervisor, which may be a safety officer in some businesses. The first report of an industrial injury submitted by the employer and the physician is required by law in most states. The employer sends an Employer's Report of Occupational Injury or Illness Form (Figure 15–10) to the insurance company. The time limit on submission of this form varies from immediately to as long as 30 days in different states (see Table 15.1). Many states have adopted the form shown

Fracture	Definition		Fracture	Definition	
Closed or simple	Broken bone is contained within intact skin.		Pathologic	Results from weakening of bone by disease	
Open or compound	Skin is broken above the fracture, which is thus open to the external environment, resulting in potential for infection.		Nondisplaced	Bone ends remain in alignment	
Longitudinal	Fracture extends along the length of the bone.		Displaced	Bone ends are out of alignment	
Transverse	Produced by direct force applied perpendicularly to a bone		Spiral	Have long, sharp, pointed bone ends; produced by twisting or rotary forces	
Oblique	Produced by a twisting force with an upward thrust; fracture ends are short and run at an oblique angle across the bone		Compression	Produced by transmitted forces that drive bones together	
Greenstick	Produced by compression or angulation forces in long bones of children younger than 10. Bone is cracked on one side and intact on the other due to softness.		Avulsion	Produced by forceful contraction of a muscle against resistance, with a bone fragment tearing at the site of muscle insertion	
Comminuted	Has multiple fragments and is produced by severe direct violence		Depression	Bone fragments of the skull are driven inward	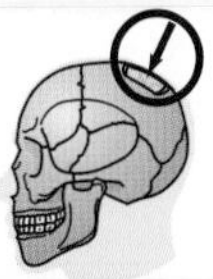
Impacted	Produced by strong forces that drive bone fragments firmly together				

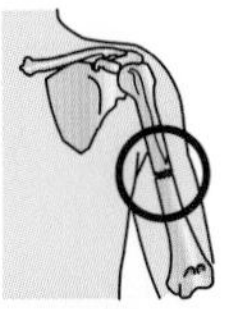

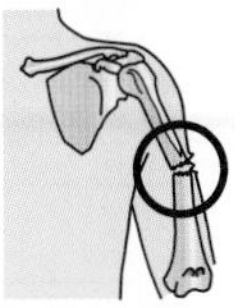

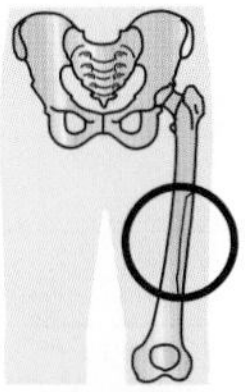

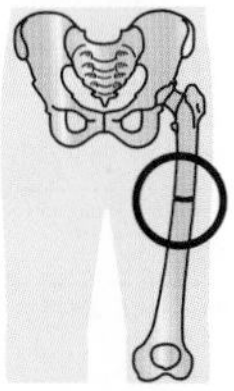

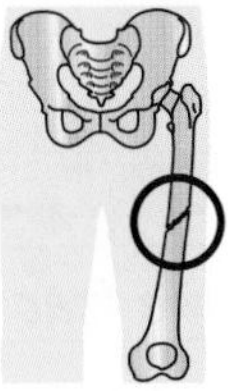

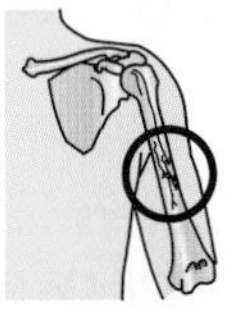

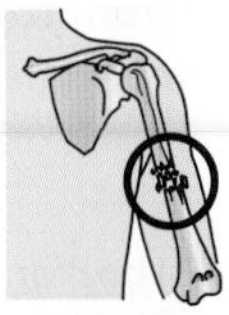

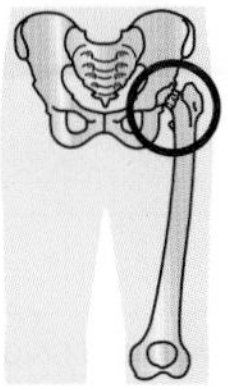

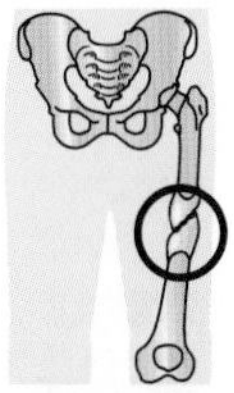

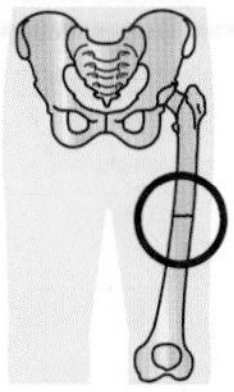

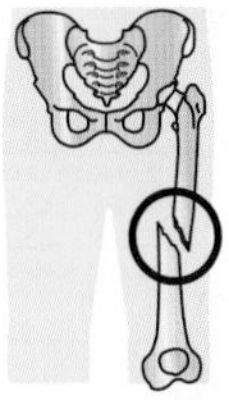

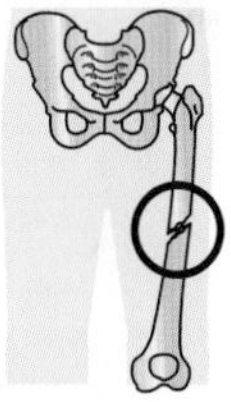

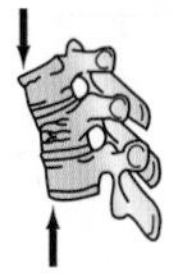

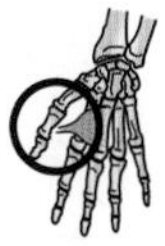

FIGURE 15–9 Terminology and illustration of different types of fractures. (*From Chester GA: Modern Medical Assisting. Philadelphia, Saunders, 1998.*)

State of California	Please complete in triplicate (type, if possible). Mail two copies to:	OSHA
EMPLOYER'S REPORT OF OCCUPATIONAL INJURY OR ILLNESS	XYZ Insurance Company PO Box 5 Woodland Hills, XY 12345	Case No. **# 18** ☐ Fatality

Any person who makes or causes to be made any knowingly false or fraudulent material statement or material representation for the purpose of obtaining or denying workers' compensation benefits or payments is guilty of a felony.

NOTICE: California law requires employers to report within **five days** of knowledge every occupational injury or illness which results in lost time beyond the date of the incident **OR** requires medical treatment beyond first aid. If an employee subsequently dies as a result of a previously reported injury or illness, the employer must file within **five days** of knowledge an amended report indicating death. In addition, every serious injury/illness, or death must be reported **immediately** by telephone or telegraph to the nearest office of the California Division of Occupational Safety and Health.

EMPLOYER

1. FIRM NAME
The Conk Out Company

1A. POLICY NUMBER
B12345

DO NOT USE THIS COLUMN

2. MAILING ADDRESS (Number and Street, City, ZIP)
45 South Gorman St. Woodland Hills, XY 12345

2A. PHONE NUMBER
555-430-3488

Case No.

3. LOCATION, IF DIFFERENT FROM MAILING ADDRESS (Number and Street, City, ZIP)

3A. LOCATION CODE

Ownership

4. NATURE OF BUSINESS, e.g., painting contractor, wholesale grocer, sawmill, hotel, etc.
Plumbing Repair

5. STATE UNEMPLOYMENT INSURANCE ACCT. NO.

Industry

6. TYPE OF EMPLOYER
[X] PRIVATE　☐ STATE　☐ CITY　☐ COUNTY　☐ SCHOOL DIST.　☐ OTHER GOVERNMENT - SPECIFY _____

Occupation

EMPLOYEE

7. EMPLOYEE NAME
Ima B. Hurt

8. SOCIAL SECURITY NUMBER
120-XX-6542

9. DATE OF BIRTH (mm/dd/yy)
3-4-66

Sex

10. HOME ADDRESS (Number and Street, City, ZIP)
300 E.Central Ave. Woodland Hills, XY 12345

10A. PHONE NUMBER
555-476-9899

Age

11. SEX
☐ MALE　[X] FEMALE

12. OCCUPATION (Regular job title — NO initials, abbreviations or numbers)
Clerk Typist

13. DATE OF HIRE (mm/dd/yy)
1-20-86

Daily Hours

14. EMPLOYEE USUALLY WORKS
8 hours per day　*5* days per week　*40* total weekly hours

14A. EMPLOYMENT STATUS (check applicable status at time of injury)
[X] regular full-time　___ part-time　___ temporary　___ seasonal

14B. Under what class code of your policy were wages assigned?
7219

Days per week

15. GROSS WAGES/SALARY
$ *700.00* per *week*

16. OTHER PAYMENTS NOT REPORTED AS WAGES/SALARY (e.g. tips, meals, lodging, overtime, bonuses, etc.)?
☐ YES $ _____ PER _____　[X] NO

Weekly hours

INJURY OR ILLNESS

17. DATE OF INJURY OR ONSET OF ILLNESS (mm/dd/yy)
4-3-XX

18. TIME INJURY/ILLNESS OCCURRED
___ A.M. *2:00* P.M.

19. TIME EMPLOYEE BEGAN WORK
8:00 A.M. ___ P.M.

20. IF EMPLOYEE DIED, DATE OF DEATH (mm/dd/yy)

Weekly wage

21. UNABLE TO WORK AT LEAST ONE FULL DAY AFTER DATE OF INJURY?
[X] YES　☐ NO

22. DATE LAST WORKED (mm/dd/yy)
4-3-XX

23. DATE RETURNED TO WORK (mm/dd/yy)

24. IF STILL OFF WORK, CHECK THIS BOX
[X]

County

25. PAID FULL WAGES FOR DAY OF INJURY OR LAST DAY WORKED?
[X] YES　☐ NO

26. SALARY BEING CONTINUED?
☐ YES　[X] NO

27. DATE OF EMPLOYER'S KNOWLEDGE/NOTICE OF INJURY/ILLNESS (mm/dd/yy)
4-3-XX

28. DATE EMPLOYEE WAS PROVIDED
4-3-XX

Nature of injury

29. SPECIFIC INJURY/ILLNESS AND PART OF BODY AFFECTED, MEDICAL DIAGNOSIS, if available, e.g., second degree burns on right arm, tendonitis of left elbow, lead poisoning.
ankle injury swelling, possible fracture

Part of body

30. LOCATION WHERE EVENT OR EXPOSURE OCCURRED (Number, Street, City)
45 South Gorman St. Woodland Hills, XY 12345

30B. ON EMPLOYERS PREMISES?
[X] YES　☐ NO

Source

31. DEPARTMENT WHERE EVENT OR EXPOSURE OCCURRED, e.g., shipping department, machine shop.
stock room

32. OTHER WORKERS INJURED/ILL IN THIS EVENT?
☐ YES　[X] NO

Event

33. EQUIPMENT, MATERIALS AND CHEMICALS THE EMPLOYEE WAS USING WHEN EVENT OR EXPOSURE OCCURRED, e.g., acetylene, welding torch, farm tractor, scaffold.
6 foot ladder

Sec. Source

34. SPECIFY ACTIVITY THE EMPLOYEE WAS PERFORMING WHEN EVENT OR EXPOSURE OCCURRED, e.g., welding seams of metal forms, loading boxes onto truck.
climbed ladder to remove a ream of paper from shelf; fell

Extent of injury

35. HOW INJURY/ILLNESS OCCURRED. DESCRIBE SEQUENCE OF EVENTS. SPECIFY OBJECT OR EXPOSURE WHICH DIRECTLY PRODUCED THE INJURY/ILLNESS, e.g., worker stepped back to inspect work and slipped on scrap material. As he fell, he brushed against fresh weld, and burned hand. USE SEPARATE SHEET IF NECESSARY.
worker climbed ladder to remove a ream of paper from top shelf in stock room. She was descending and mis-stepped falling to the floor. She tried to land upright, and her left leg took the brunt of the fall.

36. NAME AND ADDRESS OF PHYSICIAN (Number and Street, City, ZIP)
Raymond Skeleton, MD 4567 Broad Ave., Woodland Hills, XY 12345

36A. PHONE NUMBER
555-486-9002

37. IF HOSPITALIZED AS AN INPATIENT, NAME AND ADDRESS OF HOSPITAL (Number and Street, City, ZIP)

37A. PHONE NUMBER

Completed by (type or print) J.D. Hawkins	Signature *J. D. Hawkins*	Title *owner*	Date *4-3-XX*

FILING THIS REPORT IS NOT AN ADMISSION OF LIABILITY

FIGURE 15–10 Employer's Report of Occupational Injury or Illness. This form complies with OSHA requirements as well as California State Workers' Compensation laws.

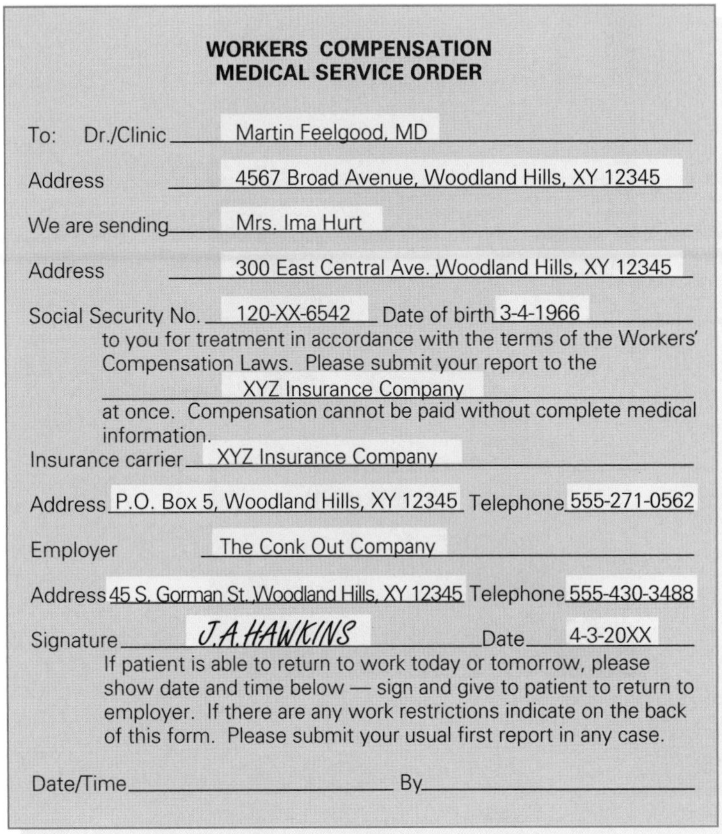

**WORKERS COMPENSATION
MEDICAL SERVICE ORDER**

To: Dr./Clinic _____ Martin Feelgood, MD _____

Address _____ 4567 Broad Avenue, Woodland Hills, XY 12345 _____

We are sending _____ Mrs. Ima Hurt _____

Address _____ 300 East Central Ave. Woodland Hills, XY 12345 _____

Social Security No. _____ 120-XX-6542 _____ Date of birth 3-4-1966 _____
    to you for treatment in accordance with the terms of the Workers'
    Compensation Laws. Please submit your report to the
    _____ XYZ Insurance Company _____
    at once. Compensation cannot be paid without complete medical
    information.
Insurance carrier _____ XYZ Insurance Company _____

Address P.O. Box 5, Woodland Hills, XY 12345 Telephone 555-271-0562

Employer _____ The Conk Out Company _____

Address 45 S. Gorman St. Woodland Hills, XY 12345 Telephone 555-430-3488

Signature _____ *J.A. HAWKINS* _____ Date _____ 4-3-20XX _____
    If patient is able to return to work today or tomorrow, please
    show date and time below — sign and give to patient to return to
    employer. If there are any work restrictions indicate on the back
    of this form. Please submit your usual first report in any case.

Date/Time _____ By _____

FIGURE 15–11   Medical service order.

in Figure 15–10 to meet the requirements of the federal OSHA of 1970 and for state statistical purposes.

Medical Service Order

In addition to the employer's report, the employer may complete and sign a **medical service order,** giving this to the injured employee to take to the physician's office (Figure 15–11). This authorizes the physician to treat the injured employee. The form should be photocopied and the copy retained for the physician's files. The original should be attached to the Doctor's First Report of Occupational Injury or Illness (preliminary report). An employer may prefer to write the service order on his or her business letterhead, on billhead, or simply on a piece of scratch paper.

Authorizations also may be obtained over the telephone. However, if a patient arrives for an appointment without written authorization, some offices prefer that the employer be telephoned and asked to have the authorized person fax the permission for treatment. Subsequently, if payment is not received or the claim is disputed, it may be easier to collect if a copy of the written authorization is included when sending collection follow-up correspondence.

The copayment should be collected when the patient has a managed care plan and neglects to bring in an authorization. It is the patient's responsibility to get the authorization if injured on the job (Figure 15–12).

A charge can be made if an appointment was arranged by the employer or insurance company for a workers' compensation patient and was not canceled 72 hours before the appointment time. Check with the insurance company because this policy may vary depending on state laws.

If outside testing or treatment is necessary, authorization should be obtained from the employer or the adjuster for the insurance company. When this is done by telephone, the name of the procedure or test and the medical necessity for it should be stated. The name and title of the person giving authorization should be obtained and written in the patient's chart and on the order form along with the date. No authorization numbers are issued in workers' compensation cases.

The insurance adjuster handling the case should be contacted if a translator is needed for a workers' compensation patient. He or she should make arrangements for an official translator to be present for all appointments. A member of the patient's family or the patient's friend

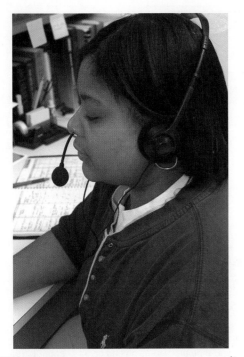

FIGURE 15–12 Receptionist receiving a medical service order via telephone for the worker to receive medical services.

should not be allowed to serve as a translator because there may be no legal recourse for the physician if miscommunicated information leads to a bad outcome.

Physician's First Report

After the physician sees the injured person, he or she sends in a completed First Treatment Medical Report (Figure 15–13) or a Doctor's First Report of Occupational Injury or Illness form (used in California; see Figure 15–20) as soon as possible.

If the physician prefers to submit a narrative letter, the medical report should include the components, if relevant, shown in Table 15.5. The time limit for filing this report varies; state requirements are provided in Table 15.1. Failure to file the report can be a misdemeanor. Copies of the report form go to the insurance carrier and the state. Some physicians also send a copy to the employer.

Because the report is a legal document, each copy *must be signed in ink* by the physician. The insurance company waits for the physician's report and bill, then issues payment to the physician. The case can be closed if there is no further treatment or disability.

Progress or Supplemental Report

In a TD case, a supplemental report is sent to the insurance carrier after 2 to 4 weeks of treatment to give information on the current status of the patient. If there is a significant change in the prognosis, a detailed progress report (sometimes called a reexamination report) is sent to the insurance carrier. Subsequent progress or supplemental reports should be sent to the insurance carrier after each hospitalization and office visit to update the progress of a case. They may be narrative and are not necessarily completed on the special forms available in most states (Figure 15–14). If the disability is ongoing over a period of time, monthly progress reports should be submitted. A follow-up report must contain the following information:

1. Date of most recent examination
2. Present condition and progress since last report
3. Measurements of function
4. X-ray or laboratory report since last examination
5. Treatment (give type and duration)
6. Work status (patient working or estimated date of return to work if patient is still temporarily disabled)
7. Permanent disability to be anticipated

The insurance carrier authorizing the examination should be furnished with the report in triplicate or quadruplicate, depending on its needs. A copy should be retained for the physician's files.

Final Report

TD ends when the physician tells the insurance carrier that the patient is able to return to work. Sometimes a physician submits a final report at the time of discharge. When the patient resumes work, the insurance carrier closes the case, and the TD benefits cease.

A physician's final report indicating any impairment or permanent disability should be sent, accompanied by a statement listing total expenses incurred (Figure 15–15).

CLAIM SUBMISSION

Financial Responsibility

As discussed in Chapter 3, the contract for treatment in a personal illness or injury case is between the physician and patient, who is responsible for the entire bill. However, when a business is self-insured, a person is under a state program for care, or an individual is being treated as a workers' compensation case, the financial responsibility exists between the physician and insurance company or state program. As long as treatment is authorized by the insurance carrier, the insurance company is responsible for payment. A physician who agrees to treat a workers' compensation case must agree to accept payment in full according to the workers' compensation fee schedule. A copayment amount cannot be

NEBRASKA WORKERS' COMPENSATION COURT
First Treatment Medical Report
(Must be filed with Compensation Court & Employer within 7 days of first treatment)
(Shaded sections are not required)

TYPE OR PRINT

PATIENT & INSURED (SUBSCRIBER) INFORMATION

1. PATIENT'S NAME (First, name, middle initial, last name)	2. PATIENT'S DATE OF BIRTH	3. INSURED'S NAME (Employer)
Lester M. Task	05 | 06 | 60	Jonas Construction Company

4. PATIENT'S ADDRESS (Street, City, State, ZIP Code)	5. PATIENT'S SEX	6. INSURED'S I.D. NO. (Include any letters)
5400 Holly Street Woodland Hills, XY 12345	[X] MALE [ ] FEMALE	B 785700

7. PATIENT'S RELATIONSHIP TO INSURED
[ ] SELF [ ] SPOUSE [ ] CHILD [X] OTHER

8 INSURED'S GROUP NO. (Or Group Name)
5601

9. OTHER HEALTH INSURANCE COVERAGE - Enter Name of Policyholder and Plan Name and Address and Policy or Medical Assistance Number	10. WAS CONDITION RELATED TO:	11. INSURED'S ADDRESS (Street, City State, ZIP Code)
	A. PATIENT'S EMPLOYMENT [X] YES [ ] NO B. AN AUTO ACCIDENT [ ] YES [ ] NO	300 Main Street Woodland Hills, XY 12345

| 12. PATIENT'S OR AUTHORIZED PERSON'S SIGNATURE
I Authorize the Release of any Medical Information Necessary to Process this Claim
SIGNED | 12A. PATIENT'S SOCIAL SECURITY NO
578 \| XX \| 1921
DATE 11-8-XX | 13. I AUTHORIZE PAYMENT OF MEDICAL BENEFITS TO UNDERSIGNED PHYSICIAN OR SUPPLIER FOR SERVICE DESCRIBED BELOW

SIGNED (Insured or Authorized Person) |

PHYSICIAN OR SUPPLIER INFORMATION

14. DATE OF: 11-8-XX ◀	ILLNESS (FIRST SYMPTOM OR INJURY (ACCIDENT)	15. DATE FIRST CONSULTED YOU FOR THIS CONDITION 11-8-XX	16. HAS PATIENT EVER HAD SAME OR SIMILAR SYMPTOMS? [ ] YES [X] NO

17. DATE PATIENT ABLE TO RETURN TO WORK	18. DATES OF TOTAL DISABILITY FROM 11-8-XX THROUGH 12-8-XX	DATES OF PARTIAL DISABILITY FROM | THROUGH

19. NAME OF REFERRING PHYSICIAN	20. FOR SERVICES RELATED TO HOSPITALIZATION GIVE HOSPITALIZATION DATES ADMITTED 11-8-XX DISCHARGED 11-10-XX

21. NAME & ADDRESS OF FACILITY WHERE SERVICES RENDERED (If other than home or office) Community Hospital, 400 Oak St., Woodland Hills, XY 12345	22. WAS LABORATORY WORK PERFORMED OUTSIDE YOUR OFFICE? [ ] YES [X] NO CHARGES:

23. DIAGNOSIS OR NATURE OF ILLNESS OR INJURY, RELATE DIAGNOSIS TO PROCEDURE IN COLUMN D BY REFERENCE TO NUMBERS 1,2,3, ETC. OR DX CODE

1. fracture of right patella   822.1
2.
3.
4.

24. A DATE OF SERVICE	B* PLACE OF SERVICE	C FULLY DESCRIBE PROCEDURES, MEDICAL SERVICE OR SUPPLIES FURNISHED FOR EACH DATE GIVEN PROCEDURE CODE (IDENTIFY:)	(EXPLAIN UNUSUAL SERVICES OR CIRCUMSTANCES)	D DIAGNOSIS CODE	E CHARGES	F
11-8-XX	1	99222	Initial hospital care	1	125 00	
11-8-XX	1	27524	Open TX patellar fracture with internal fixation	1	600 00	

24A. HISTORY. GIVE BRIEF DESCRIPTION OF WHAT OCCURRED. PATIENT'S ACCOUNT OF ACCIDENT.

Patient was up on a scaffold at a construction site and fell off of it about

8 feet hitting the ground with his right knee.

25. SIGNATURE OF PHYSICIAN OR SUPPLIER SIGNED *Gregory T. Getwell, MD* DATE 11-8-XX	26. ACCEPT ASSIGNMENT (GOVERNMENT CLAIMS ONLY) [ ] YES [ ] NO PHYSICIAN'S SOCIAL SECURITY NO.	27. TOTAL CHARGE 725.00	28. AMOUNT PAID	29. BALANCE DUE 725 | 00

32. YOUR PATIENT'S ACCOUNT NO.	33. YOUR EMPLOYER I.D. NO. 95-32089XX	31. PHYSICIAN'S OR SUPPLIER'S NAME, ADDRESS, ZIP CODE & TELEPHONE NO Gregory T. Getwell, MD 60 North State Street Woodland Hills, XY 12345 I.D. NO. A123456 555-459-0087

*PLACE OF SERVICE CODES

1—(IH) - INPATIENT HOSPITAL	4—(H) PATIENT'S HOME	7—(NH) NURSING HOME
2—(OH) - OUTPATIENT HOSPITAL	5— DAY CARE FACILITY (PSY)	8—(SNF) SKILLED NURSING FACILITY
3—(0) - DOCTOR'S OFFICE	6— NIGHT CARE FACILITY(PSY)	9— AMBULANCE

O—(OL) OTHER LOCATIONS
A—(IL) INDEPENDENT LABORATORY
B— OTHER MEDICAL/SURGICAL FACILITY

NWCC FORM 45 (Rev. 86)

reference initials

FIGURE 15-13 First Treatment Medical Report form used in Nebraska. This form follows the format of the Health Insurance Claim Form CMS-1500 developed by the American Medical Association Council on Medical Service (see Chapter 7).

Table 15.5	**Narrative Medical Report Issues, if Relevant**
History	Outline all specific details of accident, injury, or illness. Physician should state whether there is a causal connection between the accident and conditions that may appear subsequently but are not obvious **sequelae** (diseased conditions following, and usually resulting from, a previous disease). If facts were obtained by reviewing prior records or x-ray films, the source should be mentioned. When a history is obtained through an interpreter, include that person's name.
Present complaints	Usually given as subjective complaints. *Subjective* refers to statements made by the patient about symptoms and how he or she feels. Subjective disability is evaluated by • A description of the activity that produces the disability • The duration of the disability • The activities that are precluded by, and those that can be performed with, the disability • The means necessary for relief
Past history	Description of any previous, current, subsequent medical information relevant to this injury or illness and stating whether there is a preexisting defect that might entitle the injured person to benefits from the subsequent injury fund or whether this injury or illness represents the actual cause of the present condition.
Examination findings	Usually given as *objective findings*. State all significant physical or psychiatric examination, testing, laboratory, or imaging findings.
Diagnostic impression	State all diagnostic findings and opinion as to *relationship*, if any, between the injury or disease and the condition diagnosed. Use diagnostic terminology that corresponds to the diagnostic code book.
Disability/ prognosis	a. Period during which the patient has been unable to work because of the injury or illness. b. Opinion as to probable further temporary disability and a statement as to when the patient will be able to return to work or has returned to work. c. Statement indicating whether the condition is currently permanent and stationary, as well as the probability of future permanent disability. d. Statement indicating "All objective tests for organic pathology are negative. There is obviously a strong functional or emotional overlay," when a patient has multiple complaints but no clinical objective findings.
Work limitations	Description of any limitations to all activities.
Causation	Description of how the permanent disability is related to the patient's occupation and the specific injury or cumulative events causing the illness.

collected or the balance billed to the patient for any amount not covered.

If an injured worker refuses to accept the physician retained by the insurance company for the employer, the patient may be responsible for the cost of medical treatment. The employee should first contact the employer, then the insurance company, to find out if there are any provisions for a change of physicians.

Some states have a medical program wherein employers can reduce their workers' compensation rates by paying the first $1000 in medical bills. This is similar to a deductible for the employer's policy. The statement should be sent to the employer for payment in this situation.

Health insurance information should always be obtained in case services are provided that are not work related or should be billed for, or the injury or illness is declared nonindustrial. To assist in informing patients of financial responsibility for nonrelated illness, the worker should sign an agreement for nonrelated medical expenses, as shown in Figure 15–16. If the workers' compensation carrier declares the case is nonindustrial, bill the patient's health insurance, attaching a copy of the refusal by the workers' compensation carrier.

Sometimes a physician discovers a problem unrelated to the industrial injury or illness (e.g., high blood pressure) while examining an injured worker. The physician may bill the workers' compensation carrier for the examination but should code the claim carefully with regard to treatment of the injury. If treatment is initiated for the patient's high blood pressure, that portion of the examination becomes the financial obligation of the patient and not the workers' compensation carrier.

Fee Schedules

Some states have developed and adopted a workers' compensation **fee schedule,** whereas other states pay medical claims based on the Medicare fee schedule plus a certain percentage. The insurance carrier is sent the bill and no billing statements are sent to the patient. Fee schedules assist with the following:

1. They limit the fees providers can charge for standard medical procedures paid by workers' compensation companies.
2. They limit the amount that providers will be paid.
3. They make the allowable charges and procedures more consistent.
4. They provide follow-up procedures in case of a fee dispute.

ATTENDING PHYSICIAN'S REPORT

Employee: Mrs. Ima B. Hurt   Claim number: 120 XX 6542

Employer: The Conk Out Company   Date of injury(ies): 4-3-20XX   Date of next exam: 4-24-20XX

Date of this exam: 4-10-XX   Patient Social Security No: 120 XX 6542

Current diagnosis: 824.6 closed fracture; L. trimalleolar ankle
(include ICD•9 code)

PATIENT STATUS

Since the last exam, this patient's condition has:

- ☒ improved as expected.
- ☐ improved, but slower than expected.
- ☐ not improved significantly.
- ☐ worsened.
- ☐ plateaued, no further improvement is expected.
- ☐ has been determined to be non-work related.

Briefly, describe any change in objective or subjective complaint:

TREATMENT

Treatment plan: (only list changes from prior status)   ☐ No change   ☐ Patient is/was discharged from care on
Est. discharge date: 5-18-20XX   Medications: Tylenol for pain
Therapy: Type   Times per week _____ Estimated date of completion
Diagnostic studies: X-ray, L. ankle 3 views
Hospitalization/surgery:
Consult/other service:

WORK STATUS

The patient has been instructed to:

- ☐ return to full duty with no limitations or restrictions.
- ☐ remain off the rest of the day and return to work tomorrow:

    _____ with no limits or restrictions. _____ with limits listed below.

- ☐ return to work on_____
    work limitations: _____
- ☒ remain off work until 5-17-20XX — discharge exam scheduled

Estimated date patient can return full duty: 5-18-20XX

DISABILITY STATUS

- ☐ Patient discharged as cured.

Please supply a brief narrative report if any of the below apply:

- ☐ Patient will be permanently precluded from engaging in his/her usual and customary occupation.
- ☐ Patient's condition is permanent and stationary.
- ☐ Patient will have permanent residuals
- ☐ Patient will require future medical care.

Physician name: Martin Feelgood, MD   Address: 4567 Broad Avenue, Woodland Hills, XY 12345

Date: April 10, 20XX   Telephone: (555) 482-9002

Signature: Martin Feelgood, MD

reference initials

FIGURE 15–14 Physician's Supplemental Report form.

XYZ INSURANCE COMPANY

DOCTOR'S FINAL (OR MONTHLY) REPORT AND BILL

Monthly itemized bills required on all cases under continuing treatment.
Services beginning late in month and extending into succeeding month may be itemized on one statement.

CASE No. __120 XX 6542__

EMPLOYEE __Mrs. Ima B. Hurt__
DATE OF INJURY __April 3, 20XX__
EMPLOYER __The Conk Out Company__

SERVICES FOR MONTH OF __May__ 20 __XX__

Patient refused treatment _____ 20____   Patient able to return to work __May 18,__ 20 __XX__
Patient stopped treatment   Patient discharged as cured _____ 20 ____
   without orders _____ 20____   Condition at time of last visit __fracture healed__
Patient entered hospital _____ 20____
Further treatment anticipated? __X__
           (Yes)   (No)

__P.T L. Ankle 2 x wk 3 wks__
Any other charges authorized such as drugs? _____ Hospital? _____
           (Check)   (Check)

Code: O—Office: V—Home Visit: H—Hospital Visit: N—Night Visit: S—Operation: X—X-ray.

Month	1	2	3	4	5	6	7	8	9	10	11	12	13	14	15	16	17	18	19	20	21	22	23	24	25	26	27	28	29	30	31
May							O										O														

	RVS CODE	TOTALS
First aid treatment (describe) _____	# _____	$ _____
Office Visits __5/7/XX and 5/17/XX__	# __99213__	$ __40.20__
Home Visits _____	# __99213__	$ __40.20__
Hospital Visits _____	# _____	$ _____
Operations _____	# _____	$ _____
MATERIAL (Itemize at cost) __Left ankle films; complete 5/7/xx__	# __73610__	$ __34.26__
__5/17/xx__	# __73610__	$ __34.26__
	# _____	$ _____

Any charges shown above which are in excess of the scheduled fee must
be explained regarding nature of such services, indicating the date rendered.   TOTAL $ __148.92__

Make check payable to:

Doctor __Martin Feelgood, MD__   Signature __Martin Feelgood, MD__

Address __4567 Broad Avenue__   Date __May 18, 20XX__
           (Street)
__Woodland Hills, XY 12345__
     (City)   (Zip)

LEAVE BLANK	
	APPROVED
	BY _____
(Dollars) (Cents)	DATE _____

Internal Revenue Code Section 6109
requires you to furnish your Internal
Revenue Service Employer Identification
Number or Social Security Number.
Please enter the Identification Number
here __95-36640XX__

IMPORTANT—
Bills Must Be Submitted in Duplicate
MAIL ADDRESS: P.O. BOX S, WOODLAND HILLS, XY 12345

SCIF FORM 60 REV 5 78

FIGURE 15–15 Doctor's Final (or Monthly) Report and Bill form.

PATIENT AGREEMENT

Patient's Name ___James Doland___ Soc. Sec. # ___431-XX-1942___

Address ___67 Blyth Dr., Woodland Hills, XY 12345___ Tel. No. ___555-372-0101___

WC Insurance Carrier ___Industrial Indemnity Company___

Address ___30 North Dr., Woodland Hills___ Telephone No. ___555-731-7707___

Date of illness ___2-13-20XX___ Date of first visit ___2-13-20XX___

Emergency Yes ___X___ No _____

Is this condition related to employment Yes ___X___ No _____

If accident: Auto _____ Other _____

Where did injury occur? ___Construction site___

How did injury happen? ___fell 8 ft from scaffold suffering fractured right tibia___

Employee/employer who verified this information ___Scott McPherson___

Employer's name and address ___Willow Construction Company___

Employer's telephone No. ___555-526-0611___

In the event the claim for workers' compensation is declared fraudulent for this illness or condition or it is determined by the Workers' Compensation Board that the illness or injury is not a compensable workers' compensation case, I ___James Doland___ , hereby agree to pay the physician's fee for services rendered.

I have been informed that I am responsible to pay any services rendered by Dr. ___Raymond Skeleton___ with regard to the discovery and treatment of any condition not related to the workers' compensation injury or illness. I agree to pay for all services not covered by workers' compensation and all charges for treatment and personal items unrelated to my workers' compensation illness or injury.

Signed ___James Doland___ Date ___2-13-20XX___

FIGURE 15–16 Patient agreement to pay the physician's fees if the case is declared not work related or an illness is discovered and treated that is not work related.

Some workers' compensation fee schedules list maximum reimbursement levels for physicians and other non-hospital providers. However, the physician generally is expected to accept payment by the insurance company as payment in full when reimbursement is based on a fee schedule. If the fee charged is more than the amount listed, the following factors may be considered:

- Provider's medical training, qualifications, and time in practice
- Nature of services provided
- Fees usually charged by the provider
- Fees usually charged by others in the region where services were given
- Other relevant economic factors of the provider's practice
- Any unusual circumstances in the case

The insurance carrier may pay the additional amount if documentation is sent validating the fee and noting the aforementioned facts.

Types of Fee Schedules

Types of fee schedules include the following:

- *Percentile of charge schedule,* which is designed to set fees at a percentile of the providers' usual and customary fee.
- *Relative value scale schedule,* which takes into account the time, skills, and extent of the service provided by the physician. Each procedure is rated on how difficult it is, how long it takes, the training a physician must have to perform it, and expenses the physician incurs, including the cost of malpractice insurance. Many of the fee schedules are similar to the CPT format in regard to sections (e.g., evaluation and management; anesthesia; surgery; radiology, nuclear medicine, and diagnostic ultrasound; pathology and laboratory; and medicine).

A *conversion factor* that uses a specific dollar amount is used for each of the sections of the fee schedule. Conversion factors may be adjusted to reflect regional differences and in some states are recalculated annually.

1999 Conversion Factors for Workers' Compensation in California	
$8.50/unit	Evaluation and management section
$34.50/unit	Anesthesia section
$153.00/unit	Surgery section
$12.50/unit	Radiology section (total unit value column)
$1.95/unit	Radiology section (professional component)
$1.50/unit	Radiology section (technical component)
$1.50/unit	Pathology section (technical component)
$6.15/unit	Medicine section

Actual covered procedures, descriptions, modifiers, global periods, and other elements of a fee guideline may significantly differ from those used for other plans or programs. Sometimes a schedule includes modifiers and code numbers not listed in the CPT code book. The workers' compensation codes should be used regardless of what is done for other insurance plans. Some states have their fee schedules posted at their state Web site. If it is not available online, telephone your state's program to obtain a copy.

Reviews or audits may be performed by the following entities to enforce fee schedules:

- The state agency or state fund responsible for overseeing workers' compensation (bill review)
- The payer, employer, or insurance carrier (bill review)
- The payer (bill review) and state agency (compliance audit)

Helpful Billing Tips

The following are helpful hints for billing workers' compensation claims.

1. Ask whether the injury occurred within the scope of employment and verify insurance information with the benefits coordinator for the employer. This will promote filing initial claims with the correct insurance carrier.
2. Either ask the employer the name of the claims adjuster or request that the patient obtain the claim number of his or her case when he or she comes in for the initial visit.
3. Ask the workers' compensation carrier who is going to review the claim. Sometimes there are independent third-party billing vendors that work for the insurance carriers. Get the name and contact information.
4. Educate the patient with regard to the medical practice's billing policies for workers' compensation cases by having him or her complete the patient agreement form shown in Figure 15–16.
5. Verify whether prior authorization is necessary before a surgical procedure is performed.

6. Document in a telephone log or patient's record all data for authorization of examination, diagnostic studies, or surgery (e.g., date, name of individual who authorizes, and response).
7. Obtain the workers' compensation fee schedule for the relevant state.
8. Use appropriate five-digit code numbers and modifiers to ensure prompt and accurate payment for services rendered.
9. Complete the Doctor's First Report of Occupational Injury or Illness form for the relevant state and submit it within the time limit shown in Table 15.1. Some states (e.g., California) allow a late fee if payment is not received within 30 to 45 days.
10. Ask whether there is a state-specific insurance form or if the CMS-1500 form is acceptable.
11. Ask what year CPT and ICD-9-CM code books the insurance carrier uses. Some carriers use 2003 or earlier books, which means they do not reflect the deletion or addition of some procedure and diagnostic codes.
12. Submit a monthly itemized statement or bill on the termination of treatment for nondisability claims.
13. Clearly define any charges in excess of the fee schedule. Attach any x-ray reports, operative reports, discharge summaries, pathology reports, and so forth to clarify such excess charges or when **by report (BR)** is shown for a code selected from the workers' compensation procedure code book.
14. Itemize in detail and send invoices for drugs and dressings furnished by the physician. Bill medical supplies on a separate claim or statement and do not bill with services because this may be routed to a different claims processing department.
15. Call the insurance carrier and talk with the **claims examiner** (also known as the claims adjuster) who is familiar with the patient's case, if there is a question about the fee.
16. Search the Internet for a Web site or write to the workers' compensation state plan office in each state for booklets, bulletins, forms, and legislation information. See Appendix A for the workers' compensation address in each state.
17. Find out if the insurance carrier uses "usual and customary" payments tied to the physician's ZIP code. Most carriers use fee schedules.
18. Follow up and track the date the claim was filed. If no payment has been received or payment has been received beyond the 30- to 45-day deadline, determine whether it meets eligibility requirements for interest.

Billing Claims

For efficiency in processing industrial claims, many insurance carriers have developed their own forms for workers' compensation cases, whereas others allow use of the

CMS-1500 claim form. Some carriers have made slight modifications to the CMS-1500 claim form as depicted in Figure 15–13.

Figure 7–15 is an illustration of a completed workers' compensation case on a nonmodified CMS-1500 claim form.

Electronic Claims Submission and Reports

Uniform data processing codes and universal electronic injury report forms have been developed by the American National Standards Institute (ANSI) and the International Association of Industrial Accident Boards and Commissions (IAIABC). ANSI is a national organization founded in 1918 to coordinate the development of voluntary business standards in the United States. Texas is one of the first states to establish an insurance regulation requiring workers' compensation carriers to use universal electronic transmission for first report of injury forms and subsequent reports developed by IAIABC.

Electronic Data Systems, Inc., (EDS) in Dallas, Texas, and Insurance Value-Added Network Services (IVANS) in Greenwich, CT, introduced the nation's first coast-to-coast electronic claims processing and report-filing network, called Workers' Compensation Reporting Service. EDS processes all claims and follow-up reports. IVANS provides the network service and marketing of software to employers. This system is operational in many states.

Some workers' compensation insurance companies are using telephone reporting of claims. Employers report injuries occurring on the job by calling a toll-free number. Calls go to a regional center where service representatives document the first report of injury and electronically transmit it to the local claim office handling workers' compensation insurance. Employers avoid tardiness of reporting when using this system. Employers neglecting prompt report of injuries could delay payments to physicians.

Because workers' compensation is operated under state laws, each state is required to report financial data, statistics on injuries and illnesses, and other information to state insurance regulators. In the states that use telephone reporting service, workers' compensation payers use the system to reduce the paper processing costs that have escalated out of proportion and to improve administrative efficiency.

Out-of-State Claims

When billing for an out-of-state claim, insurance billing specialists must follow all workers' compensation regulations from the jurisdiction (state) in which the injured was hired and not the state where the injury occurred.

Companies that have employees who travel to other states are required to obtain workers' compensation insurance in those states unless they have a policy that covers out-of-state employees. Sometimes a patient may seek care from a physician in an adjacent state because he or she feels the physician provides a higher quality of care or the patient needs a specialized type of surgery, expensive diagnostic tests, or treatment. Referral requirements should be met before the patient is seen (e.g., letter of referral or preauthorization from the managing doctor with a copy to the workers' compensation carrier). Nine states hold the injured employee responsible for unauthorized care (Alabama, Alaska, Arkansas, New Jersey, North Dakota, Ohio, Washington, West Virginia, and Wisconsin). When a patient crosses a state line for treatment, he or she may be liable for some balance billing, and the patient should be informed of this fact. The date the employer subcontracts with another company to have the work performed must be researched. Many times the injured employee states that he or she works for ABC Company. The claim is denied because the employee is actually working for XYZ Company, which has subcontracted with ABC Company. This also happens with hospitals. One may think a hospital employee is being treated when an employee working for a company hired by the hospital actually is being treated. In these cases, extra time is spent identifying the subcontractor, and it may be discovered that the subcontractor does not have workers' compensation insurance and expected the hiring company to provide the coverage. In another scenario, a cruise ship employee injured at sea does not fall under state workers' compensation laws and is not required to have insurance in the state. Many cruise ships have maritime companies that settle these types of claims. Normally the claim should be paid in full, but many of these companies try to negotiate a much lower rate. This rate can be accepted in lieu of futile attempts to collect from the patient.

When the claim is billed, the out-of-state fee schedule should be obtained to determine the proper procedure codes, modifiers, and amounts. It should be determined whether the claimant's jurisdiction accepts electronic submission of the CMS-1500 claim form or another form and whether other documents (e.g., the operative report) are required to be submitted with the bill.

Delinquent or Slow Pay Claims

If payment of a workers' compensation claim is slow or the claim becomes delinquent, the insurance billing

Martin Feelgood, MD
4567 Broad Avenue
Woodland Hills, XY 12345
555-486-9002

June 20, 20XX

XYZ Insurance Company
P. O. Box S
Woodland Hills, XY 12345

Dear Madam or Sir:

Re: Case No.:   120 XX 6542
        Injured: Mrs. Ima B. Hurt
        Date of Injury: April 3, 20XX
        Employer: The Conk Out Company
        Amount: $148.92

Our records indicate that our final statement for the above case
dated __5/18/20XX__ remains unpaid.

Your cooperation in furnishing us the present status of this
statement will be appreciated. A notation on the bottom of
this letter will be sufficient.

Very truly yours,

Martin Feelgood ,MD

ref initials

_____

_____No Employer's Report on file
_____No Doctor's First Report on file
_____Did not receive itemized billing statement
_____Payment was made. Check No.____Date_____
_____Other reason(s) _____

FIGURE 15–17 Letter sent to the insurance carrier when a workers' compensation claim becomes 45 days delinquent.

specialist should use an organized standard follow-up procedure:

1. Telephone the patient's employer. Note the name of the person talked to, name, address, and telephone number of the workers' compensation carrier, and the claim number. Verify the employer's address.
2. Send a copy of the claim form and an itemized copy of the financial account statement to the carrier. Send a letter and include details of the accident if necessary (see Figure 15–17). For problem claims it may be wise to obtain and complete a Certificate of Mailing form from the U.S. Postal Service. The form is initialed and postmarked at the post office and returned to the insurance biller for the office file. Because the post office does not keep a record of the mailing, this certificate costs less than certified mail. It shows proof that a special communication was mailed or sent on a certain date if a deadline is in question.

Martin Feelgood, MD
4567 Broad Avenue
Woodland Hills, XY 12345
555-486-9002

June 20, 20XX

The Conk Out Company
45 South Gorman Street
Woodland Hills, XY 12345

Dear Madam or Sir:

Re: Case No.:   120 XX 6542
        Injured: Mrs. Ima B. Hurt
        Date of Injury: April 3, 20XX

I have been informed by your workers' compensation
insurance carrier that they have not as yet received the
employer's report in regard to the above injured person.

Unless you have already done so, may I ask your cooperation
in completing and sending this report so that the case may be
closed.

Should you have any questions or if I can be of assistance to
you in any way, please do not hesitate to call on me.

Very truly yours,

Martin Feelgood , MD

ref initials

FIGURE 15–18 Letter sent to the employer when the insurance company notifies the physician's office that the employer's preliminary report of injury has not been received.

3. Telephone the insurance carrier after 45 working days and request the expected date of payment.
4. Be reminded of that payment date by using a computer automated reminder or a note on the desk calendar. If payment is not received on or before that day, call the carrier again and ask for payment on a day determined by the facility's expectations.
5. Telephone the patient's employer and explain that there is difficulty with the carrier. Ask the employer to contact the carrier and have the carrier send payment immediately. You might talk to the patient and suggest that he or she discuss the problem with their employer to see if doing so will bring positive action.
6. Send the employer a copy of the financial account statement showing the outstanding balance. If the carrier is not paying, ask the employer for payment. An employer's legal obligation to pay may vary from case to case.
7. Contact the patient only if given information by the carrier or employer that the injury is not work related.
8. Develop office policies that address when an outstanding account should be reviewed (perhaps after 90 or 120 days), whether to continue collection efforts

Martin Feelgood, MD
4567 Broad Avenue
Woodland Hills, XY 12345
555-486-9002

July 15, 20XX

Division of Industrial Accidents
State Office Building
107 South Broadway, Room 4107
Woodland Hills, XY 12345

Dear Madam or Sir:

Re: Failure of employer to follow Section No. 3760

Your office is being solicited to help secure an Employer's
Report of Work Injury from the employer listed below.

Case No.:	120 XX 6542
Name of Employer:	The Conk Out Company
Address:	45 South Gorman Street
	Woodland Hills, XY 12345
Name of Injured:	Mrs. Ima B. Hurt
Address:	300 East Central Avenue
	Woodland Hills, XY 12345
Date of Injury:	April 3, 20XX
Name of Insurance Carrier:	XYZ Insurance Company
Amount of Unpaid Bill:	$148.92

Your cooperation in this matter will be greatly appreciated. If you
need further information, please feel free to contact my office.

Sincerely yours,

Martin Feelgood   , MD

ref initials

FIGURE 15–19   Letter sent to the Workers' Compensation Board or Industrial Accident Commission in your state if the employer does not respond to your letter requesting the Employer's Report of Work Injury after 30 days have elapsed from the date of the letter.

internally, and at which point the account should be turned over to a collection agency.

It may be necessary to send subsequent letters to the employer after receiving a response from the insurance carrier. For example, a letter should be sent to the employer (Figure 15–18) if the insurance company notifies the physician's office that the employer's preliminary report of injury has not been received.

If 30 days have elapsed from the date the letter was sent requesting the Employer's Report of Work Injury and the employer has not responded, a letter should be sent to the state Workers' Compensation Board or Industrial Accidents Commission (Figure 15–19).

Refer to Chapter 9 for additional information and helpful suggestions on following up on delinquent claims.

PROCEDURE

COMPLETING THE DOCTOR'S FIRST REPORT OF OCCUPATIONAL INJURY OR ILLNESS

The submission of this form (Figure 15–20) has a deadline, from immediately to within 5 days after the patient has been seen by the physician, depending on each state's law. An original and three or four copies should be distributed as follows:

Original to the insurance carrier (unless more copies are required)

One copy to the state agency

One copy to the patient's employer

One copy retained for the physician's files in the patient's workers' compensation file folder

Continued

COMPLETING THE DOCTOR'S FIRST REPORT OF OCCUPATIONAL INJURY OR ILLNESS

STATE OF CALIFORNIA   **DOCTOR'S FIRST REPORT OF OCCUPATIONAL INJURY OR ILLNESS**

Within 5 days of your initial examination, for every occupational injury or illness, send two copies of this report to the **employer's workers' compensation insurance carrier** or the **self-insured employer.** Failure to file a timely doctor's report may result in assessment of a civil penalty. **In the case of diagnosed or suspected pesticide poisoning,** send a copy of this report to Division of Labor Statistics and Research, P.O. Box 420603, San Francisco, CA 94142-0603, and notify your local health officer by telephone within 24 hours.

	PLEASE DO NOT USE THIS COLUMN
1. **INSURER NAME AND ADDRESS** XYZ Insurance Company, P.O. Box 5, Woodland Hills, XY 12345	
2. **EMPLOYER NAME** The Conk Out Company Policy# B12345	Case No.
3. Address No. and Street City Zip 45 So. Gorman St. Woodland Hills, XY 12345	Industry
4. Nature of business (e.g., food manufacturing, building construction, retailer of women's clothes) plumbing repair	County
5. **PATIENT NAME** (first name, middle initial, last name) Ima B. Hurt 6. Sex ☐ Male ☒ Female 7. Date of birth Mo. Day Yr. 3-4-1966	Age
8. Address: No. and Street City Zip 300 East Central Ave., Woodland Hills, XY 12345 9. Telephone number (555) 476-9899	Hazard
10. Occupation (Specific job title) clerk typist 11. Social Security Number 120-XX-6542	Disease
12. Injured at: No. and street City County 45 So. Gorman St., Woodland Hills, XY 12345 Humboldt	Hospitalization
13. Date and hour of injury or onset of illness Mo. Day Yr. 4-3-20XX Hour _____ a.m. 2:00 p.m. 14. Date last worked Mo. Day Yr. 4-3-20XX	Occupation
15. Date and hour of first examination or treatment Mo. Day Yr. 4-3-20XX Hour _____ a.m. 4:00 p.m. 16. Have you (or your office) previously treated patient? ☐ Yes ☒ NO	Return date/Code

Patient please complete this portion, if able to do so. Otherwise, doctor please complete immediately. Inability or failure of a patient to complete this portion shall not affect his/her rights to workers' compensation under the California Labor Code.

17. **DESCRIBE HOW THE ACCIDENT OR EXPOSURE HAPPENED** (Give specific object, machinery or chemical. Use reverse side if more space is required.)

I climbed a ladder in the stock room and while I was coming down I missed a step, lost my balance, and fell hurting my left ankle.

18. **SUBJECTIVE COMPLAINTS** (Describe fully. Use reverse side if more space is required.)

Pain in left ankle.

19. **OBJECTIVE FINDINGS** (Use reverse side if more space is required.)

A. Physical examination

Pain, swelling and discoloration of l. ankle.

B. X-ray and laboratory results (state if none or pending.) Ankle x-ray (left) 3 views

20. **DIAGNOSIS** (if occupational illness specify etiologic agent and duration of exposure.) Chemical or toxic compounds involved? ☐ Yes ☒ No

Trimalleolar ankle fracture (left)
ICD-9 Code 824.6

21. Are your findings and diagnosis consistent with patient's account of injury or onset of illness? ☒ Yes ☐ No if "no", please explain.

22. Is there any other current condition that will impede or delay the patient's recovery? ☐ Yes ☒ No if "yes", please explain.

23. **TREATMENT RENDERED** (Use reverse side if more space is required.)

Examination, x-rays, closed treatment of trimalleolar ankle fracture (left) without manipulation. Return in one week for recheck.

24. If further treatment required, specify treatment plan/estimated duration.

25. If hospitalized as inpatient, give hospital name and location   Date admitted   Mo. Day Yr.   Estimated stay

26. WORK STATUS–Is patient able to perform usual work? ☐ Yes ☒ No
If "no", date when patient can return to: Regular work 5 / 17 /20XX
Modified work ___ / ___ / ___   Specify restrictions _____

Doctor's signature *Martin Feelgood, MD* 4-3-20XX   CA license number A 12345
Doctor name and degree (please type) Martin Feelgood, MD   IRS number 95-36640XX
Address 4567 Broad Avenue, Woodland Hills, XY 12345   Telephone number (555) 486-9002

FORM 5021 (REV. 4) 1992

Any person who makes or causes to be made any knowingly false or fraudulent material statement or material representation for the purpose of obtaining or denying workers' compensation benefits or payments is guilty of a felony.

reference initials

FIGURE 15–20 Doctor's First Report of Occupational Injury or Illness form, used in California.

PROCEDURE—CONT'D

In some states, attending physicians may file a single report directly to the insurer or self-insured employer within a specified number of days from initial treatment. The insurer or self-insured employer, in turn, is required to send a report to the state agency. This reduces paperwork and postage. Table 15.1 provides the time limit in each state during which the physician must submit the initial report.

1. Enter the insurance carrier's complete name, street address, city, state, and ZIP code.
2. Enter the employer's full name and policy number if known. Some insurance carriers file by employer and then by policy number. Sometimes the employer's telephone number is necessary on this line.
3. Enter the employer's street address, city, state, and ZIP code.
4. Enter the type of business (e.g., repairing shoes, building construction, and retailing men's clothes).
5. Enter the patient's complete first name, middle initial, and last name.
6. Enter a check mark in the appropriate box to indicate the patient's gender.
7. Enter the patient's birth date and list the year as four digits.
8. Enter the patient's street address, city, state, and ZIP code.
9. Enter the patient's home telephone number.
10. Enter the patient's specific job title. Be accurate in listing the occupation with the job title so that the insurance carrier may be certain the patient was doing the job for which he or she was insured.
11. Enter the patient's Social Security number. Some insurance carriers use the Social Security number as the industrial case number.
12. Enter the exact location where the patient was injured. Many times the injury may occur off the premises of the company or factory, depending on the type of job on which the employee was working. List the county where the patient was injured.
13. Enter the date the patient was injured and time of the injury. List the year as four digits.
14. Enter the date the patient last worked. This date should coincide with the date the patient reported to work and worked any portion of his or her shift (work day). This may be the same date of injury. This item is important because it informs the insurance carrier of the working status of the patient or whether the patient has been disabled and cannot return to work. List the year as four digits.
15. Enter the date and hour of the physician's first examination. The insurance carrier should know how soon after the accident the patient sought medical attention. List the year as four digits.
16. Enter a check mark in the appropriate box indicating whether the physician or an associate treated the patient previously.
17. Have the patient complete this section if possible in his or her own words, stating how the illness or injury occurred. The physician also may dictate this information after obtaining it from the patient.
18. Enter the answers to these questions about the patient's complaints and medical findings, which may be found in the patient's health record. List all of the patient's subjective complaints.
19. *A.* Enter all objective findings from physical examination. *B.* Enter all x-ray and laboratory results; or if none, state "none" or "pending."
20. Enter a check mark in "yes" or "no" to indicate if chemical or toxic compounds are involved. Enter the diagnosis and diagnostic code number. Specify etiologic agent and duration of exposure if occupational illness.
21. Enter a check mark in "yes" or "no" to indicate if the findings and diagnosis are consistent with the history of injury or onset of illness. Insert an explanation if "yes."
22. Enter a check mark in "yes" or "no" to indicate if there is any other current condition that will impede or delay the patient's recovery. Insert an explanation if "yes."
23. Enter a full description of what treatment was rendered.
24. Enter an explanation if further treatment is necessary and, if so, specify the treatment plan. Indicate if physical therapy is necessary and its frequency and duration.
25. Enter the name and location of the hospital, admission date, and estimated stay if the patient is to be hospitalized.
26. Enter a check mark in "yes" or "no" to indicate whether the patient is able to work as usual. If the answer is "no," give the date when it is estimated that the patient will be able to return to regular or modified work. List the year as four digits. Specify any work restrictions. It is very important for the insurance company to anticipate how long the patient will be off work so that money may be set aside for temporary disability benefits, medical benefits, and, if necessary, permanent disability benefits. If the estimated date of return to work should change after the form is submitted, a supplemental report or progress note should be sent to the insurance carrier to change the date of the disability.

Continued

PROCEDURE—CONT'D

COMPLETING THE DOCTOR'S FIRST REPORT OF OCCUPATIONAL INJURY OR ILLNESS

Bottom of Form: If not preprinted, enter the physician's name and degree (e.g., MD, DC), complete address, state license number, federal tax identification number, and telephone number. Indicate the date the report is submitted. The insurance billing specialist should type reference initials in the lower lefthand corner of the form. This form must be signed in ink by the physician. Any carbon copies or photocopies also must be signed in ink. A stamped signature will not be accepted because sometimes these cases go into litigation or are presented for a permanent disability rating. Only those documents considered original health records are acceptable; this means a handwritten signature by the attending physician is necessary.

INTERNET RESOURCES

- Contact the following for information about federal benefits:
  Department of Labor, Employment Standards Administration, Washington, DC 20210
  Web site: **http://www.dol.gov/dol/esa/welcome.html**

- Inquiry can be directed to one of the following departments:
  Division of Coal Mine Workers' Compensation
  Division of Federal Employees' Compensation
  Web site: **http://www.dol.gov/esa/contacts/owcp/fecacont.htm**

- Division Longshoremen's and Harbor Workers' Compensation
  Medicare Carriers Manual Sections 2370, 3330.6, and 330.8 (black lung and asbestos)
  Web site: **http://www.cms.gov**

- Contact the following for information about state benefits (forms, statutes, news bulletins, links to all states):
  Web site: **http://www.workerscompensation.com**
  or
  Web site: **http://www.comp.state.nc.us/ncic/pages/all50.htm**

- For railroad program information:
  Web site: **http://www.bs.org/felainfo.htm**

✔ Study Chapter 15.

✔ Answer the review questions in the *Workbook* to reinforce the theory learned in this chapter and to help prepare you for a future test.

✔ Complete the assignments in the *Workbook* for hands-on experience in completing workers' compensation insurance claim forms and reports, as well as enhanced proficiency in procedural and diagnostic coding.

✔ Turn to the glossary at the end of this textbook for a further understanding of the key terms used in this chapter.

CHAPTER OUTLINE

DISABILITY CLAIMS
HISTORY
DISABILITY INCOME INSURANCE
    Individual
    Group
FEDERAL DISABILITY
    PROGRAMS
    Workers' Compensation
    Disability Benefit Programs

STATE DISABILITY INSURANCE
    Background
    State Programs
    Funding
    Eligibility
    Benefits
    Time Limits
    Medical Examinations
    Restrictions

VOLUNTARY DISABILITY
    INSURANCE
CLAIMS SUBMISSION
    Disability Income Claims
CONCLUSION

KEY TERMS

accidental death and dismemberment

Armed Services Disability

benefit period*

Civil Service Retirement System (CSRS)

consultative examiner (CE)

cost-of-living adjustment

Disability Determination Services (DDS)

disability income insurance

double indemnity

exclusions*

Federal Employees Retirement System (FERS)

future purchase option

guaranteed renewable*

hearing

long-term disability insurance

noncancelable clause*

partial disability*

reconsideration

regional office (RO)

residual benefits*

residual disability

short-term disability insurance

Social Security Administration (SSA)

Social Security Disability Insurance (SSDI) program

State Disability Insurance (SDI)

supplemental benefits

Supplemental Security Income (SSI)

temporary disability*

temporary disability insurance (TDI)

total disability*

unemployment compensation disability (UCD)

Veterans Affairs (VA) disability program

Veterans Affairs (VA) outpatient clinic

voluntary disability insurance

waiting period*

waiver of premium*

*Some of the insurance terms presented in this chapter are shown marked with an asterisk and may seem familiar from previous chapters. However, their meanings may or may not have a slightly different connotation when referring to disability income insurance.

16

Disability Income Insurance and Disability Benefit Programs

OBJECTIVES*

After reading this chapter, you should be able to:

- Define terminology and abbreviations pertinent to disability insurance and disability benefit programs.

- Describe benefits and exclusions contained in individual and group disability income insurance.

- Define the words *temporary disability* and *permanent disability,* as related to each type of disability program.

- Name federal disability benefit programs.

- Differentiate between SSDI and SSI.

- State eligibility requirements, benefits, and limitations of SSDI and SSI.

- Explain disability benefit programs for disabled active military personnel, veterans, and their dependents.

- Name states that have state disability insurance plans.

- State eligibility requirements, benefits, and limitations of state disability plans.

- Explain voluntary disability insurance plans.

- Recognize forms used for processing state disability plans.

- Describe topics and contents of a medical history report.

- List guidelines for federal, state, individual, and group disability claim procedures.

*Performance objectives and exercises for hands-on practical experience for this chapter appear in the *Workbook.*

DISABILITY CLAIMS

Not everyone has disability insurance, but when working with patients who do have it, one may encounter some interesting and unique accidents, injuries, or illnesses. After reading these extracts or direct quotations from disability insurance claim applications, one may ask, "How in the world could something like this happen?" The following gems show just how funny some situations can appear.

Describe How Your Disability Occurred

"A hernia from pulling cork out of bottle."

"Put tire patch on Playtex girdle and it caused infection on right thigh."

"While waving goodnight to friends, fell out a two-story window."

"Back injury received from jumping off a ladder to escape being hit by a train."

One victim graphically described an experience most of us have had: "Getting on a bus, the driver started before I was all on." Can you hear them asking at the hospital, "Was this your assigned seat?"

Another victim stated, "I dislocated my shoulder swatting a fly." When asked, "Have you ever dislocated a shoulder at this sport?" He stated, "I have—I knocked over two table lamps, several high-balls, and skinned an elbow."

Because this is near the end of the course on insurance billing and a great deal of information has been covered, one may feel a bit overwhelmed by the many rules and regulations and their ever-changing nature. This introduction was intended to add a bit of levity before one delves into the world of disability insurance.

This chapter introduces various types of disability income insurance plans as well as a number of disability benefit programs. The first topic, **disability income insurance,** is a form of health insurance providing periodic payments under certain conditions when the insured is unable to work because of illness, disease, or injury—not as a result of a work-related accident or condition.

The second section describes major programs administered by the U.S. government related to industrial accidents and other disability benefit programs unrelated to work injuries.

The third part of the chapter deals with nonindustrial state disability programs administered in five states and Puerto Rico, as well as voluntary disability insurance plans.

Guidelines for federal, state, individual, and group disability claim procedures are presented at the end of the chapter.

HISTORY

Before the late 1800s, disability income insurance provided only accident protection. Some life insurance contracts had disability income riders attached to them that offered limited benefits. In the early 1880s, insurance companies began selling disability income policies that offered coverage for accident and illness. The Paul Revere Life Insurance Company introduced the first "noncancelable" disability income policy in the early 1900s. The noncancelable clause guaranteed that the contract would be in force for a certain period of time and the premium would not be increased. By 1956, Congress had enacted legislation under the Social Security program that provided disability income protection to disabled individuals older than 50 years of age. This program was expanded in 1965 to cover workers without regard to age as long as certain eligibility standards were met.

Today disability income insurance is available from private insurance companies (individual policies) and employer-sponsored plans (group policies). Government-funded and state benefit programs are also available for disabled persons. All of these plans and programs are discussed in this chapter, along with the role of the insurance billing specialist in dealing with this type of insurance.

DISABILITY INCOME INSURANCE

Individual

Individual disability income insurance is coverage that provides a specific monthly or weekly income when a person becomes unable to work, temporarily or totally, because of an illness or injury. Disability income policies do not provide medical expense benefits. The disability cannot be work related. As explained in the previous chapter, the illness or accident must be work related to be covered by workers' compensation insurance.

For individuals who are self-employed, this insurance is particularly important because a business could not meet its financial obligations if the owner became injured or too ill to work. For example, if an individual is self-employed with a home-based business, repetitive stress injuries (RSIs) would not allow that individual to use the computer for several months. The main purpose of these policies is to provide some benefits while the person is not able to work. To collect benefits, the individual must meet the policy's criteria of what constitutes partial, temporary, or total disability. These policies terminate when the individual retires or reaches a certain age, usually 65 years.

Waiting Period

The time period from the beginning of disability to receiving the first payment of benefits is called an elimination period or **waiting period.** During this initial period, a disabled individual is not eligible to receive benefits even though he or she is unable to work.

Benefit Period

A **benefit period** is the maximum amount of time that benefits will be paid to the injured or ill person for the disability (e.g., 2 years, 5 years, to age 65, or lifetime).

Benefits

Compensation paid to the insured disabled person is called *indemnity benefits* and can be received daily, weekly, monthly, or semiannually, depending on the policy. Premiums and benefits depend on several risk factors, such as age, gender, health history and physical state, income, and occupational duties. Some policies include residual or partial disability income benefits. Benefits are not taxable if premiums are paid by the individual.

Residual benefits pay a partial benefit when the insured is not totally disabled. If one becomes partially disabled or can work only part time or in a limited capacity, the residual benefits make up the difference between what an individual can earn at present and what he or she would have earned working full time.

Supplemental benefits may consist of insurance provisions that will increase monthly indemnity, such as a **future purchase option** or a **cost-of-living adjustment.** Provisions also distribute a percentage of the policy premiums if an individual keeps a policy in force for 5 or 10 years or does not file any claims.

An **accidental death and dismemberment** benefit is written into some contracts. This offers the insured person protection when loss of sight or loss of limb occurs. In some policies (e.g., life insurance), a special provision known as **double indemnity** applies if an unintended, unexpected, and unforeseeable accident occurs resulting in death. This feature provides for twice the face amount of the policy to be paid if death results from accidental causes.

Types of Disability

A disability may be partial, temporary, or total. There is no standard definition for **total disability,** and the definition stated in each disability income policy varies. For example, a liberal definition might read as follows: "The insured must be unable to perform the major duties of his or her specific occupation." Social Security has a restrictive definition presented later in this chapter.

The terms **residual disability** and **partial disability** are defined as occurring "when an illness or injury prevents an insured person from performing one or more of the functions of his or her regular job"—in other words, when a person cannot perform all of his or her job duties.

Temporary disability exists when a person cannot perform all the functions of his or her regular job for a limited period of time.

Clauses

With a **guaranteed renewable** policy, the insurer is required to renew the policy as long as premium payments are made for a specified number of years or to a specified age, such as 60, 65, or 70 years, or for life. However, the premium may be increased when it is renewed. When the policy has a **noncancelable clause,** the premium cannot be increased.

If a **waiver of premium** is included in the insurance contract, the policy pays all premiums while the employee is disabled; the employee does not have to pay. Usually this provision is used as a total and permanent disability benefit and may be available in certain other cases.

Exclusions

Exclusions are provisions written into the insurance contract denying coverage or limiting the scope of coverage. Examples are preexisting conditions; disability because of war, riot, self-inflicted injury, or attempted suicide; mental or nervous conditions; disability while legally intoxicated or under the influence of narcotics (unless prescribed by a licensed physician); conditions arising from normal pregnancy; conditions arising during the act of committing a felony; or if benefits are being received under workers' compensation or a government program. The phrase "legally intoxicated" means intoxication in an individual whose blood alcohol level, when tested, exceeds limits set by state law.

Acquired Immunodeficiency Syndrome and Human Immunodeficiency Virus Infection

States have statutes governing questions that can and cannot be asked on insurance application forms about acquired immunodeficiency syndrome (AIDS) and human immunodeficiency virus (HIV) testing; therefore each state has developed its own forms. If a private insurance company wishes to test an applicant, a consent or notice form including acceptance of pretest and posttest counseling must be signed.

Group

Some employers elect to offer group disability income insurance as a fringe benefit. These contracts are drawn up between the insurer and employer. Premiums may be paid by the employer with or without contributions from the employee. Employees hold certificates of insurance and are covered under the employer's policy; therefore they are not called policyholders. When the employee leaves the company, the insurance terminates unless the employee is disabled. A few group policies allow conversion to a limited benefit individual policy.

Benefits

Benefits vary from one plan to another but are usually for **short-term disability insurance** (13 weeks to 24 months) or **long-term disability insurance** (to age 65). To qualify for benefits, an individual must be unable to perform the major duties of his or her occupation during the initial period of disability (e.g., the first 2 years). Benefits cease when the employee returns to work, even part time. However, some of these policies offer the worker partial disability income benefits to motivate a disabled individual to return to work on a part-time basis. Monthly benefits usually are paid directly to the employee and are taxable if the employee is not making any contribution toward the premiums.

Exclusions

Disabilities commonly excluded from coverage include those seen in individual disability income insurance policies, as previously described.

FEDERAL DISABILITY PROGRAMS

Workers' Compensation

The federal government has a number of programs that cover workers from loss of income because of work-related disability. These programs are mentioned in Chapter 15 because work-related disabilities fall under workers'

compensation laws. When an individual is eligible under more than one program, coordination of benefits is used so that a worker cannot receive benefits that result in an amount greater than what the person receives when working. Coordination of benefits is a provision preventing double payment for expenses by making one of the programs the primary payer and ensuring that no more than 100% of the costs are covered.

Disability Benefit Programs

The government's major disability programs are:

- **Social Security Disability Insurance (SSDI) program**
- **Supplemental Security Income (SSI)**
- **Civil Service Retirement System (CSRS)**
- **Federal Employees Retirement System (FERS)**
- **Armed Services Disability**
- **Veterans Affairs (VA) disability program**

The **Social Security Administration (SSA)** manages two programs that pay monthly disability benefits to people younger than age 65 who cannot work for at least a year because of a severe disability: SSDI and SSI. Medical requirements are the same for both programs.

Social Security Disability Insurance Program

Background

In 1935, the Social Security Act, the Old-Age, Survivors, Disability, and Health Insurance (OASDHI) Program, was enacted. It provided benefits for death, retirement, disability, and medical care. In 1956, Congress established a program for long-term disability known as Social Security Disability Insurance (SSDI) under Title II of the Social Security Act. This is an entitlement (not welfare) program that provides monthly benefits to workers and those self-employed who meet certain conditions.

Disability Definition

Disability under Social Security has a strict definition: "Inability to engage in any substantial gainful activity by reason of any medically determinable physical or mental impairment which can be expected to result in death or which has lasted or can be expected to last for a continuous period of not less than 12 months."

Eligibility

The following is a list of individuals who meet eligibility requirements for SSDI:

- Disabled workers younger than age 65 years and their families

- Individuals who become disabled before age 22 years, if a parent (or in certain cases, a grandparent) who is covered under Social Security retires, becomes disabled, or dies
- Disabled widows or widowers, age 50 years or older, if the deceased spouse worked at least 10 years under Social Security
- Disabled surviving divorced spouses older than age 50 years, if the ex-spouse was married to the disabled person for at least 10 years
- Blind workers whose vision in the better eye cannot be corrected to better than 20/200 or whose visual field in the better eye, even with corrective lenses, is 20 degrees or less

Workers must be fully insured in accordance with standards set by the Social Security Administration in terms of age, number of quarters worked, and amount of wages earned per quarter. The processing of eligibility application forms may take up to 2 months.

Benefits

Monthly benefits are paid to qualified individuals. After 24 months of disability payments, the disabled individual also becomes eligible for Medicare. The benefits convert to retirement benefits when an individual reaches age 65.

Supplemental Security Income

Eligibility

The SSI program is under Title XVI of the Social Security Act and provides disability payments to people (adults and children) with limited income and few resources. No prior employment is needed. Many SSI recipients also qualify for Medicaid, a state assistance program. The following individuals may qualify for SSI disability payments:

- Disabled persons younger than 65 years who have very limited income and resources
- Disabled children younger than age 18 years, if the disability compares in severity with one that would keep an adult from working and has lasted or is expected to last at least 12 months or result in death
- Blind adults or children who have a visual acuity no better than 20/100 or have a visual field of 20 degrees or less in the better eye, with the use of corrective lenses

Disability Determination Process

To establish disability under SSDI or SSI, an individual calls or visits any Social Security office and completes application forms with the help of a social worker.

This triggers a determination process. A physician may be involved in the determination process in one of three ways: (1) as a treating source who provides medical evidence on behalf of his or her patient; (2) as a **consultative examiner (CE)** who is paid a fee and examines or tests the applicant; or (3) as a full- or part-time medical or psychologic consultant reviewing claims for a state or **regional office (RO)**.

In addition to a medical report from one of these sources, other criteria taken into consideration are the individual's age and vocational and educational factors that may contribute to the person's ability to work. It is possible that a person may be eligible for disability payments under one government program and not eligible under Social Security because the rules differ. The SSA may use reports that an applicant has from another agency to determine whether the person is eligible for Social Security disability payments. Many SSA state agencies have a division known as **Disability Determination Services (DDS).** Determination of disability is made by a DDS team composed of a physician or psychologist and disability examiner (DE), not by the applicant's physician.

Appeals Evaluation Process

If a claimant does not agree with the determination of disability, a four-level appeals process is available.

1. A **reconsideration,** which is a complete review of the claim by a medical or psychologic consultant or disability examiner team that did not take part in the original disability determination.
2. A **hearing** before an administrative law judge who had no part in the initial or reconsideration determinations of the claim. The hearing is held within 75 miles of the claimant's home. The claimant and his or her representative are permitted to present their case in person and present a written statement. They also are permitted to review information the judge will use to make a decision and question any witnesses.
3. A review by the Appeals Council, which considers all requests for review but may deny a request if it believes the decision by the administrative law judge was correct. If the Appeals Council decides the case should be reviewed, it will make a decision on the case or return it to an administrative law judge for further review.
4. A review by the federal court for which the claimant may file an action where he or she resides.

Disability cases are reviewed from time to time to be sure the individuals are still disabled. The frequency depends on the nature and severity of the impairment, the likelihood of improvement, rehabilitation, ability to work, and so on.

Benefits

Social Security disability programs are designed to give long-term protection and benefits to individuals totally disabled who are unable to do any type of work in the national economy. In contrast, short-term disability may be provided through workers' compensation, insurance, savings, and investments.

Work Incentives

Special rules allow disabled or blind people presently receiving Social Security or SSI to work and still receive monthly benefits as well as Medicare or Medicaid (e.g., an SSDI recipient who is given a 90-day trial of work and at the end of that time either continues to work and lose SSDI coverage or leaves the temporary employment and remains on SSDI). A limit exists as to how much the person can earn in a calendar year. These are referred to as "work incentives"; the rules are different for Social Security beneficiaries and SSI recipients. Occasionally a patient may be working as well as receiving SSDI benefits, as illustrated by the example above.

Civil Service and Federal Employees Retirement System Disability

Eligibility

Federal employees who work in civil service fall under the CSRS. This system has provisions for those who become totally disabled. This program is a combination of federal disability and Social Security disability. Both portions of the program must be applied for by the worker. The disability cannot be work related, and 5 years of service are necessary before benefits are payable. Eighteen months of service are necessary under the FERS.

Benefits

Those who qualify are entitled to benefits that are payable for life.

For example, an individual who works for the Internal Revenue Service performing clerical and filing job duties is involved in an automobile accident on the weekend. The head injuries are so severe that the person is unable to return to gainful employment at any job. He or she could apply for benefits either under the CSRS or FERS, depending on his or her eligibility status.

Armed Services Disability

Eligibility

Individuals covered under this program must be members of the armed services on active duty.

Benefits

Monthly benefits are payable for life if a disability occurs or is aggravated while the individual is serving in the military service. Benefit amounts are based on years of service, base pay, and severity of disability. This also is subject to review.

Veterans Affairs Disability

Eligibility

The VA is authorized by law to provide a wide range of benefits to both those who have served their country in the armed forces and their dependents. If a veteran who is honorably discharged files a claim for a service-connected disability within 1 year of sustaining that injury, he or she is eligible for outpatient treatment. Veterans with non–service-connected disabilities who are in receipt of housebound or aid-in-attendance benefits are eligible for treatment from a private physician if they are unable to travel to a VA facility because of geographic inaccessibility. Their identification card, benefits, and claims procedures are identical to those of veterans with service-connected disabilities who receive outpatient medical care.

Benefits

The following is a general list of veterans' medical benefits. Each benefit requires that certain criteria be met. These criteria are ever-changing and are not mentioned here. A complete up-to-date booklet listing all the benefits is available.*

- Hospital care in a VA hospital
- Nursing home care in a VA facility
- Domiciliary care
- Outpatient medical treatment at a VA facility or by a private physician
- Emergency treatment in a hospital for a service-connected condition
- Prescription drugs and medication issued by a VA pharmacy or other participating pharmacy. Only bona fide emergency prescriptions can be filled by a private pharmacy.
- Certain medical equipment, such as oxygen and prosthetics
- Travel expenses when receiving VA medical care
- Outpatient dental treatment (if the veteran files a claim within 90 days from the date that he or she was discharged from the service)

---

*Federal Benefits for Veterans and Dependents. Department of Veterans Affairs, Washington, DC 20420. The booklet is published annually and is available for a small fee from the Superintendent of Documents, U.S. Government Printing Office, Mail Stop: SSOP, Washington, DC 20402-9328.

- Treatment for "agent orange" or nuclear radiation exposure
- Alcohol and drug dependence outpatient care
- Readjustment counseling services

The physician must accept what the VA pays as payment in full for treatment of a service-connected disability and cannot bill the patient for any additional charges, even if there is a balance after the VA pays the claim. If the treatment is likely to cost more than $40 per month, the physician must obtain prior authorization from the nearest VA facility. A separate financial accounting record card must be prepared for VA benefits if the physician is also treating the patient for ailments other than a service-connected disability. Any professional service that is not related to a service-connected disability must be paid for by the veteran out of his or her own pocket. For example, a Vietnam veteran who has a long history of stump pain at the site of an amputation or suffers from old shrapnel wounds as the result of stepping on a land mine during active duty is seen and treated for acute gastroenteritis. The VA disability benefits do not apply to the episode of acute gastroenteritis and the veteran must personally pay for professional services related to that diagnosis.

Veterans with non–service-connected disabilities may have copayments when they seek treatment. For example, individuals on Medicare may be responsible for the deductible for the first 90 days of care during any 365-day period. For each additional 90 days of hospital care, the patient is charged half of the Medicare deductible, $10 a day of hospital care, and $5 a day for VA nursing home care. For outpatient care, the copayment is 20% of the cost of an average outpatient visit.

Outpatient Treatment

Veterans eligible for outpatient treatment may obtain outpatient medical care only for the disability as listed on the VA outpatient clinic card (Figure 16–1). Usually a veteran seeks care at the nearest **VA outpatient clinic.** However, when a VA facility is not within reasonable distance, when the veteran is too ill to travel to the nearest location, or when the condition needs prompt attention, the veteran can apply for and be granted medical care by a private physician through the Home Town Care Program. The VA outpatient clinic must be notified within 15 days of the treatment rendered. In such cases, the treating physician must submit evidence of medical necessity (e.g., detailed justification on the invoice) to the VA outpatient clinic. Form 10-583, Claim for Payment of Cost of Unauthorized Medical Services (Figure 16–2), generally used for hospital emergency care, also can be used for professional care if the doctor is billing after the 15-day period has elapsed. Some patients have both

Medicare and medical coverage from the VA. In such cases, Medicare is not secondary to the VA and the VA is not secondary to Medicare. The claim is to be sent where specified by the patient. The claim can be sent to Medicare, where, if the claim is processed, the patient must satisfy his or her contractual requirement to pay any deductible and copayment amounts. If the patient asks that the claim be sent to the VA instead of Medicare, the claim is processed and any payments issued are considered as payment in full. Many veterans prefer to have the claim sent to the VA.

Veterans Affairs Installations

For information on veterans' benefits or assistance in locating VA installations, go to the Veterans Affairs home Web site listed in Internet Resources at the end of this chapter.

STATE DISABILITY INSURANCE

Background

In 1944, Rhode Island began a **State Disability Insurance (SDI)** program that proved successful. This form of insurance is part of an employment security program that provides temporary cash benefits for workers suffering a wage loss because of off-the-job illness or injury. It can be referred to as **unemployment compensation disability (UCD)** or **temporary disability insurance (TDI).** California became the second state to add nonindustrial disability coverage to the Social Security protection afforded to its citizens by appending Article 10 to the Unemployment Insurance Act. This became law on May 21, 1946; when the legislation took effect on December 1, 1946, this article diverted the 1% tax formerly paid by workers for unemployment insurance to a disability insurance fund. New York and New Jersey soon followed with similar programs. Two decades later, in 1969, Puerto Rico and Hawaii passed nonindustrial disability insurance laws.

Some accidents that occur are quite serious at the time but can appear rather humorous upon review.

Unique Accident
The patient was under the kitchen sink repairing a leak when the family cat came along, watched for awhile, then playfully—but painfully—reached up and clawed him. Startled, the man threw his head back, cracked it on the bottom of the sink, and was knocked out cold. He came to as he was being carried out on a stretcher and explained to the attendants what had happened. One stretcher bearer laughed so hard, he relaxed his hold and the patient fell to the ground and broke his arm.

BILLING AND REPORTS. Bill the Station of Jurisdiction monthly. Please itemize your usual statement to include (1) patient's name; (2) identification number; (3) condition treated; (4) treatment and dates rendered; and (5) your usual and customary fee. Bills for auxiliary medical services must reflect the name of the prescribing doctor of medicine or osteopathy. Submit a brief treatment report only when the cost of urgent treatment causes the $30.00 limitation to be exceeded, or when a significant clinical change in a disability occurs.

PAYMENT. Payment by the VA for services rendered is payment in full.

IMPORTANT: Direct inquiries and any change of address to the Station of Jurisdiction.

Station of Jurisdiction:

VETERANS ADMINISTRATION
OUTPATIENT C 9044/136A6
428 SOUTH HILL ST.
LOS ANGELES CA 90013

VA OUTPATIENT MEDICAL TREATMENT INFORMATION CARD

E. Z. Slipdisk　　　　　　012-XX-5678
Beneficiary's name　　　　Identification No.

DISABILITY FOR WHICH TREATMENT IS AUTHORIZED–VALID UNTIL CANCELLED BY VA

X P. O. HERNIATED NUC. PULPOSUS

VA FORM 10-1174, FEB 1971

Front

PLEASE READ CAREFULLY

TO VETERAN — You are authorized to obtain treatment within a reasonable distance from your permanent or temporary residence for the disability shown. When treatment is required, select a doctor of medicine or osteopathy who is licensed in the State in which treatment will be rendered. This card constitutes an agreement to provide care to you as a VA beneficiary within the limitations stated. Please alert the doctor to the instructions printed on the card and be sure he has your NAME, IDENTIFICATION NO. and the ADDRESS OF THE STATION OF JURISDICTION. If a specific therapy is authorized in lieu of listing disabilities, this card authorizes ONLY that therapy. IT MAY NOT BE USED TO OBTAIN OTHER MEDICAL SERVICES, SURGICAL PROCEDURES, NON-VA HOSPITALIZATION, OR PROSTHETIC APPLIANCES. Prescriptions of a recurring nature and others not needed at once should be brought or mailed to the VA station of jurisdiction. They will be filled promptly. When it is necessary to obtain medication immediately, PLEASE REQUEST THE PRIVATE PHARMACIST TO BILL THE STATION OF JURISDICTION SHOWN ON THIS CARD.

The VA may reimburse local, round trip, travel expenses between your permanent or temporary residence and the place treatment is obtained. A mileage allowance will be paid in lieu of actual and necessary expenses of travel (including lodging and subsistence).

Your one-time, written request for travel expenses, when received within 30 days from the date you first obtain medical services, will be approved to be effective with the first visit. A claim received after that 30-day-period will be effective from the date received. Generally, travel expenses are paid for a 3-month period.

TO PHYSICIAN — The beneficiary named on this card is authorized OUTPATIENT TREATMENT for the disabilities shown by a doctor of medicine or osteopathy licensed in the state in which medical services are rendered. When treatment of these conditions requires eyeglasses, hearing aids, other prostheses, home nursing services, and/or dental services, notify the station of Jurisdiction. Items or services of this nature will be provided by the Veterans Administration. Please request additional medical or other information from the station of jurisdiction, if required.

MEDICAL SERVICES includes prescription and referral for auxiliary medical services when required. All routine treatment may not exceed a total cost of $30.00 per month without prior VA approval.

PHARMACY SERVICES: Please have Rxs filled by VA unless needed at once. Veteran may obtain stat Rx from private pharmacy if you certify Rx, "The VA has authorized me to treat the disability for which this prescription is written."

Back

FIGURE 16–1　Veterans Affairs outpatient clinic card.

State Programs

Nonindustrial disability insurance programs existed in only five states and Puerto Rico as of 2000. The law is known by a different name in each area.

Web sites for most of these programs can be found in Internet Resources at the end of this chapter.

Funding

To fund state disability insurance, a small percentage of the wage is deducted from employees' paychecks each month, or the employer may elect to pay all or part of the cost of the plan as a fringe benefit for employees. The money is then sent in quarterly installments to the state and put into a special fund.

Eligibility

To receive state disability insurance benefits, an employee must be:

● Employed full or part time or actively looking for work when disability begins
● Suffering a loss of wages because of disability
● Eligible for benefits depending on the amount withheld during a previous period before disability began
● Under the care and treatment of a physician who certifies that the employee is disabled
● Disabled at least 7 or 8 calendar days or hospitalized as an inpatient
● Filing a claim within the time limit

If the worker was employed at the time of disability, benefits are not subject to federal income tax.

Form Approved
Budget Bureau No. 76-H0325

VETERANS ADMINISTRATION
CLAIM FOR PAYMENT OF COST OF
UNAUTHORIZED MEDICAL SERVICES

Each person, firm or institution claiming payments or reimbursements must complete this form. No carbon paper is necessary. Please use typewriter or ball point pen, and submit both copies.

1A. VETERAN'S LAST NAME – FIRST – MIDDLE INITIAL	1B. CLAIM NO.	1C. SOCIAL SECURITY NO.
Thornberg, Joey T.	c–	421-XX-4182

1D. PRESENT ADDRESS (*include zip code*)

4628 Image Street, Woodland Hills, XY 12345-1290

2. NAME AND ADDRESS OF PERSON, FIRM OR INSTITUTION MAKING CLAIM (*Leave blank if same as above*)

Gerald Practon, MD 4567 Broad Ave., Woodland Hills, XY 12345-0001

3. STATEMENT OF CIRCUMSTANCES UNDER WHICH THE SERVICES WERE RENDERED (Include diagnosis, symptoms, whether emergency existed, and reason VA facilities were not used)

Patient fell on sidewalk in front of home and suffered traumatic injury of right arm.
Symptoms: Localized pain, swelling, and bruising of right arm near elbow.
AP and lateral x-rays of right elbow show anterior dislocation right radius. Negative for fracture.
Medical care rendered in Emergency Dept. at College Hospital (99282).
Patient unable to go to VA facility as this is 60 miles away.
Treatment of closed elbow dislocation without anesthesia (23400).
Diagnosis: Anterior closed dislocation right radius (Dx code No. 832.01).

4. AMOUNT CLAIMED	*Attach bills or receipts showing services furnished, dates, and charges*
$ 237.02	attached

5. COMPLETE A OR B, AS APPROPRIATE

A. Amount claimed does not exceed that charged the general public for similar services, and payment has not been received.	B. I certify that the amount claimed has been paid and reimbursement has not been made.
Gerald Practon, MD 5/11/XX	*Joey T. Thornberg* 5/11/XX
SIGNATURE AND TITLE OF PROVIDER OF SERVICE, AND DATE	SIGNATURE OF VETERAN OR REPRESENTATIVE, AND DATE

FOR VETERANS ADMINISTRATION USE ONLY

6. ACTION ☐ APPROVED $ _____ ☐ DISAPPROVED	Treatment was provided in an emergency for a service-connected or adjunct disability, any disability of a veteran who has a total disability permanent in nature from a service-connected disability, or for any illness, injury, dental condition in the case of a veteran eligible under Chapter 31 (Vocational Rehabilitation) Title 38, U. S. Code. VA facilities were not feasibly available and delay would have been hazardous.

7. SIGNATURE, CHIEF, MEDICAL ADMINISTRATION SERVICE	8. DATE	9. ADMINISTRATION VOUCHER NO.

VA FORM MAY 1974   10-583   SUPERSEDES VA FORM 10-583 FEB 1966 AND WHICH WILL NOT BE USED.

FIGURE 16–2   Veterans Affairs Form 10-583, Claim for Payment of Cost of Unauthorized Medical Services.

Table 16.1 | **State Disability Information Summary**

State	Name of State Law	Maximum Benefit Period (wk)	Time Limit for Filing Claims	2004 Deductions from Salary (%)	Benefits
California	California Unemployment Insurance Code	52	49 days from disability	0.7	Based on earnings in a 12-month base period, which begins approximately 18 months before disability
Hawaii	Temporary Disability Insurance Law	26	90 days from disability	0.5	Based on 58% of average weekly wage
New Jersey	Temporary Disability Benefits Law	26	30 days from disability	0.5	Based on average weekly wage
New York	Disability Benefits Law	26	30 days from disability	0.5 (max. 60 cents/ week)	Based on 50% of average weekly wage (max. $170/week)
Puerto Rico	Disability Benefits Act	26	3 months from disability	0.3 employee; 0.3 employer	Based on wages earned during base year
Rhode Island	Temporary Disability Insurance Act	30	1 year from disability	1.7	Based on 4.62% of wages in the base period quarter in which wages were the highest

An employee who retires is no longer eligible for the insurance. A worker may file a claim with the state seeking exemption from program participation on religious grounds.

Types of workers not covered are employees of school districts, community college districts, and churches; state workers; federal employees; interstate railroad workers; nonprofit organization employees; and domestic workers.

Benefits

Weekly benefits are determined by the wages earned in a base period or based on a percentage of average weekly wages (Table 16.1). Benefits begin after the seventh consecutive day of disability. There is no provision under the law for hospital or other medical benefits except in Hawaii and Puerto Rico, where hospital benefits are payable under a prepaid health care program if the employee meets certain eligibility requirements.

Limited Benefits

In some states, a patient may qualify for benefits if he or she is a resident of an approved alcoholic recovery facility or an approved drug-free residential facility.

Reduced Benefits

An individual may be entitled to partial benefits if he or she is receiving certain types of income:

● Sick leave
● Vacation
● Wages paid by employer
● Insurance settlement for the disability
● Workers' compensation benefits
● Unemployment benefits

Time Limits

A claim for state disability insurance should be filed within the time limit of the state laws (see Table 16.1). There is usually a grace period of 7 or 8 days after the deadline. After the claim is approved, basic benefits become payable on the eighth day of disability or the first day of hospital confinement, whichever comes first. A person may continue to draw disability insurance for a maximum of 26 weeks in Hawaii, New Jersey, New York, Puerto Rico, and Rhode Island and 52 weeks in California on the same illness or injury or overlapping disabilities. An employee is also entitled to disability benefits 15 days after recovery from a previous disability or illness. For example, if a patient is discharged by the physician to return to work and is on the job 15 calendar days and then becomes ill with the same ailment, he or she may file a new claim.

Medical Examinations

The claimant may be required to submit to an examination or examinations by an independent medical examiner to determine any mental or physical disability. Fees for such examinations are paid by the state department that handles disability insurance. Code 99450 for billing these medical examinations may be found in the Special Evaluation and Management Services section of Current Procedural Terminology.

Restrictions

There are many restrictions on disability insurance. A few of the major situations in which a claim could be denied are listed here.

1. Conditions covered by workers' compensation unless the rate is less than the disability insurance rate. In that case, the state pays the difference between the two rates.
2. Applicants receiving unemployment insurance benefits more than a certain specified amount. *Exception:* If the applicant is on unemployment insurance and then becomes ill or injured, he or she is put on temporary disability insurance until able to go on a job interview.
3. Disabilities beginning during a trade dispute. If an employee is on strike and is injured while walking a picket line, he or she is not eligible for benefits. However, if the union is on strike and an individual member remains at home and then becomes ill or injured, he or she can claim disability and will receive benefits.
4. Confinement by court order or certification in a public or private institution as an alcoholic, drug addict, or sexual psychopath.
5. When legal custody is the cause of unemployment.
6. When the employing company has a voluntary disability plan and is not paying into a state fund.
7. Religious exemption certificate on file by employee or company with no payment being made into a state fund.
8. Pregnancy-related disability, unless the pregnancy is complicated (e.g., cases in which the patient has diabetes, varicose veins, ectopic pregnancy, or cesarean section). *Exceptions:* California, Hawaii, New Jersey, and Rhode Island have maternity benefits that may be applied for at the time the physician tells the patient to stop working.

VOLUNTARY DISABILITY INSURANCE

Persons residing and working in states that do not have state disability insurance programs may elect to contact a local private insurance carrier to arrange for coverage under a **voluntary disability insurance** plan. If these persons become ill or disabled, they receive a fixed weekly or monthly income, usually for approximately 6 months. If the disability or illness is permanent and the individual is unable to return to work, there is sometimes a small monthly income for the duration of the person's life. Some of the state laws provide that a "voluntary plan" may be adopted instead of the "state plan" if a majority of company employees consent to private coverage.

CLAIMS SUBMISSION

Disability Income Claims

When the insurance billing specialist is handling disability income claim forms, he or she should note that the insured (claimant) is responsible to notify the insurance company of the disability. A proof of loss form is completed to establish disability.

The necessary facts are as follows:

- Date the disability occurred
- Date the disabled is expected to be well enough to return to work
- Description of how the disability occurred
- Name of treating physician
- Explanation of how the disability prevents the insured from work

The report must show that the patient's disability meets the policy's definition of disability, or benefits will be denied. Because the definition of disability varies among policies, the critical issues are the content and wording on the claim form.

A portion of this form is usually completed by the attending physician. The following data are necessary:

- Medical history
- Dates patient became disabled
- Subjective symptoms (patient's own words about his or her chief complaints)
- Objective findings on physical examination (e.g., rashes, lacerations, abrasions, or contusions)
- Severity of the illness or injury (range-of-motion tests)
- Photocopies of laboratory tests, x-ray studies, or hospital discharge report

- Medication
- Treatment dates
- Diagnosis
- Prognosis (outcome of the disease or injury)
- Names of any other treating physician
- Date patient expected to return to work
- Description of job duties and patient's ability to perform work

Providing the information listed above helps verify the disability. In some cases, the physician may wish to dictate a medical report and attach it to the claim form instead of completing a portion of the form. The insurance billing specialist must be prepared to extract data from source documents, such as medical and financial records, to complete the claim form. In such situations the physician should be asked to read the information carefully before signing the document. The patient should always be asked to sign an authorization form to release medical information. Reasons for denial of benefits often include improper choice of words or inadequate medical information.

The insurance company may request information from other places to justify payment of benefits, such as employer's records, employee's wage statements or tax forms, or the patient's health records from the attending physician. A company representative may interview the insured if conflicting information exists.

If disability continues, additional claim forms should be completed monthly, or more frequently, by the insured and attending physician. Other sources of information may be requested; for example, records from medical specialists or Social Security records.

If the validity of the case is in question, an independent medical examiner may be asked by the insurance company to examine the disabled individual. If the claimant neglects to return claim forms, refuses telephone calls, misses appointments, or engages in questionable activities, the insurance company will discreetly engage in surveillance of the insured through the services of a professional investigation firm.

Federal Disability Claims

The SSA division called DDS has a teledictation service so the physician or psychologist can dictate the medical report over the telephone instead of completing a medical report form. The service is available at any time, including nights and weekends. A typed transcript is sent to the physician to review, sign, and return to the SSA

state agency, or a report may be typed on the physician's stationery. The physician may photocopy relevant portions of the patient's chart and submit that information, but it should be legible. An authorization to release information, signed by the patient, should be on file. Copies of consultation reports and hospital summaries also are helpful. By law only data no more than 1 year old are allowed.

A medical report must include the following:

- Relevant medical history, past history, social history, and family history
- Subjective complaints (patient's symptoms)
- Objective findings on physical examination (e.g., results of physical or mental status examination, and blood pressure)
- Laboratory and x-ray findings
- Diagnostic studies (e.g., treadmill tests, pulmonary function tests, or electrocardiographic tracings)
- Diagnosis (statement of disease or injury based on signs and symptoms)
- Treatment prescribed, with patient's response and prognosis
- Medical prognosis about disability based on medical findings. A description of the individual's ability to perform work-related activities, such as standing, sitting, lifting, carrying, walking, handling objects, hearing, speaking, and traveling, is necessary. For cases of mental impairment, the statement should present the individual's capacity for understanding and remembering, sustained concentration and persistence, social interaction, and adaptation.

Veterans Affairs Disability Outpatient Clinic Claims

The processing of invoices from private physicians is a somewhat lengthy procedure as required by VA regulations and involves several steps. To keep the delay in payment to a minimum, private physicians are urged to bill the VA monthly. To ensure prompt processing, invoices should contain the following information:

- Patient's name as shown on the ID card, VA Form 10-1174 (see Figure 15–1).
- Patient's Social Security number.
- Condition treated, shown on every invoice, because this is the basis for approval of payment.
- Diagnosis being treated must be listed on the ID card or authorized by the statement "for any condition." Abstract the diagnosis exactly as it is stated on the ID card.

- Treatment given and dates rendered.
- Physician's usual and customary fee for services rendered.
- Name and address of private physician and his or her Social Security or Federal Taxpayer ID number. If the ID number is assigned to a group and the physician desires to be paid individually, the VA outpatient clinic must be so advised.

Private physicians, as well as veterans, are urged to read the instructions on the ID card carefully. This is sometimes neglected and can lead to misunderstanding.

If the physician does not wish to bill the VA outpatient clinic, the patient can pay the physician and then be reimbursed, but the veteran must carefully follow the instructions on the back of the VA outpatient clinic card.

State Disability Claims

Residents of a state that provides state disability benefits may call or write to the nearest office that handles state disability insurance to obtain a claim form and insurance pamphlet. See Internet Resources at the end of this chapter.

In some states, the claim form is in three parts and must be completed by the claimant, employer, and physician. In other states the form is in two parts and is completed by the claimant and physician (Figures 16–3 and 16–4). In either instance, the case must be substantiated by a physician before the applicant may begin receiving benefits. All information from the state disability insurance office should be read carefully and the directions followed precisely. The data requested should be provided, and the physician and patient should sign the forms. The form should be submitted within the stated time limits.

After the claim has been completed by all parties concerned, it is submitted to the nearest local office for processing. The most important items on the claim form are the following:

- The claimant's Social Security number; without it the claim cannot be researched properly to establish wages earned in the base period.
- The first day the patient was too sick to perform all of his or her regular work duties (item 3). This cannot be the same day the patient worked, even if the patient went home sick.

- The last day the patient worked (item 4). List the last day the patient worked even if for only part of the day.

NOTE: The two dates listed in items 2 and 3 cannot be the same; for example, if the patient went home sick on October 4, that would be considered the last day worked; October 5 would be the first day the patient was unable to work.

California has been selected as the model state for examples of the different forms used in the processing of disability insurance. To establish a claim, the First Claim for Disability Insurance Form DE 2501 must be completed by both the patient (see Figure 16–3) and the attending physician (see Figure 16–4). If an extension of disability is necessary, the Physician's Supplementary Certificate Form DE 2525XX must be completed by the physician (Figure 16–5). This accompanies the last check issued to the patient. For additional medical information that might be necessary, Forms DE 2547 and DE 2547A sometimes are sent to the attending physician for completion (Figures 16–6 and 16–7).

All follow-up correspondence should include the patient's name and Social Security number. The insurance billing specialist should promptly report any change of address, telephone number, or return-to-work date to the state disability insurance office. Patients must report any income received to the state disability insurance office because income received may affect benefits.

CONCLUSION

This chapter ends as it began—with a bit of levity. The following were taken from actual disability insurance application forms, completed by employees, that came across the desk of a claims adjuster.

Spelled as:	Should have been:
yellow "jonders"	yellow jaundice
"goalstones"	gallstones
"limp glands"	lymph glands
"falls teeth"	false teeth
"high pretension"	hypertension
"Pabst smear"	Pap smear
"wrecktum"	rectum

CLAIM STATEMENT OF EMPLOYEE   *Please read instructions on back before completing this form.*
COMPLETE *ALL* ITEMS. IF INCOMPLETE, THIS FORM WILL BE RETURNED, CAUSING A DELAY IN BENEFIT PAYMENTS

1. Print your full name: FIRST   INITIAL   LAST

  MARCIA   M.   MONROE

  Other Names (including maiden, married and ethnic surnames) Used:

  Your Mailing Address:

STREET ADDRESS, P.O. BOX OR RFD   APT. NO.   CITY OR TOWN   STATE AND ZIP CODE

  3501 Maple Street, Woodland Hills,   XY 12345

  Your Home Address: (Required if different from mailing address)
IF YOU HAVE NO STREET ADDRESS, YOU **MUST** PROVIDE SPECIFIC DIRECTIONS TO YOUR HOME

  MONTH DAY YEAR
Male ☐   Female ☒   Birthdate 03|04|1952

Do you need assistance in a language other than English? ☒ No ☐ Yes
If yes, write that language here:_____

¿Prefiere Ud. formularios escritos en español? No ☐ Sí ☐

2. **IMPORTANT:** Enter your Social Security Account Number

  5 | 4 | 0 | | X | X | | 9 | 8 | 8 | 1

2A. If you have used another Social Security number, enter that number here

  _ _ _ _ _ _ _ _ _ _

3. What was the first day you were too sick to perform all the duties of your regular or customary work, even if it was a Saturday, Sunday, holiday, or a normal day off:?

  MONTH 10 DAY 10 YEAR 20xx

4. What was the last day you worked prior to your disability?

  MONTH 10 DAY 09 YEAR 20xx

5. Current or Last Employer's Business Name: Telephone Number

  A and B Company   (555) 487-9980

  Current or Last Employer's   NUMBER AND STREET   CITY   STATE AND ZIP CODE
  Business Address   401 State Street   Woodland Hills, XY   12345

6. Your occupation with this employer. secretary   Your Badge or Payroll number: 4399

7. a. What is your usual occupation?   secretary
    b. Have you been retrained for a new occupation? If yes, please give name of that occupation: Yes ☐   No ☒

8. Are you self-employed?   Yes ☐   No ☒

9. Did you lose any time from work because of this illness or injury during the two weeks before the last day you worked as shown in item (4) above?   Yes ☐   No ☒

10. Did you stop work because of sickness, injury or pregnancy?
    If "No," please give reason: Yes ☒   No ☐

11. Have you filed for or received UNEMPLOYMENT INSURANCE benefits between the last day you worked and the first day you became disabled?   Yes ☐   No ☒

12. a. Has, or will your employer continue your pay by means of sick leave, pension, gift or other means?   Yes ☐   No ☒
    b. Do you authorize the Employment Development Department to disclose benefit eligibility information to your employer to be used only for the purpose of integrating your employer's wage continuation/sick leave program with your benefits? (This information is limited to the claim effective date; the weekly and maximum benefit amounts; and the periods covered by benefit payments.) Yes ☒   No ☐

13. Was this disability or any other disability during this claim period caused by your work?   Yes ☐   No ☒
    If "Yes," please provide: (a) The date of your work-caused injury: _____ and (b) The name and address of any insurance carrier from whom you are claiming or receiving Workers' Compensation benefits.

14. Have you recovered from your disability?
    If "Yes," enter date of recovery: Yes ☐   No ☒

15. Have you returned to work for any day, part-time or full-time, after the beginning date of your disability as shown in item (3) above?
    If "Yes," please enter such dates: Yes ☐   No ☒

16. At any time during your disability, were you, as a result of an arrest, confined to a jail, detention center, prison medical center or other correctional institution or any other place: If "Yes," give dates: Yes ☐   No ☒

I hereby claim benefits and certify that for the period covered by this claim I was unemployed and disabled, that the foregoing statements, including any accompanying statements, are to the best of my knowledge and belief true, correct and complete. I hereby authorize my attending physician, practitioner, hospital, vocational rehabilitation counselor, employer, and California Department of Industrial Relations to furnish and disclose all facts concerning my disability and wages or earnings that are within their knowledge and to allow inspection of and provide copies of any medical, vocational rehabilitation, and billing records concerning my disability that are under their control. I understand that authorizations contained in this claim statement are granted for a period of five years from the date of my signature or the effective date of the claim, whichever is later. I agree that a photocopy of this authorization shall be as valid as the original.

Claim signed on: MONTH DAY YEAR
▶   10   12   20xx

Under Section 2101 of the California Unemployment Insurance Code, it is a violation to willfully make a false statement or knowingly conceal a material fact in order to obtain the payment of any benefits, such violation being punishable by imprisonment and/or by a fine not exceeding $20,000 or both.

Claimant's signature: (DO NOT PRINT)   Telephone Number
                                (555) 487-9980
                             ▶

If your signature is made by mark (X) it must be attested by two witnesses with their addresses.
SIGNATURE-WITNESS   SIGNATURE-WITNESS

ADDRESS   ADDRESS

If an authorized agent is filing for benefits for an INCAPACITATED or DECEASED claimant, or a spouse is filing for a MENTALLY INCAPACITATED individual, contact the office below for the required forms and instructions.

FIGURE 16–3 Form DE 2501, Claim Statement of Employee. This side of the two-part form is completed by the claimant.

DOCTOR'S CERTIFICATE

Certification may be made by a licensed medical or osteopathic physician and surgeon, chiropractor, dentist, podiatrist, optometrist, designated psychologist or an authorized medical officer of a United States Government facility. Certification may also be made by a licensed nurse-midwife or nurse practitioner for the purposes of disability related to normal pregnancy or childbirth. All items on this sheet must be completed legibly.

Patient File No.	Name	Social Security Number
	MARCIA M. MONROE	540-XX-9881

17. I attended the patient for the present medical problem

	MONTH DAY YEAR	MONTH DAY YEAR
from:	10-12-20XX	To present	At intervals of: two visits to date

18. Are you completing this form for the sole purpose of referral or recommendation to an alcoholic recovery home or drug-free facility?
Yes ☐ No ☒ If yes, please enter facility name and address in item #28.

19. History:
cough of 2 wks duration, chest pain, 100°F

Objective Findings/Detailed Statement of Symptoms

Diagnosis:
(REQUIRED)
bilateral pneumonitis

bilateral pneumonitis

ICD-9 Disease Code, Primary: 486
(REQUIRED)

ICD-9 Disease Code, Secondary:

Type of treatment and/or medication rendered to patient:
Bed rest   Rx   antibiotic

20. Diagnosis confirmed by: **(Specify type of test or X-ray)**
AP and lateral chest x-rays

21. Is this patient now pregnant or has she been pregnant since the date of treatment as reported above?
Yes ☐ No ☒   If "Yes," date pregnancy terminated or future EDC.

Is the pregnancy normal?
Yes ☐ No ☐   If "No," state the abnormal and involuntary complication causing maternal disability:

22. Operation: Date performed or to be performed   DNA
Type of Operation:
ICD-9 Procedutre Code:
(REQUIRED)

23. Was or is patient confined as a registered bed patient in a hospital?   Yes ☐   No ☒
If "Yes," please provide dates:
Entered hospital on —————————— , 20——
Discharged from hospital on —————————— , 20——

24. Has the patient at any time during your attendance for this medical problem, been incapable of performing his or her regular work as a —————————— ?   Yes ☒ No ☐ If "Yes" the disability commenced on: 10-10-20XX

25. APPROXIMATE date, based on your examination of patient, disability (if any) should end or has ended sufficiently to permit the patient to resume regular or customary work. Even if considerable question exists, make SOME "esti-mate." This is a requirement of the Code, and the claim will be delayed if such date is not entered. Such answers as "Indefinite" or "don't know" will not suffice.
(ENTER DATE)
10-30-20XX

26. Based on your examination of patient, is this disability the result of "occupation" either as an "industrial accident" or as an "occupational disease"?
Yes ☐   No ☒   This should include aggravation of pre-existing conditions by occupation.

27. Have you reported this OR A CONCURRENT DISABILITY to any insurance carrier as a Workers' Compensation Claim?
Yes ☐   No ☒   If "Yes," to whom?
(Name of carrier or firm)

28. Was or is patient a resident in an alcoholic recovery home or drug-free residential facility?   Yes ☐   No ☒
If "Yes," please provide name and address:

29. Would the disclosure of this information to your patient be medically or psychologically detrimental to the patient?
Yes ☐   No ☒

I hereby certify that, based on my examination, the above statements truly describe the patient's disability (if any) and the estimated duration thereof, and that I am a MD | GP licensed to practice by the State of California
(TYPE OF DOCTOR)   (SPECIALTY, IF ANY)

▶ David W. Smith, MD   ▶
PRINT OR TYPE DOCTOR'S NAME AS SHOWN ON LICENSE

ORIGINAL SIGNATURE OF ATTENDING DOCTOR
- RUBBER STAMP IS NOT ACCEPTABLE -

▶ 4567 Broad Ave., Woodland Hills, XY   12345   ▶ C 14020   (555) 486-9002   10-19-20XX
NO. AND STREET   CITY   ZIP CODE   STATE LICENSE NUMBER   TELEPHONE   DATE OF SIGNING THIS FORM

Under Section 2116 of the California Unemployment Insurance Code, it is a violation for any individual who, with the intent to defraud, falsely certifies the medical condition of any person in order to obtain disability insurance benefits, whether for the maker or for any other person, and is punishable by imprisonment and/or a fine not exceeding twenty thousand dollars. Section 1143 requires additional administrative penalties.

FIGURE 16-4 Form DE 2501, Doctor's Certificate. This side of the form is completed by the attending physician. It is submitted within a set time period, determined by the beginning date of disability, to initiate benefits. If the patient is seen by a second physician, this form is mailed to the claimant to secure the certification of a new physician or to clarify a specific claimed period of disability.

NOTICE OF FINAL PAYMENT

The information contained in your claim for Disability Insurance indicates that you are now able to work; therefore, this is the final check that you will receive on this claim.

IF YOU ARE **STILL** DISABLED: You should complete the Claimant's Certification portion of this form and contact your doctor immediately to have him/her complete the Physician's Supplementary Certificate below.

IF YOU BECOME DISABLED **AGAIN:** File a new Disability Insurance claim form.

IF YOU ARE UNEMPLOYED AND AVAILABLE FOR WORK: Report to the nearest Unemployment Insurance office of the Department for assistance in finding work and to determine your entitlement to Unemployment Insurance Benefits.

This determination is final unless you file an appeal within twenty (20) days from the date of mailing of this notification. You may appeal by giving a detailed statement as to why you believe the determination is in error. All communications regarding this Disability Insurance claim should include your Social Security Account Number and be addressed to the office shown.

CLAIMANT'S CERTIFICATION

I certify that I continue to be disabled and incapable of doing my regular work, and that I have reported all wages, Workers' Compensation benefits and other monies received during the claim period to the Employment Development Department.

ENTER YOUR SOCIAL SECURITY NUMBER _540_ _XX_ _9881_

Sign Your Name _Marcia M. Monroe_   Date signed _October_ _29_ 20 _xx_

PHYSICIAN'S SUPPLEMENTARY CERTIFICATE

Department Use Only

1. Are you still treating patient? _Yes_ Date of last treatment _October_ _29_ 20 _xx_

2. What present condition continues to make the patient disabled?

bilateral pneumonitis; infiltrate still present

3. Date patient recovered, or will recover sufficiently (even if under treatment) to be able to perform his/her regular and customary work _November_ _7_ 20 _xx_   Please enter a specific or estimated recovery date.

4. Would the disclosure of this information to your patient be medically or psychologically detrimental to the patient?

Yes ☐   No ☒

I hereby certify that the above statements in my opinion truly describe the claimant's condition and the estimated duration thereof.

Date _October_ _29_ 20 _xx_   Doctor's Signature _David W. Smith M.D._

                                                Phone Number _555-486-9002_

DE 2525XX Rev. 13 (3-86)   —Version en español el dorso—

FIGURE 16–5 Notice of Final Payment/Physician's Supplementary Certificate Form DE 2525XX. This form indicates that the period of disability is "closed" or terminated with the accompanying check, based on information in the claim records. Benefits will cease unless the reverse side of the form is completed by the claimant's physician, extending the duration of disability. This form is pink. One side of the form is in English, and the other is in Spanish.

STATE OF CALIFORNIA
EMPLOYMENT DEVELOPMENT DEPARTMENT

FOR DEPT. USE ONLY

REFER TO

4920 – Our File No.
Marcia M. Monroe – Your Patient
Secretary – Regular or Customary Work

REQUEST FOR ADDITIONAL
MEDICAL INFORMATION

David W. Smith, MD
4567 Broad Avenue
Woodland Hills, XY 12345

The original basic information and estimate of duration of your patient's disability have been carefully evaluated. At the present time, the following additional information based upon the progress and present condition of this patient is requested. This will assist the Department in determining eligibility for further disability insurance benefits. Return of the completed form as soon as possible will be appreciated.

WM. C. SCHMIDT, M.D., MEDICAL DIRECTOR

CLAIMS EXAMINER   *DOCTOR: Please complete either Part A or B, date and sign.*

PART A IF YOUR PATIENT HAS RECOVERED SUFFICIENTLY TO BE ABLE TO RETURN TO HIS/HER REGULAR OR CUSTOMARY WORK LISTED ABOVE, PLEASE GIVE THE DATE, _____ 20_____.

PART B THIS PART REFERS TO PATIENT WHO IS STILL DISABLED.

Are you still treating the patient?   YES ☒   NO ☐   _November____15___, 20 _xx_
                                                       DATE OF LAST TREATMENT

What are the medical circumstances which continue to make your patient disabled?

Bilateral pneumonitis. Patient has had continual fever 100°F to 102°F, productive cough, chest pains, and lethargy

What is your present estimate of the date your patient will be able to perform his/her regular or customary work listed above? Date _November___30_ 20_ _xx_ .

Further Comments: _____

Would the disclosure of this information to your patient be medically or psychologically detrimental to the patient?   YES ☐   NO ☒

Date _November____17_ 20__ _xx_

David W. Smith M.D.
DOCTOR'S SIGNATURE

David W. Smith, MD

SE
ENCLOSED IS A STAMPED PREADDRESSED ENVELOPE FOR YOUR CONVENIENCE.

DE 2547 R v. 18 (8-84)

FIGURE 16–6 Request for Additional Medical Information Form DE 2547. This form is mailed to the physician when the normal expectancy date of the disability is reached, provided that the physician has requested a longer than normal duration without complications as indicated.

STATE OF CALIFORNIA

EMPLOYMENT DEVELOPMENT DEPARTMENT
P.O. Box 1529, Santa Barbara, CA 93102
(555) 963-9611

For Dept. Use Only

REFER TO

4920   - Our File No.   MEDICAL INQUIRY
Marcia M. Monroe   - Your Patient
Secretary   - Regular Work

David W. Smith, MD
4567 Broad Avenue
Woodland Hills, XY 12345

A review of the medical certificate received in conjunction with a claim
for disability insurance benefits filed by your patient, named above,
reveals that some additional information is needed in order to evaluate
the claim properly. Your cooperation in answering the question or
questions below and returning the form in the enclosed stamped and
addressed envelope will be appreciated.

WM. C. SCHMIDT, MD, MEDICAL DIRECTOR

CLAIMS EXAMINER

What is the name and address of the facility that took the x-rays on
this patient?

Speedy Radiology Service
4598 Main Street
Woodland Hills, XY 12345

Would the disclosure of this information to your patient be medically or
psychologically detrimental to the patient: Yes ☐   No ☒

October 24   20XX   *David W. Smith MD*
        Date   Doctor's Signature
SE   David W. Smith, MD

DE 2547A Rev. 10 (9-84)

FIGURE 16–7   Medical Inquiry Form DE 2547A. This form is mailed to the physician at any time during the life of the claim if any questions need to be answered or if the physician has failed to enter a prognosis date.

RESOURCES

INTERNET

Web sites pertaining to the law for nonindustrial disability insurance programs:

- California Unemployment Insurance Code
  Web site: **www.edd.ca.gov/**

- Hawaii Temporary Disability Laws
  Web site: **www.uhwo.hawaii.edu/clearHRS392.html**
  Rules: Web site: **d/ir.state.hi.us/rule/12-11.pdf**

- New Jersey Temporary Disability Benefits Law
  Web site: **www.nj.gov/labor**

- New York Disability Benefits Law
  Web site: **www.web.state.ny.us**

- Rhode Island Temporary Disability Insurance Act
  Web site: **www.state.ri.u**s
  (Puerto Rico does not have a Web site.)

- Department of Veterans Affairs Facility Directory
  Web site: **http://www1.va.gov/directory/guide/home.asp?isFlash=1**

  Click on "Facility Locator" at the bottom of the screen. Click on the state initials within the U.S. map to view facilities in that state. Many states have toll-free telephone services to the Department of Veterans Affairs from communities in the state. Consult the local telephone directory or directory assistance operator for the latest listing of these numbers.

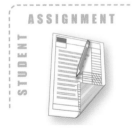

ASSIGNMENT

STUDENT

✔ Study Chapter 16.

✔ Answer the review questions in the *Workbook* to reinforce the theory learned in this chapter and to help prepare you for a future test.

✔ Complete the assignments in the *Workbook*. These assignments will provide you with hands-on experience in working with patient histories and completing disability insurance claim forms described in this chapter.

✔ Turn to the glossary at the end of this textbook for a further understanding of the key terms used in this chapter.

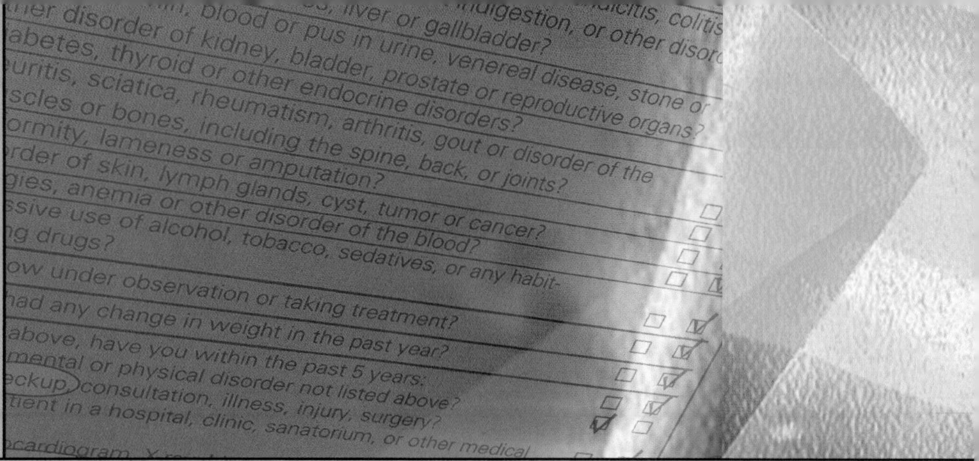

UNIT 4

Inpatient and Outpatient Billing

CHAPTER OUTLINE

PATIENT SERVICE
  REPRESENTATIVE
    Qualifications
    Primary Functions and
      Competencies
    Principal Responsibilities
MEDICOLEGAL
  CONFIDENTIALITY ISSUES
    Documents
    Verbal Communication
    Computer Security
ADMISSIONS PROCEDURES
    Appropriateness Evaluation
      Protocols
    Admitting Procedures for Major
      Insurance Programs
    Preadmission Testing
COMPLIANCE SAFEGUARDS
UTILIZATION REVIEW
    Quality Improvement
      Organization Program
CODING HOSPITAL
  PROCEDURES
    Outpatient—Reason for Visit
    Inpatient—Principal Diagnosis
CODING INPATIENT
  PROCEDURES
    ICD-9-CM Volume 3 Procedures

CODING OUTPATIENT
  PROCEDURES
    Current Procedural
      Terminology
    Health Care Common
      Procedure Coding System
    Modifiers
INPATIENT BILLING PROCESS
    Admitting Clerk
    Insurance Verifier
    Attending Physician, Nursing
      Staff, and Medical
      Transcriptionist
    Discharge Analyst
    Charge Description Master
    Code Specialist
    Insurance Billing Editor
    Nurse Auditor
REIMBURSEMENT PROCESS
    Reimbursement Methods
    Electronic Data Interchange
    Hard Copy Billing
    Receiving Payment
OUTPATIENT INSURANCE
  CLAIMS
    Hospital Professional Services
BILLING PROBLEMS
    Duplicate Statements

    Double Billing
    Phantom Charges
HOSPITAL BILLING CLAIM FORM
    Uniform Bill Inpatient and
      Outpatient Paper or
      Electronic Claim Form
DIAGNOSIS-RELATED GROUPS
    History
    The Diagnosis-Related Groups
      System
    Diagnosis-Related Groups and
      the Physician's Office
OUTPATIENT CLASSIFICATION
    Ambulatory Payment
      Classification System
PROCEDURE: NEW PATIENT
  ADMISSION AND INSURANCE
  VERIFICATION
PROCEDURE: CODING FROM
  ICD-9-CM VOLUME 3
PROCEDURE: EDITING A
  UNIFORM BILL (UB-92) PAPER
  OR ELECTRONIC CLAIM FORM
PROCEDURE: COMPLETING THE
  UB-92 PAPER OR ELECTRONIC
  CLAIM FORM

KEY TERMS

admission review

ambulatory payment
  classifications (APCs)

appropriateness evaluation
  protocols (AEPs)

capitation

case rate

charge description master (CDM)

charges

clinical outliers

code sequence

comorbidity

cost outlier

cost outlier review

day outlier review

diagnosis-related groups (DRGs)

DRG validation

DRG creep

elective surgery

grouper

inpatient

*International Classification of
  Diseases, Ninth Revision, Clinical
  Modification* (ICD-9-CM)

looping

major diagnostic categories
  (MDCs)

outpatient

percentage of revenue

per diem

preadmission testing (PAT)

principal diagnosis

procedure review

quality improvement organization
  (QIO) program

readmission review

scrubbing

stop loss

transfer review

Uniform Bill (UB-92) paper or
  electronic claim form

utilization review (UR)

17

Hospital Billing

OBJECTIVES*

After reading this chapter, you should be able to:

- Name qualifications necessary to work in the financial section of a hospital.

- Define appropriateness evaluation protocols.

- List criteria used for admission screening.

- Define the 72-hour rule.

- Describe the quality improvement organization and its role in the hospital reimbursement system.

- Define common terms related to hospital billing.

- List instances of breach of confidentiality in a hospital setting.

- State the role of ICD-9-CM Volume 3 in hospital billing.

- Identify categories in ICD-9-CM Volume 3.

- State reimbursement methods made to hospitals under managed care contracts.

- Explain the sequence of an inpatient hospital stay from billing through receipt of payment.

- Describe the charge description master.

- State when the Uniform Bill (UB-92) paper or electronic claim form may and may not be used.

- Edit and complete insurance claims in both hospital inpatient and outpatient settings to minimize their rejection by insurance carriers.

- State the general guidelines for completion of the paper (Uniform Bill [UB-92]) and transmission of the electronic claim form.

- Describe the history and purpose of diagnosis-related groups.

- Identify how payment is made based on diagnosis-related groups.

- State how payment is made based on the ambulatory payment classification system.

- Name the four types of ambulatory payment classifications.

---

*Performance objectives and exercises for hands-on practical experience for this chapter appear in the *Workbook*.

Service

Learn to be courteous in all interactions with co-workers and patients so patients sense an atmosphere of high morale in the working environment. Be watchful about observing how patients and co-workers react to you and to hospital policies and procedures so communication ends up as positive patient encounter. Make sure you are educated about your job duties and hospital policy, otherwise responses to the patient may vary from employee to employee when training is not thorough. Always look and act as a professional and respond immediately to patients' questions and problems.

PATIENT SERVICE REPRESENTATIVE

Qualifications

A variety of jobs are available in the financial department and health information management (HIM) department, formerly known as the medical record department, of hospitals; therefore this chapter focuses on hospital inpatient and outpatient insurance billing and coding. Individuals who desire a position in a hospital facility business department should have knowledge and competence in the following subjects:

- ICD-9-CM diagnostic codes
- CPT and HCPCS procedure codes
- Paper or electronic CMS-1500 insurance claim form
- Paper or electronic Uniform Bill (UB-92) insurance claim form
- Explanation of benefits and remittance advice document
- Medical terminology
- Major health insurance programs
- Managed care plans
- Insurance claim submission
- Denied and delinquent claims

A hospital facility is larger than a clinic or private physician's office, so there is greater opportunity for advancement. An individual may be hired as an entry level coder, file clerk, or insurance verifier and advance from junior to senior clerk, insurance clerk, or patient service representative. He or she may continue to advance to an administrative position. Most hospital facilities have policies that encourage career growth by promoting jobs from within. Additional personal and physical qualifications are shown in Figure 17–1. Also refer to Chapter 1 for details on educational and training requirements and ethics and Chapter 18 for information on certification.

Primary Functions and Competencies

A generic job description for a patient service representative in a hospital business office whose primary function is to file hospital inpatient and outpatient claims with third-party payers is shown in Figure 17–1. Competencies for inpatient coding that were approved by the American Hospital Association (AHA), American Health Information Management Association (AHIMA), Centers for Medicare and Medicaid Services (CMS; formerly Health Care Financing Administration), and the National Center for Health Statistics are shown in Box 17–1.

Principal Responsibilities

Because of the diversity in reimbursement methods, the insurance billing specialist must have basic knowledge of insurance programs and know how to use summary or "cheat sheets," which give summaries of the contracts to correctly process each insurance claim. Accurate claim processing is essential for obtaining maximum reimbursement from the insurance company and when collecting payment from the patient. To remain an asset to employers, an insurance billing specialist must continually update his or her knowledge of coding and insurance program policies by attending seminars, workshops, classes, and in-house training. See Figure 17–1 for a list of principal responsibilities for a patient service representative.

MEDICOLEGAL CONFIDENTIALITY ISSUES

Documents

The patient's financial and medical records and any photographs are legal documents and must be kept confidential (see Chapter 4). They may not be released unless a patient has signed an authorization form to make the information public. An exception is when a medical record is subpoenaed by the court. Chapter 4 contains information on confidentiality when facsimile communication is used. When work is done in a sensitive area of a facility, document shredders should be used to destroy unwanted documents and prevent violations of confidentiality.

Examples 17.1 and 17.2 show breaches of confidentiality with medical and financial records.

Verbal Communication

Verbal breaches of confidentiality in a hospital setting, much like in a provider's office, could result in an insurance billing specialist being held liable and the facility being sued by a patient. Also, HIPAA violations carry monetary penalties and may include a jail sentence. New employees must be trained in confidentiality and asked to sign an

POSITION DESCRIPTION

Title: Patient Service Representative
Department: Business Office
Reports to: Patient Accounts Supervisor

Job Number: 215
Effective Date: 3/1/04
Revision Date: 11/1/04

Primary Function:
To promptly file hospital inpatient and outpatient claims with third-party payers, following up in a timely and efficient manner, to ensure maximum reimbursement is received for services provided. To assist the public in obtaining full benefits from their coverage and in understanding billing procedures, always maintaining good public relations.

Principal Responsibilities:
1. Processes claims within assigned responsibility in a timely and efficient manner, performing all associated duties in order to ensure completeness and correctness of all claims information, facilitating maximum reimbursement.
   a. Analyzes, updates and corrects claim data according to established procedure.
   b. Inputs data accurately, efficiently and consistently.
   c. Performs work as scheduled, prioritizing as required for maximizing cash flow.
   d. Demonstrates thorough knowledge of third-party payers, claims requirements, UB-92 requirements by payer, computer capabilities as related to claims production, and admitting/medical records input as it affects claims.
2. Handles phone, mail and personal inquiries from and regarding patient accounts.
   a. Assists each person promptly, efficiently and courteously.
   b. Follows through on all issues identified as requiring action as a result of inquiry.
   c. Performs duties with a minimum of supervision, exhibits innovation and good judgment as well as thorough knowledge of ethical and legal billing procedures.
3. Performs related business office responsibilities as assigned by patient accounts manager.
   a. Follows hospital and department policies and procedures.
   b. Observes confidentiality in all matters.
   c. Maintains all documentation and records in accordance with federal and state regulations.
   d. Maintains good interdepartmental relations.
4. Provides coverage for A/R specialist 2 position for vacation and illness.
   a. Demonstrates knowledge of and ability to perform all duties and functions.
5. Participates in educational opportunities offered by hospital for job and personal development.
   a. Attends classes, workshops and seminars relating to billing/collection functions.
   b. Participates actively in such seminars, classes and workshops.
   c. Takes advantage of opportunities for personal growth and development as offered.
6. Takes an active role in facilitating team approach to functions within the department.
   a. Attends departmental meetings.
   b. Actively participates as team member in resolution of problems as they are identified.
   c. Analyzes current procedures, bringing suggestions for improvement to the attention of team members and supervisor for consideration.

Direction of Others:
Provides some direction to student learner. Number of persons supervised —1.

Qualifications:
High school graduation with 1–3 years experience in claims processing, business or accounting. Experience in health care field desirable.

Physical Qualifications:
These requirements may be met with the aid of mechanical devices and are those minimally necessary for safe completion of duties. They are not intended to discriminate against handicapped persons, only to ensure safe working conditions for all persons.
1. Must be able to enter data into a computer and effectively operate a 10-key adding machine.
2. Must be able to communicate in a pleasant and tactful manner to other employees and patients.
3. Must pass a pre-employment physical examination.

Working Conditions:
Normal office working conditions.

Department approval: _____ Date: _____

Administrative approval: _____ Date: _____

Human resources approval: _____ Date: _____

FIGURE 17–1 Job description for patient service representative (hospital biller). (From Goselin L. *Questions and Answers: Job Descriptions Provide Guidelines for Employees/Managers: Get It in Writing, Health Care Biller,* vol 4, no 6. New York, Aspen Publishers, 1995.)

Box 17.1 | **American Health Information Management Association CCS Coding Competencies—ICD-9-CM and CPT/HCPCS Procedural Coding**

DATA IDENTIFICATION

1. Read and interpret health record documentation to identify all diagnoses and procedures that affect the current inpatient stay or outpatient encounter visit.
2. Assess the adequacy of health record documentation to ensure that it supports all diagnoses and procedures to which codes are assigned.
3. Apply knowledge of anatomy and physiology, clinical disease processes, pharmacology, and diagnostic and procedural terminology to assign accurate codes to diagnoses and procedures.
4. Apply knowledge of disease processes and surgical procedures to assign nonindexed medical terms to the appropriate class in the classification/nomenclature system.

CODING GUIDELINES

1. Apply knowledge of current approved ICD-9-CM coding guidelines to assign and sequence the correct diagnosis and procedure codes for hospital inpatient services.
2. Apply knowledge of current diagnostic coding and reporting guidelines for outpatient services.
3. Apply knowledge of CPT format, guidelines, and notes to locate the correct codes for all services and procedures performed during the encounter/visit and sequence them correctly.
4. Apply knowledge of procedural terminology to recognize when an unlisted procedure code must be used in CPT.

REGULATORY GUIDELINES

1. Apply Uniform Hospital Discharge Data Set definitions to select the principal diagnosis, principal procedure, complications and comorbid conditions, other diagnoses, and significant procedures that require coding.
2. Select the appropriate principal diagnosis for episodes of care in which determination of principal diagnosis is not clear because the patient has multiple problems.
3. Apply knowledge of the Prospective Payment System to confirm DRG assignment that ensures optimal reimbursement.
4. Refuse to fraudulently maximize reimbursement by assigning codes that do not conform to approved coding principles/guidelines.
5. Refuse to unfairly maximize reimbursement by unbundling services and codes that do not conform to CPT basic coding principles.
6. Apply knowledge of the Ambulatory Surgery Center Payment Groups to confirm ASC assignment that ensures optimal reimbursement.
7. Apply policies and procedures on health record documentation, coding and claims processing, and appeal.
8. Use the HCFA Common Procedural Coding System (HCPCS) to appropriately assign HCPCS codes for outpatient Medicare reimbursement.

CODING

1. Exclude from coding diagnoses, conditions, problems, and procedures related to an earlier episode of care that have no bearing on the current episode of care.
2. Exclude from coding ICD-9-CM nonsurgical, noninvasive procedures that carry no operative or anesthetic risk.
3. Exclude from coding information such as symptoms or signs characteristic of the diagnosis, findings from diagnostic studies, or localized conditions that have no bearing on the current management of the patient.
4. Apply knowledge of ICD-9-CM instructional notations and conventions to locate and assign the correct diagnostic and procedural codes and sequence them correctly.
5. Facilitate data retrieval by recognizing when more than one code is required to adequately classify a given condition.
6. Exclude from coding procedures that are component parts of an already assigned CPT procedure code.

DATA QUALITY

1. Clarify conflicting, ambiguous, or nonspecific information appearing in a health record by consulting the appropriate physician.
2. Participate in quality assessment to ensure continuous improvement in ICD-9-CM and CPT coding and collection of quality health data.
3. Demonstrate ability to recognize potential coding quality issues from an array of data.
4. Apply policies and procedures on health record documentation and coding that are consistent with official coding guidelines.
5. Contribute to development of facility-specific coding policies and procedures.

MEDICOLEGAL CONFIDENTIALITY ISSUES—cont'd

Example 17.1 Medical Record Scenario

An insurance billing specialist working at home has a sister who was hospitalized to undergo major surgery and wants to help his or her parents better understand the medical condition. The specialist calls a friend in the hospital billing department and asks that person to make photocopies of a document in the medical record.

Comment

Remember that all medical reports are confidential, so the employee must deny the request unless the sister signs a release of information that would authorize her family to have copies of the document.

Example 17.2 Financial Record Scenario

An experienced insurance billing specialist applies for a job. At an interview, he or she presents some samples of typed insurance claims that include hospital and patient names.

Comment

This indicates that the prospective employee has taken data from a former employer's facility and violated the patient's confidentiality by not removing the names in the samples.

Example 17.3 Verbal Breach of Confidentiality Scenario

A coding clerk overhears two hospital employees discussing a patient by name. Because the clerk had been working on the medical record of that patient and is now familiar with the patient's history, he or she realizes that the information being discussed is not accurate. The coding clerk then interrupts, making a comment about the patient's diagnosis.

Comment

Information should not be discussed with co-workers or other hospital employees and must never be related to anyone other than a person who has a valid need to provide care for the patient.

Example 17.4 Verbal Breach of Confidentiality Scenario

A Marilyn Monroe impersonator is discharged from the hospital after receiving plastic surgery. Over dinner at home, an insurance billing specialist relates the diagnosis and name of the surgery to his or her spouse.

Comment

Never discuss confidential information about patients to family or friends.

Example 17.5 Verbal Breach of Confidentiality Scenario

In reviewing an insurance claim before it is mailed, the insurance billing specialist realizes that he or she knows the individual who has a diagnosis that indicates a mental condition. The specialist discusses this with a co-worker.

Comment

This is a violation because a hospital employee must never give anyone information on a patient's diagnosis.

Example 17.6 Verbal Breach of Confidentiality Scenario

A physician in private practice calls via cellular telephone to the billing clerk to answer a question about the diagnosis to be listed on a patient's insurance claim.

Comment

Cellular transmission may be intercepted by anyone with inexpensive eavesdropping equipment. In this scenario, a traditional telephone line must be used when relating confidential information about a patient's diagnosis. The physician should verify whether he or she is speaking to the billing clerk.

Computer Security

As learned in Chapter 8 in regard to computer security, when using a computer, adhere to hospital policies with respect to the following:

- Use of passwords and other encryption methods
- Policies for composition and transmission of electronic mail
- Policies for use of the fax machine
- Downloading of computer data from one department to another
- Length of time that documents may be retained on computer hard drives by employees
- Procedures for deletion of confidential information
- Procedures for archiving of data
- Closing out when leaving a workstation or desk

understanding of confidentiality statement. This statement should emphasize that the employee may be subject to immediate termination in the event of a violation. Any one of the following scenarios in which the patient's right to privacy has been breached in the hospital setting may be encountered by an insurance billing specialist (Examples 17.3 through 17.6).

ADMISSIONS PROCEDURES

Appropriateness Evaluation Protocols

A patient is considered an **inpatient** on admission to the hospital for an overnight stay for observation care or for an extended stay for inpatient services. **Appropriateness evaluation protocols (AEPs)** by the hospital's utilization review (UR) department must be met to certify that the patient's complaints warrant admittance to the hospital. In addition, the hospital may have specific rules for observation status dictated by the American Hospital Association (AHA), the hospital administration, and the hospital medical staff's specific rules. Specific criteria are used by the insurance company for admission screening. The Medicare Prospective Payment System (PPS) requires that all patients meet at least one severity of illness (SI) or intensity of service (IS) criterion, unless otherwise indicated, to be certified for reimbursement. Within the first 24 hours, the hospital's UR department analyzes the documentation on the medical record, which must reflect how the patient meets these criteria. UR is discussed in detail later in this chapter. A list of AEPs is provided in Figure 17–2.

Admitting Procedures for Major Insurance Programs

The admitting process varies according to rules set down by the patient's insurance plan and hospital rules based on guidelines from the American Hospital Association. Following are basic admitting procedures and preadmission authorization requirements for the major insurance programs.

Private Insurance (Group or Individual)

It is the responsibility of the outpatient and inpatient admitting personnel to obtain complete and accurate information during initial registration of the patient. The patient must provide a current insurance card or cards. Obtain photocopies of the front and back of all cards. Some hospital facilities employ an insurance verification clerk. He or she has the responsibility of contacting the insurance company or the insured individual's employer to verify the type of health insurance. The clerk also must call the insurance company to verify eligibility and benefits and determine whether prior authorization is needed.

Managed Care

There may be restrictions and various policies and procedures to follow when admitting a patient who has a managed care health

APPROPRIATENESS EVALUATION PROTOCOL CRITERIA FOR ADMISSION CERTIFICATION

An admission may be certified if one of the following criteria is met:

SEVERITY OF ILLNESS (SI)
1. Sudden onset of unconsciousness or disorientation (coma or unresponsiveness).
2. Pulse rate <50 or >140.
3. Systolic blood pressure <80 or >200 mm Hg. Diastolic blood pressure <60 or >120 mm Hg.
4. Sudden onset of loss of sight or hearing.
5. History of persistent fever ≥ 100° F (orally) or 101° F (rectally) for more than 5 days or with white blood cell count >15,000/mm³.
6. Sudden onset of motor function loss of any body part.
7. Active, uncontrolled bleeding.
8. Electrolyte or blood gas abnormality of serum K+: <2.5, >6.0; serum Na+ <123, >156; CO_2 <20 mEq/L, >36 mEq/L (new findings).
9. Acute or progressive sensory, motor, circulatory, or respiratory embarrassment sufficient to incapacitate the patient (one of the IS criteria must also be met).
10. Electrocardiographic evidence of acute ischemia with suspicion of new myocardial infarction.
11. Wound dehiscence or evisceration.

INTENSITY OF SERVICE (IS)
12. Administration and monitoring of intravenous medications and/or fluid replacement (does not include tube feeding).
13. Surgery or procedure scheduled within 24 hours requiring general or regional anesthesia with use of equipment and facilities available only in a hospital.
14. Vital sign monitoring at least every 2 hours, including telemetry and bedside cardiac monitoring.
15. Use of chemotherapeutic agents that require continuous observation for a life-threatening toxic reaction.
16. Treatment in intensive/coronary care unit.
17. Administration of intramuscular antibiotics at least every 8 hours.
18. Intermittent or continuous respirator use at least every 8 hours.
19. Documentation on the medical record by the attending physician that the patient has been unsuccessfully treated as an outpatient *with* further documentation of how the patient is now to be treated as an inpatient.

FIGURE 17–2 Appropriateness evaluation protocol criteria for admission certification listing severity of illness and intensity of service.

maintenance organization (HMO) or preferred provider organization (PPO) type of insurance. Obtain photocopies of the front and back sides of the identification card. Several types of patient admissions to the hospital are recognized by managed care plans. See Chapter 11 for further information on this subject.

Emergency Inpatient Admission

Hospital with Contract. A patient is seen in the emergency department, and the physician determines that it is necessary to admit the patient to the hospital. The managed care program should be notified the next working day or within 48 hours to obtain an authorization number. The plan authorizes the first days of the admission automatically and approves subsequent days based on utilization review. The review organization determines the emergency status and may send written notification to the hospital and physician. The patient may have a deductible and copayment requirement. Emergency department charges are billed with charges for the inpatient stay on the electronic or paper (Uniform Bill [UB]-92) claim form. This form is also known as the 837i (institutional) and is being redesigned. The physician's professional services for a patient seen in the emergency department are submitted as outpatient billing on the CMS-1500 insurance claim form. This form is also known, but less commonly, as the 837p (professional).

Hospital without Contract. The managed care program of emergency admission should be notified on the next working day to obtain an authorization number. The patient should be prepared for transfer to a contracting hospital if necessary. The patient may have the option of staying and paying the deductible, copayment, or entire bill and not file a claim with the managed care plan. The managed care plan may or may not cover any charges depending on the type of plan. However, some plans with deductibles and copayments cover certain charges.

Nonemergency Inpatient Admission

Hospital with Contract. The patient must be referred by his or her primary care physician and obtain authorization for the length of the hospital stay. The patient may have a copayment requirement.

Hospital without Contract. The patient may request authorization with a noncontracted hospital; however, the patient may be responsible for a higher deductible and copayment or the entire bill.

Elective Admission to a Participating Hospital

An attending participating physician contacts the insurance plan at least 3 days before admission to give notification of a member's proposed elective admission. If a preadmission review is necessary, the physician is responsible for obtaining prior authorization from the review organization or the managed care plan. The physician calls the hospital to relay information about the patient for admitting purposes.

Elective Admission to a Nonparticipating Hospital

An attending physician contacts the designated review organization for admission approval in a nonemergency situation. Within 1 working day of approved requests for prior authorization, the review organization calls the physician and hospital and assigns a control number that certifies approval of the admission. The review organization furnishes the physician and hospital with an approved preadmission or referral request form.

Medicaid

In most states, a treatment authorization request form should be approved before elective admissions. For an emergency, preapproval is not necessary; however, a retroactive form is needed before the claim is billed. Photocopies of the front and back of the patient's identification card should be obtained or eligibility verified via touchtone telephone, modem, or specialized Medicaid terminal equipment. See Chapter 13 for additional information.

Medicare

Medicare patients do not need prior approval for admission to a hospital. However, their admittance should be certified by AEPs, as previously discussed in this chapter. Photocopies of the front and back of the patient's identification cards should be obtained for Medicare and any supplemental or secondary insurance policies. A common working file is used to verify coverage, look up information, and bill Medicare. For patients who receive both Medicare and Medicaid or other secondary insurance benefits, the claims are considered crossover claims. The claim form is processed automatically by Medicaid (in California Medi-Cal) after processing is completed by Medicare. See Chapter 12 for detailed data on the Medicare program.

TRICARE and CHAMPVA

As stated in Chapter 14, all admissions to a civilian hospital and ambulatory surgical facility except emergency cases require precertification. The health care finder assists with this process when a military treatment hospital is not available. Precertification should be verified; photocopies of the front and back of the patient's identification card should be obtained or eligibility verified via touchtone telephone or modem. See Chapter 14 for additional information.

Workers' Compensation

 The patient does not have an insurance card in a workers' compensation case. When the patient is seen on an emergency basis, an employer's report of injury must be completed and sent to the insurance company and the state industrial accident board before a hospital or physician's insurance claim may be submitted. A case number is assigned. Appropriate information relating to the injured patient, industrial accident, insurance carrier, and employer must be obtained. The insurance adjuster must authorize admission, length of stay, and all surgical procedures for an elective admission. See Chapter 15 for further details on this subject.

Preadmission Testing

To obtain necessary diagnostic information, reduce inpatient expenses, and eliminate extra hospital days, a patient is usually sent to the hospital for **preadmission testing (PAT)** before being admitted for major surgery. Preadmission tests include diagnostic studies, such as laboratory tests, chest x-ray films, and electrocardiography. When a laboratory panel of tests is performed, each separate test must be itemized and must show the clinical benefit for each test performed based on the patient's diagnosis. In elective surgical cases, preadmission services (e.g., history and physical examination) are done in the physician's office and are bundled with hospital services instead of appearing as separate charges on inpatient or outpatient bills.

Medicare 3-Day Payment Window Rule or 72-Hour Rule

One of the most important regulations in hospital billing is compliance with the CMS's 72-hour rule, also called the 3-day payment window rule because it is 3 calendar days rather than 72 hours. The Medicare rule states that if a patient receives diagnostic tests and hospital outpatient services within 72 hours of admission to a hospital (3-day payment window), then all such tests and services are combined (bundled) with inpatient services only if services are related to the admission. However, unrelated therapeutic service is paid. The preadmission services become part of the diagnosis-related group (DRG) payment to the hospital and may not be billed or paid separately. This is valid if the services (including emergency department services) are considered related to the reason for admission. If a hospital owns or operates a physician's office that provides diagnostic or other services related

to the admission within 3 days of subsequent inpatient admission, the services must be included in the DRG payment. If this rule is not followed, fraud and abuse may be considered and a penalty in the form of a fine or imprisonment may be carried out.

Exceptions to the 72-Hour Rule

The following are exceptions to the 72-hour rule:

● Services provided by home health agencies, hospice, nursing facilities (NFs), and ambulance services
● Physician's professional portion of a diagnostic service (the technical portion of a diagnostic service must be included in the inpatient bill)
● Preadmission testing at an independent laboratory when the laboratory has no formal agreement with the health care facility

For patients with private insurance (non–Medicare) receiving tests within 24 hours of hospital admission, include such tests with inpatient billing.

COMPLIANCE SAFEGUARDS

Many times a patient is seen in the physician's office (outpatient service), which leads the provider to admit the patient to the hospital as an inpatient; therefore, services related to both outpatient and inpatient cases are performed. Problems may develop when billing for the physician's office that is done on a separate billing system, making it difficult to match the outpatient services with subsequent inpatient hospital admission billed by the hospital's system. Ideally a facility should have a computer editing program that searches for any outpatient services given within the time frame before admission, or both sides (provider and hospital) should have integrated information systems. If not an integrated system, the hospital should have a relationship with the provider's office to obtain the minimum necessary information to treat the patient and bill for services. The hospital admitting clerk can also ask patients if they have received any medical service in the past 3 days; however, a patient may not be feeling well and not be able to recall or communicate the correct dates. Another solution is to use a post claim submission review program that searches outpatient claims and generates a weekly report identifying the outpatient and inpatient accounts that overlap. This should be manually reviewed by a billing department supervisor or manager. Identified overpayments must be promptly documented and refunded to the insurance program.

UTILIZATION REVIEW

Each hospital should have a **utilization review (UR)** department that conducts an admission and concurrent review and prepares a discharge plan on all cases. This process determines whether admissions are justified, anticipates length of stay (LOS), and concludes the expected discharge date. If the admission is found to be necessary, it is certified.

UR companies provide utilization review and case management services for self-insured employers, third-party administrators, and insurance companies. They furnish data to the person who buys their services to achieve cost savings, and they generate reports on how much money has been saved.

Quality Improvement Organization Program

CMS administers the **quality improvement organization (QIO) program,** which is designed to monitor and improve the usage and quality of care for Medicare beneficiaries. The program consists of a national network of 53 QIOs (formerly known as professional or peer review organizations) responsible for each state, territory, and the District of Columbia. QIO is governed by Titles XI and XVIII of the Social Security Act and is an organization contracting with CMS to review medical necessity, reasonableness, appropriateness, and completeness and adequacy of inpatient hospital care for which additional payment is sought under the outlier provisions of the PPS. QIOs are required to review all written quality of service complaints submitted by Medicare beneficiaries. The review addresses whether the services met professionally recognized standards of health care and may include whether the appropriate services were or were not provided in appropriate settings. The QIO's professional medical staff performs these reviews. The results of the reviews are submitted to CMS. The QIOs are responsible for the following types of review:

● **Admission review** for appropriateness and necessity of admissions.
● **Readmission review** on patients readmitted within 7 days with problems related to the first admission to determine whether the first discharge was premature or the second admission is medically necessary.
● **Procedure review** of diagnostic and therapeutic procedures in cases in which past abuses have been found, to determine appropriateness.
● **Day outlier review** of short or unusually long length of hospital stays to determine the number of days before the day outlier threshold is reached as well as the number of days beyond the threshold. This process

is done to certify necessity of admission and medical necessity of services for additional Medicare reimbursement.
● **Cost outlier review** of cases not eligible for day outlier review to determine the necessity of admission and the necessity and appropriateness of services rendered.
● **DRG validation** to find out whether the diagnostic and procedural information affecting DRG assignment is substantiated by the clinical information in the patient's chart. DRGs are discussed later in this chapter.
● **Transfer review** of cases involving a transfer to a distinct part or unit of the same hospital or other hospitals.

CODING HOSPITAL PROCEDURES

Current Procedural Terminology (CPT), Medicare's Health Care Common Procedure Coding System (HCPCS), and the three volumes of *International Classification of Diseases, Ninth Revision, Clinical Modification* **(ICD-9-CM)** are used to list codes on hospital insurance claims. In lieu of the books, computer software programs contain the same data to locate the codes accurately, quickly, and easily. Different code books are used to code an insurance claim when a patient receives services as an outpatient or inpatient. They are the following:

● *Outpatient* hospital insurance claims use CPT and HCPCS codes for procedures and ICD-9-CM, Volumes 1 and 2, for diagnoses.
● *Inpatient* hospital insurance claims use ICD-9-CM, Volumes 1 and 2, for diagnoses and Volume 3 for procedures. (Some private insurance companies are requesting CPT codes.)

Chapter 5 gives basic information and instructions on how to use Volumes 1 and 2. This chapter explains the use of Volume 3. Chapter 6 gives information on CPT and HCPCS procedure codes.

Outpatient—Reason for Visit

The patient's reason for the visit is listed for outpatient claims rather than the patient's principal diagnosis; for example, the reason for the outpatient visit may be chest pain but anxiety could be listed as the final outpatient diagnosis.

Inpatient—Principal Diagnosis

The **principal diagnosis** is the condition that is assigned a code representing the diagnosis established after study that is chiefly responsible for the admission of the patient to the hospital. This is the most important code, so be sure the code for the principal diagnosis is listed first. For example, heart disease is the principal diagnosis if a patient initially comes in for heart transplantation. However, pneumonia is the principal diagnosis if the heart transplant patient goes home and then comes back to the hospital with pneumonia. Subsequent diagnostic codes should be used for any current coexisting concurrent condition (comorbidity), that is, a condition that coexists with the principal condition, complicating the treatment and management of the principal disorder and that is documented in the record. These codes are sequenced after the principal diagnosis. Codes for conditions that were previously treated and no longer exist should not be included. A secondary diagnosis is one that may contribute to the condition, treatment, or recovery from the condition shown as the principal diagnosis. It also may define the need for a higher level of care but is not the underlying cause. The diagnostic **code sequence** (correct order) is very important in billing of hospital inpatient cases because maximum reimbursement is based on the DRGs system. This is explained in detail at the end of this chapter.

Rules for Coding Inpatient Diagnoses

Coding diagnoses for inpatient and outpatient cases can differ. One important difference is how uncertain diagnoses are coded. For inpatient cases, code all "rule out," "suspected," "likely," "questionable," "possible," or "still to be ruled out" as if it existed. For example, the physician documents upper abdominal pain, rule out cholecystitis. Assign code 575.0 (cholecystitis) for this diagnosis. This rule applies to inpatient records only.

In addition, the following rules and examples should be noted about the principal diagnosis.

● Codes for signs and symptoms of ICD-9-CM are not reported as principal diagnoses (Example 17.7).
● When two or more conditions meet the definition of principal diagnosis, either condition may be sequenced first unless otherwise indicated by the circumstances of admission or the therapy provided (Example 17.8).

Example 17.7   Principal Diagnosis/Signs and Symptoms

Mr. Brown was admitted to the hospital with fever, severe abdominal pain, nausea, and vomiting.

Diagnosis: Acute appendicitis
Dx Code: 540.9 (acute appendicitis without peritonitis)

NOTE: Symptoms are considered integral to the condition so the condition should be coded.

Example 17.8   Two Medical Conditions

Mrs. Sanchez was admitted with acute congestive heart failure (CHF) and unstable angina. Both conditions are treated.

Diagnosis: CHF and unstable angina
Dx Code: 428.0 (CHF) or 411.1 (unstable angina) Either code may be used.

NOTE: This is the focus of many compliance reviews.

Example 17.9   Symptom as Principal Diagnosis

Miss Chan was admitted with acute epigastric abdominal pain.

Diagnosis: Epigastric abdominal pain, acute pyelonephritis versus acute gastritis.
Dx Code: 789.06 (epigastric abdominal pain)
             590.10 (acute pyelonephritis)
             535.00 (acute gastritis without hemorrhage)

NOTE: Code symptoms first followed by conditional diagnoses.

● When a symptom is followed by a contrasting comparative diagnosis, sequence the symptom code first (Example 17.9).

Conditions that are an integral part of a documented disease process should not be coded; abnormal findings should not be coded unless the physician indicates their clinical significance.

The physician should be made aware that certain principal diagnoses are subject to 100% review by the review agency. The physician should pay special attention in using the following as principal diagnoses:

● Arteriosclerotic heart disease (ASHD)—acceptable as a diagnosis only when cardiac catheterization or open heart surgery is performed
● Diabetes mellitus without complications
● Right or left bundle branch block
● Coronary atherosclerosis

Local hospital health information management personnel should be contacted periodically to find out whether new items have been added to this list.

CODING INPATIENT PROCEDURES

ICD-9-CM Volume 3 Procedures

ICD-9-CM Volume 3, which is not used in physician's offices or outpatient hospital billing, is used for the inpatient hospital setting. This volume combines both the alphabetic and tabular lists for the classification of surgical and nonsurgical procedures and miscellaneous therapeutic and diagnostic procedures. Some editions of ICD-9-CM may contain Volumes 1, 2, and 3 in one book.

Currently, ICD-10 guidelines have been developed but not yet adopted, so training has not yet begun. The most likely implementation date is October 2007. The next edition of this textbook will feature how to code using ICD-10-CM. Chapter 5 has information on how the new system will work.

Tabular List

The following tabular list is divided into chapters that relate to operations or procedures for various body systems, with the last chapter referring to miscellaneous diagnostic, therapeutic, and prophylactic procedures. Procedure codes are two digits at the category code level with one or two digits beyond the decimal point. The third and fourth digits differentiate unilateral or bilateral, surgical approach or technique, and condition type (e.g., indirect and direct hernia). No alphabetic characters are used. All four digits must be listed when a three-digit code is followed by a fourth digit. Chapter categories are as follows:

Chapter 1 Operations on the Nervous System	Codes 01–05
Chapter 2 Operations on the Endocrine System	Codes 06–07
Chapter 3 Operations on the Eye	Codes 08–16
Chapter 4 Operations on the Ear	Codes 18–20
Chapter 5 Operations on the Nose, Mouth, and Pharynx	Codes 21–29
Chapter 6 Operations on the Respiratory System	Codes 30–34
Chapter 7 Operations on the Cardiovascular System	Codes 35–39
Chapter 8 Operations on the Hemic and Lymphatic System	Codes 40–41
Chapter 9 Operations on the Digestive System	Codes 42–54
Chapter 10 Operations on the Urinary System	Codes 55–59
Chapter 11 Operations on the Male Genital System	Codes 60–64
Chapter 12 Operations on the Female Genital System	Codes 65–71
Chapter 13 Obstetrical Procedures	Codes 72–75
Chapter 14 Operations on the Musculoskeletal System	Codes 76–84
Chapter 15 Operations on the Integumentary System	Codes 85–86
Chapter 16 Miscellaneous Diagnostic and Therapeutic Procedures	Codes 87–99

Alphabetic Index

The Alphabetic Index is arranged by procedure (e.g., incision, excision, graft, or implant) and not anatomic site. It is used to locate the procedure that is referred to as the main term. Read any notations that appear under the main term in bold type. A main term may be followed by modifiers (e.g., a series of subterms in parentheses) that give differences in site or surgical technique (Example 17.10).

Example 17.10   Main Diagnostic Term

Amputation (cineplastic) (closed flap) (guillotine) (kineplastic) (open) 84.91

An operation named for a person is termed an *eponym*. Such names are listed both as main terms and under the main term "operation." The description of the procedure or anatomic site follows the eponym (Example 17.11).

Example 17.11   Eponyms

Billroth II operation (partial gastrectomy with gastro-jejunostomy) 43.7
Operation
Billroth II (partial gastrectomy with gastroduodenos-tomy) 43.6

Refer to the end of this chapter to learn the step-by-step procedure for coding from ICD-9-CM Volume 3.

CODING OUTPATIENT PROCEDURES

Current Procedural Terminology

An up-to-date edition of CPT, the code book published by the American Medical Association, is used to list procedural codes on outpatient hospital insurance claims for hospital services. Chapter 6 gives basic information and instruction on how to use the code book. These codes are updated during each year. Billing software must be updated with new codes to receive maximum reimbursement.

Health Care Common Procedure Coding System

The HCPCS (pronounced "hick-picks") is used to obtain procedural codes for Medicare and some non–Medicare patients on outpatient hospital insurance claims that are not in the CPT code book (e.g., supplies, equipment rental, and drugs administered other than oral method [injectables, inhalants, and chemotherapeutics]). Chapters 6 and 12 give basic information on the three levels of this code system.

Modifiers

Refer to either Appendix A of the CPT manual or Chapter 6 of this textbook for a detailed explanation of modifier use. Selected CPT level I modifiers that generally are used for outpatient hospital billing are as follows:

● -25 Significant, separately identifiable evaluation and management (service by the same physician on the same day of the procedure or other service
● -27 Multiple outpatient hospital evaluation and management encounters on the same date
● -50 Bilateral procedure
● -52 Reduced services
● -58 Staged or related procedure or service by the same physician during the postoperative period
● -59 Distinct procedural service
● -73 Discontinued outpatient procedure before anesthesia administration
● -74 Discontinued outpatient procedure after anesthesia administration
● -76 Repeat procedure by same physician
● -77 Repeat procedure by another physician
● -78 Return to the operating room for a related procedure during the postoperative period
● -79 Unrelated procedure or service by the same physician during the postoperative period
● -91 Repeat clinical diagnostic laboratory test HCPCS level II alphanumeric modifiers

INPATIENT BILLING PROCESS

The insurance billing division is often part of the hospital's business office and may be placed near the admission department, hospital cashier, or main lobby (entry and exit) of the hospital because patients need easy access. In some facilities, the financial department may be so large that it is relocated to a building at another site. The inpatient billing process involves many people and departments in the hospital. As an introduction, Figure 17–3 shows which main departments of the hospital interact as the billing process flows from beginning to end. Following are explanations of each hospital employee's role in this process.

Admitting Clerk

An admitting clerk registers the patient by interviewing and obtaining personal (demographic) and insurance information and admitting diagnosis or symptoms. There is no law requiring that a person give his or her real name on admission. High-profile individuals often give fictitious names. In some facilities, there may be a preadmission surgery form from which data are obtained

for elective surgery. The admitting clerk position may be outsourced, and he or she may gather information via telephone from home for patients being admitted for elective procedures.

The admitting clerk has the patient sign various legal documents (e.g., consent form for an invasive procedure, insurance assignment form, blanket form for routine hospital procedures, release of information forms, arbitration agreement, verification of acknowledgment of privacy information hospital policies, or responsibility for payment form). Patients must be reminded that they may be excluded from the hospital's daily patient census, which prohibits hospital workers from releasing their condition to the media. Also, a password can be selected by or assigned to each patient being admitted, thereby allowing disclosure to family members and friends who know the password given to them by the patient.

The patient is assigned a patient control number at this time. This is a unique number given for each hospital admission, and a new number is assigned for subsequent admissions. The patient's account contains this number and all charges and payments are posted to this number for the account. Copies of the admitting face sheet, which is similar to the patient registration information form, are sent to the primary care physician or surgeon's office. Registration information, copies of all authorization and signature documents, a copy of the insurance card or cards, and a copy of the emergency department report if the patient is admitted through the emergency department are scanned in paperless facilities or assembled in a financial folder in facilities using a traditional system.

Insurance Verifier

An insurance verifier, who may work either at the hospital or from home, reads the photocopied insurance identification card and telephones the patient or physician for needed data. During or after admission, the insurance verifier's primary responsibility is to contact the insurance plan by either a computer or telephone to verify eligibility, predetermine coverage, and obtain authorization if necessary. In a workers' compensation case, the verifier may telephone the employer or insurance adjuster for needed data.

HOSPITAL BILLING PROCESS

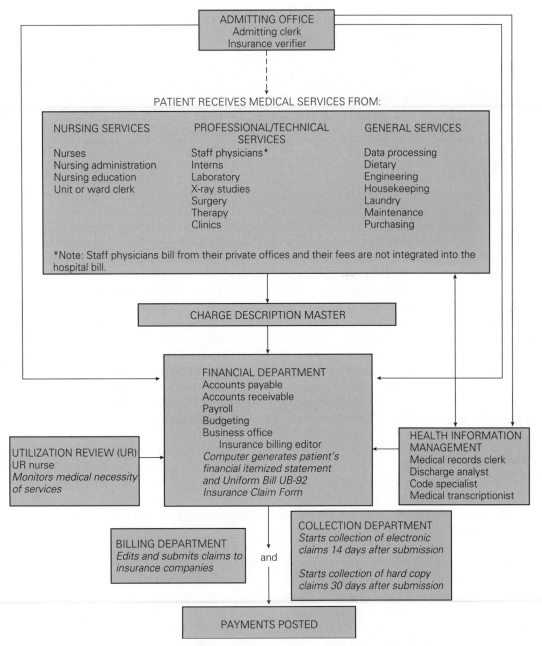

FIGURE 17–3 Basic flow of the hospital billing process for an inpatient.

Attending Physician, Nursing Staff, and Medical Transcriptionist

The patient is taken to the hospital department that is providing the outpatient service or, if an inpatient, to his or her hospital room. Generally it is the attending physician's responsibility to dictate a history and physical (H&P) on admission that lists the admitting diagnosis. A medical transcriptionist transcribes the dictation into a report form. The attending physician and nurses enter daily notations on the patient's medical record as the

patient receives medical services. A unit secretary or ward clerk inputs the physician's orders by use of a computer that electronically transmits them to other departments (e.g., pharmacy, laboratory, and radiology). A handheld computer may be used in some hospitals. If supplies are used, stickers are removed from the supply item and scanned to record data. The attending physician supplies documentation for all medical and surgical reports, ending the patient's stay with a discharge summary that sometimes is known as a *clinical resume*. A final progress note may be substituted for a discharge summary under specific instances, that is, when the inpatient stay does not exceed 48 hours for an uncomplicated condition. This document is transcribed by the medical transcriptionist and includes the course of treatment during the hospital stay, all diagnostic studies, consultations, admission and discharge diagnoses, operations performed, condition of patient at the time of discharge, instructions for continuing care and follow-up treatment, and time frame for postoperative office visit.

Discharge Analyst

A discharge analyst, usually in the medical records department, checks the completeness of each patient's medical record for dictated reports and signatures. He or she completes a deficiency sheet that is put on the medical record indicating any documentation deficiencies. Hospitals bill for services only after the discharge summary is completed and signed by the physician. Many hospitals strive to complete charts within 3 to 4 days, and no more than 14 days, after a patient is discharged; otherwise a cash flow problem will result. Per Joint Commission on Accreditation of Healthcare Organizations (JCAHO), hospital charts may be completed up to 30 days after discharge. The office receptionist (administrative medical assistant) can help by scheduling the physician's time so that medical records can be completed.

Charge Description Master

All services and items provided to the patient are keyed into a computer system to assist with a high volume of billing for services received by hospital patients. This may occur in one of two ways:

1. A designated person in each hospital department keys in all services and procedures using an internal code. This is referred to as *order entry*. The order entry automatically goes to the data processing department.
2. A charge sheet that has services and procedures checked off may be sent to the data processing department where a data processor keys in the information using the internal code. These services, coded with an internal code, link up in a computer system called a **charge description master (CDM).** This is commonly referred to as a "charge master" and includes the following data:
   a. *Procedure code.* CPT and HCPCS codes appear on detail bill, outpatient bill, outpatient paper or electronic Uniform Bill claim form UB-92, but not usually on the inpatient UB-92 claim form.
   b. *Charge.* Dollar amount for each CPT procedure or service. This is a standard fee for the item and not the actual amount paid by a third-party payer.
   c. *Revenue code.* A four-digit code number represents a specific accommodation, ancillary service, or billing

calculation related to service that is inserted in Form Locator 42 of the UB-92 claim form. For example, where the service was performed (0320 = Radiology), where the service may have been provided (0450 = ER), or the total dollar amount of the services provided for a particular time frame/bill/claim (0001 = last entry on the bill). The revenue code must be coded to the highest level of specificity. You may see a code 030X with the "X" indicating further breakdown is needed to best identify the service or supply being provided. Before using a fourth digit, confirm that the code is accepted by the payer. Some payers require the general code (three digit) instead of the four digit. Some revenue codes may indicate that a service should be put on a CMS-1500 claim form instead of a UB-92 claim form. For example, durable medical equipment (DME) code 0292 must be submitted on a CMS-1500 claim form, not on a UB-92, with the correct HCPCS and facility DME provider number. For Medicare, some revenue codes can only be used on an outpatient claim. The facility software should be able to hard-code a revenue code for inpatient but a different revenue code for outpatient for the same service/supply by financial class. An HIPAA compliance issue is that it would be fraudulent for a biller to change a revenue code so that a claim would pass edits.

The master charge list or charge description list is a computer file unique to each hospital that accommodates the charges for items and services that may be provided to patients. The content and format of the charge master varies among facilities, but the function remains the same.

Thus charges may be easily compiled via computer from all hospital departments that furnished services to the patient. For institutional facilities (e.g., inpatient and outpatient departments, rural health clinics, chronic dialysis services, and adult day health care), each patient's data consisting of revenue codes, procedure codes, descriptions, charges, and medical record data are organized by the charge description master and printed onto a hospital paper UB-92 or stored electronically for future claim transmission.

The charge master database must be kept current and accurate to obtain proper reimbursement. It must be regularly audited; otherwise negative impacts, such as overpayment, underpayment, undercharging for services, claims rejections, fines, or penalties, may result. A committee may oversee maintenance of the charge master composed of experts in coding, billing regulations, clinical procedures, and health record documentation. Because this system often is accomplished without human intervention, there is a high risk that a single coding or mapping error could replicate and many errors could occur before being identified and corrected. Duplicate reports of CPT or HCPCS level II codes for the same service, both by the department performing the service and by the HIM coding specialists, is a common billing problem. This problem may be prevented by regularly reviewing the charge master (sorted by CPT code number) with the coding staff so they are aware of the codes reported via the charge master. Category III CPT codes should be reported by only one source, either the department that charges for the service or the code specialist.

In a direct data entry (DDE) system, there is usually a lag time (e.g., from 1 to 4 days after patient discharge) before the bill is "dropped" by the charge master to be sure that all charges have been entered. The word "dropped" refers to the *dropped time*, which is the time between the discharge of the patient from the hospital and the input of the late charges to the time when the final bill is printed.

Code Specialist

The chart is given to health information management, which is directed or managed by a registered health information administrator (RHIA) or registered health information technician (RHIT). In some situations, an RHIA/RHIT may act as a consultant to several hospitals and may not be employed by one hospital. This department is also composed of discharge analysts, coding specialists, and clerical staff. A *medical record number* is assigned at this time. The medical record number never changes (even on future admits), and all records are compiled under this number.

An HIM coder abstracts procedures and diagnoses from the patient's health record and assigns the appropriate codes for the services given. It is possible that the coder may use an encoder to perform this function. As learned, an encoder is a computer software program that assigns a code to represent data. Refer to Chapter 8 for detailed information.

Coding Credentials

Accuracy of coding impacts the financial viability of acute care hospitals. The coder, whose job is highly analytical, not only should abstract information from the medical record and assign the correct code but also should guard against the most common errors of transposing numbers and leaving off fourth and fifth digits from diagnostic codes. A majority of coders in the hospital setting have credentials and often have earned a certificate or degree from an educational institute. A number of different

professional organizations that offer certification for coders are mentioned in Chapter 18.

Insurance Billing Editor

The UB-92 electronic claim form is then generated and reviewed by an insurance billing editor before it is generated as a paper claim or transmitted electronically to the appropriate insurance company to obtain payment. Editing claims is a vital skill that is gained from hands-on experience. Information from the patient's financial data may be compared to verify insurance information. The UB-92 is considered a *summary statement*, which compiles all charges, and is accompanied by a *detailed statement*, which shows itemized charges. The detailed statement, which is sent to the patient, lists dates of services, codes, descriptions, and fees for individual services. The CMS-1500 claim form is used for physicians' professional outpatient claims.

A systematic approach should be established when editing a claim, and the same procedure should be used each time. The procedure of learning to edit a UB-92 is presented at the end of this chapter. This helps train the editor to notice errors or omitted information. Insurance personnel should understand coding, but in a hospital setting it is not their job to assign codes. Final code selection is done by clinical coding specialists. Reviewing form locators (FL) 42 through 47 is the most time-consuming portion of the editing process and the area that requires experience to master. This is the area where most of the errors and omissions occur.

Refer to the procedure at the end of this chapter for a suggested sequence of steps in editing a UB-92 claim.

The claim form may go back to the health information management department after it is edited (where the coder verifies all codes) and to the contract department (where a contractor matches the bill with the insurance type). An adjustment to the account is posted, indicating the dollar amount above that which the insurance carrier will pay according to the contract. This adjustment is done after the insurance payment is received in the majority of hospitals. However, a small number of hospitals are able to write off the portion of the bill that is not covered by the insurance plan before receipt of payment. This transaction is referred to as *relieving the accounts receivable on the front end* and is desirable because the accounts receivable does not appear inflated.

Electronically transmit or mail all claim forms to the insurance carrier for payment and retain computer files or copies for the office files. Document the patient's file with the date mailed and the address to which the insurance claim was filed. The claim may be rejected or delayed if errors are not caught, leading to slow payment or nonpayment. See Chapter 7 for a list of common reasons why claims are rejected or delayed.

Nurse Auditor

Registered nurses (RNs) work as nurse auditors and verify the doctor's orders and the medical record against each charge item on the bill. They may be onsite employees or hired offsite to come in periodically. The nurse must have clinical and financial expertise. A *clean bill* has no errors. An *under bill* has services that have been provided and not billed. An *over bill* has charged items that have not been documented in the chart. A report goes to the health information management department if a coding error or omission occurs. All such accounts have coding priority. Several types of audits follow:

- *Random internal audit.* This occurs continually. Blind charts are pulled and audited to maintain quality control.
- *Audit by request.* The patient can request an audit to verify charges.
- *Defense audit.* The insurance company requests an audit. The insurance auditor may or may not (but should) meet with a hospital auditor, depending on the circumstances. Charts are pulled and audited.

REIMBURSEMENT PROCESS

Generally a hospital bill for inpatient care is much larger than the bill for services rendered in a physician's office. Individuals are admitted to hospitals for severe health problems, and many require major surgery, resulting in considerable expense to the patient. Hospitals use and maintain highly sophisticated, expensive equipment, are located in large facilities, and employ large numbers of personnel, many of whom are state licensed and specialized. Salaries and operating costs must be recovered through patient billing. The majority of hospital reimbursement is from insurance companies. However, working parents with families, elderly people, and jobless persons (even those who have insurance) have found it increasingly difficult to pay their share of the hospital bills. Consequently, accurate and timely hospital billing and good follow-up and collection techniques are in demand.

Reimbursement Methods

Growing numbers of the population are being served by a variety of managed health care programs. All of these programs operate under varying contracts, policies, and guidelines, depending on individual state and federal laws. In negotiating a reimbursement arrangement, the managed care plan administrator tries to obtain discount rates for participation by a hospital in the plan in exchange for an increased volume of patients. These programs use any one or a combination of various payment methods. However, as health care costs escalate, some of these payment methods have been discontinued. Refer to Chapter 11 for definitions on types of managed care plans. A brief description of some reimbursement methods follows:

- *Ambulatory payment classifications.* An outpatient classification system developed by Health Systems International is **ambulatory payment classifications (APCs).** This method is based on procedures rather than diagnoses. For Medicare patients, services associated with a specific procedure or visit are bundled into the APC reimbursement. More than one APC may be billed if more than one procedure is performed, but discounts may be applied to any additional APCs. This topic is discussed in detail at the end of this chapter.
- *Bed leasing.* A managed care plan leases beds from a facility (e.g., payment to the hospital of $300 per bed for 20 beds, regardless of whether those beds are used).
- *Capitation or percentage of revenue.* **Capitation** means reimbursement to the hospital on a per-member per-month basis regardless of whether the patient is hospitalized. **Percentage of revenue** means a fixed percentage paid to the hospital to cover charges.
- *Case rate.* **Case rate** is an averaging after a flat rate (set amount paid for a service) has been given to certain categories of procedures (e.g., normal vaginal delivery is $1800 and cesarean section is $2300). Utilization is expected to be 80% vaginal deliveries and 20% cesarean section; therefore the case rate is $1900 for all deliveries. Specialty procedures also may be given a case rate (e.g., coronary artery bypass graft surgery or heart transplantation). *Bundled case rate* means an all-inclusive rate is paid for both institutional and professional services; for example, for coronary artery bypass graft surgery, a rate is used to pay all who provide services connected with that procedure. Bundled case rates are seen in teaching facilities in which a faculty practice plan works closely with the hospital.
- *Diagnosis-related groups.* A classification system called **diagnosis-related groups (DRGs)** categorizes patients who are medically related with respect to diagnosis and treatment and are statistically similar in length of hospital stay. Medicare and some private hospital insurance payments are based on fixed dollar amounts determined by DRGs. DRGs are discussed in detail later in the chapter.
- *Differential by day in hospital.* The first day of the hospital stay is paid at a higher rate (e.g., the first day may be paid at $1000 and each subsequent day at $500). Most hospitalizations are more expensive on the first day.

This type of reimbursement method may be combined with a per diem arrangement.

- *Differential by service type.* The hospital receives a flat per-admission reimbursement for the service to which the patient is admitted. A prorated payment may be made (e.g., 50% for intensive care and 50% medicine) if services are mixed. Service types are defined in the contract (e.g., medicine, surgery, intensive care, neonatal intensive care, psychiatry, and obstetrics).
- *Fee schedule.* A comprehensive listing of charges based on procedure codes, under a fee-for-service (FFS) arrangement, or discounted FFS, states fee maximums paid by the health plan within the period of the managed care contract. Usually the fee schedule is based on CPT codes. For industrial cases, whether managed care or not, this listing may be called a workers' compensation fee schedule. This document also may be known as a fee maximum schedule or fee allowance schedule.
- *Flat rate.* A set amount (single charge) per hospital admission is paid by the managed care plan, regardless of the cost of the actual services the patient receives.
- *Per diem.* **Per diem** is a single charge for a day in the hospital regardless of actual charges or costs incurred (e.g., a plan that pays $800 for each day regardless of the actual cost of service).
- *Periodic interim payments (PIPs) and cash advances.* These are methods in which the plan advances cash to cover expected claims to the hospital. The fund is replenished periodically. Insurance claims may be applied to the cash advance or may be paid outside it. Generally this is done by Medicare.
- *Withhold.* In this method, part of the plan's payment to the hospital may be withheld or set aside in a bonus pool. If the hospital meets or exceeds the criteria set down, the hospital receives its withhold or bonus; other terms used are bonus pools, capitation, risk pools, or withhold pools.
- *Managed care stop loss outliers.* **Stop loss** is a form of guarantee that may be written into a contract using one of a variety of methods. The purpose is to limit the exposure of cost to a reasonable level to prevent excessive loss. Stop loss is the least understood of reimbursement issues and can leave many thousands of dollars uncollected. There are a number of different ways stop loss can be applied; each contract is different. Become familiar with each contract and the stop loss provisions in it. Following are some methods that may be encountered.
  - *Case-based stop loss.* This is the most common stop loss and can apply to the physician, on a smaller case basis, as well as to the individual hospital claim. For example, the hospital bill may run more than $1 million in cases of premature infants of extremely low birth weight babies. The contract may pay $2000 to $3000 per day, which may reimburse the

hospital several hundred thousand dollars, but the hospital must absorb the excess. Stop loss provisions may pay 65% of the excess over $100,000. Thus the hospital and the insurance carrier share the loss.
  - *Reinsurance stop loss.* The hospital buys insurance to protect against lost revenue and receives less of a capitation fee; the amount they do not receive helps pay for the insurance. For example, after a case reaches $100,000, the plan may receive 80% of expenses in excess of $100,000 from the reinsurance company for the remainder of the year.
  - *Percentage stop loss.* Some managed care contracts pay a percentage of charges when the total charge exceeds $65,000.
  - *Medicare stop loss.* Medicare provides stop loss called *outliers* in its regulations. The *day outliers* for patients who remain in the hospital for long spells of illness no longer apply. Medicare provides cost outliers for those cases in which charges exceed the DRG or $30,000. DRGs are discussed at the end of this chapter.

Some reimbursement methods that are not used very much follow:

- *Charges.* In a managed care plan, **charges** are the dollar amounts owed to a participating provider for health care services rendered to a plan member, according to a fee schedule set by the managed care plan. This is the most expensive and least desirable type of reimbursement contract, so not many of these contracts exist.
- *Discounts in the form of sliding scale.* This is a form of discount with a limit in which the percentage amount increases, based on hospital numbers. For example, a 10% reduction in charges for 0 to 500 total bed days per year with incremental increases in the discount up to a maximum percentage.
- *Sliding scales for discounts and per diems.* Based on total volume of business generated, this is a reimbursement method in which an interim per diem is paid for each day in the hospital. For example, a lump sum is either added to or withheld from the payment due at the end of each year to adjust for actual hospital usage. This is difficult to administer because it can be done either monthly or annually.

Electronic Data Interchange

As early as the 1980s, large hospitals began submitting electronic claims for payment to third-party payers instead of printing out the UB-92 claim form. Just as in the health care provider's office, the use of electronic data interchange (EDI) allows the claim to arrive at the insurance company the same day it is generated to allow for an expeditious payment. Confirmation of claim transmission and receipt is received within minutes or hours. Use of computer software assists the insurance billing editor in checking for errors before forwarding the claim to the proper claims office. This is called **scrubbing** or *cleaning the bill*. Medicare, Medicaid, group health carriers, many managed care plans, and some workers' compensation carriers mandate use of EDI. All hospital electronic billing goes through a clearinghouse where additional edits are made and claims are batched and sent electronically to insurance companies. Billing can be set up according to days or dollar amounts, typically every 30 days. If a Medicare patient remains in an acute care hospital, he or she may be billed on the 60th day and not again until discharge. Refer to Chapter 8 for detailed information on this topic.

Hard Copy Billing

A printed paper copy of the UB-92 that is generated from the computer system is referred to as a *hard copy*. The same edits are made and the claim is cleaned (scrubbed) before it is sent. Some insurance companies are not capable of receiving electronic claims, so billing by hard copy is mandatory. All secondary insurance companies and claims that require attachments also fit into this category.

Receiving Payment

Timeliness of payment may be included in a contract to encourage a hospital to join a plan (e.g., an additional 4% discount for paying a clean claim within 14 days of receipt), or a hospital may demand a penalty for clean claims not processed within 30 days. Some states require this payment by law.

After receipt of payment from insurance and managed care plans, the patient is sent a net bill that lists any owed deductible, coinsurance amount, and charges for services not covered under the insurance policy. Standard bookkeeping procedures are used to post entries showing payments and adjustments. Financial management for managed care programs is discussed and shown in figures in Chapter 11.

OUTPATIENT INSURANCE CLAIMS

The term **outpatient** is used when an individual receives medical service in a section or department of the hospital and goes home the same day. If an individual has an accident, injury, or acute illness, he or she may seek the services of medical personnel in the emergency department of the hospital. When seen in this department, a patient is considered an outpatient unless he or she is admitted for overnight hospital stay. Many elective surgeries are done on an outpatient surgery basis. **Elective surgery** indicates a surgical procedure that can be scheduled in advance, is not an emergency, and is discretionary on the part of the physician and patient. Elective procedures are those that are deferrable, which means that the patient will not experience serious consequences if the operation is postponed or there is failure to undergo the operation. Some insurance policies require a second opinion for elective surgery. The insurance company may not pay if the patient does not seek a second opinion and chooses to undergo surgery. See Chapter 12 for elective surgery in regard to the Medicare program. Patients may receive certain types of therapy and diagnostic testing services on an outpatient basis.

Hospital Professional Services

Although physicians make daily hospital visits to their patients, perform surgeries, discharge patients from the hospital, and are called to the hospital to provide consultations and emergency department treatment, their professional services are submitted on the CMS-1500 insurance claim form by the physician and not by the hospital billing department. Only services provided by the hospital should be submitted by the hospital unless the hospital is billing for physicians who are on the hospital payroll. Such hospital services include the following:

● Emergency department (ED) facility fee (supplies)
● Laboratory (technical component)
● Radiology (technical component)
● Physical and occupational therapy facility fee

Personnel who work in these departments (e.g., ED physician, pathologist, radiologist, and physical therapist) might be employees of the hospital. The hospital submits bills for professional services in that situation. The professional charges are billed independently if the physician is not an employee.

Using the hospital for surgical or medical consultations that could be done in a specialist's office should be avoided unless the patient physically requires admission. This necessity should be documented. If a patient is admitted for consultation only, the entire payment for hospital admission will be denied as will any physician fees involved.

BILLING PROBLEMS

Most hospitals routinely send the patient an itemized list of all charges. Many times, patients are stunned by the total balance due and are unable to make sense of specific items, abbreviations, or codes on the statement. A bill should never show unexplained codes or items without descriptions. A brief hospital stay may translate into hundreds of individual charges. A patient has the right to request, examine, and question a detailed statement, as mentioned in the Patient's Bill of Rights—a nationally recognized code of conduct published by the American Hospital Association. If the bill lumps charges together under broad categories such as pharmacy, surgical supplies, and radiology and the patient requests an itemized invoice, it should be provided at no cost to the patient. In fact, consumer advocates and policies governing the Medicare program encourage consumers to scrutinize their hospital bills for mistakes. The hospital may receive a call or letter from the patient asking for an explanation of the charges if the charges seem exorbitant. Sometimes hospital billing personnel, a hospital patient representative or advocate, the attending physician, and his or her staff may be able to satisfactorily explain a confusing charge.

Common billing errors follow:

● Incorrect name. Use of maiden name instead of married name
● Wrong subscriber. Patient's name listed in error
● Covered days versus noncovered days

Duplicate Statements

Duplicate billings, which may confuse the patient, can occur when a patient receives inpatient and outpatient preadmission tests or services. Perhaps a test was canceled and rescheduled, and a charge is shown for the canceled test; or several physicians may have consulted on a case, and each ordered the same test or therapy. Possibly a technician took the incorrect amount of blood or produced an unclear radiograph, submitted a charge for the service performed in error, as well as for the correct service, and thereby generated two charges for one test. These examples are hospital personnel errors; patients should not have to pay for such mistakes.

Double Billing

Another example involving a violation of Medicare policy is double billing, which results when a patient undergoes routine outpatient testing for a specific diagnosis and then develops unanticipated problems related to that diagnosis that require hospital admission. Outpatient personnel may not be aware that the patient was later admitted, and inpatient personnel may not know that the patient had undergone outpatient testing within the previous 72 hours. A hospital that bills for such services may be fined because it is in violation of the Medicare 3-day window rule. Such charges must be bundled into the inpatient DRG payment. Therefore it is imperative that the hospital billing department develop procedures to check for potential double-billing problems.

Phantom Charges

Physicians order admission procedures for each patient who enters the hospital. If a patient refuses some of these tests, the charges should be deleted from the financial records before the bill is sent out. Similarly, a patient should not be charged for refused medication. The hospital may offer a standard kit of supplies on admission or a new-mother packet when appropriate. A patient should not have to pay for supplies that he or she refuses. If a patient requests a semiprivate room but is sent to a private room because all semiprivate rooms are occupied, the patient should not be billed at the higher rate. Phantom charges may appear if a scheduled test is canceled by a physician or the patient is released early, making it imperative to check the dates and times of admission and discharge. Charges that should appear on a patient's itemized statement may be missing because the charges were transferred to the wrong patient's bill. This requires a review of the patient's medical records. The charge should be deleted from the bill when a charge cannot be accounted for by a review of the patient's medical record or by talking to the attending physician.

HOSPITAL BILLING CLAIM FORM

Uniform Bill Inpatient and Outpatient Paper or Electronic Claim Form

In 1982 the UB-82 claim form was developed for hospital claims and was printed in green ink. A revision was issued in 1992 because it was determined that an update of this form was needed. The **Uniform Bill (UB-92) paper or electronic claim form** is also known as the CMS-1450. This form is considered a summary document supported by an itemized or detailed bill. It is used by institutional facilities (e.g., inpatient and outpatient departments, rural health clinics, chronic dialysis services, and adult day health care) to submit claims for inpatient and outpatient services. This paper claim form is printed in red ink on white paper for processing with optical scanning equipment. Figure 17–4 illustrates a completed UB-92 paper claim form. Dates of service and monetary values are entered without spaces or decimal points (e.g., $200 should be shown as 20000, and June 23, 1995, should be shown as 062395). Dates of birth are entered using two sets of two-digit numbers for the month and day and a four-digit number for the year (e.g., June 23, 1995, should be shown as 06231995). (See Chapter 6 for information on how to complete the CMS-1500 Claim Form for professional services.)

The UB-04 is intended to replace the UB-92, with an implementation date of March 2007 for payers and vendors and May 2007 for providers.

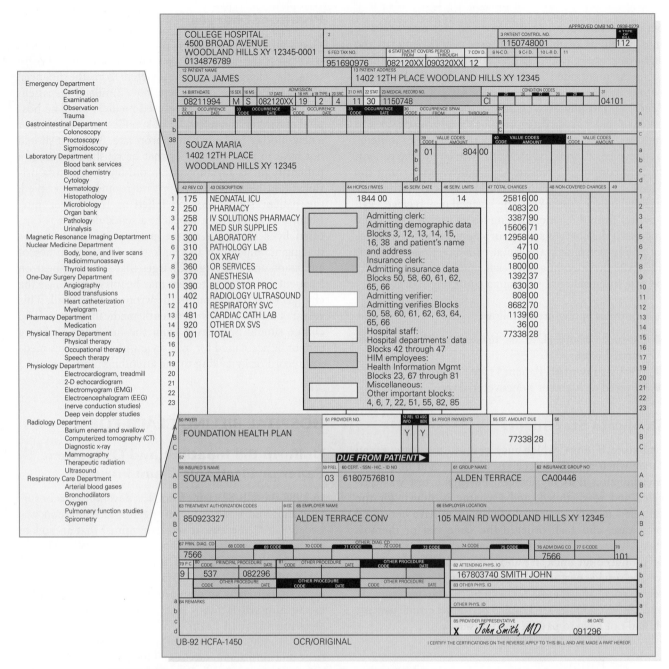

FIGURE 17–4 Scannable (red ink) Uniform Bill (UB-92) insurance paper claim form completed for an inpatient showing hospital departments that input data for hospital services. Colored blocks indicate data obtained by various hospital personnel. Job titles and the exact data each person obtains may vary from facility to facility. Form locator guidelines vary and may not always follow the visual guide presented here.

DIAGNOSIS-RELATED GROUPS

History

The concept of DRGs was developed by Professors John D. Thompson and Robert B. Fetter at Yale University and tested in New Jersey from 1977 to 1979. The goal was to develop a scheme of patient classification to be used in UR.* Soon other applications were found in such areas as budgeting, planning, and reimbursement.

Because of inconsistencies and inadequacies in the original concept, a second set of DRGs was developed and has been used in New Jersey since 1982. Under the Medicare PPS, the DRGs were implemented nationwide for all hospitalizations after the Tax Equity and Fiscal Responsibility Act of 1982 (TEFRA) was passed.

---

*Review of hospital admissions to determine whether they are justified; this is discussed at the beginning of the chapter.

The purpose of a DRG-based system used for Medicare reimbursement is to hold down rising health care costs. Therefore Medicare reimbursement as a whole is expected to decrease significantly under the DRG payment system.

The Diagnosis-Related Groups System

The DRG system is a patient classification method that categorizes patients who are medically related with respect to diagnosis and treatment and who are statistically similar in length of stay. It is used to both classify past cases to measure the relative resources hospitals have expanded to treat patients with similar illnesses and to classify current cases to determine payment. This system changed hospital reimbursement from a fee-for-service system to a lump sum, fixed-fee payment based on the diagnoses rather than on time or services rendered. The fees were fixed by a research team, which determined a national "average" fee for each of the principal discharge diagnoses. The classifications were formed from more than 10,000 ICD-9-CM codes that were divided into 25 basic **major diagnostic categories (MDCs).** These diagnoses were assigned a specific DRG number from 001 to 511 (as of the printing of this edition) and specific values commensurate with geographic areas, types of hospitals, depreciation values, teaching status, and other specific criteria. To obtain DRG information, go to the *Federal Register's* Web site each September for the update, which is mentioned in the Internet Resources at the end of this chapter. TRICARE and other private insurance that use DRGs use DRG numbers 600 to 900. Most MDCs are based on a particular organ system of the body. Within MDCs, DRGs are either medical or surgical. Seven variables are responsible for DRG classifications:

- Principal diagnosis
- Secondary diagnosis (up to eight)
- Surgical procedures (up to six)
- Comorbidity and complications
- Age and sex
- Discharge status
- Trim points (number of hospital days for a specific diagnosis)

At the time of the initial admission review, the physician establishes a tentative diagnosis so that a tentative DRG can be assigned. The tentative DRG is assigned based on: (1) admission diagnosis; (2) scheduled procedures; (3) age; and (4) known secondary diagnoses. An individual in the health information management department obtains the pertinent patient case history information listed in the preceding and codes the principal and secondary diagnoses and operative procedures. Using a computer software program called a **grouper,** this information is keyed in and the program calculates and assigns the DRG payment group. The grouper is not able to consider any differences between chronic and acute conditions. **Looping** is the grouper process of searching all listed diagnoses for the presence of any comorbid condition or complication or searching all procedures for operating room procedures or more specific procedures. If any factors that affect the DRG assignment change or are added, the new information is entered and the case is assigned to the new DRG.

The following is an example of the case of a patient with chronic bronchitis who is admitted to the hospital with pneumonia; his medical record shows that he has had emphysema for many years. Refer to Figure 17–5, which lists the chronic obstructive lung disease diagnostic code as the principal diagnosis, with pneumonia as a secondary diagnosis (inaccurate DRG assignment). This entitles the hospital to receive $2723.66. However, if the pneumonia diagnostic code was listed as the principal diagnosis with two secondary diagnostic codes, emphysema and chronic bronchitis, then the hospital would be entitled to $3294.17—$570 additional reimbursement with the use of the correct DRG assignment.

A case that cannot be assigned to an appropriate DRG because of an atypical situation is called a **cost outlier.** These atypical situations are as follows:

1. Clinical outliers:
   a. Unique combinations of diagnoses and surgeries causing high costs
   b. Very rare conditions
2. Long length of stay, or *day outliers,* no longer apply
3. Low-volume DRGs
4. Inliers (hospital case falls below the mean average or expected length of stay)
5. Death
6. Leaving against medical advice (AMA)
7. Admitted and discharged on the same day

The current federal plan for outliers is the full DRG rate plus an additional payment for the services provided. An unethical practice, **DRG creep,** is to code a patient's DRG category for a more severe diagnosis than indicated by the patient's condition. This is also called *upcoding.*

In hospital billing, *downcoding* can also erroneously occur when sequencing several diagnoses (e.g., listing a normal pregnancy as the primary diagnosis for payment and complications in the secondary position when the patient remained in the hospital for an extended number of days). Additional examples are discussed in Chapter 6.

The amount of payment may be increased by documenting in the patient's medical record any comorbid conditions or complications. When referring to DRGs, the abbreviation CC is used to indicate such complications or comorbidities (not the more common interpretation

SAMPLE CASE HISTORY	
CORRECT DRG ASSIGNMENT	**INACCURATE DRG ASSIGNMENT**

CORRECT DRG ASSIGNMENT		INACCURATE DRG ASSIGNMENT	
MDC 4: Respiratory System		MDC 4: Respiratory System	
Principal Diagnosis	Pneumonia (ICD9CM-486)	Principal Diagnosis	COPID (ICD9CM-496)
Secondary Diagnosis	Emphysema (ICD9CM-492.8)	Secondary Diagnosis	Pneumonia (ICD9CM-486)
Secondary Diagnosis	Chronic Bronchitis (ICD9CM-491.2)	Principal Operative Procedure	None
Principal Operative Procedure	None	Principal Operative Procedure	None
Secondary Operative Procedure	None	Secondary Operative Procedure	None
Age	69 Years	Age	69 Years
Discharge Status	Routine	Discharge Status	Routine
Sex	Male	Sex	Male
Length of Stay	15 Days	Length of Stay	15 Days
DRG	89	DRG	88
Trim Points	4-22 Days	Trim Points	3-19 Days
Rate	$3294.17	Rate	$2723.66

FIGURE 17–5   Case history showing correct and incorrect DRG assignment and the difference in payment between the two.

found in patient charting, Chief Complaint). **Comorbidity** is defined as a preexisting condition that, because of its effect on the specific principal diagnosis, will require more intensive therapy or cause an increase in length of stay by at least 1 day in approximately 75% of cases.

If a patient is admitted because of two or more conditions and the physician fails to indicate the "most resource-intensive" or "most specific" diagnosis as the principal diagnosis, the DRG assessment will be incorrect, resulting in decreased reimbursement to the health care facility (Examples 17.12 and 17.13). It is the responsibility of the attending physician to decide on a principal diagnosis based on his or her best judgment.

Both examples warrant additional payment because of comorbid conditions and complications.

Example 17.12   Comorbid Condition and Complication

A patient has had congestive heart failure for several years and is admitted with an admitting diagnosis of chest pain and principal diagnosis of anterior wall myocardial infarction (MI). While hospitalized, the patient experiences atrial fibrillation.

Principal diagnosis: 410.11 anterior wall myocardial infarction, initial episode

Comorbid condition (CC): 428.0   congestive heart failure

Complication: 427.31   atrial fibrillation

Example 17.13   Comorbid Condition and Complication

A patient has had chronic obstructive pulmonary disease (COPD) for the last 6 months and is admitted with an admitting diagnosis of chest pain and a principal diagnosis of anterior wall myocardial infarction (MI). While hospitalized, the patient experiences respiratory failure.

Principal diagnosis: 410.11   anterior wall myocardial infarction

Comorbid condition: 496   chronic obstructive pulmonary disease

Complication: 799.1   respiratory failure

The *DRG/ICD-9-CM Code Book* is a good reference and code book presented in an easy-to-use binder and containing Volumes 1, 2, and 3 of ICD-9-CM. Sections are color-highlighted for maximum payment. Refer to Appendix B to locate publishers of ICD-9-CM code books.

Diagnosis-Related Groups and the Physician's Office

Even though DRGs affect Medicare hospital payments, the individual in a physician's office who communicates the admitting diagnosis to the hospital can greatly affect the DRG assignment. Remember the following points:

1. Give all of the diagnoses authorized by the physician, if there are more than one, when calling the hospital

to admit a patient so the hospital personnel can use their expertise in listing the primary and secondary diagnoses.

2. Ask the physician to review the treatment or procedure in question when a hospital representative calls about a test, length of stay, or treatments ordered by the attending physician. The hospital needs this information to justify a higher-than-average bill to Medicare.

3. Get to know the hospital personnel on a first-name basis so that when the physician or patients have DRG-related questions, you can call on this hospital expert.

When the DRG system is implemented by other third-party payers or segments of the population other than Medicare patients, you should contact them locally to assist you. Records and hospital insurance claims must contain the correct principal diagnosis, detailed facts to support the principal diagnosis and complications, medical data to justify all procedures performed, patient's age, and discharge diagnosis.

OUTPATIENT CLASSIFICATION

In late 2000 under the requirements of the Balanced Budget Act of 1997, the CMS implemented a PPS for Medicare beneficiaries. This was a move from a cost-based reimbursement system to a line-item billing system for ambulatory surgery centers and hospital outpatient services. The CMS has categorized outpatient services into an ambulatory payment classification system. Some Medicaid programs and private payers have embraced this system because of the escalation of outpatient costs.

Ambulatory Payment Classification System

Originally, ambulatory visit groups (AVGs) and then ambulatory patient groups (APGs) were developed as outpatient classification systems by Health Systems International (HSI). These groups were based on patient classifications (ICD-9-CM diagnoses, CPT and HCPCS procedures, age, and gender) rather than disease classifications. Ambulatory surgery categories (ASCs) were then adopted, replacing APGs for outpatient or 1-day surgery cases that were derived from the surgery section of the CPT. ASCs used disease and procedural coding classification systems to supply the input to the computer program to assign ASCs.

Recently the General Accounting Office (GAO) ordered Congress to begin conversion of surgical, radiologic, and other diagnostic services to an APC system effective August 1, 2000, which replaced ASCs. The more than 500 APCs are continually being modified (added to)

and deleted. Because of this constant state of change, APC information is updated and released twice a year in the *Federal Register*.

APCs are applied to the following:

● Ambulatory surgical procedures
● Chemotherapy
● Clinic visits
● Diagnostic services and diagnostic tests
● Emergency department visits
● Implants
● Outpatient services furnished to nursing facility patients not packaged into nursing facility consolidated billing (services commonly furnished by hospital outpatient departments that nursing facilities are not able to provide [computed tomography, magnetic resonance imaging, or ambulatory surgery)
● Partial hospitalization services for community mental health centers (CMHCs)
● Preventive services (colorectal cancer screening)
● Radiology, including radiation therapy
● Services for patients who have exhausted Part A benefits
● Services to hospice patient for treatment of a nonterminal illness
● Surgical pathology

Hospital Outpatient Prospective Payment System

The development process for APCs is similar to that used for DRGs; however, the procedure code is the primary axis of classification, not the diagnosis code. The reimbursement methodology is based on median costs of services and facility cost to determine charge ratios in addition to copayment amounts. There is also an adjustment for area wage differences, which is based on the hospital wage index currently used for inpatient services. This hospital Outpatient Prospective Payment System (OPPS) may be updated annually, not periodically. An APC group may have a number of services or items packaged within it so that separate payment cannot be obtained.

APC Status

Categories of services have payment status indicators consisting of alpha code letters or symbols. These are the following:

Category	Payment Status Indicator
A	Durable medical equipment, prosthetics and orthotics
A	Physical, occupational and speech therapy
A	Ambulance
A	EPO for ESRD patients

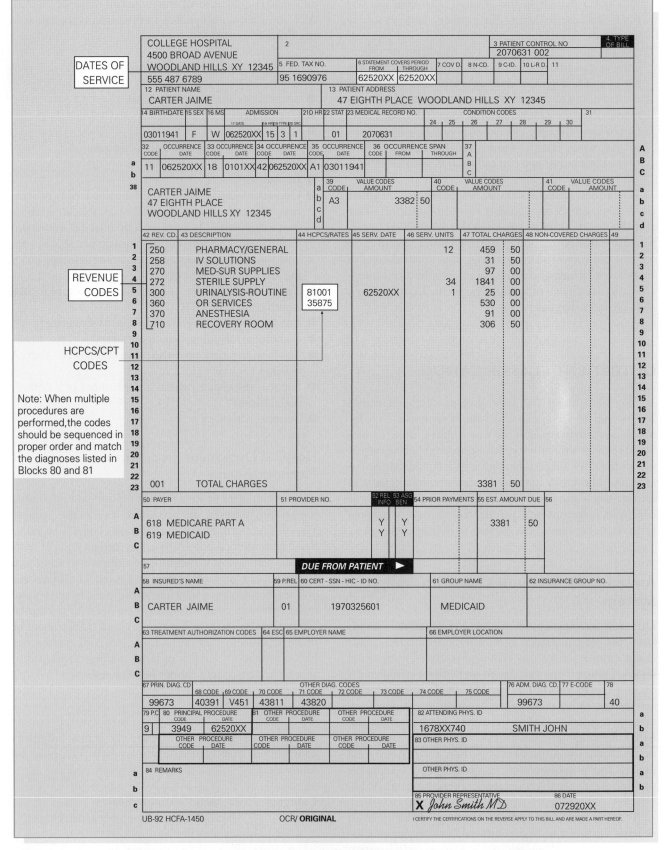

FIGURE 17-6 Scannable (red ink) Uniform Bill (UB-92) insurance paper claim form showing placement of APC data for an outpatient for submission to insurance company.

A	Clinical diagnostic laboratory services
A	Physician services for ESRD patients
A	Screening mammography
C	Inpatient procedures
E	Noncovered items and services
F	Acquisition of corneal tissue
G	Drug/biological pass-through payment
H	Device pass-through payment
K	Non pass-through drug/biological
N	Incidental services, packaged into APC rate
P	Partial hospitalization
S	Significant procedure, not discounted when multiple
T	Significant procedure, multiple procedure reduction applies
V	Visit to clinic or emergency department
X	Ancillary service

Partial hospitalization refers to a distinct and organized intensive psychiatric outpatient day treatment program designed to provide patients with profound and disabling mental health conditions with an individual, coordinated, comprehensive, and multidisciplinary treatment program.

Types of APCs

The four types of APCs follow:

1. *Surgical procedure APCs.* These are surgical procedures for which payment is allowed under the PPS (e.g., cataract removal, endoscopies, and biopsies). Surgical APCs are assigned based on CPT codes.
2. *Significant procedure APCs.* These consist of nonsurgical procedures that are the main reason for the visit and account for the majority of the time and services used during the visit (e.g., psychotherapy, computed tomography and magnetic resonance imaging, radiation therapy, chemotherapy administration, and partial hospitalization). Significant procedure APCs are selected based on CPT codes.
3. *Medical APCs.* These include encounters with a health care professional for evaluation and management services. The medical APC is determined by site of service (clinic or ED), level of the evaluation and management service (CPT code), and diagnosis from one of 20 diagnostic categories (ICD-9-CM code).
4. *Ancillary APCs.* These involve diagnostic tests or treatments not considered to be significant procedure APCs (e.g., plain x-ray film, electrocardiograms, and cardiac rehabilitation). Ancillary APCs are assigned based on CPT codes.

It is possible that multiple APCs can be used when billing for a visit. Use of CPT modifiers for hospital outpatient visits affects APC payments; therefore it is very important to accurately apply correct modifiers when applicable.

Most hospitals use a type of computer encoder program in which the CPT code is input and an APC group code number is assigned. For example, if CPT code number 99282 is input for a low-level emergency department visit, the encoder assigns APC Group 610. Use of an unbundling reference book may be of help in assigning a CPT code; it is preferable to use the code that will generate the highest APC payment.

The data that hospitals submit during the first years of implementation of the APC system are vitally important to the revision of weights and other adjustments that affect payment in future years. The APC data that appear on the UB-92 paper claim form are shown in Figure 17–6.

PROCEDURE

NEW PATIENT ADMISSION AND INSURANCE VERIFICATION

1. Interview the patient and obtain complete and accurate information during initial registration. If an emergency inpatient admission, the managed care program should be notified the next working day or within 48 hours to obtain an authorization number.
2. Write down the information from the physician's office who has telephoned for admittance of the patient.
3. Make photocopies of the front and back of all insurance cards.
4. Contact the insurance company or the insured individual's employer to verify the type of health insurance or telephone the insurance company to verify eligibility and benefits and determine whether prior authorization is needed.
5. Obtain an approved signed treatment authorization request for elective admissions for a Medicaid or TRICARE patient.
6. Collect any copayment or deductible.
7. Obtain information relating to the injured patient, industrial accident, insurance carrier, and employer for a patient injured on the job.
8. Get an authorization for admission, length of stay, and all surgical procedures for an elective admission of a patient injured on the job from the workers' compensation insurance adjuster.
9. Ask the patient to read and sign the necessary hospital admitting documents (e.g., Notice of Privacy document, surgical consent form, financial agreement, and so on).

PROCEDURE

CODING FROM ICD-9-CM VOLUME 3

Basic steps in coding from Volume 3 of ICD-9-CM code book are as follows:

1. Locate the main term (procedure) in the Alphabetical Index.
2. Read all modifiers (descriptive notations relating to the condition).
3. Obtain the code number and refer to the Tabular List (Volume 3) to verify that the code number selected matches the description of the procedure. Never code using only the Alphabetical Index because important instructions may appear in the Tabular List.
4. Note any exclusions, inclusions, remarks concerning fourth digits, colons, and any other information that may affect the choice of codes. Notice "code also" and "omit code" instructions.

5. Select the appropriate code number. Use fourth digit codes and, if necessary, apply two or more code numbers to completely describe a procedure (Example 17.14).

Example 17.14

Procedure: Complete vaginal hysterectomy with bilateral salpingectomy

CODE	DESCRIPTION
68.5	Vaginal hysterectomy
66.51	Removal of both fallopian tubes at same operative episode

---

PROCEDURE

EDITING A UNIFORM BILL (UB-92) PAPER OR ELECTRONIC CLAIM FORM

Each field or block is called a Form Locator (FL).

1. Review the top left corner to determine if the facility information is printed (FLs 1 and 5).
2. Determine whether it is an inpatient (11X) or outpatient (13X) type of bill (FL 4).
3. Scan the UB-92 claim form to determine who the patient is (FL 12), the responsible party (FL 38), the insured (FL 58), and the patient's relationship to the insured (FL 59).
4. Check the birth date of the patient (FL 14); it should be printed in eight digits.
5. Confirm the gender of the patient (FL 15), comparing it with the patient's name (FL 12). If the patient's name could be used for either gender, verify the sex by reviewing the patient's insurance identification card, patient's medical record, or handwritten admitting record.
6. Verify the insurance information including the payer (FL 50), certificate, Social Security, or insurance identification number (FL 60), group name (FL 61), insurance group number (FL 62), employer name (FL 65), and employer location (FL 66). FLs 50 and 60 are mandatory.
7. Confirm that data are present by reviewing the following: principal diagnostic code (FL 67), admitting diagnostic code (FL 76), and DRG number (FL 78) if applicable.
8. Verify that there is a principal procedure code with date (FL 80) and all other procedures with date(s) or service (FL 81). These should match the sequence and services provided and should appear in FL 43.

9. Verify that there is an attending, referring, or prescribing physician with identification number listed (FL 82). A physician other than the attending physician should be listed (FL 83).
10. Cross-check the third digit in FL 4, indicating the bill type with statement from and through dates (FL 6), admission date (FL 17), and occurrence date (FL 32) to determine whether this is the first bill. If it is not, look at the original bill so all entries are understood.
11. Inpatient: Verify the number of hospital days for semiprivate or coronary care unit (CCU) room charges (FL 42 through 47). Compare the number of units (FL 46) with the total number of inpatient days (FL 7). These should match. Look at the hour the patient was admitted (FL 18) and the hour of discharge (FL 21) if there is a discrepancy.
12. Correlate the room rates (FL 47) with the preceding services, making sure the per diem is based on the revenue. The computer software program takes the number of days and multiplies that by the room rate, and this figure equals the amount of the revenue shown.
13. Review all of the patient's services listed (FL 42) line by line. Each service listed must show a unit value (FL 46). Search for any revenue codes that may be used for a special type of service that may be itemized and charged separately (e.g., 0274 through 0279 implants or 0258 through 0259 special drugs).
14. Outpatient: Verify that each service described (FL 43) has a CPT or HCPCS code (FL 44) and a date of service listed (FL 45).

PROCEDURE—CONT'D

15. Check the detailed patient's health record (chart) if there is a question about a service listed. All services must be listed by hospital department.
16. Verify the total amount due by adding all amounts (FL 47) and comparing them with the last line item

in FL 42 (001), Fl 43 (Total), and final totaled amount as the last line entry in FL 47.
17. Determine whether the estimated amount due from the insurance company is calculated and shown (FL 55).
18. Sign and date (FLs 85 and 86).

PROCEDURE

COMPLETING THE UB-92 PAPER OR ELECTRONIC CLAIM FORM

Only general guidelines for completing the UB-92 claim form are mentioned here. The medical hospital manual and, if available, the local UB-92 manual should always be consulted to determine whether billing guidelines pertain to a particular region. No guidelines had been published about insertion of the APC group number for outpatient claims at the time this edition was printed. The recommendation is to use either FL 75 or 84 for this purpose. The UB-92 claim form is in the process of being revised, and guidelines will be released when that becomes available. Some facilities are grouping claims in-house that relate to APCs before submitting them to the fiscal intermediaries. The following color screens, item numbers, and descriptions correspond to Figure 17–4, which shows a completed UB-92 paper claim form for inpatient claims.

FL 1.
Field Name/Description. Enter the provider name, address, city, state, and ZIP code on the first three lines. Enter telephone number, fax number, or county code applicable to the provider on the fourth line. Medicaid, Medi-Cal, and Medicare: The fourth line is optional. TRICARE: The fourth line is required.

FL 2.
Untitled. Leave blank.

FL 3.
Patient Control Number. This is an optional form locator that can be used to identify an individual patient account. It is the patient's medical record number or account number in some facilities. Medicare: Required.

FL 4.
Type of Bill. Enter the appropriate three-digit bill code as specified in the UB-92 Manual Billing Procedures. The digits indicate the following:
First digit (type of facility)
   1 = Hospital (acute)
   2 = Skilled nursing facility
   3 = Home health
Second digit (bill classification)
   1 = Inpatient
   3 = Outpatient

Third digit (frequency). Use of this digit may change according to facility.
   1 = Admit to discharge
   2 = Interim—First claim
   3 = Interim—Continuing claim
   4 = Interim—Last claim
   5 = Late charge bill
Medi-Cal: Optional. Medicare: Required.

FL 5.
Federal Tax Number. Enter the facility's provider federal tax number. This number is also called a tax identification number (TIN) or employer identification number (EIN). Medi-Cal and Medicare: Not required. Private payers and TRICARE: Required. Some Medicaid programs: A number in this field may be required.

FL 6.
Statement Covers Period. Enter beginning and ending dates of service for the period shown on the bill (e.g., 011820XX to 012020XX). The electronic version requires an eight-character date listing year, month, and day: 20XX0118 to 20XX0120. Medicare and Private payers: Required. Medi-Cal: Not required.

FL 7.
Covered Days. Enter number of inpatient days covered by primary insurance carrier. Medicare: Required. Private payers and Medicaid: Depending on plan or state policies, may be required. Medi-Cal and TRICARE: Not required.

FL 8.
Noncovered Days. Enter the days of care not covered by the primary insurance carrier. Medicare: Required. Private payers and Medicaid: Depending on plan or state policies, may be required. Medi-Cal and TRICARE: Not required.

FL 9.
Coinsurance Days. Medicare: Enter inpatient days occurring after the 60th day and before the 91st day of one illness. Medicare/Medicaid and Medicare/supplemental insurance: Required. Medi-Cal and TRICARE: Not required.

Continued

PROCEDURE—CONT'D

COMPLETING THE UB-92 PAPER OR ELECTRONIC CLAIM FORM

FL 10.

Lifetime Reserve Days. Under Medicare, each beneficiary has a lifetime reserve of 60 additional days of inpatient hospital services after using 90 days of inpatient hospital services during an occurrence of illness. Medicare: Required. Medicare/ Medicaid and Medicare/supplemental insurance: Must be completed for patients. Medicaid, Medi-Cal, and TRICARE: Not required.

FL 11.

Reserved for State Assignment. Leave blank.

FL 12.

Patient's Name. Enter the patient's last name, first name, and middle initial. Avoid nicknames or aliases.

FL 13.

Patient's Address. Enter the patient's street address, city, state, and ZIP code. Private payers, some Medicaid programs, Medicare, and TRICARE: Required. Medi-Cal: Not required.

FL 14.

Patient's Birth Date. Enter the patient's date of birth in an eight-digit format (e.g., June 1, 20XX, becomes 060120XX). Private payers and Medicare: Required.

FL 15.

Patient's Sex. Enter a capital "M" for male, or "F" for female. Private payers and Medicare: Required.

FL 16.

Patient's Marital Status. S indicates single; M, married; P, life partner (also called domestic partner and significant other); D, divorced; W, widowed; X, legally separated; and U, unknown. Some private payers and TRICARE: Enter marital status of the patient on date of registration as an in patient or outpatient or at the start of care. Medicaid, Medi-Cal, and Medicare: Not required.

FL 17.

Admission/Start of Care Date. Enter admission or start of care date. The electronic version requires an eight-character date in this format: 20XX 0710. Medi-Cal: Not required. Medicaid, Medicare, third-party payers, and TRICARE: Required.

FL 18.

Admission Hour. Enter the hour during which the patient was admitted for inpatient or outpatient care in two numeric characters using the 24-hour clock (e.g., midnight is 00 and noon is 12, 1 to 1:59 AM is 01, 1 to 1:59 PM is 13, 11:59 is shown as 23; Figure 17-7). Private payers and TRICARE: Required. Medicare and Medicare/Medi-Cal: Not required.

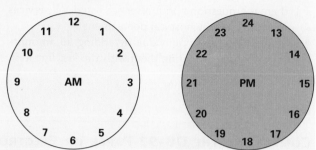

FIGURE 17-7   Clock face depicting standard AM time and clock face depicting PM military time.

FL 19.

Admission Type. Enter the code indicating the priority of the inpatient admission. Coding structure: 1 = indicates emergency; 2 = urgent; 3 = elective; 4 = newborn; and 9 = information not available. Private payers, some Medicaid programs, Medicare, and TRICARE: Required when inpatient claim submitted. Medi-Cal: Not required.

FL 20.

Source of Admission. Enter the code indicating the source of the admission or outpatient service. Medicare, private payers, and TRICARE: Required. Medicaid and Medi-Cal: Not required. Code as follows:

Source of Admission Codes	
1	Physician referral
2	Clinic referral
3	Health maintenance organization (HMO) referral
4	Transfer from a hospital
5	Transfer from a skilled nursing facility (SNF)
6	Transfer from another health care facility
7	Emergency department
8	Court/law enforcement
9	Information not available
A	Transfer from a critical access hospital
B	Transfer from another home health agency
C	Readmission to some home health agency
D-Z	Reserved for national assignment

Newborn Codes	
1	Normal delivery
2	Premature delivery
3	Sick baby
4	Extramural birth
5-8	Reserved for national assignment
9	Information not available

PROCEDURE—CONT'D

FL 21.

Discharge Hour. Enter hour when patient was discharged from inpatient care. Hours are indicated by two numeric characters using the 24-hour clock (e.g., midnight is 00 and noon is 12, 1 to 1:59 AM is 01, 1 to 1:59 PM is 13, 11:59 is 23; see Figure 17–8). Medicaid: May be required. Private payers and TRICARE: Required. Medi-Cal and Medicare: Not required.

FL 22.

Patient Status. Enter a code indicating the patient's disposition as of the ending date of service for the period of care reported. Private payers, Medicaid, Medicare, and TRICARE: Required for inpatient claims. Medi-Cal: Not required.

Patient Status Codes	
01	Discharged to home or self-care (routine discharge)
02	Discharged/transferred to another short-term general hospital for inpatient care
03	Discharged or transferred to SNF with Medicare certification
04	Discharged or transferred to an intermediate care facility
05	Discharged or transferred to a non-Medicare PPS children's hospital or non-Medicare PPS cancer hospital for inpatient care
06	Discharged or transferred to home under care of organized home health service organization
07	Left against medical advice or discontinued care
08	Discharged or transferred to home under care of home intravenous therapy provider
09	Admitted as an inpatient to this hospital
10-19	Reserved for national assignment
20	Expired
21-29	Reserved for national assignment
30	Still a patient
31-39	Reserved for national assignment
40	Expired at home (for hospice care)
41	Expired in a medical facility such as a hospital, SNF, intermediate care facility, or freestanding hospice (for hospice care)
42	Expired, place unknown (for hospice care)
43	Discharged or transferred to a federal health care facility
44-49	Reserved for national assignment
50	Discharged to hospice or home
51	Discharged to hospice or medical facility
52-60	Reserved for national assignment
61	Discharged/transferred within this institution to a hospital-based Medicare-approved swing bed
62	Discharged or transferred to an inpatient rehabilitation facility (IRF) including rehabilitation distinct part units of a hospital
63	Discharged or transferred to a Medicare certified long term care hospital (LTCH)
64	Discharged or transferred to a nursing facility certified under Medicaid but not certified under Medicare
65	Discharged or transferred to a psychiatric hospital or psychiatric distinct part unit of a hospital
66-70	Reserved for national assignment
71	Reserved for national assignment
72	Reserved for national assignment
73-99	Reserved for national assignment

FL 23.

Medical Record Number. Enter the number assigned by the provider to the patient's medical record. Private payers, Medicare, and TRICARE: Required. Some Medicaid programs: May be required.

FLs 24-30.

Condition Codes. The codes help determine patient eligibility and benefits from primary or secondary insurance coverage and affect payer processing.

Condition Codes	
01	Military service related
02	Condition is employment related
03	Patient is covered by insurance not reflected here
04	Information only bill
05	Lien has been filed
06	End-stage renal disease (ESRD) patient in first 18 months of entitlement covered by employer group health insurance
07	Treatment of nonterminal condition for hospice patient
08	Beneficiary will not provide information concerning other insurance coverage
09	Neither patient nor spouse is employed
10	Patient or spouse is employed but no employer group health plan (EGHP) coverage exists
11	Disabled beneficiary, but no large group health plan (LGHP) coverage exists
12-16	Reserved for payer use only

Continued

PROCEDURE—CONT'D

COMPLETING THE UB-92 PAPER OR ELECTRONIC CLAIM FORM

17	Patient is homeless
18	Maiden name retained
19	Child retains mother's name
20	Beneficiary requested billing
21	Billing for denial notice
22	Patient is on multiple drug regimens
23	Home caregiver is available
24	Home intravenous therapy patient also receiving home health agency (HHA) services
25	Patient is a non–U.S. resident
26	Veterans Affairs—eligible patient chooses to receive services in Medicare–certified facility
27	Patient is referred to a sole community hospital for a diagnostic laboratory test
28	Patient or spouse's EGHP is secondary to Medicare
29	Disabled beneficiary or family member's LGHP is secondary to Medicare
30	Non-research services provided to patients enrolled in a qualified clinical trial
31	Patient is student (full-time day)
32	Patient is student (cooperative or work study program)
33	Patient is student (full-time night)
34	Patient is student (part-time)
35	Reserved for national assignment
36	General care patient is in a special unit
37	Ward accommodation at patient's request
38	Semiprivate room is not available
39	Private room is medically necessary
40	Same-day transfer
41	Partial hospitalization
42	Continuing care is not related to inpatient admission
43	Continuing care is not provided within prescribed postdischarge window
44	Inpatient admission changed to outpatient
45	Reserved for national assignment
46	TRICARE Nonavailability Statement on file
47	Reserved for TRICARE
48	Claims submitted by a TRICARE–authorized psychiatric residential treatment center (RTC) for children and adolescents
49-54	Reserved for national assignment.
55	SNF bed is not available
56	Medical appropriateness. SNF admission was delayed more than 30 days after hospital discharge
57	SNF readmission
58	Terminated Medicare and choice organization enrollee

59	Nonprimary ESRD facility
60	Reports the stay was a day outlier
61	Requests additional payment for the stay as a cost outlier
62	Payer code indicating bill was paid under a DRG
63	Incarcerated beneficiaries
64-65	Payer only codes
66	Provider does not wish cost outlier payment
67	Beneficiary elects not to use lifetime reserve (LTR) days
68	Beneficiary elects to use LTR days
69	Operating indirect medical education (IME) payment only
70	Self-administered epoetin (EPO) for home dialysis patient
71	Full care in dialysis unit
72	Self-care in dialysis unit
73	Self-care in dialysis training
74	Patient receiving dialysis services at home
75	Home dialysis—100% payment
76	Backup in-facility dialysis
77	Provider accepts or is obligated or required because a contractual arrangement or law to accept payment by a primary payer as payment in full
78	New coverage not implemented by HMO
79	Comprehensive outpatient rehabilitation facility (CORF) services provided offsite
80-99	Reserved for state assignment
A0	TRICARE External Partnership Program
A1	Early Periodic Screening Diagnosis Treatment/Child Health Assurance Program (EPSDT/CHAP)
A2	Physically handicapped children's program
A3	Special federal funding
A4	Family planning
A5	Disability
A6	Medicare pneumococcal pneumonia vaccine (PPV) services; influenza virus vaccine
A7-A8	Reserved for national assignment
A9	Second opinion surgery
AA	Abortion performed due to rape
AB	Abortion performed due to incest
AC	Abortion performed due to serious fetal genetic defect, deformity, or abnormality
AD	Abortion performed due to a life-endangering physical condition caused by, arising from, or exacerbated by the pregnancy itself
AE	Abortion performed due to physical health of mother that is not life endangering

PROCEDURE—CONT'D

AF	Abortion performed due to emotional or psychological health of the mother
AG	Abortion performed due to social or economic reasons
AH	Elective abortion
AI	Sterilization
AJ	Payer responsible for copayment
AK	Air ambulance required
AL	Specialized treatment or bed unavailable
B4-BZ	Reserved for national assignment
C0	Reserved for national assignment
C1	Approved as billed
C2	Automatic approval as billed based on focused review
C3	Partial approval
C4	Admission or services denied
C5	Postpayment review applicable
C6	Admission preauthorization
C7	Extended authorization
C8-CZ	Reserved for national assignment
D0	Change to services dates
D1	Change to charges
D2	Changes in revenue codes or HCPCS or HIPPS rate codes
D3	Second or subsequent interim prospective payment system bill
D4	Change in ICD-9-CM diagnosis and/or procedure codes
D5	Cancel to correct health insurance claim number (HICN) or provider identification number
D6	Cancel only to repay a duplicate or Office of the Inspector General (OIG) overpayment
D7	Change to make Medicare the secondary payer
D8	Change to make Medicare the primary payer
D9	Any other change
E0	Change in patient status
E1-E9	Reserved for national assignment
GI-G9	Reserved for national assignment
HO	Delayed filing, statement of intent submitted
H1-LZ	Reserved for national assignment
MO-MZ	Reserved for payer assignment
NO-WZ	Reserved for national assignment
XO-ZZ	Reserved for national assignment

FL 31.
Reserved for National Assignment.

FLs 32-35.
Occurrence Codes and Dates. Occurrence codes and dates are used to identify significant events relating to a

bill that may affect payer processing (e.g., determination of liability, coordination of benefits, or administration of subrogation clauses in benefit programs). The electronic version requires an eight-character date listing year, month, and day: 20XX0328. A total of seven occurrence codes and dates may be reported on a UB-92. Private payers or Medicare: Required.

Occurrence Codes and Dates	
01	Auto accident or medical coverage
02	No-fault insurance involved including auto accident or other
03	Accident—tort liability
04	Accident—employment related
05	Accident or no medical or liability coverage
06	Crime victim
07-08	Reserved for national assignment
09	Start of infertility treatment cycle
10	Last menstrual period
11	Onset of symptoms or illness
12	Date of onset for a chronically dependent individual (CDI) (HHA claims only)
13-15	Reserved for national assignment
16	Date of last therapy
17	Date outpatient occupational therapy plan established or last reviewed
18	Date of retirement of patient and beneficiary
19	Date of retirement of spouse
20	Guarantee of payment began
21	UR notice received
22	Date active care ended
23	Date of cancellation of hospice election period
24	Date insurance denied
25	Date benefits terminated by primary payer
26	Date SNF bed became available
27	Date of hospice certification or recertification
28	Date comprehensive outpatient rehabilitation plan established or last reviewed
29	Date outpatient physical therapy plan established or last reviewed
30	Date outpatient speech pathology plan established or last reviewed
31	Date beneficiary notified of intent to bill (accommodations)
32	Date beneficiary notified of intent to bill (diagnostic procedures or treatments)
33	First day of the Medicare coordination period for ESRD beneficiaries covered by an EGHP
34	Date of election of extended care services
35	Date treatment started for physical therapy

Continued

PROCEDURE—CONT'D

COMPLETING THE UB-92 PAPER OR ELECTRONIC CLAIM FORM

36	Date of inpatient hospital discharge for covered transplant patient
37	Date of inpatient hospital discharge for noncovered transplant patient
38	Date treatment started for home intravenous therapy
39	Date discharged on a continuous course of intravenous therapy
40	Scheduled date of admission
41	Date of first test for preadmission testing
42	Date of discharge (hospice only)
43	Scheduled date of canceled surgery
44	Date treatment started for occupational therapy
45	Date treatment started for speech therapy
46	Date treatment started for cardiac rehabilitation
47	Date cost outlier status begins
48-49	Payer codes
50-69	Reserved for national assignment
70-99	Reserved for occurrence span codes
A0	Reserved for national assignment
A1	Birthdate—insured A
A2	Effective date—insured A policy
A3	Benefits exhausted
A4	Split Bill date
A5-AZ	Reserved for national assignment
B0	Reserved for national assignment
B1	Birthdate—insured B
B2	Effective date—insured B policy
B3	Benefits exhausted
B4-BZ	Reserved for national assignment
C0	Reserved for national assignment
C1	Birthdate—insured C
C2	Effective date—insured C policy
C3	Benefits exhausted
C4-CZ	Reserved for national assignment
D0-DZ	Reserved for national assignment
E0	Reserved for national assignment
E1	Birthdate—insured D
E2	Effective date—insured D policy
E3	Benefits exhausted
E4-EZ	Reserved for national assignment
F0	Reserved for national assignment
F1	Birthdate—insured E
F2	Effective date—insured E policy
F3	Benefits exhausted
F4-FZ	Reserved for national assignment
G0	Reserved for national assignment
G1	Birthdate—insured F
G2	Effective date—insured F policy

G3	Benefits exhausted
G4-GZ	Reserved for national assignment
H0-IZ	Reserved for national assignment
J0-LZ	Reserved for national assignment
M0-ZZ	See FL 36 occurrence span codes

FL 36.

Occurrence Span Codes and Dates. Enter code identifying occurrence that happened over a span of time. The electronic version requires an eight-character date listing year, month, and day (20XX0812). Medicaid: Complete when required. Private payer, Medicare, and TRICARE: Required.

Occurrence Span Codes and Dates

70	Qualifying stay dates (for SNF use only)
71	Prior stay dates
72	First and last visits
73	Benefit eligibility period
74	Noncovered level of care or leave of absence (LOA)
75	SNF level of care
76	Patient liability period
77	Provider liability period
78	SNF prior stay dates
79	Payer code
80-99	Reserved for national assignment
MO	PRO/UR approved stay dates (partial approval)
M1	Provider liability—no utilization
M2	Dates of inpatient respite care
M3	ICF level of care
M4	Residential level of care
M5-WZ	Reserved for national assignment
XO-ZZ	Reserved for national assignment

FL 37.

Internal Control Number (ICN)/Document Control Number (DCN). Enter the ICN or DCN assigned to the original bill by the payer or the payer's intermediary. Medicaid: May be required depending on contract requirements. Medi-Cal and private payers: Not required. Medicare: Required. TRICARE: For reporting claim changes.

FL 38.

Responsible Party Name and Address. Enter the name and address of the party responsible for the bill. Private payers: Required. Medicaid, Medi-Cal, Medicare, or TRICARE: Not required.

PROCEDURE—CONT'D

FLs 39-41.

Value Codes and Amounts. Enter codes that have related dollar amounts that identify monetary data required for processing claims. Medicaid: May be required depending on state policy. Private payer, Medicare, and TRICARE: Complete when applicable. Enter the value codes as described in the following:

Value Codes	
01	Most common semiprivate room rate
02	Hospital has no semiprivate rooms
03	Reserved for national assignment
04	Inpatient professional component charges that are combined billed
05	Professional component included in charges and also billed separately to carrier
06	Medicare blood deductible amount
07	Reserved for national assignment
08	Medicare lifetime reserve amount in the first calendar year
09	Medicare coinsurance amount in the first calendar year in billing period
10	Medicare lifetime reserve amount in the second calendar year
11	Medicare coinsurance amount for second calendar year
12	Working aged beneficiary or spouse with EGHP
13	ESRD in a Medicare coordination period for an EGHP
14	No-fault insurance, including auto or other
15	Workers' compensation
16	Public health service (PHS) or other federal agency
17	Outlier amount
18	Disproportionate share amount
19	Indirect medical education amount
20	Total prospective payment system capital payment amount
21	Catastrophic
22	Surplus
23	Recurring monthly income
24	Medicaid rate code
25	Offset to the patient-payment amount—prescription drugs
26	Offset to the patient-payment amount—hearing and ear services
27	Offset to the patient-payment amount—vision and eye services
28	Offset to the patient-payment amount—dental services
29	Offset to the patient-payment amount—chiropractic services
30	Preadmission testing
31	Patient liability amount
32	Multiple patient ambulance transport
33	Offset to the patient-payment amount—podiatric services
34	Offset to the patient-payment amount—other medical services
35	Offset to the patient-payment amount—health insurance premiums
36	Reserved for national assignment
37	Pints of blood furnished
38	Blood deductible pints
39	Pints of blood replaced
40	New coverage not implemented by HMO (for inpatient claims only)
41	Black lung
42	Veterans affairs
43	Disabled beneficiary under age 65 with LGHP
44	Amount provider agreed to accept from primary insurer when this amount is less than total charges but greater than the primary insurer's payment
45	Accident hour
46	Number of grace days
47	Any liability insurance
48	Hemoglobin reading
49	Hematocrit reading
50	Physical therapy visits
51	Occupational therapy visits
52	Speech therapy visits
53	Cardiac rehabilitation visits
54	Newborn birth weight in grams
55	Eligibility threshold for charity care
56	Skilled nurse—home visit hours (HHA only)
57	Home health aide—home visit hours (HHA only)
58	Arterial blood gas (PO_2/PA_2)
59	Oxygen saturation (O_2 SAT/oximetry)
60	HHA branch metropolitan statistical area (MSA)
61	Location where service is furnished (HHA and hospice)
62	HHA visits—Part A
63	HHA visits—Part B
64	HHA reimbursement—Part A
65	HHA reimbursement—Part B
66	Medicaid spend down amount
67	Peritoneal dialysis
68	EPO—drug
69	State charity care percent

Continued

PROCEDURE—CONT'D

COMPLETING THE UB-92 PAPER OR ELECTRONIC CLAIM FORM

70-72	Payer codes
73	Drug deductible; payer code
74	Drug coinsurance; payer code
75-76	Gramm-Rudman-Hollings reduction—for payers use only
77	Payer code; new technology add-on payment
78-79	Payer codes
80-99	Reserved for state assignment
A0	Special zip code reporting
A1	Deductible payer A
A2	Coinsurance payer A
A3	Estimated responsibility payer A
A4	Covered self-administrable drugs—emergency
A5	Covered self-administrable drugs—not self administered in form and situation furnished to patient
A6	Covered self-administrable drugs—diagnostic study and other
A7	Copayment payer A
A8	Patient weight
A9	Patient height
AA	Regulatory surcharges, assessments, allowances or health care related taxes payer A
AB	Other assessments or allowances (e.g., medical education) payer A
AC-AZ	Reserved for national assignment
B0	Reserved for national assignment
B1	Deductible payer B
B2	Coinsurance payer B
B3	Estimated responsibility payer B
B4-B6	Reserved for national assignment
B7	Copayment payer B
B8-B9	Reserved for national assignment
BA	Regulatory surcharges, assessments, allowances or health care related taxes payer B
BB	Other assessments or allowances (e.g., medical educational) payer B
C0	Reserved for national assignment
C1	Deductible payer C
C2	Coinsurance payer C
C3	Estimated responsibility payer C
C4-C6	Reserved for national assignment
C7	Copayment payer C
C8-C9	Reserved for national assignment
CA	Regulatory surcharges, assessments, allowances, or health care related taxes payer C
CB	Other assessments or allowances (e.g., medical education) payer C

CC-CZ	Reserved for national assignment
D0-D2	Reserved for national assignment
D3	Estimated responsibility patient
D4-DZ	Reserved for national assignment
E0	Reserved for national assignment
E1	Deductible payer D
E2	Coinsurance payer D
E3	Estimated responsibility payer D
E4-E6	Reserved for national assignment
E7	Copayment payer D
E8-E9	Reserved for national assignment
EA	Regulatory surcharges, assessments, allowances or health care related taxes payer D
EB	Other assessments or allowances (e.g., medical educational) payer D
EC-EZ	Reserved for national assignment
F0	Reserved for national assignment
F1	Deductible payer E
F2	Coinsurance payer E
F3	Estimated responsibility payer E
F4-F6	Reserved for national assignment
F7	Copayment payer E
F8-F9	Reserved for national assignment
FA	Regulatory surcharges, assessments, allowances or health care related taxes payer E
FB	Other assessments or allowances (e.g., medical education) payer E
FC-FZ	Reserved for national assignment
G0	Reserved for national assignment
G1	Deductible payer F
G2	Coinsurance payer F
G3	Estimated responsibility payer F
G4-G6	Reserved for national assignment
G7	Copayment payer F
G8-G9	Reserved for national assignment
GA	Regulatory surcharges, assessments, allowances or health care related taxes payer F
GB	Other assessments or allowances (e.g., medical education) payer F
GC-GZ	Reserved for national assignment
H0-YZ	Reserved for national assignment
X0-ZZ	Reserved for national assignment

FL 42.

Revenue Code. Enter a four-digit code corresponding to each narrative description or standard abbreviation that identifies a specific accommodation, ancillary service, or billing calculation related to services billed.

PROCEDURE—CONT'D

Revenue code 0001 indicating a total must be the final entry on all bills. Revenue codes are an important factor when payment is considered by managed care contractors or private payers. Billing guidelines for revenue codes are extensive, so refer to the UB-92 manual for detailed information. Managed care: Required because payment may be based on diagnosis, procedure, and revenue codes. For example, codes 0274, 0275, 0276, and 0278 relate to implant of a pacemaker, lens, pin, or bolt. If the correct code is not used, payment will not be made for implant item if the cost is buried in supplies. Other items to be sure to code are special drugs for chemotherapy, cardiac balloons, cardiac catheters, and so on. Medicare: Required. All revenue codes from 001 to 999 must be preceded with an "0." The leading "0" is added automatically for electronic claims. Basic revenue codes end in "0." Detailed revenue codes end in 1 through 9. List revenue codes in ascending order. Do not repeat revenue codes on the same claim except when required by field or for coding more than one HCPCS code for the same revenue code item. Medi-Cal: Not required for outpatient services except when code 0001 is used to indicate Total Charge line.

FL 43.
Revenue Description. This optional form locator helps separate and identify descriptions of each service. The description must identify the particular service code indicated in FL 44, the HCPCS/Rates form locator. Third-party payers and TRICARE: Required Medicare: Not required. Medicaid: May be required depending on contract.

FL 44.
HCPCS/Rates/Health Insurance Prospective Payment System (HIPPS) Rate Codes. Enter the applicable CPT or HCPCS code number and modifier (applicable to ancillary services for outpatient claims), HIPPS rate code, and two-digit modifier, or the accommodation rate for inpatient claims. Dollar values must include whole dollars, the decimal, and cents (e.g., $999.99). Medicare: Required. Medicaid and private payers: May be required depending on contract.

FL 45.
Service Date. Enter the date the service was rendered for outpatient services in eight digits (e.g., 062320XX). See the patient's itemized bill for dates. The electronic version requires an eight-character date listing year, month, and day (e.g., 20XX0128). Inpatient dates are not required in this form locator. Medicare: Required. Medicaid and private payers: May be required depending on contract.

FL 46.
Service Units. Enter the number of accommodation days, ancillary units, or visits when appropriate for each revenue code. This is itemized on the patient's detail bill. Medicare and private payers: Required.

FL 47.
Total Charges. Enter the total charge pertaining to the related revenue codes (Example 17.15). Medicare and private payers: Required.

FL 48.
Noncovered Charges. Enter total noncovered charges for the primary payer pertaining to a particular revenue code. Personal items are not covered. Medicaid, Medicare, and private payers: Required. Medi-Cal and TRICARE: Not required.

FL 49.
Unlabeled form locator. Reserved for national assignment.

FL 50.
Payer Identification. Enter name and number identifying each payer organization from which the provider may expect some payment for the bill. Line 50A is used to report the primary payer. Line 50B is used for the secondary payer. Line 50C is used for the tertiary payer. Medicaid, Medicare, private payers, and TRICARE: Required. Medi-Cal: Enter "O/P MEDI-CAL" to indicate the type of claim and payer.

FL 51.
Provider Number. Enter the number assigned to the provider by the payer. Medicaid, Medicare, and private payers: Required. TRICARE: Requires the ZIP code of the physical location of the provider plus the four-digit subidentification number.

FL 52.
Release Information Certification Indicator. Enter code indicating if provider has patient's signature on file permitting release of data. Y (yes); R (restricted or modified release); and N (no release). Medicaid: May be required depending on contract. Medicare, private payers, and TRICARE: Required. Medi-Cal: Not required.

FL 53.
Assignment of Benefits. Enter Y (yes, benefits assigned) or N (no, benefits not assigned). Private payers and TRICARE: Required. Medicaid, Medi-Cal, and Medicare: Not required.

FL 54.
Prior Payments/Payers and Patient. Enter the amount of payment received on this bill before the billing date. If payment has been received from other coverage, enter the amount on the same line as the other coverage

Continued

PROCEDURE—CONT'D

COMPLETING THE UB-92 PAPER OR ELECTRONIC CLAIM FORM

Example 17.15

	42 REV. CD.	43 DESCRIPTION	44 HCPCS/RATES	45 SERV. DATE	46 SERV. UNITS	47 TOTAL CHARGES	48 NONCOVERED CHARGES 49	
1	0175	Neonatal ICU	1844.00		14	25816.00		1
2	0250	Pharmacy				4083.20		2
3	0258	IV Solutions–Pharmacy				3387.90		3
4	0270	Med-Sur Supplies				15606.71		4
5	0300	Laboratory				12958.40		5
6	0310	Pathology Lab				47.10		6
7	0320	OX X-Ray				950.00		7
8	0360	OR Services				1800.00		8
9	0370	Anesthesia				1392.37		9
10	0390	Blood/Stor-Proc				630.30		10
11	0402	Radiology Ultrasound				808.00		11
12	0410	Respiratory SVC			22	8682.70		12
13	0481	Cardiac Cath Lab				1139.60		13
14	0920	Other DX SVS				36.00		14
15								15
16								16
17								17
18								18
19								19
20								20
21								21
22								22
23	001	Total				77338.28		23

PROCEDURE—CONT'D

"payer" listed in FL 50 (e.g., $100 should be entered as 100 00). Do not enter Medicare payments in this form locator; leave blank if not applicable. Medicaid, Medi-Cal and Medicare: Required.

FL 55.

Estimated Amount Due. Enter the estimated amount due from the indicated payer according to the contract. Medicaid, Medi-Cal, Medicare, private payers, and TRICARE: Not required.

FL 56.

Untitled form locator. Reserved for state assignment.

FL 57.

Untitled form locator. Reserved for national assignment.

FL 58.

Insured's Name. Enter name of the patient or insured individual in whose name the insurance is issued. If billing for an infant, use the mother's name. If billing for an organ donor, enter the recipient's name and the patient's relationship to the recipient in FL 59. Otherwise leave blank. Medicaid, Medicare, private payers, and TRICARE: Required.

FL 59.

Patient's Relationship to Insured. Enter code number indicating relationship of the patient to the insured individual identified in FL 58. Medicaid, Medicare, private payers, and TRICARE: Required.

Patient Relationship Codes	
01	Spouse
04	Grandfather or grandmother
05	Grandson or granddaughter
07	Nephew or niece
10	Foster child
15	Ward
17	Stepson or stepdaughter
18	Self
19	Child
20	Employee
21	Unknown
22	Handicapped dependent
23	Sponsored dependent
24	Dependent or a minor dependent
29	Significant other
32	Mother
33	Father
36	Emancipated minor
39	Organ donor
40	Cadaver donor
41	Injured plaintiff

43	Child where insured has no financial responsibility
53	Life partner
G8	Other relationship

FL 60.

Certificate/Social Security Number/Health Insurance Claim/Identification Number. Enter the insured's identification number assigned by the payer organization. Required by all programs.

FL 61.

Group Name. Enter the group name or plan through which the health insurance coverage is provided to the insured. Medicare and private payers: Required. Medi-Cal: Not required. TRICARE: Enter the sponsor's branch of service (e.g., USAF).

FL 62.

Insurance Group Number. Enter the insurance group number. Private payers: Required. Medi-Cal and Medicare: Not required. TRICARE: Enter the sponsor's military status and pay grade codes. CHAMPVA: Enter the veteran's military status code (e.g., "ACT" for active or "RET" for retired).

FL 63.

Treatment Authorization Codes. Enter the treatment authorization request (TAR) number provided by the payer. Medicare, private payers, and TRICARE: Required. Medi-Cal: For services requiring a TAR, enter the 11-digit TAR Control Number. It is not necessary to attach a copy of the TAR to the claim.

FL 64.

Employment Status Code. Enter the employment status code of the insured individual identified in FL 58. Some Medicaid programs: May be required. Medi-Cal: Not required. Medicare and private payers: Required. TRICARE: Enter the code that describes the employment status of the individual identified in FL 58.

Employment Status Codes	
1	Employed full-time
2	Employed part-time
3	Not employed
4	Self-employed
5	Retired
6	On active military duty
7-8	Reserved for national assignment
9	Unknown

Continued

PROCEDURE—CONT'D

COMPLETING THE UB-92 PAPER OR ELECTRONIC CLAIM FORM

FL 65.

Employer Name. Enter the employer's name for the individual listed in FL 58. Medicaid: May be required. Medi-Cal: Not required. Medicare, private payers, and TRICARE: Required.

FL 66.

Employer Location. Enter the employer's location of the insured individual identified in FL 58. Some Medicaid programs: May be required. Medi-Cal: Not required. Medicare, private payers, and TRICARE: Required.

FL 67.

Principal Diagnosis Code. Enter all numbers and letters of the ICD-9-CM code for the principal diagnosis, including fourth and fifth digits. Do not insert a decimal point. Required for all programs.

FLs 68-75.

Other Diagnosis Codes. Enter all numbers and letters of the ICD-9-CM codes that correspond to the patient's additional conditions that coexist at the time of admission or develop subsequently and have an effect on the treatment received or length of stay. Required for all programs. Medi-Cal: Not required.

FL 76.

Admitting Diagnosis Code/Patient's Reason for Visit. Enter admitting diagnosis code, including fourth and fifth digits as stated by the physician at the time of admission for inpatient claims. For outpatient claims, enter the patient's stated reason for seeking care. Required for all programs.

FL 77.

External Cause of Injury Code. If there is an external cause of injury, poisoning, or adverse effect, enter the diagnostic E code, including the third and fourth digits. Medicare and private payers: Not required.

FL 78.

Unlabeled form locator. Reserved for state assignment.

FL 79.

Procedure Coding Method Used. Enter appropriate code to identify the coding system used. Medicaid, private payers, and TRICARE: Required. Medicare: Not required.

Coding System Codes	
1-3	Reserved for state assignment
4	CPT procedure codes
5	HCPCS codes
6-8	Reserved for national assignment
9	ICD-9-CM procedure codes

FL 80.

Principal Procedure Codes and Date. Enter the procedure code for the principal procedure and date performed. The electronic version requires an eight-character date listing year, month, and day (20XX0425). Medicaid, Medicare, private payers, and TRICARE: Required.

FL 81.

Other Procedure Codes and Dates. Enter one or two additional major procedure codes and dates performed to identify significant procedures other than the principal procedure and corresponding dates when procedures were performed. The electronic version requires an eight-character date listing year, month, and day (20XX0215). Medicare, private payers, and TRICARE: Required. Medicaid: May be required depending on contract.

FL 82.

Attending Physician ID. Enter the name or provider number for the physician who has primary responsibility for the patient's care and treatment. This form locator is mandatory for radiologists. If the physician is a Medicaid or Medi-Cal provider, enter the state license number. Do not use a group provider number. Required by all programs.

FL 83.

Other Physician ID. Enter the name or identification number of the licensed physician other than the attending physician. Required for all programs. Medi-Cal: On the upper line of FL 83, enter the individual nine-digit Medi-Cal provider number for the physician actually providing services. Do not use a group provider number or state license number.

FL 84.

Remarks. Use this area to fulfill any reporting requirements, such as procedures that require additional information, justification for services, an emergency certification statement, or as an optional form locator for DRG group number for inpatient claims if not entered in FL 75. If it will not fit in this area, attach the statement to the claim. Required for all programs.

FL 85.

Provider Representative Signature. Provider or authorized signer must sign and date claim. Medicare, Medicaid, private payers, and TRICARE: Required. For Medicare, a stamped signature is acceptable. For other programs, a facsimile signature may be acceptable after approval.

FL 86.

Date Bill Submitted. Insert the date the claim is submitted to the insurance company or fiscal intermediary.

PROCEDURE—CONT'D

Medicaid, private payers, and TRICARE: Required. Medicare: Not required.

Taking the hospital billing process a step further, Figure 17–5 illustrates which form locator of the UB-92 claim form is affected by the hospital department and employee. To become familiar with the UB-92 claim form, an assignment is presented in the *Workbook* asking that the 86 form locators of information be divided into six categories according to departmental input.

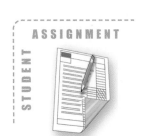

RESOURCES

INTERNET

- Refer to the *Federal Register* Web site for up-to-date guidelines and policies at:
  Web site: **www.cms.gov**

ASSIGNMENT

STUDENT

✔ Study Chapter 17.

✔ Answer the review questions in the *Workbook* to reinforce the theory learned in this chapter and to help prepare you for a future test.

✔ Complete the assignments in the *Workbook* to gain hands-on experience in analyzing and editing information from computer-generated UB-92 claim forms for inpatient and outpatient hospital billing. One of the assignments will assist you in further enhancing your diagnostic coding skills in relation to DRGs. These problems point out the value of coding properly in terms of proper diagnostic sequence, indicating the variance in payment.

✔ Turn to the glossary at the end of this textbook for a further understanding of the key terms used in this chapter.

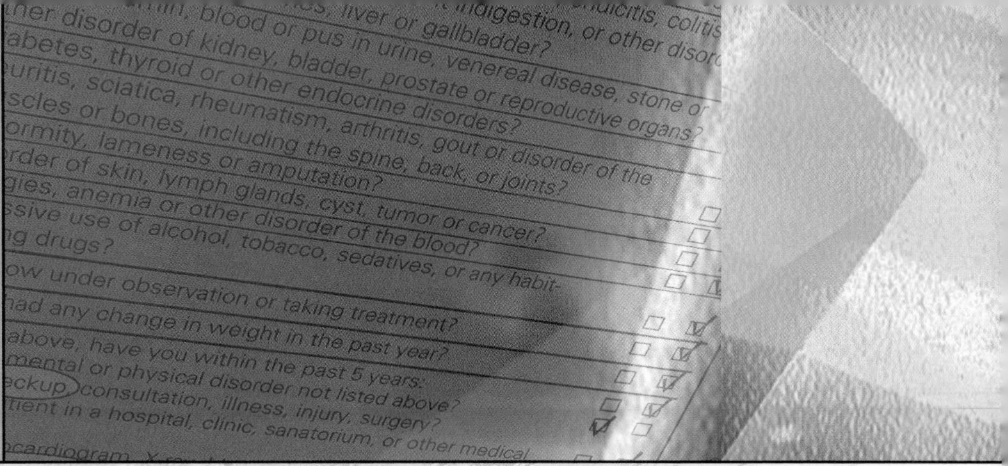

UNIT 5

Employment

CHAPTER OUTLINE

EMPLOYMENT OPPORTUNITIES
  Insurance Billing Specialist
  Claims Assistance
    Professional
JOB SEARCH
  Online Job Search
  Job Fairs
  Application
  Letter of Introduction

Resume
Interview
Follow-Up Letter
SELF-EMPLOYMENT
  Setting Up an Office
  Finances to Consider
  Marketing, Advertising,
    Promotion, and Public
    Relations

Documentation
Mentor
Networking
PROCEDURE: CREATING
  AN ELECTRONIC RESUME
PROCEDURE: PREPARING
  A RESUME IN ASCII

KEY TERMS

alien

application form

blind mailing

business associate agreement

certification

Certified Coding Specialist (CCS)

Certified Coding Specialist-
  Physician (CCS-P)

Certified Medical Assistant
  (CMA)

Certified Medical Billing Specialist
  (CMBS)

Certified Professional Coder
  (CPC, CPC-A, CPC-H)

chronologic resume

claims assistance professional
  (CAP)

combination resume

continuing education

cover letter

electronic claims processor (ECP)

employment agency

functional resume

interview

mentor

National Certified Insurance
  and Coding Specialist
  (NCICS)

networking

portfolio

Professional Association of
  Health Care Office Managers
  (PAHCOM)

Registered Medical Assistant
  (RMA)

Registered Medical Coder (RMC)

registration

resume

self-employment

service contract

18

Seeking a Job and Attaining Professional Advancement

OBJECTIVES*

After reading this chapter, you should be able to:

- Prepare to find a position as an insurance billing specialist, claims assistance professional, or electronic claims processor.

- Conduct a job search by listing prospective employers.

- Compose a letter of introduction to accompany the resume.

- Analyze education and experience to prepare a resume.

- Identify illegal interview questions.

- Prepare responses to interview questions.

- Assess responsibilities assigned to insurance billing and coding specialists, electronic claims processors, and claims assistance professionals.

- Contact computerized job search databases for online services.

- Explore the business aspects of self-employment.

- Search online for employment opportunities.

- State types of certification and registration available to insurance billers, coders, and administrative medical assistants.

*Performance objectives and exercises for hands-on practical experience for this chapter appear in the *Workbook*.

Service

An insurance billing specialist has other service-oriented positions, such as collection manager, claims assistant professional for elderly patients, insurance counselor, and so on, which focus on attention to patient needs. Whatever you decide to specialize in as far as a career related to insurance billing and coding, remember that the most important aspect of your job is patient care.

EMPLOYMENT OPPORTUNITIES

Insurance Billing Specialist

Employment opportunities are available throughout the United States for insurance billing specialists who attain coding skills, knowledge of insurance programs, and expertise in completing insurance claims accurately. In addition to the skills necessary for performance on the job, ask yourself the following questions to determine whether you need to sharpen your job-seeking techniques:

● Are you motivated and interested in finding a job?
● Can you communicate effectively in an interview?
● Do you enjoy good health?
● Are you mature?
● Do you have good grooming and manners?

The increase in the knowledge necessary and volume of paperwork associated with insurance claims, medical record keeping, and state and government agencies means a corresponding increase in the need for an insurance billing specialist. Because an individual can choose a number of different types of positions, this chapter provides information on each.

There are two ways to work—either employed by someone or self-employed after a number of years of experience (Figure 18–1). The following are some of the choices in this career field:

● Insurance billing specialist
● **Electronic claims processor (ECP)**
● Medicare or Medicaid billing specialist
● Claims assistance professional
● Coding specialist (freelance or employed)

Some hospital facilities and physicians prefer credentialed coders or insurance billers and advertise for the following:

● Certified medical billing specialist (CMBS)
● Certified medical reimbursement specialist (CMRS)
● Certified professional coder-hospital (CPC-H or CPC)
● Certified coding specialist (CCS)
● Certified coding specialist-physician (CCS-P)
● Certified electronic claims processor (CECP)

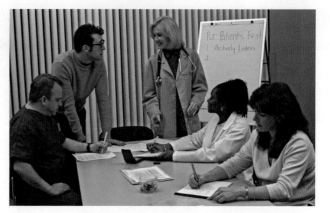

FIGURE 18–1   Staff conference discussing applicants for potential interviews.

● Certified claims assistance professional (CCAP)
● Health care reimbursement specialist (HRS)
● National certified insurance and coding specialist (NCICS)
● Registered medical coder (RMC)

Becoming certified is certainly an essential goal if one seeks career advancement, and the steps to accomplish this as well as certification in other careers allied to this one are detailed at the end of this chapter.

Claims Assistance Professional

Contact local hospitals to determine whether they have patients who require insurance help if you wish to establish yourself as a self-employed **claims assistance professional (CAP)** (in addition to some of the aforementioned positions). Also call on small employers to determine whether they need assistance in explanation of their health insurance policies or enhancement of insurance benefits.

JOB SEARCH

There are several ways to seek employment. You may wish to be employed by a physician, hospital, medical facility, insurance company, or managed care organization. You may choose to be self-employed if you have had a number of years of experience or you may even choose some type of combination situation. Here are suggested ways to search for a job.

1. Join a professional organization, as mentioned later in this chapter, to network with others in the same career field and to hear about job openings (Figure 18–2). Put a notice about your availability in the chapter newsletter.
2. Attend meetings and workshops in this career field to keep up-to-date and network with others.

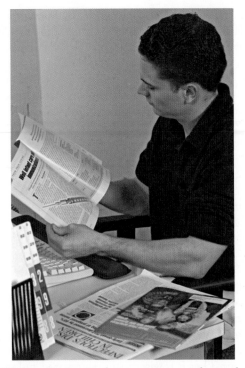

FIGURE 18–2 Student scanning a professional journal for job leads.

3. Contact the school placement personnel, complete the necessary paperwork, and leave a resume on file if you have just completed a course at a community college or trade school.

4. Spread the word to those who work in medical settings and those who might hear of openings in medical facilities, such as classmates, instructors, school counselors, relatives, and friends.

5. Contact pharmaceutical representatives who visit physicians' offices and hospitals for employment information or leads.

6. Visit public and private **employment agencies,** including temporary and temporary to permanent agencies. Before signing up with an agency, ask whether the employer or applicant pays the agency fee.

7. Inquire at state and federal government offices and their employment agencies.

8. Look for part-time employment that might lead to a permanent full-time position.

9. Check bulletin boards frequently in personnel offices of hospitals and clinics for posted job offerings.

10. Go to your local medical society to see determine whether it has a provision for supplying job leads.

11. Consult the *Yellow Pages* of the telephone directory or medical society roster for names of professional offices and hospitals to contact with an introductory telephone call or letter.

12. Send a **blind mailing** of the resume, including a cover letter, to possible prospects. A blind mailing means to send information to employers whom you do not

know personally and who have not advertised for a job opening. This may result in a positive response with either a request to complete an application form or an invitation for an interview.

13. Go to the local library and look through Dun and Bradstreet's *Million Dollar Directory* and the *Middle Market Directory* for information on potential employers in many cities.

14. Visit the chamber of commerce and ask for some of their publications that contain membership directories, names of major professional employers in specific areas, and brochures describing regional facts.

15. Subscribe to the principal newspaper of the city where employment is desired. Read help wanted ads in the classified section especially in the Sunday newspaper. Positions of interest might be listed as insurance billing specialist, reimbursement manager, insurance claims manager, insurance coordinator, insurance biller, coding/reimbursement specialist, reimbursement coordinator, coder/abstracter, electronic claims processor, and so on. Do not be discouraged by specific requirements in an advertisement but apply anyway. Send your resume and a cover letter the next day. Some employers give priority to candidates who respond within the first 3 or 4 days after a job announcement because they believe it is an indication that someone is truly interested in the position. Many jobs are not advertised and there could be an opening available for which you qualify.

16. Telephone job hot lines of large medical clinics in your area.

17. Visit unannounced ("cold calls") at job locations.

18. Explore the Internet's World Wide Web. See Internet Resources at the end of this chapter.

Online Job Search

Because of vast communication available via the Internet's World Wide Web, newspaper and magazine classified advertisements may become resources of the past. An individual with a computer and modem can access online services. Many Web sites on the Internet incorporate text, sound, graphics, animation, and video. It is possible to locate potential employers at their Web sites who are offering jobs to health care workers by using various search engines. At some sites, you can find detailed descriptions of posted positions and locate opportunity postings by location or employer. You may be able to find and respond to a specific job of interest by delivering an online resume, attaching a cover letter, and updating your posting as often as needed. Some Web sites allow you to receive e-mailed job alerts.

There are several ways to gain access to the Internet. Your school may allow you to access the Internet on campus. Many libraries have computers with free

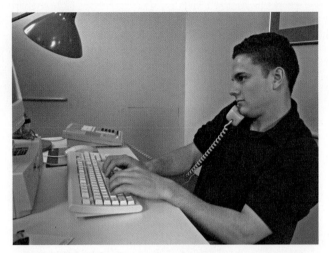

FIGURE 18–3   Student doing an online job search.

Internet service. If you have a computer at home, you may wish to subscribe to either a commercial online service (e.g., America Online) with Internet access or an Internet service in your locale (Figure 18–3).

Internet

Once online, go to a Web index to locate a search engine that lists different options to explore, such as Yahoo (www.yahoo.com), Google (www.google.com), Infoseek (www.infoseek.go.com), or Alta Vista (www.altavista.com). One of the resources is Career Magazine (www.careermag.com/careermag/), which lets you browse through hundreds of national job openings in a variety of fields. Check out America's Job Bank (www.ajb.dni.us) and E-Span Employment Database Search (www.espan.com/), which have job postings that you can browse according to field, location, and career type. Go to PracticeNet (www.practice-net.com), which provides descriptions of medical practice opportunities. This 24-hour service names the recruiter, location, and an 800 number to contact. MedSearch America is another health employment service that posts jobs for hospitals, managed care organizations (MCOs), and pharmaceutical companies. Job seekers can send their resumes via e-mail for free online posting. Contact MedSearch online at www. medsearch.com.

If you subscribe monthly to a commercial online service, you can network by posting a notice on a bulletin board with your resume or a note that you are looking for a particular type of position in a given locale.

Register with a computerized job search company. The firm American Computerized Employment Service (Irvine, California),* has entered the job placement field

---

*American Computerized Employment Service, 17801 Main Street, Suite A, Irvine, CA 92714. Telephone 714-250-0221.

with a trademarked system called TeleRecruiting. Job candidates may register without charge and complete an extensive profile questionnaire listing experience, skills, job-related factors, maximum commuting distance, and flex-time requirements. The firm acts as a liaison between employers and applicants. Employers use a touchtone telephone to access the computer and search for candidates. They pay an annual subscription, pay-per-search, or package search fee.

Career options on the Internet are discussed in a book by Joyce Lain Kennedy entitled, *Hook Up, Get Hired! The Internet Job Search Revolution*, published by John Wiley & Sons, New York.

Job Fairs

Annual community events feature job fairs at community colleges and technical trade schools or sponsored by professional associations. Job recruiters set up booths with information about their companies and available positions; however, they do not have much time to spend with each job seeker. Thus it is wise to come prepared and practice a 30-second introduction before attending. This introduction should consist of a quick overview of your career goals, experience, skills, training, education, and personal strengths. Be sure to explain what you can offer the employer. These are usually day-long events and you may wish to investigate a number of participating employers' booths.

Go prepared by carrying a binder or folder with plenty of copies of your resume to give to the company representatives you meet. Resumes should be neat, clean, and not folded, wrinkled, or coffee-stained. Take a pen, pencil, and notepad to obtain information. Research the employers attending so you know which ones you will visit and can appear confident, enthusiastic, interested, and knowledgeable to the job recruiter.

Take home the business card and brochure of anyone you talk to who genuinely interests you. After the fair, send that person a follow-up letter to reaffirm your interest.

Application

When visiting a potential employer, ask for an **application form** to complete and inquire whether the facility keeps potential job applicants on file and for how long (Figure 18–4). Study each question carefully before answering because the employer may evaluate the application itself to determine whether the applicant can follow instructions. Furnish as much information as possible, and if a question does not apply or cannot be answered, insert "no," "none," "NA" (not applicable), or "DNA" (does not apply). When visiting a potential employer for

APPLICATION FOR POSITION / Medical or Dental Office
AN EQUAL OPPORTUNITY EMPLOYER

(in answering questions, use extra blank sheet if necessary)

No employee, applicant, or candidate for promotion, training or other advantage shall be dicriminated against (or given preference) because of race, color, religion, sex, age, physical handicap, veteran status, or national origin.

PLEASE READ CAREFULLY AND WRITE OR PRINT ANSWERS TO ALL QUESTIONS. DO NOT TYPE.

Date of application: 7-2-XX

A. PERSONAL INFORMATION

Name - Last	First	Middle	Social Security No.	Area code/phone no.
Velasquez,	Jennifer	M.	361 XX 4915	(555) 439-9800

Present address: Street (Apt.#)	State	Zip	How long at this address?:
1234 Martin Street, Woodland Hills	XY	12345	10 years

Previous address: Street City State Zip | Person to notify in case of emergency or accident - name: John Velasquez
From: To: | Address: Telephone: 555-439-9800

B. EMPLOYMENT INFORMATION

For what position are you applying?: ☒Full-time ☐Part-time ☐Either	Date available for employment?: 7-6-XX	Wage/salary expectations: negotiable
insurance biller		

List hrs./days you prefer to work: M-F 8-5PM | List any hrs./days you are not available: (Except for times required for religious practices or observances) | Can you work overtime, if necessary? ☒Yes ☐No

Are you employed now? ☐Yes ☒No | If so, may we inquire of your present employer?: ☐No ☐Yes, if yes: Name of employer: | Phone number: ( )

Have you ever been bonded? ☐Yes ☒No | If required for position, are you bondable? ☒Yes ☐No ☐Uncertain | Have you applied for a position with this office before? ☒No ☐Yes If Yes, when?:

Referred by / or where did you learn of this job?:

Can you, upon employment, submit verification of your legal right to work in the United States? ☒Yes ☐No
Submit proof that you meet legal age requirement for employment? ☒Yes ☐No

Language(s) applicant speaks or writes (if use of a language other than English is relevant to the job for which the applicant is applying: Spanish

C. EDUCATION HISTORY

	Name and address of schools attended (include current)	Dates From — Thru	Highest grade/level completed	Diploma/degree(s) obtained/areas of study
High school	ABC High School, Woodland Hills, XY	1990–1994	12	Diploma
College	Vocational-Tech School	1995		Degree/major Certificate
Post graduate	Montana State University	1995-97		Degree/major 24 credits
Other				Course/diploma/license/certificate

Specific training, education, or experiences which will assist you in the job for which you have applied. See résumé

Future educational plans: Continuing education-preparing for certification

D. SPECIAL SKILLS

CHECK BELOW THE KINDS OF WORK YOU HAVE DONE:

		☒ MEDICAL INSURANCE FORMS	☐ RECEPTIONIST
☐ BLOOD COUNTS	☐ DENTAL ASSISTANT	☒ MEDICAL TERMINOLOGY	☒ TELEPHONES
☐ BOOKKEEPING	☐ DENTAL HYGIENIST	☐ MEDICAL TRANSCRIPTION	☒ TYPING
☒ COLLECTIONS	☐ FILING	☐ NURSING	☐ STENOGRAPHY
☒ COMPOSING LETTERS	☐ INJECTIONS	☐ PHLEBOTOMY(draw blood)	☐ URINALYSIS
☐ COMPUTER INPUT	☐ INSTRUMENT STERILIZATION	☒ POSTING	☐ X-RAY
OFFICE EQUIPMENT USED: ☒ COMPUTER	☐ DICTATING EQUIPMENT	☒ WORD PROCESSOR	☒ OTHER calculator

Other kinds of tasks performed or skills that may be applicable to position:	Typing speed 60 wpm	Shorthand speed

ORDER # 72-110 • © 1976 BIBBERO SYSTEMS, INC. • PETALUMA, CA. • (Rev. 1/95)
TO REORDER CALL TOLL FREE: (800) BIBBERO (800-242-2376) OR FAX (800) 242-9330

Mᴼᴳ Iɴ U.S.A.

(PLEASE COMPLETE OTHER SIDE)

FIGURE 18–4 Application for Position/Medical or Dental Office form. *(From Bibbero Systems, Inc., Petaluma, Calif.)* *Continued*

E. EMPLOYMENT RECORD

LIST MOST RECENT EMPLOYMENT FIRST   May we contact your previous employer(s) for a reference?   ☒Yes   ☐No

1) Employer *St. John's Outpatient Clinic*	Worked performed. Be specific: *ins biller–see résumé*

Address: Street   City   State   Zip code
24 Center St. Woodland Hills, XY   12345

Phone number   *(555)782-0155*

Type of business *outpt hospital/clinic*	Dates Mo. Yr. Mo. Yr. From 2 | 97 To 8 | 2000
Your position *ins billing specialist*	Hourly rate/salary Starting *$9/hr* Final *$11.50/hr*

Supervisor's name   *Candice Johnson*

Reason for leaving   *Professional advancement*

1) Employer *Eastern Airlines*	Worked performed. Be specific:

Address: Street   City   State   Zip code
Orlando, Florida

Phone number *(555)350-7000*	Dates Mo. Yr. Mo. Yr. From 1 | 88 To 12 | 89
Type of business *airline transportation*	Hourly rate/salary Starting Final

Your position   *receptionist*

Supervisor's name   *Gary Stevens*

Reason for leaving   *career change*

1) Employer	Worked performed. Be specific:

Address: Street   City   State   Zip code

Phone number ( )	Dates Mo. Yr. Mo. Yr. From To
Type of business	Hourly rate/salary Starting Final

Your position

Supervisor's name

Reason for leaving

F. REFERENCES — FRIENDS / ACQUAINTANCES NON-RELATED

(1) _*furnished upon request*_
    Name   Address   Telephone number   (☐Work ☐Home)   Occupation   Years acquainted

(1) _____
    Name   Address   Telephone number   (☐Work ☐Home)   Occupation   Years acquainted

Please feel free to add any information which you feel will help us consider you for employment

READ THE FOLLOWING CAREFULLY, THEN SIGN AND DATE THE APPLICATION

"I certify that all answers given by me on this application are true, correct and complete to the best of my knowledge. I acknowledge notice that the information contained in this application is subject to check. I agree that, if hired, my continued employment may be contingent upon the accuracy of that information. If employed, I further agree to comply with Company/Office rules and regulations."

Signature: *Jennifer M. Velasquez* _____   Date: *7-2-XX*

FIGURE 18–4, cont'd   Application for Position/Medical or Dental Office form.
(From Bibbero Systems, Inc., Petaluma, Calif.)

an application form, be sure you have prepared in advance for an interview in case an opportunity arises on that first visit.

Follow these guidelines when completing an application form:

1. Read the whole application form because some instructions may appear on the last page or last line.
2. Read the fine print and instructions: "Please print," "Put last name first," or "Complete in your own handwriting." This indicates ability to follow directions or instructions.
3. Print if your handwriting is poor, and abbreviate only when there is lack of space.
4. Complete the application in black ink unless pencil is specified.
5. Refer to data from a portfolio, sample application form, or resume that has been checked for accuracy; use this information to copy onto each new application form. Be neat.
6. List correct dates of previous employment so that it will be accurate if the employer seeks verification. If a question is presented asking the reason for leaving a position, leave it blank and discuss this during the interview.
7. Name specific skills, such as procedural coding, diagnostic coding, knowledge of insurance programs, completing the CMS-1500 claim form, typing or keyboarding (number of words per minute), and speaking a second language.
8. When a question is asked about salary amount, write in "negotiable" or "flexible" and then discuss this during the interview.
9. Sign the application after completion.
10. Reread the entire form, word for word, to find any errors of omission or commission. This avoids having to apologize during an interview for a mistake.

Letter of Introduction

Individuals spend days perfecting a resume but throw together a *letter of introduction* or *cover letter* in minutes. This is a mistake. The main goal of the **cover letter** is to get the employer to take notice of the potential employee and resume so an interview appointment can be made. Letters should be typed, addressed to a specific person, and customized to each potential employer. If the advertisement gives a telephone number, call and ask for the name of the person doing the interviewing so the letter can include that person's name. When the name is unknown, use "Dear Sir or Madam" or "To Whom It May Concern," or a less formal "Hello" or "Good Morning."

Do not repeat everything in the resume. Begin with an attention grabber, and get right to the point so the employer knows what you want and why. The letter should explain how the applicant's qualifications and skills would benefit the employer. Use key words that appear in the "position wanted" ad. End the letter by requesting an interview and be sure to enclose a resume. Always include a telephone number and the time of day when you are available.

Reread the letter for typos and errors in grammar, punctuation, and spelling. Avoid the use of "I" in the sentence structure (Figure 18–5).

Resume

A **resume** is a data sheet designed to sell job qualifications to prospective employers. There are several formats from which to choose:

- **Chronologic resume** gives recent experiences first with dates and descriptive data for each job.
- **Functional resume** states the qualifications or skills an individual is able to perform.
- **Combination resume** summarizes the applicant's job skills as well as educational and employment history. The combination style is the best choice for an insurance billing specialist (Figure 18–6).

A results-oriented resume focuses on results, not characteristics. It helps prospective employers reduce the risks that are associated with hiring because it shows what the job seeker has accomplished and his or her attitude toward work.

The ideal length for a resume is one page. It can be typed on an $8\frac{1}{2}$- × 14-inch page and reduced to letter size. The resume should be keyed or typed, not handwritten, on high-quality, wrinkle-free bond off-white or white paper; single spaced internally with double spacing between main headings; and balanced spacing for all four margins. Laser-printed resumes give a professional appearance. You might want to have a longer (two-page maximum) resume on hand to offer during an interview.

Under the Civil Rights Act of 1964, enforced by the Equal Employment Opportunity Commission, information about height, weight, birth date, marital status, Social Security number, and physical condition may be omitted. Additional items to omit are salary requirements, reason for leaving jobs, date of resume preparation, date available to begin work, references, and vague references to time gaps. Questions about these items might be asked

Street Address
City, State, ZIP code
Date of letter

John Doe, MD or
Personnel Director
Street Address
City, State, ZIP code

Dear Dr. Doe:

Paragraph 1: Explain where you heard about the position and say you are writing for a position mentioned in the advertisement.

Paragraph 2: Name two or more qualifications of great interest to the prospective employer. State reasons you are interested in this specialty, location, or type of work. Mention if experienced or trained for this career field.

Paragraph 3: Refer the reader to the resume or application form enclosed.

Paragraph 4: Close the letter by asking for an interview and suggesting a date and time or that you will call for an appointment. If requesting further information about the job opening, enclose a self-addressed, stamped envelope as a courtesy. Do not end the letter with a vague statement but give the reader a specific action to take.

Sincerely yours,

(handwritten signature)

Type name

Enclosure

FIGURE 18–5   Suggested content for a letter of introduction to accompany a resume.

by the interviewer during an interview. Hobbies and outside interests that relate to the profession might be included. Membership or leadership positions held in professional organizations related to the medical field might be mentioned. A photograph is not necessary but might be included if it will be of value to the interviewer for recall purposes (Figure 18–7).

The format may include the following:

- Title. Resume, personal data sheet, biographic sketch, or curriculum vitae.
- Heading. At the beginning of the resume, the applicant's name, address, e-mail address, and telephone and fax numbers.
- Summary. This may be a statement as to why the employer should be interested in this applicant. Use action words as shown in Figure 18–6 and avoid the personal pronoun.
- Education. Name high school, college, any business school attended, and **continuing education** classes, city and state, degree, and date received. List in reverse chronologic order. Grade average and awards or scholastic honors may be included.

- Professional experience. Name all employers in reverse chronologic order with addresses, telephone numbers, and dates of employment. Include summer, full-time, part-time, and temporary jobs as well as externship and volunteer work.
- Skills. List typing or keyboarding words per minute, computer equipment operated, experience in medical software programs, accurate procedure and diagnostic coding, expertise in insurance claims completion and submission, knowledge of medical terminology and insurance terminology, bookkeeping (posting charges, payments, and adjustments to accounts receivable journal), experience in preparing appeals for denied claims, resubmittal of delinquent claims, ability to explain insurance programs and plans (e.g., benefits, requirements, and submission of claims), ability to abstract information from patients' medical and financial records, and ability to review insurance payments. If you are fluent in another language, insert this information. Telephone and reception skills also might be mentioned.
- References. Type in the phrase "Furnished upon request." Prepare approximately five references on a separate sheet and be sure to contact the persons referenced before an interview.

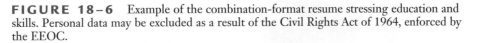

It is optional to type RESUME or CURRICULUM VITAE. Every personnel manager knows what a resume looks like.

One error can kill your chances for a job. Proofread carefully.

Shows recent education to learn personal computers. Employers sense extra initiative and new skills.

Although no degree was awarded, listing the number of credits earned and highlighting some business and medical courses may help broaden an employer's interest.

Listing and bulleting skills are vital when applying for work as an insurance billing specialist.

Cover letter can explain why no job was held in years because a person had to raise a family or was ill.

This section not only gives job titles but also emphasizes accomplishments.

It is not necessary to list references.

RESUME

Jennifer M. Velasquez
1234 Martin Street
Woodland Hills, XY 12345-0001

Telephone/Fax 555-439-9800
E-mail: VelasquezJ@aol.com

CAREER
OBJECTIVE: Insurance billing specialist

EDUCATION: ABC HIGH SCHOOL, Woodland Hills, XY.
                  Graduated 1994. Diploma awarded.

                  VOCATIONAL-TECH SCHOOL, Woodland Hills, XY (1995)
                  Certificate awarded for personal computer word processing and
                  spread sheet programs.

                  MONTANA STATE UNIVERSITY, Woodland Hills, XY (1997)
                  24 credits (1995-97). Medical classes including insurance,
                  medical terminology, anatomy and physiology, and other core
                  courses.

CONTINUING
EDUCATION: Preparing for certification.

SKILLS: • Ability to code diagnoses and procedures proficiently
                  • Key 60 words per minute
                  • Operate computer: File management, Internet, E-mail, word
                    processing, spreadsheet, database management
                  • Operate photocopy and calculator equipment
                  • Knowledge of insurance programs, completing CMS-1500,
                    medical terminology, diseases, surgeries, and insurance terms
                  • Ability to speak Spanish fluently
                  • Excellent proofreader, good oral and writing communication
                    skills, including grammar, punctuation, and style

EMPLOYMENT: EASTERN AIRLINES, Orlando, Florida
                  RECEPTIONIST–1988 to 1989

                  ST. JOHN'S OUTPATIENT CLINIC, Woodland Hills, XY
                  INSURANCE BILLING SPECIALIST – February 1997 to
                  August 2000
                  Began as a part-time billing clerk and worked into a full-time
                  position developing skills in diagnostic and procedural coding and
                  insurance claims completion. Received bonus for keeping
                  delinquent claims affecting accounts receivable below previous
                  year's total.

REFERENCES: Furnished upon request.

FIGURE 18–6 Example of the combination-format resume stressing education and skills. Personal data may be excluded as a result of the Civil Rights Act of 1964, enforced by the EEOC.

● Final details. It is acceptable to fax a resume to an employer who advertises a job opening but gives no guidelines on how to submit the resume. It is wise to use every advantage possible in a competitive employment market where time is of the essence (Figure 18–8).

Proofread the resume carefully for spelling, punctuation, grammar, and typographic errors. Ask a friend or professional individual with excellent English skills to read and critique it. Remember that the resume is only a foot in the door and not what is going to land that job for you—you are!

Interview

After looking for a potential employer, preparing a resume, and completing an application, the final step in landing a job is the face-to-face interview. An **interview** is a formal consultation with questions by an employer to evaluate the qualifications of a prospective job applicant (Figure 18–9). Make the best impression possible on the prospective employer as soon as you walk through the door. It is a well-known fact that the first 30 seconds makes either a positive or negative impression. Hiring depends on positive qualities. Concentrate on good grooming and a fresh, relaxed appearance. Display a

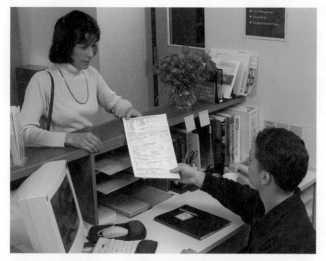

FIGURE 18–7   Student delivering a resume to a potential job site.

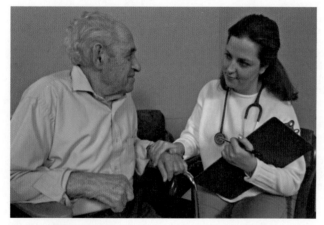

FIGURE 18–8   Insurance billing student at an externship site.

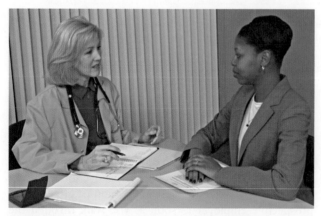

FIGURE 18–9   Student being interviewed for an insurance billing position.

warm, positive attitude. Use proper grammar, avoid using slang, and maintain eye contact.

A female applicant should wear a clean skirt, dress, or tailored suit and nylon stockings with low-heeled pumps. A male applicant should wear a clean dark suit or sport coat, conservative necktie, white shirt, plain slacks, plain socks, and well-shined shoes. A man should avoid a lot of facial hair, long hair, earrings, and heavy after-shave lotion. A woman should have a conservative hair style, wear jewelry sparingly, and avoid heavy makeup, a low-cut neckline, a sleeveless dress, strong perfume, and dark or bright nail polish. Do not smoke or chew gum. Use a proper deodorant. Eliminate nervous habits. It has been found that when applicants have similar skills and education, the decision to hire has been based on physical appearance at the interview.

Figure 18–10 is an example of an interview evaluation and reference investigation form. This form points out the areas an interviewer observes and how impressions are rated.

Research beforehand to know whether the salary (when offered) is acceptable. If you wish to ask questions about fringe benefits, do not appear to be overly interested in them.

Choose the right time for the interview and arrive promptly. It has been found that late Monday and Friday afternoons between 4:00 and 5:00 PM are not good times for interviews because Mondays are usually catch-up, heavily scheduled days and Fridays are getaway days. Research has proved that the likelihood of hiring the last person interviewed for a position is greater than that of hiring those interviewed first. Carry something in your hand (e.g., portfolio with notepad, resume, and other documents) so you are not showing nervousness or anxiety, which might detract and be detrimental during the interview.

Role playing is a good method to use to prepare for an interview. Give a friend a list of questions to ask you, then try to answer the questions spontaneously without stumbling. Videotape or audiotape the session, if possible, to see or hear what the employer will experience.

Questions an interviewer might ask about personal life (marital status), family planning, pregnancy, provision for child care, religious preference, club memberships, height, weight, dependents, age (birth date), ethnic background, maiden name, native language, physical or psychiatric problems, spouse's employment and earnings, credit rating, and home and automobile ownership are illegal and do not have to be answered. (It is not considered discriminatory if an employer wishes to know

INTERVIEW EVALUATION AND REFERENCE INVESTIGATION FORM, MEDICAL or DENTAL OFFICE	SUMMARY OF EVALUATION	
	POINTS FROM APPLICATION AND INTERVIEW	
	POINTS FROM REFERENCES	
	TOTAL POINTS	

NAME OF APPLICANT	DATE	OVERALL IMPRESSION	

RATING: GOOD – 2 POINTS
FAIR – 1 POINT
POOR – 0 POINTS

POSITION APPLIED FOR:			
FROM APPLICATION FOR POSITION, GAUGE APPLICANT IN FOLLOWING AREAS	GOOD	FAIR	POOR
1. STABILITY (REMAINED IN ONE PLACE OF RESIDENCE AND ONE JOB FOR A REASONABLE LENGTH OF TIME)?			
2. HEALTH?			
3. THE PROPER EDUCATIONAL BACKGROUND TO FILL THE POSITION?			
4. LEGIBLE HANDWRITING?			
5. AN EMPLOYMENT HISTORY THAT POINTS TOWARD DEPENDABILITY?			
6. LIMITATION ON WORKING HOURS?			
7. THE PROPER EXPERIENCE AND / OR SKILLS TO FILL THE POSITION?			
8. SALARY REQUIREMENT COMMENSURATE WITH POSITION?			
FROM THE PERSONAL INTERVIEW – (SHOULD BE SPECIFIC QUALITIES – OBJECTIVE)			
9. SUFFICIENT CAPABILITY TO HANDLE ANY SITUATION THAT MAY ARISE WHEN ALONE IN OFFICE?			
10. AN APPROPRIATE ATTITUDE TOWARD WORK?			
11. AN APPROPRIATE VOICE, DICTION, GRAMMAR?			
12. POISE?			
13. SELF CONFIDENCE (NOT OVER-CONFIDENCE)?			
14. TACT?			
15. SUFFICIENT MATURITY FOR JOB?			
16. AN ABILITY TO EXPRESS ONESELF WELL?			
17. AN INITIATIVE OR INTEREST IN LEARNING?			
18. APPROPRIATE APPEARANCE (NEAT, CLEAN; SUITABLE TO BUSINESS)			
19. ENERGY, VITALITY AND PERCEIVED ABILITY TO HANDLE PRESSURE OF POSITION?			
20. EAGERNESS TO OBTAIN THE POSITION IN QUESTION?			
COLUMNAR TOTALS			
GRAND TOTAL			

Left vertical label: APPLICATION SECTION / REFERENCE

DIRECTIONS FOR USE OF FORM:
1. Look over your ratings. A zero score on any one VITAL question should automatically eliminate applicant. Add up the total rating points and enter in the SUMMARY OF EVALUATION BLOCK in the upper right-hand corner of this page.
2. After finishing all interviews, choose the "best bets" and check their references using the reverse side of this form.
3. Enter, as above, the results of your reference check and then your overall impression. (E – Excellent, G – Good, F – Fair, P – Poor)

FORM # 72-120 © 1987 BIBBERO SYSTEMS, INC. • PETALUMA, CA. • TO REORDER CALL TOLL FREE: (800) BIBBERO (800-242-2376) OR FAX (800) 242-9330 (REV. 7/87)

FIGURE 18–10 Example of an interview evaluation and reference investigation form. *(From Bibbero Systems, Inc., Petaluma, Calif.)* *Continued*

NOTES:

REFERENCE INVESTIGATION			
1. OFFICE CONTACTED		PHONE: ( )	DATE
PERSON CONTACTED			
HOW LONG HAVE YOU KNOWN THIS PERSON?			
BETWEEN WHAT DATES WAS THIS PERSON EMPLOYED BY YOU?		FROM	TO
WHAT TYPE OF WORK DID THIS PERSON DO FOR YOU?		TITLE OF POSITION:	SATISFACTORILY?
WAS THIS PERSON CONSISTENTLY COOPERATIVE?		WHAT WERE SHORTCOMINGS?	
DID THIS PERSON GET ALONG WELL WITH OTHERS?			
WAS THIS PERSON TRUSTWORTHY / DEPENDABLE?			ATTENDANCE RECORD:
WHY DID THIS PERSON LEAVE YOUR EMPLOY?			SALARY LEVEL:
WOULD YOU REHIRE THIS PERSON?			
NOTES:			
			RATING:
2. OFFICE CONTACTED		PHONE: ( )	DATE
PERSON CONTACTED			
HOW LONG HAVE YOU KNOWN THIS PERSON?			
BETWEEN WHAT DATES WAS THIS PERSON EMPLOYED BY YOU?		FROM	TO
WHAT TYPE OF WORK DID THIS PERSON DO FOR YOU?		TITLE OF POSITION:	SATISFACTORILY?
WAS THIS PERSON CONSISTENTLY COOPERATIVE?		WHAT WERE SHORTCOMINGS?	
DID THIS PERSON GET ALONG WELL WITH OTHERS?			
WAS THIS PERSON TRUSTWORTHY / DEPENDABLE?			ATTENDANCE RECORD:
WHY DID THIS PERSON LEAVE YOUR EMPLOY?			SALARY LEVEL:
WOULD YOU REHIRE THIS PERSON?			
NOTES:			
			RATING:
3. OFFICE CONTACTED		PHONE: ( )	DATE
PERSON CONTACTED			
HOW LONG HAVE YOU KNOWN THIS PERSON?			
BETWEEN WHAT DATES WAS THIS PERSON EMPLOYED BY YOU?		FROM	TO
WHAT TYPE OF WORK DID THIS PERSON DO FOR YOU?		TITLE OF POSITION:	SATISFACTORILY?
WAS THIS PERSON CONSISTENTLY COOPERATIVE?		WHAT WERE SHORTCOMINGS?	
DID THIS PERSON GET ALONG WELL WITH OTHERS?			
WAS THIS PERSON TRUSTWORTHY / DEPENDABLE?			ATTENDANCE RECORD:
WHY DID THIS PERSON LEAVE YOUR EMPLOY?			SALARY LEVEL:
WOULD YOU REHIRE THIS PERSON?			
NOTES:			
			RATING:

INTERVIEWER _____   DATE: _____

FIGURE 18–10, cont'd   Example of an interview evaluation and reference investigation form. *(From Bibbero Systems, Inc., Petaluma, Calif.)*

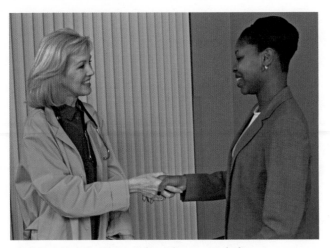

FIGURE 18–11 Job applicant concluding an interview with an office manager.

whether an applicant smokes.) Three suggestions for handling an illegal question follow:

1. Answer the question and ignore the fact that you know it is illegal.
2. Answer with, "I think the question is not relevant to the requirements of this position."
3. Refuse to answer and contact the nearest Equal Employment Opportunity Commission (EEOC) office.

Shake the interviewer's hand at the conclusion of the meeting (Figure 18–11). Ask how long it will be before a job offer or denial is forthcoming, and then leave with a "thank you." If the job is offered at the interview and the applicant is not sure about accepting, ask, "How soon do you need to know?" This will allow time to think and compare job offers before making a commitment.

Portfolio

Prepare in advance for the interview by organizing a **portfolio.** Assemble letters of recommendation (from former employers, teachers, family physician, professional friends, community leaders), school diplomas or degrees, transcripts, certificates, names and addresses of references, extra copies of the resume, Social Security card, timed typing test certified by an instructor, some neatly typed insurance claim forms with evidence of coding skills, and any other items related to prior education and work experience.

Alien

Any **alien** employee must have an Employment Eligibility Verification Form I-9 on file with his or her employer. This form can be obtained by writing to the Immigration and Naturalization Service (INS) at 425 I Street, NW,

Washington, DC 20536. Within 3 days of hiring an alien, the employee must show one of the following: a naturalization certification (citizen papers), an alien registration receipt card, a temporary resident receipt card, or an employment authorization card. One of these items should be in the portfolio in the event it is requested by the prospective employer during the interview.

Follow-Up Letter

Write a follow-up letter indicating thanks for the interview and restating interest in the position (Figure 18–12). This keeps the applicant's name before the potential employer. Telephone to express continued interest in the position if no response is heard within the time frame given.

SELF-EMPLOYMENT

Setting Up an Office

When an individual wishes to be his or her own boss **(self-employed),** it is usually wise to become educated and have some experience in the chosen career before undertaking this task. Having a positive and effective rapport with the public, as well as a strong background in insurance, is desirable for the individual who wants to work independently as a billing specialist. Outpatient hospital and physician billing experience in several specialties is important if you choose to focus on outpatient billing/coding services. If you specialize in hospital services billing/coding, experience is necessary, especially because it is not common for a hospital to outsource

The HIPAA security rules indicate that working from home requires security policies and practices the same as working in the office. However, there are no specific policies given. It is up to each covered entity to establish these documents based on their security risk assessment. Security measures should address the technical setup. For example, typical security policy might stipulate that the telecommuter use a dedicated computer with a virtual private network solution, antivirus software, and a firewall if the computer is connected to the Internet and the office. Management of work papers and disks and the computer work environment (protected from family and visitors) might also be indicated. Additionally, privacy compliance policies apply at home just as they do when working in an office.

Street Address
City, State, ZIP code
Date of letter

John Doe, MD or
Personnel Director
Street Address
City, State, ZIP code

Dear Dr. Doe:

Thank you for spending your valuable time yesterday to interview me for
the insurance billing specialist position in your clinic.

I hope that you will allow me the opportunity to prove my abilities as I feel
that I am able to perform the work with expertise. Meeting your staff was
most enjoyable, and it would certainly be pleasurable working with them as
a team.

I am looking forward to hearing from you in the near future.

Sincerely yours,

(handwritten signature)

Type name

FIGURE 18–12 Example of a thank-you letter sent after an interview.

these services to a small billing company. If coding services are to be part of the billing company's offerings, the coding professional should be certified by a reputable organization such as American Academy of Professional Coders (AAPC) or American Health Information Management Association (AHIMA).

One must have something to offer clients when marketing and selling one's services and skills. This knowledge and expertise can only be gained with years of experience and persistence. Full-time commitment, hard work, dedication, and many long hours to obtain clients are encountered when beginning a business.

If you work awhile before striking out independently, you will make contacts on the job that may help build clientele. Networking is extremely important and may open up many opportunities when starting and growing a successful business. Many times it is who the individual knows that may get a foot in the potential client's door.

An insurance billing specialist can work as an independent contractor to have flexible hours, work from home, and reduce a medical practice's overhead. Some communities prohibit residents from telecommuting or operating a home-based business, although most allow it with restrictions. Working at home requires self-discipline, and one must develop a schedule and stick to it. Good time management is essential. It takes additional hours to advertise, obtain clients, bill, and perform the bookkeeping tasks. Box 18.1 is a checklist of tasks that must be done to establish a new business.

Planning Your Business

Every successful business endeavor begins with a smart business plan. This is a roadmap that will guide your business from start-up to continuous success. A business plan addresses facts and figures pertinent to your business and financial abilities as well as assesses your objectives and goals. Visit Web site http://www.entrepreneur.com/howto/bizplan/ for a complete guide on writing a business plan.

Professional Mailing Address

No doubt you will receive mail, so it is important to establish a professional address. It is always wise to rent a post office box. Doing this creates a business-oriented mailing address, helps maintain confidentiality in mailings you receive about clients and patient accounts, and protects you from unwanted visitors to your home. Visit Web site http://www.irs.gov/businesses/small/ for the IRS's "Small Business and Self-Employed One-Stop Resource."

Finances to Consider

Taxes

You must decide on what form of business entity you will be, that is, sole proprietor, partnership, or corporation. It is advisable to seek the services of a lawyer, accountant, or both before legally establishing a business and making appropriate selection of the tax options involved. Set up detailed financial records from the beginning, even if an accountant is to be hired. Obtain simplified bookkeeping software for use on the computer. Expert advice is

Box 18.1 | New Business Checklist

The following is a checklist to help you in starting a new home business. This is not a complete list of items to consider nor the exact order to accomplish them in; however, important points are covered in this list.

- Define your services and construct a business plan. Make sure you forecast for success. Will this business be viable? Can you accomplish the services you will promise to carry out? Can you financially afford this endeavor?
- Research whether you need to obtain a business license from the business license section of your city hall. Regulations vary in each city licensing office. You might have to obtain a home occupation permit from the planning department and have it signed by your landlord if you are renting. The city may have guidelines on hours of business, pedestrian and vehicular activity, noise, and so on in the residential area. Determine whether your county has rules on operating a small business from home.
- Consider a name for your business. File a fictitious business name (doing business as, or DBA) at the county clerk's office by obtaining the proper form for completion. If you use your given name, you do not have to file a fictitious business name.
- Decide what address to use. You may want to obtain a post office box number instead of using your home address. This will help with a professional mailing address as well as protect you from unexpected visitors to your home.
- Consult with an accountant for advice on tax structure of your company, for example sole proprietor, corporation, and so on. Learn about what expenses are deductible. Depending on how you set up your business, some possible tax breaks are depreciation of office equipment; declaring a room of your home as an office; subscriptions to professional publications; dues to professional associations; expenses associated with your automobile; telephone, photocopying, and office supplies (e.g., stationery, books, photocopy and fax paper); promotion and advertising (e.g., postage, meals with business associates); and any expenses pertaining to meetings, conventions, workshops, or seminars (e.g., registration fees, lodging, meals, transportation, parking).

Visit Web site http:www.irs.gov to learn more about how taxes will affect your business.

- Obtain the insurance that you need; health insurance, disability insurance, life insurance, liability insurance, workers' compensation (if you have employees), and so on. Insurance called "release of information insurance" or "errors and omissions insurance" with a "hold harmless" clause is available to protect you against loss of material. You might want to consider a retirement plan, such as an individual retirement account or a Keogh plan.
- Obtain a separate telephone number and possibly fax number to separate "home" from "business." However, you might consider using your existing telephone number and switching to a business listing. Having a business listing allows you to be listed in the yellow pages of your telephone directory. Remember that advertising can be expensive, so be sure this falls within your budget.
- Open a bank account. Many banks offer small business accounts with nominal monthly fees. For example, you can open an account "Jane Doe DBA 123 Claims Service."
- Create a professional image through business cards, stationery, and invoice billing forms. You can find resources on the Internet or in software programs to print your own.
- Stay current in the industry with up-to-date reference books. Begin to assemble a library to include a good medical dictionary, procedural and diagnostic code books, compliance handbooks, trade journals, and so on.
- Start a contact database and begin to advertise your business by some of the following methods: visiting offices, mailing flyers, advertising in trade journals or your local newspaper, sending announcements, putting up signs (be sure to get permission), and sending personalized letters to prospects (hospitals, clinics, and physician's offices).
- If you have opened an office at a location outside of your home, make sure you have reviewed a proper lease before signing it, and consider the finances needed for items such as utility deposits (i.e., water, gas, and electricity). Rent, renovation, and janitorial or trash services must also be considered.

essential and helps develop a successful business; a business could fail without it.

Establishing a business in a home may result in some deductions, so obtain all the information you can from your accountant and the Internal Revenue Service (IRS) regarding important laws concerning small business and self-employment taxes. Keep receipts and complete records of income and expenses because these are extremely important for IRS purposes.

Check stubs, copies of hours worked, and identifying data on clients must be retained for the period of time stipulated by the IRS. The following is a record retention schedule.

- Bank statements and canceled checks: 7 years
- Expired contracts: 7 years
- Financial statements: permanently
- General correspondence: 1 to 5 years

- Payroll records and summaries: 7 years
- Income tax returns: permanently
- Worksheets and supporting documents: 7 years

Keep a record of business travel expenses and document mileage. Travel log books are available at stationery stores.

Start-Up Expenses

In addition, money is needed for equipment, computer software, overhead, taxes, stationery, preprinted statements and forms, and a myriad of other expenses. It is vital to have sufficient funds to run the business for a period of 1 year or more. It is imperative that this be accrued before vacating a full-time job. This will help eliminate a lot of fear and anxiety over not having enough business clients. A common reason for business failure is running out of the money necessary to keep the business going. It may take a year or more to begin seeing a profit, so one must be patient. This is where the business plan becomes a useful resource!

If an individual has had no business management experience, courses may be taken to gain knowledge and instill confidence in these areas before beginning a business. Attend workshops and lectures on starting a business that are offered by financial institutions, universities, community colleges, or private institutions.

Bank Account

Open a bank account that is separate from your own personal checking account. This smart approach saves a lot of time in the future when it comes to sorting out expenses and working on taxes. Also, think about the professional image that a business check will convey. Most banks have small business account services, including those for the self-employed. Shop around and visit several banks, if you do not already have a preference, and compare monthly fees and transaction capabilities.

Business Name, Plan, and License

Some towns or counties require a business license to operate a business. This may include working from your home office. Check with your local offices to determine whether an application or fee is required. This is the time to choose an appropriate business name and get applicable town and county licenses.

A business name should be easy to remember and explain what your company does. For example, ABC's #1 Medical Billing Service will tell potential clients that the company works with health care related to billing and insurance claims.

A successful business must start with a smart business plan. This guides and helps your small business with financial and business strategies. It would be wise to meet with an accountant, an attorney, or a business consultant to help get your start up company off in the right direction.

For more information about business planning, visit the U.S. Small Business Association at Web site http://www.sba.gov.

Insurance

It may be necessary and sometimes required that business owners protect income and property from unexpected loss. Some types of insurance to investigate are as follows:

● Professional liability/errors and omissions. Protects you and your company from claims if your client holds you responsible for errors, or the failure of your work

to perform as promised in your service contract. Coverage can include legal costs and may pay for resulting judgments against you.
● Property insurance in case of fire, theft, or a disaster. Protects your assets and may help you in the recovery of data.
● Disability insurance if one becomes unable to work because of illness or injury. This can include yourself and/or an employee.
● Health and life insurance. Health coverage for yourself and/or employee as well as life insurance.

Business Associate Under HIPAA

HIPAA rules apply to most billing companies as a business associate when a relationship is formed with one or more health care providers for whom you perform billing services.

Business associate: (Sect: 160.103)

A person (or organization) who, on behalf of such covered performs, or assists in the performance of a function or activity involving the use or disclosure of individually identifiable health information, including claims processing or administration, data analysis, processing or administration, utilization review, quality assurance, billing, benefit management, practice management, and repricing;
or
(ii) Provides, other than in the capacity of a member of the workforce of such covered entity, legal, actuarial, accounting, consulting, data aggregation, management, administrative, accreditation, or financial services, where the provision of the service involves the disclosure of individually identifiable health information from such covered entity or arrangement, or from another business associate of such covered entity or arrangement, to the person.

Therefore, if your billing company gets PHI from a covered entity to perform a function or activity on behalf of that covered entity, your relationship is likely that of a business associate and your responsibilities must be defined with a Business Associate Agreement.

The Business Associate Agreement and the Service Contract

The **business associate agreement** must give "satisfactory assurances" to the covered entity on whose behalf it performs services and must include, according to HIPAA rule, the following terms as set forth in the regulation:

Obligations and Activities of Business Associate

● Business Associate agrees to not use or disclose Protected Health Information other than as permitted or required by the Agreement or as Required By Law.
● Business Associate agrees to use appropriate safeguards to prevent use or disclosure of the Protected Health Information other than as provided for by this Agreement.

- Business Associate agrees to mitigate, to the extent practicable, any harmful effect that is known to Business Associate of a use or disclosure of Protected Health Information by Business Associate in violation of the requirements of this Agreement. [This provision may be included if it is appropriate for the Covered Entity to pass on its duty to mitigate damages to a Business Associate.]
- Business Associate agrees to report to Covered Entity any use or disclosure of the Protected Health Information not provided for by this Agreement of which it becomes aware.
- Business Associate agrees to ensure that any agent, including a subcontractor, to whom it provides Protected Health Information received from, or created or received by Business Associate on behalf of Covered Entity agrees to the same restrictions and conditions that apply through this Agreement to Business Associate with respect to such information.
- Business Associate agrees to provide access, at the request of Covered Entity, and in the time and manner [Insert negotiated terms], to Protected Health Information in a Designated Record Set, to Covered Entity or, as directed by Covered Entity, to an Individual in order to meet the requirements under 45 CFR § 164.524. [Not necessary if business associate does not have protected health information in a designated record set.]
- Business Associate agrees to make any amendment(s) to Protected Health Information in a Designated Record Set that the Covered Entity directs or agrees to pursuant to 45 CFR § 164.526 at the request of Covered Entity or an Individual, and in the time and manner [Insert negotiated terms]. [Not necessary if business associate does not have protected health information in a designated record set.]
- Business Associate agrees to make internal practices, books, and records, including policies and procedures and Protected Health Information, relating to the use and disclosure of Protected Health Information received from, or created or received by Business Associate on behalf of, Covered Entity available [to the Covered Entity, or] to the Secretary, in a time and manner [Insert negotiated terms] or designated by the Secretary, for purposes of the Secretary determining Covered Entity's compliance with the Privacy Rule.
- Business Associate agrees to document such disclosures of Protected Health Information and information related to such disclosures as would be required for Covered Entity to respond to a request by an Individual for an accounting of disclosures of Protected Health Information in accordance with 45 CFR § 164.528.
- Business Associate agrees to provide to Covered Entity or an Individual, in time and manner [Insert negotiated terms], information collected in accordance with

Section [Insert Section Number in Contract Where Provision (i) Appears] of this Agreement, to permit Covered Entity to respond to a request by an Individual for an accounting of disclosures of Protected Health Information in accordance with 45 CFR § 164.528.

Service Contract

The **service contract** is a separate document from the business associate agreement. The service contract is a necessary document that defines the duties and obligations of each party involved in the business relationship as far as who is responsible for what duty or task that carries out the purpose of the service contract agreement. Contracts or agreements should be made in writing, signed, and notarized. For example, a contract should define the following:

- Who is responsible for the coding (the physician or the billing service)?
- What will be the routine for claim submission?
- Is there a per-claim processing fee or is there a flat monthly fee?
- Who is responsible for follow-up on collection procedures (telephone calls or letters)?
- Who pays for rebilling, photocopying of records, mailing fees, and clearinghouse charges? Is this included in a flat monthly service fee?
- Under whose name will bills be sent to patients (the physician or the billing service)?
- Will the billing service telephone number appear on the statement, or will a toll-free or local number be used?
- How will the telephone be answered?
- What are the charges for coding consultation services?
- What are the coverage arrangements for absence or illness?
- How will information be protected and handled between client and billing company?

If there is any change in the terms of the agreements, write an addendum to the original agreement and have both parties sign to acknowledge the change. Be sure all agreements and contracts have proper effective and termination dates. Remember that renegotiation is in order when the contract expires.

HIPAA Compliance Alert

Some contracts may include a statement on confidentiality assuring the contracting facility that all patient data will be handled in a confidential manner.

Pricing Your Services

Define your services and work out a structured fee schedule making sure to review state laws regarding percentage billing (it is illegal in some states). Get legal advice when creating contracts and agreements.

A variety of methods are used to price services, such as a percentage of reimbursement or an annual, hourly, or per-claim fee. Deciding on which method depends on the type of client being served and the work to be done. For example, a claims assistance professional may bill in 15-minute increments. Telephone other billing and insurance services, preferably outside the area, to learn what they are charging because in-area competitors may be reluctant to divulge that information.

Setting Up Your Office

The most important consideration is privacy and security of the health information and business documents you will handle and be responsible for. Review the security suggestions as outlined in Chapter 8.

An initial equipment checklist may include the following:

- Computer
- Laser and/or ink jet printer
- Paper
- Current billing and coding manuals and books
- Desk supplies such as stapler, paper clips, self-adhesive notes, and so on.
- Locking file cabinets
- Fax machine

Also consider using separate computer backup protection (e.g., a surge protector with battery power) to guard against faulty wiring or power failure. This gives more than 10 minutes to back up your current project and then shut down. These are available at office stores for about $100.

Shop smart. Research upcoming sales and lease programs, rebates, upgrade trade-ins, and service plans.

Research the various medical billing software programs asking for demo software before purchasing. Also, look for a reputable clearinghouse. Compare functionality, customer service, technical support, and prices.

Marketing, Advertising, Promotion, and Public Relations

Marketing refers to how a business is presented or advertised to promote sales. Marketing strategies vary depending on the section of the public that is targeted.

When promoting a medical billing service, develop a well-organized marketing plan and follow basic guidelines to reach a specific target audience.

Ways to market a business and the reasons for marketing strategies are presented in Table 18.1.

At this point you should be ready to get out there and start marketing your business. If you are creative, you can certainly design your own business cards and get them printed. A classic white card with black font (print) depicts professionalism. You can also find matching stationery sets. Create flyers, brochures, newsletters, surveys, and so on. Obtain financial data to help convince clients that the service you are offering is better and can do more for their business than what they presently have. Save them time and money! Stress being honest, reliable, committed, efficient, and professional, and offer them something they cannot do for themselves.

Put yourself in front of the office managers and health care providers to advertise your services. Consider visiting the health care offices in your area and be sure to follow up with visits and calls. Be careful with offices that have a sign stating "No Soliciting." If you see this sign, respect it and jot the address down to mail them literature instead. Also note that solicitation by fax is illegal according to the Federal Communications Commission: "Enacted by Congress in 1991, the Telephone Consumer Protection Act (TCPA) restricts the use of the telephone and facsimile machine to deliver unsolicited advertisements. Under the TCPA, one may not send an unsolicited advertisement to a fax machine. In addition, those sending fax messages or transmitting artificial or prerecorded voice messages are subject to certain identification requirements."

Marketing can be tough and intimidating. Networking with other colleagues and professions along with persistence will pay off.

Documentation

Besides keeping documentation received from your client, keep written records of the numbers of hours worked, the quantity of work done each day, and the corrections applied to the work by officials in the contracting facility or hospital. Retain any written coding guideline from the contracting facility or hospital.

Trends for Success with Professional Associations, Certification, and Registration

More exacting professional requirements have evolved because of specialization in the allied health careers. Certification and registration are two ways of exhibiting

Table 18.1 Business Marketing and Strategies

Strategy	Reason
Obtain professionally printed stationery and business cards.	Enhances professional image.
Pass out business cards at professional meetings.	Advertises availability and services. Helps with networking.
Develop a business name and logo for the company.	Enables potential clients to identify you are in your business.
Ensure accuracy of all printed materials.	When items are not professionally assembled or proofread to eliminate typographic errors, a potential client receives a doubtful or negative image of the company.
Develop a professional flyer and distribute it to medical facilities and physicians' offices.	Introduces company name, advertises services, and describes benefits.
Follow up with a personal visit or telephone call.	A friendly voice and professional image offer personal services and let potential clients know you are available and interested.
Advertise in the journal or newsletter of the county medical society and state medical association.	Potential clients read such publications and advertisements of this nature lend to your credibility.
Place an advertisement in the newspaper or on cable television.	Circulates business within the county.
Put an ad in the *Yellow Pages*.	Solicits wider range of prospective clients.
Network with members of professional organizations.	Word of mouth advertising can be the best public relations tool, especially if done by professional peers.
Network via computer using the Internet's discussion and career boards, such as America Online and Yahoo.	Offers wide range of contacts.
Promote your business with a professionally developed Web site.	Search engines will help find you. Web sites deliver immediate, detailed information about your company.
Check with established businesses to determine whether they are overloaded with work, the owner needs a vacation, or help is needed in a temporary situation because of illness.	Present your services as a help, not a threat, to current office staff.

professional standards (Table 18.2). **Certification** is a statement issued by a board or association verifying that a person meets professional standards. **Registration** may be accomplished in two methods, as an entry in an official registry or record that lists names of persons in an occupation who have satisfied specific requirements or by attaining a certain level of education and paying a registration fee. In the latter, if there are certain requirements for registration, then an unregistered person may be prevented from working in a career for which he or she is otherwise qualified.

Membership in professional organizations helps in keeping up-to-date. Most of these associations have student as well as active and associate membership categories. You can inquire whether there is a local chapter or state organization affiliated with the national association. Benefits of belonging to a professional organization, in addition to certification and recertification, include problem solving, continuing education, and employment opportunities. Local meetings can keep you knowledgeable by providing guest speakers on topics of current interest. The newsletters and journals published by these organizations keep you abreast of current trends either as a subscriber or as a benefit when becoming a member.

Mentor

A valuable vehicle for career development is to find a **mentor** in the business. A mentor is a guide or teacher who offers advice, criticism, wisdom, guidance, and perspective to an inexperienced but promising protégé to help reach a life goal. Decide what kind of help you want, such as technical, general feedback, managerial, and so on. Then look for a mentor whose background, values, and style are similar to yours. Be willing to face criticism with a positive attitude and express gratitude when excellence is praised.

Networking

Another avenue to pursue for career development is to *network*. **Networking** is the exchange of information or services among individuals, groups, or institutions and making use of professional contacts. To do this, join as many organizations as possible because it can be difficult to keep abreast of ongoing changes in the insurance industry when you are self-employed. Many of the professional organizations publish monthly newsletters or quarterly journals, offer certification, and plan national conventions, state conferences, and regional meetings.

Claims assistance professionals should attend local meetings for Medicare recipients. Join local volunteer service organizations and the chamber of commerce to network with others. Contact the LEADS Club at (800) 783-3761 or The National Association of Female Executives at (800) 669-1002 for potential client leads and networking.

Table 18.2 Certification and Registration

Title/Abbreviation	Description to Obtain Certification or Registration	Professional Association Mailing Address	Telephone Number	Web Site	E-Mail Address
Certified bookkeeper (CB)	Self-study program and employment experience; pass three tests	American Institute of Professional Bookkeepers 6001 Montrose Road, Suite 207 Rockville, MD 20852	(800) 622-0121	www.aipb.org	Visit Web site
Certified coding associate (CCA) **Certified coding specialist (CCS)** **Certified coding specialist-physician based (CCS-P)** Certified in health care privacy (CHP)	Self-study program; pass certification examination	American Health Information Management Association (AHIMA) 233 N. Michigan Ave., Suite 2150 Chicago, IL 60601-5800	(800) 335-5535	www.ahima.org	info@ahima.org
Certified health care financial professional (CHFP)	60 hours college/university and complete core examination and one specialty examination within 2-year period	Healthcare Financial Management Association (HFMA) 2 Westbrook Corporate Center, Suite 700 Westchester, IL 60154-5700	(800) 252-4362	www.hfma.org	webmaster@hfma.com
Certified electronic claims professional (CECP)	Self-study program; pass certification examination	Alliance of Claims Assistance Professionals (ACAP) 873 Brentwood Drive West Chicago, IL 60185		www.claims.org	askacap@charter.net
Certified health care billing and management executive (CHBME)	Complete comprehensive program; pass proficiency test	Healthcare Billing and Management Association (HMBA) 1550 South Coast Highway, Suite 201 Laguna Beach, CA 92651	(877) 640-4262	www.hbma.com	info@hbma.com
Certified in health care compliance (CHC)	Have work experience, continuing education, and pass examination	Health Care Compliance Association	(888) 580-8373	www.hcca-info.org	info@hcca-info.org
Certified in health care privacy (CHP) Certified in health care privacy and security (CHPS) Certified in health care security (CHS)	Eligibility requirements and pass examination Pass CHP and CHS examinations	American Health Information Management Assn. (AHIMA) PO Box 97349 Chicago, IL 60690-7349	(800) 335-5535	www.ahima.org	info@ahima.mhs. compuserve.com
Certified information systems security professional (CISSP) Certified HIPAA security professional (CHSP) Systems security certified practitioner (SSCP)	Pass examination and submit endorsement form	International Information Systems Security Certifications Consortium, Inc.	(866) 278-1994	www.isc2.org	Isc2@asestores.com

Certification	Requirements	Organization	Phone	Website	Visit Web site
Certified medical assistant (CMA)	Graduate from accredited medical assisting program; apply to take national certifying examination	American Association of Medical Assistants (AAMA) 20 North Wacker Drive Chicago, IL 60606	(800) 228-2262	www.aama.ntl.org	
Certified medical biller (CMB)	Pass 2-hour examination written for physician's office billers and other outpatient facilities	American Association of Medical Billers (AAMB) PO Box 44614 Los Angeles, CA 90044-0614	(323) 778-4352 Fax: (323) 778-2814	Billers.com/aamb/page2.html	AAMB@aol.com
Certified medical billing specialist (CMBS)	Pass 3-hour examination written for physician's office billers and other outpatient facilities	American Association of Medical Billers (AAMB) PO Box 44614 Los Angeles, CA 90044-0614	(323) 778-4352 Fax: (323) 778-2814	www.billers.com/aamb/page2.html	AAMB@aol.com
Certified medical billing specialist (CMBS)	Complete six courses and provide evaluation of billing performance by supervisor	Medical Association of Billers (MAB) 2441 Tech Center Court, Suite 108 Las Vegas, NV 89128	(702) 240-8519 Fax: (702) 243-0359	www.physicianswebsites.com	mailroom@physicianswebsites.com
Certified medical office manager (CMOM)	Examination for supervisors or managers of small group and solo practices	**Professional Association of Health Care Office Managers (PAHCOM)** 461 East Ten Mile Road Pensacola, FL 32534-9712	(800) 451-9311	www.pahcom.com	pahcom@pahcom.com
Certified medical practice executive (CMPE) Nominee 1st level 2nd level Fellow 3rd level	1st level—Eligible group managers join; membership/nominee 2nd level—Complete 6- to 7-hour examination 3rd level—Mentoring project or thesis	Medical Group Management Association (MGMA), American College of Medical Practice Executives (affiliate) 104 Inverness Terrace East Englewood, CO 80112	(303) 397-7869	www.mgma.com/acmpe	acmpe@mgma.com
Certified medical reimbursement specialist (CMRS)	Self-study program; successfully pass 18 sections of examination	American Medical Billing Association (AMBA) 4297 Forrest Drive Sulphur, OK 73086	(580) 622-2624	www.ambanet.net/cmrs.htm	larry@brightok.net
Certified medical transcriptionist (CMT)	Self-study program and successfully pass written and practical examinations offered by Medical Transcription Certification Commission (MTCC)	American Association for Medical Transcription 100 Sycamore Avenue Modesto, CA 95354-0550	(800) 982-2182	www.aamt.org	Visit Web site
Certified patient account technician (CPAT) Certified clinic account technician (CCAT) Certified clinic account manager (CCAM)	Complete self-study course; pass standard examination administered twice yearly	American Association of Healthcare Administrative Management (AAHAM) National Certification Examination Program 11240 Waples Mill Road, Suite 200 Fairfax, VA 22030	(703) 281-4043	www.aaham.org/aaham.cfm	debra@statmarket.com

Continued

Table 18.2 Certification and Registration—cont'd

Title/Abbreviation	Description to Obtain Certification or Registration	Professional Association Mailing Address	Telephone Number	Web Site	E-Mail Address
Certified professional coder (CPC) Certified professional coder-apprentice (CPC-A) Certified professional coder-hospital (CPC-H)	Independent study program; examination approximately 5 hours (CPC) and 8 hours (CPC-H)	American Academy of Professional Coders (AAPC) 309 West 700 South Salt Lake City, UT 84101	(800) 626-CODE	www.aapc.com	info@aapc.com
Certified claims assistance professional (CCAP)	Self-study program; pass certification examination	Alliance of Claims Assistance Professionals (ACAP) 873 Brentwood Drive West Chicago, IL 60185	No listing	www.claims.org	askus@claims.org
Health care reimbursement specialist (HRS)	Successfully complete open-book examination	National Electronic Biller's Alliance (NEBA) 2226-A Westborough Blvd. #504 South San Francisco, CA 94080	(650) 359-4419 Fax: (650) 355-8683	http://www.nebazone.com	mmedical@aol.com
National certified insurance and coding specialist (NCICS)	Graduate from an insurance program; sit for certification examination given by independent testing agency at many school sites across the nation	National Center for Competency Testing 7007 College Blvd., Suite 250 Overland Park, KS 66211	(800) 875-4404 Fax: (913) 498-1243	www.ncctinc.com	Visit Web site
Registered medical assistant (RMA)	Certification offered by the American Medical Technologist (AMT)	Registered Medical Assistant (AMT) 710 Higgins Road Park Ridge, IL 60068-5765	(847) 823-5169	www.amt1.com	amtmail@aol.com
Registered medical coder (RMC)	Yearly correspondence program governed by the National Coding Standards Committee; pass an examination	Medical Management Institute 1125 Cambridge Square Alpharetta, GA 30004-5724	(800) 334-5724	www.the-institute.com	bobby.carvell @ipractice.md
Utilization Review Accreditation Commission (URAC)-accredited consultant	Application	Utilization Review Accreditation Commission 1220 L Street, NW, Suite 400 Washington, DC 20005	(202) 216-9010	www.urac.org	ita@urac.org
Certified in health care compliance (CHC)	Examination, work experience, and continuing education	Health Care Compliance Association 5780 Lincoln Drive, Suite 120 Minneapolis, MN 55436	(888) 580-8373	www.hcca-info.org	info@hcca-info.org
Systems security certified practitioner (SSCP)	Pass examination and submit endorsement form	International Information Systems Security Certifications Consortium, Inc. 2494 Bayshore Blvd., Suite 201 Dunedin, FL 34698	(888) 333-4458	www.isc2.org	isc2@asestores.com

Reassess and Continue with Success

Once your billing service is under way, you will find it necessary to routinely assess the overall health of the business. Review your business plans and make sure you are following the guidelines. Make changes where applicable and revise strategies and goals. Running your own successful business is challenging and highly rewarding both emotionally and financially. Good luck!

PROCEDURE

CREATING AN ELECTRONIC RESUME

Once a medical position has been discovered, the basic steps for putting out an online resume are as follows:

1. Compose a resume using a word processor with accurate spelling features and be sure to keep it simple. Then save the electronic resume in a job search file.
2. Discard traditional resume-writing techniques, such as focusing on action verbs. Instead, think descriptive nouns, such as medical biller, education, experience, skills, knowledge, and abilities.
3. Avoid the use of decorative graphics and complex typefaces, bulleted lists, complicated page formatting, symbols, underlining, or italics. These features may not appear the same on an employer's computer online.
4. Forget the one-page rule; electronic resumes may be three to four pages.
5. Refer to the word processor manual to convert the cover letter and resume to ASCII (American Standard Code for Information Interchange; pronounced AS-kee), or plain text, which can be read by most personal computers.
6. Study online guides presenting special procedures for sending e-mail and files. Some e-mail programs allow binary files to be sent, whereas others only allow ASCII text files.
7. Use the word processing software's "copy and paste" feature and enter the information into e-mail or "attach a file" to the e-mail message.
8. Do not post a letter of introduction when posting a resume to a bulletin board.
9. Upload the resume to post online using the file transfer feature of the software following the computer manual directions. The ASCII file is all that is necessary when sending the resume over an online service or from a computer to a dial-direct bulletin board.
10. After you send a resume electronically, mail a hard copy and call the hiring manager directly to follow up. Be aggressive.

PROCEDURE

PREPARING A RESUME IN ASCII

If the file is sent across the Internet, it should be doctored up in a technical form—encoded by the sender and decoded by the receiver. Take the following steps to prepare a plain ASCII text file.

1. Create the message using WordPerfect or Word software. Make certain all lines are no more than 65 characters in length. Put a space at the beginning of each blank line between paragraphs.
2. Proofread the resume and save it as plain ASCII text, referring to the word processing software manual for directions.
3. Log onto the bulletin board to upload the ASCII text. Go to the message menu and follow the bulletin board's directions.
4. Select or type "All" or "Resume posting" from the bulletin board's message menu for the recipient and subject.
5. Upload the resume, following the software manual's directions for the communications program being used.
6. Customize the resume by typing in additional information related to the specific job. Depending on the bulletin board, a "Message Edit" menu or the next available line will appear, issuing message-editing commands.

Advance for Careers is a Web site designed to facilitate the job-seeking process. Go to Web site: www.Advanceweb.com and click on "Need to find a job."

- Google (search engine)
  Web site: **www.google.com**

- Yahoo (search engine)
  Web site: **www.yahoo.com/**

- Infoseek (search engine)
  Web site: **www.infoseek.go.com**

- Alta Vista (search engine)
  Web site: **www.altavista.com**

- Ask Jeeves (search engine)
  Web site: **www.ask.com**

- Teoma (search engine)
  Web site: **www.teoma.com**

- Kanoodle (search engine)
  Web site: **www.kanoodle.com**

- Lycos (search engine)
  Web site: **www.lycos.com**

- Career Magazine
  Web site: **www.careermag.com/careermag/**

- America's Job Bank
  Web site: **www.ajbb.dni.us**

- E-Span Employment Database Search
  Web site: **www.espan.com/**

- MedSearch
  Web site: **www.medsearch.com**

Refer to Table 18.2 for professional organization Web sites.

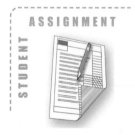

STUDENT **ASSIGNMENT**

✔ Study Chapter 18.

✔ Answer the review questions in the *Workbook* to reinforce the theory learned in this chapter and help prepare you for a future test.

✔ Complete the assignments in the *Workbook* to give you hands-on experience in completing an application for a position as an insurance billing specialist, preparing and typing a resume, composing a cover letter to go with the resume, having someone evaluate you during an interview, and typing a follow-up thank-you letter after being interviewed.

✔ Turn to the glossary at the end of this textbook for a further understanding of the key terms used in this chapter.

A

Resources for Audiotapes, Books, Newsletters, Periodicals, Software, and Videotapes

Technical data changes quickly in the field of insurance billing and coding and because of this the need for current editions and titles is imperative. From the following list, either telephone the toll-free numbers or go to the Web sites to access the most up-to-date information on audiotapes, books, certification, newsletters, periodicals, software, and videotapes.

America's Health Insurance Plans (health insurance glossary book, disability income insurance book, audiocassette tapes for education and training)
    601 Pennsylvania Avenue, NW, South Building, Suite 500, Washington DC 20004
    (202) 778-8471
    Web site: www.ahip.org

American Academy of Orthopaedic Surgeons (books, diagnostic and procedural)
    6300 N. River Road, Rosemont, IL 60018-4262
    Phone: (800) 346-AAOS or (847) 823-7186
    Fax: (847) 823-8125
    Web site: www.aaos.org

American Academy of Pediatrics (books, diagnostic and procedural)
    141 N.W. Point Boulevard, Elk Grove Village, IL 60007-1098
    (847) 434-4000
    Web site: www.aap.org

American Academy of Professional Coders (certification study guides)
    309 West 700 South, Salt Lake City, UT 84101
    (800) 626-CODE
    Web site: www.aapc.com

American Association of Medical Assistants (education and training code books)
    20 N. Wacker Drive, Suite 1575, Chicago, IL 60606
    (800) 228-2262
    Web site: www.aama-natl.org

American College of Emergency Physicians (books, diagnostic and procedural)
    P.O. Box 619911, Dallas, TX 75261
    (800) 798-1822
    Web site: www.acep.org

American College of Radiology (RVS book)
    1891 Preston White Drive, Reston, VA 22090
    (703) 648-8900
    Web site: www.acr.org

American College of Rheumatology (books, diagnostic and procedural)
    1800 Century Place, Suite 250 Atlanta, GA 30345-4300
    (404) 633-3777

American Health Information Management Association (Books, certification information, medical documentation, publications, and education and training code books and seminars)
    233 North Michigan Avenue, Suite 2150 Chicago, IL 60601-5800
    (312) 233-1100 or (800) 335-5535
    Web site: www.ahima.org

American Hospital Association
    AHA Resource Center
    One North Franklin
    Chicago, IL 60606
    (312) 422-2050
    Web site: http://aharc.library.net

American Medical Association (books, diagnostic and procedural, code journals, code software, fraud and abuse compliance book, law and ethics books)
    515 N. State Street, P.O. Box 10946, Chicago, IL 60610-0946
    (800) 621-8335
    Web site: www.ama-assn.org

American Psychiatric Publishing, Inc. (books, diagnostic and procedural)
    1000 Wilson Building, Suite 1825, Arlington, VA 22209-3901
    (800) 368-5777 or (703) 907-7322
    Web site: www.appi.org

Appeal Solutions (collection software)
    P.O. Box 1087, Blanchard, OK 73010
    (888) 399-4925
    Web site: www.appealsolutions.com

Aspen Publishers, Inc. (books, newsletters, compliance books, medical documentation book, healthcare software source book, reference guides)
    7201 McKinney Circle (21704) P.O. Box 990, Frederick, MD 21705-9727
    (800) 638-8437
    Web site: www.aspenpub.com

California Health Information Association (education and training code books)
    1915 North Fine Avenue, Suite 104, Fresno, CA 93727-1510
    (800) 247-8907
    Web site: www.californiahia.org

Channel Publishing, Ltd. (books, diagnostic and procedural, code software)
    4750 Longley Lane, Suite 110, Reno, NV 89502
    (800) 248-2882
    Web site: www.channelpublishing.com

ChartCare (books, diagnostic and procedural)
    7403 Lakewood Dr. West, Suite 12, Lakewood,
    WA 98499
    (800) 438-1277
    Web site: www.chartcare.com

Commerce Clearing House, Inc. (disability,
unemployment, and managed care newsletters, Medicare
and Medicaid books and newsletters, and CDs)
    4025 West Peterson Avenue (60646), P.O. Box 5490,
    Chicago, IL 60680-9882
    (800) 835-5224
    Web site: www.cch.com

Conomikes Associates, Inc. (collection handbook,
Medicare RVU Scale handbook, newsletters, and
seminars)
    12233 West Olympic Blvd., Suite 116, Los Angeles,
    CA 90064
    (800) 421-6512
    Web site: www.conomikes.com

Captiva Context (code software)
    601 Oakmont Lane, Suite 200, Westmont, IL 60559
    (800) 783-3378 or (630) 654-8800
    Web site: www.captivacontext.com

DiagnostIC Data, Inc. (code software)
    20 Balfour Drive, West Hartford, CT 06117
    (800) 999-6405
    Web site: www.diagdata.com

Elsevier/Mosby/Saunders (books, diagnostic and
procedural, education and training code and insurance
books, medical dictionaries)
    11830 Westline Industrial Drive, St. Louis,
    MO 63146
    Phone: (800) 633-6699
    Fax: (314) 432-1380
    Web site: www.elsevier.com

F.A. Davis Company/Publishers (medical dictionaries)
    1915 Arch Street, Philadelphia, PA 19103
    (800) 523-4049 (editorial office); 800-323-3555
    (distribution)
    Web site: www.fadavis.com

Faulkner & Gray, Thomson Financial (electronic health
records compliance book, electronic data interchange
book)
    11 Penn Plaza, 17th floor, New York,
    NY 10117-0373
    (800) 535-8403
    Web site: www.thomsonmedia.com

Glencoe/McGraw-Hill (education and training code
and insurance books, law and ethics books)
    P.O. Box 545, Blacklick, OH 43004
    (800) 722-4726
    Web site: www.glencoe.com

Information Handling Services (IHS) Regulatory
Products (Medicare and Medicaid books)
    6160 S. Syracuse Way, Englewood, CO 80110
    (800) 525-5539 or (303) 267-0543
    Web site: www.ihshealth.com

Ingenix Publishing Group (books, diagnostic and
procedural code books, RVS code books, newsletters,
research and review services, code hotlines, compliance
books, DRG books, medical documentation book,
education and training books, fee schedules for
specialties, hospital insurance claims, DRG, RBRVS fee
schedule, APC, and insurance directory)
    5225 Wiley Post Way, Suite 500 (84116-2889),
    P.O. Box 27116, Salt Lake City, UT 84152-6180
    Phone: (800) 464-3649
    Fax: (801) 983-4033
    Web site: www.ingenixonline.com
    Ingenix seminars:
    Web site: www.ingenix.com

Lexi-Comp (diagnostic and procedure handbooks for
terminology)
    1100 Terex Road, Hudson, OH 44236
    (800) 837-5394 (sales)
    Web site: www.lexi.com

Lippincott Williams & Wilkins (medical dictionaries)
    530 Walnut Street, Philadelphia, PA 19106-3621
    (800) 777-2295
    Web site: www.lww.com

Magmutual (specialty software for fees and fee and
coding guide)
    3025 Breckinridge Blvd., Suite 120, Duluth, GA 30096
    Phone: (800) 253-4945
    Web site: www.coderscentral.com

McGraw-Hill Healthcare Management Group
(books, diagnostic and procedural)
    1221 Avenue of the Americas, New York, NY 10020
    (877) 833-5524
    Web site: http://books.mcgraw-hill.com

MedBooks (education and training code books)
    101 West Buckingham Road, Richardson, TX 75081
    (800) 443-7397
    Web site: www.medbooks.com

Medical Economics Publishing
(practice management articles)
    P.O. Box 6085, Duluth, MN 55806-9810
    (800) 432-4570
    Web site: www.memag.com (click on practice
    management to get to billing topics)

Medical Learning Incorporated
(books, diagnostic and procedural)
    287 East Sixth Street, Suite 400, St. Paul, MN 55101
    (800) 252-1578
    Web site: www.medlearn.com

Medical Management Institute (books, diagnostic and procedural, compliance books, and seminars)
  MMI Campus Bookstore
  11405 Old Roswell Road, Alpharetta, Georgia 30004
  (800) 334-5724 ext. 1
  Web site: www.codingbooks.com

Opus Communications (newsletters, code software)
  100 Hoods Lane, P.O. Box 1168, Marblehead,
  MA 01945
  (877) 727-1728
  Web site: www.hcpro.com

Practice Management Information Corporation (books, diagnostic and procedural, collection books, fee books, insurance directory)
  4727 Wiltshire Boulevard, Los Angeles,
  CA 90010
  (800) MED-SHOP
  Web site: www.pmiconline.com

Rayve Productions, Inc. (independent medical coding book)
  P.O. Box 726, Windsor, CA 95492
  (800) 852-4890
  Web site: www.rayveproductions.com

Shannon Publications, Inc. (Medicare monthly newsletter)
  6380 LBJ Freeway, Suite 286, Dallas,
  TX 75240
  (800) 578-4888

The Society of Interventional Radiology (books, diagnostic and procedural)
  10201 Lee Highway, Suite 500, Fairfax,
  VA 22030
  (703) 691-1805
  Web site: www.sirweb.org

Society of Thoracic Surgeons (books, diagnostic and procedural)
  633 N. Saint Clair St., Suite 2320, Chicago,
  IL 60611-3658
  (312) 202-5800
  Web site: www.sts.org

State of California, Department of Industrial Relations, Division of Workers' Compensation (California Medical Fee Schedule)
  455 Golden Gate Avenue, Room 5182,
  San Francisco, CA 94102

Thomson American Health Consultants (books, diagnostic and procedural and managed care newsletters)
  P.O. Box 105109, Department 1203, Atlanta, GA 30348
  (800) 688-2421
  Web site: www.ahcpub.com/online.html

Thomson Delmar Learning (education and training code and insurance books, law and ethics books)
  P.O. Box 6904, Florence, KY 41022
  (800) 347-7707
  Web site: www.delmarlearning.com

Thomson West (fee manual and law and ethics books and software)
  620 Opperman Drive, P.O. Box 64526, Eagan,
  MN 55123-1396
  (800) 328-9352
  Web site: www.west.thomson.com

Unicor Medical, Inc. (books, diagnostic and procedural, code newsletters, code software)
  4160 Carmichael Road, Suite 101, Montgomery,
  AL 36106
  (800) 825-7421
  Web site: www.unicormed.com

United Communications Group (billing books, newsletters, RBRVS code book, and code software)
  11300 Rockville Pike, Suite 1100 (20852),
  P.O. Box 90608, Washington, DC 20077-7637
  (800) 929-4824
  Web site: www.ucg.com

United States Government Printing Office (books on fraud and abuse, Medicare and RBRVS fee schedule in *Federal Register*)
  Superintendent of Documents, Washington,
  DC 20402
  Web site: http://bookstore.gpo.gov

Wasserman Medical Publishers, Limited (physicians' fee reference book and disk and HCPCS code books, insurance directory)

3036 S. 92nd Street, P.O. Box 27365, West Allis, WI 53227

(800) 669-3337

Web site: www.medfees.com

Zhealth Publishing (code books about interventional radiology and cardiology)

330 Franklin Road, Suite 135A, Brentwood, TN 37027

(615) 778-4927

Web site: www.zhealthpublishing.com

Karen Zupko & Associates (forms and downloads)

980 N. Michigan Avenue, #1325, Chicago, IL 60611

(312) 642-5616

Web site: www.karenzupko.com

APPENDIX OUTLINE

TYPES OF MEDI-CAL PLANS
Managed Care Plans
Descriptions of Managed Care
  Plans
MEDI-CAL ELIGIBILITY
Share of Cost
Identification Card
Eligibility Verification
MEDI-CAL BENEFITS
Medi-Services
PRIOR APPROVAL
Telecommunications Networks
Treatment Authorization
  Request
CLAIM PROCEDURE
Fiscal Intermediaries
Copayment

Time Limit
Helpful Billing Tips
Medi-Cal and Other
  Coverage
Computer Media Claims
UNIFORM BILL (UB-92)
OUTPATIENT CLAIM
FORM
Instructions for
  Completing the UB-92
  Claim Form
AFTER CLAIM SUBMISSION
Remittance Advice Details
Resubmission Turnaround
  Document
Claims Inquiry Form
Appeal Process

PROCEDURE: COMPLETING
  A TREATMENT
  AUTHORIZATION
  REQUEST FORM 50-1
PROCEDURE: INSTRUCTIONS
  FOR COMPLETING THE
  CMS-1500 CLAIM FORM
  FOR THE MEDI-CAL
  PROGRAM
PROCEDURE: COMPLETING
  THE RESUBMISSION
  TURNAROUND DOCUMENT
PROCEDURE: COMPLETING
  THE CLAIMS INQUIRY
  FORM
PROCEDURE: COMPLETING
  AN APPEAL FORM

KEY TERMS

Medi-Cal terms are used when reading updates to the program policy manuals, which are available via the Internet or in hard copy by annual subscription. However, abbreviations are used rather than complete terms or phrases during lectures and in some publications about the Medi-Cal program. Therefore study both thoroughly. In addition to the key terms given in Chapter 13 used for Medicaid and Other State Programs, the following key terms and abbreviations are emphasized for study from Appendix B that are specific to the Medi-Cal program.

accounts receivable (A/R) transaction

Aid to the Blind (AB)

Aid to Families with Dependent Children (AFDC)

Aid to the (permanently) Disabled (ATD)

automated eligibility verification system (AEVS)

benefits identification card (BIC)

California Children's Services (CCS)

Child Health and Disability Prevention Program (CHDP)

claim control number (CCN)

claims and eligibility real-time software (CERTS)

Claims Inquiry Form (CIF)

Comprehensive Perinatal Services Program (CPSP)

computer media claims (CMC)

County Medical Services Program (CMSP)

Department of Health Services (DHS)

durable medical equipment (DME)

Electronic Data Systems (EDS) Corporation

electronic funds transfer (EFT)

eligibility verification confirmation (EVC)

Genetically Handicapped Persons Program (GHPP)

medically indigent (MI)

medically needy (MN)

nursing facility (NF)

Old Age Survivors, Health and Disability Insurance (OASHDI) Program

point-of-service (POS) device or network

presumptive eligibility (PE)

Provider Telecommunications Network (PTN)

Remittance Advice Details (RAD)

Resubmission Turnaround Document (RTD)

share of cost (SOC)

Treatment Authorization Request (TAR) Form

Voice Drug TAR System (VDTS)

B
Medi-Cal

OBJECTIVES*

After reading this appendix, you should be able to:

- Define key terms and abbreviations inherent to Medi-Cal.

- Identify the patient's Medi-Cal benefits identification card and list important information to obtain from the card.

- Describe the point-of-service device and state how it relates to the recipient's eligibility and share of cost.

- List important information to obtain from the patient's Medi-Cal identification card.

- State how to verify a patient's Medi-Cal eligibility.

- Explain how to identify patients covered by Medi-Cal prepaid health plans.

- Understand the benefits and nonbenefits of Medi-Cal.

- Explain when it is necessary to use and how to complete a Treatment Authorization Request form.

- List basic Medi-Cal claim procedure guidelines.

- State how to collect information and process claim forms for Medi-Cal patients who have additional coverage.

- Explain how to minimize the number of insurance forms rejected because of improper completion.

- Identify the Medi-Cal time limit for submitting claims.

- Identify when an OOY Medi-Cal claim will be accepted by the fiscal intermediary.

- Edit the Uniform Bill (UB-92) Outpatient Claim Form.

- Explain entries shown on a Remittance Advice Details document.

- Identify information on a Resubmission Turnaround Document.

- State when to use and how to complete a Claims Inquiry Form.

*Performance objectives and exercises for hands-on practical experience for this chapter appear in the *Workbook*.

For the history of Medicaid and basic knowledge about how the welfare system works, read Chapter 13 before reading Appendix B. As mentioned in Chapter 13, in California the Medicaid program is known as Medi-Cal and became effective on March 1, 1966. Medi-Cal is administered by the California State **Department of Health Services (DHS),** a department of the California State Human Relations Agency. The information in this appendix is a brief overview of the Medi-Cal program with basic guidelines for most regions in California. For additional current detailed information on policies and procedures supplied by the current fiscal intermediary, refer to either an updated *Medi-Cal Provider Manual for Medical Services* or see Internet Resources at the end of this appendix and go online to obtain the information.

TYPES OF MEDI-CAL PLANS

Managed Care Plans

The Medi-Cal program has evolved into health care plans (HCPs) that fall into one of several managed care plan (MCP) models:

- MCP: county organized health system (COHS)
- MCP: fee-for-service/managed care (FFS/MC)
- MCP: geographic managed care (GMC)
- MCP: prepaid health plan (PHP)
- MCP: primary care case management (PCCM)
- MCP: special projects
- MCP: two-plan model

Individuals covered under these plans must seek treatment from facilities contracted under the MCP, except in emergencies. Otherwise services will not be reimbursed by Medi-Cal. If service is not available through contracted facilities and the patient seeks care outside of the plan, a denial letter from the health plan must accompany the Medi-Cal claim.

Descriptions of Managed Care Plans

The MCP: COHS is a local agency created by a county board of supervisors to contract with the Medi-Cal program. Enrolled recipients choose their health care provider from among all COHS providers.

The MCP: FFS/MC program requires specific Medi-Cal recipients to enroll in state-contracted FFS/MC networks (FFS/MCNs) administered by selected rural counties. Enrollees may select a primary care provider (PCP) who will manage their health care. The PCP provides primary care services and referrals for all necessary specialty services through an ongoing patient–physician relationship. The county is paid a case management fee for creating the provider network, establishing enrollee outreach services, and monitoring use.

The MCP: GMC program model was established to provide medical and dental care for Medi-Cal recipients in specified aid code categories for a capitated fee. Each county may have different guidelines as to the delivery of the dental care; that is, a recipient either may choose between various dental MCPs or may receive dental care on a fee-for-service basis.

The MCP: PHP was established to allow Medi-Cal recipients to enroll in health maintenance organizations (HMOs) as an alternative to the Medi-Cal fee-for-service program. PHPs are required to render, on a capitated at-risk basis, all basic Medi-Cal covered benefits. PHPs provide case management, prevention, and health maintenance services. These plans have membership services and member grievance procedures. PHPs render care to privately insured individuals as well as Medi-Cal recipients.

The MCP: PCCM program contractors case manage medical care for a voluntarily enrolled population of Medi-Cal recipients. PCCM plans are capitated for most outpatient services. Prior approval requests must be obtained for noncapitated services that require authorization under the fee-for-service program, with the exception of acute inpatient facility psychiatric services and adult day health care (ADHC) services. PCCM contractors also assume an additional responsibility to arrange and authorize inpatient services, which are reimbursed fee-for-service by Medi-Cal. Contracts participate in program savings through a savings sharing agreement with the DHS.

The MCP: special projects are new managed care county programs or pilot projects to extend coordinated, competent care to identified populations. These special projects are designed to improve recipients' health status and avoid unnecessary costs.

With the MCP: two-plan model, the DHS contracts with two managed care plans in each of 12 California counties to provide medical services to most Medi-Cal recipients in each county. Each county offers both a local initiative plan and a commercial plan. Local initiative plans are operated by a locally developed comprehensive managed care organization. Commercial plans are operated by nongovernmental managed health care organizations. Medi-Cal recipients may enroll in either plan.

MEDI-CAL ELIGIBILITY

Individuals in the following groups are entitled to benefits under the Medi-Cal program:

- Californians who qualify for **Old Age Survivors, Health and Disability Insurance (OASHDI) program**
- **Aid to Families with Dependent Children (AFDC)**

- **Aid to the Blind (AB)**
- **Aid to the (permanently) Disabled (ATD)**
- **Medically needy (MN)** people whose incomes are above the assistance level but who are unable to provide mainstream medical care and are eligible as **medically indigent (MI).**

Share of Cost

Some medically needy patients have a dollar amount (liability) to meet each month called **share of cost (SOC).** This is the amount of money that must be paid by the patient each month before any Medi-Cal benefits will begin.

Identification Card

The State of California Department of Health Services issues a plastic **benefits identification card (BIC)** to each Medi-Cal recipient when the individual is declared eligible for benefits (Figure B–1). County welfare departments may issue paper Medi-Cal cards in exceptional cases for temporary use (e.g., retroactive eligibility). A person may have a Medi-Cal card, but this does not indicate proof of eligibility.

Eligibility Verification

It is the provider's responsibility to verify that the person to receive care is eligible during the month service is rendered and is the individual to whom the card was issued. Eligibility, which is verified at the first of the month, is valid for the entire month of service. Inspect the card and look for the following key points.

- The recipient's identification number may be numeric or alphanumeric.
- The issue date on the card must match the issue date on the recipient's master file accessed through the Medi-Cal point-of-service (POS) network.
- The recipient's date of birth on the card must match the recipient's date of birth on the recipient's master file, accessed through the point-of-service network.
- The recipient's signature located on the back of the BIC is used to verify the recipient's identification. This should be compared with the signature on a valid California driver's license, a California identification card issued by the Department of Motor Vehicles, another acceptable picture identification card, or another credible document of identification.

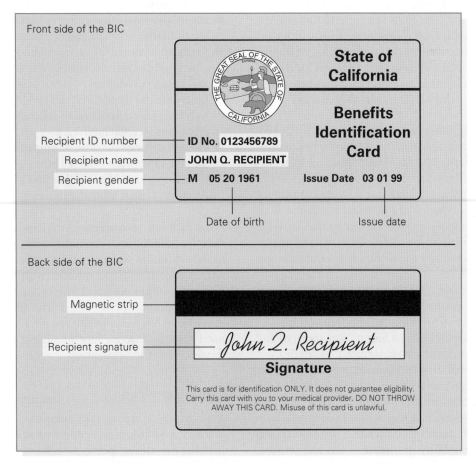

FIGURE B–1 Medi-Cal sample plastic benefits identification card. This is a white card with blue letters on the front and black letters on the back.

Verification Methods

Methods by which to verify eligibility and perform SOC and Medi-Service transactions are listed in the following:

● **POS device.** This is a piece of equipment interfaced with an analog telephone line. It has swipe card capabilities, or data may be manually input. It is used to identify recipient eligibility, obtain SOC liability status, key in SOC payment toward balance, reserve Medi-Services, perform Family PACT (planning, access, care, and treatment) client eligibility transactions, and submit pharmacy or CMS-1500 insurance claims.

An **eligibility verification confirmation (EVC)** number on a printout from the POS device verifies that an inquiry was received and eligibility information was transmitted. The insurance billing specialist should keep the eligibility verification confirmation number in the recipient's file and use it as proof of eligibility for the entire month. When a Medi-Cal recipient is limited to receive certain medical services, a restriction message is returned from the Medi-Cal host computer after verification of eligibility. Document that the services relate to the applicable restriction (e.g., date of service and name of provider who prescribed limited services). Never bill Medi-Cal for the SOC that a patient pays. Instead enter the amount paid into the POS system and indicate the amount on the CMS-1500 claim form. This will let the Medi-Cal fiscal intermediary know that the patient has paid and clear the SOC, allowing the recipient to become eligible for Medi-Cal benefits. Figure B–2 illustrates SOC and Medi-Service printouts from the POS device.

● **Claims and eligibility real-time software (CERTS).** This is computer software that allows providers to electronically verify recipient eligibility, clear SOC liability, reserve Medi-Services, perform Family PACT client eligibility transactions, and submit pharmacy or CMS-1500 claims by use of a personal computer. Both a modem and telephone line are necessary. An EVC number on a printout from the software verifies that an inquiry was received and eligibility information was transmitted.
● Computer software. This may be existing software modified by a vendor or a vendor-supplied software package capable of performing the transactions. An EVC number verifies that an inquiry was received and eligibility information was transmitted.
● **Automated eligibility verification system (AEVS).** This is an interactive voice response system allowing providers to access recipient eligibility, clear SOC, or reserve a Medi-Service. A touch-tone telephone is necessary. An EVC number verifies that an inquiry was received and eligibility information was transmitted.

However, this system is not able to perform SOC or Medi-Service transactions.

Receipt of an EVC number does not guarantee claim payment. Carefully review all information returned with the eligibility response to ensure that services are covered under the recipient eligibility.

MEDI-CAL BENEFITS

The basic medical benefits provided under Medi-Cal include the following:

● Physician services
● Inpatient or outpatient hospital services in any approved hospital
● Laboratory and x-ray services
● Nursing home services
● Home health care
● Private duty nursing
● Outpatient clinic services
● Dental services (through Delta Dental, called Denti-Cal)
● Hearing aids
● Drugs and medical supplies
● Optometric services and eye appliances
● Physical therapy and other diagnostic, preventive, or rehabilitative services and equipment
● Medicare deductible and premium payment. Medi-Cal also pays the full deductible under Medicare Part A and buys into Medicare Part B by paying the monthly premiums for those who are older than 65, disabled, or blind. These persons are called Medicare/Medi-Cal recipients (see Chapter 12).
● Obstetric services. The **Comprehensive Perinatal Services Program (CPSP)** offers a wide range of services to pregnant Medi-Cal recipients from conception through 60 days after the month of delivery.

In addition to maternity services, certified providers may be reimbursed for nutritional, psychosocial, and health education services; case coordination; client orientation; and vitamin and mineral supplements. A federal or state program designed to ease access to prenatal care is called **presumptive eligibility (PE)**. It allows the provider to offer immediate temporary coverage for prenatal care to low-income pregnant women pending a formal Medi-Cal application.

Medi-Services

Medi-Services are certain services supplied by chiropractors, psychologists, acupuncturists, podiatrists, occupational therapists, speech pathologists, and audiologists.

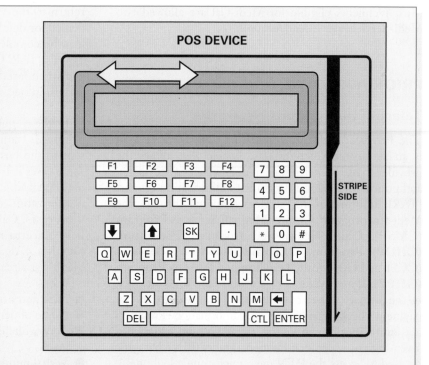

POS DEVICE: SHARE OF COST PRINTOUT

EDS TRAINING 3213 PROSPECT PARK TERMINAL

XX-02-15
01:44:35

PROVIDER NUMBER:
HSC3017XX

TRANSACTION TYPE: SHARE OF COST

RECIPIENT ID:
607357101

YEAR AND MONTH OF BIRTH:
1964-10

DATE OF ISSUE:
XX-02-01

DATE OF SERVICE:
XX-02-15

CASE NUMBER:

PROCEDURE CODE:
90945

PATIENT APPLIED AMOUNT:
$50.00

TOTAL BILLED AMOUNT:
$100.00

LAST NAME: JOHNSO.
AMOUNT DEDUCTED: $50.00
SHARE OF COST HAS BEEN MET.

POS DEVICE: MEDI-SERVICE PRINTOUT

EDS 10050 OLSON DRIVE TERMINAL T309006

XX-02-15
17:16:36

PROVIDER NUMBER:
HSC3017XX

TRANSACTION TYPE: MEDI-SERVICES

RECIPIENT ID:
607357101

YEAR AND MONTH OF BIRTH:
1966-12

DATE OF ISSUE:
XX-02-01

DATE OF SERVICE:
XX-02-15

PROCEDURE CODE:
A2000

LAST NAME: JOHNSO. MEDI SVC
RESERVATION APPLIED.

FIGURE B–2 Point-of-service device and two examples of printouts: Share of cost and Medi-Service.

Most recipients eligible for Medi-Cal are allowed two Medi-Services per calendar month.

PRIOR APPROVAL

Telecommunications Networks

The **Provider Telecommunications Network (PTN)** is an automated voice-response system that allows the provider to use the telephone to obtain checkwrite, claim, and prior authorization (treatment authorization request [TAR]) information for services rendered through the Medi-Cal program, **County Medical Services Program (CMSP), Child Health and Disability Prevention (CHDP) Program, California Children's Services (CCS),** and **Genetically Handicapped Persons Program (GHPP).** If a provider chooses to use the PTN, it must be the primary source of checkwrite (issuing of Medi-Cal payment check), claim, and TAR information. Providers are automatically enrolled in the PTN and assigned a seven-digit provider identification number (PIN) that must be used to access the PTN on a touch-tone telephone.

Treatment Authorization Request

Certain procedures and services require prior approval from the Medi-Cal field office consultant. The approval process is begun by either completing a **TAR Form** 50-1 or accessing the Medi-Cal Web site via the Internet to electronically transmit an e-TAR.

To find out whether a particular service requires a TAR, refer to the *Medi-Cal Provider Manual for Medical Services* or go to the Medi-Cal Web site mentioned in Internet Resources at the end of this appendix. Find the TAR benefit and nonbenefit list that indicates what services require a TAR or are not a benefit. Some of the TAR-required services are as follows:

- Long-term care facility services
- Some vision services
- Inpatient hospital services
- Home health agency services
- Chronic hemodialysis services
- Some transportation services
- Some **durable medical equipment (DME),** medical supplies, or prosthetic/orthotic appliances
- Hearing aids
- Some pharmacy services
- Some surgical procedures

Response to a form-generated TAR takes 10 to 15 days, but an e-TAR has a quicker response time. Once an e-TAR is submitted, it is electronically routed to the appropriate field office for a decision (adjudication). Providers can return to the Web site to check TAR status (approved, denied, or deferred). A TAR Transmittal Form MC3020 may be completed to help track submitted TARs or to appeal a TAR. Check with the field office to determine if and when faxed TARs will be accepted, because policies vary from one office to another.

If the request for hospitalization of a patient is approved, a copy of the approved TAR should be faxed or sent to the hospital before admission of the patient. In some cases it is not possible to obtain a TAR in advance of hospital admission or initiation of a treatment program. Authorization may be obtained by telephone or fax in these cases. Call the local department of health services field office to receive approval, and then complete and submit a TAR Form 50-1 to the field office, indicating that it was already authorized by including the following:

- Date authorized
- Name of person who gave authorization
- Approximate time of day at which authorization was given
- Verbal number stated by the field office

Do not bill the fiscal intermediary with the verbal TAR number.

A **Voice Drug TAR System (VDTS)** is also available and linked to the Medi-Cal Drug Units to permit the processing of TARs after completion of a recording. VDTS can *only* be used to request *urgent* and *initial* drug TARs, inquire about the status of previously entered drug TARs, or inquire whether a patient is receiving continual care with a drug.

CLAIM PROCEDURE

Fiscal Intermediaries

Two fiscal intermediaries are contracted by the state of California to receive and audit claims for payment of medical services and make payments to providers of services. When the contract expires, these intermediaries may change, but at present they are (1) **Electronic Data Systems (EDS) Corporation** in Sacramento, California, for hospital billing and outpatient professional services and (2) Delta Dental (formerly California Dental Services) for dental services under Denti-Cal. For the address of EDS, refer to the Medi-Cal Web site mentioned in Internet Resources at the end of this appendix.

Copayment

Current law requires Medi-Cal recipients to make a nominal copayment for most outpatient services, some emergency department services, and some prescribed drugs. Copayment is never necessary for the following:

- Any person 18 years of age or younger
- Any woman receiving perinatal care
- Any child in AFDC foster care
- Any person who is an inpatient in a health facility (e.g., hospital, skilled nursing facility, or intermediate care facility)
- Any service for which payment by Medi-Cal is $10 or less

Emergency services or family planning services and supplies; the health care provider has the option to collect or not collect copayment at the time at which emergency service is rendered. Figure B–3 lists the services subject to copayment, copayment fees, and exclusions.

Time Limit

Medi-Cal claims must be submitted within 6 months from the end of the month of service to be reimbursed at 100% of the Medi-Cal maximum allowable. To be eligible for full reimbursement on late claims, one of the approved billing limit exception codes (1-8 or A) shown in the provider manual must be used in Field 22 of the CMS-1500 claim form. Claims submitted more than

6 months after the month of service are reimbursed at the following reduced rates:

100%	1 to 6 months after the month of service
75%	7 to 9 months after the month of service
50%	10 to 12 months after the month of service
0%	Over 1 year from the month of service

An Over-One-Year (OOY) claim may be submitted with appropriate documentation or justification attached using exception code 8 for one of the following reasons:

- Retroactive eligibility
- Court order
- State of administrative hearing
- County error
- Department of Health Services approval
- Reversal of decision on appealed TAR
- Medicare or other health coverage

Helpful Billing Tips

When submitting an insurance claim for surgical procedures performed, the Medi-Cal global fee includes the preoperative visit 7 days before surgery, the surgical procedure, and the postoperative care (0, 10, 30, or 90 days).

MEDI-CAL COPAYMENT CRITERIA

Services Subject to Copayment	Copay-ment Fee	Exceptions to Fee
NONEMERGENCY SERVICES PROVIDED IN AN EMERGENCY ROOM A nonemergency service is defined as "any service not required for alleviation of severe pain or in the immediate diagnosis and treatment of severe medical conditions which, if not immediately diagnosed and treated, would lead to disability or death." Such services provided in an emergency room are subject to copayment.	$5.00	1. Persons age 18 or under. 2. Any woman during pregnancy and the postpartum period (through the end of the month in which the 60-day period following termination of pregnancy ends) 3. Persons who are inpatients in a health facility (hospital, skilled nursing facility or intermediate care facility)
OUTPATIENT SERVICES Physician, optometric, chiropractic, psychology, speech therapy, audiology, acupuncture, occupational therapy, podiatric, surgical center, hospital or outpatient clinic, physical therapy.	$1.00	4. Any child in AFDC-foster care 5. Any service for which the program's payment is $10 or less
DRUG PRESCRIPTIONS Each drug prescription or refill.	$1.00	6. Any hospice patient 7. Family planning services and supplies

FIGURE B–3 Medi-Cal copayment criteria.

This differs from standard surgical and Medicare global package policies.

Medi-Cal and Other Coverage

Medi-Cal and Private Insurance

Medi-Cal is considered the payer of last resort, and the physician must bill all other insurance carriers first and then Medi-Cal. Have the patient sign an assignment of benefits form for the other insurance. After payment is received from the other insurance carrier, include a copy of the other insurance EOB when submitting the Medi-Cal claim.

Medi-Cal and Medicare

Outpatient claims for recipients eligible for both Medicare and Medi-Cal coverage must always be billed to Medicare before Medi-Cal. These claims may be referred to as *crossover claims* because after being processed by Medicare, claims are automatically crossed over to the Medi-Cal fiscal intermediary for final processing unless 100% of the claim was paid by Medicare. The claim *must be assigned* or it will not be crossed over. Hard copy billing instructions for Medicare Part B crossover claims

are different from the instructions for submitting standard Medicare or Medi-Cal claims. When submitting a crossover claim, enter an "X" in both the Medicaid and Medicare boxes of Block 1 on the CMS-1500 claim form to identify the claim as a crossover. Enter the Medicare claim number from the identification card in Block 1a. Include the Medi-Cal recipient identification number in either Block 9a or Block 32, depending on the circumstances of the case (Figure B–4). The Medi-Cal provider identification number appears in Block 31.

Medi-Cal and TRICARE

Bill TRICARE first if a Medi-Cal patient is also covered by TRICARE. Then bill Medi-Cal and attach the TRICARE Summary Payment Voucher to the claim form (see Chapter 14).

Computer Media Claims

The **computer media claims (CMC)** system permits submission of Medi-Cal claims via telecommunication through magnetic tape or diskette and modem. A variety of computer software formats are acceptable. *The Medi-Cal CMC Technical Manual* and the Medi-Cal Web

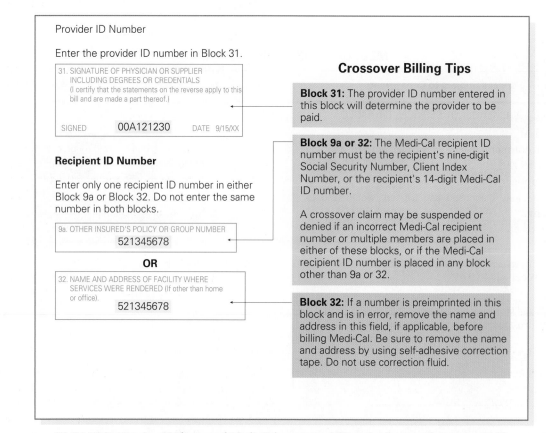

FIGURE B–4 Medicare and Medi-Cal crossover billing tips for completing the CMS-1500 insurance claim form.

site contain the latest specifications to update existing systems.

UNIFORM BILL (UB-92) 0UTPATIENT CLAIM FORM

The Uniform Bill (UB-92) claim form is used by institutional facilities (e.g., inpatient and outpatient departments, rural health clinics, chronic dialysis services, and adult day health care) to submit claims for outpatient services.

Instructions for Completing the UB-92 Claim Form

When editing a computer-generated UB-92 claim form, refer to basic Medi-Cal block-by-block information about completion of the UB-92 claim form in Chapter 17. Figure 17–5 shows a completed UB-92 claim form; however, because Medi-Cal guidelines vary from the block-by-block illustration shown, refer to the block-by-block Medi-Cal instructions in that chapter. Outpatient claims are submitted in an orange envelope, and inpatient claims are submitted in a red envelope provided by the EDS.

AFTER CLAIM SUBMISSION

Remittance Advice Details

A **Remittance Advice Details (RAD),** formerly known as Explanation of Benefits and Remittance Advice (EOB/RA), accompanies all Medi-Cal payment vouchers (checks) sent to the physician. Five categories of adjudicated claims appear on an RAD:

1. Adjustments
2. Payments or approvals
3. Denials
4. Suspends
5. Accounts receivable (A/R) transactions.

Some categories of adjudicated claims are shown in Figure 13–8, illustrating the Medicaid resolution process.

Electronic RADs are transmitted via computer to providers who have individual agreements with the fiscal intermediary. The State Controller's Office also sends a hard copy of the RAD.

Providers receiving RADs should reconcile each claim transaction to their records. Claim payments are posted as credits to the patient's financial accounting record card. Negative adjustments are posted as debits to the patient's financial accounting record card. Each claim being reported, or not reported, must be accounted for, the necessary follow-up performed, and all the rules governing timelines followed.

Adjustments

When overpayments or underpayments occur, an adjustment is initiated and two lines appear on the RAD. The first line indicates a "take back" of the original payment (original CCN); the second line reflects the correct payment of the claim (new CCN). The net amount between the two lines is the adjustment. CCNs are assigned to identify and track claims as they move through the claims processing system.

Approvals or Payments

If an original claim or a previously denied claim is approved for payment, it is listed on the RAD. If a reduction in the billed amount is warranted, the explanation will be given by means of a three-digit code.

Electronic Funds Transfer

Through **electronic funds transfer (EFT),** providers may have their payments deposited directly into their bank accounts, and paper warrants will not be generated. However, the provider will receive an RAD document. This system will be phased in to enrollees, so keep abreast of the latest information through Medi-Cal bulletins.

Denials

Denial of claims is shown only on the RAD. Review denied claims to ensure they are correct. If a physician believes that the claim was incorrectly denied, he or she should submit a Claims Inquiry Form (CIF) for reconsideration of the claim. Until the claim is resubmitted for processing, it is no longer in the system. When the claim is resubmitted, it will be given a new CCN and be processed as a new claim in the system. For translations of the RAD codes and billing tips on how to correct denied claims, refer to the *Medi-Cal Provider Manual for Medical Services.*

Suspends

A claim requiring special handling or correction of errors is placed in temporary suspense and may be referred to as a *suspend.* Claims in suspense for 30 days or more are listed. Suspends should be referenced to determine whether an RTD was issued. There are several general explanation codes for suspended claims. Such a listing does not explain the reason but lets the physician know that the claim was received by the fiscal intermediary. *Do not* send CIFs for claims that have been temporarily suspended.

Accounts Receivable Transactions

An **A/R transaction** is a miscellaneous transaction as a result of a cost settlement, state audit, or refund check received by the fiscal intermediary. A three-digit code indicates the reason for the A/R transaction. A/R transactions show when it is necessary to recover funds from a provider or, in certain situations, to pay funds to a provider. The A/R system is used in financial transactions pertaining to:

● Recoupment of interim payments
● Withholds against payments to providers according to state instructions
● Payments to providers according to state instructions

Amounts may be either positive or negative amounts that correspond to the increase or decrease in the amount of the Medi-Cal voucher (check). An adjustment may be initiated by the provider, fiscal intermediary, or the state. Some adjustments refer to previously paid claims that may be adjusted if an error in payment occurred. A/R transactions are posted to the appropriate suspense account.

Resubmission Turnaround Document

The fiscal intermediary sends a **Resubmission Turnaround Document (RTD),** the RTD 65-1, to providers when the submitted claim form has questionable or missing information. This document eliminates the need for providers to resubmit the entire claim form to correct a limited number of errors. The RTD must be completed and returned to the fiscal intermediary by the date specified on the RTD.

Claims Inquiry Form

A **Claims Inquiry Form (CIF)** 60-1 is used when tracing a claim, resubmitting a claim after a denial, or requesting an adjustment for underpaid or overpaid claims. This form also may be used to request SOC reimbursement for a previously paid claim, but such cases must be submitted separately. CIFs should be submitted within 6 months of the date of the RAD and mailed in a black and white envelope provided by the EDS.

Providers wishing to refund an incorrect payment may complete a CIF, noting the overpayment, and forward the refund to the fiscal intermediary. Attach a photocopy of the RAD. It should be mentioned that if an overpayment is received and an insurer presses the provider of service for a refund, the insurance plan can always recoup the money requested from the next check. This happens frequently with refunds owed to Medicare, Medicaid, and other government payers.

For denial and adjustment requests, complete a CIF and attach a legible copy of the corrected claim form, a copy of the RAD on which the claim is listed, and any other pertinent information.

A CIF may be used to trace claims submitted to the fiscal intermediary more than 45 days previously that have not appeared on the RAD as approved or denied and that are not indicated on the most recent RAD as suspended. When submitting a tracer, leave the CCN box blank.

As many as eight claims may be listed on a single CIF when tracing. Do not attach claim copies or any other documentation to a tracer. The CIF request for tracing a claim will automatically review the recipient's history and generate a response letter showing the results of the review. Based on the information in the letter, a CIF may be resubmitted for denial reconsideration, adjustment, or proof of previous timely submission.

Appeal Process

A provider with a grievance or complaint about payment of claims must direct this grievance or complaint to the fiscal intermediary *within* 90 days of the action causing the grievance or complaint. The appeal is subject to automatic denial if the 90-day limit is not met. Appeals must be submitted using the Appeal Form 90-1 and should include legible copies of supporting documentation (e.g., claim forms, RADs, CIFs, and TARs). Appeals are sent in a lavender envelope provided by the EDS. The fiscal intermediary will send an acknowledgment within 15 days of receipt and make a decision within 30 days from the date of the acknowledgment. If the appealed claim is approved for reprocessing, it will appear on a RAD. A subsequent appeal may be made if the provider is not satisfied with the decision. Judicial remedy no later than 1 year after receipt of the decision may be undertaken if the provider is still not satisfied with the decision.

PROCEDURE

COMPLETING A TREATMENT AUTHORIZATION REQUEST FORM 50-1

The following item numbers and descriptions correspond to Figure B–5.

1. Leave blank.

1A. The fiscal intermediary inserts a **claim control number (CCN)** in this box.

1B. Verbal Control Number is generally left blank unless this number is obtained by telephone.

2. Enter an "X" in the appropriate boxes to show Drug or Other, Retroactive Request, or Medicare eligibility status.

2A. Enter the provider's area code and telephone number.

2B. Enter the provider's name and complete address.

3. Enter the nine-digit Medi-Cal rendering provider number. When requesting authorization for an elective hospital admission, the hospital provider number must be entered in this box. The hospital name may be placed in the Medical Justification area.

4. Enter the patient's last name, first name, middle initial, address, and telephone number.

5. Enter the recipient's Medi-Cal identification number from the BIC. The county code and aid code must be entered above this box. Do not use any characters (dashes, hyphens, or special characters) in the remaining blank positions of the Medi-Cal ID field or in the Check Digit box (Figure B–6).

6. Insert the letter P to indicate pending if the patient's Medi-Cal eligibility is not yet established and the Medi-Cal number is unknown.

7. Use a capital M for male or F for female, obtained from the BIC. Enter the patient's age in the AGE box.

8. Enter the recipient's date of birth in six-digit format. If not available, enter the year of the recipient's birth preceded by "0101."

8A. Patient's status: Enter an "X" if patient is an inpatient in a **nursing facility** level A (NF-A) or nursing facility level B (NF-B). Enter the name of the facility in the Medical Justification area of the form.

8B. Diagnosis: Enter the description of the diagnosis and its code from the diagnostic code book.

8C. Medical justification: Provide sufficient supporting information for the consultant to determine whether the service is medically justified. Attach documentation if necessary. Enter name of the hospital or nursing facility level A or B. Requests by nonmedical providers must include the name and telephone number of the prescriber (placed in the lower left corner of this box).

9. Leave blank. Consultant will indicate if the service line item is authorized.

10. Approved Units. Leave blank. Consultant will indicate the number of times the procedure, item, or days have been authorized.

10A. Specific Services Requested: Indicate the name of the procedure, item, or service requested.

10B. Units of Service: Leave blank.

11. Enter the procedure code (five-digit CPT with two-digit modifier or five-character HCPCS when necessary). When requesting hospital days, the stay must be requested on the first line of the TAR with the provider entering the word "DAY(S)."

12. Enter the number of times a procedure or service is requested or the number of hospital days requested.

12A. Indicate the dollar amount of the provider's usual and customary charge for the service(s) requested.

13 to 32. Additional TAR lines 2 through 6.

32A. Enter the name and address of the patient's authorized representative, representative payee, conservator over the person, legal representative, or other representative handling the recipient's medical and personal affairs, if applicable.

33 to 36. Leave blank. Consultant's determination and comments will be entered in this section. The TAR must show the consultant's signature. Comments and Explanation lines: List the approved procedures or any further information the provider must submit with the CMS-1500 claim.

37 to 38. Leave blank. Consultant will indicate valid dates of authorization.

39A. Signature of physician or provider: the provider or authorized representative must sign and date the form.

39B. Leave blank. Medi-Cal field office consultant will enter a two-digit prefix and a one-digit suffix to the preprinted eight-digit number. This 11-digit number must be entered on the CMS-1500 claim form when the service is billed, indicating prior authorization has been obtained. PI means pricing information and is to be left blank. *Do not attach a copy of the TAR to the CMS-1500 claim form.*

40 to 43. Leave blank.

Continued

COMPLETING A TREATMENT AUTHORIZATION REQUEST FORM 50-1

① STATE USE ONLY
SERVICE CATEGORY

①A CONFIDENTIAL PATIENT INFORMATION
FOR F.I. USE ONLY

C C N

TREATMENT AUTHORIZATION REQUEST
STATE OF CALIFORNIA DEPARTMENT OF HEALTH SERVICES

TYPEWRITER ALIGNMENT — Elite / Pica

F.I. USE ONLY ④⓪ ④① ④② ④③
TYPEWRITER ALIGNMENT — Elite / Pica

(PLEASE TYPE) FOR PROVIDER USE **②A** (PLEASE TYPE)

①B VERBAL CONTROL NO.

② TYPE OF SERVICE REQUESTED — DRUG / [X] OTHER

REQUEST IS RETROACTIVE? — YES / [X] NO

IS PATIENT MEDICARE ELIGIBLE? — YES / [X] NO

PROVIDER PHONE NO. AREA (555) 555-1111

③②A PATIENT'S AUTHORIZED REPRESENTATIVE (IF ANY) ENTER NAME AND ADDRESS

②B PROVIDER NAME AND ADDRESS
PLEASE TYPE YOUR NAME AND ADDRESS HERE
SMITH, SUSAN MD
727 ELM BLVD
ANYTOWN, CA 90101

③ PROVIDER NO.
HSC12345F

30 83

FOR STATE USE

③③ PROVIDER; YOUR REQUEST IS:
1 — APPROVED AS REQUESTED / DENIED / DEFERRED
2 — APPROVED AS MODIFIED (ITEMS MARKED BELOW AS AUTHORIZED MAY BE CLAIMED) / JACKSON VS RANK PARAGRAPH CODE

BY *John Doe* MEDI-CAL CONSULTANT

NAME AND ADDRESS OF PATIENT
PATIENT NAME (LAST, FIRST, M. I.)
④ APPLEGATE, NANCY

⑤ MEDI-CAL IDENTIFICATION NO. 253971060 CHECK DIGIT

⑥

STREET ADDRESS
1515 RIVER ROAD

⑦ SEX F AGE 32 **⑧** DATE OF BIRTH 06 18 65

I.D. # **③④** 01 **③⑤** DATE 08 20 X X 44 REVIEW COMMENTS INDICATOR

CITY, STATE, ZIP CODE
SACRAMENTO, CA 95822

⑧A PATIENT STATUS: [X] HOME / BOARD AND CARE / SNF/ICF / ACUTE HOSPITAL

COMMENTS/ EXPLANATION

PHONE NUMBER AREA
(555) 545-1123

DIAGNOSIS DESCRIPTION:
ENDOMETRIOSIS

⑧B ICD-9-CM DIAGNOSIS CODE
617.9

⑧C MEDICAL JUSTIFICATION:
VISTA HOSPITAL - 1200 MAPLE ST., ANYTOWN, CA

UNCONTROLLABLE ENDOMETRIOSIS

RETROACTIVE AUTHORIZATION GRANTED IN ACCORDANCE WITH SECTION 51003 (B)
③⑥ 1 2 3 4 5 6

	AUTHORIZED YES / NO	APPROVED UNITS	SPECIFIC SERVICES REQUESTED	UNITS OF SERVICE	PROCEDURE OR DRUG CODE	QUANTITY	CHARGES
1	**⑨** [X]	**⑩** 3	**⑩A** DAYS: 3 HOSPITAL DAYS REQUESTED	**⑩B**	**⑪**	**⑫** 3	$ **⑫A**
2	**⑬** [X]	**⑭** 1	HYSTERECTOMY	1	15 5815070	16 1	$ 1300.00
3	17	18			19	20	$
4	21	22			23	24	$
5	25	26			27	28	$
6	29	30			31	32	$

TO THE BEST OF MY KNOWLEDGE, THE ABOVE INFORMATION IS TRUE, ACCURATE AND COMPLETE AND THE REQUESTED SERVICES ARE MEDICALLY INDICATED AND NECESSARY TO THE HEALTH OF THE PATIENT.

③⑨A SIGNATURE OF PHYSICIAN OR PROVIDER *Susan Smith* TITLE MD DATE 8-10-XX

AUTHORIZATION IS VALID FOR SERVICES PROVIDED
③⑦ FROM DATE 09 01 XX **③⑧** TO DATE 09 30 XX

TAR CONTROL NUMBER
③⑨B OFFICE 12 SEQUENCE NUMBER 61240229 PI 0

NOTE: AUTHORIZATION DOES NOT GUARANTEE PAYMENT. PAYMENT IS SUBJECT TO PATIENT'S ELIGIBILITY. BE SURE THE IDENTIFICATION CARD IS CURRENT BEFORE RENDERING SERVICE. SEND TO FIELD SERVICES (F.I. COPY)

SEE YOUR PROVIDER MANUAL FOR ASSISTANCE REGARDING THE COMPLETION OF THIS FORM. 50-1 12/87

FIGURE B-5 Example of a Medi-Cal Treatment Authorization Request form completed by a primary care physician for preauthorization of a professional service.

PROCEDURE—CONT'D

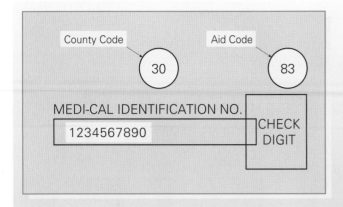

FIGURE B–6 Block 5 of the Treatment Authorization Request (50-1) form. Leave Check Digit block blank. This example shows placement of the county code and aid code on the form above block 5.

PROCEDURE

INSTRUCTIONS FOR COMPLETING THE CMS-1500 CLAIM FORM FOR THE MEDI-CAL PROGRAM

Complete an CMS-1500 claim form and mail it to the fiscal intermediary in the blue and white envelope provided by EDS after verifying Medi-Cal eligibility using one of the aforementioned methods.

Refer to these OCR guidelines and the Medi-Cal template shown in Figure B–7.

Top of the form. Do not type to the right of the bar code because the fiscal intermediary inserts a claim number in that space.

Block 1. Check Medicaid box for Medi-Cal claims.

Block 1a. Enter the Medi-Cal number in the left portion of the block. Do not enter dashes or other special characters in this block.

Block 2. Enter the last name, first name, and middle initial of the patient as shown on the patient's identification card. Do not use any punctuation.

Block 3. Enter the patient's birth date using six digits and indicate gender.

Block 4. Complete only if the patient has not been issued an identification card and is covered under another person (e.g., infant younger than 2 months of age); otherwise leave blank.

Block 5. Enter the patient's mailing address and residential telephone number.

Block 6. Generally, leave blank. Check "child" for a claim submitted for a child younger than 2 months of age using the mother's identification card.

Block 7. Leave blank.

Block 8. Leave blank.

Blocks 9, 9a, 9b, 9c, and 9d. Leave blank; for crossover claims, list the Medi-Cal identification number in Block 9a or in Block 32.

Block 10a. Check "yes" if applicable; otherwise leave blank.

Block 10b. Leave blank.

Block 10c. Leave blank.

Block 10d. Enter the amount of the patient's SOC for the procedure, service, or supply. Do not enter a decimal point (.) or dollar sign ($); for example, $95.00 should be shown as 9500.

Blocks 11, 11a, 11b, and 11c. Leave blank.

Block 11d. Check "Yes" if recipient has other health coverage (OHC); otherwise leave blank. OHC includes private insurance carriers, PHPs, and HMOs. Eligibility under Medicare or Medi-Cal MCP is *not* considered Other Health Coverage. If OHC has paid, enter the amount in the right side of this block (e.g., $50.00 should be shown as 5000).

Block 12. Leave blank.

Block 13. No signature required; however, the EVC number may be entered here.

Block 14. Complete if applicable.

Blocks 15 and 16. Leave blank.

Block 17. Enter complete name and degree of referring physician, when applicable.

Block 17a. Enter the Medi-Cal nine-digit provider number or state license number (not UPIN) of the referring provider or nonphysician practitioner working under the supervision of a physician.

Block 18. Enter dates of hospital confinement and discharge as six digits if service is related to inpatient hospitalization.

Block 19. Enter remarks or a statement certifying the claim includes emergency services.

Block 20. Leave blank if not applicable. Check "Yes" if the claim includes fees for outside laboratory tests and state in Block 19 that a specimen was sent to an unaffiliated laboratory.

Block 21. List up to two diagnostic codes (primary and secondary).

Continued

Instructions for Completing the CMS-1500 Claim Form for the Medi-Cal Program

APPROVED OMB 0936-006

PLEASE DO NOT STAPLE IN THIS AREA

CARRIER

HEALTH INSURANCE CLAIM FORM

6 Digits

1. MEDICARE (Medicare #) | MEDICAID (Medicaid #) [X] | CHAMPUS (Sponsor's SSN) | CHAMPVA (VA File #) | GROUP HEALTH PLAN (SSN or ID) | FECA BLK LUNG (SSN) | OTHER (ID)

1a. INSURED'S I.D. NUMBER (FOR PROGRAM IN ITEM 1): MEDI-CAL ID NUMBER

2. PATIENT'S NAME (Last Name, First Name, Middle Initial): PATIENT'S COMPLETE NAME

3. PATIENT'S BIRTH DATE MM DD YYYY / SEX M F: DATE OF BIRTH / SEX

4. INSURED'S NAME (Last Name, First Name, Middle Initial): MOTHER'S NAME FOR NEWBORN

5. PATIENT'S ADDRESS (No., Street): PATIENT'S COMPLETE ADDRESS

CITY: PATIENT'S CITY — STATE: ST

ZIP CODE: PATIENT'S ZIP — TELEPHONE (include Area Code): ( )PATIENT'S PHONE

6. PATIENT RELATIONSHIP TO INSURED: Self / Spouse / Child / Other

7. INSURED'S ADDRESS (No., Street): N/A — CITY: N/A — STATE: N/A — ZIP CODE: N/A — TELEPHONE (Include Area Code): ( ) N/A

8. PATIENT STATUS: N/A — Single / Married / Other — Employed / Full-Time Student / Part-Time Student

9. OTHER INSURED'S NAME (Last Name, First Name, Middle Initial): N/A

a. OTHER INSURED'S POLICY OR GROUP NUMBER: N/A

b. OTHER INSURED'S DATE OF BIRTH MM DD YYYY: N/A — SEX M F: N/A

c. EMPLOYER'S NAME OR SCHOOL NAME: N/A

d. INSURANCE PLAN NAME OR PROGRAM NAME: N/A

10. IS PATIENT'S CONDITION RELATED TO:

a. EMPLOYMENT? (CURRENT OR PREVIOUS) YES / NO

b. AUTO ACCIDENT? N/A YES / NO — PLACE (State) N/A

c. OTHER ACCIDENT? N/A YES / NO

10d. RESERVED FOR LOCAL USE: PATIENT'S SHARE OF COST

11. INSURED'S POLICY GROUP OR FECA NUMBER: N/A

a. INSURED'S DATE OF BIRTH MM DD YYYY: N/A — SEX M F

b. EMPLOYER'S NAME OR SCHOOL NAME: N/A

c. INSURANCE PLAN NAME OR PROGRAM NAME: N/A

d. IS THERE ANOTHER HEALTH BENEFIT PLAN? YES / NO — *If yes, return to and complete item 9 a-d.*: OTHER COVERAGE/DOLLAR AMOUNT

READ BACK OF FORM BEFORE COMPLETING AND SIGNING THIS FORM.

12. PATIENT'S OR AUTHORIZED PERSON'S SIGNATURE I authorize the release of any medical or other information necessary to process this claim. I also request payment of government benefits either to myself or to the party who accepts assignment below.

SIGNED N/A DATE N/A

13. INSURED'S OR AUTHORIZED PERSON'S SIGNATURE I authorize payment of medical benefits to the undersigned physician or supplier for services described below.

SIGNED EVC Number

PATIENT AND INSURED INFORMATION

14. DATE OF CURRENT: ILLNESS (First symptom) OR INJURY (Accident) OR PREGNANCY (LMP) MM DD YYYY: DATE OF ONSET

15. IF PATIENT HAS HAD SAME OR SIMILAR ILLNESS GIVE FIRST DATE MM DD YYYY: N/A

16. DATES PATIENT UNABLE TO WORK IN CURRENT OCCUPATION FROM MM DD YYYY N/A TO MM DD YYYY

17. NAME OF REFERRING PHYSICIAN OR OTHER SOURCE: NAME OF REFERRING PROVIDER

17a. I.D. NUMBER OF REFERRING PHYSICIAN: REFERRING PROVIDER NUMBER

18. HOSPITALIZATION DATES RELATED TO CURRENT SERVICES FROM MM DD YYYY FROM DOS TO MM DD YYYY THRU DOS

19. RESERVED FOR LOCAL USE: REMARKS/EMERGENCY CERTIFICATION STATEMENT

20. OUTSIDE LAB? YES / NO — $ CHARGES: OUTSIDE LAB — N/A — N/A

21. DIAGNOSIS OR NATURE OF ILLNESS OR INJURY (RELATE ITEMS 1,2,3 OR 4 TO ITEM 24E BY LINE)

1. PRIMARY ICD 9-CM
2. SECONDARY ICD 9-CM
3. N/A
4. N/A

22. MEDICAID RESUBMISSION CODE: MEDICARE STATUS ZONE — ORIGINAL REF. NO.: N/A

23. PRIOR AUTHORIZATION NUMBER: TAR CONTROL NUMBER — 11-digit

24. A DATE(S) OF SERVICE From MM DD YYYY	To MM DD YYYY	B Place of Service	C Type of Service	D PROCEDURES, SERVICES, OR SUPPLIES (Explain Unusual Circumstances) CPT/HCPCS	MODIFIER	E DIAGNOSIS CODE	F $ CHARGES	G DAYS OR UNITS	H EPSDT Family Plan	I EMG	J COB	K RESERVED FOR LOCAL USE
DATE OF SERVICE FROM 6 Digits	DATE OF SERVICE	POS	N/A	PRO-CEDURE CODE	MOD N/A	N/A	SERVICE CHARGES	QUANTITY	FP/CHDP	EMER CERT	BILLING LIMIT	RENDERING PROVIDER NUMBER

25. FEDERAL TAX I.D. NUMBER SSN EIN: N/A

26. PATIENT'S ACCOUNT NO.: PATIENT ACCOUNT NUMBER

27. ACCEPT ASSIGNMENT? (For govt. claims, see back) YES / NO: N/A

28. TOTAL CHARGE $: TOTAL CHARGES

29. AMOUNT PAID $: TOTAL DEDUCTIONS

30. BALANCE DUE $: NET AMT BILLED

31. SIGNATURE OF PHYSICIAN OR SUPPLIER INCLUDING DEGREES OR CREDENTIALS (I certify that the statements on the reverse apply to this bill and are made a part thereof.): SIGNATURE OF PROVIDER OR PERSON AUTHORIZED — SIGNED DATE

32. NAME AND ADDRESS OF FACILITY WHERE SERVICES WERE RENDERED (if other than home or office): FACILITY PROVIDER NUMBER

33. PHYSICIAN'S, SUPPLIER'S BILLING NAME, ADDRESS, ZIP CODE AND PHONE #: PROVIDER NAME, ADDRESS, CITY, STATE, ZIP, PROVIDER PHONE NUMBER — MEDI-CAL PROVIDER # — GRP# N/A

PHYSICIAN OR SUPPLIER INFORMATION

(APPROVED BY AMA COUNCIL ON MEDICAL SERVICE 8/88) — *PLEASE PRINT OR TYPE* — FORM HCFA (12 90) FORM OCWP 1500 FORM RRB 1500

REORDER FROM STANDARD REGISTER FORM NO HC0901B-2

FIGURE B-7 CMS-1500 claim form illustrating Medi-Cal required fields.

Block 22. Medicare status codes are required for Charpentier claims. In all other circumstances, these codes are optional. The Medicare status codes are as follows:

Code Explanation

0 Younger than 65; does not have Medicare coverage

*1 Benefits exhausted

*2 Utilization committee denial or physician noncertification

*3 No prior hospital stay

*4 Facility denial

*5 Noneligible provider

*6 Noneligible recipient

*7 Medicare benefits denied or cut short by Medicare intermediary

8 Noncovered services

*9 PSRO denial

*L Medi/Medi Charpentier (rebill): Benefit limitations

*R Medi/Medi Charpentier (rebill): Rates

*T Medi/Medi Charpentier (rebill): Both rates and benefit limitations

NOTE: A permanent injunction (*Charpentier v. Belshe [Coye/Kizer]*) filed December 29, 1994, allows providers to rebill Medi-Cal for supplemental payment for Medicare/Medi-Cal Part B services, excluding physician services (e.g., G0001 venipuncture or laboratory tests). All Charpentier rebilled claims must have been first processed as Medi/Medi crossover claims.

Block 23. Enter the 11-digit TAR control number, if applicable.

Block 24A. Enter date of service, using six digits.

Block 24B. Enter POS code (refer to Figure 7-4.)

Block 24C. Leave blank.

Block 24D. Enter the appropriate CPT/HCPCS code for each procedure, service, or supply and applicable modifier without a hyphen.

Block 24E. Leave blank.

Block 24F. Enter the fee for each listed service from the fee schedule. Do not enter dollar signs or decimal points. Always include cents.

Block 24G. Each service must be listed on separate lines (no date ranging). Indicate that each service was performed one time by listing "1" in this block.

Block 24H. Enter code for family planning (FP) or CHDP services. Leave blank if not applicable.

Code Description

1 Family planning/sterilization (sterilization consent form must be attached)

2 Family planning/other

3 CHDP screening related

Block 24I. Enter an "X" if the claim includes emergency services taking place in a hospital emergency department, and attach an emergency certification statement or enter a statement in Block 19.

Block 24J. Enter code that corresponds with billing limit exception and include the required documentation (see Medi-Cal provider manual).

Block 24K. Enter the nine-digit Medi-Cal provider number of the rendering provider if part of a group practice or different from the billing provider number in Block 33.

Block 25. Leave blank.

Block 26. Enter the patient's account number assigned by the physician's accounting system. Do not use dashes or slashes.

Block 27. Leave blank.

Block 28. Enter total charges for services listed in Block(s) 24F.

Block 29. Enter only the payment on claim if applicable (e.g., SOC).

Block 30. Enter balance due on claim (Block 28 less Block 29).

Block 31. Type the provider's name and show the signature of the physician or the physician's representative above or below the name. Enter the six-digit date the form was prepared. On crossover claims, enter the provider number.

Block 32. Enter only the facility's nine-digit provider number. Do not include the name and address of the facility. For crossover claims, list the Medi-Cal identification number here and in Block 9a.

Block 33. Enter the name and address of the physician or group billing for services and the individual or group nine-character Medi-Cal provider number in the PIN# area as shown in Figure B–8.

To delete specific information from Blocks 24A through K on the CMS-1500 claim form, draw a thin black line through the entire line but do not obliterate. Enter the correct information on another line. Use white paper tape or dry line tape to block out and correct a typed error in all other blocks. There is no need to write "See Attachments" because the equipment stamps the same assigned claim number on all accompanying sheets until the equipment recognizes another bar code. Keep the small printout from the POS device for the physician's records and, in general, do not use this receipt as an attachment. If for some reason the printout is sent to the fiscal intermediary, attach it to a standard-size sheet of paper, noting the EVC number in Block 13.

33. PHYSICIAN'S, SUPPLIER'S BILLING NAME, ADDRESS, ZIP CODE AND PHONE #

COLLEGE CLINIC
4567 BROAD AVENUE
WOODLAND HILLS XY 12345 0001
013 486 9002

PIN# ZZR12005F GRP#

FIGURE B–8 Block 33 of the CMS-1500 insurance claim form indicating the location for insertion of an individual or group nine-character Medi-Cal provider number.

*Documentation required.

PROCEDURE

COMPLETING THE RESUBMISSION TURNAROUND DOCUMENT

Part A of the RTD describes the information that requires correction, and part B corrects the suspended claim. To complete an RTD, either type or handwrite the correct data on the appropriate line in the Correct Information section of Part B. The data should be entered exactly as required on the claim form (e.g., no dashes, all dates in six-digit format). If a line is correct, it is not necessary to repeat the data; leave blank that line of the Correct Information section. Providers must return Part B of the RTD to the fiscal intermediary, but do not mail RTDs in the same envelope with claims. Refer to the *Medi-Cal Medical Services Provider Manual* for the address. Figure B–9 shows a correctly completed RTD, and the following item numbers and descriptions correspond to the figure. The top of the form contains instructions for completing the form.

1. Information block: The name of the claim form box in question.
2. Submitted information: Questionable or missing information on the claim as entered into the Medi-Cal system.
3. Service code: Procedure code, medical supply code, or drug code for the services under inquiry.
4. Error code: See Item 7. RTD error codes are *not* the same as the remittance advice denial codes. Note that 0012 indicates that "the number given on the claim as the TAR control number is not numeric or has an incorrect number of digits."
5. Beginning date of service: Date the service was rendered.
6. Corrected information: If the information in Item 2 should be corrected, the correct information may be noted here for the provider's records. The actual correction of the information that is sent to the fiscal intermediary is entered in Item 21.

7. Error description: This is the full explanation of the code that appears in Item 4. Compare this with your copy of the claim to assist you in identifying the error; the error description will be helpful.
8. Provider's name and address.
9. Provider's identification number.
10. Final notice: This is for the fiscal intermediary's use only.
11. Date of notice.
12. Number of pages in RTD.
13. Service date(s) and provider reference number.
14. Preprinted information that identifies the patient, Medi-Cal identification number, medical records number, total charges, and specific CCN.
15. Correspondence reference number: leave blank.
16. Provider's identification number.
17. Provider's name.
18. Patient's Medi-Cal identification number entered by the provider on the original claim.
19. Patient's name.
20. For fiscal intermediary's use only.
21. Enter correct information (Part B of the RTD) in the numbered box that corresponds with the error line in the Information Block (Item 1 in Part A). If the information in Part A is correct, leave the corresponding line blank. When entering correct information, enter all characters (numbers and letters) exactly as they would be entered on the claim. Corrected information on the RTD must be the same alphabetic or numeric format required on the claim form (e.g., date of birth: June 6, 1968, would be entered 060668). Claims cannot be processed if the corrected information is not accurate or is not shown in the required format.
22. Signature. All RTDs must be signed and dated by the provider or an authorized representative.
23. Blocks 1 through 6 are no longer used.

PROCEDURE—CONT'D

RESUBMISSION TURNAROUND DOCUMENT

INSTRUCTIONS: Listed in Section "A" are error(s) found on the original claim. To expedite payment, type the correct information in the numbered Box of Section "B" that corresponds to numbered line in Section "A", sign and date the form, and return Section "B" (bottom portion) to F.I. Please respond promptly as the claim cannot be paid unless your corrections are received by October 30, 1999. See your provider manual for assistance regarding the completion of this form.

INFORMATION BLOCK	SUBMITTED INFORMATION	SERVICE CODE	ERROR CODE	BEG DOS - PATIENT NAME - COR INFO
1 TAR CONTROL NUMBER A1123456789			0012	XX/08/01 Smith, Mike
①	②	③	④	⑤ ⑥

ERROR DESCRIPTION

⑦ 0012 - THE NUMBER GIVEN ON THE CLAIM AS THE TAR CONTROL NUMBER IS NOT NUMERIC OR HAS AN INCORRECT NUMBER OF DIGITS

PROVIDER NAME AND ADDRESS

⑨ PROVIDER NUMBER XXXXXXXX   FINAL NOTICE ⑩

ABC PROVIDER
123 ANY STREET
ANYTOWN, CA 95000
⑧

⑪ DATE August 30, 20XX   PAGE 1 ⑫ OF 1

SERVICE DATE(S) / PROVIDER REFERENCE NO.
August 15, 20XX ⑬

RETAIN THIS PORTION

PATIENT NAME ⑭	MEDI-CAL ID NUMBER	MEDICAL RECORDS NO.	TOTAL CHARGES	CLAIM CONTROL NUMBER
SMITH, MIKE	1234567899	123455	$1575.00	0170626097022

DETACH AND RETURN TO APPROPRIATE F.I.

DO NOT STAPLE IN BAR AREA

CORRESPONDENCE REFERENCE NUMBER - F.I. USE ONLY

⑮

PROVIDER NUMBER
XXXXXXXX ⑯   FINAL NOTICE AUGUST 30, 1999

PROVIDER NAME
ABC PROVIDER ⑰

PATIENT MEDI-CAL ID NO.
1234567899 ⑱

PATIENT NAME
SMITH, MIKE ⑲

F.I. USE ONLY

CORRECT INFORMATION MUST BE ENTERED ON THE SAME LINE AS THE ERROR SHOWN IN SECTION "A"

CCN 0170626097022	CLAIM TYPE	PAGE 1 OF	PAGES 1	

CORRECT INFORMATION

SUBMITTED INFORMATION A1123456789	ERROR CODE 0012	LINE 01	FIELD 012	LABEL

⑳

☐ 1 ㉑ 11234567899
☐ 2
☐ 3
☐ 4
☐ 5
☐ 6

This is to certify that the correct information is true, accurate and complete and that the provider has read, understands, and agrees to be bound by and comply with the statements and conditions contained on the back of this form.

㉒

Signature of provider or person authorized by provider to bind provider by above signature to statements and conditions contained on this form.   DATE

IF SPECIFICALLY REQUESTED, PLACE LABEL IN THE BOX INDICATED BELOW. THIS SPACE MAY ALSO BE USED FOR COMMENTS.

1	**2** ㉓	**3**
4	**5**	**6**

FIGURE B–9 Completed Medi-Cal Resubmission Turnaround Document Form 65-1.

PROCEDURE

COMPLETING THE CLAIMS INQUIRY FORM

Each line on the CIF corresponds to a single line on the CMS-1500 claim form. Complete the lines on the CIF according to the type of inquiry you wish to make. Adjustment and denial reconsideration requests may be combined on one CIF. Tracer requests must be submitted separately.

The correct number of characters must be entered in the spaces provided on the form. Any time a reference is made to a claim previously adjudicated, be certain to indicate the previous CCN and attach a copy of the corrected claim and RAD. *Do not* submit CIFs for claims that are listed under the Suspends heading on the RAD. Each numbered item refers to the numbers on the CIF (Figure B–10).

1. Correspondence reference number: Leave blank. The fiscal intermediary will assign a number.
2. Document number: A preprinted number identifying the CIF.
3. Provider's name and address: Enter provider's name, street address, city, state, and ZIP code.
4. Provider's number: Enter the nine-character provider identification number, plus optional Check Digit, assigned by the Department of Health Services.
5. Claim type: Enter an "X" in the box indicating the claim type. Check only one box.
6. Delete: Enter an "X" to delete the entire line. Enter the correct billing information on another line.
7. Patient's name or medical record number: Enter up to the first 10 letters of the patient's last name or the first 10 characters of the patient's medical record number.
8. Patient's Medi-Cal identification number: Enter the recipient's identification number that appears on the RAD showing adjudication of that claim.
9. CCN: Enter the 13-digit number assigned by the fiscal intermediary to the claim line in question. This may be found on the RAD. If this line is blank, the inquiry will be considered a tracer request.
10. Date of service: Enter the date in six-digit format (e.g., 0606XX), on which the service was rendered. For consecutive date ranges (block-billed claims), enter the "From" date of service.
11. NDC/UPC or procedure code: Enter the appropriate procedure code, modifier, and drug or supply code if applicable. Codes of less than 11 digits should be left-justified. *Long-term care and inpatient providers may leave this box blank.*
12. Amount billed: Enter the amount originally billed, using the two boxes to the right of the decimal point to reflect cents.
13. Attachment: Enter an "X" when attaching documentation and when resubmitting a denied claim. All CIFs should have attachments except when submitting a tracer.
14. Underpayment: Enter an "X" for an underpayment adjustment of a paid claim. *Do not* mark if the claim was denied.
15. Overpayment: Enter an "X" if all or part of the claim was overpaid. *Do not* mark if the claim was denied.
16. Remarks: Use this area to state the reason for submitting a CIF and include the corresponding line number if listing multiple claim lines on the CIF.
17. Signature: The provider or an authorized representative must sign the CIF.

PROCEDURE—CONT'D

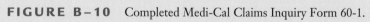

DO NOT STAPLE IN BAR AREA

(1) CORRESPONDENCE REFERENCE NUMBER • FOR F.I. USE ONLY

(1)

FASTEN HERE

7

READ INSTRUCTIONS ON REVERSE PRIOR TO COMPLETING AND SIGNING THIS FORM. DO NOT TYPE/MARK IN SHADED AREAS.

(2) DOCUMENT NUMBER

39377390

CLAIMS INQUIRY

SEE YOUR PROVIDER MANUAL FOR ASSISTANCE REGARDING THE COMPLETION OF THIS FORM.

TYPEWRITER ALIGNMENT

Elite   Pica

TYPEWRITER ALIGNMENT

(2)

Elite   Pica

(3) PROVIDER NAME/ADDRESS

(3)

(4) PROVIDER NUMBER XXXXXXXXX   CHECK **5** DIGIT

ABC PROVIDER
123 ANY STREET
ANYTOWN, CA 90000

(5) CLAIM CHECK
CHECK ONE BOX ONLY

01 ☐ PHARMACY
02 ☐ LTC
03 ☐ HOSPITAL INPATIENT

04 ☐ HOSPITAL OUTPATIENT CLINIC
05 ☐ PHYSICIAN/ALLIED
07 ☐ VISION

(5)

check the appropriate claim type

PLEASE FILL IN ALL APPLICABLE INFORMATION REQUESTED BELOW

(6) DELETE	(7) PATIENT'S NAME OR MEDICAL RECORD NO.	(8) PATIENT'S MEDI-CAL I.D. NO.	(9) CLAIM CONTROL NO. LINE	(10) DATE OF SERVICE	(11) NDC/UPC OR PROCEDURE CODE	(12) AMOUNT BILLED	(13) ATTACHMENT	(14) UNDERPAYMENT	(15) OVERPAYMENT
01	JONES	123456789	42513434567 02 TRACER-NO CCN				X		
02	BROWN	987654321	42503878934 01 TRACER-NO CCN				X	X	
03	SMITH	345678912	42559327678 01 TRACER-NO CCN				X		X
04			TRACER-NO CCN						
05			TRACER-NO CCN						
06			TRACER-NO CCN						
07			TRACER-NO CCN						
08			TRACER-NO CCN						

REMARKS: (CORRECTIONS OR ADDITIONAL INFORMATION NECESSARY TO RESUBMIT A DENIED CLAIM, OR REQUEST AN ADJUSTMENT FOR AN UNDERPAYMENT OR AN OVERPAYMENT.) (16)

LINE 1   CLAIM DENIED 001 BECAUSE RECIPIENT WAS INELIGIBLE FOR MONTH OF SERVICE. RETROACTIVE ELIGIBILITY INFORMATION RECEIVED AUG. 3. PLEASE RECONSIDER.

LINE 2   WE BILLED FOR $5.00 INSTEAD OF $50.00. SEE CORRECTED CLAIM. PLEASE ADJUST.

LINE 3   CLAIM BILLED IN ERROR. INSURANCE PAID. PLEASE RECOUP PAYMENT OF $22.00.

This is to certify that the information contained above is true, accurate and complete, and that the provider has read, understands, and agrees to be bound by and comply with the statements and conditions contained on the back of this form.

(17)

Chris Neill   *9/15/XX*

Signature of provider or person authorized to bind provider by above signature to statements and conditions contained on this form.   DATE

FORWARD TO APPROPRIATE F.I.   60-1 08/93

FIGURE B–10   Completed Medi-Cal Claims Inquiry Form 60-1.

PROCEDURE

COMPLETING AN APPEAL FORM

Each numbered item refers to the numbers on the Appeal Form shown in Figure B–11.

1. Appeal reference number: Leave blank. The fiscal intermediary will assign a number.
2. Document number: A preprinted number is used when requesting information about the status of an appeal.
3. Provider's name and address: Enter the provider's name, street address, city, state, and ZIP code.
4. Provider's number: Enter the nine-character provider's identification number, plus Check Digit, assigned by the Department of Health Services. Appeal acknowledgment may be delayed without the correct provider number.
5. Claim type: Enter an "X" in the box indicating the claim type. Check only one box.
6. Statement of appeal: This is for information purposes only.
7. Patient's name or medical record number: Enter up to the first 10 letters of the patient's last name or the first 10 characters of the patient's medical record number.
8. Patient's Medi-Cal identification number and Social Security Number (SSN): Enter the recipient's identification number that appears on the plastic BIC or paper Medi-Cal card.
9. Delete: Enter an "X" to delete the corresponding line. Enter correct billing information on another line.
10. CCN: For adjudicated claims, enter the 13-digit number assigned by the fiscal intermediary to the claim line in question. This number appears on the RAD. When appealing a nonadjudicated claim (e.g., a traced claim that could not be located), the CCN field is not required.
11. Date of service: Enter the date the service was rendered in six-digit format (0102XX). For claims billed in a "From-Through" format, enter the "From" date of service.
12. RAD code or EOB/RA code: Enter the RAD message code for the claim line (e.g., 010, 072, or 401) when appealing an adjudicated claim.
13. Reason for appeal: Indicate the specific reason for filing an appeal. Remember to attach all supporting documentation.
14. Common appeal reason: Check one of the boxes if applicable. Include a copy of the claim and supporting documents (e.g., TAR or RAD). Box 13 may be left blank if this box is used.
15. Signature: The provider or an authorized representative must sign.

PROCEDURE—CONT'D

FIGURE B–11 Completed Medi-Cal Appeal Form 90-1 to be used for denial resubmissions, underpayment reconsiderations, and overpayment returns.

RESOURCES

INTERNET

- Job search resources:
  Federal Register
  Web site: **http://www.archives.gov**

- Medicaid
  Web site: **http://www.cms.gov/Medicaid**

- Medi-Cal
  Web site: **http://www.medi-cal.ca.gov**

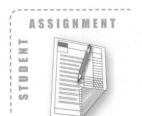

ASSIGNMENT

STUDENT

✔ Study Chapter 13 and this appendix.

✔ Answer the self-study review questions in the *Workbook* to reinforce the theory learned in these portions of the text and help prepare you for a future test.

✔ Complete the assignments in the *Workbook* to give you experience abstracting from case histories, posting to financial accounting record cards, and completing forms pertinent to the Medi-Cal program.

✔ Turn to the glossary at the end of this textbook for a further understanding of the key terms used in this chapter.

Chapter number(s) is shown in parentheses after each term.

Abuse (2): Incidents or practices, not usually considered fraudulent, that are inconsistent with accepted sound medical business or fiscal practices.

Accident (15): An unexpected happening, causing injury traceable to a definite time and place.

Accidental death and dismemberment (16): An insurance policy provision that protects the insured if he or she suffers loss of sight or loss of limb(s) or death by accident.

Accounts receivable (A/R) (10): The total amount of money owed for professional services rendered.

Accounts receivable management (3): The organization and administration of coding and billing in a medical practice.

Accounts receivable (A/R) transaction (B): A miscellaneous Medi-Cal accounting transaction that results from cost settlements, state audits, or refund checks received by the fiscal intermediary.

Accredited Standards Committee × 12 (ASC × 12) (8): The U.S. standards body formed by the American National Standards Institute (ANSI) for cross-industry development, maintenance, and publication of electronic data exchange standards.

Active duty service member (ADSM) (14): An active member of the United States government military services (e.g., Army, Navy, Air Force, Marines, or Coast Guard).

Acute (4): A medical condition that runs a short but relatively severe course.

Adjudication (15): The final determination of the issues involving settlement of an insurance claim; also known as a claim settlement.

Admission review (17): A review for appropriateness and necessity of admissions.

Advance beneficiary notice (ABN) (12): An agreement given to the patient to read and sign before rendering a service if the participating physician thinks that it may be denied for payment because of medical necessity or limitation of liability by Medicare. The patient agrees to pay for the service; also known as a waiver of liability agreement or responsibility statement.

Adverse effect (5): An unfavorable, detrimental, or pathologic reaction to a drug that occurs when appropriate doses are given to humans for prophylaxis (prevention of disease), diagnosis, and therapy.

Age analysis (10): The procedure of systematically arranging the accounts receivable, by age, from the date of service.

Aid to the Blind (AB) (B): A group entitled to benefits under the Medi-Cal program.

Aid to Families with Dependent Children (AFDC) (B): A group entitled to benefits under the Medi-Cal program.

Aid to the (permanently) Disabled (ATD) (B): A group entitled to benefits under the Medi-Cal program.

Alien (18): An individual belonging to another country or people; a foreigner.

Allowable charge (14): An amount on which TRICARE figures the patient's cost-share for covered care. This is based on 75% to 80% of the *allowable* charge.

Alternative billing codes (ABCs) (6): A code system for integrative health care products and services consisting of five-character alphabetic symbols with appended two-character practitioner modifiers that represent the practitioner type.

AMA Code of Medical Ethics (10): A code of medical ethics formulated by the American Medical Association and adopted in 1847.

Ambulatory payment classifications (APCs) (17): A system of outpatient hospital reimbursement based on procedures rather than diagnoses.

American Health Information Management Association (AHIMA) (1): A national professional organization for promoting the art and science of medical record management and improving the quality of comprehensive health information for the welfare of the public.

American Medical Association (AMA) (1): A national professional society of physicians.

Ancillary services (11): Supportive services other than routine hospital services provided by the facility, such as x-ray films and laboratory tests.

Appeal (9): A request for a review of an insurance claim that has been underpaid or denied by an insurance company to receive additional payment.

Applicant (3): A person applying for insurance coverage.

Application form (18): A request form to be completed with pertinent data when applying for employment.

Application service provider (ASP) (8): A practice management system available over the Internet in which data are housed on the server of the ASP but the accounts are managed by the health care provider's staff.

Appropriateness evaluation protocols (AEPs) (17): Nineteen criteria for admission under the prospective payment system, separated into two categories: severity and intensity of illness. To allow a patient admission to an acute care facility, one criterion from each category must be met.

Approved charges (12): A fee that Medicare decides the medical service is worth, which may or may not be the same as the actual amount billed. The patient may or may not be responsible for the difference.

Armed Services Disability (16): A disability occurring or aggravated while the patient is in military service.

Assignment (3, 12): A transfer, after an event insured against, or an individual's legal right to collect an amount payable under an insurance contract. For Medicare, an agreement in which a patient assigns to the physician the right to receive payment from the fiscal intermediary. Under this agreement, the physician must agree to accept 80% of the allowed amount as payment in full once the deductible has been met. For TRICARE, providers who accept assignment agree to accept 75% or 80% of the TRICARE allowable charge as the full fee, collecting the deductible and 20% or 25% of the allowable charge from the patient. With other carriers, accepting assignment means that, in return for payment of the claim, the provider accepts the terms of the contract between the patient and carrier. The provider also accepts the payment from the carrier as payment in full with no balance billing of the patient.

Attending physician (4): A medical staff member who is legally responsible for the care and treatment given to a patient.

Authorization form (2): A document signed by the patient that is needed for use and disclosure of protected health information that is not included in any existing consent form agreements.

Authorized provider (14): A physician or other individual authorized provider of care or a hospital or supplier approved by TRICARE to provide medical care and supplies.

Automated eligibility verification system (AEVS) (B): An interactive voice-response system in the Medi-Cal program that allows providers to access recipient eligibility, clear share of cost, or reserve a Medi-Service.

Automatic stay (10): A court order that goes into effect once a bankruptcy petition is filed; all other legal actions are halted, such as attachments and foreclosures.

Backup (8): A duplicate data file: tape, CD-ROM, disk, or ZIP disk used to record data; it may be used to complete or redo the operation if the primary equipment fails.

Balance (10): An amount owed on a credit transaction; also known as the outstanding or unpaid balance.

Bankruptcy (10): A condition under which a person or corporation is declared unable to pay debts.

Batch (8): A group of claims for different patients from one office submitted in one computer transmission.

Beneficiary (14): An individual entitled to receive insurance policy or government program health care benefits. Also known as *participant, subscriber, dependent, enrollee,* or *member.*

Benefit period (12, 16): A period of time for which payments for Medicare inpatient hospital benefits are available. A benefit period begins the first day an enrollee is given inpatient hospital care (nursing care or rehabilitation services) by a qualified provider and ends when the enrollee has not been an inpatient for 60 consecutive days. In workers' compensation cases, it is the maximum amount of time that benefits will be paid to the injured or ill person for the disability. For disability insurance, it is the maximum amount of time that benefits will be paid to the injured or ill person for a disability.

Benefits identification card (BIC) (B): A Medi-Cal identification card.

Benign tumor (5): An abnormal growth that does not have the properties of invasion and metastasis and is usually surrounded by a fibrous capsule; also called a *neoplasm.*

Bilateral (6): When coding surgical procedures, this term refers to both sides of the body.

Blanket contract (3): Comprehensive group insurance coverage through plans sponsored by professional associations for their members.

Blind mailing (18): To send a resume with cover letter to possible prospects whom the individual does not know personally and who have not advertised for a job opening.

Bonding (10): An insurance contract by which, in return for a stated fee, a bonding agency guarantees payment of a certain sum to an employer in the event of a financial loss to the employer by the act of a specified employee or by some contingency over which the employer has no control.

Breach of confidential communication (2): "Breach" means breaking or violation of a law or agreement. In the context of the medical office it means the unauthorized release of information about the patient.

Buffing (11): A physician's justifying the transference of sick, high-cost patients to other physicians in a managed care plan.

Bundled codes (6): To group more than one component (service or procedure) into one CPT code.

Business associate (2): A person who, on behalf of the covered entity, performs or assists in the performance of a function or activity involving the use or disclosure of individually identifiable health information, including claims processing or administration, data analysis, processing or administration, utilization review, quality assurance, billing, benefit management, practice management, and repricing.

Business associate agreement (8, 18): Contract between the provider and a clearinghouse that submits the electronic claims on behalf of the provider

By report (BR) (15): A report must be submitted with the claim when the notation BR follows the procedure code description. This term is sometimes seen in workers' compensation fee schedules.

Cable modem (8): A modem used to connect a computer to a cable television system that offers online services.

California Children's Services (CCS) (B): A state program for disabled children.

Capitation (3, 11, 17): A system of payment used by managed care plans in which physicians and hospitals are paid a fixed per capita amount for each patient enrolled over a stated period of time, regardless of the type and number of services provided; reimbursement to the hospital on a per-member/per-month basis to cover costs for the members of the plan. Capitation also can mean a set amount to be paid per claim.

Carve outs (11): Medical services not included within the capitation rate as benefits of a managed care contract and may be contracted for separately.

Case rate (17): An averaging after a flat rate is given to certain categories of procedures.

Cash flow (1, 10): In a medical practice, the amount of *actual* cash generated and available for use by the medical practice within a given period of time.

Catastrophic cap (14): The maximum dollar amount that a member has to pay under TRICARE or CHAMPVA in any fiscal year or enrollment period for covered medical bills.

Catchment area (14): In the TRICARE program, an area, defined by ZIP codes, that is approximately 40 miles in radius surrounding each United States military treatment facility.

Categorically needy (13): Aged, blind, or disabled individuals or families and children who meet financial eligibility requirements for Aid to Families with Dependent Children, Supplemental Security Income, or an optional state supplement.

Centers for Medicare and Medicaid Services (CMS) (12): Formerly known as the Health Care Financing Administration

(HCFA), CMS divides responsibilities among three divisions: the Center for Medicare Management, the Center for Beneficiary Choices, and the Center for Medicaid and State Operations.

Certification (18): A statement issued by a board or association verifying that a person meets professional standards.

Certified Coding Specialist (CCS) (18): A title received by a person after appropriate training and by passing a certification examination administered by the American Health Information Management Association for hospital-based coding.

Certified Coding Specialist-Physician (CCS-P) (18): A title received by a person after appropriate training and by passing a certification examination administered by the American Health Information Management Association for physician-based coding.

Certified Medical Assistant (CMA) (18): A title received by a person after appropriate training and by passing a certification examination administered by the American Association of Medical Assistants, Inc.

Certified Medical Billing Specialist (CMBS) (18): A title received by a person after appropriate training and by passing a certification examination administered either by the American Association of Medical Billers in Los Angeles or the Medical Association of Billers in Las Vegas.

Certified Professional Coder (CPC) (18): A title received by a person after appropriate training and by passing a certification examination administered by the American Academy of Professional Coders.

CHAMPVA (3, 14): *See* The Civilian Health and Medical Program of the Department of Veterans Affairs.

Charge description master (CDM) (17): A computer program that is linked to various hospital departments and includes procedure codes, procedure descriptions, service descriptions, fees, and revenue codes; also known as *charge master*.

Charges (17): The dollar amount a hospital bills an outlier case based on the itemized bill.

Chief complaint (CC) (4, 5): A patient's statement describing symptoms, problems, or conditions as the reason for seeking health care services from a physician.

Child Health and Disability Prevention Program (CHDP) (B): A state health and disability prevention program for children.

Chronic (4): A medical condition persisting over a long period of time.

Chronologic resume (18): A data sheet that outlines experience and education by dates.

Churning (11): Physicians' seeing of a high volume of patients—more than medically necessary—to increase revenue. May be seen in fee-for-service or managed care environments.

Civil Service Retirement System (CSRS) (16): A program for federal employees hired before 1984.

Claim (3): A bill sent to an insurance carrier requesting payment for services rendered; also known as *encounter record*.

Claim control number (CCN) (B): A number assigned by the Medi-Cal fiscal intermediary on a Treatment Authorization Request and used for reference when processing the request.

Claims assistance professional (CAP) (18): A practitioner who works for the consumer and helps patients organize, complete, file, and negotiate health insurance claims of all types to obtain maximum benefits as well as tell patients what checks to write to providers to eliminate overpayment.

Claims and eligibility real-time software (CERTS) (B): Computer software that allows Medi-Cal providers to electronically verify recipient eligibility, clear share of cost liability, reserve Medi-Services, perform family PACT (planning, access, care, treatment) client eligibility transactions, and submit pharmacy or CMS-1500 claims using a personal computer.

Claims examiner (15): In industrial cases, a representative of the insurer who authorizes treatment and investigates, evaluates, and negotiates the patient's insurance claim and acts for the company in the settlement of claims; also known as *claims adjuster, claim representative,* and *claims administrator.*

Claims Inquiry Form (CIF) (B): A Medi-Cal form used for tracing a claim, resubmitting a claim after a denial, or when requesting an adjustment for underpaid or overpaid claims.

Claims—review type of foundation (11): A type of foundation that provides peer review by physicians to the numerous fiscal agents or carriers involved in its area.

Clean claim (7): A completed insurance claim form submitted within the program time limit that contains all the necessary information without deficiencies so it can be processed and paid promptly.

Clearinghouse (2, 8): A third-party administrator (TPA) that receives insurance claims from the physician's office, performs software edits, and redistributes the claims electronically to various insurance carriers.

Clinical outliers (17): Cases that cannot adequately be assigned to an appropriate DRG owing to unique combinations of diagnoses and surgeries, very rare conditions, or other unique clinical reasons. Such cases are grouped together into clinical outlier DRGs and therefore are considered *outliers.*

Closed panel program (11): A form of HMO that limits the patient's choice of personal physicians to those doctors practicing in the HMO group practice within the geographic location or facility. A physician must meet very narrow criteria to join a closed panel.

Code of Medical Ethics (10): A code of medical ethics written by Thomas Percival in 1803.

Code sequence (17): The correct order of diagnostic codes (1, 2, 3, 4) when submitting an insurance claim that affects maximum reimbursement. Other factors affecting maximum reimbursement are accurate diagnostic code selection and linking the proper service or procedures provided to the patient.

Code set (2, 8): Any set of codes with their descriptions used to encode data elements, such as tables of terms, medical concepts, medical diagnostic codes, or medical procedure codes.

Coinsurance (3): A cost-sharing requirement under a health insurance policy providing that the insured will assume a percentage of the costs for covered services; for Medicare, after application of the yearly cash deductible, the portion of the reasonable charges (20%) for which the beneficiary is responsible.

Collateral (10): Any possession, such as an automobile, furniture, stocks, or bonds, that secures or guarantees the discharge of an obligation.

Collection ratio (10): The relationship between the amount of money owed and the amount of money collected in reference to the doctor's accounts receivable.

Combination code (5): A code from one section of the procedural code book combined with a code from another section that is used to completely describe a procedure performed; in diagnostic coding, a single five-digit code used to identify etiology and secondary process (manifestation) or complication of a disease.

Combination resume (18): A data sheet that combines specific dates or work experience with educational skills.

Comorbidity (4, 17): An ongoing condition that exists along with the condition for which the patient is receiving treatment; in regard to DRGs, a preexisting condition that, because of its presence with a certain principal diagnosis, will cause an increase in length of stay by at least 1 day in approximately 75% of cases. Also known as *substantial comorbidity.*

Competitive Medical Plan (CMP) (3): A state licensed health plan similar to a health maintenance organization (HMO) that delivers comprehensive, coordinated services to voluntarily enrolled members on a prepaid capitated basis. CMP status may be granted by the federal government for the enrollment of Medicare beneficiaries into managed care plans, without having to qualify as an HMO.

Compliance (2): A process of meeting regulations, recommendations, and expectations of federal and state agencies that pay for health care services and regulate the industry.

Compliance plan (2): A management plan composed of policies and procedures to accomplish uniformity, consistency, and conformity in medical record keeping that fulfills official requirements.

Complication (5): A disease or condition arising during the course of, or as a result of, another disease modifying medical care requirements; for DRGs, a condition that arises during the hospital stay that prolongs the length of stay by at least 1 day in approximately 75% of cases. Also known as *substantial complication.*

Comprehensive (C) (4): A term used to describe a level of history or physical examination.

Comprehensive code (6): A single procedural code that describes or covers two or more CPT component codes that are bundled together as one unit.

Comprehensive Perinatal Services Program (CPSP) (B): A program that offers a wide range of services to pregnant Medi-Cal recipients.

Comprehensive type of foundation (11): A type of foundation that designs and sponsors prepaid health programs or sets minimum benefits of coverage.

Compromise and release (C and R) (15): An agreement arrived at, whether in or out of court, for settling a workers' compensation case after the patient has been declared permanent and stationary.

Computer media claims (CMC) (B): A system that permits submission of Medi-Cal claims via telecommunication through magnetic tape or diskette and modem.

Concurrent care (4): The provision of similar services (e.g., hospital visits) to the same patient by more than one physician on the same day. Usually there is the presence of a separate physical disorder.

Conditionally renewable (3): An insurance policy renewal provision that grants the insurer a limited right to refuse to renew a health insurance policy at the end of a premium payment period.

Confidential communication (2): A privileged communication that may be disclosed only with the patient's permission.

Confidentiality (2): The state of treating privately or secretly, and not disclosing to other individuals or for public knowledge, the patient's conversations or medical records.

Consent form (2): A document that *is not* required *before* physicians use or disclose protected health information for treatment, payment, or routine health care operations of the patient. For other purposes, see Authorization form.

Consultation (4): Services rendered by a physician whose opinion or advice is requested by another physician or agency in the evaluation or treatment of a patient's illness or suspected problem.

Consultative examiner (CE) (16): A physician who is paid a fee to examine or test a person for disability under either the SSDI or SSI program.

Consulting physician (4): A provider whose opinion or advice about evaluation or management of a specific problem is requested by another physician.

Continuing education (CE) (18): Formal education pursued by a working professional and intended to improve or maintain professional competence.

Continuity of care (4): When a physician sees a patient who has received treatment for a condition and is referred by the previous doctor for treatment of the same condition.

Contract (3): A legally enforceable agreement when relating to an insurance policy; for workers' compensation cases, an agreement involving two or more parties in which each is obligated to the other to fulfill promises made. (The contract exists between the physician and the insurance carrier.)

Conversion factor (6): The dollars and cents amount that is established for one unit as applied to a procedure or service rendered. This unit is then used to convert various procedures into fee-schedule payment amounts by multiplying the relative value unit by the conversion factor.

Cooperative care (14): A term used when a patient is seen by a civilian physician or hospital for services cost-shared by TRICARE.

Coordination of benefits (14): Two insurance carriers working together and coordinating the payment of their benefits, so that there is no duplication of benefits paid between the primary and secondary insurance carriers. In TRICARE, the coordination of the payment of TRICARE benefits with the payment of benefits made by the double coverage plan, so that there is no duplication of benefits paid between the double coverage plan and TRICARE; likewise applied to disability programs.

Copayment (copay) (11): A patient's payment (e.g., 20% of a bill or flat fee of $10 per visit) of a portion of the cost at the time the service is rendered. Also referred to as *coinsurance.*

Correct coding initiative (CCI) (12): Federal legislation that attempts to eliminate unbundling or other inappropriate reporting of procedural codes for professional medical services rendered to patients.

Cost-of-living adjustment (16): A disability insurance provision to increase monthly benefits.

Cost outlier (17): A typical case that has an extraordinarily high cost when compared with most discharges classified to the same DRG.

Cost outlier review (17): A review by a Professional Review Organization (PRO) for the necessity of a patient's hospital admission and to determine whether all services rendered were medically necessary. Cost outlier cases are recognized only if the case is not eligible for day outlier status.

Cost-share (14): The portion of the allowable charges (20% or 25%) after the deductible has been met that the TRICARE patient is responsible for.

Counseling (4): A discussion between the physician and a patient, family, or both concerning the diagnosis, recommended studies or tests, prognosis, risks, and benefits of treatment, treatment options, patient and family education, and so on.

County Medical Services Program (CMSP) (B): A county program for medical services.

Cover letter (18): A letter of introduction prepared to accompany a resume when seeking a job.

Covered entity (CE) (2, 8): An entity that transmits health information in *electronic form* in connection with a *transaction* covered by HIPAA. The covered entity may be (1) a health care coverage carrier such as Blue Cross/Blue Shield, (2) a health care clearinghouse through which claims are submitted, or (3) a health care provider such as the primary care physician.

Covered services (13): Specific services and supplies for which Medicaid will provide reimbursement; these consist of a combination of mandatory and optional services stated in the plan.

CPT (6): See *Current Procedural Terminology.*

Credit (10): 1. From the Latin *credere*, meaning "to believe" or "to trust"; trust in regard to financial obligation. 2. Accounting entry reflecting payment by a debtor (patient) of a sum received on his or her account.

Credit card (10): A card issued by an organization and devised for the purpose of obtaining money, property, labor, or services on credit.

Creditor (10): A person to whom money is owed.

Critical care (4): In reference to coding professional services, this phrase relates to intensive care provided in a variety of acute life-threatening conditions requiring constant bedside attention by a physician.

Crossover claim (12): A bill for services rendered to a patient receiving benefits simultaneously from Medicare and Medicaid or from Medicare and a Medigap plan. Medicare pays first and then determines the amounts of unmet Medicare deductible and coinsurance to be paid by the secondary insurance carrier. The claim is automatically transferred (electronically) to the secondary insurance carrier for additional payment; also known as *claims transfer.*

***Current Procedural Terminology* (CPT) (6):** A reference procedural code book using a five-digit numerical system to identify and code procedures established by the American Medical Association.

Customary fee (6): The amount that a physician usually charges most of her or his patients.

Cycle billing (10): A system of billing accounts at spaced intervals during the month based on breakdown of accounts by alphabet, account number, insurance type, or date of first service.

Data elements (8): *Medical codes sets* used uniformly to document why patients are seen (diagnosis, ICD-9-CM) and what is done to them during their encounter (procedure, CPT-4, HCPCS).

Day outlier review (17): A review of potential day outliers (short or unusually long length of hospital stay) to determine the necessity of admission and number of days before the day outlier threshold is reached as well as the number of days beyond the threshold. The PRO determines the certification of additional days.

Daysheet (3): A register for recording daily business transactions (charges, payments, or adjustments); also known as *daybook, daily log,* or *daily record sheet.*

Debit card (10): A card permitting bank customers to withdraw from any affiliated automated teller machine (ATM) and make cashless purchases from funds on deposit without incurring revolving finance charges for credit.

Debt (10): A legal obligation to pay money.

Debtor (10): A person owing money.

Deductible (2, 11): A specific dollar amount that must be paid by the insured before a medical insurance plan or government program begins covering health care costs.

Defense Enrollment Eligibility Reporting System (DEERS) (14): An electronic database used to verify beneficiary eligibility for those individuals in the TRICARE programs.

Delinquent claim (9): An insurance claim submitted to an insurance company, for which payment is overdue.

Denied paper or electronic claim (9): An insurance claim submitted to an insurance company in which payment has been rejected owing to a technical error or because of medical coverage policy issues.

Department of Health Services (DHS) (B): Medi-Cal is administered by this state department, which is a department of the California State Human Relations Agency.

Deposition (15): The process of taking sworn testimony from a witness out of court. This is usually done by an attorney.

Detailed (D) (4): A term used to describe a level of history or physical examination.

Diagnosis-related groups (DRGs) (17): A patient classification system that categorizes patients who are medically related with respect to diagnosis and treatment and statistically similar in length of hospital stay. Medicare hospital insurance payments are based on fixed dollar amounts for a principal diagnosis as listed in DRGs.

Diagnostic cost groups (DCGs) (12): A system of Medicare reimbursement for HMOs with risk contracts in which enrollees are classified into various DCGs on the basis of each beneficiary's prior 12-month hospitalization history.

Diagnostic creep (17): Coding that is inappropriately altered to obtain a higher payment rate. Also known as *coding creep, DRG creep,* or *upcoding.*

Direct data entry (DDE) (8): Keying claim information directly into the payer system by accessing over modem dial-up or DSL. This is a technology to directly enter the information into the payer system via the access whether it is dial-up or DSL.

Digital subscriber line (DSL) (8): A high-speed connection through a telephone line jack and usually a means of accessing the Internet.

Direct referral (11): Certain services in a managed care plan may not require preauthorization. The authorization request form is completed and signed by the physician and handed to the patient (e.g., obstetric care or dermatology) to be done directly.

Dirty claim (7): A claim submitted with errors or one that requires manual processing to resolve problems or is rejected for payment.

Disability Determination Services (DDS) (16): A state Social Security division office that assesses a case for disability benefits.

Disability income insurance (3, 16): A form of health insurance that provides periodic payments to replace income when the insured is unable to work as a result of illness, injury, or disease—not as a result of a work-related accident or condition.

Disabled (12): For purposes of enrollment under Medicare, individuals younger than 65 years of age who have been entitled to disability benefits under the Social Security Act or the railroad retirement system for at least 24 months are considered disabled and are entitled to Medicare.

Disclosure (2): The release, transfer, provision of access to, or divulging in any other manner of information outside the entity holding the information.

Discount (10): A reduction of a normal charge based on a specific amount of money or a percentage of the charge.

Disenrollment (11): A member's voluntary cancellation of membership in a managed care plan.

Documentation (4): A chronologic detailed recording of pertinent facts and observations about a patient's health as seen in chart notes and medical reports; entries in the medical record such as prescription refills, telephone calls, and other pertinent data. For computer software, a user's guide to a program or piece of equipment.

Double indemnity (16): A feature in some life and disability insurance policies that provides for twice the face amount of the policy to be paid if death results to the insured from accidental causes.

Downcoding (6): This occurs when the coding system used by the physician's office on a claim does not match the coding system used by the insurance company receiving the claim. The insurance company computer system converts the code submitted to the closest code in use, which is usually down one level from the submitted code, generating decreased payment.

DRG creep (17): See Diagnostic creep.

DRG validation (17): To find out whether the diagnostic and procedural information affecting DRG assignment is substantiated by the clinical information in the patient's chart.

Dun message (10): A message or phrase to inform or remind a patient about a delinquent account.

Durable medical equipment (DME) (B): A billing phrase used to specify medical supplies, devices, and equipment to Medicare and Medi-Cal fiscal intermediaries for reimbursement.

Durable medical equipment (DME) number (7): A group or individual provider number used when submitting bills for specific medical supplies, devices, and equipment to the Medicare fiscal intermediary for reimbursement.

E codes (5): A classification of ICD-9-CM coding used to describe environmental events, circumstances, and conditions as the external cause of injury, poisoning, and other adverse effects. E codes are also used in coding adverse reactions to medications.

Early and Periodic Screening, Diagnosis, and Treatment (EPSDT) (13): The EPSDT program covers screening and diagnostic services to determine physical or mental defects in recipients younger than 21 years of age and health care, treatment, and other measures to correct or ameliorate any defects and chronic conditions discovered. In New York, this is called the Child Health Assurance Program (CHAP).

E-Health information management (e-HIM) (2): A term coined by the American Health Information Management Association's eHealth Task Force to describe any and all transactions in which health care information is accessed, processed, stored, and transferred using electronic technologies.

Elective surgery (17): A surgical procedure that may be scheduled in advance, is not an emergency, and is discretionary on the part of the physician and patient.

Electronic claim (7): An insurance claim submitted to the insurance carrier via a central processing unit (CPU), tape, diskette, direct data entry, direct wire, dial-in telephone, digital fax, or personal computer download or upload.

Electronic claims processor (ECP) (18): An individual who converts insurance claims to standardized electronic format and transmits electronic insurance claims data to the insurance carrier or clearinghouse to help the physician receive payment. Sometimes referred to as *electronic claims professional.*

Electronic data interchange (EDI) (8): The process by which understandable data items are sent back and forth via computer linkages between two or more entities that function alternatively as sender and receiver.

Electronic Data Systems (EDS) Corporation (B): The Medi-Cal fiscal intermediary in the state of California.

Electronic funds transfer (EFT) (8, B): A paperless computerized system enabling funds to be debited, credited, or transferred, eliminating the need for personal handling of checks.

Electronic health record (EHR) (4): A patient record that is created using a computer with software. A template is brought up and by answering a series of questions data are entered.

Electronic media (2): The mode of electronic transmission (e.g., Internet, Extranet, leased phone or dial-up phone lines, fax modems).

Electronic remittance advice (ERA) (8): An online transaction about the status of a claim.

Electronic signature (3): An individualized computer access and identification system (e.g., a series of numbers, letters, electronic writing, voice, computer key, and fingerprint transmission [biometric system]) accepted by both parties to show intent, approval of, or responsibility for computer document content.

Eligibility (3): Qualifying factors that must be met before a patient receives benefits (medical services) under a specified insurance plan, government program, or managed care plan.

Eligibility verification confirmation (EVC) (B): A reference number on a printout from the Medi-Cal point-of-service device that verifies that an inquiry was received and eligibility information was transmitted.

Emancipated minor (3): A person younger than 18 years of age who lives independently, is totally self-supporting, and possesses decision-making rights.

Embezzlement (2, 10): A willful act by an employee of taking possession of an employer's money.

Emergency (14): A sudden and unexpected medical condition, or the worsening of a condition, that poses a threat to life, limb, or sight and requires immediate treatment to alleviate suffering (e.g., shortness of breath, chest pain, or drug overdose).

Emergency care (4): Health care services provided to prevent serious impairment of bodily functions or serious dysfunction to any body organ or part. Advanced life support may be necessary. Not all care provided in an emergency department of a hospital can be termed "emergency care."

Employer identification number (EIN) (7): An individual's federal tax identification number issued by the Internal Revenue Service for income tax purposes.

Employment agency (18): A business organization that refers job applicants to potential employers.

Encoder (8): An add-on software to practice management systems that can reduce the time it takes to build or review insurance claims before batch transmission to the carrier.

Encounter form (3): See Multipurpose billing form.

Encryption (8): To assign a code to represent data. This is done for security purposes.

End-stage renal disease (ESRD) (12): Individuals who have chronic kidney disease requiring dialysis or kidney transplant are considered to have ESRD. To qualify for Medicare coverage, an individual must be fully or currently insured under Social Security or the railroad retirement system or be the dependent of an insured person. Eligibility for Medicare coverage begins with the third month after beginning a course of renal dialysis. Coverage may commence sooner if the patient participates in a self-care dialysis training program or receives a kidney transplant without dialysis.

Eponym (4): The name of a disease, anatomic structure, operation, or procedure, usually derived from the name of a place where it first occurred or a person who discovered or first described it.

Ergonomic (15): Science and technology that seeks to fit the anatomic and physical needs of the worker to the workplace.

Established patient (4): An individual who has received professional services within the past 3 years from the physician or another physician of the same specialty who belongs to the same group practice.

Estate administrator (10): One who takes possession of the assets of a decedent, pays the expenses of administration and the claims of creditors, and disposes of the balance of an estate in accordance with the statutes governing the distribution of decedents' estates.

Estate executor (10): One who takes possession of the assets of a decedent, pays the expenses of administration and the claims of creditors, and disposes of the balance of an estate in accordance with the decedent's will.

Ethics (1): Standards of conduct generally accepted as a moral guide for behavior by which an insurance billing or coding specialist may determine the appropriateness of his or her conduct in a relationship with patients, the physician, co-workers, the government, and insurance companies.

Etiology (5): The cause of disease; the study of the cause of a disease.

Etiquette (1): Customs, rules of conduct, courtesy, and manners of the medical profession.

Exclusion(s) (3, 16): Provisions written into the insurance contract denying coverage or limiting the scope of coverage.

Exclusive provider organization (EPO) (3, 11): A type of managed health care plan that combines features of HMOs and PPOs. It is referred to as exclusive because it is offered to large employers who agree not to contract with any other plan. EPOs are regulated under state health insurance laws.

Expanded problem focused (EPF) (4): A phrase used to describe a level of history or physical examination.

Explanation of benefits (EOB) (9): A document detailing services billed and describing payment determinations; also known in Medicare, Medicaid, and some other programs as a *remittance advice*. In the TRICARE program, it is called a *summary payment voucher.*

Explanation of Medicare benefits (EOMB): See Remittance advice.

Expressed contract (3): A verbal or written agreement.

Extended (3): To carry forward the balance of an individual financial accounting record.

External audit (4): A review done after claims have been submitted (retrospective review) of medical and financial records by an insurance company or Medicare representative to investigate suspected fraud or abusive billing practices.

Extraterritorial (15): State laws effective outside the state by either specific provision or court decision. In workers' compensation cases, benefits under the state law that apply to a compensable injury of an employee hired in one state but injured outside that state.

Facility provider number (7): A facility's (hospital, laboratory, radiology office, nursing facility) provider number to be used by the facility to bill for services, or by the performing physician to report services done at that location.

Facsimile (4): An electronic process for transmitting graphic and written documents over telephone lines and sometimes referred to as fax.

Family history (FH) (4): A review of medical events in the patient's family, including diseases that may be hereditary or place the patient at risk.

Federal Employees' Compensation Act (FECA) (15): An act instituted in 1908 providing benefits for on-the-job injuries to all federal employees.

Federal Employees Retirement System (FERS) (16): A program for federal employees hired after 1984 or those hired before 1984 who switched from CSRS to FERS.

Fee for service (11): A method of payment in which the patient pays the physician for each professional service performed from an established schedule of fees.

Fee schedule (6, 10, 15): A list of charges or established allowances for specific medical services and procedures. See also Relative value studies (RVS).

Financial accounting record (3, 10): An individual record indicating charges, payments, adjustments, and balances owed for services rendered; also known as a ledger.

Fiscal agent (13): An organization under contract to the state to process claims for a state Medicaid program; insurance carrier handling claims from physicians and other suppliers of service for Medicare Part B; also referred to as *fiscal intermediary.*

Fiscal intermediary (FI) (12, 14): An organization under contract to the government that handles claims under Medicare Part A from hospitals, skilled nursing facilities, home health agencies, or providers of medical services and supplies. For TRICARE and CHAMPVA, the insurance company that handles the claims for care received within a particular state or country. Also known as *fiscal agent, fiscal carrier,* and *claims processor.*

Formal referral (11): An authorization request (telephone, fax, or completed form) required by the managed care organization contract to determine medical necessity and grant permission before services are rendered or procedures performed.

Foundation for medical care (FMC) (3, 11): An organization of physicians sponsored by a state or local medical association concerned with the development and delivery of medical services and the cost of health care.

Fraud (2): An intentional misrepresentation of the facts to deceive or mislead another.

Functional resume (18): A data sheet that highlights qualifications and skills.

Future purchase option (16): See Cost-of-living adjustment.

Garnishment (10): A court order attaching a debtor's property or wages to pay off a debt.

Gatekeeper (11): In the managed care system, this is the physician who controls patient access to specialists and diagnostic testing services.

Genetically Handicapped Persons Program (GHPP) (B): A state program for genetically disabled children.

Global surgery policy (6): A Medicare policy relating to surgical procedures in which preoperative and postoperative visits (24 hours before [major] and day of [minor]), usual, intraoperative services, and complications not requiring additional trips to the operating room are included in one fee.

Group provider number (7): A number assigned to a group of physicians submitting insurance claims under the group name and reporting income under one name; used instead of the individual's physician's number (PIN) for the performing provider.

Grouper (17): The computer software program that assigns DRGs of discharged patients using the following information: patient's age, sex, principal diagnosis, complications/comorbid conditions, principal procedure, and discharge status.

Guaranteed renewable (3, 16): A clause in an insurance policy that means the insurance company must renew the policy as long as premium payments are made. However, the premium may be increased when it is renewed. These policies may have age limits of 60, 65, or 70 years or may be renewable for life.

Guarantor (3): An individual who promises to pay the medical bill by signing a form agreeing to pay or who accepts treatment, which constitutes an expressed promise.

Health benefits advisor (HBA) (14): An individual at military hospitals or clinics who is there to help TRICARE beneficiaries obtain medical care through the military and through TRICARE.

Health Care Financing Administration (HCFA) (12): See Centers for Medicare and Medicaid Services (CMS).

Healthcare Common Procedure Coding System (HCPCS) (6): The CMS's Common Procedure Coding System. A three-tier national uniform coding system developed by the Centers for Medicare and Medicaid Services (CMS), formerly HCFA, used for reporting physician or supplier services and procedures under the Medicare program. Level I codes are national CPT codes. Level II codes are HCPCS national codes used to report items not covered under CPT. Level III codes are HCPCS regional or local codes used to identify new procedures or items for which there is no national code. Pronounced "hick-picks."

Health Care Finder (HCF) (14): A health care professional, generally a registered nurse, who is located at TRICARE Service Centers to act as a liaison between military and civilian providers, verify eligibility, determine availability of services, coordinate care, facilitate the transfer of records, and perform first-level medical review.

Health care provider (2): A provider of medical or health services and any other person or organization who furnishes bills or is paid for health care in the normal course of business.

Health insurance (3): A contract between the policyholder or member and insurance carrier or government program to reimburse the policy holder or member for all or a portion of the cost of medical care rendered by health care professionals; generic term applying to lost income arising from illness or injury; also known as *accident and health insurance* or *disability income insurance*.

Health Insurance Claim Form (CMS-1500) (7): Now known as CMS-1500. A universal insurance claim form developed and approved by the American Medical Association Council on Medical Service and the Centers for Medicare and Medicaid Services. It is used by physicians and other professionals to bill outpatient services and supplies to TRICARE, Medicare, and some Medicaid programs as well as some private insurance carriers and managed care plans.

Health maintenance organization (HMO) (3, 11): The oldest of all prepaid health plans. A comprehensive health care financing and delivery organization that provides a wide range of health care services with an emphasis on preventive medicine to enrollees within a geographic area through a panel of providers. Primary care physician "gatekeepers" are usually reimbursed via capitation. In general, enrollees do not receive coverage for the services from providers who are not in the HMO network, except for emergency services.

Health record (4): Written or graphic information documenting facts and events during the rendering of patient care. Also known as *medical record*.

Hearing (16): The second level of the appeal process for an individual applying for SSDI or SSI. This is a hearing before an administrative law judge who had no part in the initial or reconsideration disability determination.

High complexity (HC) (4): A phrase used to describe a type of medical decision making when a patient is seen for an E/M service.

High risk (3): A high chance of loss.

HIPAA Transaction and Code Set (TCS) rule (8): This regulation under HIPAA defines the standardized methods for transmitting electronic health information. The TCS process includes any set of HIPAA-approved codes with their descriptions used to encode data elements, such as tables of terms, medical concepts, medical diagnostic codes, or medical procedure codes. TCS regulations were implemented to streamline electronic data interchange.

History of present illness (HPI) (4): A chronologic description of the development of the patient's present illness from the first sign or symptom or from the previous encounter to the present.

Hospice (12): A public agency or private organization primarily engaged in providing pain relief, symptom management, and supportive services to terminally ill patients and their families in their own homes or in a homelike center.

Hospital insurance (12): Known as Medicare Part A. A program providing basic protection against the costs of hospital and related after-hospital services for individuals eligible under the Medicare program.

Implied contract (3): A contract between physician and patient not manifested by direct words but implied or deduced from the circumstance, general language, or conduct of the patient.

In-area (11): Within the geographic boundaries defined by an HMO as the area in which it will provide medical services to its members.

Incomplete claim (7): Any Medicare claim missing necessary information; such claims are identified to the provider so they may be resubmitted.

Indemnity (3): Benefits paid to an insured while disabled; also known as reimbursement.

Independent (or Individual) Practice Association (IPA) (3, 11): A type of HMO in which a program administrator contracts with a number of physicians who agree to provide treatment to subscribers in their own offices. Physicians are not employees of the MCO and are not paid salaries. They receive reimbursement on a capitation or fee-for-service basis; also referred to as a *medical capitation plan.*

Individually identifiable health information (IIHI) (2): Any part of an individual's health information, including demographic information (e.g., address, date of birth) collected from the individual, that is created or received by a covered entity.

Injury (15): In a workers' compensation policy, this term signifies any trauma or damage to a body part or disease sustained, arising out of, and in the course of employment, including injury to artificial members and medical braces of all types.

Inpatient (17): A term used when a patient is admitted to the hospital for overnight stay.

Inquiry (9): See Tracer.

In situ (5): A description applied to a malignant growth confined to the site of origin without invasion of neighboring tissues.

Insurance adjuster (15): An individual at the workers' compensation insurance carrier overseeing an industrial case, authorizing diagnostic testing and medical treatment, and communicating with the provider of medical care.

Insurance balance billing (10): A statement sent to the patient after his or her insurance company has paid its portion of the claim.

Insurance billing specialist (1): A practitioner who carries out claims completion, coding, and billing responsibilities and may or may not perform managerial and supervisory functions; also known as an *insurance claims processor, reimbursement specialist, medical billing representative,* or *senior billing representative.*

Insured (3): An individual or organization protected in case of loss under the terms of an insurance policy.

Intelligent character recognition (ICR) (7): Same as Optical character recognition.

Intermediate care facilities (ICFs) (12): Institutions furnishing health-related care and services to individuals who do not require the degree of care provided by acute care hospitals or nursing facilities.

Internal review (4): The process of going over financial documents before and after billing to insurance carriers to determine documentation deficiencies or errors.

***International Classification of Diseases, Ninth Revision, Clinical Modification* (ICD-9-CM) (5, 17):** A diagnostic code book that uses a system for classifying diseases and operations to facilitate collection of uniform and comparable health information. A code system to replace this is ICD-10, which is being modified for use in the United States.

Interview (18): Meeting an individual face-to-face for evaluating and questioning a job applicant.

Intoxication (5): A diagnostic coding term that relates to an adverse effect rather than a poisoning when drugs such as digitalis, steroid agents, and so on are involved.

Invalid claim (7): Any Medicare claim that contains complete, necessary information but is illogical or incorrect (e.g., listing an incorrect provider number for a referring physician).

Invalid claims are identified to the provider and may be resubmitted.

Italicized code (5): A diagnostic code in ICD-9-CM, Volume 1, Tabular list, that may never be sequenced as the principal diagnosis.

Itemized statement (10): A detailed summary of all transactions of a patient's account: dates of service, detailed charges, payments (copayments and deductibles), date the insurance claim was submitted, adjustments, and account balance.

Late effect (5): An inactive residual effect or condition produced after the acute phase of an illness or injury has ended.

Ledger card (3, 10): See Financial accounting record.

Lien (10, 15): A claim on the property of another as security for a debt. In litigation cases, it is a legal promise to satisfy a debt owed by the patient to the physician out of any proceeds received on the case.

Limiting charge (12): A percentage limit on fees, specified by legislation, that nonparticipating physicians may bill Medicare beneficiaries above the fee schedule amount.

List service (listserv) (1): An online computer service run from a Web site where questions may be posted by subscribers.

Long-term disability insurance (16): A provision to pay benefits to a covered disabled person as long as he or she remains disabled, up to a specified period exceeding 2 years.

Looping (17): The automated grouper (computer software program that assigns DRGs) process of searching all listed diagnoses for the presence of any comorbid condition or complication, or searching all procedures for operating room procedures or other specific procedures.

Lost claim (9): An insurance claim that cannot be located after sending it to an insurer.

Low complexity (LC) (4): Phrase used to describe a type of medical decision making when a patient is seen for an E/M service.

Major diagnostic categories (MDCs) (17): A broad classifications of diagnoses. There are 83 coding system–oriented MDCs in the original DRGs and 23 body system–oriented MDCs in the revised set of DRGs.

Major medical (3): A health insurance policy designed to offset heavy medical expenses resulting from catastrophic or prolonged illness or injury.

Malignant tumor (5): An abnormal growth that has the properties of invasion and metastasis (e.g., transfer of diseases from one organ to another). The word "carcinoma" (CA) refers to a cancerous or malignant tumor.

Managed care organizations (MCOs) (11): A generic term applied to a managed care plan. May apply to EPO, HMO, PPO, integrated delivery system, or other different managed care arrangement. MCOs are usually prepaid group plans, and physicians are typically paid by the capitation method.

Manual billing (10): Processing statements by hand; may involve typing statements or photocopying the patient's financial accounting record and placing it in a window envelope, which then becomes the statement.

Maternal and Child Health Program (MCHP) (3, 13): A state service organization to assist children younger than 21 years of age who have conditions leading to health problems.

Medicaid (MCD) (3, 13): A federally aided, state-operated and -administered program that provides medical benefits for certain low-income persons in need of health and medical care. California's Medicaid program is known as *Medi-Cal.*

Medi-Cal (13): California's version of the nationwide program known as Medicaid. See Medicaid.

Medical billing representative (1): See Insurance billing specialist.

Medical necessity (4, 12): The performance of services and procedures that are consistent with the diagnosis in accordance with standards of good medical practice, performed at the proper level, and provided in the most appropriate setting. Medical necessity must be established (via diagnostic or other information presented on the individual claim under consideration) before the carrier may make payment.

Medical record (4): Written or graphic information documenting facts and events during the rendering of patient care. Also known as *health record.*

Medical report (4): A permanent, legal document (letter or report format) that formally states the consequences of the patient's examination or treatment.

Medical service order (15): An authorization given to the physician, either written or verbal, to treat the injured or ill employee.

Medically indigent (MI) (B): See Medically needy.

Medically (or psychologically) necessary (14): Medical or psychologic services considered appropriate care and generally accepted by qualified professionals to be reasonable and adequate for the diagnosis and treatment of illness, injury, pregnancy, and mental disorders, or that are reasonable and adequate for well-baby care.

Medically needy (MN) (13, B): Persons in need of financial assistance or whose income and resources will not allow them to pay for the costs of medical care; also called *Medically indigent* in some states.

Medicare (M) (3, 12): A nationwide health insurance program for persons age 65 years of age and older and certain disabled or blind persons regardless of income, administered by HCFA. Local Social Security offices take applications and supply information about the program.

Medicare/Medicaid (Medi-Medi) (3, 12): Refers to an individual who receives medical or disability benefits from both Medicare and Medicaid programs; sometimes referred to as a *Medi-Medi case* or *crossover.*

Medicare Part A (12): Hospital benefits of a nationwide health insurance program for persons age 65 years of age and older and certain disabled individuals regardless of income, administered by CMS. Local Social Security offices take applications and supply information about the program.

Medicare Part B (12): Medical insurance of a nationwide health insurance program for persons age 65 years of age and older and certain disabled individuals regardless of income, administered by CMS. Local Social Security offices take applications and supply information about the program.

Medicare Part C (12): Medicare + Choice plans offer a number of health care options in addition to those available under Medicare Part A and Part B. Plans may include health maintenance organizations, fee-for-service plans, provider-sponsored organizations, religious fraternal benefit societies, and Medicare medical savings accounts.

Medicare Secondary Payer (MSP) (12): The primary insurance plan of a Medicare beneficiary that must pay for any medical care or services first before Medicare is sent a claim.

Medicare Summary Notice (MSN) (12): A document received by the patient explaining amount charged, Medicare approved, deductible, and coinsurance for medical services rendered.

Medigap (MG) (12): A specialized supplemental insurance policy devised for the Medicare beneficiary that covers the deductible and copayment amounts typically not covered under the main Medicare policy written by a nongovernmental third-party payer. Also known as *Medifill.*

Member (3): Person covered under an insurance program's contract, including: (1) the subscriber or contract holder who is the person named on the membership identification card; and (2) in the case of (a) two-person coverage, (b) one adult-one child coverage, or (c) family coverage (eligible family dependents enrolled under the subscriber's contract).

Mentor (18): Guide or teacher who offers advice, criticism, wisdom, guidance, and perspective to an inexperienced but promising protégé to help reach a life goal.

Military treatment facility (MTF) (14): All uniformed service hospitals or health clinics; also known as *military hospitals* or *uniformed service hospitals.*

Moderate complexity (MC) (4): A phrase used to describe a type of medical decision making when a patient is seen for an E/M service.

Modifier (6): In CPT coding, a two-digit add-on number placed after the usual procedure code number to indicate a procedure or service has been altered by specific circumstances. The two-digit modifier may be separated by a hyphen. In HCPCS level II coding, one-digit or two-digit add-on alpha characters, placed after the usual procedure code number (Example G.1).

Example G.1

27372-51 (typed on one line)

Multipurpose billing form (3): An all-encompassing billing form personalized to the practice of the physician, it may be used when a patient submits an insurance billing; also called *charge slip, communicator, encounter form, fee ticket, patient service slip, routing form, superbill,* and *transaction slip.*

Multiskilled health practitioner (MSHP) (1): An individual cross trained to provide more than one function, often in more than one discipline. These combined functions can be found in a broad spectrum of health-related jobs, ranging in complexity including both clinical and administrative functions. The additional skills added to the original health care worker's job may be of a higher, lower, or parallel level. The terms *multiskilled, multicompetent,* and *cross trained* can be used interchangeably.

National alphanumeric codes (12): Alphanumeric codes developed by HCFA. See Health Care Financing Administration Common Procedure Coding System (HCPCS).

National Certified Insurance and Coding Specialist (NCICS) (18): An insurance and coding certification that is awarded by an independent testing agency, the National Center for Competency Testing (NCCT).

National provider identifier (NPI) (7): A Medicare lifetime 10-digit number issued to providers. When adopted, it will be recognized by Medicaid, Medicare, TRICARE, and CHAMPVA programs and eventually may be used by private insurance carriers.

National standard format (NSF) (8): The name of the standardization of data to reduce paper and have more accurate information and efficient organization.

Netback (10): Evaluating a collection agency's performance by taking the amount of monies collected and subtracting the agency's fees.

Networking (18): Exchanging information or services among individuals, groups, or institutions and making use of professional contacts.

New patient (NP) (4): An individual who has not received any professional services from the physician or another physician of the same specialty who belongs to the same group practice within the past 3 years.

No charge (NC) (10): Waiving the entire fee owed for professional care.

Noncancelable clause or policy (3, 16): An insurance policy clause that means the insurance company cannot increase premium rates and must renew the policy until the insured reaches the age stated in the contract. Some disability income policies have noncancelable terms.

Nondisability (ND) claim (15): A claim for an on-the-job injury that requires medical care but does not result in loss of working time or income.

Nonexempt assets (10): One's total property (in bankruptcy cases) not falling in the exemption category; including money, automobile equity, and property, more than a specified amount, depending on the state in which the person lives.

Nonparticipating physician (nonpar) (12): A provider who does not have a signed agreement with Medicare and has an option about assignment. The physician may not accept assignment for all services or has the option of accepting assignment for some services and collecting from the patient for other services performed at the same time and place.

Nonparticipating provider (nonpar) (3, 14): A provider who decides not to accept the determined allowable charge from an insurance plan as the full fee for care. Payment goes directly to the patient in this case, and the patient is usually responsible to pay the bill in full.

Nonprivileged information (2): Information consisting of ordinary facts unrelated to the treatment of the patient. The patient's authorization is not required to disclose the data unless the record is in a specialty hospital or in a special service unit of a general hospital, such as the psychiatric unit.

Not elsewhere classifiable (NEC) (5): This term is used in the ICD-9-CM diagnostic coding system when the code lacks the information necessary to code the term in a more specific category.

Not otherwise specified (NOS) (5): Unspecified. Used in ICD-9-CM numeric code system for coding diagnoses.

Nursing facility (NF) (12, B): A specially qualified facility that has the staff and equipment to provide skilled nursing care and related services that are medically necessary to a patient's recovery; formerly known as a *skilled nursing facility.*

Occupational illness (or disease) (15): An abnormal condition or disorder caused by environmental factors associated with employment. It may be caused by inhalation, absorption, ingestion, or direct contact.

Occupational Safety and Health Administration (OSHA) (15): A federal agency that regulates and investigates safety and health standards in work locations.

Old Age Survivors, Health and Disability Insurance (OASHDI) Program (B): A group that is entitled to benefits under the Medi-Cal program.

Optical character recognition (OCR) (7): A device that can read typed characters at very high speed and convert them to digitized files that can be saved on disk. Also known as *intelligent character recognition* (ICR).

Optionally renewable (3): An insurance policy renewal provision in which the insurer has the right to refuse to renew the policy on a date and may add coverage limitations or increase premium rates.

Ordering physician (4): The physician ordering non-physician services for a patient (e.g., diagnostic laboratory tests, pharmaceutical services, or durable medical equipment) when an insurance claim is submitted by a nonphysician supplier of services. The ordering physician also may be the treating or performing physician.

"Other" claims (7): Medicare claims not considered "clean" claims that require investigation or development on a prepayment basis to determine if Medicare is the primary or secondary carrier.

Other health insurance (OHI) (14): Health care coverage for TRICARE beneficiaries through an employer, an association, or a private insurer. A student in the family may have a health care plan through school.

Outpatient (17): A patient who receives services in a health care facility, such as a physician's office, clinic, urgent care center, emergency department, or ambulatory surgical center and goes home the same day.

Overpayment (9): Money paid over and above the amount due by the insurer or patient.

Paper claim (7): An insurance claim submitted on paper, including those optically scanned and converted to an electronic form by the insurance carrier.

Partial disability (16): A disability from an illness or injury that prevents an insured person from performing one or more of the functions of his or her regular job.

Participating physician (11): 1. A physician who contracts with an HMO or other insurance company to provide services. 2. A physician who has agreed to accept a plan's payments for services to subscribers (e.g., some Blue plans). Eighty percent of practicing American physicians are participating physicians.

Participating physician (par) (12): A physician who agrees to accept payment from Medicare (80% of the approved charges) plus payment from the patient (20% of approved charges) after the $100 deductible has been met.

Participating provider (par) (3, 14): One who accepts TRICARE assignment. Payment in this case goes directly to the provider. The patient must still pay the cost-share outpatient deductible and the cost of care not covered by TRICARE. See *Assignment.*

Partnership program (14): A program that lets TRICARE–eligible individuals receive inpatient or outpatient treatment from civilian providers of care in a military hospital or from uniformed services providers of care in civilian facilities.

Password (8): A combination of letters and numbers that each individual is assigned to access computer data.

Past history (PH) (4): A patient's past experiences with illnesses, operations, injuries, and treatments.

Patient registration form (3): A questionnaire designed to collect demographic data and essential facts about medical insurance coverage for each patient seen for professional services; also called *patient information form.*

Peer review (9): The review of a patient's case by one or more physicians using federal guidelines to evaluate another physician in regard to the quality and efficiency of medical care. This is done to discover overutilization or misutilization of a plan's benefits.

Peer review organization (PRO) (12): A state-based group of practicing physicians paid by the federal government to review hospital care of Medicare patients to determine appropriateness and quality of care.

Pending claim (7): An insurance claim held in suspense because of review or other reason. These claims may be cleared for payment or denied.

Per capita (11): See Capitation

Percentage of revenue (17): The fixed percentage of the collected premium rate that is paid to the hospital to cover services.

Per diem (17): A single charge for a day in the hospital regardless of any actual charges or costs incurred.

Permanent and stationary (P and S) (15): A phrase used when a workers' compensation patient's condition has become stabilized and no improvement is expected. It is only after this declaration that a case can be rated for a compromise and release.

Permanent disability (PD) (15): An illness or injury (impairment of the normal use of a body part) expected to continue for the lifetime of the injured worker that prevents the person from performing the functions of his or her regular occupation, therefore impairing his or her earning capacity.

Personal insurance (3): An insurance plan issued to an individual (or his or her dependents). Also known as *individual contract.*

Petition (15): A formal written request commonly used to indicate an appeal; also means any request for relief other than an application.

Phantom billing (2): Billing for services not performed.

Physical examination (PE or PX) (4): Objective inspection or testing of organ systems or body areas of a patient by a physician.

Physically clean claim (7): Insurance claims with no staples or highlighted areas. The bar code area has not been deformed.

Physician provider group (PPG) (11): A physician-owned business that has the flexibility to deal with all forms of contract medicine and still offer its own packages to business groups, unions, and the general public.

Physician's fee profile (5): A compilation of each physician's charges and the payments made to him or her over a given period of time for each specific professional service rendered to a patient.

Point-of-service (POS) device or network (B): A piece of equipment interfaced with an analog telephone line used to identify Medi-Cal recipient eligibility, obtain share of cost liability status, key in share of cost payment toward balance, reserve Medi-Services, perform family PACT (planning, access, care, and treatment) client eligibility transactions, and submit pharmacy or CMS-1500 insurance claims.

Point-of-service (POS) option (14): Individuals under the TRICARE program can choose to get TRICARE–covered nonemergency services outside the prime network of providers without a referral from the primary care manager and without authorization from a health care finder.

Point-of-service (POS) plan (3, 11): A managed care plan in which members are given a choice as to how to receive services, whether through an HMO, PPO, or fee-for-service plan. The decision is made at the time the service is needed (e.g., "at the point of service"); sometimes referred to as open-ended HMOs, swing-out HMOs, self-referral options, or multiple option plans.

Poisoning (5): A condition resulting from an overdose of drugs or chemical substances or from the wrong drug or agent given or taken in error.

Portfolio (18): A compilation of items that represents a job applicant's skills.

Posted (3): To record or transfer financial entries, debit or credit, to an account (e.g., daysheet, financial account record [ledger], bank deposit slip, check register, or journal).

Preadmission testing (PAT) (17): Treatment, tests, and procedures done 48 to 72 hours before admission of a patient into the hospital. This is done to eliminate extra hospital days.

Preauthorization (3, 14): A requirement of some health insurance plans to obtain permission for a service or procedure before it is done and to see whether the insurance program agrees it is medically necessary.

Precertification (3): To find out whether treatment (surgery, tests, or hospitalization) is covered under a patient's health insurance policy.

Predetermination (3): To determine before treatment the maximum dollar amount the insurance company will pay for surgery, consultations, postoperative care, and so forth.

Preferred provider organization (PPO) (3, 11): A type of health benefit program in which enrollees receive the highest level of benefits when they obtain services from a physician, hospital, or other health care provider designated by their program as a "preferred provider." Enrollees may receive substantial, although reduced, benefits when they obtain care from a provider of their own choosing who is not designated as a "preferred provider" by their program.

Premium (3, 12): The cost of insurance coverage paid annually, semiannually, or monthly to keep the policy in force. In the Medicare program, monthly fee that enrollees pay for Medicare Part B medical insurance. This fee is updated annually to reflect changes in program costs.

Prepaid group practice model (11): A plan under which specified health services are rendered by participating physicians to an enrolled group of persons, with fixed periodic payments made in advance, by or on behalf of each person or family. If a health insurance carrier is involved, it contracts to pay in advance for the full range of health services to which the insured is entitled under the terms of the health insurance contract. Such a plan is one form of a *health maintenance organization.*

Presumptive eligibility (PE) (B): A federal/state program designed to ease access to prenatal care offering immediate temporary coverage to low-income women pending a formal Medi-Cal application.

Primary care manager (PCM) (14): A physician who is responsible for coordinating and managing all the TRICARE beneficiary's health care unless there is an emergency.

Primary care physician (PCP) (4, 11): A physician (e.g., family practitioner, general practitioner, pediatrician, obstetrician/gynecologist, or general internist) who oversees the care of patients in a managed health care plan (HMO or PPO) and refers patients to see specialists (e.g., cardiologists, oncologists, or surgeons) for services as needed. Also known as a *gatekeeper.*

Primary diagnosis (5): Initial identification of the condition or chief complaint for which the patient is treated for outpatient medical care.

Principal diagnosis (5, 17): A condition established after study that is chiefly responsible for the admission of the patient to the hospital.

Prior approval (13): The evaluation of a provider request for a specific service to determine the medical necessity and appropriateness of the care requested for a patient. Also called *prior authorization* in some states.

Privacy (2): The condition of being secluded from the presence or view of others.

Privacy officer, privacy official (2): An individual designated to help the provider remain in compliance by setting policies and procedures in place, and by training and managing the staff regarding HIPAA and patient rights; usually the contact person for questions and complaints.

Privileged information (2): Data related to the treatment and progress of the patient that can be released only when written authorization of the patient or guardian is obtained.

Problem focused (PF) (4): A phrase used to describe a type of medical decision making when a patient is seen for an E/M service.

Procedure code numbers (6): Five-digit numeric codes that describe each service the physician renders to a patient.

Procedure review (17): A review of diagnostic and therapeutic procedures to determine appropriateness.

Professional Association of Health Care Office Managers (PAHCOM) (18): A nationwide organization dedicated to providing a strong professional network for health care office managers.

Professional component (PC) (6): That portion of a test or procedure (containing both a professional and technical component) which the physician performs (e.g., interpreting an electrocardiogram [ECG], reading an x-ray, or making an observation and determination using a microscope).

Professional courtesy (10): A discount or exemption from charges given to certain people at the discretion of the physician rendering the service. It is rarely used in current medicine.

Prospective payment system (PPS) (12): A method of payment for Medicare hospital insurance based on diagnosis-related groups (DRGs) (a fixed dollar amount for a principal diagnosis).

Prospective review (4): The process of going over financial documents before billing is submitted to the insurance company to determine documentation deficiencies and errors.

Protected health information (PHI) (2): Any data that identify an individual and describes his or her health status, age, sex, ethnicity, or other demographic characteristics, whether or not that information is stored or transmitted electronically.

Provider identification number (PIN) (7): A carrier-assigned number that every physician uses who renders services to patients when submitting insurance claims.

Provider Telecommunications Network (PTN) (B): An automated voice-response system that allows the provider to use the telephone to obtain checkwrite, claim, and prior authorization information for services rendered through the Medi-Cal program and several other state programs.

Quality assurance program (14): A plan that continually assesses the effectiveness of inpatient and outpatient care in the TRICARE and CHAMPVA programs.

Quality improvement organization (QIO) program (17): A program designed to monitor and improve the usage and quality of care for Medicare beneficiaries.

Qui tam action (12): An action to recover a penalty, brought by an informer in a situation in which one portion of the recovery goes to the informer and the other portion to the state or government.

Readmission review (17): A review of patients readmitted to a hospital within 7 days with problems related to the first admission, to determine whether the first discharge was premature or the second admission is medically necessary.

Real time (8): Online interactive communication between two computer systems allowing instant transfer of information.

Reasonable fee (6, 12): A charge is considered reasonable if it is deemed acceptable after peer review even though it does not meet the *customary* or *prevailing* criteria. This includes unusual circumstances or complications requiring additional time, skill, or experience in connection with a particular service or procedure. In Medicare, the amount on which payment is based for participating physicians.

Rebill (resubmit) (9): To send another request for payment for an overdue bill to either the insurance company or patient.

Recertification (18): A renewal of certification after a specified time.

Recipient (13): A person certified by the local welfare department to receive the benefits of Medicaid under one of the specific aid categories; an individual certified to receive Medicare benefits.

Reconsideration (16): The first level of appeal process for an individual applying for SSDI or SSI. It is a complete review of the claim by a medical or psychologic consultant or disability examiner team who did not take part in the original disability determination.

Referral (4): The transfer of the total or specific care of a patient from one physician to another. In managed care, a request for authorization for a specific service.

Referring physician (4): A physician who sends the patient for testing or treatment noted on the insurance claim when it is submitted by the physician performing the service.

Regional office (RO) (16): A Social Security state office.

Registered Medical Assistant (RMA) (18): A title earned by completing appropriate training and passing a registry examination administered by the American Medical Technologists (AMT).

Registered Medical Coder (RMC) (18): A registered title awarded after completion of coursework given by the Medical Management Institute (MMI) with recertification requirements.

Registration (18): Entry in an official registry or record that lists names of persons in an occupation who have satisfied specific requirements or by attaining a certain level of education and paying a registration fee.

Reimbursement (10): Repayment; the term used when insurance payment is pending.

Reimbursement specialist (1): See Insurance billing specialist.

Rejected claim (7, 9): An insurance claim submitted to an insurance carrier that is discarded by the system because of a technical error (omission or erroneous information) or because it does not follow Medicare instructions. It is returned to the provider for correction or change so that it may be processed properly for payment.

Relative value studies (scale) (RVS) (6): A list of procedure codes for professional services and procedures that are assigned unit values that indicate the relative value of one procedure over another.

Relative value unit (RVU) (6, 12): A monetary value assigned to each service based on the amount of physician work, practice expenses, and the cost of professional liability insurance. These three RVUs are then adjusted according to geographic area and used in a formula to determine Medicare fees.

Remittance advice (RA) (9, 12): A document detailing services billed and describing payment determination issued to providers of the Medicare or Medicaid program; also known in some programs as an *explanation of benefits*.

Remittance Advice Details (RAD) (B): A document that accompanies all Medi-Cal payment vouchers (checks) sent to providers of medical services.

Resident physician (4): A physician who has finished medical school and is performing one or more years of training in a specialty area on the job at a hospital (medical center).

Residual benefits (16): A term used in disability income insurance for disability that is not work related. It is the payment of partial benefits when the insured is not totally disabled.

Residual disability (16): A disability from an illness or injury that prevents an insured person from performing one or more of the functions of his or her regular job. This is sometimes referred to as *partial disability*. See also *partial disability*.

Resource-based relative value scale (RBRVS) (6, 12): A system that ranks physician services by units and provides a formula to determine a Medicare fee schedule.

Respite care (12): A short-term hospice inpatient stay for a terminally ill patient to give temporary relief to the person who regularly assists with home care of a patient.

***Respondeat superior* (1):** "Let the master answer." Refers to a physician's liability in certain cases for the wrongful acts of his of her assistant(s) or employee(s).

Resubmission Turnaround Document (RTD) (B): A document that the Medi-Cal fiscal intermediary sends to providers when a claim form has questionable or missing information.

Resume (18): A summary of education, skills, and work experience, usually in outline form.

Retrospective review (4): The process of going over financial documents after billing an insurance carrier to determine documentation deficiencies and errors.

Review (9): To look over a claim to assess how much payment should be made.

Review of systems (ROS) (4): An inventory of body systems obtained through a series of questions used to identify signs or symptoms that the patient might be experiencing or has experienced.

Running balance (3): An amount owed on a credit transaction; also known as *outstanding* or *unpaid balance*.

Scrubbing (17): The process in which computer software checks for errors before a claim is submitted to an insurance carrier for payment; also known as edit check or cleaning the bill.

Second-injury fund (15): See Subsequent injury fund.

Secondary diagnosis (5): A second reason to the primary diagnosis for an office or hospital encounter that may contribute to the condition or define the need for a higher level of care but is not the underlying cause. There may be more than one secondary diagnosis.

Secured debt (10): A debt (an amount owed) in which a debtor pledges certain property (collateral), in a written security agreement, to the repayment of the debt.

Self-employment (18): Working for oneself, with direct control over work, services, and fees.

Self-referral (11): A patient in a managed care plan that refers himself or herself to a specialist. The patient may be required to inform the primary care physician.

Senior billing representative (1): See Insurance billing specialist.

Sequelae (15): Diseased conditions after, and usually resulting from, a previous disease.

Service area (11): The geographic area defined by an HMO as the locale in which it will provide health care services to its members directly through its own resources or arrangements with other providers in the area.

Service benefit program (14): A program (e.g., TRICARE) that provides benefits without a contract guaranteeing the indemnification of an insured party against a specific loss; there are no premiums. TRICARE Standard is considered a service benefit program.

Service-connected injury (14): Injury incurred by a service member while on active duty.

Service contract (18): A document that enumerates the obligations of a billing service and a medical practice stating the responsible party for each specific duty and task.

Service retiree (14): An individual who is retired from a career in the armed forces; also known as a *military retiree*.

Share of cost (13, B): The amount the patient must pay each month before he or she can be eligible for Medicaid. Also known as *liability* or *spend down*.

Short-term disability insurance (16): A provision to pay benefits to a covered disabled person as long as he or she remains disabled, up to a specified period not exceeding 2 years.

Skip (10): A debtor who has moved and neglected to give a forwarding address (e.g., skipped town).

Slanted brackets (5): A symbol used with a diagnostic code in ICD-9-CM, Volume 2, Alphabetic Index, indicating the code may never be sequenced as the principal diagnosis.

Social history (SH) (4): An age-appropriate review of a patient's past and current activities (e.g., smoking, diet intake, and alcohol use).

Social Security Administration (SSA) (16): Administers SSDI and SSI programs for disabled persons.

Social Security Disability Insurance (SSDI) (16): Entitlement program for disabled workers or self-employed individuals.

Social Security Disability Insurance (SSDI) program (16): A federal entitlement program for long-term disability under Title II of the Social Security Act. It provides monthly benefits to workers and those self-employed who meet certain conditions.

Social Security number (SSN) (7): An individual's tax identification number issued by the federal government.

Sponsor (14): For the TRICARE program, the service person (active duty, retired, or deceased) whose relationship makes the patient (dependent) eligible for TRICARE.

Staff model (11): The type of HMO in which the health plan hires physicians directly and pays them a salary.

Standard (2): A rule, condition, or requirement.

Standard transactions (8): The electronic files in which medical data are compiled to produce a specific format.

State Children's Health Insurance Program (SCHIP) (13): A state child health program that operates with federal grant support under Title V of the Social Security Act. In some states this program may be known as Maternal and Child Health Program (MCHP) or Children's Special Health Care Services (CSHCS).

State Disability Insurance (SDI) (3, 16): See Unemployment Compensation Disability.

State license number (7): A number issued to a physician who has passed the state medical examination indicating his or her right to practice medicine in the state where issued.

State preemption (2): A complex technical issue not within the scope of the health care provider's role; refers to instances when state law takes precedence over federal law.

Statute of limitations (10): A time limit established for filing lawsuits; may vary from state to state.

Stop loss (11, 17): An agreement between a managed care company and a reinsurer in which absorption of prepaid patient expenses is limited; or limiting losses on an individual expensive hospital claim or professional services claim; form of reinsurance by which the managed care program limits the losses of an individual expensive hospital claim.

Straightforward (SF) (4): Phrase used to describe a type of medical decision making when a patient is seen for an E/M service.

Subpoena (4): "Under penalty." A writ that commands a witness to appear at a trial or other proceeding and give testimony.

Subpoena duces tecum **(4):** "In his possession." A subpoena that requires the appearance of a witness with his or her records. Sometimes the judge permits the mailing of records and it is not necessary for the physician to appear in court.

Sub rosa films (15): Videotapes made without the knowledge of the subject; used to investigate suspicious claims in workers' compensation cases.

Subscriber (3): The contract holder covered by an insurance program or managed care plan, who either has coverage through his or her place of employment or has purchased coverage directly from the plan or affiliate. This term is used primarily in Blue Cross and Blue Shield plans.

Subsequent injury fund (SIF) (15): A special fund that assumes all or part of the liability for benefits provided to a worker because of the combined effect of a work-related impairment and a preexisting condition; also known as second-injury fund.

Summary payment voucher (14): The document the fiscal agent sends to the provider or beneficiary, showing the service or supplies received, allowable charges, amount billed, the amount TRICARE paid, how much deductible has been paid, and the patient's cost-share.

Supplemental benefits (16): Disability insurance provisions that allow benefits to the insured to increase the monthly indemnity or receive a percentage of the policy premiums if an individual keeps a policy in force for 5 or 10 years or does not file any claims.

Supplemental Security Income (SSI) (12, 13, 16): A program of income support for low-income aged, blind, and disabled persons established by Title XVI of the Social Security Act.

Supplementary medical insurance (SMI) (12): Part B—medical benefits of Medicare program.

Surgical package (6): Unstarred surgical procedure code numbers include the operation; local infiltration, digital block, or topical anesthesia; and normal, uncomplicated postoperative care. This is referred to as a "package," and one fee covers the whole package.

Suspended claim (9): An insurance claim that is processed by the insurance carrier but held in an indeterminate (pending) state about payment either because of an error or the need for additional information.

Suspense (9): The pending indeterminate state of an insurance claim because of an error or need for more information.

Syndrome (5): Another name for a symptom complex (a set of complex signs, symptoms, or other manifestations resulting from a common cause or appearing in combination, presenting a distinct clinical picture of a disease or inherited abnormality).

T-1 (8): A T-carrier channel that can transmit voice or data channels quickly.

Taxonomy codes (8): Numeric and alpha provider *specialty* codes that are assigned and classify each health care provider when transmitting electronic insurance claims.

Teaching physician (4): A physician who has responsibilities for training and supervising medical students, interns, or residents and who takes them to the bedsides of patients in a teaching hospital to review course and treatment.

Technical component (6): That portion of a test or procedure (containing both a technical and a professional component) that pertains to the use of the equipment and the operator who performs it (e.g., ECG machine and technician, radiography machine and technician, and microscope and technician).

Temporary disability (TD) (15, 16): The recovery period after a work-related injury during which the employee is unable to work and the condition has not stabilized; a schedule of benefits payable for the temporary disability.

Temporary disability insurance (TDI) (16): See Unemployment Compensation Disability.

Tertiary care (11): Services requested by a specialist from another specialist (e.g., neurosurgeons, thoracic surgeons, and intensive care units).

The Civilian Health and Medical Program of the Department of Veterans Affairs (CHAMPVA) (3, 14): The Civilian Health and Medical Program of the Department of Veterans Affairs, a program for veterans with total, permanent, service-connected disabilities or surviving spouses and dependents of veterans who died of service-connected disabilities.

Third-party liability (15): Third-party liability exists if an entity is liable to pay the medical cost for injury, disease, or disability of a person hurt during the performance of his or her occupation and the injury is caused by an entity not connected with the employer.

Third-party subrogation (15): The legal process by which an insurance company seeks from a third party, who has caused a loss, recovery of the amount paid to the policyholder.

Total disability (16): A term that varies in meaning from one disability insurance policy to another. An example of a liberal definition might read, "The insured must be unable to perform the major duties of his or her specific occupation."

Total, permanent service-connected disability (14): A total permanent disability incurred by a service member while on active duty.

Tracer (9): An inquiry made to an insurance company to locate the status of an insurance claim (e.g., claim in review, claim never received, and so forth).

Trading partner agreement (TPA) (8): See Business associate agreement.

Transaction (2): The transmission of information between two parties to carry out financial or administrative activities related to health care.

Transfer review (17): Review of transfers to different areas of the same hospital that are exempted from prospective payment.

Treating or performing physician (4): A provider who renders a service to a patient.

Treating practitioner (4): A nurse practitioner, clinical nurse specialist, or physician assistant who furnish a consultation or treat a Medicare beneficiary for a specific medical problem and uses the results of a diagnostic test in the management of the beneficiary's specific medical problem.

Treatment Authorization Request (TAR) form (B): A Medi-Cal form that must be completed by a provider for certain procedures and services that require prior approval.

TRICARE (3): A three-option managed health care program offered to spouses and dependents of service personnel with uniform benefits and fees implemented nationwide by the federal government.

TRICARE Extra (14): A PPO–type of TRICARE option in which the individual does not have to enroll or pay an annual fee. On a visit-by-visit basis, the individual may seek care from an authorized network provider and receive a discount on services and reduced cost-share (copayment).

TRICARE for Life (14): A health care program that offers additional TRICARE benefits as a supplementary payer to Medicare for uniformed service retirees, their spouses, and survivors age 65 years of age or older.

TRICARE Prime (14): A voluntary HMO-type option for TRICARE beneficiaries.

TRICARE Service Center (14): An office staffed by TRICARE Health Care Finders and beneficiary service representatives.

Turfing (11): Transferring the sickest, high-cost patients to other physicians so the provider appears as a low-utilizer in a managed care setting.

Unbundling (6): The practice of using numerous CPT codes to identify procedures normally covered by a single code; also known as *itemizing, fragmented billing, exploding,* or *a la carte medicine*; billing under Medicare Part B for nonphysician services to hospital inpatients furnished to the hospital by an outside supplier or another provider. Under the new law, unbundling is prohibited, and all nonphysician services provided in an inpatient setting will be paid as hospital services.

Unemployment Compensation Disability (UCD) (3, 16): Insurance that covers off-the-job injury or sickness and is paid for by deductions from a person's paycheck. This program is administered by a state agency and is sometimes also known as *State Disability Insurance (SDI) or temporary disability insurance (TDI).*

Uniform Bill (UB-92) paper or electronic claim form (17): A Uniform Bill insurance claim form developed by the National Uniform Billing Committee for hospital inpatient billing and payment transactions.

Unique provider identification number (UPIN) (7): A number issued by the Medicare fiscal intermediary to each physician who renders medical services to Medicare recipients; used for identification purposes on the CMS-1500 claim form.

Unsecured debt (10): Any debt (amount owed) that is not secured or backed by any form of collateral.

Upcoding (6): Deliberate manipulation of CPT codes for increased payment.

Urgent care (14): Medically necessary treatment that is required for illness or injury that would result in further disability or death if not treated immediately.

Use (2): The sharing, employment, application, utilization, examination, or analysis of individually identifiable health information (IHII) within an organization that holds such information.

Usual, customary, and reasonable (UCR) (6): A method used by insurance companies to establish their fee schedules in which three fees are considered in calculating payment: (1) the usual fee is the fee typically submitted by the physician; (2) the customary fee falls within the range of usual fees charged by providers of similar training in a geographic area; and (3) the reasonable fee meets the aforementioned criteria or is considered justifiable because of special circumstances. UCR uses the conversion factor method of establishing maximums; the method of reimbursement used under Medicaid by which state Medicaid programs set reimbursement rates using the Medicare method or a fee schedule, whichever is lower.

Utilization review (UR) (11, 17): A process, based on established criteria, of reviewing and controlling the medical necessity for services and providers' use of medical care resources. Reviews are carried out by allied health personnel at predetermined times during the hospital stay to assess the need for the full facilities of an acute care hospital. In managed care systems, such as an HMO, reviews are done to establish medical necessity, thus curbing costs. Also called *utilization* or *management control.*

V codes (5): A subclassification of ICD-9-CM coding used to identify health care encounters that occur for reasons other than illness or injury and to identify patients whose injury or illness is influenced by special circumstances or problems.

Verbal referral (11): A primary care physician informs the patient and telephones to the referring physician that the patient is being referred for an appointment.

Veteran (14): Any person who has served in the armed forces of the United States, especially in time of war; is no longer in the service; and has received an honorable discharge.

Veterans Affairs (VA) disability program (16): A program for honorably discharged veterans who file claim for a service-connected disability.

Veterans Affairs (VA) outpatient clinic (3, 16): A clinic where medical and dental services are rendered to veterans who have service-related disabilities.

Voice Drug TAR System (VDTS) (B): A Medi-Cal telecommunication system for processing urgent and initial drug Treatment Authorization Requests, to inquire about the status of previously entered drug TARs, or to inquire whether a patient is receiving continual care with a drug.

Volume performance standard (VPS) (12): The desired growth rate for spending on Medicare Part B physician services, set each year by Congress.

Voluntary disability insurance (16): A majority of employees of an employer voluntarily consent to be covered by an insured or self-insured disability insurance plan instead of a state plan.

Waiting period (WP) (15, 16): For disability insurance, the initial period of time when a disabled individual is not eligible to receive benefits even though unable to work; for workers' compensation, the days that must elapse before workers' compensation weekly benefits become payable.

Waiver of premium (16): A disability insurance policy provision that an employee does not have to pay any premiums while disabled. Also known as *elimination period*.

Whistleblowers (12): Informants who report physicians suspected of defrauding the federal government.

Withhold (11): A portion of the monthly capitation payment to physicians retained by the HMO until the end of the year to create an incentive for efficient care. If the physician exceeds utilization norms, he or she will not receive it.

Workers' Compensation Appeals Board (WCAB) (15): The board that handles workers' compensation liens and appeals.

Workers' compensation (WC) insurance (3, 15): A contract that insures a person against on-the-job injury or illness. The employer pays the premium for his or her employees.

Work hardening (15): An individualized program of therapy using simulated or real job duties to build up strength and improve the worker's endurance to be able to work up to 8 hours per day. Sometimes work site modifications are instituted to get the employee back to gainful employment.

Write-off (10): Assets or debts that have been determined to be uncollectable and therefore are adjusted off the accounting books as a loss.

Index

A

Abbreviations
  collection, 358, 358t
  diagnostic, 107-108
Abortion, coding for, 140-141
Abuse, medical billing, 46b
Accident
  definition of, 59
  industrial
    definition of, 480
    reporting requirements for, 482t-483t
Accidental death and dismemberment benefit,
  in disability insurance, 521
Accord and satisfaction theory, 342-343
Accounting, in role of insurance billing
  specialist, 5
Accounts receivable (A/R), 334-335
  management of, 14, 68
Accreditation, of HMOs, 381
Accredited Standards Committee X12
  (ASC X12), 276
Acquired immunodeficiency syndrome (AIDS),
  disability income insurance and, 522
Acute, definition of, 108
Adjudication, of workers' compensation
  case, 487
Administrative law judge hearing, in
  Medicare review and redetermination
  process, 323
Administrative safeguards, 43
  for electronic claims, 296
Administrative simplification, under HIPAA,
  27-28
Administrative simplification enforcement tool
  (ASET), 292, 296
Admitting diagnoses, coding in, 141
Advance Beneficiary Notice (ABN),
  417-418, 417f
  completing, procedure for, 432
Adverse effects of drugs, 135, 136b
AEPs (appropriateness evaluation protocols),
  546, 546f
Age analysis, 346-347
Aging reports, 84
  age analysis by, 346-347
  in claim management, 308
Aliens
  job searches for, 595
  Medicaid for, claims for, 445
  Medicare for, 403
Alliance of Claims Assistance Professionals
  (ACAP), 297, 298f
Allowable charge, under TRICARE, 455
Alphabetic index, for *International Classification
  of Diseases*, 551

Alternative billing codes (ABCs), 153-154
Ambulatory payment classifications (APCs),
  556, 563, 565
American Association of Medical Assistants
  (AAMA), 14
  principles of medical ethics of, 20b, 21f
American Computerized Employment
  Service, 586
American Health Information Management
  Association (AHIMA), 16-17
  procedure coding and, 152
American Hospital Association (AHA)
  policy of, on abbreviations, 108
  procedural coding and, 152
American Managed Care and Review
  Association (AMCRA), 384
American Medical Association (AMA)
  claim forms and, 196
  Code of Ethics of, 20, 339
  terminology changes by, for documentation,
    93-94
America's Job Bank, 586
Ancillary services, 395
Annual alpha files, 85
Anti-Kickback Statute, 47
Appeal, definition of, 319
Appeal and review process
  Medi-Cal, 622
  Medicaid, 447
  TRICARE, 323, 326-328
Application service provider (ASP), for
  electronic claim transmission, 292
Applications
  insurance policy, 58
  job, 586, 587f-588f, 589
Appointment scheduling, managed care,
  391-392
Appropriateness evaluation protocols (AEPs),
  546, 546f
Armed services disability, 524
Arteriosclerotic cardiovascular disease, coding
  for, 139
Arteriosclerotic heart disease, coding
  for, 139
ASP (application service provider), for
  electronic claim transmission, 292
Assignment, Medicare, 414
Assignment of benefits, 77-78
Attending physician, roles of, 93
Auditing, internal, in compliance plan, 49
Audits
  external, 94, 113b-114b
  by nurse auditors, 556
  prevention of, 114b
  software edit checks and, 115-116

Authority, verification of, in protecting patient
  rights, 39-40
Authorization for Release of Information, 31f
Authorization form, definition of, 30
Automobile liability insurance, Medicare
  and, 411

B

Balance, running, calculation of, 81
Bank deposits, 85
Bankruptcy, 367-368, 367t
  of managed care organization, 396
Batch, definition of, 270
Bed leasing, in hospital reimbursement, 556
Behavior of insurance billing specialists, 19
Beneficiary, TRICARE, 451
Beneficiary representative, for Medicare,
  425-426, 427f-430f
Benefit period, Medicare, 404
Benefits
  coordination of, 60
  explanation of, 307-309, 308f
Bilateral, definition of, 111
Billing
  cycle, 371
  forms for, multipurpose, in electronic
    claims, 281-822
  hospital, 4, 539-579
    admission procedures and, 546-548
    coding procedures and, 549-552
      inpatient, 549-551
      outpatient, 549, 551-552
    double, 559
    duplicate statements and, 559
    hard copy, 558
    inpatient, 552-558. See also Inpatient
      billing process.
    patient service representative in, 542, 543f
    phantom changes in, 559
    problems with, 558-559
    professional versus, 4
    utilization review and, 549
  methods of, 348
  procedural guidelines for, 371
  of workers' compensation claims, 510-511
Birthday law, 60
Black Lung Benefits Act, 480
Blanket contracts, 61
Blind mailing, in job search, 585
Blue Cross/Blue Shield plans, 380
Bonding, 370-371
Bookkeeping, in role of insurance billing
  specialist, 5
Bookkeeping-financial accounting records, 79
Buffing, 386

Page numbers followed by b indicate boxes; f, figures; t, tables.

Bundled codes, 173-174
Burns, coding in, 141, 142f
Business associate, definition of, 28

C

Cable modems, for electronic claim
    transmission, 289
Capitation, 65, 381, 396
    contact, in managed care, 393
    in hospital reimbursement, 556
    verses fee-for-service, 396, 397f
Career advantages for insurance billing
    specialists, 17
Carrier, 60
Carrier Dealing Prepayment Organizations, 412
Carrier-direct systems, 292
Case management requirements, 61
Case rating pricing, 393
    in hospital reimbursement, 556
Cash discounts, 337
Cash flow, 8, 334-336
Catastrophic cap, under TRICARE, 456
Catchment areas, in TRICARE, 451
Categorically needy, under Medicaid, 438, 438b
Centers for Medicare and Medicaid Services
    (CMS), 319
    divisions of, 402
    regional offices of, in Medicare review and
        redetermination process, 323
    rule of, on professional courtesy, 339
    72-hour rule of, 548
Certification, of insurance billing specialists,
    601, 602t-604t
Challenged policies, 57
CHAMPVA. See Civilian Health and Medical
    Program of the Department of
    Veterans Affairs (CHAMPVA).
Charge description master (CDM), 554-555
Charging entries, in role of insurance billing
    specialist, 5
Check, payments by, 342-345
    electronic, 350
CHEDDAR, 96, 97f
Chief complaint (CC), 98
    in diagnostic coding, 128
Child Health Assurance Program (CHAP),
    Medicaid and, 436
Chronic, definition of, 108
Chronic rheumatic heart disease, coding
    for, 139
Churning, 386
CIGNA Healthplans of California, 381
Circulatory system conditions, coding for,
    138-139
Civil Monetary Penalties Law, 46-47
Civil Service and Federal Employees
    Retirement System Disability, 524
Civilian Health and Medical Program of the
    Department of Veterans Affairs
    (CHAMPVA), 65, 462-474
    admission procedures for, 547-548
    benefits of, 463
    claim form for, completing, 471-474
    claims procedure for, 463-466, 467-468
    eligibility for, 462
    enrollment in, 462
    Explanation of Benefits Document for,
        468, 470f
    Health Insurance Claim Form for
        example of, 266f
        instructions for, 210-256
    identification card for, 462-463, 463f
    preauthorization for, 463
    provider for, 463

Civilian Health and Medical Program of the
    Uniformed Services (CHAMPUS).
    See TRICARE.
Claim policy provisions, 304-305
Claims, insurance, 59-60
    CHAMPVA, 463-466, 467, 468
    clean, 197
    clearinghouses for, 292, 293f-295f
    cover letter accompanying, 198
    delayed, reasons for, 207
    denied
        problem solving for, 313-315
        review of, letter requesting, 308, 310f
    dirty, 197-198
    disability income, 529-531, 532f-536f
    electronic, 268-301. See also Electronic
        claims.
    filing of, 81-83
    forms for, 202-205
    history of, 196
    incomplete, 197
    inquiries into, 308, 310, 310f, 311f
    invalid, 197
    lost, problem solving for, 312
    mailing, 85
    management techniques for, 307-308
    Medi-Cal, 618-622
    Medicaid, 443-447
    Medicare, 422-425
    outpatient, 558
    overpayments of, problem solving for,
        316-317
    paper, submission of, Medicare
        requirements for, 287t
    pending, tracking, 84-85
    physician identification numbers for, 203
    problem solving for, 311-317
    problems with, 302-331. See also Problems.
    procedures for, 68-88
    provider identification numbers for, 203-204
    register, 84-85
    rejected, 197
        problem solving for, 313
        reasons for, 205-207
    review and appeal process for, 319-328
    status of, 197-198
    submission of, follow-up after, 304
    suspended, 307
    TRICARE, 463-467
    types of, 196-198
    Uniform Bill (UB-92), 555, 559, 564f
        for Medi-Cal, 621
    workers' compensation, 504-513
Claims adjudicator, 60
Claims assistance professionals (CAPs), 5, 584.
        See also Insurance billing specialists.
    employment opportunities for, 584
    scope of practice of, 22
Clearinghouse, 28
    for electronic claims, 270-271, 292,
        293f-295f
Clinical Laboratory Improvement
        Amendment, 413-414
Closed panel program, 381
CMS-1500, 196, 202-267. See also Health
        Insurance Claim Form (CMS-1500).
CMS (Centers for Medicare and Medicaid
        Services). See Centers for Medicare
        and Medicaid Services (CMS).
Code edits, coding guidelines for, 172-176
Code of Medical Ethics, 339
Code sets, 272-275
    medical, 273, 274t
    supporting, HIPAA, 276b

Code specialist, in inpatient billing process, 555
Coding
    diagnostic, 126-129, 126-149. See also
        Diagnostic coding.
    procedural, 150-193. See also Procedural
        coding.
Coding procedures. See also Current Procedural
        Terminology (CPT); International
        Classification of Diseases (ICD-9-CM).
Coinsurance payments, 359
Coinsurance requirements, 59
Collection ratio, 335
Collections
    abbreviations used in, 358, 358t
    agencies for, 361-363
    controls over, 370-371
    counseling on, preappointment, 341
    fees and, 336-348. See also Fees.
    insurance, 358-361
    laws on, 351-354
    letters in, 355-358, 356f, 357f
    litigation and, 368
    patient education and, 335-336
    patient registration forms and, 336
    procedural guidelines for, 371
    process for, 354-371
    skip tracing and, 365-366
    telephone in, 354-355
        plan for, 372-373
Communication, open lines of, developing,
    50-51
Communication of fees, 340
Comorbidity, 104, 562
Competitive Medical Plans (CMPs), 65
Complaints, in protecting patient rights, 41
Complex lacerations, definition of, 110
Compliance
    definition of, 26
    implementing, 49-50
    privacy, HIPAA, guidelines for, 43-44
Compliance officer/contact, designating, 50
Compliance plan
    basic components of, 49-51
    for individual and small group physician
        practices, 48-49
Component codes, 173
Comprehensive codes, 173
Computer media claims (CMC) system, for
        Medi-Cal, 620-621
Computer system, office, selection of, 299
Computerized signatures, 83
Computers
    billing, 348
    confidentiality and, 297-298
    records management using, 299-300
    skip tracing using, 366
Concurrent care, 106-107
Conditionally renewable insurance
        policies, 59
Confidential communication(s)
    breach of, 32
    definition of, 34-35
    right to request, 36-37
Confidential information, 30, 32
    de-identification of, definition of, 37b
    ensuring security of, in protecting patient
        rights, 41
Confidentiality
    definition of, 30
    of medical records, 116, 494-495,
        542-545
Consecutive dates, on claim form, 203
Consent for Release of Information, 32f
Consent form, definition of, 30

Consolidated Omnibus Budget Reconciliation
   Act of 1985 (COBRA), 61
   employed elderly Medicare benefits
      and, 409
   in payment monitoring, 393
Consultations, 104
   coding for, 160, 166t-167t
Consultative examiner, in SSI program, 523
Consulting physician, roles of, 93
Contact capitation, in managed care, 393
Continuity of care, 107
Contract(s)
   blanket, 61
   expressed, 57
   implied, 57
   insurance, 57. *See also* Policy(ies), health
      insurance.
Contract payment time limits in managed
   care, 393
Conversion factor (CF)
   determining, 190
   in relative value unit formula, 156-157
Conversion privileges, 61
Cooperative care, with TRICARE, 452
Coordination of benefits, 60
Copayments, 393
   definition of, 59
   Medi-Cal, 618-619, 619f
   Medicaid, 443
   TRICARE, 455
   waivers, 339
Correct Coding Initiative (CCI), 48
   Medicare, 420-421
Corrective action, developing, 50
Cost-of-living adjustment, in disability
   insurance, 521
Cost outlier, 561
Cost-share, under TRICARE, 455
Counseling, 107
   coding or, 163
   credit, 363-364
Courtesy adjustments, 338
Covered entity, definition of, 28
CPT. *See Current Procedural Terminology* (CPT).
Credit
   arrangements for, 348-350, 349f, 351f
   bureaus for, 363
   cards, 349-350
   counseling on, 363-364
   definition of, 334
   laws affecting, 351-354
Creditor, 342
Criminal False Claims Act, 47
Critical care, 107
   coding for, 160-161
   pediatric, coding for, 161-162
Current Procedural Terminology (CPT)
   adjunct codes in, 177
   bundled codes in, 173-174
   categories and subcategories of, 163, 167
   code book symbols in, 158-159, 159f
   code edits and, 172-176
   code modifiers in, 177-190, 177t-183t
   in coding from operating reports, 167-168
   coding skills using, 152-153
   component codes in, 173
   comprehensive codes in, 173
   consultation codes in, 160, 166t-167t
   critical care codes in, 160-161
   downcoding in, 175
   drug and injection codes in, 176-177
   emergency care codes in, 162-163
   evaluation and management section of,
      159-167, 164f, 164t-167t

Current Procedural Terminology—cont'd
   hospital coding using, 549-552
      outpatient, 549, 551-552
   how to use, 157-158
   life or disability evaluation services codes in,
      177
   mutually exclusive code denials and, 173
   neonatal and pediatric critical care codes in,
      161-612
   office visit codes in, 176
   preventive medicine in, 163
   in procedural coding, 152
   prolonged services, detention, or standby
      codes in, 172
   surgery section of, 167-172
   surgical package codes in, 168-169
   unbundling and, 174-175
   unlisted procedures in, 172
   upcoding in, 175-176
Customary fee, 155
Cycle billing, 371

D

Data elements
   medical, 273, 274t
   required, 274-275
   situational, 274-275
Data exchange, electronic, streamlining,
      transaction and code set regulations
      in, 41-43, 42t
Data storage, for electronic claims, 299
Dates, on claim form, 203
Daysheets, 81
DCGs (diagnostic cost groups), 412
DDE (direct data entry), for electronic claim
      transmission, 292
DDS (Disability Determination Services), 523
De-identification, of confidential information,
      definition of, 37b
Debit cards, 350
Debtor, communication with, 341
Deceased patients, 120
   Medicare claims for, 424-425
Deductibles, insurance, 59, 392
   TRICARE, 455
DEERS (Defense Enrollment Eligibility
      Reporting System), 451
Defense Enrollment Eligibility Reporting
      System (DEERS), 451
Deficit Reduction Act of 1984 (DEFRA)
   employed elderly Medicare benefits and, 409
   Medicaid and, 436
   Medicare reimbursement and, 421
Delinquent claims
   definition of, 311
   problem solving for, 311-312
   workers' compensation, 511-513, 512f, 513f
Delivery, coding in, 140-141
Denied claims
   Medi-Cal, appeal process for, 622
   problem solving for, 313-315
   review of, letter requesting, 308, 310f
Depositions, workers' compensation and, 491
Diabetes mellitus, coding for, 139-140, 140f
Diagnosis, on claim form, 202
Diagnosis-related groups (DRGs)
   in hospital billing, 560-563
   in hospital reimbursement, 556
   physician's office and, 562-563
Diagnostic coding, 126-149. *See also*
      *International Classification of Diseases
      (ICD-9-CM).*
   development of, reasons for, 128-129
   history of, 129-130

Diagnostic coding—cont'd
   for psychiatric disorders, 130
   system for, 128-129
   types of codes in, 128
Diagnostic cost groups (DCGs), 412
Diagnostic terminology and abbreviations,
      107-108
Diagnostic tests and managed care, 390
Digital signatures, 83
Digital subscriber line (DSL), for electronic
      claim transmission, 289
Direct data entry (DDE), for electronic claim
      transmission, 292
Direct referrals, 387
Directional terms, 108, 495, 496f
Disability Determination Services (DDS), 523
Disability income insurance, 65, 518-537
   AIDS/HIV and, 522
   benefits of
      group, 522
      individual, 521
   claims for, 529-531, 532f-536f
   clauses in, 521
   examinations for, 58
      coding for, 177
   exclusions under, 521
   federal, 522-525
   group, 522
   history of, 520
   individual, 520-522
   state, 67, 525-529, 528t
      workers' compensation and, 484
   types of disability covered by, 521
Disabled, Medicare and, 402
Discharge analysts, 554
Disciplinary standards, enforcing, 51
Disclosure, definition of, 30
Discounted fees, 336-338
Discounts, cash, 337
Diseases
   coding of, history of, 129-130
   international classification of, 130
Disenrollment, 391
Disputes, payment, 342-343
Documentation
   medical, 90-125. *See also* Health record(s).
      for evaluation and management services,
         95-98
      general principles of, 93-94
      legal, 93
      legalities of, 94
      process of, 92-93
      reasons for, 93
   in role of insurance billing specialist, 4-5
Documenters, 92-93
Double indemnity, in disability insurance, 521
Downcoding, 175, 561
   problem solving for, 315-316
DRG creep, 561
Drugs, coding for, 176-177
DSL (digital subscriber line), for electronic
      claim transmission, 289
Dun messages, 347-348
Durable medical equipment number, 204

E

E-checks, 350
E codes, 134-136, 135f
E-health information management (eHIM), 26
E-Span Employment Database, 586
Early and Periodic Screening, Diagnosis,
      and Treatment (EPSDT), Medicaid
      and, 442
EDI. *See* Electronic data interchange (EDI).

Edit checks, software, 115-116
Education, in compliance plan, conducting, 50
Educational and training requirements for
        insurance billing specialists, 14, 16-17
EFT (electronic funds transfer), 288
EHR (electronic health record), 92
EIN (employer identification number)
    in electronic claims, 277, 279
    of physician, 203
Elective surgery
    Medicare and, 418-419
    outpatient insurance claims for, 558
Electronic claim
    completing, procedure for, 567-579
    editing procedure for, 566-567
Electronic claims. *See also* Claims, insurance.
    administrative simplification enforcement
        tool for, 292, 296
    advantages of, 270
    attachments standards for, 277-
    billing and account management schedule
        for, 292, 295t
    building, 281-288
        encoder in, 287-288
        encounter forms in, 281-282
            scannable, 282, 283f
        keying insurance data in, for claim
            transmission, 282, 284f-285f, 285,
            286f, 287, 287t
        multipurpose billing forms in, 281-282
        signature requirements in, 288
    clearinghouses for, 270-271
    computer system selection for, 299
    data storage for, 299
    definition of, 197
    driving data in, 289
    Health Insurance Portability and, 271-275,
        273f, 274t, 275t, 276b
    history of, 270
    interactive transactions in, 288
    Medicaid, 445
    Medicare requirements when submitting, 424
    multipurpose billing forms in, 281-282
    optical scanned format guidelines for, 207-210
    problem solving for, 311-317
    processing problems with, 292
    processors of, 584
        job description for, 10f-11f
    records management for, 299-300
    remittance advice statements in, 289
    security rule for, 296
    signature requirements for, 287-288
    submission of
        clean, 288
        Medicare requirements for, 287, 287t
    transmission reports for, 292, 293f-295f
    workers' compensation, submission of, 511
Electronic data interchange (EDI), 268-301
    in hospital reimbursement, 557-558
    streamlining, transaction and code set
        regulations in, 41-43, 42t
Electronic environment, signature guidelines
        for, 78
Electronic funds transfer (EFT), 288
Electronic health record (EHR), 92
Electronic power protection, 299
Electronic remittance advice (ERA), 289,
        290f-291f
Electronic signatures, 83
Electronic technologies, health information
        using, 26-27
Eligibility requirements
    for health insurance, 61
    for Medi-Cal, 614-616

Eligibility requirements—cont'd
    for Medicaid, 438-442
    for Medicare, 402-403
    for TRICARE, 450-451
Elimination periods, 59
Emancipated minors, 57-58
Embezzlement, 47
    precautions for, 370
Emergency care, 107
    admission for, under managed care, 547
    coding for, 162-163
    TRICARE for, 451
Employees. *See also* Disability income
        insurance; Workers' compensation
        insurance.
    confidentiality statements, 34f
    liability of, 2
    minor, workers' compensation and, 481
    Occupational Safety and Health
        Administration and, 489-490
    reporting requirements regarding, 500,
        502f-503f, 503-504
    volunteer, workers' compensation and, 481
Employer, reporting requirements for, under
        workers' compensation, 500, 502f, 503
Employer identification number (EIN)
    in electronic claims, 277, 279
    of physician, 203
Employer professional liability, 21-22
Employment, 581-606
    opportunities for, 584
    seeking. *See* Job searches.
Employment examinations, 58
Encoder(s)
    in building electronic claims, 287-288
    electronic claims, 287-288
Encounter forms, 79, 80f, 81f
    in electronic claims, 281-282
    fee collection and, 342, 343f
    in managed care, 392
    scannable, in electronic claims, 282, 283f
Encryption, 270
End-stage renal disease (ESRD), Medicare
        and, 402
Endorsement, restrictive, 370
EOB (explanation of benefits), 307-309, 308f
Epigastric, definition of, 108
Equal Credit Opportunity Act, 351-352
ERA (electronic remittance advice), 289,
        290f-291f
Ergonomics, workers' compensation and, 486
Errors and omissions insurance, 22
Estate claims, 368
    filing, 374
Ethics, medical, 20-21
Etiology, in diagnostic coding, 128
Etiquette, medical, 19-20
Evaluation and management section of
        Current Procedural Terminology
        (CPT) codes, 159-167, 164f,
        164t-167t
Evaluation and management services, code
        modifiers for, 186-187, 188f
Exclusion program, 48
Exclusions, insurance policy, 60
Exclusive provider organizations (EPOs),
        65, 384
Explanation of benefits (EOB), 305-307, 306f
Explanation of benefits (EOB) forms, 394f
    EHAMPVA, 468, 470f
Expressed contract, 57
Extending, of account balance, 81
External audits, 113b-114b
    point systems for, 94

F
Facility provider number, 204
Facsimiles (faxes), 116-119, 117f
    patient confidentiality and, 116
FACT (Fair and Accurate Credit Transactions)
        Act, 351
Fair and Accurate Credit Transactions (FACT)
        Act, 351
Fair Credit Billing Act, 352
Fair Credit Reporting Act, 351, 352, 363
Fair Debt Collection Practices Act,
        353-354, 353b
Fairs, job, 586
False Claims Act (FCA), 45-46
Family history (FH), 101
FCA. *See* False Claims Act (FCA).
Federal Coal Mine Health and Safety Act, 480
Federal Deposit Insurance Corporation
        (FDIC) Mail and Wire Fraud
        provisions, 47-48
Federal disability income insurance, 522-525
    claims submission for, 530
Federal Employees' Compensation Act, 480
Federal False Claims Amendment Act, 413
Federal Trade Commission (FTC), 328
Fees
    adjustments of, 336-340
    collecting, 346-348
    communicating, 340
    customary, 155
    determination of, 79
    discounted, 336-338
    late payment, 353
    netback, 362
    reasonable, 155
        under Medicare, 421
    reduced, 340
    relative value studies (RVs) and, 156, 157
    schedules of, 154-155, 336
        development of, using relative value
            studies conversion factors, 157
        Medicare, 157
        workers' compensation, 506, 509-510
    for service accounts, 394-395, 396, 397f
    usual, customary, and reasonable (UCR),
        155-157, 155f
Fetter, Robert B., 560
Filing, in role of insurance billing specialist, 5
Financial accounting records, 79, 81, 82f,
        336-337, 337f, 345
    in managed care, 394
    Medicare, 427f
    preparing and posting, 88
    retention of, 120
Financial agreement forms, 341f
    creating, 373
Financial hardship, determining, 337-338
Financial management of managed care plans,
        392-396
Financial protection, precautions for, 370
Financial responsibility, 57
    in workers' compensation case, 504, 506, 509f
Fiscal agent, Medicaid, 443
Fiscal intermediaries (FIs), 422
    for Medi-Cal, 618
    in TRICARE Standard and CHAMPVA
        programs, 463-464
Flexible spending account (FSA), 62
Forgery, check, 342
Formal referrals, 387
Formal review, in TRICARE review and
        appeal process, 328
Forms, insurance claim, 203
    Medicaid, 443, 445

Foundation for medical care (FMC), 65, 384
Fractures, types of, 497, 498f-500f, 501f
Franklin Health Assurance Company, 56
Fraud, 22
　examples of, 46b
　Health Care, in Criminal False Claims
　　Act, 47
　laws on, 45
　Medicaid, 115, 447
　workers' compensation, 487-489, 488f,
　　489b-490b
Fundraising, definition of, 37b
Future purchase option, in disability
　insurance, 521

G

Garfield, Sidney R., 381
Garnishments, wage, 365
Gatekeepers, in HMOs, 382
Grace period, definition of, 59
Group contracts, 61-65
　disability income, 522
Group health insurance, Medicaid and, 445
Group insurance, 202
Group provider number, 204
Groupers, electronic claims, 288
Guaranteed renewable insurance
　policies, 59
　disability, 521
Guarantors, 57

H

Hardship, financial, determining, 337-338
Hardware, computer, selection of, 299
HCPCS. *See* Healthcare Common Procedure
　Coding System (HCPCS).
Health Care Financing Administration
　(HCFA), 153
Health care finder, TRICARE, 455
Health care provider, definition of, 29
Health information, using electronic
　technologies, 26-27
Health information record keeping, 495
Health insurance
　applications for, abstracting from medical
　　records fro, 159-163
　definition of, 56
　history of, 56
　legal principles of, 56-57
Health Insurance Association of America
　(HIAA), 196
Health Insurance Claim Form (CMS-1500),
　172-236, 196, 202-267
　dates in, 203
　diagnosis in, 202
　guidelines for submitting, 202-205
　history of, 196
　insurance biller's initials in, 205
　in Medi-Cal, 625-627
　no charge in, 203
　office pending file and, 205
　paper, transition from, to electronic
　　standard HIPAA 837P, 276, 277t
　physicians' identification numbers in,
　　203-204
　physician's signature on, 204-205
　proofreading, 205
　provider identification numbers in,
　　203-204
　standard transaction format 837P compared
　　with, 276, 277t-279t
　supporting documents for, 205
Health insurance contracts, 57. *See also*
　Policy(ies), health insurance.

Health Insurance Portability and
　Accountability Act (HIPAA), 27-29
　administrative simplification in, 27-28
　application of, to practice setting, 43-44
　claim form issues related to, 196, 197
　coding compliance plan under, 152
　compliance program of, 114
　compliance with, workers' compensation
　　and, 478
　computer confidentiality and, 297-298, 465
　confidentiality and, 21, 29-39, 465, 542-545
　electronic claims and, 271-275, 273f, 274t,
　　275t, 276b
　electronic security standards and, 92
　employee liability and, 21-22
　exceptions to, 32-35
　insurance policies and, 61-62
　insurance reform in, 27
　Medicaid fraud control, 447
　Medicare billing compliance and, 413
　noncompliance with, consequences of, 44-45
　patient confidentiality and, 116
　patient rights under, 36-39
　in practice setting, 29
　on privacy and confidentiality related to
　　medical reports, 494-495
　release of information and, 77f
　self-employed insurance billing specialist as
　　business associate under, 598
Health Level Seven (HL7), 26-27
Health Maintenance Organization Act of
　1973, 381
Health maintenance organizations (HMOs)
　accreditation of, 381
　admission procedures for, 546-547
　eligibility for, 381-382
　encounter forms, 392
　financial management of, 392-396
　Medicare, 411-412
　models of, 65, 383
　plan administration, 390-392
　plan management, 386-391
　primary care physicians in, 382
　TRICARE and, 462
　year-end evaluations in, 395-396
Health record(s)
　abstracting from, 198, 199f-201f
　confidentiality of, 116, 297, 542-545
　definition of, 92
　electronic, 92
　external audit point systems for, 94
　faxing of, 116, 117f
　guidelines for, for evaluation and
　　management services, 95-98
　history documentation in, 98
　of medical decision-making complexity,
　　103-104
　of physical examinations, 101-103, 102f
　process of, 92-93
　reasons for, 93
　retention of, 119, 119t
　review and audit of, 113-123
　terminology for, 104, 106-111, 109f, 110f,
　　111f, 111t-112t, 495, 495b, 496f,
　　496t, 497f-500f, 501f
Health Reimbursement Account (HRA), 64
Health savings accounts (HSAs), 63-64
Healthcare Common Procedure Coding
　System (HCPCS), 153
　codes of
　　applicability of, 153
　　modifiers as, 189-190, 189f
　Medicare and, 421
　in outpatient coding procedures, 551

Hearing
　administrative law judge, in Medicare review
　　and redetermination process, 323
　in SSI program, 523
　in TRICARE review and appeal
　　process, 328
Heart disease, coding for, 139
Hemorrhage, definition of, 111
High blood pressure, coding for, 139
HIPAA. *See* Health Insurance Portability and
　Accountability Act (HIPAA).
History
　of accounts, in insurance collection, 359
　documentation of, 98-104
　of present illness (HPI), 99-101
Honesty bond, 370-371
Hook up, Get Hired!, 586
Hospice care
　definition of, 404
　Medicare and, 404
Hospice program, TRICARE, 461-462
Hospital(s)
　admission procedures for, 546-548
　billing procedures for, 539-579. *See also*
　　Billing, hospital.
　inpatient billing process for, 552-558
　inpatient coding for, 549-551
　outpatient classification for, 563, 564
　outpatient coding for, 549, 551-552
　outpatient insurance claims, 558
　preadmission testing for, 548
　procedure coding for, 549-552
　reimbursement process for, 556-558
　Uniform Bill (UB-92) claim form, 555, 559,
　　564f. *See also* Uniform Bill (UB-62)
　　claim form.
　utilization review and, 549
Hospital coders, job description for, 12f-13f
Hsiao, William, 156
Human immunodeficiency virus (HIV)
　disability income insurance and, 522
　life insurance applications and, 198
Hypertension, coding for, 130
Hypogastric, definition of, 108

I

*ICD-9-CM. See International Classification of
　Diseases (ICD-9-CM).*
Identification cards
　CHAMPVA, 462-463, 463f
　health insurance, 75, 76f
　Medi-Cal, 615, 615f
　Medicaid and Medicare, 403-404, 403f
　Medicare, 440, 440f
　Supplemental Health Care Program, 461
　TRICARE Extra, 456
　TRICARE for Life, 459
　TRICARE Plus, 459
　TRICARE Prime, 457
　TRICARE Prime Remote Program, 461
　TRICARE Standard, 451, 452f
Identifiers, unique, standard, 277, 279-280
Identity, verification of, in protecting patient
　rights, 39-40
Image copy recognition (ICR), 207
Implied contracts, 57
Income continuation benefits, 61
Incontestability, 57
Indemnity, 60
Independent contractor, insurance billing
　specialist as, 17
　job description for, 8f-9f
Independent or individual practice associations
　(IPAs), 66, 384

Individual and Small Group Physician Practices,
   compliance program guidance for,
   48-49
Individual contracts, 65
Individually identifiable health information
   (IIHI), definition of, 30
Industrial accidents and occupational illnesses
   defining, 480
   employer's reports on, 500, 502f, 503
   final report on, 504, 508f
   legal situations involving, 491-494
   medical service orders and, 503-504, 503f
   physician's first report on, 504, 505f, 506t
   progress or supplemental report on, 504, 507f
   reporting requirements for, 482t-483t, 500,
      502f-503f, 503-504
Information, release of, 77
Injections, coding for, 176-177
Injuries and late effects coding, 141-143, 142t
Inpatient billing process, 552-558
   admitting clerk in, 552
   attending physician in, 553
   charge description master in, 554-555
   code specialist in, 555
   coding credentials in, 555
   discharge analyst in, 554
   insurance billing editor in, 555-556
   insurance verifier in, 552
   medical transcriptionist in, 553
   nurse auditor in, 556
   nursing staff in, 553
Inpatients, coding for, 549-551
Insurance
   reform of, under HIPAA, 27
   for self-employed insurance billing
      specialists, 598
   verification of, procedure for, 565
Insurance adjuster, workers' compensation, 485
Insurance balance billing, 348
Insurance billing editor, 555-556
Insurance billing specialists
   attributes of, *18*
   behavior of, 19
   career advantages, 17
   certification and registration for, 601,
      602t-604t
   confidentiality statement for, 21
   disabled, 17
   educational and training requirements, 14,
      16-17
   employee liability and, 21-22
   employment opportunities for, 584
   ethics, 20-21
   example cases for, 67-68
   flexible hours for, 17
   future challenges for, 22
   as independent contractors, 17
   job responsibilities of, 5, 6f-13f, 8-9, 14
   mentors and, 601
   networking by, 601
   personal image of, 18-19, 19f
   procedures of, 68-88
   professional associations for, 601
   qualifications of, 18-19
   Role Delineation Chart, 14, *14t-15t*
   roles of, 2-23, 584
   scope of practice, 22
   self-employed, 17, 595-605
      advertising by, 600
      bank account for, 598
      business associate agreement for, 598-599
      business name, plan and license for, 598
      documentation by, 600
      finances for, 596-598

Insurance billing specialists—cont'd
   self-employed—cont'd
      insurance for, 598
      marketing by, 600, 601t
      planning business for, 596
      pricing services by, 600
      professional mailing address for, 596
      promotion by, 600
      public relations by, 600
      service contract for, 599
      setting up office by, 595-596, 600
      trends in, 600-601
   skills of, 18
Insurance carriers
   payment histories of, in claim
      management, 308
   private. *See* Private insurance.
   regulation of, 328
   suing, 361
   types of, 65-67
Insurance claims register, 307
Insurance contracts, 57. *See also* Policy(ies),
   health insurance.
Insurance verifier, 552
Insured
   claim policy provisions governing, 304
   definition of, 58
Intelligent character recognition (ICR), 207
Interactive transactions, in claims
      processing, 288
Intermediate care facilities (ICFs), 422
Intermediate lacerations, definition of, 110
Internal monitoring, in compliance plan, 49
Internal reviews, 113
*International Classification of Diseases, 10th
      Revision (ICD-10-CM),* diagnosis and
      procedure codes of, 143-149
*International Classification of Diseases
      (ICD-9-CM). See also* Diagnostic
      coding.
   abortion coding in, 140-141
   admitting diagnoses coding in, 141
   alphabetic index for, 551
   basic steps in coding, 132-134
   burn coding in, 141, 142f
   circulatory system coding in, 138-139
   coding competencies, 544b
   coding numbers in, 132-133
   coding rules for, 136-143
   contents of, 130, 131t-132t
   diabetes mellitus coding in, 139-140, 140f
   downcoding and, 316
   E codes in, 134-136, 135f
   electronic claims and, 273, 274
   history of, 130
   hospital coding using, 549-552
   injuries and late effects coding in, 141-143,
      142t
   main terms in, 132
   neoplasm coding in, 137-138, 138t
   organization and format of, 130
   pregnancy coding in, 140-141
   proper use of, 130, 132-136
   signs and symptoms in, 136-137
   sterilization coding in, 137
   system replacing, 143-149
   terminology of, 130-132, 131b-132b
   V codes in, 134
Interview, job, 591-595, 592f, 593-594f, 595f
Intimidation, refraining from, in protecting
      patient rights, 41
Intoxication, 132
Italicized code, 132
Itemized patient statements, 345-348

J
Job fairs, 586
Job searches
   applications in, 586, 587f-588f, 589
   blind mailing in, 585
   employment agencies in, 585
   interviews in, 591-595, 592f, 593f-594f, 595f
   letters of introduction in, 589, 590f
   methods for, 584-595
   online, 585-586
   resumes in, 589-591, 591f
Judicial review, in Medicare review and
      redetermination process, 323

K
Kaiser, Henry J., 381
Kaiser Industries, 56
Kaiser Permanente Medical Care Program, 381
Knox-Keene Health Care Service Plan Act of
      1975, 396

L
Lacerations
   repair of, coding for, 170-171
   terminology for, 110
Late effects coding, 143
Late payment charges, 353
LCD (Local Coverage Determination), under
      Medicare, 422
Ledger card, 336-337, 337f
Left hypochondriac, definition of, 108
Left inguinal, definition of, 108
Left lower quadrant, definition of, 108
Left upper quadrant, definition of, 108
Legal documents, faxing of, 118
Legal problems, prevention of, 123, 123b
Legislation
   credit and collection, 351-354
   estate claim, 368
   on health care reform, 382-383
   insurance, 56
   Medicare, 409, 413-414
   on Occupational Safety and Health
      Administration, 489-490
   small claims court, 364
   workers' compensation, 479-480,
      480-484
Letters
   collection, 355-358, 356f, 357f
   of introduction, 589, 590f
Liability
   limited, under Medicare, 417-418
   professional, 21-22
   third-party
      TRICARE and, 468
      in workers' compensation cases, 494
Liability insurance, Medicare and, 411
Liens, 338, 369f
   filing of, in workers' compensation cases,
      491-494, 492b, 493f
Life insurance examination services
   abstracting from medical records for, 198,
      199f-201f
   coding for, 177
Limitations, insurance policy, 60-61
Limiting charge, 414-415
Litigation, for collections, 368
Local Coverage Determination (LCD), under
      Medicare, 422
Longshoremen's and Harbor Workers'
      Compensation Act, 480
Looping, 561
Loos, H. Clifford, 381
Lost claims, problem solving for, 312

Low-income Medicare recipients, 437
Lumbar, right and left, definition of, 108

M

Major diagnostic categories, 561
Malignant hypertension, 139
Malpractice issues, reduced fees and, 340
Managed care
    accounting in, 394-395
    admission procedures for, 546-547
    appointment scheduling, 391-392
    assignment of benefits in, 77
    bankruptcy in, 396
    carve outs, 387
    collection procedures for, 360
    contracts, 58, 386
    diagnostic tests and, 390
    encounter forms in, 392
    financial management in, 392-396
    guide to, 390
    health maintenance organization (HMO) as, 65, 383-384
    history of, 56, 380-381
    management of plans in, 386-391
    Medi-Cal and, 614
    Medicaid, 442-443
    medical records management in, 391
    medical review and, 385-386
    Medicare patients and, 410-411
    Medicare plus choice program and, 408
    overpayments made by, problem solving for, 317
    patient information letters on, 390-391, 392f
    payments for, 392-393
    plan administration in, 390-392
    preauthorization or prior approval requirements, 387, 388f-389f, 390
    stop loss outliers in, 557
    types of, 383-385
    withholds in, 395-396
    workers' compensation insurance and, 480
    year-end evaluations in, 395-396
Managed care plans, payment release by, 304-305
Management service organizations (MSOs), 5
Manual billing, 348
Marketing, definition of, 37b
Maternal and Child Health Programs (MCHPs), 66, 436-437
    claims under, 445
    eligibility for, 439
McCarran Act, 328
MCHPs. See Maternal and Child Health Programs (MCHPs).
Medi-Cal, 426, 612-634
    appeals process for, 622
    benefits of, 616, 618
    claim procedure for, 618-622
    eligibility for, 614-616
    Health Insurance Claim Form (CMS-1500) and, 625-627
    managed care plans and, 614
    Medicare and, 620, 620f
    prior approval requirements in, 618
    private insurance and, 620
    remittance advice details in, 621-622
    Resubmission Turnaround Documents for, 622, 628
    treatment authorization form for, completing, 623, 624-625f
    treatment authorization request in, 618
    Uniform Bill (UB-92) claim form and, 621
Medi-Cal CMC Technical Manual, 620-621

Medicaid, 434-447
    admission procedures for, 547
    appeals, 447
    assignment of benefits and, 78
    benefits under, 442, 442b
    in California. See Medi-Cal.
    carrier-direct system and, 292
    claim procedure under, 443-447
    electronic claims, 445
    eligibility for, 438-442
    fraud in, 115, 447
    government programs and, 445
    health care reform and, 382
    Health Insurance Claim Form for
        example of, 260f, 262f
        instructions for, 210-256
    history of, 436
    identification cards for, 440, 440f
    low-income Medicare recipients and, 437
    managed care, 442-443
    Maternal and Child Health Programs (MCHP) of, 66, 436-437
    with Medicare, claims under, 424
    Medicare and, 409-410
    patients on, accepting, 439-440
    policies and regulations of, 21, 56, 66
        on assignment of benefits, 78
    programs of, 436-437
    Qualified Medicare Beneficiary Program (MQMB), 437
    Qualifying Individuals Program (QI), 437
    remittance advice statements, 446-447
    TRICARE/CHAMPVA and, claims procedure for, 467
Medical billing representative, 5. See also Insurance billing specialist.
Medical code sets, 42, 42t, 273, 274t
Medical decision-making complexity documentation, 103-104
Medical ethics, 20-21
Medical etiquette, 19-20
Medical evaluator, for workers' compensation, 491
Medical necessities, 94, 95f
Medical records. See Health record(s).
Medical report(s), 494-497, 495b, 496f, 496t, 497f-500f
    confidentiality of, 494-495
    contents of, 98-104
    definition of, 92
    privacy and confidentiality of, 494-495
Medical review, 385-386
Medical savings accounts (MSAs), 61-63
Medical service orders, on workers' compensation case, 503-504, 503f
Medical testimony, in workers' compensation cases, 491, 492f
Medical transcriptionist, in inpatient billing process, 553
Medically needy, under Medicaid, 438-439, 438b
Medicare, 400-433
    admission procedures for, 547
    advance beneficiary notice (ABN) and, 417-418, 417f, 418f
    alien eligibility for, 403
    assignment of benefits and, 78
    beneficiary representatives for, 425-426, 427f-430f
    benefits and nonbenefits of, 404-409, 405f, 406f, 407t
    bundled codes and, 174

Medicare—cont'd
    Carrier Dealing Prepayment Organizations, 412
    carrier-direct system and, 292
    CHAMPVA and, claims procedure for, 467
    claims under
        for deceased patients, 424-425
        electronic, 424
        Medicaid and, 424
        Medigap and, 424
        paper, 423-424
        status of, 197-198
        submission of, 422-425
            procedures after, 425
        time limit for, 423
    Clinical Laboratory Improvement Amendment and, 413-414
    collection procedures for, 360
    copay requirements under, 59
    Correct Coding Initiative (CCI) of, 420-421
    double billing and, 559
    elective surgery and, 418-419
    eligibility requirements for, 402-403
    employed elderly benefits of, 409
    enrollment status in, 404
    faxing documents related to, 117
    Federal False Claims Amendment Act and, 413
    fee schedule for, 157
    fees under, 421
    fiscal intermediaries (FI) and, 422
    global surgery policies of, 169-170, 169f
    Health Insurance Claim Form for
        example of, 261f-264f
        instructions for, 210-256
    Health Insurance Portability and Accountability Act and, 413
    Health Maintenance Organizations and, 411-412
    Healthcare Common Procedure Coding System (HCPCS) for, 153, 421
    history of, 56, 402
    hospital benefits of, 404-405, 405f
    insurance cards for, 403-404, 403f
    Local Coverage Determination under, 422
    Medi-Cal and, 620, 620f
    Medicaid and, 409-410, 436
    medical benefits of, 405-408, 406f, 407t
    medical ethics and, 21
    Medigap and, 323, 360, 409-410, 410f
    non-participating physicians in, 414-415
    noncontracted physicians and, 412
    noncovered services payment under, 418
    overpayments made by, problem solving for, 317
    participating physicians in, 414
    payment fundamentals for, 414-421
    plus choice program, 408
    policies and regulations of, 66, 402-409, 403f, 405f, 406f, 407t
        on assignment of benefits, 78
        on signatures, 79
    posting payments under, 426
    prepayment screens for, 419-420
    as primary and secondary insurance, determining, 431
    prior authorizations and, 415
    provider identification numbers in, 422
    quality improvement organization program of, 549
    railroad retirement benefits, 408-409
    reasonable fees under, 421
    reimbursement under, 421

Medicare—cont'd
  remittance advice statements of, 425, 428f-429f
  requirements when submitting paper and electronic claims, 287, 287t
  resource-based relative value scale (RBRVS) and, 421
  review and redetermination process of, 320-323, 320t, 324f-326f, 426
  Secondary Payer (MSP), 410-411
  72-hour rule of, 548
  signature requirements under, 422-423
  Summary Notice of, 425
  supplemental coverage and, 424
  3-day payment window rule of, 548
  TRICARE and, claims procedure for, 467
  utilization and quality control for, 412-414
  waiver of liability provision, 417-418
Medicare Integrity Program (MIP), 48
Medicare medical savings account, 63
Medifill, 409
Medigap, 409-410, 410f
  collection procedures for, 360
  Health Insurance Claim Form for, example of, 263f
  with Medicare, claims under, 424
  in Medicare review and redetermination process, 323
MedSearch America, 586
Member, definition of, 58
Mentors, 601
Military retiree, TRICARE and, 451
Minimum necessary, definition of, 37b
Minors
  coordination of benefits regarding, 60
  emancipated, 57-58
  workers' compensation and, 481
Mitigation, in protecting patient rights, 41
Modems, 289
Modifiers, CPT code, 177-190, 177t-183t
Monthly statements, 86
Morbidity, 103, 104
Mortality, 103, 104
Multiple procedures, coding modifiers for, 184-185, 187f
Multipurpose billing forms
  in electronic claims, 281-282
  fee collection and, 342
Multiskilled health practitioners (MSHPs), 5
Mutually exclusive code denials, 173
Myocardial infarctions, coding for, 139

N

National alphanumeric codes, of Healthcare Common Procedure Coding System, 421
National Health Information Infrastructure (NHII), 26, 27b
National Provider Identifier (NPI), 204
  for electronic claims, 279-280
National Standard Format (NSF), 272
NEMB (Notice of Exclusions of Medicare Benefits), 418, 419f
Neonatal critical care, coding for, 161-162
Neoplasms, coding for, 137-138, 138t
Netback fees, 362
Network HMOs, 383
Networking, 601
New versus established patients, 104
No charge (NC) visits, 339-340
  on claim form, 203
Nonavailability statements (NAS), TRICARE and, 451
Noncancelable insurance policies, 59

Noncompliance, with HIPAA, consequences of, 44-45
Nondisability claim, workers' compensation, 485
Nonparticipating provider (nonpar), 77
  under TRICARE, 456
Nonpayer excuses, 342, 344t
Nonprivileged information, 35
Notice of Exclusions of Medicare Benefits (NEMB), 418, 419f
Notice of Privacy Practices (NPP), 72
NPI (National Provider Identifier), 204
  for electronic claims, 279-280
NSF (National Standard Format), 272
Nurse auditors, in hospital reimbursement, 556
Nursing facility, Medicare benefits and, 404
Nursing staff, in inpatient billing process, 553

O

Occupational illness/disease, definition of, 480
Occupational illnesses. See Industrial accidents and occupational illnesses.
Occupational Safety and Health Administration (OSHA) Act of 1970, 489-490
OCR (optical character recognition), 207-210
Offenses, detected, responding appropriately to, 50
Office of Civilian Health and Medical Program of the Uniformed Services (OCHAMPUS), 196
Office of Inspector General (OIG), 45-48
Office visits, coding for, 176
Omnibus Budget Reconciliation Act (OBRA)
  employed elderly Medicare benefits and, 409
  Medicare reimbursement under, 421
Online job search, 585-586
Operation Restore Trust (OR|T), 48
Optical character recognition (OCR), 207-210
Optical scanned format guidelines, 207-210
Optionally renewable insurance policies, 59
Ordering physician, roles of, 93
Outpatients
  classification of, 563, 565
  coding for, 549, 551-552
  insurance claims for, 558
Overpayments, problem solving for, 316-317

P

Paper claims, 194-267
Paper environment, signature guidelines for, 79
Paper trail, never-ending, 86-87
Partial disabilities, 521
Participating provider (par), 77
  in TRICARE, 455-456
Partnership program, of TRICARE, 452
Past histories (PH), 101
PAT (preadmission testing), 548
Patient(s)
  bankrupt, 367-368, 367t
  classification of, diagnosis-related groups in, 561-563
  complaints of, 338-369
  confidentiality for, 116, 542-545
  contracts of, with physicians, 57-58
  deceased, 120
    Medicare claims for, 424-425
    reduced fees for, 340
  education of, on payment policies, 335-336
  excuses of, for nonpayment, 342, 344t
  financial accounting records of, 79, 81, 82f, 336-337, 337f, 345
    preparing and posting, 88
  financial hardship and, 337-338

Patient(s)—cont'd
  guarantors for, 57
  in-. See Inpatients.
  information letters, 390-391, 392f
  insurance payments made to, 360
    problem solving for, 316
  itemized statements for, 345-348
  liens against, 338, 369f
  minor, 57-58, 60
    workers' compensation and, 481
  new versus established, 104
  nonprivileged information related to, 35
  out-. See Outpatients.
  privileged information related to, 35
  rebilling of, 319
  referrals of, 387
  registration forms for, 72, 73f-75f, 336
  rights of, 35
    to privacy, 35
    protecting, organization and staff responsibilities in, 39-41
  self-pay, 14
  signatures of, requirements for, 78-79
    in electronic claims, 288
    under Medicare, 422-423
  terminally ill, 368
  termination of care of, 120-123, 120f, 121f-122f
  workers' compensation, 58
Patient identifier, standard unique, for electronic claims, 280
Patient services representatives, 542, 543f
Payment(s)
  check, 342-345
  coinsurance, 359
  credit arrangements for, 348-350, 349f, 351f
  disputed, 342-343
  fee schedules and, 154-155
  in managed care, 392-393
  Medicare, 414-421
  methods of, 154-157
  plans fixed prosthodontics, 350, 351f
  in Supplemental Health Care Program, 461
  time limits on, 304-305
  at time of service, 340-342
  in TRICARE Extra, 456
  in TRICARE for Life, 459
  in TRICARE Plus, 459
  in TRICARE Prime, 457
  in TRICARE Prime Remote Program, 461
Pediatric critical care, coding for, 161-162
Peer review organizations (PROs), 412
Pending claim, problem solving for, 311-312
Per diem, in hospital reimbursement, 557
Percentage of revenue, in hospital reimbursement, 556
Percival, Thomas, 339
Performing physician, roles of, 93
Permanent disability claims, workers' compensation, 486-487
Permission, patient, validating, in protecting patient rights, 40-41
Personal image for insurance billing specialists, 18-19
Phantom charges, 559
PHI. See Protected health information (PHI).
Physical examinations, documentation of, 101-103, 102f
Physical safeguards, 43
  for electronic claims, 296
Physician(s)
  attending, in inpatient billing process, 553
  contracts of, with patients, 57-58
  of documenters, 93

Physician(s)—cont'd
  fee profiles of, 129
  first report of, on industrial accident or
     occupational illness, 504, 505f, 506t
     completing, procedure for, 513-516, 514f
  identification numbers, 203
  medical testimony by, in workers'
     compensation cases, 491, 492f
  non-participating, 412, 414-415
  participating, 414
  primary care
    in HMOs, 382
    in TRICARE Prime, 457
  professional courtesy and, 339
  provider groups of (PPGs), 385
  referrals, 387
  signatures of, 79, 204-205
    requirements for, in electronic claims, 288
  termination of cases by, 120-123, 120f,
    121f-122f
  in workers' compensation evaluation, 491
Physicians' Current Procedural Terminology, 152.
    See also Current Procedural
    Terminology (CPT).
PMS (practice management system), 280-281
Point-of-service (POS) device machine in
    Medicaid, 440, 441f
Point-of-service (POS) plans, 66, 385
Poisoning, 135-136, 136b
Policy(ies)
  assignment of benefits and, 77-78
  case management requirements for, 61
  choices of, 61-65
  conversion privileges, 61
  group, 61-65
  health insurance, 58-61
    applications for, 58
    exclusions in, 60
    limitations of, 60-61
    renewal provisions for, 58-59
    terms of, 59-60
  identification cards, 75, 76f
  individual, 65
  private carriers of, assignment of benefits
    under, 77
  types of, 65-67
Portfolio, for job interview, 595
Posting of daily transactions, 81
Power protection, electronic, 299
Practice management system (PMS), 280-281
Practice setting, HIPAA in, 29
Practice standards, implementing, 49-50
PracticeNet, 586
Preadmission testing (PAT), 548
Preapprovals and preauthorizations
  CHAMPVA, 463
  managed care, 387, 388f-389f, 390
  Medi-Cal, 618
  Medicaid, 443
  requirements for, 61
  Supplemental Health Care Program, 461
  TRICARE Extra, 456
  TRICARE for Life, 459
  TRICARE Prime, 457
  TRICARE Prime Remote Program, 461
  TRICARE Standard, 455
Precertification, 61, 62f
Predetermination, 61, 63f
Preferred provider organizations (PPOs), 66,
    384-385
Pregnancy, coding for, 139
Premiums, insurance, 59
Prepaid group practice model, 383
Prepaid group practice plans, 381-382

Prepaid health plan, 65
Prepayment screens, for Medicare, 419-420
Preregistration, patient, 68, 72
Present illness, history of, 99-101
Prevention of legal problems, 123, 123b
Preventive medicine, coding for, 163
Primary care manager, in TRICARE Prime, 457
Primary care physician, roles of, 93
Primary diagnosis, in diagnostic coding,
    128, 128b
Privacy
  definition of, 30
  right to, 35
Privacy compliance, HIPAA, guidelines for,
    43-44
Privacy officer, definition of, 29
Privacy official, definition of, 29
Privacy rule, 29-39
Private carriers, assignment of benefits and, 77
Private contractor, insurance billing specialist
    as, 17
  job description for, 8f-9f
Private insurance
  admission procedures for, 546
  Blue Cross/Blue Shield (BCBS), 380
  Health Insurance Claim Form for, example
    of, 258f-259f
  Health Insurance Claim Form instructions
    for, 210-256
  Medi-Cal and, 620
  overpayment by, problem solving for, 317
  payment time limits for, 304
  secondary and, 202
Privileged information, 35
Problems
  claim. *See also* Claims, insurance.
  claim management techniques and, 307-308
  claim policy provisions and, 304-305
  collection agencies and, 361-363
  collection letters for, 355-358, 356f, 357f
  delinquent, pending, or suspense, problem
    solving or, 311-312
  estate, 368
  explanation of benefits (EOB) and,
    305-307, 306f
  insurance collections and, 358-361
  insurance company payment histories
    and, 308
  small claims court and, 364-365
  state insurance commissioners and, 328-330
  telephone collections for, 354-355, 372-373
  "tickler files" for, 307-308
  types of, 310-317
Procedural coding, 150-193
  alternative billing codes in, 153-154
  code modifiers in, 177-190, 177t-183t
  Current Procedural Terminology in, 152-153,
    157-176. *See also Current Procedural*
    Terminology (CPT); Current Procedural
    Terminology (CPT).
  definition of, 152
  HCPCS codes in, 153
  helpful hints in, 176-177
  payment methods and, 154-157
  skills in, 152-154
Procedure code numbers, 153
Procedures
  admission, 546-548
  for bookkeeping-financial accounting, 79,
    81, 82f
  for CHAMPVA claim form, 471-474
  for claim form submission, 85
  conversion factor determination for,
    156-157

Procedures—cont'd
  for determining if Medicare is primary or
    secondary, 431
  for disability claim submission, 529-531,
    532f-536f
  for encounter form, 79, 80f
  for estate claim, 368
  for fee determination, 79
  for Health Insurance Claim Form
    (CMS-1500), 210-256
  for ICD-9-CM coding, 130-149
  insurance identification card, 75, 76f
  for insurance payments, 85
  for Medicaid claim, 443-447
  for monthly statements, 86
  for official appeal, 319-328
  for patient signature, 78-79
  for physician's signature, 79
  for preregistration-patient registration, 68,
    72-75
  for Resubmission Turnaround
    Documents, 626
  for resume creation, 605
  for small claims court, 364-365
  for telephone collection, 354-355, 372-373
  for tracking claim and insurance claims
    register, 84-85
Professional associations, 601
Professional billing, 4
Professional component, 184
Professional courtesy, 339
Prospective payment system (PPS), 421
Prospective reviews, 113
Protected health information (PHI)
  accounting of disclosures of, right to
    receive, 39
  amendment of, right to request, 38
  definition of, 30
  right to access, inspect, and obtain, 37-38
  uses and disclosures of, 40t
Provider identification numbers, 203-204, 204
  for electronic claims, 279-280
Provider Telecommunications Network
    (PTN), 618
Providers, signature guidelines for, 83-84

Q
Quality assurance program, for TRICARE-
    managed care programs, 468
Quality Improvement Organization (QIO),
    385-386
  Medicare and, 412-413
Quality Improvement Organization (QIO)
    program, 549
Quality Improvement System for Managed
    Care (QISMC), 386
Qui tam action, 413
Qui tam "whistleblower," 46

R
RA (remittance advice), 307
Railroad retirement benefits, 408-409
RBRVS. *See* Resource-based relative value
    scale (RBRVS).
Real time, in electronic claims processing, 288
Reasonable fee, 155
Rebilling, 317-319
Reciprocity, Medicaid, 443
Reconsideration
  in Medicare review and redetermination
    process, 321-323
  in SSI program, 523
  in TRICARE review and appeal process,
    326-328

Record keeping, health information, 495
Records management, for electronic claims, 299-300
Redeterminations
definition of, 319
in Medicare review and redetermination process, 320
Reduced fees, 340
Reduced services, coding modifiers for, 185
Referrals, 104, 387
in Supplemental Health Care Program, 461
in TRICARE for Life, 402459
in TRICARE Prime Remote Program, 461
Referring physician, roles of, 93
Reform, health care, 382-383
Registration
of insurance billing specialists, 601, 602t-604t
patient, 72-75, 336
of patients, in role of insurance billing specialist, 4
Reimbursement
definition of, 334
Medicare, 421
Reimbursement specialists, 5. *See also* Insurance billing specialists.
Rejected claims, 197
reasons for, 313
Rejection of claim forms, reasons for, 205-207
Relative value studies (RVS), 152
conversion factors in, fee schedule development using, 157
fees and, 156
Relative value unit (RVU) formula, 156-157
Remittance, statements of, 394
Remittance advice
Medicaid, 446-447
Medicare, 425, 428f-429f
Remittance advice (RA), 307
Remittance advice statements, for Medi-Cal, 621-622
Renewal provisions, insurance policy, 58-59
Reporting requirements for industrial accidents, 500, 502f-503f, 503-504
Representative payee, for Medicare, 425-426, 427f-430f
Resident physician, roles of, 93
Residual disability, 521
Resource-based relative value scale (RBRVS), 152
fees and, 156-157
Medicare and, 421
Resources, 607-611
Respite care, Medicare and, 404
Respondeat superior, 21-22
Restrictive endorsement, 370
Resubmission Turnaround Documents, 622, 628
Resumes, 589-591, 591f
electronic, creating, procedure for, 605
Retaliatory acts, refraining from, in protecting patient rights, 41
Retention
of financial documents, 120
of health records, 119, 119t
Retroactive eligibility, for Medicaid, 442
Retrospective reviews, 113
Returned checks, 344-345
Review
Medicare, 320-323, 320t, 324f-326f, 426
professional, 385-386
of systems (ROS), 101
TRICARE, 323, 326-328
utilization, 386
Rheumatic heart disease, chronic, coding for, 139

Right
to access, inspect, and obtain PHI, 37-38
to Notice of Privacy Practices, 36
to privacy, 35
to receive an accounting of disclosures of PHI, 39
to request amendment of PHI, 38
to request confidential communications, 36-37
to request restrictions on certain uses and disclosures of protected health information, 36
Right and left lumbar, definition of, 108
Right hypochondriac, definition of, 108
Right inguinal, definition of, 108
Right lower quadrant, definition of, 108
Right upper quadrant, definition of, 108
Ross, Donald E., 381
Ross-Loos Medical Group, 381
Running balance, calculation of, 81
RVS. *See* Relative value studies (RVS).
RVS (relative value studies), 152
RVU (relative value unit) formula, 156-157

S

Safe harbors, 47
Safeguards
administrative, 43
for electronic claims, 296
physical, 43
in protecting patient rights, 41, 41b
technical, 43
Scannable encounter forms, 282, 283f
Scheduling, in role of insurance billing specialist, 4
SCHIP (State Children's Health Insurance Program), 436
Scrubbing, in hospital reimbursement, 557
Second-injury fund (SIF), workers' compensation and, 481, 484
Secondary diagnosis, in diagnostic coding, 128, 128b
Secondary insurance, 196, 202
Security rule, 42
for electronic claims, 296
Self-employed insurance billing specialists, 17, 595-605. *See also* Insurance billing specialists, self-employed.
Self-insurance by employers, 479
Self-pay patients, 14
Self-referrals, 387
Senior billing representative, 5. *See also* Insurance billing specialist.
Service contract, for self-employed insurance billing specialists, 599
Service dates, on claim form, 203
Service retiree, TRICARE and, 451
72-hour rule, 548
SHCP (Supplemental Health Care Program), 461
Signature(s)
digital, 83
electronic, 83
provider, guidelines for, 83-84
Signature guidelines, patient, 78-79
Signature log, 96, 96f
HIPAA compliance and, 98
Signature requirements, 204-205
for electronic claims, 287-288, 288
under Medicare, 422-423
physician's, 79
physician's representative, 83
provider's, 83-84
Simple lacerations, definition of, 110

Skip tracing, 365-366
SLMB (Specified Low-Income Medical Beneficiary) Program, 437
Small claims court, 364-365
filing claim in, 373-374
SMI (supplementary medical insurance), 405
SOAP, 96, 96f
Social history (SH), 101
Social Security Act, Section 1128(b) of, fees and, 154
Social Security Administration
Disability Insurance Program of, 522-523
Medicare and, 402
Medicare reimbursement and, 421
Social Security number, of physician, 203
Software, edit checks, 115-116
Specified Low-Income Medicare Beneficiary (SLMB) Program, 437
Sponsor, TRICARE, 451
SSI (Supplemental Security Income), 402
Stamps, signature, 83-84, 85f
Standard, definition of, 26
Standard transactions, 272-275
Standard unique identifiers, in streamlining electronic data exchange, 42-43
Stark Laws, 47
State Children's Health Insurance Program (SCHIP), 436
State disability insurance (SDI), 67, 525-529, 528t. *See also* Disability income insurance.
claims submission for, 531, 532f-536f
workers' compensation and, 484
State insurance commissioners, 328-330
State license number, of physician, 203
State preemption, definition of, 29
Statute of limitations, 351
Sterilization, coding for, 137
Stop loss, in hospital reimbursement, 557
Stop-loss limits, 393
Sub rosa films, in rating workers' compensation case, 487
Subpoenas, 118-119
Subrogation, third-party, in workers' compensation cases, 494
Subscribers, 58
Supplemental Health Care Program (SHCP), 461
Supplemental Security Income (SSI), 402, 523-524
Medicaid eligibility and, 438
Supplementary medical insurance (SMI), 405
Surge suppressors, 299
Surgeons, multiple, coding modifiers for, 188-189
Surgery
decision for, coding modifiers for, 185-186, 188f
elective
Medicare and, 418-419
outpatient insurance claims for, 558
Medicare global policies for, 169-170, 169f
terminology for, 110-111, 111f
Surgery section of *Current Procedural Terminology* codes, 167-172
for coding from operative report, 167-168
follow-up days in, 170
incident-to services in, 171-172
Medicare global package of, 169, 169f
multiple lesions in, 171
repair of lacerations in, 170-171
supplies in, 171
surgical package of, 168-169, 169f
Surgical package, coding for, 168-169, 169f

Surveillance, in rating workers' compensation case, 487
Suspended claim, 307
Suspense claim, problem solving for, 312
Systematized Nomenclature of Human and Veterinary Medicine (SNOMED) International, 27

T

T-1, for electronic claim transmission, 292
Tax Equity and Fiscal Responsibility Act (TEFRA)
  employed elderly Medicare benefits and, 409
  Medicaid and, 436
Tax identification number, of physician, 203
Tax Reform Act, employed elderly Medicare benefits and, 409
Taxes, for self-employed insurance billing specialist, 596-597
Taxonomy codes, 275
TCS regulations. *See* Transaction and Code Set (TCS) regulations.
TCS (transaction and code set), 271-275, 272t
Teaching physician, roles of, 93
Technical component, 184
Technical safeguards, 43
  for electronic claims, 296
Telephone debt collection, 354-355
  plan for, 372-373
Telephone review, in Medicare review and redetermination process, 320
Temporary disability claims, 521
  Workers' compensation, 485-486
Temporary disability insurance, 525
Terminally ill patients, 368
Termination of cases, 120-123, 120f, 121f-122f
Terminology
  body activity, 496t
  in coding procedure, 111t-112t
  diagnostic, 107-108
  directional, 108, 495, 496f
  documentation, 104, 106-111, 109f, 110f, 111f, 111t-112t
  for fracture types, 497, 498f-500f, 501f
  for range of motion of extremities, 497
  surgical, 110-111, 111f
Terms, insurance policy, 59-60
Tertiary care, 387
Testimony, medical, in workers' compensation cases, 491, 492f
Theft, in Criminal False Claims Act, 47
Third-party subrogation, in workers' compensation cases, 494
3-day payment window rule, 548
"Tickler" files, 84, 86f
  in claims management, 307-308
Time limit
  definition of, 59
  for Medi-Cal claim, 619
Total disability, 521
Tracer, insurance claim, 308, 309f
Training
  in compliance plan, conducting, 50
  in protecting patient rights, 41
Transaction(s)
  definition of, 29
  interactive, in claims processing, 288
  standard, 272-275
Transaction and Code Set (TCS), 271-275, 272t
  regulations on, in streamlining electronic data exchange, 41-43, 42t
Transaction format, standard, 837P, 276, 277t
  CMS-1500 compared with, 276, 277t-279t

Transaction functions and formats, HIPAA, 275t
Treating physician, roles of, 93
Treating practitioner, roles of, 93
Treatment authorization form, for Medi-Cal, 623, 624-625f
TRICARE
  admission procedures for, 547-548
  assignment of benefits and, 78
  carrier-direct system and, 292
  claim form adopted by, 196
  eligibility for, 450-451
  Health Insurance Claim Form for
    example of, 265f
    instructions for, 210-256
  Health Maintenance Organizations (HMOs) and, 462
  history of, 450
  Medi-Cal and, 620
  participating provider, 455-456
  policies and regulations of, 21, 56, 66
    on assignment of benefits, 78
    on signatures, 79
  programs of, 450-451
  review and appeal process of, 323, 326-328
  Summary Payment Voucher for, 468, 469f
  Supplemental Health Care Program of, 461
    claims procedure for, 466-467
TRICARE/CHAMPVA, claims procedure for, 467
TRICARE Extra, 456
  claims procedure for, 466
TRICARE for Life, 458-459
  claims procedure for, 467
TRICARE hospice program, 461-462
TRICARE Plus, 459-460
TRICARE Prime, 457
  claims procedure for, 466
TRICARE Prime Remote Program, 461
  claims procedure for, 466-467
TRICARE Standard, 451-456
  authorized providers for, 453
  benefits of, 451-452
  claims procedure for, 464-466
  fiscal year of, 452-453
  identification cards for, 451, 452f
  nonavailability statements and, 451
  preauthorization for, 455
Triple-option health plans, 385
Truth in Lending Act, 352
Truth in Lending Consumer Credit Cost Disclosure, 353
Turfing, 386
Two-party checks, problem solving for, 316

U

UCR (usual, customary and reasonable) fees, 155-157, 155f
Umbilical, definition of, 108
Unbundling, 174-175
Unemployment compensation disability (UCD), 67, 525
Uniform Bill (UB-92) claim form, 555, 559, 564f
  completing, procedure for, 567-579
  editing procedure for, 566-567
  for Medi-Cal, 621
Unique identifiers, standard, 277, 279-280
Unique provider identification number, 204
Unlisted procedures, coding for, 172
Unsigned checks, 344
Upcoding, 175-176, 561
Urgent care, TRICARE for, 451

Use, definition of, 30
Usual, customary, and reasonable fees (UCR), 155-157, 155f
Utilization review (UR), 386
  hospital, 549

V

V codes, 134
Verbal referrals, 387
Verification, check, 342
Veterans affairs (VA)
  disability, 524-525, 526f, 527f
  outpatient clinic of, 67, 525
    claims submission for, 530-531
Vicarious liability, 21-2
Vocational rehabilitation, workers' compensation and, 486
Voice Drug (TAR) System, 618
Volume performance standard (VPS), Medicare fees and, 426
Voluntary disability insurance, 529
Volunteer workers, workers' compensation and, 481
VPS (volume performance standard), Medicare fees and, 426

W

Wage garnishments, 364
Waiting periods, 59
  for disability income insurance, 521
  for workers' compensation, 484, 485t
Waiver
  copayment, 339
  of premium, in disability insurance, 521
Whistleblowers, Federal False Claims Amendment Act and, 413
Withholds, 395-396, 557
Work hardening, workers' compensation and, 486
Work incentives, in SSI program, 524
Workers' compensation insurance, 67, 476-517
  administration of, 58
  admission procedures for, 548
  assignment of benefits under, 78
  benefits of, 484-485
    coordination of, with federal disability programs, 522
  claims in
    billing, 510-511
    delinquent or slow pay, 511-513, 512f, 513f
    electronic, submission of, 511
    out-of-state, 511
    submission of, 504-513
  collection procedures for, 360-361
  coverage under, 480-484, 482t-483t
  eligibility for, 480
  fraud and abuse in, 487-489, 488f, 489b-490b
  funding of, 481
  Health Insurance Claim Form for
    example of, 267f
    instructions for, 210-256
  HIPAA compliance and, 478
  history of, 478-479
  industrial accidents and, 480, 482t-483t
  laws governing
    federal, 480
    interstate, 481
    state, 480-484
  legal situations involving, 491-494
  legislation on, 479-480, 480-484
  medical service orders and, 503-504, 503f
  minimum number of employees for, 484t
  occupational illness and, 480

Workers' compensation insurance—cont'd
  OSHA and, 489-490
  rating case in, 487
  reform of, 478-479
  reporting requirements for, 500, 502f-503f,
    503-504
  second-injury fund and, 481, 484
  state disability and, 484
  statutes on, 478
  surveillance and, 487
  TRICARE/CHAMPVA and, claims
    procedure for, 468
  waiting periods for, 484, 485t

Workers' compensation insurance Appeals
  Board, 487
Workmen's Compensation Law of the District
  of Columbia, 480
Write-offs, 338
Written estimates for services, 61, 64

Y

Year-end evaluations, in managed care,
  395-396